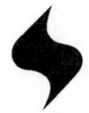

Stedman's

ORTHOPAEDIC & REHAB

WORDS

INCLUDES
CHIROPRACTIC, OCCUPATIONAL THERAPY, PHYSICAL THERAPY, PODIATRIC, & SPORTS MEDICINE
Sixth Edition

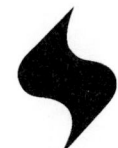

Stedman's

ORTHOPAEDIC & REHAB
WORDS

INCLUDES
CHIROPRACTIC, OCCUPATIONAL THERAPY, PHYSICAL THERAPY, PODIATRIC, & SPORTS MEDICINE
Sixth Edition

Wolters Kluwer | Lippincott Williams & Wilkins
Health

Philadelphia • Baltimore • New York • London
Buenos Aires • Hong Kong • Sydney • Tokyo

Senior Publisher: Julie K. Stegman
Editorial Manager: Eric Branger
Associate Managing Editor: Erin M. Cosyn
Typesetter: Aptara, Inc.
Printer & Binder: Data Reproductions Corporation

Copyright © 2009 Lippincott Williams & Wilkins
351 West Camden Street
Baltimore, Maryland 21201-2436

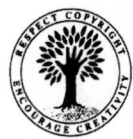

Printed in the United States of America

Sixth Edition, 2009

Library of Congress Cataloging-in-Publication Data

Stedman's orthopaedic & rehab words : includes chiropractic, occupational therapy, physical therapy, podiatric, & sports medicine. – 6th ed.
    p. ; cm.
Developed from the database of Stedman's medical dictionary, 28th ed., and supplemented by terminology found in current medical literature
    Includes bibliographical references.
    ISBN 978-0-7817-9726-9
1. Orthopedics–Terminology. 2. People with disabilities–Rehabilitation–Terminology.
I. Stedman, Thomas Lathrop, 1853-1938. II. Stedman, Thomas Lathrop, 1853-1938. Stedman's medical dictionary. III. Title: Stedman's orthopaedic and rehab words. IV. Title: Orthopaedic & rehab words.
    [DNLM: 1. Orthopedic Procedures–Terminology–English. 2. Athletic Injuries–Terminology–English. 3. Foot Diseases–Terminology–English. 4. Manipulation, Chiropractic–Terminology–English. 5. Physical Therapy Modalities–Terminology–English. 6. Rehabilitation–Terminology–English. WE 15 S812 2009]
RD723.S74 2009
616.7001′4–dc22

                                                                    2009001585

                                                            09 10 11 12
                                            1 2 3 4 5 6 7 8 9 10

Contents

Acknowledgments

An important part of our editorial process is the involvement of medical transcriptionists—as advisors, reviewers, and/or editors.

We extend special thanks to Ellen Atwood and Stacy Letho, CMT for editing the manuscript, helping to resolve many difficult questions, and contributing material for the appendix sections. We are grateful to our MT Editorial Advisory Board members: Jenifer Walker, Janice Deal, Cheryl Ackerman, Robin Koza, and Robin Snider, who were instrumental in the development of this reference. They recommended sources and shared their valuable judgment, insight, and perspective.

We also extend additional thanks to Janet West for updating and revising the appendices. Additional thanks to Jeanne Bock, CSR, MT for performing the final prepublication review. For their invaluable work in culling new terminology for this edition we extend thanks to Jeanne Bock, CSR, MT; Shemah Fletcher; Rhonda S. Hase; Robin Koza; and Beverly S. Oberline, CMT.

As with all our *Stedman's* word references, this resource incorporates the suggestions and expertise of our many contacts in the medical transcriptionist community. Thanks to all of our advisory board participants, reviewers, and editors; AAMT meeting attendees; and others who have written us with requests and comments—keep talking, and we'll keep listening.

Editor's Preface

Civilization, they say, is characterized by the lack of barbarous behavior and the keeping of written records. In fact, a hallmark of civilization is the healing of the sick. What is more demonstrative of humanity than supplying an ill individual the food, shelter, comfort, and support necessary to enable full recovery of productive health? Way back when, before infectious disease got such a foothold in towns and cities, broken bones were considered the most frequent cause of death. Surprisingly, broken bones showing evidence of healing are frequently found in the buried-with-care skeletons of the ancients, even pre-civilization. Was the setting of bones, as the auto insurance commercial insists, so easy a caveman could do it? Or, was this skill learned because it was so necessary to preserve the life of individuals comprising the community of persons living vigorous and dangerous outdoor lives?

When we fast forward to the time of writing things down, we see that the earliest known written records dealt with trauma surgery, with head-down observations for surgical and orthopaedic interventions for fractures. Of the 48 extant recorded cases in the Edwin Smith papyrus, about a third deal with head, vertebral, and skeletal bony defects. Smashed heads and torsos were more often brought to the attention of the healers, along with open fractures. Perhaps closed bony injuries were commonly dealt with at home. Even today in third world countries, crooked limbs as a result of improperly set, healed fractures are much too common.

Broken bones and little children with limb, feet, and spine malformations were tops on the list of medical problems for many centuries. Ever-increasing efforts to mend these problems have brought us to the sophistication of the 21st century, where surgery barely makes a dent in the skin; broken or malformed bones can be remodeled with glue made of living bone; and the creation of prostheses is wending its way toward the 70s ideal of bionic persons, just in time for the baby boomers to need wholesale lots of joint replacements.

Medical language has evolved along with the way it is recorded. Scratching away on wet clay, papyrus, or vellum sounds like a very tedious way to make a living. No wonder there are so few medical documents left. The line count was probably atrocious. Today's Internet and the quirks involved in electronic publishing have lent themselves to a dizzying rate of changes in usage and style preferences, retaining its splintered personality of extremely formal language interspersed with short forms, abbreviations, and slang. Despite interdictions against using certain abbreviations, most doctors still use cc, q.h.s., and others, all the while making up new short forms for evolving technologies.

To add to our burden of keeping up with the changes, equipment manufacturers like to name their products with the common terms and abbreviations of a specialty: a new splint is unveiled and called, for example the ROM-rite Immobilizer, and of course everyone is using a wound VAC. Or is that the V.A.C.? Some days the inside of my head feels like one of those lottery machines, where the numbered balls tumble furiously on bursts of air. Quick! Pick the right word for the anatomy, the procedure, the manufacturer. Should it be all cap, initial cap, or none at all? Oh, wait, it is at the beginning of a sentence, so it must be capitalized.

So, too, preparing a word book manuscript requires sifting through mounds of right and wrong words, slotting them into the preferred style and allowable space, and juggling the preferences of Stedman's scholars and other experts. All the while, editors have to keep in mind the temperament of medical language specialists, who by their very nature are people who want to do it right, with little tolerance for error. Civilized behavior now includes acceptance of differences and preferences: you say to-may-toe and I say to-mah-toe.

Appropriate to orthopaedics (or is that orthopedics?), variant forms are rampant. Chief among the variant terms that polarize the MLS community is the endlessly discussed disc versus disk. AHDI's 3rd edition of their *Book of Style for Medical Transcription* prefers disk. Stedman's prefers disc.

So in Stedman's word books you will see:

disc, disk

and

disk (*var. of* disc)

This format indicates that both are correct. Use whichever you or your employer or client prefers. For some, this will mean using one form for one specialty and the different form for another.

In the end, the goal is to communicate effectively in the 21st century's vastly complicated civilization, doing our part to provide excellent medical care to the community.

Ellen Atwood

Publisher's Preface

Stedman's Orthopaedic & Rehab Words, Includes Chiropractic, Occupational Therapy, Physical Therapy, Podiatric, & Sports Medicine, Sixth Edition offers an authoritative assurance of quality and exactness to the wordsmiths of the healthcare professions—medical transcriptionists, medical editors and copyeditors, health information management personnel, court reporters, and the many other users and producers of medical documentation.

We have received many requests to update this title. As a result, we have published this new edition that includes orthopaedic, rehabilitation, chiropractic, occupational therapy, physical therapy, and sports medicine terminology. In this new edition, we have expanded and revised all terminology, particularly in the areas of chiropractic and podiatric terminology.

In *Stedman's Orthopaedic & Rehab Words, Sixth Edition* users will find protocols, diagnoses, and therapeutic procedures, new techniques, lab tests, and clinical research terms, as well as abbreviations with their expansions pertinent to orthopaedics, rehabilitation, chiropractic, occupational therapy, physical therapy, and sports medicine. The appendix sections provide anatomical illustrations with useful captions and labels; fracture illustrations; a table of muscles and cranial nerves; a table of ligaments and tendons; professional organizations, associations, and titles; sample reports; common terms by procedure; and drugs by indication. New appendices to this edition are common chiropractic terms; common pain management terms; and common physical therapy and sports medicine terms.

This compilation of more than 90,000 new and revised entries, fully cross-indexed for quick access, was built from a base vocabulary of approximately 66,000 medical words, phrases, abbreviations, and acronyms. The extensive A–Z list was developed from the database of *Stedman's Medical Dictionary, 28th Edition,* and supplemented by terminology found in current medical literature (see References on page xix).

We at Lippincott Williams & Wilkins strive to provide you with the most up-to-date and accurate word references available. Your use of this word book will prompt new editions, which we will publish as often as updates and revisions justify. We welcome your suggestions for improvements, changes, corrections, and additions—whatever will make this *Stedman's* product more useful to you.

Explanatory Notes

Medical transcription is an art as well as a science. Both approaches are needed to correctly interpret the dictation of a physician, whose language is a product of education, training, and experience. This variety in medical language means that there are several acceptable ways to express certain terms, including jargon. *Stedman's Orthopaedic & Rehab Words, Sixth Edition* provides variant spellings and phrasings for many terms. These elements, in addition to complete cross-indexing, make *Stedman's Orthopaedic & Rehab Words, Sixth Edition* a valuable resource for determining the validity of terms as they are encountered.

Alphabetical Organization
Alphabetization of main entries is letter by letter as spelled, ignoring punctuation, spaces, prefixed numbers, or other characters. For example:

Nancy nailing
nandrolone
nanocolloid

Terms beginning or ending with Greek letters show the Greek letters spelled out and listed alphabetically. For example:

gamma
  g. camera

In subentry alphabetization, the abbreviated singular form or the spelled-out plural form of the noun main entry word is ignored.

Format and Style
All main entries are in **boldface** to expedite locating a sought-after term, to enhance distinction between main entries and subentries, and to relieve the textual density of the pages.

Irregular plurals and variant spellings are shown on the same line as the singular or preferred form of the word. For example:

foot, pl. feet
orthopaedist, orthopedist

Hyphenation

As a rule of style, multiple eponyms (e.g., Mears-Rubash approach) are hyphenated. Also, hyphens have been added between a manufacturer and one or more eponyms (e.g., Vital-Metzenbaum dissecting scissors). Please note that in many cases, hyphenation is a question of style, not of accuracy, and thus is a matter of choice.

Possessives

Possessive forms have been dropped in this reference for the sake of consistency and conformance with the guidelines of the Association for Healthcare Documentation Integrity (AHDI, formerly AAMT) and other groups. Please note, however, that in many cases, retaining the possessive, like hyphenating, is a question of style, not of accuracy, and thus is a matter of choice. To form the possessive of a word, simply add the apostrophe or apostrophe "s" to the end of the word.

Cross-indexing

The word list is in an index-like main entry-subentry format that contains two combined alphabetical listings:

(1) A *noun* main entry-subentry organization, which is typical of the A–Z section of medical dictionaries like *Stedman's*:

Spenco
   S. arch support
   S. boot
   S. insole

shoe
   Canfield s.
   cast s.
   Comed postoperative s.

(2) An *adjective* main entry-subentry organization, which lists words and phrases as you hear them. The main entries are the adjectives or modifiers in a multiword term. The subentries are the nouns around which the terms are constructed and to which the adjectives or modifiers pertain:

anterior
   a. cavus
   a. cervical approach
   a. cervical body fusion

bicipital
   b. muscle
   b. rib
   b. sulcus

This format provides the user with more than one way to locate and identify a multiword term. For example:

block
   Bier b.

Bier
   B. block

aquatic
   a. exercise

exercise
   aquatic e.

It also allows the user to see together all terms that contain a particular descriptor, as well as all types, kinds, or variations of a noun entity. For example:

magnetic
   m. resonance arthrograpy
   m. retriever
   m. sensor

patellar
   p. edge
   p. fat pad
   p. fossa

Wherever possible, abbreviations are separately defined and cross-referenced. For example:

IOM
   interosseous membrane

interosseous
   i. membrane (IOM)

membrane
   interosseous m. (IOM)

References

In addition to the manufacturers' literature we gather at various medical meetings, scientific reports from hospitals, and the lists of our MT Editorial Advisory Board members (from their daily transcription work), we used the following sources for new terms in *Stedman's Orthopaedic & Rehab Words, Sixth Edition.*

Books

Adelaar, R.S. *Complex Foot & Ankle Trauma.* Philadelphia: Lippincott Williams & Wilkins, 1999.

Banks, A.S., M.S. Downey, D.E. Martin, and S.J. Miller. *Foot and Ankle Surgery, Third Edition.* Philadelphia: Lippincott Williams & Wilkins, 2001.

Banks, A.S., M.S. Downey, D.E. Martin, and S.J. Miller. *McGlamry's Forefoot Surgery.* Philadelphia: Lippincott Williams & Wilkins, 2004.

Blauvelt, C.T. and F.R.T. Nelson. *A Manual of Orthopaedic Terminology, Sixth Edition.* Philadelphia: Mosby-Yearbook, 1998.

Bracker, M.D. *The 5-Minute Sports Medicine Consult.* Philadelphia: Lippincott Williams & Wilkins, 2001.

Brammer, C.M. and M.C. Spires. *Manual of Physical Medicine & Rehabilitation.* Philadelphia: Hanley & Belfus, Inc., 2002.

Chang, T.J., ed. *Master Techniques in Podiatric Surgery: The Foot and Ankle.* Baltimore: Lippincott Williams & Wilkins, 2005.

Crepeau E.B., E.S. Cohn and B.A.B. Schell, eds. *Williard and Spackman's Occupational Therapy, Tenth Edition.* Philadelphia: Lippincott Williams & Wilkins, 2003.

Crim J.R., A. Cracchiolo and R.L. Hall. *Imaging of the Foot and Ankle.* Philadelphia: Lippincott Williams & Wilkins, 1996.

DeLisa J.A., B.M. Gans, and N.E. Walsh, eds. *Physical Medicine and Rehabilitation, Fourth Edition.* Philadelphia: Lippincott Williams & Wilkins, 2004.

Dorland's Orthopedic Word Book for Medical Transcriptionists. Philadelphia: Saunders, 2002.

Drake E. Sloane's Medical Word Book, Fourth Edition. Philadelphia: Saunders, 2001.

Ebnezar, J. *Step by Step Injection Techniques in Orthopaedics.* Philadelphia: Lippincott Williams & Wilkins, 2007.

ElAttrache, N.S., C.D. Harnder, R. Mirzayan and J.K. Sekiya, eds. *Surgical Techniques in Sports Medicine.* Philadelphia: Lippincott Williams & Wilkins, 2006.

Garrison, S.J., ed. *Handbook of Physical Medicine and Rehabilitation Basics, Second Edition.* Philadelphia: Lippincott Williams & Wilkins, 2003.

Gatterman, M. *Chiropractic Management of Spine Related Disorders, Second Edition.* Baltimore: Lippincott Williams & Wilkins, 2003.

Greenspan, A. *Orthopedic Imaging: A Practical Approach, Fourth Edition.* Philadelphia: Lippincott Williams & Wilkins, 2004.

Herkowitz, H.N. *The Lumbar Spine, Third Edition.* Philadelphia: Lippincott Williams & Wilkins, 2004.

Hoppenfeld, S. and P. deBoer. *Surgical Exposures in Orthopaedics: The Anatomic Approach, Third Edition.* Philadelphia: Lippincott Williams & Wilkins, 2003.

Johnson, D.H. and R.A. Pedowitz, eds. *Practical Orthopaedic Sports Medicine & Arthroscopy.* Philadelphia: Lippincott Williams & Wilkins, 2006.

Karageanes, S.J. *Principles of Manual Sports Medicine.* Philadelphia: Lippincott Williams & Wilkins, 2005.

Lance, L.L. *Quick Look Drug Book.* Baltimore: Lippincott Williams & Wilkins, 2008.

Leach, R.A. *The Chiropractic Theories, Fourth Edition.* Philadelphia: Lippincott Williams & Wilkins, 2003.

Liebenson, C. *Rehabilitation of the Spine: A Practitioner's Manual, Second Edition.* Philadelphia: Lippincott Williams & Wilkins, 2006.

McKeag, D.B. and J.L. Moeller, eds. *ACSM's Primary Care Sports Medicine, Second Edition.* Philadelphia: Lippincott Williams & Wilkins, 2007.

Mow, V.C. and R. Huskies, eds. *Basic Orthopaedic Biomechanics and Mechano-Biology, Third Edition.* Philadelphia: Lippincott Williams & Wilkins, 2004.

Oatis, C.A. *Kinesiology: The Mechanics & Pathomechanics of Human Movement, Second Edition.* Philadelphia: Lippincott Williams & Wilkins, 2008.

Olson, T. *A.D.A.M. Student Atlas of Anatomy.* Philadelphia: Lippincott Williams & Wilkins, 1996.

Orthopedic/Neurology Words and Phrases, Second Edition. Modesto, CA: Health Professions Institute, 2000.

Safran, M.R., D.B. McKeag, and S.P. Van Camp. *Manual of Sports Medicine.* Philadelphia: Lippincott Williams & Wilkins, 1998.

Sponseller, P.D., F.J. Frassica, and J.F. Wenz. *The 5-Minute Orthopaedic Consult.* Philadelphia: Lippincott Williams & Wilkins, 2000.

Stedman's Medical Dictionary, 28th Edition. Baltimore: Lippincott Williams & Wilkins, 2006.

Stedman's Orthopaedic & Rehab Words, Fifth Edition. Baltimore: Lippincott Williams & Wilkins, 2006.

Tessier, C. *The AAMT Book of Style*. Modesto, CA: AAMT, 1995.

Thordarson, D.B., ed. *Foot and Ankle*. Philadelphia: Lippincott Williams & Wilkins, 2004.

Vera Pyle's Current Medical Terminology, Ninth Edition. Modesto, CA: Health Professions Institute, 2003.

Images

Agur, A.M.R. and M.J. Lee. *Grant's Atlas of Anatomy, Tenth Edition*. Baltimore: Lippincott Williams & Wilkins, 1999.

Blackbourne, L.H., MD. *Advanced Surgical Recall, Second Edition*. Baltimore: Lippincott Williams & Wilkins, 2004.

Koval, K.J. and J.D. Zuckerman. *Atlas of Orthopaedic Surgery: A Multimedia Reference*. Philadelphia: Lippincott Williams & Wilkins, 2004.

LifeART Super Anatomy Collection 1–3, 5, 7 CD-ROM. Baltimore: Lippincott Williams & Wilkins.

MediClip Human Anatomy 1–3, CD-ROM. Baltimore: Lippincott, Williams & Wilkins.

MediClip Manual Medicine II, CD-ROM. Baltimore: Lippincott Williams & Wilkins.

Hardy, Neil O. Westport, CT. From *Stedman's Medical Dictionary, 27th Edition*. Baltimore: Lippincott Williams & Wilkins, 2000.

Saurerland, E. and W. Saurerland. *Grant's Dissector, Twelfth Edition*. Baltimore: Lippincott Williams & Wilkins, 1999.

Smeltzer, S.C. and B.G. Bare. *Textbook of Medical-Surgical Nursing, Ninth Edition*. Philadelphia: Lippincott Williams & Wilkins, 2000.

Stedman's Orthopedic & Rehab Words, 5th Edition. Baltimore: Lippincott Williams & Wilkins, 2006.

Journals

ACSM's Health & Fitness Journal. Baltimore: Lippincott Williams & Wilkins, 1999–2000.

Chiropractic Products. Los Angeles: Medical World Communications, Inc., 2000.

Clinical Journal of Sports Medicine. Philadelphia: Lippincott Williams & Wilkins, 2001–2008.

Current Opinion in Orthopaedics. Philadelphia: Lippincott Willaims & Wilkins, 2001–2002.

Foot & Ankle International. Philadelphia: Lippincott Willaims & Wilkins, 1999–2002.

Journal of the American Association for Medical Transcription. Modesto, CA: American Association for Medical Transcription, 2000–2001.

Journal of Bone & Joint Surgery. Needham, MA: The Journal of Bone & Joint Surgery, Inc. 1999–2008.

Journal of Foot & Ankle Surgery. Park Ridge, IL: American College of Foot and Ankle Surgeons, 1999–2005.

Journal of Orthopaedic Trauma. Philadelphia: Lippincott Williams & Wilkins, 2006–2008.

Journal of Pediatric Orthopaedics B. Philadelphia: Lippincott Williams & Wilkins, 2007–2008.

Journal of Prosthetics and Orthotics. Philadelphia: Lippincott Williams & Wilkins, 2007–2008.

Journal of Spinal Disorders and Techniques. Philadelphia: Lippincott Williams & Wilkins, 2006–2008.

Latest Word. Philadelphia: Saunders, 1999–2005.

O & P Almanac. Alexandria, VA: American Orthotic and Prosthetic Association, 1999–2000.

OrthoKinetic Review. Los Angeles: MWC/Allied Healthcare Group, 2001.

Perspectives on the Medical Transcription Profession. Modesto, CA: Health Professions Institute, 2001.

Physical Therapy Products. Los Angeles: MWC/Allied Healthcare Group, 1998–1999.

Podiatric Products. Los Angeles: MWC/Allied Healthcare Group, 1999–2000.

Spine. Philadelphia: Lippincott Williams & Wilkins, 2006–2008.

Sports Medicine Digest. Philadelphia: Lippincott Williams & Wilkins, 2001–2002.

Websites

http://www.accessdata.fda.gov/scripts/cdrh/cfdocs/cfTopic/MDA/mda-list.cfm?list+1

http://www.aaos.org

http://www.aota.org

http://www.aotf.org

http://www.apma.org

http://www.askdrwalker.com/index/professional.organizations.htm

http://www.bonehome.com/Home/Topics/orthopedics/orthopedics.html

http://www.chiroweb.com

http://www.fda.gov
http://www.hpisum.com
http://www.mtaccstudent.com
http://www.mtdaily.com
http://www.mtdesk.com
http://www.mtmonthly.com
http://www.orthonurse.org/education/links.cfm
http://www.podiatrychannel.com
http://www.seaspine.com

A
> A bands
> A pin
> A wave

a
> arteria

aa
> arteriae

aa.
> arteries

AAA
> autolyzed antigen-extracted allogenic
> diagnostic arthroscopy, operative arthroscopy, possible operative arthrotomy
>> AAA bone
>> AAA bone graft

AAD
> atlantoaxial dislocation

AAE
> active-assistive exercise

AAHKS
> American Association of Hip and Knee Surgeons

AAHS
> American Association for Hand Surgery

AAI
> activating adjusting instrument
> atlantoaxial instability
> axial acetabular index

AAL
> anterior axillary line

AANA
> Arthroscopy Association of North America

AAOS
> American Academy of Orthopaedic Surgeons
>> AAOS acetabular abnormality classification
>> AAOS Knee Society Clinical Rating Score

AARF
> atlantoaxial rotatory fixation

AAROM
> active-assisted range of motion
> active-assistive range of motion

Aarskog-Scott syndrome

AAS
> atlantoaxial subluxation

AAT
> animal-assisted therapy

AB/AD
> abduction/adduction
> abductor/adductor

AB:AD
> abduction-to-adduction ratio
> abductor-to-adductor ratio

abarthrosis

abarticular

abarticulation

abasia
> atactic a.
> choreic a.
> spastic a.
> a. trepidans

abasia-astasia

abasic, abatic

abatement

abatic (*var. of* abasic)

Abbe operation

Abbott
> A. brace
> A. gouge
> A. method
> A. operation
> A. posterior knee approach
> A. splint

Abbott-Carpenter posterior knee approach

Abbott-Fischer-Lucas hip arthrodesis

Abbott-Gill
> A.-G. epiphysial plate exposure
> A.-G. epiphysiodesis
> A.-G. osteotomy

Abbott-Lucas
> A.-L. arthrodesis
> A.-L. shoulder operation

abbreviated injury scale (AIS)

ABC
> aneurysmal bone cyst
> Assessment Battery for Children

ABCOP
> American Board for Certification in Orthotics and Prosthetics and Pedorthics

ABCS
> anatomic appearance and alignment, bony mineralization and texture, cartilage, and soft tissue abnormalities

ABD
> abdomen
> abduction
>> ABD sterile abdominal pad

abdomen (ABD)
abdominal
    a. binder
    a. dressing
    a. flap
    a. lap pad
    a. muscle
    a. view
abdominis
    transverse a.
abduct
abducted thumb
abduction (ABD)
    a. and external rotation (ABER)
    a. and external rotation view
    a. angle
    a. bolster
    a. brace
    a. contracture
    Cruiser hip a.
    a. cushion
    a. deformity
    a. external rotation test
    a. finger splint
    hinge a.
    hip a.
    a. hip orthosis
    a. humeral splint
    humerothoracic a.
    index finger a.
    a. knee separator
    a. load and shift test
    a. osteotomy
    a. pillow
    a. pillow cover splint
    a. sign
    a. stress test
    a. thumb splint
    a. traction technique
    a. wedge
abduction/adduction (AB/AD)
abduction-external
    a.-e. rotation (AER)
    a.-e. rotation fracture
abduction-to-adduction ratio
(AB:AD)
abductor
    a. digiti minimi (ADM)
    a. digiti minimi muscle
    a. digiti minimi nerve
    a. digiti minimi opponensplasty
    a. digiti quinti (ADQ)
    a. digiti quinti muscle
    a. digiti quinti opponensplasty
    a. digiti quinti tendon
    a. hallucis longus flap
    a. hallucis muscle
    a. hallucis oblique head
    a. hallucis tendon

    a. hallucis transverse head
    a. insufficiency
    a. lever arm
    a. lurch
    a. lurch gait
    a. mechanism
    a. pollicis brevis
    a. pollicis brevis muscle
    a. pollicis brevis tendon
    a. pollicis longus (APL)
    a. pollicis longus muscle
    a. pollicis longus tendon
    side-lying hip a.
    a. slide technique
    a. tendinitis
abductor/adductor (AB/AD, AB:AD)
abductorplasty
    flexor pollicis longus a.
    Smith flexor pollicis longus a.
abductor-to-adductor ratio
(AB:AD)
abductory
    a. midfoot osteotomy
    a. wedge osteotomy
abductovalgus
    adolescent hallux a.
    hallux a. (HAV)
abductus
    forefoot a.
    hallux interphalangeal a.
    metatarsus a.
    pes a.
    pollex a.
ABER
    abduction and external rotation
    ABER view
Abernethy fascia
aberrant movement
aberration
    hypokinetic a.
ABG cement-free hip system
ABI
    acquired brain injury
ability
    abstracting a.
    bathing and dressing a.
    conceptual a.
    constructional a.
    fluid absorption a.
    general a.
    McCarthy Scale of Children's
      Abilities
    positive a.
    self-help a.
    squatting a.
ablation
    cartilage a.
    cyst a.
    nerve rootlet a.

radical nail bed a.
surgical a.
Zadik total nail bed a.

ablative
a. arthroplasty
a. laser therapy
a. surgery

ablator
Concept a.

Ableware Volumeter

abnormal
a. fixation
a. instantaneous axis of
   rotation
A. Involuntary Movement Scale
   (AIMS)
a. motor control (AMC)
a. posterior talar process
a. shoe wear

abnormality
alignment a.
anatomic appearance and alignment,
   bony mineralization and texture,
   cartilage, and soft tissue
   abnormalities (ABCS)
biochemical a.
bony a.
bulbar a.
cranial nerve a.
cytoarchitectonic a.
dislocation contour a.
engulfment a.
fibropathic a.
frontal plane growth a.
neural axis a.
sensorineural a.
soft tissue a.
sonographic a.
spinal cord injury without
   radiographic a. (SCIWORA)
tissue texture a. (TTA)
torsional a.

Abouna mallet finger splint

above
a. elbow (AE)
a. knee (AK)

above-elbow
a.-e. amputation (AEA)
a.-e. cast

above-knee
a.-k. amputation (AKA)
a.-k. prosthesis
a.-k. suction enhancement
   system

ABPTS
American Board of Physical Therapy
   Specialist

abrader
cartilage a.

abrasion
a. arthroplasty
a. chondroplasty
graft-bony tunnel wall a.

Abrikossoff tumor

abscess
arthrifluent a.
bone a.
Brodie a.
bursal a.
button a.
cold a.
collar-button a.
epidural a.
growth plate a.
gummatous a.
horseshoe a.
hypostatic a.
intraosseous a.
ischiorectal a.
lumbar a.
metaphysial a.
midpalmar a.
ossifluent a.
paraspinal a.
paravertebral a.
pelvic a.
periarticular a.
posterior pharyngeal a.
Pott a.
prevertebral a.
psoas a.
retropharyngeal a.
retrosternal a.
sacrococcygeal a.
serous a.
shirt-stud a.
soft tissue a.
spinal a.
subaponeurotic a.
subcutaneous a.
subfascial a.
subgaleal a.
subperiosteal a.
subphrenic a.
subplatysmal a.
subungual a.
supralevator a.
suture a.
syphilitic a.
thecal a.
traumatic a.

abscessogram

absconsio

absence
congenital intercalary
   limb a.
congenital terminal limb a.
limb a.

absent
- a. patella
- a. radius
- a. reflex
- a. spinous process
- a. tibia
- a. ulna

absolute
- A. absorbable screw
- a. refractory period
- a. scotoma

absorbable
- a. biomaterial
- a. collagen paste
- a. gelatin sponge
- a. polymeric pin
- a. polyparadioxanone pin
- a. suture anchor

Absorbine
- A. antifungal foot powder
- A. Jr. Antifungal

absorptiometry
- dual-energy x-ray a. (DEXA, DXA)
- dual-photon a. (DPA, DPX)
- peripheral dual-energy x-ray a. (pDXA)

absorption
- bone a.
- bony a.
- a. cavity
- energy a.
- lysosomal a.
- shock a.

absorptive dressing
abstracting ability
Abumi screw insertion technique
abundant potential
abut
abutment
- calcaneofibular a.
- a. splint
- ulnocarpal a.

Abzorb cushioning
AC
- acromioclavicular
- adrenal cortex
- AC joint
- AC joint separation

ACA
- augmentative communication aid

acampsia
acantha
acanthoma
- clear cell a.
- epidermolytic a.

acanthosis nigricans
acanthotic
Acapella chest physical therapy device

acathisia (*var. of* akathisia)
accelerated
- a. bone maturation
- a. chondral wear

acceleration
- angular a.
- a. injury
- swing-phase a.
- tibial a.

acceleration/deceleration injury
accelerator
- Bevatron a.
- linear a. (LINAC)
- Philips linear a.
- Siemens linear a.

accelerometer
- piezoelectric a.

Accell
- A. Connexus bone matrix
- A. Evo3 matrix
- A. 100 matrix
- A. TBM
- A. total bone matrix

acceptance
- weight a.

access
- eccentric a.
- A. Ostase
- southern a.

accessiflexor
accessory
- a. abductor hallucis
- a. atlantoaxial ligament
- Auto Glide walker a.
- a. bone
- a. cartilage
- a. communicating tendon
- a. digit
- a. epiphysis
- Isola spinal implant system a.
- a. lateral collateral ligament
- a. motion
- a. movement technique
- a. navicular
- a. navicular avulsion
- a. navicular cast
- a. navicular fracture
- a. navicular pain syndrome
- a. nerve
- a. nerve injury
- a. ossicle
- a. ossicle fracture
- a. ossification center
- a. ossification center of calcaneus
- a. phalanx
- pneumatic drill a.
- portal a.
- a. portion
- a. sesamoid

a. soleus
a. soleus muscle
AccessTrainer exerciser
accident
cerebrovascular a. (CVA)
compensable a.
motorcycle a. (MCA)
motor vehicle a. (MVA)
pedestrian a.
vascular a.
acclimate
acclivity
Accolade hip prosthesis
accommodation
accommodative
a. brace
a. equipment
a. orthosis
a. shoe
Accommodator arch support
accordion test
accoucheur hand
ACCR
American Chiropractic College of
Radiology
Accu-Back back support
Accu-Cut
A.-C. osteotomy guide
A.-C. osteotomy guide system
accuDEXA bone densitometer
Accuflate tourniquet
Accu-Flo
A.-F. polyethylene bur hole cover
A.-F. silicone rubber bur hole
cover
A.-F. ultrafiltration system
Accugraft
A. allograft
Puros A.
AccuGuide injection monitor
**Aculength arthroplasty measuring
system**
Accu-Line
A.-L. dual pivot
A.-L. femoral resector
A.-L. guide
A.-L. knee instrument
A.-L. knee instrumentation
A.-L. tibial resector
accumulation
blood lactate a.
onset of blood lactate a.
(OBLA)
AccuPressure heel cup
**Accurate Surgical and Scientific
Instruments Corporation (ASSI)**
**AccuSharp carpal tunnel release
instrument**
AccuSpan tissue expander

Accu-SPINA
A.-S. cervical decompression
machine
A.-S. cervical decompression system
AccuSway
A. balance measurement
A. balance measurement system
AccuTread shoe
Accu-Tron microcurrent machine
Accuvac smoke evacuation attachment
ACDF
anterior cervical discectomy and fusion
ACDS
acrocephalopolysyndactyly
ace
A. adherent bandage
A. bandage reduction
A. brace
A. intramedullary (AIM)
A. intramedullary femoral nail
system
A. Pelvic Stabilizer
A. pin
A. screw
A. Unifix fixation
A. Unifix fixation apparatus
A. Unifix fixation device
A. wrap
Ace-Colles
A.-C. external fixator
A.-C. fixation
A.-C. fracture frame
A.-C. frame for radial dysplasia
repair technique
A.-C. half ring
Ace-Fischer
A.-F. external fixator
A.-F. fixation
A.-F. fracture frame
A.-F. ring frame
Ace/Normed osteodistractor
Acephen
acepromazine
ACET
aquatic cardiac evaluation and testing
ACET system
Aceta
acetabula (*pl. of* acetabulum)
acetabular
a. allograft
a. angle
a. angle of Sharp
a. anteversion
a. augmentation graft
a. bone
a. branch
a. cap
a. cement compactor
a. component

acetabular (*continued*)
    a. component loosening
    a. cup
    a. cup arthroplasty
    a. cup holder
    a. cup peg drill guide
    a. cup positioner
    a. cup system
    a. cup template
    a. cyst
    a. defect
    a. deficiency
    a. depth
    a. depth to femoral head diameter ratio (AD:FHD)
    a. dysplasia
    a. endoprosthesis
    a. expander
    a. extensile approach
    a. fossa
    a. gauge
    a. head index (AHI)
    a. head quotient
    a. index
    a. knee
    a. knife
    a. labrum
    a. line
    a. liner
    a. notch
    a. osteolysis
    a. posterior wall fracture
    a. pressurizer
    a. prosthesis
    a. prosthesis system
    a. prosthetic interface
    a. prosthetic liner
    a. protrusion deformity
    a. reamer
    a. recess
    a. reconstruction plate
    a. reinforcement
    a. reinforcement device
    a. rim
    a. rim fracture
    a. rim syndrome
    a. roof
    a. round chisel
    a. seating hole
    a. shelf osteotomy
    a. shell
    a. slot
    a. spacer
    a. trial set
acetabulectomy
acetabuli (*gen. of* acetabulum)
    arteria a.
    deep-shelled acetabulum
    dysplastic acetabulum

    false acetabulum
    floor of acetabulum
    lip of acetabulum
    malunited acetabulum
    protrusio a.
    true acetabulum
acetabuloplasty
    Albee a.
    Lance a.
    Pemberton a.
    San Diego spastic hip a.
    shelf a.
acetabulum, *pl.* **acetabula,** *gen.* **acetabuli**
acetaminophen
    a. and codeine
    a. and dextromethorphan
    a. and diphenhydramine
    a. and phenyltoloxamine
    acetaminophen, aspirin, caffeine
    hydrocodone and a.
    oxycodone and a.
    propoxyphene and a.
acetate
    compression-molded ethylene vinyl a. (CM EVA)
    Cortone A.
    ethylene vinyl a. (EVA)
    glatiramer a.
    Hydrocortone A.
    mafenide a.
    methylprednisolone a.
    paramethasone a.
    triamcinolone a.
acetic acid
acetonide
    fluocinolone a.
    triamcinolone a.
acetylsalicylic acid (ASA)
ACF
    anterior cervical fusion
ACFS
    anterior cervical plate fixation system
    Dogbone ACFS
ache
    theater a.
    weather a.
acheiria
acheiropodia
aches and pains
achieve
    A. computer-assisted instruments
    A. software
Achilles
    A. bulge sign
    A. bursitis
    A. heel pad
    A. jerk
    A. peritendinitis
    A. Plus Ultrasound bone densitometer

A. squeeze test
A. tendinitis
A. tendinopathy
A. tendon
A. tendon advancement
A. tendon bursa
A. tendon bursitis
A. tendon contracture
A. tendon enthesis
A. tendon enthesis calcification
A. tendon lengthening
A. tendon pain
A. tendon repair (ATR)
A. tendon resurfacing
A. tendon rupture (ATR)
A. tendon rupture repair
  comparison
A. tendon shortening
A. tendon taping technique
A. tendon test
A. tendon V-Y turndown technique
A. tendon xanthoma
A. tendon Z-lengthening
A. tenotomy
A. triangle
Achillis
Banks open slide lengthening of
  tendo A.
tendo A.
White slide lengthening of
  tendo A.
achillobursitis
achillodynia
Albert a.
achillogram
Achillon instrument guide
achillorrhaphy
achillotenotomy
plastic a.
achillotomy
Achillotrain
A. active Achilles tendon support
Bauerfeind A.
aching
interscapular a.
a. pain
achondrogenesis
achondroplasia
achondroplast
adult a.
immature a.
skeletally immature a.
achondroplastic
a. dwarfism
a. pelvis
a. spine
a. stenosis
achondroplasty
achromatopsia, achromatopsy

achromatopsy (*var. of* achromatopsia)
Achromycin Topical
ACI
autologous chondrocyte implantation
acid
acetic a.
acetylsalicylic a. (ASA)
benzoic acid and salicylic a.
bichloracetic a.
carbolic a.
clavulanic a.
conjugated linoleic a.
essential fatty a.
fenamic a.
folic a.
gadolinium-diethylenetriamine
  pentaacetic a. (gadolinium-DTPA)
gadolinium-labeled diethylenetriamine
  pentaacetic a.
gamma aminobutyric a.
indoleacetic a.
lactic a.
mefenamic a.
methylmalonic a.
oleic a.
paraaminosalicylic a.
peracetic a.
PhysioLogics Alpha
  Lipoic A.
polyglycolic a. (PGA)
polyglycolic acid-polylactic a.
  (PGA-PLA)
polylactic a.
polylevolactic a. (PLLA)
poly-L-lactic a. (PLLA)
poly-L-lactide a. (PLLA)
propionic a.
salicylic a.
salicylic acid and lactic a.
salicylsalicylic a.
self-reinforcing polylevolactic a.
  (SR-PLLA)
tranexamic a.
trans fat elaidic a.
trans unsaturated fatty a.
a. treatment
undecylenic a.
valproic a.
acid-citrate-dextrose solution
acidosis
lactic a.
Acinetobacter
A. *anitratus*
A. *wolffii*
ACIS
Assessment of Communication and
  Interaction Skills
ACJ
acromioclavicular joint

Ackerman
    A. bone biopsy set
    A. criteria for osteomyelitis
    A. osteomyelitis criteria
ACL
    anterior cruciate ligament
    ACL drill
    ACL drill guide
    ACL graft
    ACL graft knife
    ACL guide set
    ACL Lite functional knee
      brace
    ACL reconstruction
    ACL repair
    ACL Screen
Acland
    A. clamp-applying forceps
    A. clamp approximator
    A. double-clamp approximator
    A. microvascular clamp
aclasia
aclasis
    diaphysial a.
    metaphysial a.
    tarsoepiphysial a.
aclastic
ACL-deficient knee
ACLR
    anterior capsulolabral reconstruction
ACLS
    Allen Cognitive Level Screen
acnemia, aknemia
acnes
    Propionibacterium a.
Acoma scanner
acorn
    Midas Rex a.
    a. reamer
acorn-tipped bur
Acor Quikform I, II shoe
acoustical shadowing
acoustic myography
ACP
    anterior cervical plate
AC-PC
    anterior commissure-posterior
    commissure
    AC-PC line
    AC-PC plane
acquired
    a. brain injury (ABI)
    a. clubfoot
    a. digital fibrokeratoma
    a. flatfoot
    a. myopathy
    a. tarsal coalition
    a. thumb flexion contracture
    a. torticollis

acquisita
    myotonia a.
ACR
    American College of Rheumatology
    ACR juvenile arthritis classification
    ACR osteoarthritis of hand
      classification
    ACR osteoarthritis of hip
      classification
    ACR Reiter syndrome classification
    ACR rheumatic diseases
      classification
Acra-Cut wire pass drill
acral
    a. digital fibrokeratoma
    a. lentiginous melanoma
Acrel ganglion
acroarthritis
acroataxia
acrocephalopolysyndactyly (ACDS)
acrocephalosyndactylia (*var. of*
    acrocephalosyndactyly)
acrocephalosyndactylism
acrocephalosyndactyly,
    acrocephalosyndactylia
acrochordon
AcroContin drug delivery system
acrocontracture
acrocyanosis
acrodysesthesia
acrodysostosis
acrodysplasia
Acro-Flex artificial disc
acrokeratoelastoidosis
acrokinesia
acromacria
AcroMed
    A. screw
    A. VSP fixation system
    A. VSP plate
acromegalia (*var. of* acromegaly)
acromegalic
    a. arthralgia
    a. arthritis
    a. facies
acromegalogigantism
acromegaloidism
acromegaly, acromegalia
acromelia
acromelic dwarfism
acromesomelia
acromesomelic
    a. dwarfism
    a. dysplasia
acrometagenesis
acromial
    a. angle
    a. bone
    a. end of clavicle

a. extremity of clavicle
a. profile
a. spur
a. spur index (ASI)
acromiale
os a.
acromioclavicular (AC)
a. arthroplasty
a. articulation
a. cyst
a. disc
a. immobilizer
a. injury classification
a. joint (ACJ)
a. joint compression test
a. joint dislocation
a. joint distraction test
a. joint injury
a. joint repair
a. ligament
a. separation
a. sprain
acromiocoracoid ligament
acromiohumeral interval (AHI)
acromion
hooked a.
a. process
acromionectomy
Armstrong a.
McLaughlin a.
acromionizer tip
acromioplasty
anterior a.
arthroscopic a.
decompressive a.
McShane-Leinberry-Fenlin
open a.
Neer a.
Rockwood anterior a.
acromioscapular
acromyotonia, acromyotonus
acromyotonus (*var. of* acromyotonia)
acroosteolysis
frostbite a.
acroosteosclerosis
acropachy
acropachyderma
acroparalysis
acroparesthesia
Nothnagel a.
Schultze a.
acropathology
acropathy
amyotrophic a.
ulcerative mutilating a.
acropectorovertebral dysplasia
acroscleroderma (*var. of* acrosclerosis)
acrosclerosis, acroscleroderma
acrostealgia

acrosyndactyly
Apert a.
Acrotorque hand engine
acrylate drill guide
acrylic
a. bar prosthesis
a. bone cement
a. cap splint
a. implant material
a. orthotic device
a. template splint
Acryl-X-II bone cement removal system
Acryl-X orthopaedic cement removal system
ACS
anterior compartment syndrome
ACS Gemini prosthesis
ACS Profile prosthesis
ACS Star prosthesis
ACSM
American College of Sports Medicine
ACSM Guidelines for Exercise Testing and Prescription
act
A. joint support
A. knee support
ACTH
adrenocorticotropic hormone
Acthar
Actifuse bone graft material
Actimove Mitella
actinic keratosis
actinomycosis
action
concentric muscle a.
a. current
double-pendulum a.
eccentric muscle a.
A. elbow wrap
inversion of muscle a.
A. Jr. wheelchair
a. line
Marshall Hall theory of reflex a.
a. myoclonus
a. potential (AP)
reflex a.
A. ThumSling
A. traction system
a. tremor
A. wrist wrap
ActivaScrew
activated partial thromboplastin time (aPTT)
activating adjusting instrument (AAI)
activation
antagonistic a.
electromyographic a.
a. force
latency of a.

activation (*continued*)
    order of a.
    volitional a.
activator
    tissue-type plasminogen a.
active
    a. and passive range of motion
    A. ankle brace
    a. ankle joint complex range of motion
    A. Ankle support
    a. back exercise
    a. bending test
    a. contraction
    a. dorsiflexion
    a. electrode
    a. flexion
    a. hip movement
    a. insufficiency
    a. integral range of motion (AIROM)
    a. knee extension (AKE)
    a. knee extension test
    a. mobility
    a. motion testing (AMT)
    a. movement testing
    a. muscle co-contraction
    a. physiotherapy
    a. range of motion (AROM)
    a. range of motion exercise
    a. release shoulder test
    a. restraint
    A. sock
    a. splint
    A. support and brace
    a. treatment
active-assisted
    a.-a. range of motion (AAROM)
    a.-a. range of motion exercise
active-assistive
    a.-a. exercise (AAE)
    a.-a. motion therapy
    a.-a. range of motion (AAROM)
active-release technique (ART)
ActiVin
activity
    a. adaptation
    a. analysis
    ankylosing spondylitis spine MRI score for a.
    biphasic endplate a.
    a. configuration
    discrete a.
    diversional a.
    endplate a.
    functional a.
    a. grading
    a. group

    high-altitude a.
    high-impact a.
    A. Index and Meaningfulness of Activity Scale
    insertional a.
    involuntary a.
    level of a.
    A. Loss Assessment (ALA)
    mechanoreceptor a.
    monophasic endplate a.
    motion a.
    motor a.
    a. of daily living (ADL)
    activities of daily living index
    opsonic a. (OA)
    physical a.
    pivoting and cutting a.
    pivot sport a.
    prolonged insertional a.
    purposeful a.
    push-pull a.
    spontaneous a.
    sudomotor a.
    a. synthesis
    a. training (AT)
    volitional a.
    voluntary a.
Activity-Lite knee brace
activity-pattern analysis
Activ slideboard
actomyosin
Actonel
Actovegin
Actron
actual leg length test
actuator
    NYU-Hosmer prehension a.
ACU-derm wound dressing
AcuDriver osteotome
ACU-dyne antiseptic
Acufex
    A. alignment guide
    A. ankle distractor
    A. arthroscopic instrument
    A. arthroscopic instrumentation
    A. bioabsorbable fixation device
    A. bioabsorbable Suretac suture
    A. bioabsorbable suture anchor
    A. convex rasp
    A. curette
    A. curved basket forceps
    A. distractor pin
    A. double-lumen arthroscopic cannula
    A. drill
    A. drill-guide
    A. Edge
    A. gouge
    A. grasper

A

A. knee laxity arthrometer
A. mallet
A. meniscal basket
A. meniscal stitcher
A. microsurgical rear-entry or front-entry femoral guide system
A. microsurgical tendon stripper
A. MosaicPlasty instrument
A. nerve hook
A. osteotome
A. probe
A. rotary biting basket forceps
A. rotary punch
A. scissors
A. tensiometer
A. T-Fix suture anchor
A. tibial guide

AcuFix anterior cervical plate system
Acuforce 7.0 therapy tool
Acu-Magnet therapy
AcuMatch

A. A, L, M Series acetabular component
A. integrated hip system
A. L Series cemented femoral stem component
A. M Series modular femoral hip prosthesis

Acumed

A. congruent clavicle plate
A. great toe system
A. suture anchor

Acupoint stimulator
AcuPressor myotherapy tool
acupressure

neiguan point a.

Acu-Pressure slipper
acupuncture

Korean hand a.
laser a.
a. needle
a. point

Acuson imaging system
AcuSpark piezoelectric device
Acustar surgical navigation system
acute

a. angular kyphosis
a. avulsion fracture
a. brachial radiculitis
a. calcific tendinitis
a. exertional compartment syndrome (AECS)
a. foot strain
a. gout
a. hematogenous arthritis
a. hematogenous osteomyelitis (AHO)
a. inflammatory demyelinating polyradiculoneuropathy (AIDP)
a. inflammatory polyradiculopathy

a. inflammatory response
a. ischemic contracture
a. locked-back syndrome
a. low back syndrome
a. meniscal tear
a. pain
a. phase rehabilitation
A. Physiology and Chronic Health Evaluation (APACHE)
a. progressive myositis
a. reflex bone atrophy
a. repetitive seizure (ARS)
a. spinal arthritis
a. stretch injury
a. transverse myelitis
a. traumatic hemarthrosis
a. traumatic lesion
a. whiplash

AcuTENS transcutaneous nerve stimulator
Acutrak

A. fusion system
A. headless compression screw system
A. screw system
A. small bone fixation system

Acu-Treat electroacupuncture
AcuVibe massager
AD

anterodistal

ADA

atlantodental articulation

adactylia, adactyly
adactylous
adactyly (*var. of* adactylia)

partial a.

Adair-Dighton

A.-D. osteogenesis imperfecta
A.-D. syndrome

Adair screw compressor
Adalat CC
Adam and Eve rib belt splint
Adamantiades-Behçet syndrome
adamantinoma

a. of long bone
tibial a.

Adamkiewicz artery
Adams

A. forward-bending test
A. hallux valgus interphalangeus correction procedure
A. hip operation
A. position test
A. saw
A. scoliosis test
A. shoulder view
A. splint
A. transmalleolar arthrodesis

Adapin
Adapta physical therapy table

adaptation
    activity a.
    high-altitude a.
adapted stroller
adapter, adaptor
    Christmas tree a.
    chuck a.
    collet screwdriver a.
    French a.
    Grace plate 4-hole a.
    Hudson chuck a.
    Jacobs chuck a.
    Leksell a.
    Lloyd a.
    Mayfield a.
    SACH foot a.
    Smith-Petersen nail with Lloyd a.
    Trinkle brace and a.
    Trinkle chuck a.
Adapteur multifunctional drill guide
Adaptic
    A. crown
    A. dressing
    A. gauze
    A. pack
    A. packing
    A. sponge
adaptive equipment
adaptor (*var. of* adapter)
Adcon adhesive control gel
Adcon-L anti-adhesion barrier gel
Add-A-Clamp
    Hex-Fix A.-A-C.
adducent
adduct
adducta
    coxa a.
adducted thumb
adduction
    a. contracture
    a. deformity
    Edgarton-Grand thumb a.
    a. fracture
    a. load and shift test
    a. osteotomy
    a. sign
    a. stress test
    a. stress to finger
    a. traction technique
adduction-internal rotation
adductocavus
    metatarsus a.
adductor
    a. aponeurosis
    a. hallucis longus
    a. hallucis muscle
    a. hallucis tendon
    a. hamstring tightness
    a. hiatus

    a. longus muscle rupture
    a. magnus
    a. magnus adductor flap
    a. muscle group
    a. origin
    a. pollicis
    a. pollicis brevis tendon
    a. pollicis muscle
    a. pollicis paralysis
    a. reflex
    a. sweep of thumb
    a. tendinitis
    a. tendon and lateral capsular
      release
    a. tenotomy
    a. tenotomy and obturator
      neurectomy (ATON)
    a. tubercle
    a. tubercle of femur
    a. tuberosity
adductovarus
    a. deformity
    forefoot a.
    metatarsus a.
adductus
    compensated metatarsus a.
    congenital metatarsus a.
    digitus a.
    dynamic metatarsus a.
    forefoot a.
    metatarsus a. (MTA)
    metatarsus primus a. (MPA)
    midfoot a.
    pes a.
    pes equinovarus a.
    simple metatarsus a.
    true metatarsus a.
Adelaar-Williams-Gould 10-point scale
Adelmann hand operation
A-delta fiber
adenine arabinoside
adenoma, *pl.* **adenomas,** *pl.* **adenomata**
    papillary a.
adenomas (*pl. of* adenoma)
adenomata (*pl. of* adenoma)
adenomyosis
adenosine thallium scan
AD:FHD
    acetabular depth to femoral head
      diameter ratio
adherence
    skin a.
adherent
    a. profundus tendon
    Tuf-Skin tape a.
adhesion
    bandlike a.
    capsular a.
    fibrous a.

filmy a.
a. formation
intraarticular a.
subacromial bursa a.
subdeltoid bursa a.
adhesion/cohesion mechanism
adhesive
APR cement fixation a.
a. arachnoiditis
Aron Alpha a.
benzoin a.
Biobrane a.
a. capsulitis
Coe-pak paste a.
Coverlet a.
Cover-Roll gauze a.
cyanoacrylate a.
a. drape
a. dressing
fibrin glue a.
Fix-Sil silicone a.
Histoacryl glue a.
hydroxyapatite a.
Implast a.
ligand a.
LLPS hydroxyapatite a.
Mastisol liquid a.
medical a.
methyl methacrylate a.
a. neuralgia
Orthomite II a.
Palacos cement a.
Simplex cement a.
a. strapping
Superglue a.
Surfit a.
Surgical Simplex P a.
a. tenosynovitis
T-Stick a.
Zimmer low-viscosity a.
ADI
atlantodens interval
adipofascial flap
adipose
a. ligament
a. tissue (AT)
ADJ
adjustable dynamic joint
adjacent segment degeneration (ASD)
adjoining pedicle
adjunct
walking a.
adjunctive screw fixation
Adjustaback wheelchair backrest system
adjustability
3D positional a.
adjustable
A. Advanced Reciprocating Gait
Orthosis (ARGO)

a. aiming apparatus
a. aiming device
a. angle guide
a. brace
a. cane
a. cane board
a. dynamic joint (ADJ)
a. leg and ankle repositioning
mechanism (ALARM)
a. nail
a. pedicle connector
a. 2-point caliper sensory
assessment device
a. posterior upright (APU)
a. postoperative protective prosthetic
socket (APOPPS)
a. splint
Adjusta-Wrist
A.-W. hinge
A.-W. splint
adjuster
DonJoy OA a.
adjusting
computer-assisted mechanical
instrument a.
mechanical instrument a.
a. table
adjustive
a. thrust
a. treatment
adjustment
anticipatory posture a.
atlas a.
chiropractic spinal a.
a. disorder
a. equipment
figure-of-8 a.
general a.
level-specific chiropractic a.
manual a.
a. of spine
osseous a.
psychological a.
set-hold a.
side-specific chiropractic a.
specific a.
toggle-recoil a.
vectored a.
vertebral a.
adjuvant chemotherapy
adjuvant-induced arthritis (AIA)
Adkins
A. spinal arthrodesis
A. spinal fusion
ADL
activity of daily living
adrenoleukodystrophy
ADL index
extended ADLs

ADL (*continued*)
  hierarchial scale of ADLs
  instrumental ADLs
  Northwick Park Index of
    Independence in ADL
Adlone injection
ADM
  abductor digiti minimi
  Allen Diagnostic Module
admixed epinephrine
adolescent
  A. and Pediatric Pain Tool
    (APPT)
  A. and Pediatric Pain Tool
    Scale
  a. back pain
  a. condylar blade-plate
  a. growth spurt
  a. hallux abductovalgus
  a. idiopathic scoliosis (AIS)
  a. kyphosis
  a. rigid foot
  A. Role Assessment (ARA)
  a. round back
  a. scoliosis
  a. tibia vara
adolescentium
  apophysitis tibialis a.
Adprin-B
  Extra Strength A.-B
ADQ
  abductor digiti quinti
adrenal
  a. cortex (AC)
  a. disorder
adrenergic
  beta a.
  a. vagal function
adrenocorticotropic hormone (ACTH)
adrenoleukodystrophy (ADL)
adrenomedullin
Adriamycin PFS
ADROM
  ankle dorsiflexion range of motion
adromia
Adson
  A. bur
  A. cerebellar retractor
  A. clip-introducing forceps
  A. conductor
  A. drill guide
  A. drill guide forceps
  A. enlarging bur
  A. hemilaminectomy retractor
  A. hypophysial forceps
  A. laminectomy chisel
  A. perforating bur
  A. periosteal elevator
  A. radial pulse loss sign

A. rongeur
A. saw guide
A. spiral drill
A. suction tube
A. thoracic outlet maneuver
A. thoracic outlet test
A. twist drill
A. wire saw
Adson-Rogers perforating drill
ADT
  anterior drawer test
adult
  a. achondroplast
  a. acquired flatfoot
  a. congregate living facility
  a. flatfoot correction
  a. gait
  A. Nowicki Strickland Internal
    External Control Scale (ANSIE)
  A. Playfulness Scale
  a. pseudohypertrophic muscular
    dystrophy
  a. rickets
  a. scoliosis
  a. scoliosis surgery
  Test of Visual-Motor Skills: Upper
    Level Adolescents and A.'s
    (TVMS:UL)
  Test of Visual-Perceptual Skills:
    Upper Level Adolescents and A.'s
    (TVPS:UL)
  a. tethered cord syndrome
adult-acquired flatfoot deformity
aduncus
  unguis a.
advance
  A. PS total knee prosthesis
  A. PS total knee system
advanced
  a. mobile-bearing knee implant
  a. mobile-bearing prosthesis
advancement
  Achilles tendon a.
  Atasoy V-Y a.
  Baker patellar a.
  calcaneonavicular ligament-tibialis
    posterior tendon a.
  Chandler patellar a.
  en bloc a.
  a. flap
  a. flap graft
  frontoorbital a.
  heel cord a. (HCA)
  Johnson pronator a.
  Lloyd-Roberts-Swann trochanteric a.
  Maquet tibial tuberosity a.
  Murphy Achilles tendon a.
  Murphy heel cord a.
  patellar a.

plantar calcaneonavicular
ligament-tibialis posterior tendon a.
profundus a.
tendon a.
tongue-in-groove a.
trochanteric a.
vastus medialis a. (VMA)
Wagner profundus a.
Wagner trochanteric a.
advancer
advancing wedge appearance
Advanta Orthopaedics
Advantim
A. revision knee system
A. total knee prosthesis
A. total knee system
A. unconstrained prosthesis
adventitia
adventitial
a. forceps
a. scissors
adventitious
a. bursa
a. cyst
a. movement
adverse neurodynamic tension (ANDT)
adversive
a. attack
a. movement
advisor
Schwinn Fitness A.
advocacy
National Association for Rights,
Protection, and A.
Advocate electric flexion distraction table
AE
above elbow
AE amputation
AEA
above-elbow amputation
Aeby muscle
AECS
acute exertional compartment
syndrome
AEP
auditory evoked potential
Aequalis
A. humeral head
A. humeral prosthesis
A. reamer
A. reversed shoulder prosthesis
A. shoulder prosthesis
A. stem
A. system
AER
abduction-external rotation
aerate
aeration
Aeroaid

aerobic
a. bacteria
a. boxing
a. capacity (VO$_2$, VO$_2$max)
a. cellulitis
a. conditioning
a. conditioning functional
assessment
a. exercise
a. infection
karate-inspired a.'s
a. walking
AerobiCycle
Universal A.
Aerodyne
Aerodyn orthotic
Aeromonas hydrophilia
aeroplane (*var. of* airplane)
Aeroplast dressing
aeruginosa
Pseudomonas a.
Aesculap
A. ABC cervical plating system
A. bipolar cautery
A. bipolar cautery forceps
A. clamp
A. drill
A. headholder
A. saw
**Aesculap-PM noncemented femoral
prosthesis**
aesthesia (*var. of* esthesia)
aesthesiometry (*var. of* esthesiometry)
AF
antifungal
arcuate fasciculus
Restore AF
affection
patellar a.
afferent
a. fiber
a. nerve impulse
Affinity Anterior Cervical Cage System
AFG ankle/foot gauntlet
Aflexa
AFO
ankle-foot orthosis
articulated AFO
AFO brace sock
AFO molded
AFO pediatric brace
AFO posterior leaf-spring
sliding AFO
AFO standard shell
AFO (Type C-50, C-90)
A-Force dorsal night splint
A-frame
A-f. notch
A-f. orthosis

AFT
anconeus flap transolecranon
AFT approach
Aftate for Athlete's Foot
afterdrop
after-potential (*var. of* afterpotential)
afterpotential, after-potential
negative a.
positive a.
Ag
silver
AGC
anatomically graduated component
AGC Biomet total knee system
AGC femoral prosthesis
AGC knee prosthesis
AGC knee replacement system
AGC tibial prosthesis
AGE
angle of greatest extension
age
bone a.
Greulich-Pyle bone a.
skeletal a.
age-associated degenerative change
Agee
A. carpal tunnel release
A. carpal tunnel release technique
A. endoscopic carpal tunnel release
A. force-couple splint reduction
A. 4-pin fixation device
Agee-WristJack
A.-W. external fixator
A.-W. fracture reduction system
agency
A. for Healthcare Research and
Quality (AHRQ)
A. for Healthcare Research and
Quality guidelines for treatment of
acute low back pain
agenesis
Bayne classification of radial a.
(I-IV)
caudal spinal a.
lumbar a.
odontoid a.
radial a.
sacral a.
agenetic fracture
agent
Albunex ultrasound imaging a.
anabolic a.
antifungal a.
antimicrobial a.
antiosteoclastic a.
antipyretic a.
Cara Klenz cleansing a.
cellulose hemostatic a.
chondroprotective a.

chymopapain blocking a.
contrast a.
enzymatic débriding a.
fibrinolytic a.
keratolytic a.
mechanical a.
nociceptor a.
phlogistic a.
physical a.
thermal a.
uricosuric a.
water-soluble contrast a.
AGF
angle of greatest flexion
autologous growth factor
agglomerans
Enterobacter a.
aggressive
a. infantile fibromatosis
a. solitary plasmacytoma
a. tumor
agility
a. drill
A. total ankle system
agitans
paralysis a.
AGL
anterior glenoid labrum
Agliette
A. measurement
A. supracondylar osteotomy
Agnew splint
AgNO3
silver nitrate
agnosia
finger a.
agonist
gamma-aminobutyric acid a.
a. muscle
agonist-antagonist
agonistic muscle
agrammatism
agraphia
atactic a.
AHCPR (*see* **AHRQ**)
Ahern trochanteric débridement
AHI
acetabular head index
acromiohumeral interval
Arthritis Helplessness Index
Ahlbäck grade classification (1–5)
AHO
acute hematogenous osteomyelitis
AHP
American Hand Prosthetics
AHP digital prosthesis
AHRQ
Agency for Healthcare Research and
Quality (formerly AHCPR)

AHRQ guidelines
AHRQ guidelines for treatment of acute low back pain
AHSC
Arizona Health Science Center
AHSC elbow prosthesis
AHSC-Volz
AHSC-V. elbow prosthesis
AHSC-V. hinge
A-hydroCort
AI
anterior and inferior
anterior-inferior
anteroinferior
AIA
adjuvant-induced arthritis
aid
augmentative communication a. (ACA)
Carex ambulatory a.
Compoz Nighttime Sleep A.
ergogenic a.
extension a.
mobility a.
OrthoTurn standing transfer a.
prosthetic speech a.
seating a.
sock a.
speech a.
StraddleSitter seating a.
transfer a.
Turn-Easy transfer a.
ultrasonic mobility a.
walking a.
AIDP
acute inflammatory demyelinating polyradiculoneuropathy
AIIS
anterior inferior iliac spine
AIIS avulsion fracture
AIM
Ace intramedullary
AIM continuous passive motion
AIM CPM
AIM femoral nail system
aimer
Arthrotek femoral a.
tibial a.
aiming
a. bow
a. guide
AIMS
Abnormal Involuntary Movement Scale
Alberta Infant Motor Scales
Arthritis Impact Measurement Scale
ainhum
Ainslie acrylic splint

Ainsworth modification of Massie nail
air
a. arthrography
a. band
a. bed
a. bicycle
a. compression osteotome
a. contrast
a. cylinder
A. DonJoy patellofemoral brace
a. drill
a. embolism
a. flow mat
a. inflation system
a. myelography
a. plasma spray (APS)
a. pressure splint
a. sinus
a. splint
A. Townsend brace
a. walker
Air-Back spinal system
airborne bacteria
Aircast
A. ankle brace
A. Cryo/Cuff
A. Cryo/Cuff brace
A. fracture brace
A. Knee System
A. leg brace
A. Pneumatic Air Stirrup brace
A. pneumatic walker
A. Rolimeter
A. Swivel-Strap
A. Swivel-Strap brace
A. walking brace
air-contrast study
air-driven
a.-d. bur
a.-d. oscillating saw
Air-Drop chiropractic table
Air-Dyne bicycle
Airex
A. balance pad
A. mat
AirFlex carpal tunnel splint
Air-Flex chiropractic table
air-flow enclosure
Airfoam splint
AirGEL ankle brace
Air-Limb amputation protector
Airlite
A. alignable ankle block
A. prosthesis
A. support pad
AIROM
active integral range of motion

airplane, aeroplane
    a. cast
    a. shears
    a. splint
    a. splint orthosis
    a. splint shoulder brace
air-powered cutting drill
Airprene
    A. Action knee brace
    A. hinged knee prosthesis
Air-Soft Splint
AirStance pylon
Air-Stirrup ankle training brace
Airtrac ambulatory cervical/lumbar
  traction system
airway management
AIS
    abbreviated injury scale
    adolescent idiopathic scoliosis
Aitken
    A. classification of epiphysial
      fracture
    A. epiphysial fracture classification
    A. femoral deficiency
AJC
    ankle joint complex
AK
    above knee
    AK prosthesis
AKA
    above-knee amputation
akathisia, acathisia
AKE
    active knee extension
    AKE test
Akin
    A. bunionectomy
    A. operation
    A. procedure
    A. proximal phalangeal osteotomy
akinesia amnestica
aknemia (*var. of* acnemia)
Akne-Mycin Topical
Akron midtarsal osteotomy
Akros
    A. extended care mattress
    A. pressure mattress
AkroTech mattress
AK-Taine
Al
    aluminum
ALA
    Activity Loss Assessment
ala, *pl.* and *gen.* **alae**
    a. ossis ilii
    sacral a.
alae (*pl.* and *gen. of* ala)
AlamarBlue osteoblast proliferation assay
Alanson amputation

alar
    a. bone
    a. cartilage
    a. chest
    a. creaking
    a. crease
    a. dysgenesis
    a. ligament
    a. plate
    a. rim
    a. scapula
    a. screw
    a. spine
alaria
ALARM
    adjustable leg and ankle repositioning
    mechanism
alarm cushion
alata
    scapula a.
ALB
    Assessment of Ludic Behaviors
Albee
    A. acetabuloplasty
    A. bone graft
    A. drill
    A. hip arthrodesis
    A. lumbar spinal fusion
    A. olive-shaped bur
    A. operation
    A. orthopaedic table
    A. osteotome
    A. shelf procedure
Albee-Delbert operation
Albers-Schönberg
    A.-S. disease
    A.-S. marble bone
Albert
    A. achillodynia
    A. disease
    A. knee operation
Alberta Infant Motor Scales (AIMS)
Albinus muscle
Albizzia
    A. intramedullary nail
    A. leg-lengthening procedure
    A. minimally invasive intramedullary
      nail femoral lengthening technique
Albrecht bone
Albright
    A. disease
    A. hereditary osteodystrophy
    A. syndrome
    A. synovectomy
Albright-Chase palmar shelf arthroplasty
Albright-McCune-Sternberg syndrome
Albunex ultrasound imaging agent
Alcaine
Alcock canal

alcohol
- a. cauterization
- denatured a.
- a. fat embolism syndrome
- a. injection
- a. neurolysis
- polyvinyl a.
- A. Use Disorders Identification test

alcoholic
- a. avascular necrosis
- a. neuropathy

Alcon
- A. Closure System
- A. Instrument Delivery System tray

Alden CDI orthotic
aldolase
aldose reductase inhibitor
Alemdaroglu splint
alendronate
Aleve
Alexander
- A. acromioclavicular joint view
- A. chisel
- A. costal osteotome
- A. costal periosteotome
- A. gouge
- A. musculoskeletal relaxation technique
- A. periosteal elevator
- A. rasp

Alexander-Farabeuf
- A.-F. periosteotome
- A.-F. rasp

alexia
Alexian Brothers overhead frame
alfacalcidol
Alfenta injection
alfentanil hydrochloride
algesidystrophy
algesimeter
- Aly a.
- Björnström a.

alginate dressing
algiomotor
algiomuscular
AlgiSite alginate wound dressing
algodystrophy
AlgoMed infusion system
algometer
- pressure a.

algometry
algoneurodystrophy
algorithm
- injury a.
- polytrauma a.
- Tile polytrauma a.

AliCool splint spray
AliCork Foot Orthosis

alien hand sign
ALIF
- anterior lumbar interbody fusion
- BERG ALIF

aligner
- Charnley femoral inlay a.
- femoral a.
- patellar a.
- tibial a.

alignment
- a. abnormality
- anatomic a.
- angular a.
- atlantoaxial a.
- calcaneus a.
- cervical sagittal a.
- colinear a.
- dynamic a.
- extramedullary a.
- foot a.
- a. guide
- a. guide rod
- a. index
- integrity and a.
- a. measurement
- a. of fracture fragments
- a. of vertebral bodies
- optimal a.
- patellar a.
- patellofemoral a.
- a. pin
- poor a.
- rotational a.
- sagittal a.
- sagittal anatomic a.
- static a.
- talocrural a.
- talus a.
- thoracolumbar junction a.
- tibiofemoral a.
- toe a.
- torsional a.
- transfemoral a.
- transverse plane a.

AliMed
- A. Conductive Patient Shifter
- A. diabetic night splint
- A. hemi arm sling
- A. insert
- A. orthosis
- A. putty
- A. sensor floor mat
- A. turnbuckle elbow splint
- A. wrist/thumb support

AliMed-Freedom arthritis support
alimentary osteopathy
Aliplast
- A. blank
- A. custom-molded foot orthosis

Aliplast (*continued*)
 A. insole
 A. pad
Alisoft splinting material
AliStrap Velcro-type strapping
Alivium
 A. implant metal
 A. implant metal prosthesis
alk phos
alkaline phosphatase (alk phos)
alkaloid
 opium a.
Alka-Mints
Alkeran
Alkphase-B immunoassay
ALL
 anterior longitudinal ligament
all
 a. median-nerve hand prosthesis
 A. Poly Deltafit keel
all-alumina socket
Allen
 A. arthroscopic elbow positioner
 A. arthroscopic knee positioner
 A. arthroscopic wrist positioner
 A. blood supply to hand test
 A. Cognitive Battery
 A. Cognitive Level Screen (ACLS)
 A. Diagnostic Module (ADM)
 A. hand/arm surgery table
 A. head screwdriver
 A. lung volume reduction
 A. open reduction of calcaneal
 fracture
 A. scalenous anterior syndrome
 maneuver
 A. Semantic Differential Scale
 A. shoulder arthroscopy
 A. shoulder/wrist arthroscopy
 traction system
 A. sign
 A. spinal system
 A. stirrup
 A. wrench
Allen-Brown prosthesis
Allender vertical laminar flow room
Allen-Ferguson Galveston pelvic fixation
Allen-Kocher clamp
allergenic arthritis
AllerMax Oral
Allevyn
 A. island dressing
 A. wound dressing
Allgöwer
 A. apparatus
 A. stitch
 A. suture technique
Allgöwer-Donati suture
Alliance rehabilitation system

alligator
 a. bone-reduction forceps
 a. grasping forceps
all-inside repair
Allis
 A. clamp
 A. hip dislocation maneuver
 A. leg length test
 A. sign
 A. tissue forceps
Allman
 A. acromioclavicular injury
 classification (1-3)
 A. modification of Evans ankle
 reconstruction
**Allman-Tossy acromioclavicular injury
 classification (1–3)**
AlloAnchor
 A. RC allograft
 A. RC allograft device
AlloCraft
 A. bone spacer substitute
 A. PL allograft spacer
allodynia
 heat a.
 mechanical a.
Allofit acetabular cup system
Allofix
 A. freeze-dried bone
 A. freeze-dried cortical bone pin
allogeneic (*var. of* allogenic)
allogenic, allogeneic
 antigen-extracted a.
 autolyzed antigen-extracted a. (AAA)
 a. bone graft
 a. lyophilized bone graft implant
 material
allograft
 Accugraft a.
 acetabular a.
 AlloAnchor RC a.
 autologous bone-tissue a.
 bone a.
 a. bone graft
 bone-tendon-bone a.
 a. bone vise
 calcaneus a.
 a. coronary artery disease
 a. cortical bone
 dense cancellous a.
 femoral cortical ring a.
 femoral diaphysial a.
 fibular ring a.
 freeze-dried cancellous a.
 fresh-frozen nonirradiated
 bone-patellar tendon-bone a.
 HTO wedge human donor tissue a.
 a. iliac bone
 intercalary diaphysial a.

intramedullary fibular a.
large composite a.
a. ligament replacement
MiCOR machine bone a.
MiCOR precision bone a.
napkin ring calcar a.
osteoarticular a.
osteochondral a.
a. paste
a. reconstruction
a. reconstruction of fibular collateral
ligament
Red Cross freeze-dried a.
shell a.
tendon-bone a.
a. transplant
whole bone fresh-frozen a.
whole fresh-frozen calcaneal a.

allograft-host junction
AlloGrip bone vise
AlloGro bone graft material
alloimplant
AlloMatrix
A. bone graft putty
A. injectable putty
A. injectable putty bone graft
substitute

allopathic medicine
alloplastic
a. graft
a. material

Allo-Pro hip system
allopurinol
alloy
cobalt-based a.
cobalt-chromium a.
Eligoy metal a.
GADS vitallium a.
NiTi a.
shape memory a. (SMA)
stainless steel a.
titanium a.

all-polyethylene socket
Allport retractor
All-Pro ScanX-12 digital imaging system
all-purpose
all-screw construct
all-terrain vehicle
All-Tronics scanner
Allurion foot prosthesis
Alm wound retractor
Aloe Grande creme
Alora Transdermal
Alouette
A. amputation
A. operation

ALP
ankle ligament protector
ALP Plus ankle brace

Alpers
A. progressive infantile
poliodystrophy
A. syndrome

alpha (α)
a. antagonist
a. chymotrypsin
A. cushion liner
A. flat sheet
a. index
A. suction attachment block kit

alphabet board
alpha-BSM bone repair material
alphaprodine
AlphaStar table
alpha-sympathomimetic
Alphatec
A. mini lag-screw system
A. small fragment system

alprazolam
ALPS
anterior locking plate system
Amset ALPS
ALPS CustomPro custom liner
ALPS EasyLiner

ALPSA
anterior labrum periosteal sleeve
avulsion
ALPSA lesion

ALRI
anterolateral rotary instability
ALRI test

ALS
amyotrophic lateral sclerosis

ALSAR
Assessment of Living Skills and
Resources

Alsberg
A. angle
A. triangle

alta
A. advance tibial/humeral rod
A. cancellous screw
A. CFX reconstruction rod
A. condylar buttress plate
A. cortical screw
A. cross-locking screw
A. distal fracture plate
A. lag screw
A. modular trauma system
patella a.
A. supracondylar screw
A. tibial-humeral rod
A. tibial nail
A. transverse screw

altered
a. intervertebral mechanics
a. regional mechanics
a. sensation

alternating
    a. pressure pad
    a. range of motion (ARM)
alternative
    graft material a.
    a. medicine
altitude syndrome
altitudinal anopsia
Altius
    A. M-INI occipitocervicothoracic
    spinal fixation system
    A. M-INI spinal fixation system
Alumafoam splint
alumina
    a. bioceramic joint replacement
    a. cemented total hip prosthesis
    a. ceramic
alumina-on-alumina total hip prosthesis
aluminum (Al)
    a. bridge splint
    a. contouring template set
    a. fence splint
    a. finger cot splint
    a. foam splint
    a. hand splint
    implant alloy a.
    a. master rod
    a. oxide arthroplasty material
    a. oxide ceramic coating
    a. toxicity
    a. wire splint
Alvarado
    A. collateral ligament protector
    A. knee holder
    A. legholder
    A. Orthopaedic Research
Alvar condylar bolt
alvei
    Hafnia a.
alveolar
    a. bone fracture
    a. osteitis
    a. rhabdomyosarcoma
    a. soft part sarcoma (ASPS)
    a. supporting bone
Aly algesimeter
Alzet continuous infusion osmotic pump
Alznner orthotic
amalgam
amantadine
Ambi
    A. compression hip screw system
    A. fixation
    A. hip screw
    A. wrist brace
ambidextrous
Ambien

AMBRI
    atraumatic multidirectional bilateral
    rehabilitation inferior
    AMBRI glenohumeral instability
ambulant (*var. of* ambulatory)
ambulate with assistance
ambulation
    assisted a.
    brace-free a.
    crutch a.
    functional a.
    a. index
    prosthetic a.
    a. skills
    a. training orthosis
ambulator
    Apex A.
    A. biomechanical footwear
    A. Bio-Rocker sole
    A. Chukka Boot
    A. conform footwear
    A. H1200 healing shoe
ambulatory, ambulant
    a. function
    household a.
    a. shoe
    a. status
    a. traction
AMC
    abnormal motor control
    AMC total wrist prosthesis
AMD
    arthroscopic microdiscectomy
    articular motion device
AME
    American Medical Electronics
    Austin Medical Equipment
    AME bone growth stimulator
    AME microcurrent TENS unit
    AME pin site shield
amebiasis
amelanotic
amelia
    brachial a.
    complete a.
amenorrhea, amenorrhoea
    athletic a.
    exercise-induced a.
amenorrhoea (*var. of* amenorrhea)
America
    Arthroscopy Association of North
    A. (AANA)
    Rehabilitation Engineering and
    Assistive Technology Society of
    North A. (RESNA)
American
    A. Academy of Orthopaedic
    Surgeons (AAOS)

A. Academy of Orthopaedic Surgeons classification of acetabular deficiency
A. Academy of Orthopaedic Surgeons/Hip Society Questionnaire
A. Academy of Orthopaedic Surgeons Pediatrics Outcomes Instrument
A. Association for Hand Surgery (AAHS)
A. Association of Hip and Knee Surgeons (AAHKS)
A. Board for Certification in Orthotics and Prosthetics and Pedorthics (ABCOP)
A. Board of Physical Therapy Specialist (ABPTS)
A. Chiropractic College of Radiology (ACCR)
A. College of Rheumatology (ACR)
A. College of Rheumatology classification
A. College of Sports Medicine (ACSM)
A. Hand Prosthetics (AHP)
A. Heyer-Schulte chin prosthesis
A. Heyer-Schulte Radovan tissue expander prosthesis
A. Joint Commission on Cancer
A. Medical Electronics (AME)
A. Medical Society for Sports Medicine (AMSSM)
A. Orthopaedic Association (AOA)
A. Orthopaedic Association halo cervical traction
A. Orthopaedic Foot and Ankle Society (AOFAS)
A. Orthopaedic Foot and Ankle Society Ankle-Hindfoot Scale
A. Orthopaedic Society for Sports Medicine (AOSSM)
A. Research Circulation Osseous Osteonecrosis classification
A. Rheumatism Association rheumatoid arthritis classification
A. Seating Access-O-Matic bed
A. Shoulder and Elbow Surgeons (ASES)
A. Shoulder and Elbow Surgeons questionnaire
A. Society for Surgery of the Hand (ASSH)
A. Society for Testing and Materials (ASTM)
A. Society of Anesthesiologists
A. Spinal Cord Injury Association classification

A. Spinal Injury Association (ASIA)
A. Spinal Injury Association impairment scale
A. Spinal Injury Association standard neurological classification of spinal cord injury
Amerigel
A-methaPred Injection
AMFH
    angiomatoid malignant fibrous histiocytoma
Amfit
    A. custom orthosis
    A. digitizer
    A. orthotic
Amico drill
Amigo mechanical wheelchair
Amigos
    Rancho Los A.
amikacin
aminoglycoside
aminoglycoside-impregnated methyl methacrylate bead
aminohydroxypropylidene diphosphonate
aminophylline
Amipaque contrast medium
amiprilose hydrochloride
AMIS
    anterior minimally invasive surgery
    AMIS extension table
Amitone
amitriptyline
AMK
    anatomic modular knee
    AMK fixed bearing knee system
    AMK total knee system
    AMK unconstrained prosthesis
AML
    anatomic medullary locking
    AML Plus prosthesis
    AML socket
    AML tang femoral prosthesis
    AML total hip prosthesis
    AML total hip system
    AML trial hip component
AmLactin
    A. cream
    A. lotion
Ammens foot powder
AM-MI orthopaedic table
amnesia
    posttraumatic a. (PTA)
amnestica
    akinesia a.
amobarbital and secobarbital
amorphous eosinophilic material
Amoss sign
amphetamine

amphiarthrodial
    a. disc
    a. symphysis
amphiarthrosis
amphidiarthrodial joint
ampicillin and sulbactam
ampicillin/sulbactam
Amplatz anchor system
amplifier
    Omniace RT3200N
    electromyographic a.
amplitude
    high velocity, low a.
amplitude-summation
    a.-s. interferential current
    a.-s. interferential current therapy
    (ASICT)
Ampoxen sling
AMPS
    Assessment of Motor and Process
    Skills
amputation
    above-elbow a. (AEA)
    above-knee a. (AKA)
    AE a.
    Alanson a.
    Alouette a.
    Anderson a.
    ankle disarticulation a.
    aperiosteal a.
    BE a.
    Béclard partial foot a.
    below-elbow a. (BEA)
    below-knee a. (BKA)
    Berger interscapular a.
    Bier a.
    bilateral a.
    bloodless a.
    border ray a.
    Boyd ankle a.
    Bunge a.
    Burgess below-knee a.
    button toe a.
    Callander knee disarticulation a.
    Carden a.
    central a.
    central ray a.
    Chopart hindfoot a.
    cinematic a.
    cineplastic a.
    circular open a.
    circular supracondylar a.
    closed flap a.
    coat-sleeve a.
    complete a.
    congenital above-elbow a.
    congenital below-elbow a.
    consecutive a.'s
    cutaneous a.

diaclastic a.
Dieffenbach a.
digital a.
disarticulation a.
distal thigh a.
double-flap a.
dry a.
Dupuytren a.
eccentric a.
elliptical a.
end-bearing a.
excentric a.
Farabeuf a.
femoral head a.
finger a.
fingertip a.
fishmouth a.
flap a.
flapless a.
forearm a.
forefoot digital a.
forequarter a.
Foucher classification of digital a.
Gordon-Taylor hindquarter a.
great toe a.
Gritti a.
Gritti-Stokes a.
guillotine a.
Guyon a.
Hancock a.
hand a.
Hey a.
hindfoot a.
hindquarter a.
immediate a.
incomplete a.
a. in contiguity
a. in continuity
index ray a.
interilioabdominal a.
interinnominoabdominal a.
intermediary a.
intermediate a.
interpelviabdominal a.
interphalangeal a.
interscapular a.
interscapulothoracic forequarter a.
intrapyretic a.
Jaboulay a.
kineplastic a.
King-Steelquist hindquarter a.
Kirk distal thigh a.
knee disarticulation a.
a. knife
Krukenberg a.
Langenbeck a.
Larrey a.
Le Fort a.
linear a.

Lisfranc a.
lower extremity a. (LEA)
Mackenzie a.
Maisonneuve a.
major a.
Malgaigne a.
McKittrick transmetatarsal a.
mediotarsal a.
metacarpal a.
middle finger a.
midthigh a.
Mikulicz-Vladimiroff a.
minor a.
mixed a.
modified Boyd a.
multiple ray a.
musculocutaneous a.
nonreplantable a.
oblique a.
open a.
osteoplastic a.
oval a.
partial hand a.
pathologic a.
periosteoplastic a.
phalangophalangeal a.
Pirogoff a.
primary a.
provisional a.
proximal level a.
pulp a.
quadruple a.
racket a.
ray a.
rectangular a.
replantable a.
a. retractor
Ricard a.
a. saw
secondary a.
semicircular flap a.
shoulder a.
spontaneous a.
1-stage a.
2-stage Syme a.
Stokes a.
a. stump
a. stump neuroma
subastragalar a.
subperiosteal a.
supracondylar a.
supramalleolar open a.
Syme ankle disarticulation a.
tarsal a.
tarsometatarsal a. (TMA)
tarsotibial a.
Teale a.
tertiary a.
through-the-knee a.

toe a.
transcarpal a.
transcondylar a.
transfemoral a.
transfixation a.
transhumeral a.
transiliac a.
translumbar a.
transmetacarpal a.
transmetaphysial a.
transpelvic a.
transphalangeal a.
transtibial a.
transverse a.
traumatic a.
traverse a.
Tripier foot a.
Vladimiroff-Mikulcz foot a.
Wagner modification of Syme a.
Wagner 2-stage Syme a.

amputation-related bone pain

amputee
a. athlete
child a.
a. cushion
transfemoral a.

Amrex
A. muscle stimulator
A. SynchroSonic muscle
stimulation-ultrasound
A. therapeutic ultrasound

AMS
antimigration system
AMS intramedullary fixation

Amsco fracture table

Amset
A. ALPS
A. anterior locking plate system
A. R-F fixation system
A. R-F rod
A. R-F screw

Amspacher-Messenbaugh closing wedge osteotomy

AMSSM
American Medical Society for Sports
Medicine

Amstutz
A. cemented hip prosthesis
A. femoral component
A. hip resurfacing arthroplasty
technique
A. reattachment
A. resurfacing
A. resurfacing operation
A. total hip replacement

Amstutz-Wilson osteotomy

AMT
active motion testing

AMX knee brace

amyloid neuropathy
amyloidosis
    beta-2-microglobulin a.
    skeletal a.
amyoplasia congenita
amyostasia
amyostatic
amyosthenia
amyosthenic
amyotaxia (*var. of* amyotaxy)
amyotaxy, amyotaxia
amyotonia
    a. congenita
    Oppenheim a.
amyotrophia (*var. of* amyotrophy)
amyotrophic
    a. acropathy
    a. lateral sclerosis (ALS)
amyotrophy, amyotrophia
    Aran-Duchenne a.
    diabetic a.
    hemiplegic a.
    neuralgic a.
    neuritic a.
    primary progressive a.
    progressive nuclear a.
    progressive spinal a.
    syphilitic a.
amyous
Amytal
ANA
    antinuclear antibody
anabolic
    a. agent
    a. steroid
Anacin
anaemia (*var. of* anemia)
anaerobic, anaerobiotic
    a. bacteria
    a. cellulitis
    a. exercise
    a. infection
    a. osteomyelitis
    a. threshold (AT)
anaerobiotic (*var. of* anaerobic)
anaesthesia (*var. of* anesthesia)
anaesthesiologist (*var. of* anesthesiologist)
anaesthetic (*var. of* anesthetic)
Anafranil
anal
    a. reflex
    a. triangle
    a. wink
analgesia
    patient-controlled a. (PCA)
    preemptive a.
analgesic, analgetic
    nonnarcotic a.
analgetic (*var. of* analgesic)

analgia
analog (*var. of* analogue)
analogous signal detector
analogue, analog
    a. neurotrophic factor
analyses (*pl. of* analysis)
analysis, *pl.* **analyses**
    activity a.
    activity-pattern a.
    bioelectrical impedance a. (BIA)
    biomechanical a.
    cerebrospinal fluid a.
    chiropractic a.
    computer-aided joint space a. (CAJSA)
    computerized gait a.
    computerized musculoskeletal a.
    deformity a.
    DeLee radiographic a.
    3-dimensional a.
    fiber a.
    footprint a.
    force plate foot a.
    frequency a.
    F-Scan foot pressure a.
    gait a.
    high-resolution a.
    job task a. (JTA)
    Khan-Lewis phonological a.
    kinetic gait a.
    lateral flexion dynamic visual a.
    muscle a.
    musculoskeletal a.
    occipital-fiber a.
    peak-pressure a.
    pedobarographic a.
    phonological a.
    plumb line a.
    postural a.
    prognostic a.
    rasterstereographic a.
    roentgen stereophotogrammetric a. (RSA)
    spinal a.
    trapezius fiber a.
    video-dimensional a. (VDA)
    video-gate a.
analyzer, analyzor
    Arthrodial Protractor range of motion a.
    CA-6000 spine motion a.
    Elite Plus motion a.
    Futrex body fat a.
    Metrecom spinal a.
    NordicTrack Motion A.
    Pediatric Ultrasound Bone A.
    Sam Jr. posture a.
    Stride A.
    Tanita Professional Body Composition A.

analyzor (*var. of* analyzer)
anametric
    a. total knee arthroplasty
    a. total knee prosthesis
anaphylaxis
    exercise-induced a.
    latex a.
anapophysis
Anaprox DS
anarrhexis
anarthritic rheumatoid disease
anastomoses (*pl. of* anastomosis)
anastomosis, *pl.* **anastomoses**
    extradural a.
    fishmouth a.
    flexor tendon a.
    gastrointestinal a. (GIA)
    intradural a.
    Martin-Gruber a.
    microvascular surgical a.
    peroneus brevis to longus a.
    Riche-Cannieu a.
    surgical a.
anatomic, anatomical
    a. alignment
    anatomic appearance and alignment, bony mineralization and texture, cartilage, and soft tissue abnormalities (ABCS)
    a. axis
    a. barrier
    a. fracture reduction principle
    a. hook
    a. insertion
    a. intermetatarsal angle
    a. landmark
    a. leg length inequality
    a. loading
    a. medullary locking (AML)
    a. medullary locking hip system
    a. medullary locking socket
    a. modular knee (AMK)
    a. neck fracture
    a. nerve trunk
    a. plane
    porous-coated a. (PCA)
    a. porous replacement (APR)
    a. porous replacement hemispheric acetabular component
    a. position
    A. Precoat hip prosthesis
    a. reduction
    a. short leg
    a. snuffbox
    a. surface prosthesis
anatomical (*var. of* anatomic)
    a. classification system of Severin
    a. hip center of rotation
    a. vertical

anatomically
    a. based exercise system
    a. graduated component (AGC)
anatomopathological study
Anatomotor traction/massage table
anatomy
    cervicothoracic pedicle a.
    cross-sectional a.
    Daseler-Anson classification of plantaris muscle a.
    designed after natural a. (DANA)
    developmental a.
    dorsalis pedis artery a.
    neurovascular a.
    nonobscured a.
    pedicle a.
Ancef
anchor
    absorbable suture a.
    Acufex bioabsorbable suture a.
    Acufex T-Fix suture a.
    Acumed suture a.
    Anspach suture a.
    Arthrex bone a.
    Arthrex TwistLoc suture a.
    AxyaWeld bone a.
    Bio-Anchor suture a.
    Bio-FASTak a.
    Biologically Quiet Mini-Screw suture a.
    Biomet bone a.
    Bio-Phase suture a.
    BioROC a.
    BioSphere suture a.
    bone a.
    Bone Bullet suture a.
    Bone Button orthopaedic suture a.
    buttress and button a.
    Catera suture a.
    compression locking a.
    a. connector
    Corkscrew suture a.
    CurvTek drill bone a.
    FASTak suture a.
    Fastin suture a.
    Fastin threaded a.
    GLS suture a.
    Harpoon suture a.
    a. hole
    Howmedica bone a.
    implantable bone a.
    Innovasive bone a.
    intraosseous suture a.
    Isola spinal implant system a.
    ligament a.
    Linvatec bone a.
    MicroLite suture a.
    MicroMite suture a.

anchor (*continued*)
    Mini Bio-Phase suture a.
    Mini GLS a.
    Mini-Revo Screws suture a.
    Mini-ROC a.
    Mitek absorbable a.
    Mitek bone a.
    Mitek Fastin threaded a.
    Mitek GII easy a.
    Mitek GL a.
    Mitek knotless a.
    Mitek ligament a.
    Mitek micro a.
    Mitek Mini GLS a.
    Mitek Panalok RC a.
    Mitek rotator cuff a.
    Mitek Tacit QuickAnchor
      suture a.
    Mitek Tacit threaded a.
    Ogden bone a.
    Orthofix Ogden a.
    Panalok absorbable suture a.
    PLA a.
    a. plate
    PLLA a.
    Revo suture a.
    ROC EZ a.
    RotorloC absorbable rotator cuff
      suture a.
    a. screw
    Sherlock threaded suture a.
    a. splint
    Stealth a.
    suture a.
    Tacit threaded a.
    Therap-Loop door a.
    threaded suture a.
    traction a.
    UltraFix MicroMite suture a.
    UltraFix RC suture a.
    UltraSorb suture a.
    Wright Medical bone a.
    Zimmer Statak a.
anchorage-dependent growth
anchoring
    anterior cervical a.
    a. hole
    a. peg
    a. point
    a. tendon
anchovy
    a. tendon interposition
      procedure
    tensor fasciae latae a.
ancient tuberculous arthritis
ancillary muscle group
anconeus
    a. arthroplasty
    a. epitrochlearis

    a. flap transolecranon (AFT)
    a. flap transolecranon approach
    a. muscle
anconitis
anconoid
Anderson
    A. acetabular prosthesis
    A. amputation
    A. ankle fusion
    A. distractor
    A. fixation apparatus
    A. fixation device
    A. frame
    A. leg-lengthening apparatus
    A. leg-lengthening device
    A. medial-lateral grind test
    A. modeling
    A. modification of Berndt-Harty
      osteochondral talar lesion
      classification
    A. operation
    A. pin fixation
    A. screw placement technique
    A. splint
    A. system
    A. tibial lengthening
    A. tibial pseudarthrosis
      classification
    A. traction
Anderson-D'Alonzo odontoid fracture
classification
Anderson-Fowler paralytic clawhand
correction procedure
Anderson-Green growth prediction
Anderson-Hutchins unstable tibial shaft
fracture
andersoni
    Dermacentor a.
Anderson-Neivert osteotome
Andersson hip outcome assessment
Andren-von Rosen line
André-Thomas ulnar nerve paralysis
sign
Andrews
    A. anterior instability test
    A. gouge
    A. iliotibial band reconstruction
    A. iliotibial band tenodesis
    A. lateral tenodesis
    A. osteotome
    A. spinal surgery frame
    A. spinal surgery table
    A. SST-3000 spinal surgery table
    A. technique
androgenic-enhancing substance
androstenediol
androstenione
ANDT
    adverse neurodynamic tension

anemia, anaemia
 blood loss a.
 Fanconi a.
 foot-strike hemolysis a.
 iron deficiency a.
 sickle-cell a.
 sports a.
anergy
aneroid gauge
Anestacon
anesthesia, anaesthesia
 ankle block a.
 Bier block a.
 bulbar a.
 compression a.
 continuous intravenous regional a.
  (CIVRA)
 crash induction of a.
 digital block a.
 dissociative a.
 epidural a.
 field block a.
 gauntlet a.
 general endotracheal a.
 glove a.
 glove-and-stocking a.
 graded spinal a.
 hypotensive a.
 inhalant a.
 inhalation a.
 intrathecal a.
 intravenous block a.
 intravenous regional a. (IVRA)
 local standby a.
 lumbar a.
 Madajet XL local a.
 Mayo block a.
 patient-controlled a. (PCA)
 peripheral nerve block a.
 regional a.
 ring block a.
 saddle block a.
 short-acting block a.
 spinal a.
 supraclavicular brachial block a.
 tactile a.
 thermal a.
 toe block a.
anesthesiologist, anaesthesiologist
 American Society of A.'s
anesthetic, anaesthetic
 DermaFreeze topical a.
 eutectic mixture of local a.'s
  (EMLA)
 foot a.
 instillation of a.
 Lido-Gel topical a.
aneurysm
 arterial a.

 benign bone a.
 brachial artery a.
 clavicular fracture a.
 false a.
 Park a.
aneurysmal bone cyst (ABC)
aneurysmorrhaphy
Anexsia
ANF
 atrial natriuretic factor
Angeles
 Los A.
 University of California Los A.
  (UCLA)
Angell
 A. James dissector
 A. James hypophysectomy forceps
angel wing
Anghelescu vertebral tuberculosis sign
angina cruris
angioblastoma
angiodysplasia
angioendotheliomatosis
angiofibroblastic
 a. hyperplasia tendinosis
 a. proliferation
angiofibroma
angiogram
 biplane a.
angiography
 digital subtraction a. (DSA)
 spinal cord a.
 vertebral a.
angiokeratoma
 diffuse a.
angioleiomyoma
angiolipoma
angioma, *pl.* **angiomata, angiomas**
 cirsoid a.
angiomas (*pl. of* angioma)
angiomata (*pl. of* angioma)
angiomatoid malignant fibrous
 histiocytoma (AMFH)
angiosarcoma
angiosclerotica
 dysbasia a.
 myasthenia a.
angiospasm
angiospastica
angiotropic lymphoma
angle
 abduction a.
 acetabular a.
 acromial a.
 Alsberg a.
 anatomic intermetatarsal a.
 antegonial a.
 anteroposterior talocalcaneal a.
 antetorsion a.

angle (*continued*)
arch a.
articular facet a.
articular set a.
Baumann supracondylar fracture a.
Beatson radiographic combined
  talocalcaneal a.
bimalleolar a.
Böhler calcaneal a.
Böhler lumbosacral a.
Bowman lateral condyle a.
Bragg x-ray a.
C a.
calcaneal inclination a. (CIA)
calcaneal pitch a. (CPA)
calcaneal-second metatarsal a.
calcaneoplantar a.
calcaneotibial a.
capital epiphysial a.
capitolunate a.
carrying a.
CCD a.
CE a.
center-edge a.
central collodiaphysial a.
cervicothoracic pedicle a.
Citelli sinodural a.
Clarke arch a.
Cobb scoliosis spinal curve a.
Codman osteosarcoma radiological a.
collodiaphysial a.
condylar a.
condylar plateau a. (CPA)
congruence a.
costal a.
costolumbar a.
costophrenic a.
costosternal a.
costovertebral a. (CVA)
craniofacial a.
cuboid abduction a.
cuboid declination a.
declination a.
distal articular set a. (DASA)
distal metatarsal articular a.
dorsiflexion a. (DFA)
dorsoplantar talometatarsal a.
dorsoplantar talonavicular a.
Drennan metaphysial-epiphysial a.
elevation a.
Engel hand x-ray a.
epiphysial a.
Euler a.
eulerian a.
facet a.
femoral trunk a.
femorotibial a. (FTA)
Ferguson sacral base a.
a. finder

finger a.
first–fifth intermetatarsal a.
first–second intermetatarsal a.
flexion a.
foot a.
foot progression a. (FPA)
Fowler-Philip back of heel a.
functional intermetatarsal a.
Garden femoral neck fracture a.
gastrocnemius a.
Gissane calcaneal x-ray a.
gonial a.
hallux valgus a. (HVA)
hallux valgus interphalangeus a.
head-shaft a.
Hibbs metatarsocalcaneal a.
Hilgenreiner acetabular a.
hip joint a. (HJA)
hip-knee-ankle a.
HKA a.
humeroulnar a.
IM a.
inclination a.
increased carrying a.
inferior a.
intermetatarsal a. (IMA)
intrascaphoid a.
a. isometric testing
Kite talocalcaneal index a.
kyphotic a.
lateral deviation a.
lateral distal femoral a.
lateral patellofemoral a.
lateral plantarflexion talar a.
lateral plantar metatarsal a.
lateral slip a.
lateral talar-first metatarsal a.
lateral talocalcaneal a.
lateral tarsometatarsal a.
Laurin lateral patellofemoral a.
Levine and Drennan metaphysial to
  diaphysial a.
Lisfranc articular set a.
  (LASA)
Lovibond nail fold and plate a.
Ludwig sternal a.
lumbosacral joint a.
lumbosacral segmental a.
mandibular a.
manubriosternal a.
Meary metatarsotalar a.
medial proximal tibial a.
mediolateral radiocarpal a.
Merchant congruence a.
metaphysial-diaphysial a.
metaphysial-epiphysial a.
metatarsal base a.
metatarsal phalangeal a.
metatarsocalcaneal a.

metatarsocuneiform a.
metatarsotalar a.
metatarsus adductus a.
metatarsus primus declination a.
Mikulicz knee a.
navicular to first metatarsal a.
neck-shaft a. (NSA)
negative congruence a.
neutral a.
occipitocervical a.
a. of antetorsion
a. of anteversion
a. of convergence
a. of declination
a. of divergence
a. of gait
a. of greatest extension (AGE)
a. of greatest flexion (AGF)
a. of incongruity
a. of retroversion
a. of thoracic inclination
a. of torsion
a. of Wiberg
patellofemoral a.
Pauwels vertical sheet vector a.
pedicle axis a.
pelvic a.
pelvic-femoral a.
pelvic frontal obliquity a.
pennation a.
physial a.
plantar metatarsal a.
popliteal a.
proximal articular facet a.
proximal articular set a.
  (PASA)
Q a.
quadriceps a. (Q-angle)
quadriceps neutral a. (QNA)
radiocarpal a.
resting forefoot supination a.
rib-vertebral a.
sacral base a.
sacrofemoral a.
sacrohorizontal a.
sacrovertebral a.
sagittal pedicle a.
salient a.
scapholunate a.
scoliosis a.
set a.
Sharp acetabular a.
slip a.
Southwick lateral slip a.
spinographic a.
spinolaminar a.
a. splint
stance a.
sternoclavicular a.

subscapular a.
sulcus a.
talar axis-first metatarsal base a.
  (TAMBA)
talar declination a.
talar tilt a.
talocalcaneal a. (TCA)
talocrural a.
talometatarsal a.
talonavicular a.
tarsometatarsal a.
thigh-foot a. (TFA)
tibiofemoral a. (TFA)
tibiotalar a.
toe-out a.
Toygar a.
transverse pedicle a.
tuber a.
tuber-joint a.
tuberosity joint a.
ulnohumeral a.
valgus a.
varus MTP a.
vertebral wedge a.
Wiberg center-edge a.
Wiberg fracture a.
Wiltse a.

angled
a. arthroscope
a. awl
a. bearing insert
a. blade-plate fixation
a. compression plate
a. DeBakey clamp
a. dissector
a. jaw rongeur
a. Lowman-type bone clamp
a. pituitary rongeur
a. probe
a. rasp
a. Scoville curette
angled-down forceps
angled-up forceps
angry backfiring C nociceptor
angular
a. acceleration
a. alignment
a. bone rongeur
a. curvature
a. deviation
a. displacement
a. elevator
a. hinge clamp
a. momentum
a. motion
a. osteotomy
a. parameter
a. position
a. process of orbit

angular (*continued*)
    a. screw stability
    a. spine
    a. tilt
angularity
angulated fracture
angulation
    anterior a.
    apex anterior a.
    apex dorsal a.
    apex posterior a.
    cephalic a.
    a. deformity
    degrees of valgus a.
    degrees of varus a.
    forefoot a.
    kyphotic a.
    limb length a.
    a. motion
    a. osteotomy
    plantar a.
    posttraumatic a.
    radius of a.
    screw a.
    spinal a.
    valgus a.
    varus-valgus a.
angulatory malunion
Angus-Cowell scale
anhidrosis, anidrosis
anhydrous ethanol
anidrosis (*var. of* anhidrosis)
animal-assisted therapy (AAT)
animal beanbag exerciser
anion transport inhibitor
anisomelia
anisospondyly
anisotropy
    architectural a.
anitratus
    Acinetobacter a.
Ank-L-Aid brace
ankle
    a. arthrodesis
    a. arthrography
    a. arthroplasty
    a. arthroscopy
    autologous reverse graft to a.
    a. block
    a. block anesthesia
    a. bone
    a. clonus
    a. clonus test
    a. contracture orthosis
    a. disarticulation
    a. disarticulation amputation
    a. disc device
    disc of a.
    a. disc training

a. dislocation
a. dorsiflexion range of motion (ADROM)
a. dorsiflexion test
a. effusion
a. equinus
a. eversion
a. exercise machine
footballer's a.
a. fracture classification
fused a.
a. fusion
giving way of a.
a. guard
a. hitch
a. immobilizer
a. impingement
a. infectious arthritis
a. inferior transverse ligament
a. injury
a. instability
instability of the a.
internal fixation compression arthrodesis of a.
a. inversion
a. inversion-eversion
a. inversion-eversion range of motion
Irvine a.
A. Isolator
A. Isolator ankle rehabilitator
A. Isolator foot and ankle exerciser
a. jerk
a. jerk reflex
a. joint
a. joint complex (AJC)
a. joint leg-curl
a. laxity
a. ligament protector (ALP)
a. ligament protector brace
a. loose body
a. magnet
a. mortise
a. mortise diastasis
a. mortise fracture
a. mortise widening
multiaxis a.
neuropathic a.
New Jersey a.
a. orthosis
a. osteoarthritis
a. osteomyelitis
a. portal
posterior knee a. (PKA)
pronation-eversion-external rotation injury of a.
a. prosthesis
a. reconstruction

a. rehabilitation pump
R-Hab lighter weight a.
a. rheumatoid arthritis
Rincoe human action bionic a.
a. scoring system of Baird and
  Jackson
snowboarder's a.
a. sprain
a. stability
a. stabilizer
a. stabilizing orthosis
  (ASO)
a. stabilizing orthosis support
a. stirrup brace
syndesmosis sprain of a.
synthetic graft bypass to a.
a. systolic pressure
tailor's a.
tendon Z-lengthening around knee
  and a.
a. traction bandage
transmalleolar a.
USMC multiaxis a.
a. weight
Wiltse osteotomy of a.
Wolin meniscoid lesion of a.
ankle-brachial pressure ratio
ankle-foot
a.-f. electrogoniometer
a.-f. orthosis (AFO)
a.-f. orthosis brace sock
a.-f. orthotic splint
a.-f. plastic orthosis
ankle-hindfoot scale
ankle-level arteriotomy
ankle-pump exercise
ankleRAP
orthoRAP a.
a. postsurgical wound wrap
AnkleTough rehabilitation system
ankylodactylia
ankylodactyly, ankylodactylia
ankylopoietic
ankylose
ankylosed
ankylosing
a. spinal hyperostosis
a. spinal stenosis
a. spondylitis
a. spondylitis spine MRI score for
  activity
ankylosis
artificial a.
bony a.
capsular a.
carpal bone fracture a.
extraarticular a.
extracapsular a.
false a.

fibrous a.
intracapsular a.
ligamentous a.
operative a.
partial a.
shoulder a.
spurious a.
true a.
unsound a.
vertebral a.
ankylotic
anlage, *pl.* **anlagen**
cartilaginous a.
fibular a.
radial head a.
ulnar a.
anlagen (*pl. of* anlage)
Anna-Dote Positioning Support
Annandale operation
Ann Arbor double towel
  clamp
anneal
annular (*var. of* anular)
annulare (*var. of* anulare)
annulotomy
annulus (*var. of* anulus)
anodal block
Anodynos-DHC
anomalous
a. fibular nutrient artery
a. insertion
anomaly
congenital a. (CA)
facet a.
hand a.
Kimerle a.
Poland a.
root a.
vertebral segmentation a.
anonychia, anonychosis
anonychosis (*var. of* anonychia)
anopsia
altitudinal a.
anoscope
anosteoplasia
anoxia
ANP
atrial natriuretic peptide
ANS
autonomic nervous system
Ansaid Oral
anserine
a. bursa
a. bursitis
anserinus
pes a.
ANSIE
Adult Nowicki Strickland Internal
External Control Scale

Anspach
    A. cementome
    A. 65K Universal instrument system
    A. power drill
    A. reamer
    A. suture anchor
antagonist
    alpha a.
    opiate receptor a.
    opioid a. (OA)
    reversal of a. (ROA)
antagonistic
    a. activation
    a. muscle
    a. reflex
antalgic
    a. gait
    a. lean
    a. limp
antarthritic
antasthenic
Ant-Cer
    A.-C. cervical plate
    A.-C. dynamic cervical plate
anteater
    a. nose
    a. nose sign
antebrachial
    a. cutaneous nerve
    a. fascia
    a. fascial graft
antebrachium
antecedent sign
antecubital fossa
anteflex
anteflexion
antegonial angle
antegrade
    a. femoral nail
    a. method
    a. nailing
antegrade/retrograde compression nail
antenatal dislocation
antenna procedure
Antense antitension device
anterior
    a. acromioplasty
    a. acromioplasty approach
    a. acute flexion elbow splint
    a. advancement of tendo calcaneus
    a. and inferior (AI)
    a. and posterior (AP)
    a. and posterior fusion
    a. and superior (AS)
    a. angulation
    a. ankle impingement
    a. ankle shift operation
    a. apprehension shoulder test

    a. aspiration
    a. atlantooccipital membrane
    a. atlantoodontoid interval
    a. axillary approach
    a. axillary line (AAL)
    a. bending moment
    a. calcaneal lateral column lengthening
    a. calcaneal osteotomy
    a. calcaneal process fracture
    a. capsule
    a. capsulectomy
    a. capsulolabral reconstruction (ACLR)
    a. capsulotomy
    a. cavus
    a. cervical anchoring
    a. cervical approach
    a. cervical body fusion
    a. cervical cord syndrome
    a. cervical discectomy
    a. cervical discectomy and fusion (ACDF)
    a. cervical fascia
    a. cervical fixation
    a. cervical fusion (ACF)
    a. cervical plate (ACP)
    a. cervical plate fixation system (ACFS)
    a. cervicothoracic junction surgery
    a. collateral ligament
    a. column
    a. column disruption
    a. column fracture
    a. column of spine
    a. column osteosynthesis
    a. commissure-posterior commissure (AC-PC)
    a. compartment
    a. compartment syndrome (ACS)
    a. construct
    a. cord compression
    a. cord impingement
    a. corpectomy
    a. correction
    a. cortex penetration
    a. cruciate
    a. cruciate deficit knee
    a. cruciate ligament (ACL)
    a. cruciate ligament reconstruction
    a. cruciate ligament reconstruction using hamstrings
    a. cruciate sprain
    a. curvature
    a. cutaneous nerve entrapment
    a. decompression
    a. decompression technique
    a. distraction instrumentation
    a. drainage

a. drawer sign
a. drawer stress radiograph
a. drawer stress x-ray view
a. drawer test (ADT)
a. epineurotomy
a. equinus
a. extensile approach
a. fiber-region
a. fibular ligament
a. floating procedure
a. foot draw sign
a. forceps
a. glenoid labrum (AGL)
a. glide
a. heel
a. hiatal sign
a. hip dislocation
a. hip release
a. horn
a. horn cell
a. horn meniscal tear
a. horn of spinal cord
a. humeral line
a. iliofemoral technique
a. impingement spur
a. impingement syndrome
a. inferior iliac spine (AIIS)
a. innominate
a. innominate rotation
a. internal fixation
a. internal fixation device
a. interosseous nerve syndrome
a. interosseous syndrome
a. joint impingement
a. jugular vein
a. knee laxity
a. Kostuik-Harrington distraction system
a. kyphosis
a. labrum periosteal sleeve avulsion (ALPSA)
a. labrum periosteal sleeve avulsion lesion
a. locking plate system (ALPS)
a. longitudinal ligament (ALL)
a. long toe flexor
a. lower cervical spine surgery
a. lumbar interbody fusion (ALIF)
a. lumbar translation
a. lumbar vertebral interbody fusion
a. maxillary spine
a. medial ankle ligament
a. meniscofemoral ligament
a. metallic fixation
a. metatarsal arch
a. minimally invasive surgery (AMIS)
a. myocutaneous flap
a. neutralization

a. oblique bundle
a. oblique ligament (AOL)
a. oblique meniscal tear
a. occipitocervical arthrodesis
a. occipitocervical spine
a. odontoid fixation
a. olisthesis
a. pelvic tilt
a. pes cavus
a. plate fixation
a. plate system (APS)
a. portal
a. pronator teres
a. quadriceps musculocutaneous flap technique
a. quadrilateral triplane frame
a. radial collateral artery
a. recurrent tibial artery
a. retroperitoneal decompression
a. retroperitoneal flank approach
a. rotary drawer test
a. sacrococcygeal ligament
a. sacroiliac joint plate
a. sacroiliac ligament
a. scalene muscle
a. screw fixation
a. serratus muscle
a. shear
a. shin splint
a. short-segment stabilization
a. shoulder dislocation
a. shoulder instability
a. shoulder release
a. sliding tibial graft
a. slot graft arthrodesis
a. soft tissue impingement
a. spinal artery
a. spinal fixation
a. spinal fusion
a. spinal line
a. spinocerebellar tract
a. spinothalamic tract
a. spurring
a. stabilization procedure
a. sternoclavicular joint
a. sternomastoid approach
a. strap approach
a. superior iliac spine (ASIS)
a. superior portal (ASP)
a. surgical exposure
a. talar translation (ATT)
a. talofibular ligament (ATFL)
a. talofibular ligament rupture
a. talofibular sprain
a. talotibial ligament
a. talus shift
a. tarsal resection
a. tarsal tendinitis
a. tarsal tunnel syndrome

anterior (*continued*)
a. thoracic nerve
a. tibial artery
a. tibial compartment syndrome
a. tibial fasciocutaneous flap
tibialis a.
a. tibial margin
a. tibial muscle
a. tibial nerve
a. tibial nerve dermatome
a. tibial sign
a. tibial spine
a. tibial syndrome
a. tibial tendon
a. tibial tubercle
a. tibiofibular ligament
a. tibiotalar fascicle (ATTF)
a. tibiotalar ligament
a. transfer
a. translation
a. transoral atlantoaxial
  release
a. transthoracic approach
a. triangle
a. upper spine
a. vertebral stapling
a. view
a. wedge compression fracture
a. Zielke instrumentation
anterior-inferior (AI)
a.-i. capsular ligament dysfunction
a.-i. compression
a.-i. dislocation
a.-i. fusion
a.-i. glide
a.-i. movement
anterior-posterior (AP)
a.-p. compression (APC)
a.-p. fusion with SSI
a.-p. glide
a.-p. listhesis
a.-p. movement
anterior-superior (AS)
anterocentral arthroscopic portal
anterodistal (AD)
anterograde
a. axoplasmic transport
a. AXT
anteroinferior (AI), anterior-inferior
a. glenohumeral ligament
a. portal
a. spondylolisthesis
a. tibiofibular ligament
anterolateral
a. approach
a. capsule
a. compression fracture
a. decompression
a. dislocation

a. drainage
a. femorotibial ligament tenodesis
a. fragment
a. impingement syndrome
a. portal
a. raphe
a. release
a. rotary instability (ALRI)
a. rotary knee instability
**anterolateral-anteromedial rotary
instability**
anterolisthesis
anteromedial
a. bundle
a. capsule
a. drainage
a. glenohumeral ligament
a. humeral head defect
a. incision
a. portal
a. retropharyngeal approach
a. rotary instability
a. tubercle transfer
**anteromedial-posteromedial rotary
instability**
anteroposterior (AP), anterior-posterior
a. control orthosis
a. lateral sway
a. nail
a. stress test
a. supine view
a. table
a. talocalcaneal (APTC)
a. talocalcaneal angle
a. talocalcaneal divergence
a. tilt
a. translation
a. view
anteroproximal
anterosuperior (AS)
a. external ilium (ASEX)
a. glenohumeral ligament
a. iliac spine graft
a. ilium
a. ilium major
a. internal ilium (ASIN)
a. subluxation
anterosuperior-external subluxation
anterosuperior-internal subluxation
anteroventral
antetorsion
a. angle
angle of a.
femoral a.
anteversion
acetabular a.
angle of a.
a. determination
femoral a. (FA)

femoral head-neck a.
neutral a.
a. syndrome
anthropometric
    a. caliper
    a. growth parameter
    a. measurement
    a. measuring tape
    a. method
    a. total hip (ATH)
anthropometry
antiarthritic
antibacterial pillow
antibiosis
antibiotic
    a. and saline solution
    a. bead
    a. bead pouch
    broad-spectrum a.
    a. cement-coated interlocking nail
    postoperative a.
    preoperative a.
    prophylactic a.
antibiotic-impregnated
    a.-i. bead
    a.-i. cement
    a.-i. polymethyl methacrylate
antibiotic-loaded acrylic cement
antibody
    antihistocompatibility a.
    antinuclear a. (ANA)
    T-cell receptor a.
anticavitation drill
anticentromere
anticipatory posture adjustment
anticoagulant
    lupus a.
    a. therapy
anticoagulation
    prophylactic a.
anticonvulsant therapy
antidecubitus
    a. mattress
    a. pad
antidepressant
    tricyclic a. (TCA, TCAD)
antidromic stimulation
antiembolic
    a. position
    a. stockings
antiemetic
antifungal (AF)
    Absorbine Jr. A.
    a. agent
    Breezee Mist A.
antigen
    antiproliferating cell nuclear a.
    (anti-PCNA)
    carcinoembryonic a. (CEA)

HLA B27 blood a.
human leukocyte a. (HLA)
human lymphocyte a.
transplant a.
antigen-extracted
    a.-e. allogenic
    a.-e. allogenic bone
antigenicity
antigen-induced arthritis
antiglide plate
antigravity
antihistocompatibility antibody
antiinflammatory medication
antimicrobial
    a. agent
    a. benzalkonium chloride
antimigration system (AMS)
antinuclear
    a. antibody (ANA)
    a. antibody test
antiosteoclastic agent
anti-PCNA
    antiproliferating cell nuclear antigen
**antiproliferating cell nuclear antigen
(anti-PCNA)**
antiprotrusio cage
antipyretic agent
antiretroviral
antirheumatic
antirotation
    a. cable (ARC)
    a. device
antisense gene therapy
antiseptic
    ACU-dyne a.
    colored a.
    a. solution
Antishear gel sheet
antishock garment
Anti-Shox
    A.-S. foot cushion
    A.-S. gel insole
    A.-S. heel cup
    A.-S. orthosis
    A.-S. sports orthotic
antistreptolysin O titer (ASOT)
antitension line
antithrombin
antithrombotic therapy
antithrust seat
antitipper wheelchair
antitoxin
antituberculosis drug
antivibration glove
Anturane
anular, annular
    a. cartilage
    a. constricting band syndrome
    annular elastic nail

anular (*continued*)
    a. fiber
    a. fibrosis
    a. groove
    a. injury
    a. ligament
    a. ligament entrapment
    a. ligament of radius
    a. periradial recess
    a. pulley (A1–A4)
anulare, annulare
    limbus a.
    subcutaneous granuloma a.
anularis
    digitus a.
anulospiral ending of muscle spindle
anulus, annulus
    a. degradation
    a. fibrosus
anvil
    a. bone
    Bunnell a.
    a. sign
    a. test
Anxanil oral
any-angle splint
Anywear shoe
AO
    Arbeitsgemeinschaft für
    Osteosynthesefragen
    atlantooccipital
    AO and Danis-Weber ankle fracture
    classification
    AO ankle fracture classification
    AO brace
    AO cancellous screw
    AO classification of ankle fracture
    AO compression
    AO compression apparatus
    AO condylar blade-plate
    AO contoured T plate
    AO contouring apparatus
    AO cortex screw
    AO drill bit
    AO dynamic compression plate
    AO dynamic compression plate
    construct
    AO external fixation
    AO femoral distractor
    AO fixateur interne
    AO fixateur interne instrumentation
    AO fracture pattern
    AO group
    AO group shoulder arthrodesis
    AO guidepin
    AO hook plate
    AO internal fixator
    AO lag screw
    AO minifragment set

    AO notched instrumentation
    AO plate bender
    AO procedure
    AO pseudoisochromatic color plate
    test
    AO reconstruction plate
    AO reduction forceps
    AO screw fixation
    AO semitubular plate
    AO slotted medullary nail
    AO small fragment plate
    AO spinal internal fixation
    AO spongiosa screw
    AO spoon plate
    AO surgical technique
    AO tap
    AO tension band
AOA
    American Orthopaedic Association
    AOA cervical immobilization
    brace
    AOA halo cervical traction
AO-ASIF
    Arbeitsgemeinschaft für
    Osteosynthesefragen-Association for
    Internal Fixation
    Arbeitsgemeinschaft für
    Osteosynthesefragen-Association for
    the Study of Internal Fixation
    AO-ASIF compression plate
    AO-ASIF compression technique
    AO-ASIF fixateur interne
    AO-ASIF orthopaedic implant
    AO-ASIF screw
AOF
    Assessment of Occupational
    Functioning
AOFAS
    American Orthopaedic Foot and Ankle
    Society
    AOFAS hallux rating system
    AOFAS Lesser
    Metatarsophalangeal-Interphalangeal
    Scale
    AOFAS score
AOL
    anterior oblique ligament
AO-Morscher plate
A-ONE
    Arnadottir OT-ADL Neurobehavioral
    Evaluation
AOSSM
    American Orthopaedic Society for
    Sports Medicine
AP
    action potential
    anterior and posterior
    anteroposterior
    anterior-posterior

AP fusion
AP nail
AP supine view
AP translatory motion
Apacet
APACHE
Acute Physiology and Chronic Health Evaluation
aparthrosis
APB Hi all-purpose boot
APC
anterior-posterior compression
APC hip retractor
APC proximal femoral elevator
APD
automated percutaneous discectomy
ape
a. hand
a. hand deformity
a. thumb deformity
apelike hand
aperiosteal amputation
Apert
A. acrosyndactyly
A. syndrome
aperta
spina bifida a.
aperture pad
apex, *pl.* **apices**
A. Ambulator
A. Ambulator shoe
a. anterior angulation
a. dorsal angulation
A. Energetics
A. insole
a. of head of patella
a. patellae
A. pin
a. plantar deformity
a. posterior angulation
A. Universal Drive and Irrigation System
a. vertebra
aphalangia
complete a.
congenital a.
partial a.
aphasia
Broca a.
apical
a. axis guide
a. corn
a. distraction
a. lordotic view
a. non-load-bearing bone fracture
a. segment
a. stitch
a. vertebra

apices (*pl. of* apex)
APL
abductor pollicis longus
APL Plus ankle brace
APLD
automated percutaneous lumbar discectomy
Apley
A. compression test
A. distraction test
A. examination
A. grinding test
A. knee test
A. maneuver
A. scratch shoulder test
A. sign
A. traction
Apligraf
apocope
apodia
Apofix cervical instrumentation
Apolipoprotein
Apollo
A. DXA bone densitometer
A. DXA bone densitometry system
A. hip prosthesis
A. hip system
A. hot/cold Pak
A. knee prosthesis system
A. TM electric flexion table
A. total knee system
apomorphine
aponeurectomy
aponeurorrhaphy
aponeuroses (*pl. of* aponeurosis)
aponeurosis, *pl.* **aponeuroses**
adductor a.
digital a.
meniscal a.
a. of tendon
palmar a.
plantar a.
quadriceps a.
woven gastrocnemius a.
aponeurositis
aponeurotic
a. band
a. fibroma
a. lengthening
a. reflex
a. triangle
a. troika
aponeurotome
aponeurotomy
apophysary (*var. of* apophysial)
apophyseal (*var. of* apophysial)
apophyses (*pl. of* apophysis)

apophysial, apophyseal, apophysary
   a. complex
   a. fracture
   a. joint
   a. joint capsule
   a. joint osteophyte
apophysis, *pl.* **apophyses**
   calcaneus a.
   iliac a.
   medial epicondylar a.
   slipped vertebral a.
   spinal process a.
   vertebral ring a.
apophysitis
   calcaneal a.
   iliac a.
   a. tibialis
   a. tibialis adolescentium
   traction a.
apoplexy
   delayed a.
   posttraumatic a.
APOPPS
   adjustable postoperative protective
   prosthetic socket
apoptosis
   chondrocyte a.
apparatus (*pl. of* apparatus)
   Ace Unifix fixation a.
   adjustable aiming a.
   Allgöwer a.
   Anderson fixation a.
   Anderson leg-lengthening a.
   AO compression a.
   AO contouring a.
   Arbeitsgemeinschaft für
   Osteosynthesefragen compression a.
   Arbeitsgemeinschaft für
   Osteosynthesefragen contouring a.
   Axer compression a.
   4-bar external fixation a.
   Bassett electrical stimulation a.
   Benedict-Roth a.
   Bovie electrocautery a.
   Buck convoluted traction a.
   Buck Redi-Traction a.
   Calandruccio triangular compression a.
   Cameron fracture a.
   Charnley centering a.
   Charnley compression a.
   continuous passive motion a.
   compression a.
   coracoclavicular fixation a.
   coring a.
   CPM a.
   DeWald spinal a.
   Deyerle femoral neck fixation a.
   driver tunnel locator a.
   electrocautery a.

   electronic bone stimulation a.
   a. extensor
   external skeletal fixation a.
   fixating a.
   Fox internal fixation a.
   Georgiade visor halo fixation a.
   Giliberty a.
   Golgi a.
   halo vest a.
   Hamilton a.
   Hare a.
   hinged-distraction a.
   Hoffmann-Vidal external fixation a.
   Ilizarov a.
   internal fixation a.
   isokinetic joint a.
   isokinetic resistance a.
   Kinetron muscle strengthening a.
   Kirschner a.
   Kronner external fixation a.
   Küntscher traction a.
   leg-holding a.
   McLaughlin osteosynthesis a.
   Mueller compression a.
   nail plate a.
   Nauth traction a.
   Neufeld a.
   optoelectric measuring a.
   optoelectric signal detection a.
   Orthofix a.
   Parham-Martin fracture a.
   Philips Angiodiagnostics 96 a.
   Quengel a.
   Rancho Los Amigos anklet foot
   control a.
   Redi-Trac traction a.
   Rezaian external fixation a.
   rod-mounted targeting a.
   Roger Anderson external
   fixation a.
   Sayre suspension a.
   Schneider a.
   snap-fit a.
   Southwick pin-holding a.
   spine a.
   subneural a.
   Sutter-CPM knee a.
   Taylor a.
   Telectronics electrical stimulation a.
   triplanar protractor a.
   Vidal-Adrey modified Hoffman
   external fixation device a.
   Volkov-Oganesian external
   fixation a.
   Wagner external fixation a.
   Wagner leg-lengthening a.
   Wagner-Schanz screw a.
   Zickel medullary a.
   Zickel supracondylar fixation a.

apparent leg-length discrepancy test
appearance
    advancing wedge a.
    bat-wing a.
    blade of grass a.
    bone-within-bone a.
    candle wax a.
    cotton ball a.
    crabmeatlike a.
    horseshoe a.
    mop-end a.
    mouse-ear a.
    picture-frame a.
    spongy a.
appendage clamp
appendiceal retractor
appendicular
    a. bone mass measurement
    a. skeletal muscle (ASM)
    a. skeleton
Applause Super-Hemi wheelchair
apple-shape body
appliance
    DeWald spinal a.
    Jobst a.
    Roger Anderson pin fixation a.
    therapeutic a.
application
    cast a.
    cold a.
    controlled force a.
    diversified-type force a.
    force a.
    frame a.
    Harrington rod instrumentation
      force a.
    heat a.
    ice a.
    Isola spinal implant system a.
    Kumar a.
    a. of traction device
    paraffin wax therapeutic a.
    paraspinal rod a.
    traction a.
    transverse fixator a.
applicator
    infrared a.
applied
    a. kinesiology
    a. load
applier
    bayonet clip a.
    bulldog clamp a.
    clip a.
    Ligaclip a.
    Mayfield miniature clip a.
    Mayfield temporary aneurysm
      clip a.

    mini a.
    surgical staple a.
    Vari-Angle clip a.
apposing articular surfaces
apposition
    axonal a.
    bayonet a.
    bone-to-bone a.
    bony a.
    facet a.
appositional growth
apprehension
    a. of shoulder test
    a. shoulder
    a. sign
apprentice kyphosis
approach
    Abbott-Carpenter posterior knee a.
    Abbott posterior knee a.
    acetabular extensile a.
    AFT a.
    anconeus flap transolecranon a.
    anterior acromioplasty a.
    anterior axillary a.
    anterior cervical a.
    anterior extensile a.
    anterior retroperitoneal flank a.
    anterior sternomastoid a.
    anterior strap a.
    anterior transthoracic a.
    anterolateral a.
    anteromedial retropharyngeal a.
    Aufranc lateral total hip a.
    Avila sacroiliac joint abscess
      drainage a.
    axillary a.
    Bailey-Badgley anterior cervical a.
    Banks-Laufman elbow a.
    Berger-Bookwalter posterior spine a.
    Bosworth ankle a.
    Bosworth posterior femur a.
    Boyd elbow a.
    Boyd-Sisk shoulder a.
    Brackett-Osgood knee a.
    Brackett-Osgood posterior hip a.
    Brodsky-Tullos-Gartsman posterior
      shoulder joint a.
    Broomhead medial ankle a.
    Brown knee a.
    Brown lateral knee a.
    Brügger muscle tension release
      postural a.
    Bruser lateral knee a.
    Bryan-Morrey elbow a.
    Bryan-Morrey extensive posterior
      elbow joint a.
    Callahan and Scuderi femur neck
      fracture repair a.
    Campbell elbow a.

approach (*continued*)

Campbell posterior shoulder a.
Campbell posterolateral a.
Carnesale acetabular extensile a.
Carnesale hip a.
Carroll clubfoot a.
Cave hip a.
Cave knee a.
cervical a.
Charnley-Müller lateral hip a.
Cloward cervical disc a.
Codman saber-cut shoulder a.
Colonna-Ralston medial ankle a.
combined anterior and posterior a.
combined low cervical and
    transthoracic a.
Coonse-Adams knee a.
costotransversectomy a.
Cozen transverse talonavicular
    fusion a.
Cubbins shoulder a.
curved L a.
de Andrade and MacNab anterior
    occipitocervical fusion a.
deBoer lateral knee a.
deltoid-splitting shoulder a.
deltopectoral a.
Dickinson acetabular a.
distal interphalangeal joint a.
dorsal finger a.
dorsal midline a.
dorsalward a.
dorsomedial a.
dorsoplantar a.
dorsoradial a.
dorsoulnar a.
dorsovolar a.
Downey modification of
    Fowler-Philip retrocalcaneal
    exostosis a.
DuVries plantar fasciotomy a.
endoscopic a.
extended iliofemoral a.
extensile anterior a.
extensile lateral a.
extensive posterior a.
extrabursal a.
extraperitoneal a.
extrapharyngeal a.
Fahey hip a.
femoral a.
Fernandez extensile anterior
    knee a.
Fowler-Philip retrocalcaneal
    exostosis a.
Gallie subtalar bone block
    arthrodesis a.
Gatellier-Chastang ankle a.
Gibson posterior hip a.

Gordon hip a.
Hardinge femoral hip a.
Hardinge lateral hip a.
Harmon cervical a.
Harmon modified posterolateral a.
Harmon shoulder a.
Harris anterolateral ankle a.
Harris lateral trigeminal
    neurolytic a.
Hay lateral hip a.
Henderson posterolateral tibia a.
Henderson posteromedial knee a.
Henry anterior strap a.
Henry anterolateral radial shaft a.
Henry extensile a.
Henry posterior interosseous
    nerve a.
Henry radial a.
Hirschhorn fracture compression
    plate a.
Hoffmann a.
Hoppenfeld lateral knee a.
Horwitz ankle fusion a.
Howorth a.
iliofemoral a.
ilioinguinal acetabular a.
inguinal a.
Insall anterior knee a.
intraforaminal a.
ipsilateral a.
Jones and Brackett anterior a.
keyhole a.
Kikuchi-MacNob-Moreau anterior
    cervical disectomy a.
Kocher curved-L a.
Kocher-Gibson posterolateral a.
Kocher-Langenbeck posterior
    proximal femur and acetabulum a.
Kocher lateral J a.
Langenbeck anteromedial a.
lateral deltoid-splitting a.
lateral J a.
lateral Kocher a.
lateral Ollier a.
lateral parapatellar a.
Leslie-Ryan anterior axillary a.
Letournel-Judet acetabular a.
long deltopectoral a.
low cervical a.
Ludloff medial open reduction
    hip a.
Mayo a.
McConnell extensile knee a.
McConnell median and ulnar
    nerve a.
McLaughlin a.
McWhorter posterior shoulder a.
medial parapatellar capsular a.
midlateral a.

midline medial a.
Mize-Bucholz-Grogan posterolateral femur a.
modified posterolateral a.
Moore posterior hip a.
Moore-Southern a.
multidisciplinary a.
Murphy lateral a.
muscle splitting a.
neurodevelopmental a.
Ollier a.
Ollier arthrodesis a.
Ollier lateral hip a.
open midline posterior a.
oropharyngeal a.
Osborne posterior hip a.
palmar a.
paramedian a.
parapatellar a.
pararectus a.
paraspinal a.
patella turndown a.
Perry extensile anterior distal humerus a.
Phemister medial epiphysiodesis a.
Phemister posteromedial a.
plantar a.
Pogrund lateral meniscectomy a.
posterior costotransversectomy a.
posterior interosseous nerve a.
posterior inverted-U a.
posterior midline a.
posterior occipitocervical a.
posterior shoulder a.
posterior transolecranon a.
posterolateral a.
posteromedial a.
proprioceptive neuromuscular facilitation a.
proximal interphalangeal joint a.
proximal metatarsal a.
pulp a.
Putti posterior knee a.
radical a.
Radley-Liebig-Brown ischium gluteal a.
Radley-Liebig-Brown resection of body of pubic bone a.
Reinert acetabular extensile a.
retroperitoneal a.
retropharyngeal a.
Roberts a.
Robinson-Smith anterior cervical a.
Roos transaxillary first rib resection a.
Rowe posterior shoulder a.
saber-cut a.
sacral a.
sacroiliac a.

screw-plate a.
Senegas hip a.
sensorimotor stimulation a.
Shoemaker lateral transfibular a.
Sir Henry Platt shoulder transverse a.
Smith-Petersen anterior hip a.
Smith-Robinson cervical disc a.
Somerville anterior hip a.
Southwick-Robinson anterior cervical a.
Spetzler cervical spine anterior transoral a.
split heel a.
split patellar a.
stabilization a.
Steel a.
sternum-splitting a.
subclavicular a.
supraclavicular a.
surgical a.
Swedish a.
Thompson anterolateral hip a.
Thompson anteromedial shoulder a.
Thompson posterior radial a.
thoracic a.
thoracoabdominal a.
thoracolumbar retroperitoneal a.
thoracoscopic a.
thoracotomy a.
thumb metacarpophalangeal joint a.
transacromial a.
transaxillary a.
transbrachioradialis a.
transcalcaneal a.
transclavicular a.
transfibular a.
transolecranon a.
transpedicular a.
transperitoneal a.
transsternal a.
transthoracic a.
transtrochanteric a.
transverse a.
triceps-splitting a.
triradial acetabular extensile a.
triradial transtrochanteric a.
trivector retaining a.
unilateral sacroiliac a.
Vermont Interdependent Services Team A. (VISTA)
volar a.
volarward a.
Wadsworth elbow a.
Wadsworth posterolateral a.
Wagner transfemoral total hip a.
Wagoner posterior cervical spinal a.
Watson-Jones anterolateral total hip a.

approach (*continued*)
 Wilson a.
 Wiltberger anterior cervical a.
 Wiltse paraspinal a.
 Wiltse spinal fusion
  muscle-splitting a.
 Yee posterior shoulder a.
 Young medial a.
 zigzag a.
 Z-plasty a.
approximate
approximation
approximator
 Acland clamp a.
 Acland double-clamp a.
 clamp a.
 double-clamp a.
 Henderson clamp a.
 hook a.
 Ikuta clamp a.
 Kleinert-Kutz clamp a.
 Lalonde tendon a.
 rib a.
 sternal a.
 Van Beek nerve a.
 Wolvek sternal a.
APPT
 Adolescent and Pediatric Pain Tool
APR
 anatomic porous replacement
 APR acetabular prosthesis
 APR cement fixation
 APR cement fixation adhesive
 APR femoral prosthesis
 APR hip stem
 APR I femoral stem
 APR II hip system
 APR II prosthesis
 APR total hip system
apraxia
 Bruns gait a.
 dressing a.
 Test of Oral and Limb A.
 (TOLA)
apraxic gait
ApriVera skin and hair cleanser
APRL
 Army Prosthetics Research Laboratory
 APRL hand prosthesis
 APRL prosthetic hook
apron
 quadriceps a.
apropulsive gait
APS
 air plasma spray
 anterior plate system
 APS Hi-Lo electric lift table
APTC
 anteroposterior talocalcaneal

aPTT
 activated partial thromboplastin
 time
APU
 adjustable posterior upright
 APU brace
 PRAFO APU
aqua, *pl.* **aquae**
 a. PT dry physiotherapy
 a. PT water massage
 A. Spray
 A. Spray wet nail débridement
 system
 A. Thermassage
AquaBodyCiser aquatic mat
Aqua-Cel heating pad system
Aquachloral Supprettes
Aquaciser
 A. hydrodynamic measurement
 system
 A. pool
 A. 100R underwater treadmill
 system
 A. underwater treadmill
aquae (*pl. of* aqua)
Aquaflex gel pad
AquaGaiter treadmill
AquaJogger buoyancy belt
AquaMED
 A. dry hydrotherapy
 A. dry hydrotherapy equipment
AquaMEPHYTON
AquaMotion pool
Aquanex hydrodynamic measurement system
Aquaphor gauze dressing
Aquaplast
 A. splint
 A. splinting material
Aquarelle hydrogel nucleus viscoelastic material
AquaRunners resistance footwear
AquaSens fluid monitoring system
AquaShield
 A. orthopaedic cast cover
 A. reusable cast cover
Aquasonic Transmission Gel
Aquasorb Hydrogel wound dressing
Aquatech cast pad
aquatherapy
Aquatherm bed pad
aquatic
 a. cardiac evaluation and testing
 (ACET)
 a. exercise
 a. exercise program
 a. map
 a. rehabilitation
 a. stabilization program

a. therapy
a. therapy pool
Aqua-Trainer
AquaTrek Wheelchair
Aquatrend water workout
station
Aqua/Whirl bath
ARA
Adolescent Role Assessment
ARA test
arabinoside
adenine a.
arachidonate metabolism
arachidonic
arachnodactylia (*var. of*
arachnodactyly)
arachnodactyly, arachnodactylia
arachnoid
arachnoiditis
adhesive a.
arachnoid-shape Beaver
blade
Arafiles elbow arthrodesis
Aralen Phosphate
Aran-Duchenne
A.-D. amyotrophy
A.-D. disease
Arava
Aravon footwear
Arbeitsgemeinschaft
A. für Osteosynthesefragen (AO)
A. für Osteosynthesefragen-
Association for Internal Fixation
(AO-ASIF)
A. für
Osteosynthesefragen-Association for
the Study of Internal Fixation
(AO-ASIF)
A. für Osteosynthesefragen
compression apparatus
A. für Osteosynthesefragen
contouring apparatus
arborescens
lipoma a.
ARC
antirotation cable
arc
carpal a.
flexion-extension a.
Leksell stereotactic a.
monosynaptic reflex a.
a. of motion
painful a.
reflex a.
shoulder ROM a.
stereotactic a.
arcade
Frohse ligamentous a.
a. of Frohse

a. of Struthers
superficialis a.
Arcelin petrous temporal
view
arch
a. and slouch position
a. angle
anterior metatarsal a.
axillary a.
a. binder
carpal a.
cervical a.
a. cookie
coracoacromial a.
a. cushion
deep a.
dorsal venous a.
fallen a.
a. fracture
Hapad metatarsal a.
Hapad scaphoid a.
Hillock a.
a. index
ischiopubic a.
keystone of the calcar a.
Langer axillary a.
a. loading
longitudinal plantar a.
medial longitudinal a.
metatarsal a.
a. of bone
a. of foot
a. of Frohse
palmar a.
a. peak area
pedicle of vertebral a.
plantar arterial a.
posterior a.
Roman a.
scaphoid a.
a. stress
superficial palmar a.
a. support
vertebral a.
archer's shoulder
arch-height
a.-h. index
a.-h. ratio
Archimedean drill
architectural
a. alteration of bone
a. anisotropy
architecture
bony a.
foot a.
Arch-Lok
Swede-O A.-L.
archplasty
arch-up test

Archxerciser foot exercise device
arciform
ARCO
> Association Research Circulation
> Osseous
>> ARCO classification system
>> ARCO osteonecrosis
>> ARCO osteonecrosis classification

ArCom processed polyethylene
Arctic Blaze hot/cold pack
arcuate, arciform
> a. complex
> a. fasciculus (AF)
> a. foramen
> a. movement
> a. osteotomy
> a. popliteal ligament

arcuatus
> pes a.

arcus
ardeparin sodium
area
> arch peak a.
> Broca a.
> curvilinear a.
> dorsolumbar a.
> functional cross-sectional a.
> Little a.
> odontoid-axial a.
> Patrick trigger a.
> performance a.
> pressure-sensitive a.
> problem a.
> puboischial a.
> pump bump a.
> resection a.
> a. scar
> thenar a.
> trapezial a.
> web a.

Aredia
areflexia
> detrusor a.

areola, *pl.* **areolae**
> a. of bone

areolae (*pl. of* areola)
argatroban
Argesic-SA
Arglaes antimicrobial silver film dressing
ARGO
> Adjustable Advanced Reciprocating
> Gait Orthosis

Ariat shoe
Ariel computerized exercise system
Aristocort Forte
Arixtra
Arizona
> A. ankle brace
> A. Health Science Center (AHSC)

> A. Health Sciences Center-Volz
> hinge
> A. universal leg support

ARM
> alternating range of motion
> ARM method
> ARM method of physical
> examination

arm
> abductor lever a.
> articulating a.
> artificial a.
> a. band
> a. board
> a. cuff
> a. cylinder cast
> a. drift
> a. elevator sling
> flail a.
> a. flap
> a. fossa test
> grenade thrower's a.
> a. heel-strike synchrony
> a. holder
> lever a.
> Leyla a.
> linebacker's a.
> moment a.
> MonitorMate monitor a.
> outrigger a.
> Popeye a.
> a. positioner
> a. skate
> a. swath
> tackler's a.
> Utah artificial a.
> wringer a.
> Yasargil Leyla retractor a.

armboard
armchair splint
2-arm goniometer
Armistead
> A. distraction osteogenesis
> technique
> A. ulnar lengthening
> A. ulnar lengthening operation

Armstrong
> A. acromionectomy
> A. plate

Army
> A. bone gouge
> A. osteotome
> A. Prosthetic Research Lab
> prosthetic hook
> A. Prosthetics Research Laboratory
> (APRL)

Army-Navy retractor
Arnadottir OT-ADL Neurobehavioral
Evaluation (A-ONE)

Arnold
    A. lumbar brace
    A. nerve
Arnold-Chiari
    A.-C. deformity
    A.-C. malformation
    A.-C. syndrome
AROM
    active range of motion
Aron Alpha adhesive
arotinolol
Array spinal system
arrest
    epiphysial a.
    greater trochanteric apophysial a.
    growth a.
    mechanism of growth a.
arrow
    A. absorbable meniscal repair device
    Biofix meniscus a.
    Bionx a.
    meniscal a.
    A. pin clasp
ARS
    acute repetitive seizure
    ARS disorder
ART
    active-release technique
ArtAssist arterial assist device
artefact (*var. of* artifact)
arteria (a), *pl.* **arteriae**
    a. acetabuli
arteriae (aa) (*pl. of* arteria)
arterial
    a. aneurysm
    a. flap
    a. gas embolism
    a. occlusion sign
    a. oxygen saturation (SaO_2)
    a. ring
    a. spasm
    a. trauma
arteriogram
arteriography
    femoral a.
    magnetic resonance a. (MRA)
    peripheral a.
    spinal a.
    vertebral a.
arteriosclerosis obliterans
arteriotomy
    ankle-level a.
arteriovenous (AV)
    a. fistula (AVF)
    a. malformation
arteritis
artery, arteria
    Adamkiewicz a.
    anomalous fibular nutrient a.

anterior radial collateral a.
anterior recurrent tibial a.
anterior spinal a.
anterior tibial a.
ascending cervical a.
axillary a.
basilic a.
brachial a.
carotid a.
cephalic a.
cervical a.
circumflex iliac a.
circumflex scapular a.
collateral a.
common carotid a. (CCA)
common iliac a. (CIA)
deep circumflex iliac a.
deltoid a.
digital a.
dorsal digital a. (DDA)
dorsal metatarsal a.
epiphysial a.
facial a.
femoral circumflex a.
fibular plantar marginal a.
first dorsal metacarpal a.
first dorsal metatarsal a.
  (FDMA)
first plantar metatarsal a. (FPMA)
genicular a.
gluteal a.
hypogastric a.
iliac a.
iliofemoral flap a.
iliolumbar a.
inferior thyroid a.
intercostal a.
intermetatarsal a.
internal carotid a.
internal iliac a.
interosseous a.
lateral calcaneal a.
lateral plantar a.
lingual a.
medial geniculate a.
medial plantar a.
metaphysial a.
metatarsal a.
middle sacral a.
nutrient a.
obturator a.
paramalleolar a.
perforating a.
peripheral a.
peroneal a.
persistent sciatic a. (PSA)
plantar a.
plantar metatarsal a.
popliteal a.

artery (*continued*)
    posterior inferior cerebellar a.
        (PICA)
    posterior radial collateral a.
    posterior tibial a. (PTA)
    princeps pollicis a.
    profunda brachii a.
    profunda femoris a.
    pudendal a.
    radial a.
    radicular a.
    retinacular a.
    sacral a.
    saphenous a.
    second metatarsal a.
    spinal a.
    subclavian a.
    superficial circumflex iliac a.
    superficial femoral a. (SFA)
    superficial temporal a.
    superior laryngeal a.
    superior thyroid a.
    supraclavicular fossa a.
    tarsal canal a.
    tarsal sinus a.
    thoracoacromial a.
    thrombosis radial a.
    tibial a.
    ulnar a.
    vertebral a. (VA)
    volar digital a.
Artha-G
Arth-Aid Joint Formula
arthralgia
    acromegalic a.
    intermittent a.
    migratory a.
    nonspecific a.
    periodic a.
    a. saturnina
    subtalar a.
    temporomandibular joint a.
arthralgic
arthrectomy
arthrempyesis
Arthrex
    A. Adapteur C-ring drill guide
    A. arthroscopy instrument
    A. bioabsorbable PLLA Trim-It
        system
    A. bioabsorbable Trim-It system
    A. Bio-SutureTak
    A. Bird-Beak device
    A. bone anchor
    A. coring reamer
    A. femoral guide
    A. instruments and systems
    A. meniscal dart
    A. meniscal dart gun

    A. Penetrator
    A. RetroScrew
    A. sheathed interference screw
    A. subcoracoid drill guide
    A. SutureLasso
    A. tibial guide
    A. Trim-It drill pin osteotomy
        fixation kit
    A. Trim-It screw fixation system
    A. Trim-It Spin Pin
    A. TwistLoc suture anchor
    A. zebra pin
arthrifluent abscess
arthritic
    a. ankle joint narrowing
    a. atrophy
    a. destrasis
    a. deterioration
    a. knee hemicallotasis
    a. shoe
    a. talonavicular change
arthriticum
    tuberculum a.
arthritides (*pl. of* arthritis)
arthritis, *pl.* **arthritides**
    acromegalic a.
    acute hematogenous a.
    acute spinal a.
    adjuvant-induced a. (AIA)
    allergenic a.
    ancient tuberculous a.
    ankle infectious a.
    ankle rheumatoid a.
    antigen-induced a.
    assignment criteria for rheumatoid a.
    atrophic a.
    bacterial a.
    base of thumb a.
    Bekhterev a.
    calcaneocuboid joint a.
    cervical a.
    Charcot a.
    chronic absorptive a.
    chronic villous a. (CVA)
    chylous a.
    crystal-induced a.
    cystic rheumatoid a.
    a. deformans
    degenerative a. (DA)
    elderly onset rheumatoid a.
    enteropathic a.
    erosive arthritides
    filarial a.
    A. Foundation
    A. Foundation Pain Reliever
    fungal a.
    gonococcal septic a.
    gouty a.
    A. Helplessness Index (AHI)

hemophilic a.
hypertrophic a.
hypotrophic a.
A. Impact Measurement Scale
  (AIMS)
A. Impact Measurement Scale
  classification
infectious a.
inflammatory bowel disease
  associated a.
Jaccoud a.
juvenile a. (JA)
juvenile chronic a.
juvenile-onset rheumatoid a.
juvenile rheumatoid a. (JRA)
Lyme disease a.
Marie-Strümpell a.
midfoot a.
migratory a.
monoarticular septic a.
a. mutilans
mutilans rheumatoid a.
mycobacterial a.
navicular a.
neonatal septic a.
neuropathic a.
New York diagnostic criteria for
  rheumatoid a.
a. nodosa
nonarticular a.
ochronotic a.
oligoarticular a.
pantrapezial a.
patellofemoral a.
pauciarticular a.
periosteal a.
peritrapezial a.
pisotriquetral a.
polyarticular juvenile rheumatoid a.
postinfectious a.
postmenopausal a.
posttraumatic a.
primary degenerative a.
proliferative a.
psoriatic a.
pyogenic a.
A. Quality of Life Scale
radiocarpal a.
reactive a.
rheumatoid a. (RA)
robust rheumatoid a.
Salmonella a.
sarcoid a.
septic a.
seronegative rheumatoid a.
seropositive rheumatoid a.
silicone a.
a. sock
spinal a.

staphylococcal a.
subtalar joint a.
suppurative a.
tendon bowing in a.
tibiotalar a.
Tom Smith a.
traumatic a.
tuberculous a.
vertebral a.
viral-associated a.
arthritis-associated psoriasis
Arthro-7
ArthroCare
  A. arthroscopic system
  A. electrode
  A. wand
arthrocele
arthrocentesis
arthrochalasis
arthrochondritis
arthroclasia
arthrodesed digit
arthrodesis
  Abbott-Fischer-Lucas hip a.
  Abbott-Lucas a.
  Adams transmalleolar a.
  Adkins spinal a.
  Albee hip a.
  ankle a.
  anterior occipitocervical a.
  anterior slot graft a.
  AO group shoulder a.
  Arafiles elbow a.
  arthroscopic ankle a.
  arthroscopic subtalar a.
  atlantoaxial a.
  Baciu-Filibiu dowel ankle a.
  Baciu-Filibiu transmalleolar a.
  Badgley hip a.
  Barrasso-Wile-Gage subtalar a.
  Barr-Record ankle a.
  Batchelor-Brown extraarticular
    subtalar a.
  beak modification with triple a.
  biframed distraction technique
    arthroscopic ankle a.
  bimalleolar approach to ankle a.
  Blair ankle a.
  Blair anterior a.
  Blair tibiotalar a.
  Bosworth a.
  Boyd ankle a.
  Brett a.
  Brewster triple a.
  Brittain ischiofemoral a.
  Brockman-Nissen a.
  Brooks atlantoaxial a.
  calcaneocuboid distraction a.
    (CCDA)

arthrodesis (*continued*)
calcaneopelvic a.
calcaneotibial a.
Campbell-Akbarnia a.
Campbell posterior a.
Campbell-Rinehard-Kalenak ankle a.
Carroll a.
cervical a.
Chandler a.
Chapchal knee a.
Charcot hip a.
Charnley ankle a.
Charnley compression a.
closing wedge a.
Cloward cervical a.
combined resection arthroplasty and a.
Compere-Thompson a.
compression a.
cone a.
coracoclavicular a.
cuneiform joint a.
Davis a.
Dennyson-Fulford extraarticular subtalar a.
distal fibulotalar a.
distraction bone block a.
distraction-compression bone graft a.
distraction subtalar a.
double a.
dowel a.
Dunn-Brittain triple a.
Dunn triple a.
elbow a.
Elmslie triple a.
Enneking knee a.
Enneking resection a.
excisional a.
extension injury posterior atlantoaxial a.
extraarticular a.
failed triple a.
fibulotalar a.
first cuneiform joint a.
first cuneiform-navicular joint a.
first metatarsal-first cuneiform a.
flat-cut a.
fused a.
Gallie ankle a.
Gallie atlantoaxial a.
Gant hip a.
Garceau-Brahms a.
Gill a.
Gill-Stein a.
Gissane a.
glenohumeral a.
Goldner spinal a.
Graham ankle a.
Grice extraarticular subtalar a.

Grice-Green extraarticular subtalar a.
Guttmann subtalar a.
hallux interphalangeal joint a.
hallux rigidus a.
Heiple a.
Henderson a.
Hibbs a.
hindfoot a.
Hoke triple a.
Horwitz-Adams a.
Horwitz transmalleolar a.
Huckstep nail a.
Hunt-Thompson pantalar a.
Ilizarov ankle a.
interbody a.
intercarpal a.
internal fixation compression a.
interphalangeal a.
intertransverse process a.
intraarticular a.
intramedullary a.
John C. Wilson a.
joint a.
Kapandji-Sauvé a.
Key intraarticular knee a.
Kirkaldy-Willis a.
knee a.
Küntscher modified knee a.
Lambrinudi triple a.
Lapidus a.
Lapidus modified a.
lesser tarsal a.
limited intertarsal a.
Lipscomb metatarsophalangeal a.
Lipscomb modified McKeever a.
Lisfranc a.
Lord total hip a.
lunotriquetral a.
Mann modified McKeever a.
McKeever metatarsophalangeal a.
metatarsocuneiform a.
metatarsophalangeal joint a.
midcarpal a.
midfoot a.
Millender-Nalebuff wrist a.
Moberg a.
modified Boyd ankle a.
modified Lapidus a.
Mohammed internal fixation shoulder a.
Mueller a.
Nalebuff a.
Naughton-Dunn triple a.
naviculocuneiform joint a.
non-fused a.
occipitocervical a.
panastragaloid a.
pantalar a.
paraarticular a.

Podiatry Institute procedures for ankle a.
Pontenza a.
posterior atlantoaxial a.
posterolateral a.
Potter a.
Pridie ankle a.
primary subtalar a.
Putti knee a.
radiocarpal a.
radiolunate a.
resection a.
Richards a.
Richardson subtalar a.
Robinson-Smith spinal a.
Robinson spinal a.
Ryerson triple a.
salvage ankle a.
scaphocapitolunate a.
scaphotrapeziotrapezoid a.
scapulothoracic a.
Schneider cobra head plate a.
Schneider hip a.
SCL a.
Scranton transmalleolar a.
a. screw
second metatarsophalangeal joint a.
Seoffert triple a.
shoulder a.
Simmons spinal a.
sliding a.
Smith-Robinson interbody a.
Soren foot a.
spinal a.
Staples elbow a.
Stark first metatarsophalangeal joint a.
Steindler elbow a.
stone a.
subtalar a.
talar triple a.
talonavicular a.
tarsal a.
tarsometatarsal truncated-wedge a.
thoracoscapular a.
tibiocalcaneal a.
tibiotalar joint primary a.
tibiotalocalcaneal a.
transfibular a.
transmalleolar ankle a.
triple a.
triquetrum-lunate a.
triscaphe a.
Trumble hip a.
truncated tarsometatarsal wedge a.
truncated wedge tarsometatarsal a.
Uematsu shoulder a.
ulnocarpal a.
Watson-Jones hip a.

Whitecloud-LaRocca cervical a.
White posterior occipitocervical a.
Wilson cone a.
Wolf blade plate ankle a.
arthrodial
   a. articulation
   a. cartilage
   a. protractor
   A. Protractor range of motion analyzer
arthrodiastasis
arthrodynia
arthrodynic
arthrodysplasia
arthroempyesis
arthroendoscopy
arthroereisis (*var. of* arthrorisis)
arthrofibrosis
Arthrofile orthopaedic rasp
Arthro-Flo
   A.-F. arthroscopic irrigation system
   A.-F. irrigator
Arthroforce III hand instrument
arthrogenic gait
arthrogenous
arthrogram
   double-contrast a.
   Gordon-Broström single-contrast a.
   joint a.
   nuclear a.
   saline-enhanced MR a.
   single-contrast a.
arthrographic capsular distension and rupture technique
arthrography
   air a.
   ankle a.
   contrast a.
   coronal computed tomographic a. (CCTA)
   double-contrast a.
   joint a.
   magnetic resonance a. (MRAr)
   opaque a.
   osteochondral fracture a.
   saline-enhanced a.
arthrogryposis
   a. multiplex congenita
   myopathic a.
   neurogenic a.
arthrogrypotic clubfoot
arthrokatadysis
arthrokinematic
arthrokinematics
arthrokinetic reflex
arthrokleisis
arthrolith
arthrolithiasis
Arthro-Lock system

arthrology
    zygapophysial a.
Arthro-Lok system of Beaver blade
arthrolysis
arthromeningitis
arthrometer
    Acufex knee laxity a.
    Genucom a.
    joint a.
    knee laxity a.
    knee ligament a.
    KT-1000 joint a.
    KT-1000/Jr a.
    KT-1000, 2000 knee ligament a.
    KT-1000/s surgical a.
    a. measurement
    Medmetric knee ligament a.
    Medmetric KT-1000 knee laxity a.
    Robinson a.
    stress-testing a.
    Stryker knee laxity a.
    a. test
    a. testing
arthrometric knee laxity measurement
arthrometry
arthroncus
arthroneuralgia
arthronosos
arthroonychodysplasia syndrome
arthroophthalmopathy
    hereditary progressive a.
arthroosteoonychodysplasia
Arthropan
arthropathia psoriatica
arthropathic
arthropathology
arthropathy
    Charcot a.
    crystal-induced a.
    crystal-related a.
    cuff tear a. (CTA)
    degenerative vertebral a.
    diabetic a.
    dislocating a.
    disuse a.
    facet degenerative a.
    gonococcal a.
    Heberden a.
    hemodialysis-related a.
    hemophilic a.
    inflammatory a.
    Jaccoud a.
    joint a.
    long leg a.
    midfoot a.
    neuropathic a. (NA)
    neuropathic spinal a.
    ochronotic a.
    palindromic a.

    pyrophosphate a.
    sacroiliac joint a.
    seronegative a.
    SLE a.
    static a.
    stationary a.
    tabetic a.
arthrophyte
arthroplasty
    ablative a.
    abrasion a.
    acetabular cup a.
    acromioclavicular a.
    Albright-Chase palmar shelf a.
    anametric total knee a.
    anconeus a.
    ankle a.
    Ashworth hand a.
    Ashworth implant a.
    Aufranc cup a.
    Aufranc-Turner a.
    Austin Moore a.
    autogenous interpositional
      shoulder a.
    Bankart a.
    Bechtol total hip a.
    Bechtol total knee a.
    Bigliani-Flatow total shoulder a.
    bipolar hip a.
    Bosworth a.
    Bowers radial a.
    Brain a.
    Breslow a.
    Bryan a.
    a. bur
    Campbell interpositional a.
    Campbell resection a.
    capitellocondylar total elbow a.
    capsular interposition a.
    carpometacarpal a.
    Carroll and Taber a.
    Castle-Schneider resection
      interposition a.
    a. cement
    cemented total hip a.
    cementless surface replacement a.
      (CSRA)
    cementless total hip a.
    Charcot a.
    Charnley low-friction a.
    Charnley-Müller a.
    Charnley total hip a.
    Clayton forefoot a.
    Clayton resection a.
    Colonna trochanteric a.
    condylar implant a.
    constrained ankle a.
    constrained shoulder a.
    convex condylar-implant a.

Coonrad hinged a.
Coonrad-Morrey total elbow a.
Coonrad total elbow a.
Cracchiolo forefoot a.
Cracchiolo-Sculco implant a.
Crawford-Adams acetabular cup a.
Cubbins a.
cuff tear a.
cup a.
Dewar-Barrington a.
distraction a.
DuVries a.
Eaton implant a.
Eaton volar plate a.
Eden-Hybbinette a.
elbow a.
Ewald capitellocondylar total
  elbow a.
Ewald-Walker kinematic knee a.
excision a.
extensor brevis a.
failed implant a.
fascial a.
finger joint a.
forefoot a.
Ganley modification of Keller a.
gap a.
Girdlestone resection a.
Global total shoulder a.
Gore-Tex interpositional a.
a. gouge
Green a.
Gristina-Webb total shoulder a.
Gunston a.
Gustilo-Kyle cementless total hip a.
Harrington total hip a.
Head hip a.
Helal flap a.
hemijoint a.
hemiresection interposition a.
hip a.
Hungerford-Krackow-Kenna knee a.
hydroxyapatite-coated ankle a.
ICLH double cup a.
implant a.
4-in-1 a.
Inclan-Ober a.
Inglis triaxial total elbow a.
Insall-Burstein-Freeman knee a.
interphalangeal a.
interposition a.
interpositional a.
ipsilateral total elbow a.
ipsilateral total shoulder a.
Irvine ankle a.
Jaccoud a.
Johnson resection a.
Jones resection a.
Kates forefoot a.

Keller a.
Keller-Brandes resection a.
Keller-Lelièvre a.
Keller-Mann resection a.
Keller-Mayo diabetic foot a.
Keller resection a.
knee a.
Koenig metatarsophalangeal joint a.
Lacey rotating hinge a.
Larmon forefoot a.
laser image custom a. (LICA)
Magnuson-Stack a.
Magnuson-Stack shoulder a.
Mann resection a.
Mayo ankle a.
Mayo resection a.
Mayo-Stone-Valenti hallux
  limitus/rigidus a.
Mayo total elbow a.
McKee-Farrar total hip a.
McLaughlin a.
metacarpophalangeal joint a.
metatarsophalangeal a.
Meuli a.
Millender a.
Miller-Galante knee a.
mobile-bearing knee a.
modified Keller resection a.
modified mold and surface
  replacement a.
mold acetabular a.
monospherical total shoulder a.
mosaic a.
Mould a.
Mueller hip a.
Mumford-Gurd a.
Nara a.
NEB a.
Neer unconstrained shoulder a.
Neviaser a.
New England Baptist hip a.
Nicola a.
Niebauer trapeziometacarpal a.
noncemented total hip a.
Post total shoulder a.
press-fit condylar knee a.
primary a.
A. Products Consultants foot and
  legholder
prosthetic a.
Putti-Platt a.
Regnauld modification of Keller a.
resection a.
revision a.
revision hip a.
revision of shoulder a.
Robinson a.
rotator cuff tear a.
Sauvé-Kapandji wrist a.

arthroplasty (*continued*)
- Schlein elbow a.
- Schrock hip a.
- Scott total knee revision a.
- semiconstrained total elbow a.
- shoulder a.
- silastic lunate a.
- silicone implant a.
- silicone rubber a.
- silicone wrist a.
- Smith-Petersen cup a.
- Sorrells hip a.
- Speed a.
- Stanmore shoulder a.
- Steffee thumb a.
- supine position for hip a.
- surface replacement hip a.
- Sutter silicone metacarpophalangeal joint a.
- Swanson convex condylar a.
- Swanson interpositional wrist a.
- Swanson metatarsophalangeal joint a.
- Swanson PIP joint a.
- Swanson radial head implant a.
- Swanson silicone wrist a.
- tendon interposition a.
- Thackray low friction a.
- Thompson a.
- total ankle a. (TAA)
- total articular replacement a. (TARA)
- total articular resurfacing a. (TARA)
- total elbow a. (TEA)
- total hip a. (THA)
- total joint a. (TJA)
- total knee a. (TKA)
- total patellofemoral joint a.
- total shoulder a. (TSA)
- total wrist a. (TWA)
- triaxial total elbow a.
- Trillat total knee a.
- Tupper palmar plate interposition a.
- UCLA anatomic shoulder a.
- ulnar hemiresection interposition a.
- unconstrained shoulder a.
- unicompartmental knee a. (UKA)
- Vainio metacarpal joint a.
- Valenti first metatarsophalangeal joint a.
- Valenti metatarsophalangeal a.
- van Ness rotational a.
- vitallium cup a.
- volar plate a.
- Volz total wrist a.
- Woodward scapula a.

arthropneumoradiography, arthropneumoroentgenography

arthropneumoroentgenography (*var. of* arthropneumoradiography)

Arthropor
- A. acetabular cup
- A. cup pad
- A. cup prosthesis
- A. II acetabular prosthesis
- A. II porous socket
- A. oblong cup for acetabular defect

ArthroProbe
- A. arthroscopic laser
- Contact A.
- A. laser system

arthropyosis

arthrorheumatism

arthrorisis, arthroereisis
- Maxwell-Brancheau a. (MBA)
- peg-in-hole a.
- staple a.

arthroscintigraphy

arthrosclerosis

arthroscope
- angled a.
- Baxter angled a.
- Citscope disposable a.
- disposable a.
- Dyonics a.
- Eagle a.
- Eagle straight-ahead a.
- fiberoptic a.
- GoldenEye a.
- O'Connor operating a.
- Panoview a.
- Sapphire View a.
- a. sleeve
- Storz oblique a.
- Stryker viewing a.
- triangulation technique for a.
- Trio a.
- Wolf a.

arthroscopic
- a. abrasion chondroplasty
- a. acromioplasty
- a. ankle arthrodesis
- a. augmentation
- a. Bankart repair
- a. Bankart repair using absorbable fixation device
- a. cannula
- a. capsulolateral augmentation and rotator interval
- a. cheilectomy
- a. coplaning
- a. débridement
- a. drilling
- a. drivethrough sign
- a. entry portal
- a. examination
- a. grabber
- a. knife
- a. knot

a. laser instrument
a. laser surgery
a. leg holder
a. legholder
a. meniscectomy
a. microdiscectomy (AMD)
a. mosaicplasty
a. osteotome
a. probe
a. pump
a. punch
a. resection of dorsal wrist ganglion
a. scissors
a. screw fixation
a. shaver
a. shaving
a. sheath
a. shield
a. subtalar arthrodesis
a. synovectomy
a. tourniquet
a. transglenoid suture stabilization
   procedure
a. transhumeral reconstruction
arthroscopically
a. assisted anterior cruciate ligament
   reconstruction
a. assisted synovectomy
arthroscopy
Allen shoulder a.
ankle a.
A. Association of North America
   (AANA)
a. basket forceps
calcaneonavicular joint a.
diagnostic a. (DA)
diagnostic and operative a. (DOA)
electrothermal a.
European Society of Sports
   Traumotology, Knee Surgery, and
   A. (ESSKA)
extraarticular a.
a. grasping forceps
Hawkeye suture needle for a.
knee a.
laser a.
lateral hip a.
metacarpophalangeal a.
midcarpal a.
monopolar electrothermal a.
2nd-look a.
a. of subtalar joint
operative a.
radiocarpal a.
Ringer a.
a. sleeve
wrist a.
**arthroscopy-assisted patellar tendon
   substitution**

arthroses (*pl. of* arthrosis)
ArthroSew arthroscopic suturing device
arthrosis, *pl.* **arthroses**
Charcot a.
crystal-induced a.
cystic a.
a. deformans
a. deformity
degenerative a.
Eaton and Glickel carpometacarpal
   joint a. (stage I–IV)
end-stage a.
Malleoloc anatomic ankle a.
metatarsal-sesamoid a.
posttraumatic a.
primary cystic a.
subtalar a.
trapezial a.
uncovertebral a.
winging scapula a.
Arthrosol dressing
arthrosteitis
arthrostomy
arthrosynovitis
Arthrotek
A. calibrated cylinder
A. Ellipticut hand instrumentation
A. femoral aimer
A. meniscus staple
A. tibial fixation device
arthrotome
arthrotomography
double contrast shoulder a.
arthrotomy
diagnostic arthroscopy, operative
   arthroscopy, possible operative a.
   (AAA)
Magnuson-Stack shoulder a.
medial parapatellar a.
operative a.
parapatellar a.
subtalar a.
arthrotropic
ArthroWand
bevel A.
A. device
A. disposable surgical wand
dome knee A.
Eliminator A.
meniscus A.
Microblator A.
Paragon T2 A.
RazorVac A.
Saber Bisector A.
suction A.
A. tool
arthroxerosis
arthroxesis
Arth-Support Formula

articular
- a. block
- a. blockage
- a. bone lamella
- a. bone tubercle
- a. capsule
- a. cartilage
- a. cartilage autograft
- a. cartilage autografting
- a. cartilage lesion
- a. cortex
- a. crepitus
- a. defect
- a. disc
- a. facet
- a. facet angle
- a. fragment
- a. gout
- a. insert
- a. instability
- a. labrum
- a. mass separation
- a. mass separation fracture
- a. motion device (AMD)
- a. nerve
- a. pillar
- a. pillar fracture
- a. process
- a. rheumatism
- a. sensibility
- a. set angle
- a. strain
- a. structure
- a. surface

articular-ligamentous system
articulate
articulated
- a. AFO
- a. chin implant
- a. external fixator
- a. minifixator
- a. skeleton
- a. tension device

articulating
- a. arm
- a. bone end

articulatio humeri
articulation
- acromioclavicular a.
- arthrodial a.
- atlantoaxial a.
- atlantodental a. (ADA)
- calcaneocuboid a.
- calcaneonavicular a.
- carpal a.
- carpometacarpal a.
- carporadial a.
- chondrosternal a.
- Chopart a.

condylar a.
congruent a.
coracoclavicular a.
costocentral a.
costosternal a.
costovertebral a.
coxofemoral a.
DIP a.
distal interphalangeal a.
a. disturbance
ellipsoidal a.
false a.
Goldman-Fristoe Test of A.
hinge a.
humeroradial a.
humeroulnar a.
iliosacral a.
immovable a.
incongruent a.
incudomalleolar a.
intercarpal a.
intermetacarpal a.
interphalangeal a.
lateral mass a. (LMA)
Lisfranc joint a.
manipulation of a.
metacarpophalangeal a.
metatarsocuneiform a.
occipitocervical a.
a. of foot
a. of pisiform bone
patellofemoral a.
phalangeal a.
plane-type acromioclavicular a.
proximal interphalangeal a.
proximal radioulnar a.
radiocapitellar a.
radiocarpal a.
radiohumeral a.
radioscaphoid a.
radioulnar a.
sacrococcygeal a.
sacroiliac a.
scapuloclavicular a.
slightly movable a.
sternochondral a.
sternoclavicular a.
subtalar a.
superior tibial a.
synovial a.
talocalcaneonavicular ligament a.
talofibular a.
talonavicular a.
tarsometatarsal a.
tibiofemoral a.
tibiofibular a.
transverse tarsal a.
trochoid a.
ulnolunate a.

ulnotriquetrum a.
Vermont spinal fixator a.
zygapophysial a.
articulatory
a. procedure
a. skill
a. tic
Articulose-50 Injection
artifact, artefact
electric a.
friction a.
movement a.
a. on x-ray
shock a.
stimulus a.
artifactitious (*var. of* artifactual)
artifactual, artifactitious
artificial
a. ankylosis
a. arm
a. fat pad
a. foot
a. hand
a. joint implant
a. leech
a. ligament
a. limb
a. vertebral body
Artisan cement system
Artscan
A. 200 arthroscopic cartilage
stiffness tester
A. 200 arthroscopic cartilage
stiffness testing device
arum fixation pin
arytenoid
a. cartilage
a. dislocation
a. subluxation
arytenoidectomy
arytenoiditis
arytenoidopexy
AS
anterior and superior
anterior-superior
anterosuperior
AS ilium
AS movement
AS subluxation
ASA
acetylsalicylic acid
ascending cervical artery
ascension
A. MCP finger joint implant
A. MCP total joint
A. MCP total joint implant
A. MCP total joint replacement
A. PIP total joint
A. PIP total joint replacement

Ascent total knee system
Asch
A. forceps
A. splint
Ascriptin
ASD
adjacent segment degeneration
ASE
axilla, shoulder, elbow
ASE bandage
aseptic
a. fashion
a. felon
a. hypertrophic nonunion
a. loosening
a. necrosis
ASES
American Shoulder and Elbow
Surgeons
ASES shoulder score
ASEX
anterosuperior external
ASEX ilium
ASEX movement
ASEX subluxation
**Asher physical build assessment
technique**
**Ashhurst-Bromer ankle fracture
classification**
**Ashhurst transcondylar humeral fracture
classification (I, II)**
Ashworth
A. hand arthroplasty
A. implant arthroplasty
A. scale (1–5)
A. scale of muscle spasticity score
(0-4, 1-5)
A. score of muscle spasticity (0-4,
1-5)
ASI
acromial spur index
ASIA
American Spinal Injury Association
ASIA impairment scale
ASIA standardneurological
classification of spinal cord injury
Asics Gel-MC shoe
ASICT
amplitude-summation interferential
current therapy
ASIF
Association for the Study of Internal
Fixation
ASIF broad dynamic compression
bone plate
ASIF cancellous screw
ASIF chisel
ASIF cortical screw
ASIF malleolar screw

ASIF (*continued*)
    ASIF reconstruction plate
    ASIF right-angle blade-plate
    ASIF screw fixation operation
    ASIF screw fixation technique
    ASIF screw pin
    ASIF system
    ASIF T-plate
    ASIF twist drill
ASIN
    anterosuperior internal
    ASIN ilium
    ASIN movement
    ASIN subluxation
ASIS
    anterior superior iliac spine
Asissto-Seat
    Maddapult A.-S.
Aslan endoscopic scissors
ASM
    appendicular skeletal muscle
Asnis
    A. cannulated screw fixation
      technique
    A. 3 cannulated screw system
    A. 2 guided-screw system
    A. pin
    A. pinning
ASO
    ankle stabilizing orthosis
    ASO ankle brace
    ASO support
ASOT
    antistreptolysin O titer
ASP
    anterior superior portal
aspect
    dorsal a.
    laminar cortex posterior a.
    medial a.
    posterolateral a.
    volar a.
Aspen
    A. cervical collar
    A. CTO
    A. electrocautery
aspera
    linea a.
Aspercin Extra
aspergillosis infection
Aspergillus
    A. *fumigatus*
    A. *niger*
aspirated fat
aspiration
    anterior a.
    bone marrow a.
    joint a.
    lateral a.

    medial a.
    a. needle biopsy
aspirator
    Cavitron ultrasonic surgical a.
     (CUSA)
    Sonocut ultrasonic a.
    ultrasonic a.
aspirin
    a. and codeine
    Bayer Buffered A.
    carisoprodol and a.
    Extra Strength Bayer Enteric 500
     A.
    A. Free Anacin Maximum Strength
    hydrocodone and a.
    methocarbamol and a.
    oxycodone and a.
    propoxyphene and a.
    Regular Strength Bayer Enteric 500
     A.
    St Joseph Adult Chewable A.
Asprimox
ASPS
    alveolar soft part sarcoma
assay
    AlamarBlue osteoblast proliferation
     a.
    cefazolin a.
    deoxypyridinoline crosslinks
     urine a.
    enzyme-linked immunosorbent a.
    microtiter protein kinase a.
    osteoblast proliferation fluorometric
     a.
    Pyrilinks-D urine a.
    radioisotope clearance a.
    vitamin D receptor gene serum a.
assembly
    foot-ankle a.
    Massie nail a.
    multiple hook a.
    nail a.
    nail-screw sideplate a.
    proximal drill-guide a.
assessment
    Activity Loss A. (ALA)
    Adolescent Role A. (ARA)
    aerobic conditioning functional a.
    Andersson hip outcome a.
    A. Battery for Children (ABC)
    BFM stroke impairment a.
    body composition a.
    Brunnstrom-Fugl-Meyer stroke
     impairment a.
    closed-chain functional a.
    environmental a.
    ergonomic a.
    Erhardt Developmental Prehension
     A. (EDPA)

Erhardt Developmental Vision A.
(EDVA)
a. for limiting condition
functional capacity a.
gait a.
home a.
impairment a.
injury a.
isokinetic a.
Jebsen a.
joint a.
Löwenstein Occupational Therapy
Cognitive A. (LOTCA)
Modified Dynamic Visual Processing
A. (M-DVPA)
Moire topographic scoliosis a.
motor function a.
Musculoskeletal Function A.
(MFA)
neurologic a.
A. of Communication and
Interaction Skills (ACIS)
A. of Living Skills and Resources
(ALSAR)
A. of Ludic Behaviors (ALB)
A. of Motor and Process Skills
(AMPS)
A. of Occupational Functioning
(AOF)
outcome a.
overuse injury a.
palpatory technique for joint a.
Perdriolle spinal vertebral rotation
scoliosis a.
pressure ulcer a.
rehabilitation a.
return-to-play injury a.
return-to-play musculoskeletal a.
Rivermead Motor A.
SCATBI A.
Short Musculoskeletal Function A.
(SMFA)
sideline a.
Tinetti gait a.
vascular a.
vocational a.
Assessment-Geriatric
Löwenstein Occupational Therapy
Cognitive A.-G. (LOTCA-G)
ASSH
American Society for Surgery of the
Hand
ASSI
Accurate Surgical and Scientific
Instruments Corporation
ASSI coagulator
ASSI wire-pass drill
**assignment criteria for rheumatoid
arthritis**

assimilation
atlantooccipital a.
a. pelvis
assist
Elite posterior spring a.
first dorsal interosseous a.
knee extension a.
thumb interphalangeal extension a.
assistance
ambulate with a.
assistant
assisted ambulation
assistive
a. device
a. movement
a. technology device (ATD)
Assmann disease
associated
a. movements
a. myofascial trigger point
association
American Orthopaedic A.
(AOA)
American Spinal Injury A.
(ASIA)
causal a.
A. for the Study of Internal
Fixation (ASIF)
A. for the Study of Internal
Fixation Chisel
A. for the Study of Internal
Fixation T-plate (ASIF T-plate)
Japanese Orthopaedic A.
(JOA)
National Spinal Cord Injury A.
(NSCIA)
National Stroke A.
North American Riding for
Handicapped A. (NARHA)
Orthopaedic Trauma A. (OTA)
A. Research Circulation Osseous
(ARCO)
astasia
astasia-abasia gait
astatic
astereocognosy (*var. of* astereognosis)
astereognosia (*var. of* astereognosis)
**astereognosis, astereognosia,
astereocognosy**
asterixis
asthenia
asthenic
asthma
exercise-induced a. (EIA)
ASTM
American Society for Testing and
Materials
augmented soft tissue mobilization
ASTM designation

Aston
  A. cartilage reduction
  A. patterning
astragalar bone
astragalectomy
astragalocalcaneal bone
astragalocalcanean
astragalocrural bone
astragaloid bone
astragaloscaphoid bone
astragalotibial bone
astragalus
  aviator's a.
  a. bone
Astramorph PF injection
Astroturf toe
asymmetric, asymmetrical
  asymmetrical growth
  a. incurvatum reflex
  a. skin fold
  a. subtalar joint development
  a. tonic neck reflex (ATNR)
  a. wear
asymmetrical (*var. of* asymmetric)
asymmetry
  interinnominate a.
  pure limb apraxia limb a.
asyndesis
asyndetic communication
asynergia (*var. of* asynergy)
asynergic
asynergy, asynergia
AT
  activity training
  adipose tissue
  anaerobic threshold
Atabrine
atactic (*var. of* ataxic)
atacurium
Atak knee brace
Atarax
Atasoy
  A. triangular advancement flap
  A. volar V-Y flap
  A. V-Y advancement
  A. V-Y technique
Atasoy-Kleinert hand advancement flap
Atasoy-type flap for nail injury repair
Atavi
  A. atraumatic spine fusion system
  A. atraumatic spine surgery system
  A. TiTLE rod fixation system
atavicus
  metatarsus a.
  metatarsus primus a.
atavistic
  a. cuneiform
  a. epiphysial
  a. foot

ataxia, ataxy
  Bruns a.
  cerebellar a.
  equilibratory a.
  Friedreich a.
  hereditary spinocerebellar a.
  limb a.
  locomotor a.
  spinocerebellar a.
  a. telangiectasia
  a. telangiectasia syndrome
  traumatic brain injury-related a.
  vestibulocerebellar a.
ataxiadynamia
ataxia-telangiectasia
ataxic, atactic
  atactic abasia
  atactic agraphia
  a. cerebral palsy
  a. gait
  a. paramyotonia
  a. paraplegia
ataxy (*var. of* ataxia)
ATD
  assistive technology device
atelectasis
  platelike a.
  pulmonary a.
ateliotic dwarfism
atelocollagen gel
atelomyelia
atelopodia
atelorachidia
Aten olecranon screw
ATFL
  anterior talofibular ligament
ATH
  anthropometric total hip
atherectomy
atherosclerosis
atherostenosis
athetoid cerebral palsy
athetosic, athetotic
athetosis
athetotic (*var. of* athetosic)
athlete
  amputee a.
  high-power a.
  single-organ a.
  weekend a.
athlete's
  a. foot
  a. heart
  a. pseudoanemia
athletic
  a. amenorrhea
  a. brace
  a. heart syndrome
  a. injury

a. pubalgia
a. shoe carbon fiber plate
a. trainer
Ativan
Atkin epiphysial fracture
Atkinson endoprosthesis
Atlanta
A. brace orthosis
A. hip brace
atlantal transverse ligament
Atlanta-Scottish
A.-S. Rite abduction orthosis
A.-S. Rite brace
Atlantic
A. overlap brace
A. rim brace
Atlantis
A. anterior cervical plate
A. cervical plate system
A. Vision anterior cervical plate system
atlantoaxial, atloaxoid
a. alignment
a. arthrodesis
a. articulation
a. complex
a. dislocation (AAD)
a. fracture-dislocation
a. fusion
a. impaction
a. instability (AAI)
a. interval
a. joint
a. lesion
a. ligament
a. luxation
a. osteoarthritis
a. rotary displacement
a. rotatory fixation (AARF)
a. rotatory subluxation
a. separation
a. stabilization
a. subluxation (AAS)
atlantodens interval (ADI)
atlantodental articulation (ADA)
atlantooccipital (AO), atlooccipital
a. anterior membrane
a. assimilation
a. disability
a. dislocation
a. fusion
a. joint
a. joint dislocation
a. junction
a. ligament
a. subluxation
atlantoodontoid
a. interspace
a. joint

atlas
A. adjustable stand
a. adjustment
A. cable system
a. fracture
a. laterality
A. modular humeral prosthesis
A. orthogonal percussion instrument
a. vertebral subluxation complex
atlas-axis
a.-a. complex
a.-a. movement
atlas-dens interval
atloaxoid (*var. of* atlantoaxial)
atlooccipital (*var. of* atlantooccipital)
ATNR
asymmetric tonic neck reflex
ATODC
atraumatic osteolysis of distal clavicle
ATON
adductor tenotomy and obturator neurectomy
atonia (*var. of* atony)
atony, atonia
atopic dermatitis
Ato walker
ATR
Achilles tendon repair
Achilles tendon rupture
ATR brace
atracurium besylate
atraumatic
a. forceps
a. fracture
a. multidirectional bilateral rehabilitation inferior (AMBRI)
a. multidirectional instability
a. necrosis
a. needle
a. osteolysis
a. osteolysis of distal clavicle (ATODC)
atresic (*var. of* atretic)
atretic, atresic
atrial
a. natriuretic factor (ANF)
a. natriuretic peptide (ANP)
atrophia (*var. of* atrophy)
atrophic
a. arthritis
a. fracture
a. muscular paralysis
a. neuroarthropathy
a. nonunion
atrophica
myotonia a.

atrophy, atrophia
    acute reflex bone a.
    arthritic a.
    Charcot-Marie a.
    Charcot-Marie-Tooth a.
    cortical a.
    Cruveilhier a.
    disuse a.
    Duchenne muscular a.
    Erb a.
    familial spinal muscular a.
    fascioscapulohumeral muscular a.
    fat pad a.
    Fazio-Londe a.
    gauntlet a.
    Hoffmann muscular a.
    inactivity a.
    infantile progressive spinal muscular a.
    juvenile muscular a.
    juvenile spinal muscular a. (JSMA)
    Kienböck a.
    Kugelberg-Welander juvenile spinal muscle a.
    muscular a.
    myopathic a.
    neuritic a.
    neurogenic a.
    neurotrophic a.
    peroneal muscular a. (PMA)
    progressive muscular a. (PMA)
    quadriceps a.
    scapular peroneal a.
    scapulohumeral a.
    spinal cord a.
    spinal muscular a.
    spinal muscular a. (I–III)
    Sudeck a.
    thenar a.
    thigh a.
    traction a.
    Vulpian a.
    Vulpian-Bernhardt spinal muscular a.
    Werdnig-Hoffmann spinal muscular a.
    Zimmerlin a.
A/T/S Topical
ATT
    anterior talar translation
attachment
    Accuvac smoke evacuation a.
    capsular a.
    femoral a.
    fibrous a.
    ligamentous a.
    muscle-tendon a.
    muscular a.
    osseous a.
    Pearson splint a.

    PRAFO a.
    pyramid a.
    splint a.
    tendinous a.
    tendon-bone a.
    tendon-to-bone a.
    Thomas splint with Pearson a.
    a. versatility
attack
    adversive a.
    drop a.
Attenborough total knee prosthesis
attention
    Test of Everyday A. (TEA)
attenuate
attenuation
    bone ultrasound a. (BUA)
    a. of tendon
ATTF
    anterior tibiotalar fascicle
attitude
attitudinal reflexes
ATT-300 LAT traction table
Atton disease
attrition
    ligamentous a.
    a. of tendon
    a. rupture of tendon
attritional perforation
atypical dislocation
Au
    gold
auditory evoked potential (AEP)
Aufranc
    A. awl
    A. cobra hip prosthesis
    A. cobra retractor
    A. concentric hip mold
    A. cup arthroplasty
    A. gouge
    A. lateral total hip approach
    A. modification
    A. modification of Smith-Petersen cup
    A. osteotome
    A. periosteal elevator
    A. reamer
Aufranc-Turner
    A.-T. acetabular cup
    A.-T. arthroplasty
    A.-T. cemented hip prosthesis
    A.-T. femoral component
    A.-T. operation
    A.-T. stem
Aufricht glabellar rasp
auger
augmentation
    arthroscopic a.
    bladder a.

extraarticular a.
fascial flap a.
hamstring ligament a.
iliotibial band graft a.
Leach-Schepsis-Paul a.
slotted acetabular a.
synthetic a.

augmentative communication aid (ACA)

augmented
a. reconstruction
a. repair
a. soft tissue mobilization (ASTM)
a. Tinel sign

Augustine boat nail

AuRA cemented total hip system

auranofin

aureus
methicillin-resistant *Staphylococcus a.* (MRSA)
Staphylococcus a.

aurotherapy

aurothioglucose

aurothiomalate

AUSCAN
Australian and Canadian

austenitic stainless steel

Austin
A. bunionectomy
A. chevron osteotomy fixation
A. Medical Equipment (AME)
A. Medical Equipment microcurrent TENS unit
A. Moore arthroplasty
A. Moore chisel
A. Moore extractor
A. Moore femoral head prosthesis
A. Moore hemiarthroplasty
A. Moore hook
A. Moore impactor
A. Moore pin
A. Moore rasp
A. Moore reamer
A. osteotomy

Austin-Akin bunionectomy

Australia/Canada osteoarthritis index

Australian and Canadian (AUSCAN)

auto
A. Glide walker accessory
A. Suture stapler

autoamputation

autochthonous graft

autocinesis

autoclave

autocompression plate

autodistractor

autoerythrophagocytosis

Autoflex II, III CPM unit

autofusion

autogenesis
A. automator
A. automator for Ilizarov screw

autogenic

autogenous
a. bone slurry
a. cancellous bone graft
a. cartilage transplant
a. fat
a. fibular graft
a. iliac bone
a. interpositional shoulder arthroplasty
a. meniscal cartilage replantation
a. osteocartilage transfer
a. patellar ligament graft
a. patellar tendon reconstruction
a. quadrupled hamstring tendon graft
a. semitendinosus-gracilis graft

autograft
articular cartilage a.
bone-patellar tendon-bone a.
BPTB a.
a. bridge
cartilage a.
free phalangeal bone a.
free revascularized a.
osteochondral a.
patellar bone-tendon-bone a.
Regnauld free phalangeal bone a.
Russell fibular head a.

autografting
articular cartilage a.
impaction cancellous a.

autoimmunization
surgical a.

Auto-Implant
A.-I. operation
A.-I. procedure

autokinesia, autokinesis

autokinesis (*var. of* autokinesia)

autokinetic

autologous
a. blood
a. blood transfusion
a. bone chip
a. bone-tissue allograft
a. cancellous bone graft
a. chondrocyte implantation (ACI)
a. cultured chondrocyte
a. growth factor (AGF)
a. osteochondral transplant
a. reverse graft
a. reverse graft to ankle
a. traction

autolyzed
   a. antigen-extracted allogenic (AAA)
   a. antigen-extracted allogenic bone
   a. antigen-extracted allogenic bone graft
automated
   a. disposable keratome
   a. percutaneous discectomy (APD)
   a. percutaneous lumbar discectomy (APLD)
   a. shaver
automatic
   a. neonatal walking reflex
   a. screwdriver
   a. staple
automator
   Autogenesis a.
   A. device
autonomic
   a. dysreflexia
   a. hyperreflexia
   a. nervous system (ANS)
autonomous zone
Autophor
   A. ceramic total hip prosthesis
   A. femoral prosthesis
autoplastic graft
autoreinforced polyglycolide rod
autosomal dominant mild short limb dwarfism
autotome drill
autotraction
autotransfusion suction
Autovac
   A. autotransfusion canister
   A. TC orthopaedic autotransfusion system
auxiliary power unit brace
auxiliomotor
AV
   arteriovenous
A-V
   A-V Impulse foot pump
   A-V Impulse system
   A-V Impulse System foot pump DVT prophylaxis device
   A-V Impulse System foot wrap DVT prophylaxis device
Avanta
   A. MCP joint implant finger prosthesis
   A. total wrist surface replacement prosthesis implant
   A. uHead ulnar head implant
avascular
   a. fragment
   a. necrosis (AVN)
   a. necrosis of femoral head (AVNFH)

   a. necrosis of scaphoid
   a. necrosis of talar body
   a. nonunion
   a. sequestrum
average evoked response
Averett hip prosthesis
Averill
   A. press fit prosthesis
   A. total hip replacement
AVF
   arteriovenous fistula
aviator's astragalus
Avila
   A. operation
   A. sacroiliac joint abscess drainage approach
   A. technique
Avitene
   A. flour dressing
   A. microfibrillar collagen
   A. pack
avium
   Mycobacterium a.
avium-intracellulare
   Mycobacterium a.-i. (MAI)
AVN
   avascular necrosis
AVNFH
   avascular necrosis of femoral head
avoidance gait
AVS spinal system
avulse
avulsed ligament
avulsion
   accessory navicular a.
   anterior labrum periosteal sleeve a. (ALPSA)
   bony humeral a.
   chemical nail a.
   a. chip fracture
   coracoid tip a.
   digitorum brevis a.
   a. fragment
   humeral a.
   a. injury
   isolated a.
   labral a.
   ligament a.
   nail a.
   a. of biceps tendon
   a. of nail plate
   posterior labrocapsular periosteal sleeve a. (POLPSA)
   a. stress fracture
   syndesmotic a.
   a. technique
   tibial tubercle a.
   tubercle a.
awakening trauma

awareness
> body a.
> kinesthetic a.
> sensory a.

awl
> angled a.
> Aufranc a.
> bone a.
> Carter Rowe a.
> curved a.
> DePuy a.
> Ender a.
> Ferran a.
> Kodros radiolucent a.
> Küntscher a.
> pointed a.
> radiolucent a.
> reaming a.
> rectangular a.
> Rush pin reamer a.
> square-shaped a.
> Stedman a.
> Swanson lunate a.
> Swanson scaphoid a.
> T-handled a.
> Zelicof orthopaedic a.
> Zuelzer a.

Axel wire twister

Axer
> A. compression apparatus
> A. compression device
> A. foot operation
> A. lateral opening wedge osteotomy
> A. varus derotational osteotomy

Axer-Clark muscle-tendon transfer for elbow paralysis procedure

axes (*pl. of* axis)

axial, axile
> a. acetabular index (AAI)
> a. calcaneal projection
> a. calcaneus view
> a. closed-loop hydraulic mechanical testing
> a. compression
> a. compression injury
> a. compression load
> a. compression principle
> a. compression screw
> a. compression test
> a. displacement
> a. fat-suppressed turbo spin-echo T2-weighted sequence
> a. fixation
> a. gripping strength
> a. instability
> a. loading
> a. loading injury
> a. loading of spine
> a. load teardrop fracture

> a. load test
> a. manual traction test
> a. musculature
> a. neuritis
> a. pattern flap
> a. pin technique
> a. plane
> a. plane angular deformity biomechanics
> a. plate
> a. resistance exerciser
> a. rotation
> a. sesamoid projection
> a. sesamoid view
> a. skeleton
> a. spinal system
> a. stiffness
> a. traction

axile (*var. of* axial)

axilla, *pl.* **axillae**
> a., shoulder, elbow (ASE)
> a., shoulder, elbow bandage

axillae (*pl. of* axilla)

axillary
> a. and scalene block
> a. approach
> a. arch
> a. artery
> a. block
> a. contracture
> a. crutch
> a. flap
> a. lateral view
> a. nerve
> a. nerve injury
> a. region
> a. vein

axiom
> A. modular knee system
> A. total knee
> A. total knee system

axis, *pl.* **axes**
> anatomic a.
> A. ankle brace
> bimalleolar-foot a.
> a. bone
> cardinal axes (X, Y, Z)
> deviation of atlas on a.
> distal reference a. (DRA)
> femoral shaft a.
> A. fixation system
> flexion a.
> flexion-extension a.
> foot-thigh a.
> a. guide
> HPA a.
> hypothalamic-pituitary-adrenal a.
> hypothalamoneurohypophysial a. (HNA)

axis (*continued*)
    interepicondylar a.
    leg a.
    long a.
    longitudinal a.
    longitudinal midtarsal joint a.
     (LMJA)
    mechanical a.
    metatarsal a.
    middiaphysial a.
    neural a.
    oblique midtarsal joint a.
     (OMJA)
    a. of rib motion
    a. of rotation
    proximal reference a.
    ray a.
    rotation a.
    single a.
    spinal a.
    subtalar joint a. (SJA)
    a. traction
    transcondylar a. (TCA)
    transepicondylar a.
    transverse a.
    vertical a.
    weightbearing a.
    X, Y, Z a.
axis-altering arthroereisis
 device
axle lock and bumper

axon
    a. reflex
    a. reflex test
    a. response
axonal
    a. apposition
    a. degeneration
    a. injury
axonopathy
axonotmesis
axoplasmic
    a. aberration hypothesis
    a. transport (AXT)
AXT
    axoplasmic transport
    anterograde AXT
    retrograde AXT
AXT-blocking chemical
Axxess spinal cord stimulation lead
AxyaWeld
    A. bone anchor
    A. bone anchor system
    A. instrument
    A. J-tip suture welding system
    A. product line
Ayurveda
ayurvedic herb
azathioprine
Azdone
azotemic osteodystrophy
aztreonam

B

bacitracin, neomycin, and polymyxin B
Pittsburgh Compound B (PIB)

BA

bioactive
BA bone cement

Baastrup

B. disease
B. sign
B. syndrome

Babcock

B. forceps
B. stainless steel wire
B. wire-cutting scissors

Babinski

B. percussion hammer
B. reflex
B. sign
B. test

Babinski-Fröhlich syndrome
Babinski-Nageotte syndrome
baby

b. Kocher clamp
b. Lane forceps
b. Satinsky clamp

bacampicillin
BacFix system
Baciguent Topical
bacille Calmette-Guérin (BCG)
bacitracin

b., neomycin, and polymyxin B
b., neomycin, polymyxin B, and hydrocortisone
b., neomycin, polymyxin B, and lidocaine
b. solution

Baciu-Filibiu

B.-F. dowel ankle arthrodesis
B.-F. transmalleolar arthrodesis

back

adolescent round b.
b. brace
B. Bubble gravity traction unit
B. Bull lumbar support cushion
B. Bull lumbar support system
b. creaking
b. crease
b. exercise
b. flexion
B. Hammer muscle stimulator
hollow b.
b. manipulation
old man's b.
b. pain
poker b.

b. range of motion (BROM)
b. range of motion device
b. range of motion instrument
B. Revolution Stick
B. Revolution Stick exercise
B. Revolution System
B. Revolution traction/exercise unit
rigid round b.
saddle b.
B. Seat torso-wrap brace
b. shu paraspinal point
b. slapped
B. Specialist chiropractic table
B. Specialist electric table
B. Specialist manual table
static b.
b. strain
b. stretch on ball exercise
b. support
sway b.
B. Trainer spinal exercise system

backache
Backbar device
backboard splint
backcutting osteotome
BackCycler continuous passive motion device
Back-Ease aromatherapy hot/cold pack
backfilling

bone substitute b.
b. reconstruction

backfire fracture
backfiring
Backhaus

B. towel clamp
B. towel forceps

Back-Huggar

Bodyline B.-H.
B.-H. lumbar support
B.-H. lumbar support cushion

Backjoy seat
back-knee deformity
Backnobber II massage tool
backout

screw b.

backpack

b. palsy
b. paralysis

Back-Quell
backRAP

orthoRAP b.

backside wear
back-slapping technique
backstroke

The B.

BackStrong lumbar extension machine
BackThing lumbar support
BackTracker
backward
    b. bending
    b. curvature
backward-cutting knife
baclofen
bacon
    B. bone rongeur
    B. rasp
bacterial
    b. arthritis
    b. culture
    b. flora
    b. osteomyelitis
bacterium
    aerobic bacteria
    airborne bacteria
    anaerobic bacteria
bacteriuria, bacteruria
Bacteroides
bacteruria (*var. of* bacteriuria)
Bactocill
BactoShield Topical
Bac-Track
Bactroban
badger leg
Badgley
    B. anterior cervical discectomy and
      fusion technique
    B. cervical discectomy and fusion
      combination procedure
    B. cervical spine operation
    B. hip arthrodesis
    B. iliac wing resection
    B. laminectomy retractor
    B. resection of iliac wing
    B. spinal plate
Bado Monteggia fracture classification
BADS
    Behavioral Assessment of the
      Dysexecutive Syndrome
Bad Wildungen Metz spine system
BAEP
    brainstem auditory evoked potential
BAER
    balloon-assisted endplate reduction
    brainstem auditory evoked response
Baer
    B. bone-cutting forceps
    B. bone rongeur
    B. rib shears
BaFPE
    Bay Area Functional Performance
      Evaluation
bag
    B. Bath
    containment b.

    Infusible pressure infusion b.
    Versi-Splint carry b.
Bagby
    B. and Kuslich (BAK)
    B. and Kuslich lumbar fusion cage
    B. angled compression mandibular plate
bag-of-bones technique
Bahler hinge
Bahnson appendage clamp
Bailey
    B. bur
    B. conductor
    B. drill
    B. rib contractor
    B. rib spreader
    B. saw guide
    B. wire saw
Bailey-Badgley
    B.-B. anterior cervical approach
    B.-B. cervical spine fusion
    B.-B. cervical spine interbody fusion
      technique
Bailey-Dubow
    B.-D. nail
    B.-D. rod
    B.-D. rod insertion technique
Bailey-Gibbon rib contractor
Bailey-Gigli saw guide
bail-lock
    b.-l. brace
    b.-l. knee joint
    b.-l. knee joint orthosis
baja
    patella b.
BAK
    Bagby and Kuslich
    BAK fusion cage
    BAK interbody fusion system
    BAK laparoscopic procedure
    BAK lumbar fusion cage
BAK/C Cervical Interbody Fusion
System
baker
    B. Achilles tendon lengthening
      procedure
    B. cyst
    B. lateral semitendinosus transfer
    B. patellar advancement
    B. technique
    B. tongue in groove slide
      lengthening of gastrocnemius
    B. trabecular traction
    B. translocation operation
Baker-Hill osteotomy
baker's leg
BAK/Proximity interbody fusion implant
BAK/T thoracic interbody fusion system
Balacescu closing wedge hallux valgus
  osteotomy

balance
>b. beam scale
>b. board
>b. board training
>b. bridge
>Clinical Test of Sensory Integration and B. (CTSIB)
>column b.
>dynamic b.
>dynamic standing b.
>electrolyte b.
>B. Error Scoring System (BESS)
>fluid b.
>B. hip prosthesis
>B. Master
>B. Master training and assessment system
>nitrogen b.
>b. pad
>b. padding orthosis
>postural b.
>sagittal b.

balanced
>b. forearm
>b. forearm orthosis (BFO)
>b. hemivertebra
>b. skeletal traction
>b. splint
>b. suspension
>b. suspension traction

balancing
>Chopart amputation with tendon b.

Balboa thoracolumbar fusion posterior fixation anterior buttress plate system

Balcones Sensory Integration Screening Kit

Balfour
>B. clamp
>B. self-retaining retractor

Balkan
>B. beam
>B. femoral splint
>B. fracture frame

ball
>b. bearing
>Body B.
>Bouncewell medicine b.
>b. bur
>burst resistance fitness b.
>cold-weld femoral b.
>b. dissector
>Ex-Balls medicine b.
>ExerFlex b.
>b. extractor
>Finger Fitness Spring B.
>Fitness B.
>Gertie b.
>Gripp squeeze b.
>b. guidepin

>gym b.
>Gymnastik b.
>Gymnic Plus exercise b.
>hand exercise b.
>Jurgan Fixator B.
>Jurgan Pin B.
>B. knee lock
>Ledraplastic exercise b.
>massage b.
>medicine b.
>b. of foot
>PhysioGymnic exercise b.
>Physio-Roll VisuaLiser exercise b.
>b. reamer
>R-Value exercise b.
>silastic b.
>Slo-Mo b.
>squeeze b.
>Swiss b.
>Thera-Band exercise b.
>Theragym b.
>Vari-Firm Medicine B.
>VersaBack gym b.
>vestibular b.

ball-and-socket
>b.-a.-s. ankle prosthesis
>b.-a.-s. congruity
>b.-a.-s. design
>b.-a.-s. giant pseudarthrosis
>b.-a.-s. giant pseudoarthritis
>b.-a.-s. joint
>b.-a.-s. trochanteric osteotomy

Ballantine
>B. clamp
>B. hemilaminectomy retractor

ball-catcher's view

Ballenger
>B. periosteotome
>B. swivel knife

Ballenger-Hajek chisel

ballism (*var. of* ballismus)

ballismus, ballism

ballistic injury

balloon
>b. cell nevus
>b. kyphoplasty

balloon-assisted
>b.-a. endoscopic retroperitoneal anterior lumbar interbody fusion
>b.-a. endoscopic retroperitoneal gasless (BERG)
>b.-a. endplate reduction (BAER)

ballottable
>b. patella
>b. patella test

ballottement
>patella b.
>b. test

ball-peen splint

ball-point guidepin
ball-tip
    b.-t. guidepin
    b.-t. spike
ball-tipped
    b.-t. Küntscher guide
    b.-t. pedicle sounder
ball-valve tumor
Balmoral laced shoe
balneotherapy
Baló concentric sclerosis
balsa wood filler block
Baltimore
    B. Therapeutic Equipment
    (BTE)
    B. Therapeutic Equipment work
    simulator
Bamberger-Marie
    B.-M. disease
    B.-M. syndrome
bamboo
    b. spine
    b. spine sign
banana
    b. Beaver blade
    b. finger extension splint
    b. knife
    B. Split Splint
Bancap HC
band
    A b.'s
    air b.
    AO tension b.
    aponeurotic b.
    arm b.
    big b.
    Broca diagonal b.
    calf b.
    Can-Do exercise b.
    congenital anular b.
    congenital fibrous b.
    conjoined lateral b.
    constriction b.
    deossification b.
    distal thigh b.
    ExerBand therapy b.
    exercise b.
    external b.
    fascial b.
    fibrous b.
    Fit-Lastic therapy b.
    GelBand arm b.
    Gennari b.
    iliopatellar b.
    iliotibial b. (ITB)
    internal b.
    Jobst air b.
    lateral b.
    M b.

    palpable b.
    Parham b.
    Parham-Martin b.
    Partridge b.
    patellar b.
    PDS b.
    pelvic b.
    periosteal b.
    pretendinous b.
    proximal thigh b.
    REP Bands exercise b.
    Resist-A-Band exercise b.
    Resist-A-Tube exercise b.
    rigid metal pelvic b.
    sagittal b.
    scar b.
    Simonart b.
    subsurface white b.
    taut b.
    tennis elbow arm b.
    b. tenodesis
    tension b.
    trochanteric b.
    True Blue exercise b.
    b. wire
    Xercise B.
    Z b.
bandage
    Ace adherent b.
    ankle traction b.
    ASE b.
    axilla, shoulder, elbow b.
    Barton b.
    capeline b.
    Champ elastic b.
    circular b.
    Comperm tubular elastic b.
    compression b.
    Conco elastic b.
    cotton elastic b. (CEB)
    Cover-Roll stretch b.
    cravat b.
    demigauntlet b.
    Desault wrist b.
    Dressinet netting b.
    elastic b.
    elastic foam b.
    Elastomull elastic gauze b.
    Elastoplast b.
    Esmarch b.
    Fabco gauze b.
    fiberglass b.
    figure-of-8 b.
    Flex-Foam b.
    flexible b.
    Flexilite conforming elastic b.
    Flex-Master b.
    gauntlet b.
    Gibney fixation b.

Gibson b.
gum rubber Martin b.
Hamilton jaw b.
Helenca stockinette b.
Heliodorus T b.
Hippocrates cap-shaped b.
Hueter b.
Hydron Burn B.
immobilizing b.
immovable b.
Kerlix b.
Kling elastic b.
Leukotape P stretch b.
Martin sheet rubber b.
Medi-Band b.
MPM b.
Nu Gauze b.
oblique b.
Orthoflex elastic plaster b.
Ortho-Trac adhesive skin
  traction b.
Ortho-Vent b.
Pavlik b.
plaster b.
plaster of Paris b.
Plast-O-Fit thermoplastic b.
polyurethane b.
Redigrip pressure b.
replantation b.
restrictive b.
Ribble b.
Richet b.
Robert Jones b.
roller b.
Sayre b.
scarf b.
Scultetus b.
Shur-Band self-closure elastic b.
Silesian b.
sling-and-swathe b.
spica b.
spiral b.
starch b.
stockinette b.
Thera-Boot b.
triangular b.
Tricodur compression support b.
Tricodur Epi compression b.
Tricodur Omos compression b.
Tricodur Omos elastic b.
Tricodur Talus compression b.
Tru-Support EW b.
Tru-Support SA b.
TubeGauz b.
Tubigrip b.
tubular elastic b.
Velpeau b.
Webril b.
Bandi patellofemoral pain score (1–5)

Band-It
  B.-I. magnetic elbow support
  B.-I. tennis elbow strap
bandlike
  b. adhesion
  b. pain
bandy-leg
Bane
  B. bone rongeur
  B. rongeur forceps
Bane-Hartmann bone rongeur
banjo
  b. cast
  b. splint
  b. traction
bank
  Bethesda bone b.
  Bethesda lending bone b.
  bone b.
Bankart
  B. anterior capsolabral reconstruction
  B. arthroplasty
  B. deformity
  B. dislocated shoulder capsular
    repair
  B. fracture
  B. operation
  B. procedure
  B. retractor
  B. shoulder dislocation
  B. shoulder lesion
  B. shoulder prosthesis
  B. shoulder repair set
  B. Tack implant
**Bankart-Putti-Platt dislocated shoulder
  operation**
banked
  b. bone
  b. bone graft
**Banks open slide lengthening of tendo
  Achillis**
Banks-Laufman
  B.-L. elbow approach
  B.-L. incision
Banophen Oral
bantam
  B. CDH prosthesis
  B. wire-cutting scissors
BAP
  Behavioral Assessment of Pain
BAPS
  Biomechanical Ankle Platform System
  BAPS board
Baptist
  New England B. (NEB)
4-bar
  4-b. external fixation
  4-b. external fixation apparatus
  4-b. external fixation device

4-bar (*continued*)
    4-b. link
    4-b. linkage on knee prosthesis
    4-b. linkage prosthetic knee
      mechanism
    4-b. polycentric knee prosthesis
bar
    b. bolt fixation
    bony b.
    broomstick b.
    calcaneonavicular b.
    cartilaginous b.
    congenital b.
    cross b.
    Denis Browne b.
    derotator b.
    distraction b.
    b. drill
    b. excision
    exercise grab b.
    Fillauer b.
    Gerster traction b.
    grab b.
    intramedullary b.
    Jackson intrasacral bar Jackson
      intrasacral b.
    Leyla b.
    Livingston intramedullary b.
    longitudinal spinal b.
    lumbrical b.
    medial talocalcaneal b.
    metatarsal flatfoot b.
    MT b.
    opponens b.
    patellar b.
    physial b.
    posterior thigh b.
    quad b.
    b. resection
    rigid b.
    rocker b.
    sacral b.
    screw alignment b.
    b. section
    side-cutting Swanson b.
    spacer b.
    spondylotic b.
    Sports-Grip b.
    spreader b.
    stabilizing b.
    stall b.
    Stephen spreader b.
    tarsal b.
    Thera-P exercise b.
    Thornton b.
    Tommy trapeze b.
    torsion b.
    traction b.
    trapeze b.

    unsegmented vertebral b.
    valgus b.
    vertebral b.
    Zielke derotator b.
bar-and-shoe orthosis
Bárány-Nylen vertigo maneuver
barbed
    b. broach
    b. staple
barbell
    spring angled adjustable b.
barber chair position
barber-pole
    b.-p. fashion
    b.-p. vein graft
barbotage
Barbour
    B. cervical fixation
    B. technique
Bard clamp
Bardeen primitive disc
Bardeleben bone-holding forceps
Bardenheuer
    B. extension
    B. extension fracture treatment
      method
    B. incision
Bard-Parker
    B.-P. blade
    B.-P. handle
    B.-P. knife
    B.-P. scalpel
Bareskin knee positioner
1-bar external fixator
bariatric mat table
barked
    b. injury
    b. knee
    b. shin
Barker hallux valgus operation
Barkow ligament
barlike ventral defect
Barlow
    B. cruciform infant splint
    B. developmental hip dysplasia
    B. hip dysplasia sign
    B. pediatric hip instability test
    B. provocative test
Barnes
    B. curve
    B. dystrophy
barognosis
Baron suction tube
barotrauma
    middle ear b.
    pulmonary b.
Barouk
    B. button space
    B. cannulated bone screw

B. microscrew with shortening
  osteotomy
B. microstaple
B. spacer

Barr

B. bolt
B. bolt nail
B. hook
B. open reduction and internal
  fixation
B. pin
B. tendon transfer operation
B. tibial fracture fixation
B. tibialis posterior transfer

Barraquer needle holder
Barrasso-Wile-Gage subtalar
  arthrodesis
barrel

b. bur
b. bur design
b. chest
b. crawl
b. guide
guide b.
b. plate
sideplate b.

barreled sideplate
Barré-Lieou syndrome
barrel-shaped thorax
barrel-stave skull osteotomy
barrier

anatomic b.
blood-brain b. (BBB)
calcium sulfate bone graft b.
Capset calcium sulfate bone
  graft b.
elastic b.
B. lower extremity sheet
motion b.
pathologic b.
physiologic b.
side-bending b.
b. technique

Barr-Record ankle arthrodesis
BARS

Behavior Assessment Rating Scale

Barsky

B. bilateral cleft lips repair
  technique
B. cleft hand closure
B. cleft hand closure operation
B. cleft hand repair procedure
B. macrodactyly reduction

Barthel ADL index
Bartlett

B. nail fold
B. nail fold excision
B. procedure

bar-to-bar clamp

Barton

B. bandage
B. fracture
B. sling
B. tongs
B. traction handle

Barwell knee operation
basal

b. block cervical saddle
b. bone
b. chevron osteotomy
b. closing wedge osteotomy
b. extension
b. joint
b. metabolic rate (BRM)
b. neck
b. neck fracture

BASC

Behavior Assessment System for
Children
BASC s.

base

Dycal b.
metacarpal b.
b. of finger
b. of fingernail
b. of gait
b. of neck osteotomy
b. of skull (BOS)
b. of support (BOS)
b. of thumb arthritis
plantar lateral b.
Profix nonporous tibial b.
b. wedge osteotomy (BWO)
b. wedge osteotomy/bunionectomy

baseball

b. finger
b. finger fracture
b. finger splint
b. fracture of hand
b. pitcher's elbow
b. shoulder
b. stitch
b. suture

baseline

B. Bubble inclinometer
b. capacity evaluation
B. dynamometer
b. view

basement membrane
basic

b. calcium phosphate crystal
  deposition disease
b. cranial adjusting procedure (I, II)
b. hand splint
b. Ilizarov-type frame (I-IV)
b. lamella
b. multicellular remodeling unit
b. technique

basilar, basilaris
- b. bone
- b. cartilage
- b. closing wedge metatarsal osteotomy
- b. crescentic osteotomy
- b. femoral neck fracture
- b. impression
- b. invagination
- b. plantarflexory metatarsal osteotomy
- b. region
- b. vertebra

basilaris (*var. of* basilar)
Basile hip screw
basilic artery
basioccipital
basivertebral
basket
- Acufex meniscal b.
- b. forceps
- b. rongeur
- rotary b.
- b. stockinette
- walker b.

basketball foot
basket-weave ankle taping
Basmajian iliopsoas electromyography technique
basocervical fracture
basograph
Basser migraine-vertigo syndrome
Bassett
- B. electrical stimulation apparatus
- B. electrical stimulation device
- B. electrical stimulation system
- B. sign

Basswood splint
Batchelor
- B. plaster
- B. plaster hip spica cast
- B. plate

Batchelor-Brown extraarticular subtalar arthrodesis
Batch-Spittler-McFaddin
- B.-S.-M. knee disarticulation
- B.-S.-M. through-knee amputation technique

Bateman
- B. femoral neck prosthesis
- B. finger prosthesis
- B. hemiarthroplasty
- B. shoulder operation
- B. Universal Proximal Femur prosthesis
- B. UPF II bipolar knee system
- B. UPF II bipolar prosthesis

bath
- Aqua/Whirl b.
- Bag B.
- contrast b. (CB)
- Dickson paraffin b.
- galvanic b.
- hot and cold contrast b.
- hot water b.
- mud pack b.
- Para-Care paraffin therapy b.
- paraffin b. (PB)
- whirlpool b.

Bathe Away cleanser
bathing and dressing ability
Bathlifter
- Leo B.

batrachian
- b. gait
- b. posture

Batson
- vein of B.
- B. vertebral brain system

battery
- Allen Cognitive B.
- Rand Functional Limitations B.
- Rand Physical Capacities B.

battery-driven hand drill
battery-powered instrument
batting
- Dacron b.

battledore incision
Battle skull fracture sign
bat-wing appearance
Batzdorf
- B. cervical wire passer
- B. cervical wire twister

Bauerfeind
- B. Achillotrain
- B. ankle brace
- B. Comprifix knee brace
- B. Malleolic Ankle Orthosis
- B. silicone heel pad
- B. SofSpot Heel Cup
- B. support

Bauer-Jackson traumatic chondral lesion classification
Baumann
- B. and Koch intramuscular lengthening of gastrocnemius
- B. supracondylar fracture angle

Baumgaertel and Gotzen calcaneal fracture reduction technique
Baumgard-Schwartz tennis elbow technique
Baumrucker clamp irrigator
Bavarian splint
Baxter
- B. angled arthroscope
- B. nerve release

Baxter-D'Astous proximal femoral resection-interposition arthroplasty procedure
Bay Area Functional Performance Evaluation (BaFPE)
Bayer
- B. Buffered Aspirin
- B. Low Adult Strength
- B. Select Pain Relief Formula

Bayley Scales of Infant Development
Baylor
- B. adjustable cross splint
- B. metatarsal splint

Bayne
- B. classification of radial agenesis (I-IV)
- B. radial agenesis classification (I-IV)
- B. ulnar ray deficiency classification (I-IV)

Bayne-Klug centralization
bayonet
- b. apposition
- b. clip applier
- b. dislocation
- b. fracture position
- b. knife
- b. leg
- b. nonunion
- b. osteotome
- b. position of fracture
- b. rongeur
- b. saw
- b. sign
- b. spacer

bayonet-point wire
Bazooka support surface
BB
- belly button
  - BB marker
  - BB to MM examination

BBB
- blood-brain barrier

BBC
- biceps, brachialis, coracobrachialis
  - BBC muscles

BBS
- Berg Balance Scale

BCG
- bacille Calmette-Guérin

BCP
- BiCalPhos
  - BCP synthetic bone substitute

BDD
- blistering distal dactylitis

BDH
- biologically designed hip
  - BDH prosthesis

BE
- below elbow
  - BE amputation

BEA
- below-elbow amputation

beach chair position
beachcomber
- B. prosthetic foot
- B. waterproof prosthesis

bead
- aminoglycoside-impregnated methyl methacrylate b.
- antibiotic b.
- antibiotic-impregnated b.
- copolymer starch copolymer b.
- gentamicin b.
- metallic b.
- methyl methacrylate b.
- b. pouch
- Septobal b.
- targeting b.

bead-blasted prosthesis
beaded
- b. guidewire
- b. hip pin
- b. reamer guidepin
- b. transfixion wire

beaded-pin wrench
bead-loaded wire
beak
- b. fracture
- b. ligament
- metacarpal b.
- b. modification with triple arthrodesis
- talar b.

beaked
- b. cervicomedullary junction
- b. pelvis

beaking
- b. joint
- b. of head of talus
- talar b.

beaklike osteophyte formation
Beals
- B. periarticular laceration saline load test
- B. syndrome

beam
- Balkan b.
- load b.
- primary x-ray b.
- b. theory

beanbag
bearing
- ball b.
- ceramic b.
- pretibial b. (PTB)
- radial b.
- spinal load b.

bearing (*continued*)
    Steinmann pin with ball b.
    ulnar b.
    unipolar b.
bearing-seating forceps
bear's paw hand
Beasley-Babcock forceps
3-beat clonus
Beath
    B. bone intramedullary peg
    B. needle
    B. pin
Beatson radiographic combined talocalcaneal angle
Beaty recurrent patellar dislocation lateral release
Beaufort seating orthosis
Beau line
beaver
    B. blade handle
    B. cataract knife
    B. discission blade
    B. keratome blade
    B. saw
Beaver-DeBakey
    B.-D. blade
    B.-D. knife
Bebax
    B. Bootie
    B. orthosis
    B. shoe
becaplermin
Bechterew (*var. of* Bekhterev)
Bechtol
    B. acetabular component
    B. hip prosthesis
    B. patella system
    B. patellofemoral joint prosthesis
    B. screw
    B. shoulder prosthesis
    B. system prosthesis
    B. total hip arthroplasty
    B. total hip prosthesis system
    B. total knee arthroplasty
    B. total knee prosthesis
Beckenbaugh
    B. biaxial wrist implant technique
    B. correction
Becker
    B. brace
    B. core suture
    B. hand prosthesis
    B. 655 motion control limiter
    B. muscular dystrophy (BMD)
    B. orthopaedic spinal system (BOSS)
    B. orthopaedic spinal system orthotic device
    B. orthopaedic thermoformable ankle system

    B. otoplasty technique
    B. screwdriver
    B. tendon repair
    B. variant
    B. variant of Duchenne dystrophy
Becker-type tardive muscular dystrophy
Beckman retractor
Beck-Steffee total ankle prosthesis
Béclard partial foot amputation
Becton
    B. Colles fracture plate
    B. fracture fixation technique
    B. metacarpophalangeal open reduction
bed
    air b.
    American Seating Access-O-Matic b.
    BioDyne b.
    bone graft b.
    Borg-Warner orthopaedic b.
    Burke Bariatric b.
    Chick-Foster orthopaedic b.
    circle b.
    CircOlectric b.
    Clinitron air b.
    b. cradle
    DMI orthopaedic b.
    Flexicair b.
    FluidAir b.
    Foster b.
    fracture b.
    fusion b.
    Gatch b.
    Goodman orthopaedic b.
    Hausted orthopaedic b.
    high-air-loss b.
    high muscular resistance b.
    Hill-Rom orthopaedic b.
    Hollywood b.
    Inland Super Multi-Hite orthopaedic b.
    Joerns orthopaedic b.
    Keane mobility b.
    KinAir b.
    Lapidus b.
    low-air-loss b.
    Magnum 800 b.
    Medicus b.
    Mega-Air b.
    Mega Tilt and Turn b.
    b. mobility skill
    nail b.
    obese b.
    b. of rib
    orthopaedic b.
    Plastazote foot b.
    b. rest
    Restcue b.
    b. rest-related deconditioning

Roho b.
Roto-Rest b.
Simmons Multi-Matic orthopaedic b.
Simmons Vari-Hite orthopaedic b.
skeletal b.
Skytron b.
SMI 3000, 5000 b.
Smith-Davis Converta-Hite
  orthopaedic b.
Spa B.
Stryker b.
Superior Sleeprite Hi-Lo
  orthopaedic b.
Swinger car b.
TheraPulse b.
Tilt and Turn Paragon b.
Ultraflex orthopaedic b.
b. wedge
Bed-Bar support rail
bedroom fracture
bed-to-chair transfer
Beebe wire-cutting scissors
beefburger procedure
Beery-Buktenica Developmental Test of
Visual-Motor Integration
Beery Visual Motor Integration Test
Beeson
B. cast spreader
B. plaster spreader
bee venom therapy
Beevor
B. sign
B. umbilical movement sign
behavior, behaviour
Assessment of Ludic B.'s (ALB)
B. Assessment Rating Scale
  (BARS)
B. Assessment System for Children
  (BASC)
compensatory b.
occupational b.
behavioral, behavioural
B. Assessment of Pain (BAP)
B. Assessment of Pain
  Questionnaire (P-BAP)
B. Assessment of the Dysexecutive
  Syndrome (BADS)
B. Inattention Test (BIT)
b. mapping
behaviour (*var. of* behavior)
behavioural (*var. of* behavioral)
Behçet syndrome
Behr syndrome
Beighton hypermobility syndrome criteria
Bekhterev, Bechterew
B. arthritis
B. deep reflex
B. disease
B. rheumatoid spondylitis

B. sciatica test
B. sitting test
Bekhterev-Mendel reflex
Bekhterev-Strümpell spondylitis
Belix Oral
bell
Hydro-Tone B.
B. palsy
b. rasp
B. suture
B. table
B. Tawse
B. Tawse open reduction technique
B. Tawse pediatric Monteggia
  fracture open reduction
B. Tawse radial head procedure
belladonna
b. and opium
tincture of b.
Bell-Dally
B.-D. atlas dislocation
B.-D. first cervical dislocation
Bellemore-Barrett closing wedge
osteotomy
Bellergal-S
Bellucci alligator scissors
belly
b. button (BB)
b. button to medial malleolus (BB
  to MM)
b. button to medial malleolus
  examination
muscle b.
belly-press test
Belos compression pin
below
b. elbow (BE)
b. knee (BK)
below-elbow
b.-e. amputation (BEA)
b.-e. prosthesis
below-knee
b.-k. amputation (BKA)
b.-k. prosthesis
b.-k. suspension
b.-k. walking cast (BKWC)
belt
AquaJogger buoyancy b.
Carabelt therapeutic b.
cast b.
Cool-Flex A/K suspension b.
gait b.
Meek pelvic traction b.
pelvic traction b.
Posey b.
Reed cast b.
rib b.
sacroiliac b.
Schiek b.

belt (*continued*)
  Serola sacroiliac b.
  SI b.
  Silesian b.
  Soma sacroiliac stabilization b.
  Spine Power pelvic stabilizer b.
  S'port Max sacroiliac b.
  Sports Plus II back b.
  TES b.
  Thera-Band Aqua B.
  Tri-Flex auxiliary suspension b.
  waist suspension b.
Benadryl Oral
Ben-Allergin-50 Injection
bench
  Ensolite padded transfer b.
  b. examination
  Invacare vinyl transfer b.
  Paramount 3-way press b.
  pelvic b.
  b. test
  Winco adjusting b.
bend
  deep knee b. (DKB)
  b. fracture
  sitting side b.
  standing side b.
Bend-A-Boot foot splint
bender
  AO plate b.
  Bunnell knuckle b.
  cast b.
  DePuy rod b.
  French rod b.
  Luque rod b.
  plate b.
  rod b.
  Rush b.
bending
  backward b.
  cantilever b.
  forward b.
  b. fracture
  ipsilateral side b.
  lateral b.
  b. load
  rod b.
  side b.
  b. strength
  b. stress
  b. toward the side of injury
B-endorphin
Benedek reflex
benediction
  b. attitude sign
  b. posture
Benedict-Roth apparatus
BeneFix
Benefoot & Birkenstock orthotic sandal

BeneJoint analgesic cream
Benemid
benign
  b. bone aneurysm
  b. chondroblastoma
  b. congenital myopathy
  b. cortical defect
  b. fasciculation
  b. hypermobile joint syndrome
  b. joint hypermobility syndrome
  (BJHS)
  b. subsidence
  b. transient synovitis
  b. tumor
Benink tarsal index
Bennett
  B. bone retractor
  B. elevator
  B. fracture
  B. fracture dislocation of thumb
  B. fracture of basal joint of thumb
  B. Hand Tool Dexterity Test
  B. lesion
  B. nail biopsy
  B. orthosis
  B. pain model
  B. posterior inferior glenoid lesion
  B. thumb fracture classification
  B. tibial retractor
bent
  b. Hohman retractor-narrow
  b. Hohman retractor-wide
  b. nail
  B. operation
bent-knee cast
Benton Constructional Praxis Test
benzalkonium chloride
benzedrine
benzodiazepine
benzoic acid and salicylic acid
benzoin
  b. adherent tape
  b. adhesive
  tincture of b.
benztropine mesylate
BeOK hand exercise putty
Berens osteotomy
BERG
  balloon-assisted endoscopic
  retroperitoneal gasless
  BERG ALIF
  BERG anterior lumbar interbody
  fusion
Berg
  B. Balance Scale (BBS)
  B. balance test
Berger
  B. dorsal wrist capsulodesis
  B. interscapular amputation

B

B. interscapulothoracic amputation
operation
B. paresthesia
**Berger-Bookwalter posterior spine
approach**
Bergman mallet
Bergstrom
B. cannula
B. needle
Berke clamp
Berkeley
University of California B.
(UCB)
Berliner percussion hammer
Berlin-Frankfurt-Munster (BFM)
Berman-Gartland
B.-G. forefoot procedure
B.-G. metatarsal osteotomy
Berman-Moorhead metal locator
Bermuda spica cast
Berndt-Harty
B.-H. classification of transchondral
fracture
B.-H. osteochondral fracture
classification (I-IV)
Berndt hip ruler
Bernese periacetabular osteotomy
Bernhard clamp
Berstein cast table
Bertin
B. bone
B. hip retractor
B. ligament
Bertolotti syndrome
Besnier rheumatism
BESS
Balance Error Scoring System
Bestfoam insole
besylate
atracurium b.
beta
b. adrenergic
b. blocker medication
b. index
B. Pile II, III splint strap
transforming growth factor b. (TGF
beta)
Betadine
B. dressing
B. First Aid Antibiotics +
Moisturizer
B. paint
B. scrub
B. scrub solution
B. soak
B. soap
Betadine-soaked pledget
beta-endorphin
plasma b.-e.

betamethasone
b. and clotrimazole
b. dipropionate
b. sodium phosphate
beta-2-microglobulin
b.-2-m. amyloidosis
b.-2-m. deposition
Betasept
beta-sympathomimetic
bethanechol
Bethesda
B. bone bank
B. lending bone bank
Bethune
B. periosteal elevator
B. rib shears
Bethune-Coryllos rib shears
Bevatron accelerator
bevel ArthroWand
beveled
b. chisel
b. tubular retractor
bevel-point Rush pin
Bevin shoe
Bexophene
Beyer rongeur
BF+ bone void filler
BFM
Berlin-Frankfurt-Munster
BFM impairment
BFM stroke impairment
assessment
BFO
balanced forearm orthosis
BFO Kit
BG
bone graft
BGS
bone graft substitute
BHAGL
bony humeral avulsion of
glenohumeral ligament
BHAGL lesion
BH Moore procedure
BIA
bioelectrical impedance analysis
Bi-Angular shoulder prosthesis
biarticular
b. bone-cutting forceps
b. bone shears
biarticulate
bias-cut
b.-c. stockinette
b.-c. tape
biaxial
b. compression plate fixation
b. flap
b. joint
B. Weave composite prosthesis

BiCalPhos (BCP)
    B. synthetic bone
      substitute
BICAP
    bipolar circumactive probe
    BICAP cautery
bicapsular
bicentric prosthesis
biceps (*pl. of* biceps)
    b., brachialis, coracobrachialis
      (BBC)
    b. brachialis muscle transfer
    b. brachialis tendon
    b. brachii muscle
    b. brachii tendon
    b. elevator
    b. femoris
    b. femoris muscle
    b. femoris tendon
    b. interval
    b. interval lesion (BIL)
    b. jerk reflex test
    long head of b.
    b. reflex
    short head of b.
    b. tendinitis
    b. tendon rupture repair
    b. tenodesis
bicepses (*pl. of* biceps)
Bichat ligament
bichloracetic acid
Bicillin C-R 900/300
  injection
bicipital
    b. bursitis
    b. groove
    b. muscle
    b. rib
    b. shoulder syndrome
    b. sulcus
    b. tendinitis
    b. tendon
    b. tenosynovitis
    b. tuberosity
    b. tuberosity view
Bickel
    B. intramedullary nail
    B. intramedullary rod
    B. legholder
bicolumn fracture
bicompartmental
    b. implant
    b. knee implant prosthesis
    b. replacement
    b. replacement of knee
    b. soft tissue sarcoma
biconcave
    b. deformity
    b. vertebra

bicondylar
    b. ankle prosthesis
    b. graft
    b. knee prosthesis
    b. tibial plateau
    b. T-shaped fracture
    b. Y-shaped fracture
Bicon-Plus Cup
bicorrectional Austin osteotomy
bicortical
    b. iliac bone
    b. iliac bone graft
    b. ilial strip graft
    b. screw
    b. screw fixation
bicycle, bike
    air b.
    Air-Dyne b.
    b. brace
    b. ergometer
    b. ergometry
    b. exerciser
    FES exercise b.
    b. injury
    Monark b.
    New Schwinn 900 b.
    New Schwinn elliptical b.
    recumbent b.
    Schwinn Air-Dyne b.
    Schwinn Spinner b.
    Schwinn 900 stationary b.
    b. spoke fracture
BID
    bilateral interfacetal dislocation
bidirectional traction
Bielschowsky 3–step head tilt test
Bier
    B. amputation
    B. amputation saw
    B. block
    B. block anesthesia
    B. lumbar puncture needle
    B. operation
bifid
    b. condyle
    b. foot
    b. graft
    b. hook
    b. spinous process
    b. thumb
    b. thumb deformity
bifida
    spina b.
bifilar needle recording electrode
biflanged drill
Bi-Flex
    Osteo B.-F.
biframed distraction technique
  arthroscopic ankle arthrodesis

bifrontal incision
bifurcate, bifurcated
    b. blade-plate
    b. ligament
    b. navicular
    b. vein graft for vascular
      reconstruction
bifurcated (*var. of* bifurcate)
bifurcation osteotomy
bifurcatum
    ligamentum b.
big
    b. band
    b. toe test
Bigelow
    B. ligament
    B. posterior hip dislocation
      maneuver
    B. septum
Bigliani/Flatow
    B. complete shoulder replacement
    B. shoulder system
Bigliani-Flatow total shoulder
  arthroplasty
biglycan
bike (*var. of* bicycle)
    b. ankle brace
BIL
    biceps interval lesion
bilaminar zone
bilateral
    b. acute radicular syndrome
    b. amputation
    b. arm raise back exercise
      technique
    b. chronic radicular syndrome
    b. frame
    b. hemiplegia
    b. heterotopic ossification
    b. interfacetal dislocation (BID)
    b. lateral fusion
    strength test eccentric b.
    b. talocalcaneal coalition
    b. variable screw placement
      system
    b. V-Y Kutler flap
Bilhaut-Cloquet polydactyly procedure
biloba
    Ginkgo b.
bilobed
    b. digital neurovascular island flap
    b. flap reconstruction
    b. skin flap
bilocular joint
Bilos
    B. pin
    B. pin extractor
bimalleolar
    b. angle

    b. ankle fractures
    b. approach to ankle arthrodesis
bimalleolar-foot axis
Bi-Metric
    B.-M. hip prosthesis
    B.-M. Interlok femoral prosthesis
    B.-M. porous primary femoral
      prosthesis
Bindegewebsmassage connective tissue
  massage
binder
    abdominal b.
    arch b.
    cloth b.
    Dale abdominal b.
    Helenca b.
    sacroiliac b.
    Scultetus b.
binding
    biologic b.
bind wire
binocular loupe
bioabsorbable
    b. material
    b. mesh scaffold
    b. staple
    b. tack repair
Bio-Absorbable interference screw
BioAction great toe implant
bioactive (BA)
    b. bone cement
    b. implant
Bio-Anchor suture anchor
Bio-Boot
Biobrane
    B. adhesive
    B. glove
    B. synthetic skin substitute
BioCast wrist/hand orthosis
bioceramic implant material
biochemical
    b. abnormality
    B. Ankle Platform System board
    b. integrity
    b. marker
    b. response
Bio-Chromatic hand prosthesis
Bioclad with pegs reinforced acetabular
  prosthesis
BioCleanse tissue sterilization
  process
Bioclusive select transparent film
  dressing
biocompatibility
    b. characteristic
    implant b.
biocompatible
BioCompression Pneumatic Sleeve
Biocoral bone graft substitute

Bio-Corkscrew
    headed B.-C.
biocorrosion
BioCuff
    B. bioresorbable screw and spiked
        washer implant
    B. C bioresorbable cannulated screw
    B. C bioresorbable cannulated screw
        and spike washer implant
    B. C bioresorbable spike washer
        implant
biodegradable
    b. calcium phosphate cement
    b. fixation device
    b. fixation instrumentation
    b. implant
    b. plate
    b. surgical tack
    b. synthetic polymer
Biodel implant
Bio-Dermal Hydrogel kit
BioDevices
    Paradigm B.
Biodex
    B. Balance System
    B. Balance System test
    B. cycle ergometer
    B. Gait Trainer
    B. isokinetic dynamometer
    B. isokinetic testing machine
    B. Multi-Joint System 3 MVP
    B. target balance trainer
    B. Unweighing Support System
    B. Unweighing System partial
        weight therapy
Biodine
Biodynamic Molding System
BioDyne bed
bioelectric
    b. phenomenon
    b. potential
bioelectrical
    b. impedance
    b. impedance analysis (BIA)
    b. repair
    b. repair of delayed union or
        nonunion
bioenergy imbalance syndrome (BIS)
Bio-FASTak
    B.-F. anchor
    B.-F. suture
biofeedback
    B. 5DX
    B. 5DX device
biofeedback-assisted method
BioFit Press-Fit acetabular prosthesis
Biofix
    B. absorbable fixation
    B. absorbable fixation system

B. arrow gun
B. biodegradable implant
B. meniscus arrow
B. system pin
BIOflex
    B. Magnet Back Support
    B. magnetic counterforce brace
    B. medical magnet
    B. orthotic
Bio Flote air flotation system
Biofoot orthotic
Bio-Form glove
Biofreeze
    B. Roll-On
    B. topical analgesic gel
    B. with Ilex
Bio-Gel decubitus pillow
Bioglass prosthesis
Bio-Groove
    B.-G. acetabular prosthesis
    B.-G. Macrobond HA femoral
        prosthesis
bioimplant
    OrthoBlast osteoinductive b.
Bio-Interference
    B.-I. screwdriver
    B.-I. tibial screw
biokinetic remediation
Biokinetics pedobarograph
Bio-1000 knee brace system
BioKnit garment electrode
Biolectron bone growth stimulator
biologic, biological
    b. binding
    b. dressing
    b. fixation
    b. fracture management
biological (*var. of* biologic)
biologically
    b. designed hip (BDH)
    B. Quiet interference screw
    B. Quiet Mini-Screw suture
        anchor
    B. quiet stapler
Biolox ceramic coating
biomagnet
biomarker
biomaterial
    absorbable b.
    carbon-based b.
    ceramic b.
    collagen-based b.
    PGA-PLA b.
    polymethylmethacrylate b.
biomechanical
    b. analysis
    B. Ankle Platform System
        (BAPS)
    b. control

b. deficiency
b. evaluation of foot function during stance phase of gait
b. factor
b. failure of implant
b. frame of reference
b. integrity
b. principle
b. stress
b. testing

biomechanics
axial plane angular deformity b.
bone b.
distraction instrumentation b.
Dwyer instrumentation b.
gait b.
impact b.
posterior fixation system b.
propulsion b.
soft tissue b.
walking b.

biomedium
Dynafill graft b.

BioMed TENS unit

Biomet
B. acetabular cup
B. AGC knee prosthesis
B. ankle arthrodesis nail
B. Ascent total knee
B. bone anchor
B. button
B. cement-removal hand chisel
B. custom implant
B. fracture brace
B. hip prosthesis
B. M2A metal-on-metal articulation for hip replacement system
B. MARS acetabular component
B. Maxim knee system
B. revision acetabular component
B. revision hip stem
B. revision knee system
B. Second Assistant knee positioner
B. shoulder component
B. staple
B. total toe prosthesis
B. Ultra-Drive cement remover
B. Ultra-Drive ultrasonic revision system
B. Vision FootRing system

biometal
Biometric prosthesis
Bio-Modular
B.-M. shoulder prosthesis
B.-M. total shoulder system

Bio-Moore endoprosthesis
bionic
Bionicare 1000 stimulator system

Bionx
B. absorbable cannulated screw
B. arrow
B. self-reinforced PLLA smart screw
B. servohydraulic testing machine

Bio-Oss
B.-O. collagen
B.-O. synthetic bone

biophase
b. implant metal
b. implant metal prosthesis

Bio-Phase suture anchor
biophysics
chiropractic b. (CBP)

Bioplant Surgibone
bioplastic
biopolymeric graft
BioPro ceramic TARA head
bioprosthesis
bovine collagen b.

biopsy
aspiration needle b.
Bennett nail b.
bone marrow b.
b. cannula
channel-and-core b.
closed core needle b.
cone bone b.
core needle b.
Dunn b.
excisional b.
forage b.
b. forceps
Fosnaugh nail b.
freehand CT-guided b.
incisional b.
lumbar spine b.
Michele vertebral b.
needle b.
open b.
percutaneous bone b.
percutaneous core bone b.
percutaneous muscle b.
percutaneous transpedicular b.
punch b.
Scher nail b.
spinal infection b.
synovial b.
thoracic spine b.
trephine needle b.
Turkel bone marrow b.
ultrasound-guided echo b.
ultrasound-guided stereotactic b.
Valls-Ottolenghi-Schajowicz bone neoplasm needle b.
Zaias nail b.

BioRCI bioabsorbable screw

B

bioresorbable
   b. drug delivery system
   b. implant
   b. pin
   b. screw
BioROC anchor
Bio-R-Sorb resorbable poly-L-lactic acid ministaple
BioScrew absorbable interference screw
Biosensor biomechanical testing system
BioSkin
   B. DP wrist support
   B. Q knee brace
BioSole-GEL orthotic
BioSorbFX SR self-reinforced plate and screw
BioSorb suture
BioSphere
   B. suture anchor
   B. suture anchor implant
BioStim Digital NMS muscle stimulator
BioStinger low-profile fixation device
BioStop G bone cement restrictor
Bio-SutureTak
   Arthrex B.-S.
Biosyn synthetic monofilament suture
Biotens neurostimulator
Biotex
   B. implant metal
   B. implant metal prosthesis
biothesiometer testing
Biothotic
   B. foot orthosis
   B. orthotic
   B. orthotic mold
Biotone Polar lotion
biotribology
Bio-Wick sock
BioWrap lumbosacral/sacral support
BioZone nutrition system
Biozyme-C
bipartita
   patella b.
bipartite
   b. fracture
   b. ossification
   b. patella
   b. patella operative treatment
   b. scaphoid
   b. tibial sesamoid
bipedal walking
bipedicle dorsal flap
biphasic
   b. action potential
   b. endplate activity
   b. waveform
bipivotal hinge knee brace

biplanar
   b. fixator
   b. radiography
biplane
   b. angiogram
   b. Dwyer osteotomy
   b. padding
   b. roentgenogram
   b. trochanteric osteotomy
biplaning of osteotomy
bipolar
   b. acetabular cup
   b. cauterization
   b. cautery
   b. circumactive probe (BICAP)
   b. circumactive probe cautery
   b. coagulator
   b. femoral component
   b. femoral head prosthesis
   b. forceps
   b. hip arthroplasty
   b. hip arthroplasty component
   b. hip replacement prosthesis
   b. IF waveform
   b. needle recording electrode
   b. prosthetic cup
   b. release
   b. stimulating electrode
   b. vertebral traction
Bircher
   B. bone-holding clamp
   B. cartilage clamp
   B. meniscotome
   B. meniscus knife
Bircher-Ganske cartilage forceps
birdcage splint
Bird & Cronin wrist brace
birefringent lipid crystals in tendinitis
Birkenstock
   B. Blue Footbed arch support
   B. high-flange arch support
   B. shoe
birth
   b. fracture
   b. injury
   b. trauma
BIS
   bioenergy imbalance syndrome
bisacodyl
bisacromial
Bischof myelotomy
bisector line
Bishop
   B. bone clamp
   B. chisel
   B. classification
   B. gouge
   B. saw

B

bishop's hand deformity
bisphosphonate
BIT
Behavioral Inattention Test
bit
AO drill b.
cannulated drill b.
drill b.
b. drill
femoral drill b.
Gore b.
hip fracture compaction drill b.
Howmedica Microfixation System drill b.
Leibinger Micro System drill b.
Luhr Microfixation System drill b.
Storz Microsystems drill b.
Synthes Microsystems drill b.
biter
Stille bone b.
suction b.
bite sign
bivalved
b. cast
b. cylinder cast
b. overlap brace
bizarre
b. high-frequency discharge
b. parosteal osteochondromatous proliferation (BPOP)
b. repetitive discharge
b. repetitive potential
BJHS
benign joint hypermobility syndrome
Björk
B. prosthesis
B. rib drill
Björnström algesimeter
Bjure spinal deformity formula
BK
below knee
BKA
below-knee amputation
BKWC
below-knee walking cast
black
b. heel syndrome
B. Max mid size knee component
Blackburne ratio
Blackburn-Peel
B.-P. measurement
B.-P. ratio
black-dot heel
bladder
b. augmentation
b. dysfunction
b. injury
neurogenic b. (NGB)

blade
arachnoid-shape Beaver b.
Arthro-Lok system of Beaver b.
banana Beaver b.
Bard-Parker b.
Beaver-DeBakey b.
Beaver discission b.
Beaver keratome b.
cartilage shaver b.
Caspar b.
cast b.
chisel b.
Curdy b.
curved meniscotome b.
Dynagrip handle of b.
Dyonics arthroscopic b.
Field b.
Gigli saw b.
Hebra b.
Hibbs b.
hook b.
Incisor arthroscopic b.
K b.
keratome Beaver b.
knife b.
Magnum Tiger b.
Merlin arthroscopy b.
mini-meniscus b.
3M Maxi Driver b.
narrow Assistant Free retractor b.
notchplasty b.
b. of grass appearance
Paufique b.
PowerCut drill b.
resector b.
retrograde Beaver b.
retrograde meniscal b.
rosette Beaver b.
shoulder b.
sickle-shape Beaver b.
side-cutting b.
Smillie-Beaver b.
Superblade b.
Swann-Morton surgical b.
Synovator arthroscopic b.
synovectomy b.
Taylor spinal retractor b.
Temperlite saw b.
Tiger shaver b.
triradial resector b.
Zimmer-Gigli saw b.
blade-plate, bladeplate
adolescent condylar b.-p.
AO condylar b.-p.
ASIF right-angle b.-p.
bifurcate b.-p.
Blair talar body fusion b.-p.
Blair tibiotalar arthrodesis b.-p.
b.-p. construct

blade-plate (*continued*)
 b.-p. driver
 b.-p. fixation
 fixed-angle AO b.-p.
 Giebel b.-p.
 10-hole b.-p.
 Mueller compression b.-p.
 pediatric b.-p.
 semitubular b.-p.
 Zimmer femoral condyle b.-p.
bladeplate (*var. of* blade-plate)
blade-point retractor
blade-spike retractor
Blair
 B. ankle arthrodesis
 B. ankle fusion
 B. ankle fusion in osteonecrosis
 technique
 B. anterior arthrodesis
 B. chisel
 B. elevator
 B. knife
 B. procedure
 B. saw guide
 B. talar body fusion blade-plate
 B. tibiotalar arthrodesis
 B. tibiotalar arthrodesis
 blade-plate
Blair-Brown skin graft
**Blair-Omer flexor pollicis longus
 rerouting**
Blake inverted orthotic
Blalock clamp
Blanchard
 B. traction device
 B. traction device blade
 plate
blank
 Aliplast b.
 implant b.
 Nickelplast b.
 Plastazote b.
**Blanke inverted tibialis posterior tendon
 orthotic**
blanket
 Hollister Hot/Ice knee b.
 Rowe b.
blastic
Blastomyces dermatitidis
blastomycosis
 North American b.
blastomycotic osteomyelitis
Blatt
 B. capsulodesis
 B. capsulodesis procedure
Blauth
 B. knee prosthesis
 B. thumb hypoplasia classification
 (I-V)

Blazina
 B. patellar tendinopathy
 B. prosthesis
BLE
 both lower extremities
bleb capsulodesis
Bleck
 B. iliopsoas recession
 B. metatarsus adductus classification
 B. method
 B. midcalf lengthening by recession
 technique
Bledsoe
 B. cast brace
 B. fracture brace
 B. knee brace
 B. leg brace
 B. Ultimate brace
bleeding
 b. bone
 b. point
blennorrhagica
 keratoderma b.
blind
 b. anchorage hole
 b. medullary nail
 b. medullary nailing
blink
 b. reflex
 b. response
Bliskunov implantable femoral distractor
blister
 bone b.
 b. film dressing
 fracture b.
 b. of bone
 b. of bone sign
blistering distal dactylitis (BDD)
Blis-To-Sol
Blix contractile force curve
bloc
 en b.
Blocadren
Bloch equation
block
 Airlite alignable ankle b.
 ankle b.
 anodal b.
 articular b.
 axillary b.
 axillary and scalene b.
 balsa wood filler b.
 Bier b.
 bone b.
 Boyd posterior bone b.
 brachial plexus b.
 Campbell posterior bone b.
 Chopin sacral b.
 common peroneal nerve b.

conduction b.
condyle b.
cutting b.
depolarization b.
differential spinal b.
digital b.
digital nerve b.
facet joint b.
femoral nerve b. (FNB)
field b.
filler b.
B. fixator
forefoot nerve b.
functional grip pushup b.
ganglion b.
ganglionic b.
Gill posterior bone b.
graduated-height b.
graduated spinal b. (GSB)
hand b.
Hara infiltration b.
Howard bone b.
HyProCure sinus tarsi implant b.
iliac crest bone b.
Inclan posterior bone b.
4-in-1 cutting b.
intercostal nerve b.
interscalene b.
joint b.
Kohs b.
lumbar sympathetic b.
Mayo nerve b.
median nerve b.
metacarpal b.
metatarsal b.
Mikhail bone b.
motor point b.
musculocutaneous nerve b.
nerve b.
nerve root b.
neurolytic b.
neuromuscular b.
nondepolarizing b.
b. osteotomy
parasacral b.
paravertebral b. (PVB)
patellar tendon bone b.
pelvic b.
perineural b.
peripheral nerve b.
plantar V infiltration b.
plexus b.
2-point nerve b.
popliteal b.
popliteal fossa b.
popliteal sciatic nerve b.
posterior bone b.
presacral b.
pudendal b.

push-up b.
Putti posterior bone b.
recurrent median nerve b.
regional b.
sacral b.
sacroiliac b.
scalene b.
sciatic leg b.
sciatic nerve b.
S-cutting b.
sphenopalatine ganglion b.
spinal cord b.
Steinberg infiltration b.
stellate sympathetic
    ganglion b.
Styrofoam filler b.
subarachnoid b.
sympathetic b.
b. test
tibial cutting b.
transsacral b.
ulnar nerve b.
b. vertebra
vertebral wrist b.
wrist b.
blockade
central neural b.
popliteal fossa neural b.
sympathetic b.
blockage
articular b.
extensor tendon b.
blocker
calcium channel b.
H2 b.
hook b.
blocker's exostosis
blocking
b. screw
b. wire
blood
autologous b.
b. culture
b. flow
b. lactate
b. lactate accumulation
b. loss
b. loss anemia
b. pool phase
b. pressure (BP)
b. pressure monitor (BPM)
b. pressure monitoring
b. supply
b. transfusion
b. vessel tumor
b. viscosity
b. volume pulse (BVP)
blood-borne infection
blood-brain barrier (BBB)

bloodless
   b. amputation
   b. field
bloody effusion
Bloomberg sign
Bloom-Raney modification
Bloom splint
blot test
Blount
   B. anvil retractor
   B. blade plate
   B. bone spreader
   B. brace
   B. displacement osteotomy
   B. epiphysiodesis
   B. fracture staple
   B. knee retractor
   B. knife
   B. laminar spreader
   B. osteotome
   B. pediatric bone development disease
   B. splint
   B. stapling
   B. technique for osteoclasis
   B. tracing technique
Blount-Barber disease
Blount-Schmidt Milwaukee brace
blow-in fracture
blow-out fracture
B&L pinch gauge
Blucher
   B. design
   B. laced shoe
blue
   B. Brand Therapy Putty
   b. foot syndrome
   B. Line orthotic
   B. Line ThumbStay splint
   B. Line UNO splint
   B. Line Wrist Control splint
   methylene b.
   b. nevus
   red, yellow, b. (RYB)
   Selsun B.
   b. toe syndrome
Blumensaat anterior cruciate ligament line
Blumenthal bone rongeur
Blundell-Jones
   B.-J. hip operation
   B.-J. hip osteotomy
   B.-J. varus osteotomy
blunt
   b. arthroscopic cannula
   b. caliper
   b. dissection
   b. forceps
   b. hook

   b. hook dissector
   b. nose hemostat
   b. obturator
   b. pressure testing
   b. stylet
   b. tapered T-handled reamer
   b. trocar
blunt-tip
   b.-t. iris scissors
   b.-t. probe
BMC
   bone mineral content
BMD
   Becker muscular dystrophy
   bone mineral density
BME
   brief maximal effort
BMI
   bodymass index
BMP
   bone marrow pressure
   bone morphogenetic protein
      BMP cabling and plating system
BNP
   brain natriuretic peptide
board
   adjustable cane b.
   alphabet b.
   arm b.
   balance b.
   BAPS b.
   Biochemical Ankle Platform System b.
   broad-based cane b.
   English cane b.
   Euroglide MKII slide b.
   exercise b.
   Flexisplint flexed arm b.
   glider cane b.
   grid maze b.
   Hadfield hand b.
   hand b.
   J b.
   Lowman balance b.
   manipulation b.
   memory b.
   powder b.
   quad b.
   Rock ankle exercise b.
   rocker b.
   Rock & Roller exercise b.
   spine b.
   b. splint
   Spri Xercise b.
   string drawing b.
   transfer b.
   vertical foot b.
   wobble b.
BoarderAnkle brace

boat nail
bob and weave
Bobath technique
Bobechko
    B. sliding barrel hook
    B. spreader
Bock
    B. knee prosthesis
    B. nerve
Bodenstab tourniquet
Bodnar retractor
body
    alignment of vertebral bodies
    ankle loose b.
    apple-shape b.
    B. Armor short leg walker
    B. Armor walker cast
    artificial vertebral b.
    avascular necrosis of talar b.
    b. awareness
    B. Ball
    b. building
    cartilaginous loose b.
    b. cast syndrome
    closed b.
    b. composition
    b. composition assessment
    empty vertebral b.
    b. exhaust suit
    fibrous loose b.
    foreign b.
    B. Gard neoprene support
    B. Glove orthopaedic product
    hook b.
    b. image
    intraarticular loose b.
    b. jacket
    b. jacket cast
    Kelvin b.
    b. logic rehabilitation system
    loose b. (LB)
    loose joint b.
    b. mass index (BMI)
    B. Masters MD 510 hi-lo pulley
      system
    Maxwell b.
    b. mechanics
    B. Mechanics Evaluation
      Checklist
    b. mechanics examination chart
    melon-seed b.
    navicular b.
    newtonian b.
    b. of scapula
    b. of vertebra
    open b.
    Ortho-Mold lumbar b.
    B. Oscillation Integrates
      Neuromuscular Gain (BOING)

    osteocartilaginous loose b.
    osteochondrotic loose b.
    pear-shaped b.
    B. Pedestal
    pedunculated loose b.
    Renaut b.
    B. Response system
    rice b.
    b. righting reflex
    rigid b.
    b. side integration
    B. Sport ankle brace
    B. Sticks massager
    b. sway
    talar b.
    vertebral b.
    b. weight
    b. weight/composition
BodyBilt chair
Bodyblade
bodyCushion
    SwimEx aquatic therapy b.
BodyIce
    B. cold pack
    B. cold pack wrap
Bodyline
    B. Back-Huggar
    B. sleeper mattress overlay
    B. Sports Brace
Bodymaster
Bodynapper Comfort Pillow
body-powered prosthetic device
Body-Solid exercise equipment
3-body wear
bodywork
Boeck sarcoid
bogginess
boggy
    b. consistency
    b. swelling
    b. synovitis
Böhler
    B. brace
    B. calcaneal angle
    B. calcaneal fracture reduction
      technique
    B. calcaneal view
    B. cast breaker
    B. clamp
    B. extension bow
    B. fracture frame
    B. guideline
    B. lumbosacral angle
    B. lumbosacral view
    B. nail
    B. pin
    B. reducing frame
    B. skintight cast
    B. stirrup

Böhler (*continued*)
    B. tongs
    B. tong traction
    B. wire splint
Böhler-Braun
    B.-B. frame
    B.-B. leg sling
    B.-B. splint
Böhler-Knowles hip pin
Böhler-Steinmann
    B.-S. pin
    B.-S. pin holder
Bohlman
    B. anterior cervical vertebrectomy
    B. cervical fusion technique
    B. pin
    B. triple-wire cervical fusion
        technique
    B. triple-wire fusion
Boies forceps
BOING
    Body Oscillation Integrates
    Neuromuscular Gain
        BOING arm exercise device
Bold compression screw
Boldrey brace
Bolero lift bath trolley
Bolin wedge filter system
bollard device
Bollinger knee brace
bolster
    abduction b.
    cotton b.
    finger b.
    knee b.
    padded b.
    roll control b.
    rubber b.
    Telfa b.
    tie-over b.
bolt
    Alvar condylar b.
    Barr b.
    bone lock b.
    cannulated b.
    condylar b.
    connecting b.
    b. cutter
    DePuy b.
    expansion b.
    Fenton tibial b.
    fixation b.
    b. fixation
    Hardinge expansion b.
    Harris b.
    Herzenberg b.
    hex head b.
    Holt b.
    Hubbard b.

    No-Lok b.
    Norman tibial b.
    Recon proximal drill guide b.
    Richmond b.
    slotted b.
    solid hex b.
    tibial b.
    transfixion b.
    trochanteric b.
    Webb stove b.
    Wilson b.
    wire fixation b.
    Zimmer tibial b.
bolus
bombardment by nociceptor
Bombelli-Mathys-Morscher hip prosthesis
Bombelli-Morscher femoral component
Bond arm splint
Bondek suture
bonding
    bone b.
    Poly-Lock b.
bone
    AAA b.
    b. abscess
    b. absorption
    accessory b.
    acetabular b.
    acromial b.
    adamantinoma of long b.
    b. age
    b. age according to Greulich and
      Pyle
    b. age ratio
    alar b.
    Albers-Schönberg marble b.
    Albrecht b.
    Allofix freeze-dried b.
    b. allograft
    allograft cortical b.
    allograft iliac b.
    alveolar supporting b.
    b. anchor
    b. and limb growth velocity ratios
    b. aneurysmal cyst
    ankle b.
    antigen-extracted allogenic b.
    anvil b.
    architectural alteration of b.
    arch of b.
    areola of b.
    articulation of pisiform b.
    astragalar b.
    astragalocalcaneal b.
    astragalocrural b.
    astragaloid b.
    astragaloscaphoid b.
    astragalotibial b.
    astragalus b.

b. autogenous graft
autogenous iliac b.
autolyzed antigen-extracted allogenic b.
b. awl
axis b.
b. bank
banked b.
basal b.
basilar b.
Bertin b.
bicortical iliac b.
b. biomechanics
Bio-Oss synthetic b.
b. biopsy needle
bleeding b.
b. blister
blister of b.
b. block
b. block fusion
b. block graft
b. block procedure
b. bonding
b. borer
b. bowing
bregmatic b.
Breschet b.
bridging b.
brittle b.
b. bruise
b. bruise sign
B. Bullet suture anchor
bundle b.
b. bur
B. Button orthopaedic suture anchor
cadaver b.
calcaneal b.
calcaneocuboid b.
b. callus
calvarial free b.
cancellated b.
cancellous versus cortical b.
candle wax appearance of b.
capitate b.
carpal b.
cavalry b.
b. cavity
b. cement
central b.
cervical vertebral b.
chalky b.
chevron b.
b. chip
b. chip graft
b. chisel
coalition of b.
coccygeal b.
collar b.
compact b.
b. conduction threshold

cone and socket b.
continuity of b.
convoluted b.
b. core
3-cornered b.
cortical b.
corticocancellous b.
costal b.
coxal b.
cranial b.
crazy b.
b. crisis
cuboid b.
cuneiform b.
b. curette
b. cyst
b. cyst excision
b. cyst fracture probability
b. cyst treatment
dead b.
b. debris
b. defect
demineralized b.
dense b.
b. densitometer
b. densitometry
b. density
b. density and arthritis testing
  system
b. density measurement
b. density study
b. deposition
b. depression
dermal b.
b. destructive process
detritus b.
b. development
dimple the b.
b. disease
disorganized b.
b. dissection
b. dollop
b. dowel
b. drill set
b. dysplasia
eburnated b.
ectopic b.
elbow b.
b. elevator
enchondral b.
enchondroma of b.
b. end
endochondral b.
entrapped plantar b.
eosinophilic granuloma of b.
epactal b.
epipteric b.
exercise b.
exoccipital b.

bone (*continued*)
b. extension clamp
femoral b.
b. femoral plug
fibular b.
b. file
b. fixation kit
b. fixation surface coating
flank b.
b. flap fixation plate
flat b.
B. Foam surgical patient positioning system
b. formation
fourth turbinated b.
fovea centralis of b.
fractured b.
b. fragment
fragmental b.
freeze-dried b.
freeze-dried cortical b.
freshening of b.
frontal b.
funny b.
fusiform periosteal new b.
Goethe b.
b. gouge
b. graft (BG)
b. graft bed
b. graft collapse
b. graft decompression
grafted b.
b. graft extender
b. graft extrusion
b. graft incorporation
b. graft placement
b. graft punch
b. graft putty
b. graft repair
b. graft shoe horn
b. graft substitute (BGS)
greater multangular b.
great toe b.
b. growth
growth center of b.
b. growth stimulator
hamate b.
b. hand drill
b. harvesting
b. healing
heterotopic b.
highest turbinated b.
b. holder
b. hole punch
hollow b.
b. hook
hooked b.
hook of hamate b.
b. hook with cable/wire hole

host b.
human cancellous b.
human cortical b.
humeral b.
hydroxyapatite b.
hyoid b.
hyperplastic b.
b. hypertrophy
iliac b.
immature b.
b. impactor
b. implant
b. implant material
b. in bone
b. in bone finding
Inca b.
incarial b.
incisive b.
incomplete fracture of b.
b. infarct
b. infarction
infected b.
b. infection
b. ingrowth
innominate b.
intermaxillary b.
interparietal b.
Interpore b.
b. interstitium
intrachondrial b.
irregular b.
ischial b.
b. island
b. isograft
ivory b.
jugal b.
Kiel b.
knuckle b.
Krause b.
lacrimal b.
b. lacuna
lamellar b.
lamellated b.
laminar b.
b. lavage
lenticular b.
lesser multangular b.
b. liner
b. lip
b. lock bolt
long axis of b.
b. loss
lunate b.
lunocapitate b.
luxated b.
lyophilization of b.
malar b.
b. mallet
marble b.

b. marrow
b. marrow aspiration
b. marrow biopsy
b. marrow edema
b. marrow embolism
b. marrow embolus
b. marrow graft
b. marrow pressure (BMP)
b. marrow stimulating technique
b. marrow tumor
b. mass
b. matrix
b. maturation
b. maturity
b. meal
medial metacarpal b.
membranous b.
mesocuneiform b.
b. metabolic unit
metacarpal b.
metaphysial b.
b. metastasis
metatarsal b.
b. mill
b. mineral content (BMC)
b. mineral density (BMD)
b. mineralization isotope
morcellized b.
b. morphogenetic protein (BMP)
b. mortise
B. Mulch screw
multangular b.
navicular b.
b. necrosis
necrotic b.
b. neoplasia
new b.
newly woven b.
Nicoll b.
nonlamellar b.
nonlamellated b.
nonloadbearing fractured b.
occipital b.
omovertebral b.
orbitosphenoid b.
osteoclast-mediated b.
osteonal lamellar b.
osteopenic b.
osteoporotic b.
osteotomized b.
pagetoid b.
palatine b.
parietal b.
particle of b.
b. paste
b. pathology
b. peg
b. peg epiphysiodesis
b. pegging

b. peg graft
perilesional b.
periosteal new b.
petrosal b.
petrous temporal b.
phalangeal b.
ping-pong b.
Pirie b.
pisiform b.
plantar b.
B. Plast bone replacement material
b. plate integrity
b. plate selection
b. plombage
b. plug cutter
b. plug extractor
b. plug setter
porotic b.
postulnar b.
preinterparietal b.
primary lymphoma of b. (PLB)
primitive b.
b. production
b. prosthesis
pterotic b.
pterygoid b.
pubic b.
b. punch forceps
b. punch rongeur
quadripartite b.
radial b.
raw b.
b. reamer
Recklinghausen disease of b.
b. remodeling
b. remodeling transient
b. remodeling unit
replacement b.
b. replacement graft
b. resection
b. resorption
b. resurfacing
resurrection b.
rider's b.
Riolan b.
rudimentary b.
sacral b.
b. saw
b. scan
scaphoid b.
b. scintigram
b. scintigraphy
b. sclerosis
sclerotic b.
b. screw depth gauge
b. screw ruler gauge
b. screw targeter
scroll b.
semilunar b.

B

bone (*continued*)
b. sequestrum
sesamoid b.
b. setting
b. shaft
b. shaft fracture
shank b.
shin b.
short b.
shoulder b.
b. sialoprotein
b. skid
sliver of b.
b. slurry
soft b.
b. spacer
b. spicule
spike of b.
splint b.
spongy b.
b. spreader
b. spur
squamooccipital b.
squamous-type b.
b. staple system
Steel triple osteotomy of
innominate b.
b. stock
b. strength
structured b.
stump of b.
subchondral b.
subcoracoid b.
subperiosteal new b.
b. substance
b. substitute
b. substitute backfilling
supernumerary b.
supporting b.
supraoccipital b.
suprasternal b.
b. surface lesion
b. survey
sutural b.
b. suture fixation
b. suturing wire chisel-tip wire
synthetic cortical b.
talonavicular b.
b. tamp
tarsal b.
temporal b.
thoracic b.
tibia b.
trabecular b.
b. transfer
trapezium b.
trapezoid b.
b. trephine
triangular wrist b.

tripartite b.
triquetrum b.
b. trough
b. tuberculoma
tuberosity of carpal b.
tuberosity of cuboid b.
tumor-bearing b.
b. tunnel
turbinated b.
b. turnover
b. turnover marker
tympanic b.
ulna b.
ulnar sesamoid b.
ulnar styloid b.
b. ultrasound attenuation (BUA)
unciform b.
uncinate b.
ununited b.
vascular bundle implantation
into b.
vascular metaphysial b.
vertebral b.
vesalianum b.
Vesalius b.
Vitoss synthetic b.
vomer b.
b. wax
b. wax and gelatin sponge
b. wedge
b. wire guide
wormian b.
woven b.
wrist b.
xiphoid b.
zygomatic b.
bone-biting forceps
bone-breaking forceps
bone-cement interface
bone-cutting forceps
1-bone forearm
3-bone forearm
bone-forming
b.-f. sarcoma bone imaging
b.-f. tumor
bone-graft plug
bone-grasping forceps
bone-holding
b.-h. clamp
b.-h. forceps
b.-h. instrumentation
bone-implant interface
bone-in-bone sign
bone-ingrowth fixation
bonelet
Boneloc cement
Bone-Lok device
bonemeal tablet
bone-nibbling rongeur

bone-patellar
    b.-p. tendon-bone (BPB, BPTB)
    b.-p. tendon-bone autograft
    b.-p. tendon-bone preparation
bone-peg interface
boneplast
    B. bone void filler
    Putti B.
bone-remodeling
bone-screw interface strength
BoneSource hydroxyapatite cement
bone-specific alkaline phosphatase (BSAP)
bone-splitting forceps
bone-tendon
    b.-t. exposure
    b.-t. graft
    b.-t. graft material
bone-tendon-bone (BTB)
    b.-t.-b. allograft
    b.-t.-b. graft
bone-to-bone
    b.-t.-b. apposition
    b.-t.-b. graft
bone-within-bone appearance
Bonfiglio
    B. bone graft
    B. modification
    B. modification of Phemister bone graft of femoral neck technique
bonnet
    gluteal b.
Bonney clamp
Bonney-Kessel dorsiflexionary tilt-up osteotomy
Bonola cross-arm double-flap thumb repair technique
bony
    b. abnormality
    b. absorption
    b. ankylosis
    b. apposition
    b. architecture
    b. bar
    b. bridge
    b. bridge resection
    b. consolidation
    b. crepitus
    b. deformity
    b. demineralization
    b. distal end
    b. eburnation
    b. element destruction
    b. encroachment
    b. erosion
    b. excrescence
    b. exostosis
    b. fossa
    b. hallux limitus

B

    b. healing
    b. humeral avulsion
    b. humeral avulsion of glenohumeral ligament (BHAGL)
    b. humeral avulsion of glenohumeral ligament lesion
    b. interface
    b. landmark
    b. lesion
    b. mass
    b. metastasis
    b. necrosis
    b. necrosis and destruction
    b. osteophyte
    b. overgrowth
    b. pelvis
    b. procedure
    b. process
    b. purchase
    b. resorption
    b. semicircular canal
    b. sequestrum
    b. skeleton
    b. slurry leakage
    b. spurring
    b. tenderness
    b. union
Boo-Boo Pacs
Book Butler book-grip device
boomerang wrist support
boot
    Ambulator Chukka B.
    APB Hi all-purpose b.
    b. brace
    Bunny b.
    cast b.
    Chukka b.
    clamshell AFO b.
    compression b.
    Conformer diabetic b.
    Cryo/Cuff b.
    De Lorme b.
    derotation b.
    external sequential pneumatic compression b.
    fluid barrier b.
    fracture b.
    gelatin compression b.
    Gibney b.
    Hang Ups gravity b.
    Heelift suspension b.
    Heelift traction b.
    Heel-Up Boot suspension b.
    In-Bed AFO b.
    Jobst b.
    Junod b.
    L'Nard b.
    Markell brace b.
    Markell open-toe b.

boot (*continued*)
    Moon b.
    Multi Podus b.
    Ongoing Ambulating AFO b.
    pneumatic compression b.
    Primer modified Unna b.
    quadriceps De Lorme b.
    Rik FootHugger fluid heel b.
    rocker b.
    sequential pneumatic compression b.
    SlimLine cast b.
    Sorrel-type snowboard b.
    Spenco b.
    Unna b.
    Unna paste b.
    Venodyne b.
    weight b.
    Wilke b.
    b. wrap
booth
    B. transverse humeral ligament test
    B. wire fixation of sagittal split
      mandibular osteotomy
bootie
    Bebax B.
boot-top
    b.-t. fracture
    b.-t. laceration
Boplant Surgibone bovine bone substitute
Bora
    B. centralization
    B. operation
    B. technique
borazone blade cutting machine
Borchardt olive-shaped bur
Borchgrevink traction
border
    brush b.
    coast of California (smooth) b.
    coast of Maine (irregular) b.
    cryptotic medial b.
    lateral acromial b.
    medial b.
    b. ray
    b. ray amputation
    scapular b.
    scapulovertebral b.
    superior b.
    vertebral b.
    web b.
bore needle
borer
    bone b.
    cork b.
Borg
    B. Numerical Pain Scale
    B. Scale of Rating Perceived
      Exertion

Borggreve
    B. limb rotation
    B. rotationplasty
Borggreve-Hall tibial rotation plasty technique
Borg-Warner orthopaedic bed
boring pain
Boropak astringent solution
borotannic complex
Borrelia burgdorferi
BOS
    base of skull
    base of support
Bose
    B. hip resurfacing procedure
    B. nail fold excision
BOSS
    Becker orthopaedic spinal system
boss
    carpal b.
    carpometacarpal b.
bosselated
bosselation
bossing
    frontal b.
Bostick staple
Boston
    B. bivalved cast
    B. brace thoracolumbosacral orthosis
    B. Classification System
    B. Diagnostic Aphasia examination
    B. elbow system
    B. LINAC
    B. overlap brace
    B. postoperative hip orthosis
    B. scoliosis brace
    B. soft body jacket
    B. soft corset
    B. thoracic brace
    B. thoracic splint
B&O Supprettes
Boswellia
Bosworth
    B. ankle approach
    B. arthrodesis
    B. arthroplasty
    B. bone peg insertion
    B. coracoclavicular screw
    B. crown drill
    B. femoroischial transplant
    B. fracture
    B. hip shelf operation
    B. hip shelf procedure
    B. lumbar spinal fusion
    B. posterior femur approach
    B. screwdriver
    B. spine plate
    B. splint

B. technique
B. tendo calcaneus repair
Bosworth-type reverse plasty
botfly
human b.
both
b. lower extremities (BLE)
b. upper extremities (BUE)
both-bone fracture
both-column fracture
Botox injection
botryoid sarcoma
bottleneck femoral tunnel
bottle sign
bottom
weaver's b.
Bottoms-Up posture system
Bouchard
B. node
B. nodule
B. sign
bouche de tapir
bougie
bounce home knee test
Bouncewell medicine ball
bouncing
ligamentous b.
Bourgery ligament
Bourneville disease
boutonnière
b. deformity
b. deformity sign
b. hand dislocation
b. splint
Bouvier MCP joint flexion maneuver
Bovie
B. cauterization
B. cautery
B. coagulating unit
B. electrocautery apparatus
B. electrocautery device
B. knife
underwater B.
bovine
b. collagen
b. collagen bioprosthesis
b. collagen graft
b. collagen implant
b. collagen material prosthesis
bow
aiming b.
B. & Arrow cannulated drill guide
Böhler extension b.
Cupid's b.
extension b.
finger extension b.
Framer finger extension b.
Kirschner wire traction b.
maximum radial b.

posterior b.
posteromedial b.
Schwarz finger extension b.
traction b.
wire traction b.
Bowden cable suspension system
bowed leg
bowel
b. disturbance
neurogenic b.
b. training
Bowen
B. chisel
B. disease
B. osteotome
B. periosteal elevator
B. suture drill
Bowers
B. genital reassignment technique
B. radial arthroplasty
bowing
bone b.
congenital posteromedial b.
b. deformity
b. fracture
lateral b.
tendon b.
tibial b.
Bowlby arm splint
bowl curette
bow-leg (*var. of* bowleg)
bowleg, bow-leg
b. brace
b. deformity
bowler's thumb
Bowman
B. disc
B. lateral condyle angle
B. muscle
bowstring
b. low back test
b. sign
b. tear
bowstringing
bow-tie sign
box
b. and block test of arm disability
BTE Bolt B.
b. chisel
b. curette
fracture b.
high toe b.
ligamentous b.
mirror b.
b. osteotome
sit-and-reach b.
toe b.
wide toe b.

B

box-end wrench
boxer's
- b. elbow
- b. fracture
- b. knuckle
- b. punch

boxing
- aerobic b.
- Muay Thai b.

boxwood mallet
Boyd
- B. and Griffin subtrochanteric proximal femur fracture classification (I–IV)
- B. ankle amputation
- B. ankle arthrodesis
- B. classification
- B. communicating perforation vein
- B. dual-onlay bone graft
- B. elbow approach
- B. formula
- B. hip disarticulation
- B. modification of Tardieu spastic measurement scale
- B. operation
- B. perforator
- B. podiatry chair
- B. posterior bone block
- B. side plate

Boyd-Anderson
- B.-A. biceps tendon repair
- B.-A. distal biceps tendon repair technique

Boyd-Ingram-Bourkhard treatment
Boyd-McLeod
- B.-M. tennis elbow procedure
- B.-M. tennis elbow technique

Boyd-Sisk
- B.-S. posterior capsulorrhaphy
- B.-S. shoulder approach

Boyer degenerative joint disease grade (0–4)
Boyes
- B. boutonniére deformity test
- B. brachioradialis transfer technique
- B. finger tendon transfer

Boyes-Goodfellow hook
Boyle-Davis retractor
Boytchev recurrent dislocated shoulder procedure
Bozzini light conductor
BP
- blood pressure

BPB
- bone-patellar tendon-bone
  - BPB autologous graft

BPM
- blood pressure monitor
- Laserflo BPM

BPOP
- bizarre parosteal osteochondromatous proliferation

BPTB
- bone-patellar tendon-bone
  - BPTB autograft
  - BPTB graft

BPTI
- brachial plexus traction injury

brace
- Abbott b.
- abduction b.
- accommodative b.
- Ace b.
- ACL Lite functional knee b.
- Active ankle b.
- Active support and b.
- Activity-Lite knee b.
- adjustable b.
- AFO pediatric b.
- Aircast ankle b.
- Aircast Cryo/Cuff b.
- Aircast fracture b.
- Aircast leg b.
- Aircast Pneumatic Air Stirrup b.
- Aircast Swivel-Strap b.
- Aircast walking b.
- Air DonJoy patellofemoral b.
- AirGEL ankle b.
- airplane splint shoulder b.
- Airprene Action knee b.
- Air-Stirrup ankle training b.
- Air Townsend b.
- ALP Plus ankle b.
- Ambi wrist b.
- AMX knee b.
- Ank-L-Aid b.
- ankle ligament protector b.
- ankle stirrup b.
- AO b.
- AOA cervical immobilization b.
- APL Plus ankle b.
- APU b.
- Arizona ankle b.
- Arnold lumbar b.
- ASO ankle b.
- Atak knee b.
- athletic b.
- Atlanta hip b.
- Atlanta-Scottish Rite b.
- Atlantic overlap b.
- Atlantic rim b.
- ATR b.
- auxiliary power unit b.
- Axis ankle b.
- back b.
- Back Seat torso-wrap b.
- bail-lock b.
- Bauerfeind ankle b.

B

Bauerfeind Comprifix knee b.
Becker b.
bicycle b.
bike ankle b.
BIOflex magnetic counterforce b.
Biomet fracture b.
BioSkin Q knee b.
bipivotal hinge knee b.
Bird & Cronin wrist b.
bivalved overlap b.
Bledsoe cast b.
Bledsoe fracture b.
Bledsoe knee b.
Bledsoe leg b.
Bledsoe Ultimate b.
Blount b.
Blount-Schmidt Milwaukee b.
BoarderAnkle b.
Bodyline Sports B.
Body Sport ankle b.
Böhler b.
Boldrey b.
Bollinger knee b.
boot b.
Boston overlap b.
Boston scoliosis b.
Boston thoracic b.
bowleg b.
Brite-Life wrist b.
Buck knee b.
cable-twister b.
cage-back b.
Caligamed b.
caliper b.
Callender derotational b.
Camp b.
Cam Walker ankle b.
Cam Walker leg b.
Can Am b.
canvas b.
Capener b.
Carpal Lock CTS b.
Carpal Lock wrist b.
carpenter's b.
CASH b.
cast b.
Castaway leg b.
Cast Boot polypropylene hip
  abduction b.
Castiglia ankle b.
Centec Formfit ankle b.
cervical collar b.
chairback b.
Charleston nighttime bending b.
Charleston scoliosis b.
Charnley b.
Cheetah ankle b.
Chopart b.
CI functional knee b.

Cinch Lock CTS b.
Cincinnati ACL b.
clamshell b.
CM-Band 505N b.
CM-Band silicone rubber b.
Cole hyperextension b.
collar b.
Combined Instabilities functional
  knee b.
contraflexion b.
controlled-motion b.
controlled position b. (CPB)
Cook walking b.
cool CPB b.
Cooper ankle b.
Counter Rotation System b.
Count'R-Force arch b.
cowhorn b.
CRM rehab b.
CRS b.
Cruiser hip abduction b.
Cruiser OA b.
CTi b.
CTi2 knee b.
Cunningham b.
custom-fitted b.
cutout patellar b.
Dalco Astro ankle b.
Darco back b.
DarcoGel ankle b.
Defiance functional knee b.
Dennison cervical b.
DePuy fracture b.
derotation b.
derotational b.
3D fracture walker b.
dial-lock b.
DonJoy ALP b.
DonJoy Gold Point knee b.
DonJoy Opal knee b.
DonJoy 4-point Super Sport knee b.
DonJoy Quadrant shoulder b.
DonJoy Universal ankle b.
dorsiflexion stop b.
double Becker ankle b.
double-upright short leg b.
doughnut support b.
b. drill
dropfoot b.
drop-lock knee b.
Drytex RocketSoc ankle b.
dual-lock ankle b.
Duncan shoulder b.
Dura-Flex back b.
dynamic abduction b.
dynamic hinge elbow fracture b.
Easy Lok ankle b.
Easy-On elbow b.
Eclipse Gel ankle b.

brace (*continued*)
economy ROM b.
EconoSoc ankle b.
Edge knee b.
elastic-hinge knee b.
elastic knee sleeve b.
Elite knee b.
English b.
Equalizer cast b.
Exotec b.
EZ ROM postoperative knee b.
felt b.
figure-of-8 b.
Fisher b.
Flagg fiberglass knee b.
Flex Foam b.
flexor hinge hand-splint b.
FlexTech knee b.
Floam ankle stirrup b.
Florida back b.
Florida cervical b.
Florida contraflexion b.
Florida extension b.
Florida hyperextension b.
Florida J-24, J-35, J-45, J-55 b.
Florida post-fusion b.
Florida spinal b.
foot-ankle b.
footdrop b.
Forrester cervical collar b.
Frazer carpal tunnel wrist b.
Friedman b.
functional fracture b.
functional knee b.
furniture b.
Futuro wrist b.
gait lock splint b.
Galveston metacarpal b.
Generation II 3DX b.
Generation II knee b.
Generation II Unloader ADJ
  knee b.
Generation II Unloader Select
  knee b.
Genutrain knee b.
Gillette b.
GLS b.
GoldPoint ACL functional knee b.
GoldPoint hinged knee b.
GoldPoint PCL functional knee b.
Goldthwait b.
Guilford cervical b.
halo b.
hand b.
H buttress support patellofemoral b.
head b.
Hennessy knee b.
Hessing b.
high Knight b.

high-tide walking b.
Hilgenreiner b.
hinged knee b.
Hi-Top foot/ankle b.
Hoke lumbar b.
horseshoe patellofemoral b.
Hudson-Jones knee-cage b.
Hudson TLSO b.
humeral b.
hyperextension b.
Ilfeld b.
InCare b.
Inner Lok ankle b.
internal tibial torsion b.
Intrepid functional knee b.
I-Plus system humeral fracture b.
I-Plus system ulnar fracture b.
ischial weightbearing leg b.
IsoDyn knee b.
Jewett-Benjamin cervical b.
Jones b.
J patellofemoral b.
Juzo b.
Juzo Patellaligner b.
Kallassy b.
Key wrist b.
Kicker Pavlik harness hip
  abduction b.
King cervical b.
Kleinert postoperative traction b.
Klengall b.
Klenzak spring b.
Kling cervical b.
knee cage b.
knee MD b.
KneeRanger hinged knee b.
Knight back b.
Knight-Taylor thoracic b.
knock-knee b.
KS 5 ACL b.
KSO b.
Küntscher-Hudson b.
Kydex b.
kyphosis b.
lace-on b.
lace-up RocketSoc ankle b.
lacing ankle b.
leaf-spring b.
LeCocq b.
leg b.
Legend ACL functional knee b.
Legend PCL functional knee b.
Lenox Hill derotational knee b.
Lenox Hill Spectralite knee b.
Lerman hinge b.
Liberty CMC thumb b.
ligamentous control b.
limb b.
long arm b.

long leg b.
long leg hinged b.
Lorenz b.
low-tide walking b.
LSU reciprocation-gait orthosis b.
lumbar b.
lumbosacral b.
MacAusland lumbar b.
Magnetic Support b.
M-Brace knee b.
McClintoch b.
McCollough internal tibial torsion b.
McDavid knee b.
McKee b.
MCL b.
MC walker b.
MD b.
Medical Design b.
Medipedic Multicentric knee b.
Metcalf spring drop b.
Miami fracture b.
Miami TLSO scoliosis b.
b. migration
Milwaukee scoliosis b.
Minerva cervical b.
MKS II b.
Monarch knee b.
Moon Boot b.
Mooney b.
MTA b.
Mueller ATF ankle b.
Mueller hinged knee b.
Mueller Lite ankle b.
Mueller orthopaedic shoulder b.
Mueller Ultralite b.
Mueller wrap-around knee b.
Multi-Lig knee b.
Multi-Lock knee b.
Murphy b.
Nakamura b.
neck b.
neoprene wrist b.
Nevin ankle b.
New England scoliosis b.
Newington b.
Newport MC hip orthosis b.
Nextep knee b.
night b.
nonweightbearing b.
Northville b.
no-stretch RocketSoc b.
OAdjuster knee b.
OA knee b.
OAsys knee b.
offloading knee b.
Omni knee b.
Opiela b.
Oppenheim b.
Orbital shoulder stabilizer b.

Orthomedics b.
Ortho-Mold spinal b.
Orthoplast fracture b.
Orthotech Controller knee b.
Osgood-Schlatter knee b.
OS-5/Plus 2 knee b.
OsteoArthritic knee b.
osteoarthritis padded night sleeve b.
out-of-cast ankle b.
outside-the-boot b.
oyster-shell b.
Palumbo dynamic patellar b.
Palumbo knee b.
Palumbo stabilizing b.
pantaloon b.
parachutist ankle b.
Patellaligner knee b.
patellar stabilizing b. (PSB)
patellar tendon-bearing b.
patellofemoral b.
Patten-Bottom-Perthes b.
pediatric PRAFO b.
pelvic b.
performer ultralight knee b.
Perlstein b.
PFT traction b.
Phelps b.
Philadelphia Plastizote cervical b.
piano-wire dorsiflexion b.
Playmaker functional knee b.
PlayTuf knee b.
PMT halo system b.
PneuGel ankle b.
Pneu Knee b.
Pneu-trac neck b.
4-point IROM b.
6-point knee b.
4-point SuperSport functional knee b.
Polaris knee rehab b.
2-poster b.
4-poster cervical b.
postfusion b.
Power Play knee b.
PPG-AFO b.
PPG-TLSO b.
Pro-8 ankle b.
Procase Ankle-Lock b.
progressive resistance b.
Proline Stomatex shoulder b.
Protonic b.
PTB b.
PTS knee b.
Push medical b.
Quadrant advanced shoulder b.
QualCare knee b.
Raney flexion jacket b.
range of motion b.
ratchet-type b.
reamer b.

brace (*continued*)

Rebel knee b.
Rehab TROM b.
Rhino Triangle polypropylene hip abduction b.
Richie b.
rigid postoperative b.
Ritchie b.
RocketSoc ankle b.
Rolyan TakeOff Sprint b.
Rolyan tibial fracture b.
ROM knee b.
ROM walker b.
Saltiel b.
Sarmiento fracture b.
SAS II b.
Sawa shoulder b.
Schanz collar b.
SCOI shoulder b.
scoliosis overlap b.
Scottish Rite b.
Selectively Lockable knee b.
semirigid ankle b.
Seton hip b.
short arm b.
short leg caliper b.
short leg double-upright b.
short leg walking b.
shoulder subluxation inhibitor b.
SmartBrace b.
SmartWrap elbow b.
Smedberg b.
snap-lock b.
SofTec rigid b.
SOMI b.
Speed b.
Spinal Technology bivalve TLSO b.
SpineCor nonrigid b.
Sports-Caster I, II knee b.
SSI b.
Stardox wrist b.
Stealth knee b.
Stille b.
Stimprene electrotherapy b.
stirrup b.
stop action b.
straight walker b.
Strap Lok ankle b.
Stromgren ankle b.
Stubbs 4-way clavicle b.
Sully shoulder stabilizer b.
Sure Step ankle b.
Swede-O Ankle Loc b.
Swede-O-Universal b.
Swivel-Strap ankle b.
Taylor back b.
Taylor-Knight b.
Taylor spine b.
telescoping b.

Teufel cervical b.
Teurlings wrist b.
Thermoskin b.
Thomas cervical collar b.
Thomas walking b.
thoracolumbar standing orthosis b.
TLSO b.
toe-drop b.
Toronto b.
total anatomical hinge knee b.
Townsend Air b.
Townsend Premier b.
Townsend Rebel convertible b.
Townsend Reliever b.
Tracker knee b.
Tri-Angle shoulder abduction b.
Trinkle b.
TROM knee b.
Tru-Fit b.
turnbuckle ankle b.
turnbuckle knee b.
UBC b.
UCLA functional long leg b.
ulnar b.
Ultrabrace b.
underarm b.
unilateral calcaneal b.
University of British Columbia b.
Unloader b.
Unloader ADJ OA knee b.
Unloader Bi-ComPF knee b.
Unloader Express OA knee b.
Unloader Select OA knee b.
Unloader Spirit knee b.
Value Walker b.
Varney acromioclavicular b.
Verlow b.
Victorian b.
von Lackum transection shift jacket b.
walking b.
Warm Springs b.
Watco ankle b.
weightbearing b.
Wheaton b.
Wilke boot b.
Williams b.
Wilmington scoliosis b.
Wright Universal b.
wrist b.
Yale b.
Zimmer reamer b.
Zinco Air Cam b.
Zinco Cam Walker II b.
Zinco Castaway II b.
Zinco Hi-Top b.

brace/corset

Hoke lumbar b./c.

brace-free ambulation

bracelet
    Nussbaum b.
    Q-Ray b.
    b. test
brace-type reamer
brachia (*pl. of* brachium)
brachial
    b. amelia
    b. artery
    b. artery aneurysm
    b. artery injury
    b. neuralgia
    b. neuritis
    b. plexitis
    b. plexopathy
    b. plexus
    b. plexus block
    b. plexus injury
    b. plexus neuropathy
    b. plexus palsy
    b. plexus paralysis
    b. plexus repair
    b. plexus tendon
    b. plexus tension test
    b. plexus traction injury (BPTI)
brachialgia statica paresthetica
brachialis
    b. muscle
    b. tendon
brachiocephalic vein
brachiocrural
brachiocubital
brachiogram
brachioradialis
    b. flap
    b. muscle
    b. reflex
    b. tendon
    b. transfer
    b. transfer for wrist extension
brachium, *pl.* **brachia**
brachybasia
brachybasocamptodactyly
brachybasophalangia
brachycnemic
brachydactylia (*var. of* brachydactyly)
brachydactylic
brachydactyly, brachydactylia
brachykerkic
brachymelia
brachymesophalangia
brachymetacarpalia (*var. of*
  brachymetacarpia)
brachymetacarpalism (*var. of*
  brachymetacarpia)
brachymetacarpia, brachymetacarpalia,
  brachymetacarpalism
brachymetapody
brachymetatarsia

brachyphalangia
brachypodous
brachyskelous (*var. of* bradyskelous)
brachystasis
brachysyndactyly
brachytelephalangia
bracing
    cast b.
    dynamic b.
    fracture b.
    postoperative b.
    Wiltse system cross b.
bracket
    longitudinal epiphysial b.
bracketed splint
Brackett-Osgood
    B.-O. knee approach
    B.-O. posterior hip approach
Brackett osteotomy
Braden risk assessment scale
Bradford
    B. fracture frame
    B. fusion
Bradley femoral canal preparation
  scraper
Brady
    B. balanced-suspension splint
    B. leg splint
bradycinesia (*var. of* bradykinesia)
Brady-Jewett proximal radial resection
  technique
bradykinesia, bradycinesia
bradykinetic
bradykinin
bradymetatarsalgia
bradyskelous, brachyskelous
Bragard
    B. meniscal injury sign
    B. meniscal injury test
    B. reinforcement
    B. sciatica test
Bragg-peak photon-beam therapy
Bragg x-ray angle
Brahms
    B. foot operation
    B. procedure
braid
    carbon fiber lamination b. (CFLB)
braided suture
Brailsford disease
brain
    B. arthroplasty
    b. natriuretic peptide (BNP)
    B. Pad mouth guard
    B. reflex
brainstem, brain stem
    b. auditory evoked potential (BAEP)
    b. auditory evoked response (BAER)
    transtentorial b.

B

brake
    b. lever extension
    b. phenomenon
branch
    acetabular b.
    calcaneal b.
    digital b.
    distal communicating b. (DCB)
    dorsal ulnar cutaneous b.
    interosseous b.
    motor b.
    posterior interosseous b.
    proper digital nerve b.
    proximal communicating b.
    superior laryngeal nerve
      external b.
    thenar b.
branched calculus
brand
    B. tendon-holding forceps
    B. tendon passer
    B. tendon-passing forceps
    B. tendon stripper
    B. tendon transfer technique
Branhamella catarrhalis
Brannock
    B. Device shoe sizer
    B. Foot Measuring Device
Brant aluminum splint
Brantigan interbody fusion cage
Brasseler orthopaedic power system
brassiere
    Jobst b.
Brattström condylar height ratio
Braun
    B. frame
    B. gastric procedure
    B. shoulder tenotomy
    B. skin graft
breach
    cortical b.
    naviculocuneiform b.
break
    b. point
    b. test
breakable screw
breakage
    pedicle screw b.
    rod b.
    screw b.
    tack b.
breakaway
    b. lap cushion
    b. pin
    b. weakness
breakdancer's thumb
breakdown
    skin b.

breaker
    Böhler cast b.
    cast b.
breast
    chicken b.
    funnel b.
    pigeon b.
breastbone
breaststroker's knee
breathing
    paradoxical b.
Breck
    B. pin
    B. pin cutter
Breezee Mist Antifungal
bregma
bregmatic bone
bregmatomastoid suture
Bremer
    B. AirFlo halo vest
    B. halo cervical traction
    B. Halo Crown cervical collar
    B. halo system
    B. HIFix skull pin
Breschet bone
Breschet-Gorham syndrome
Breslow
    B. arthroplasty
    B. melanoma classification
    B. melanoma thickness classification
Brett
    B. arthrodesis
    B. osteotomy
Breuerton MCP joint view
breve
    vinculum b.
brevicollis
breviflexor
Brevio nerve conduction monitor
brevis
    abductor pollicis b.
    extensor carpi radialis b. (ECRB)
    extensor digitorum b. (EDB)
    extensor pollicis b. (EPB)
    flexor digitorum b. (FDB)
    flexor digitorum quinti b. (FDQB)
    flexor hallucis b. (FHB)
    flexor pollicis b. (FPB)
    peroneus b. (PB)
    b. release
Brevital
Brewster triple arthrodesis
bridge
    autograft b.
    b. back exercise technique
    balance b.
    bony b.
    fascial b.
    b. graft

B. Hip system
iliac crest b.
b. of meniscus
osseous b.
physial b.
b. plate
b. plate fixation
skin b.
tarsal b.
tendon-bone b.

bridging
b. bone
b. callus
myocardial b.
b. of defect
b. osteophyte

bridle
b. footdrop procedure
b. posterior tibial tendon
procedure
b. posterior tibial tendon transfer
operation

Bridwell-Lenke allograft incorporation grading system

brief
b. maximal effort (BME)
B. Pain Inventory
b., small, abundant, polyphasic
potential (BSAPP)
b., small, abundant potential
(BSAP)
B. Test of Head Injury (BTHI)

Brigham prosthesis

Brighton electrical stimulation system

brim
pelvic b.
proximal medial b.
quadrilateral b.

brisement
b. forcé
b. therapy

Brissaud
B. scoliosis
B. syndrome

Bristow
B. operation
B. periosteal elevator
B. procedure
B. rasp
B. shoulder reconstruction

Bristow-Helfet recurrent shoulder dislocation procedure

Bristow-Latarjet anterior shoulder instability procedure

Bristow-May dislocated shoulder procedure

Brite-Life wrist brace

Brittain
B. chisel

B. ischiofemoral arthrodesis
B. operation

brittle
b. bone
b. bone disease
b. bone failure
b. nail

BRM
basal metabolic rate

broach
barbed b.
cemented b.
cementless b.
Charnley femoral b.
chipped-tooth b.
drilling b.
b. extractor
femoral prosthesis b.
Harris b.
Koenig metatarsal b.
orthopaedic b.
root canal b.
smooth b.
square-hole b.
Swanson metatarsal b.
Zimmer femoral canal b.

broad
b. AO dynamic compression plate
b. foot
b. thumb–big toe syndrome

broad-based
b.-b. cane
b.-b. cane board
b.-b. gait

Broadbent-Woolf 4-limb Z-plasty

broad-spectrum antibiotic

broad-toed shoe

Broberg-Morrey
B.-M. elbow function scale
B.-M. fracture

Broca
B. aphasia
B. area
B. convolution
B. diagonal band

Brockman
B. foot operation
B. incision
B. procedure

Brockman-Nissen arthrodesis

Broden
B. subtalar instability stress
examination
B. subtalar joint (I-II) view
B. subtalar stress radiography

Brodie
B. abscess
B. bursa
B. disease

Brodie (*continued*)
    B. knee
    B. ligament
Brodsky-Tullos-Gartsman posterior shoulder joint approach
BROM
    back range of motion
bromelain powder
bromfenac sodium
bromhidrosis, bromidrosis
    plantar b.
bromidrosis (*var. of* bromhidrosis)
Bromi-Lotion antiperspirant lotion
Bromi-Talc Plus antiperspirant powder
bromocriptine
bronchospasm
Brooke Army Hospital splint
Brooker
    B. classification of heterotopic
      ossification
    B. double-locking unreamed tibial
      nail
    B. femoral nail
    B. frame
    B. heterotopic bone formation
      classification (I-IV)
    B. wire
Brooker-Wills nail
Brooks
    B. atlantoaxial arthrodesis
    B. atlantoaxial technique
    B. cervical fusion
    B. cervical fusion operation
    B. sports and running shoe
Brooks-Gallie cervical fusion
Brooks-Jenkins
    B.-J. atlantoaxial fusion
    B.-J. atlantoaxial fusion technique
    B.-J. cervical fusion
Brooks-type fusion
Broomhead medial ankle approach
broomstick
    b. bar
    b. cast
    b. curl-up
Brophy periosteal elevator
Broström
    B. injection technique
    B. lateral ankle instability procedure
    B. lateral ankle ligament repair
    B. ligament reconstruction
Broström-Evans procedure
Broström-Gould ankle instability operation
Browlift Bone Bridge system
brown
    B. dermatome
    B. endoscopic carpal tunnel release
      technique

    B. fibular transfer
    B. knee approach
    B. knee approach operation
    B. knee joint reconstruction
    B. lateral knee approach
    B. periosteotome
    B. 2-portal carpal tunnel release
    B. rasp
    B. tissue forceps
    b. tumor of hyperparathyroidism
Brown-Adson forceps
Brown-Cushing forceps
Browne splint
brown-fat tumor
Brown-Mueller T-fastener set
Brown-Roberts-Wells (BRW)
    B.-R.-W. stereotactic
      frame
Brown-Séquard
    B.-S. lesion
    B.-S. syndrome
***Brucella* osteomyelitis**
brucellosis
    spinal b.
Bruce protocol
Bruck disease
Brudzinski
    B. reflex
    B. sign
Bruening chisel
Bruening-Citelli rongeur
Bruger
    cul-de-sac of B.
Brügger
    B. cogwheel analysis of posture
    B. cogwheel principle
    B. muscle tension release postural
      approach
    B. relief position exercise
    B. rocking technique
    B. sternosymphysial syndrome
Bruininks-Oseretsky Test of Motor Proficiency
bruisability
bruise
    bone b.
    reticular bone b.
Brumm technique
Brunner
    B. modified incision
    B. palmar incision
    B. rib shears
Brunn plaster shears
Brunnstrom-Fugl-Meyer
    B.-F.-M. stroke impairment
      assessment
Bruns
    B. ataxia
    B. bone curette

B. gait apraxia
B. syndrome
Brunswick-Mack rotating drill
Bruser
B. lateral knee approach
B. lateral knee technique
B. skin incision
brush
b. border
Cohort bone b.
delta b.
b. knee swelling test
Plak-Vac oral suction b.
brush-evoked pain testing
bruxing
bruxism
BRW
Brown-Roberts-Wells
BRW head ring halo
Bryan
B. arthroplasty
B. cervical disc prosthesis
B. procedure
B. total knee implant prosthesis
Bryan-Morrey
B.-M. capitellar fracture
classification (I-IV)
B.-M. elbow approach
B.-M. extensive posterior elbow
joint approach
B.-M. triceps-sparing humerus
fracture repair technique
Bryant
B. iliofemoral triangle
B. line
B. sign
B. traction
BSAP
bone-specific alkaline phosphatase
brief, small, abundant potential
BSAPP
brief, small, abundant, polyphasic
potential
BST-CarGel
BTB
bone-tendon-bone
BTE
Baltimore Therapeutic Equipment
BTE Assembly Tree
BTE Bolt Box
BTE dynamic lift
BTHI
Brief Test of Head Injury
BUA
bone ultrasound attenuation
bubbly bone lesion
buccinator
b. muscle
b. myomucosal flap

Buchanan disease
Buchholz
B. acetabular cup
B. prosthesis
buck
B. bone curette
B. convoluted traction apparatus
B. convoluted traction device
B. extension
B. extension splint
B. fascia
B. femoral cement restrictor
inserter
B. knee brace
B. method
B. neurological hammer
B. operation
B. percussion hammer
B. periosteal elevator
B. plug
B. Redi-Traction apparatus
B. traction
B. traction splint
B. traction stockinette
bucket
Denis Browne b.
Lenox b.
bucket-handle
b.-h. fracture
b.-h. fragment
b.-h. plica
b.-h. rib
b.-h. rib motion
b.-h. tear
Buck-Gramcko
B.-G. dorsal rotational advancement
flap technique
B.-G. gouge
B.-G. pollicization
buckle
b. fracture
wire-fixation b.
Buckley chisel
buckling
plantar b.
reverse b.
Bucky
B. abdominal view
B. diaphragm
B. x-ray tray
Bucy-Frazier suction cannula
bud
limb b.
buddy
b. splint
b. strap
b. taping
BuddyWrap
FoamWrap B.

B

budge
ciliospinal center of B.
Budin
B. hammertoe splint
B. joint
B. toe splint
Budin-Chandler
B.-C. anteversion determination
B.-C. femoral neck anteversion
measurement method
BUE
both upper extremities
BUE strength
Buechel-Pappas
B.-P. total ankle prosthesis
B.-P. total ankle replacement
system
**Buerger-Allen circulation of feet
exercise**
buffalo hump
Bufferin
Buffex
buffing sponge
Buffinol Extra
Buford complex
**Bugg-Boyd Achilles tendon repair
technique**
buggy
cruiser b.
Maclaren mobile b.
Buhl spirometer
Builder Grip hand exerciser
building
body b.
buildup
Elevations shoe b.
bulb
b. and thumb screw valve
b. dynamometer
irrigation b.
b. neuroma
b. suture
bulbar
b. abnormality
b. anesthesia
b. necrosis
bulbocavernosus reflex
bulge
disc b.
b. knee test
bulging
b. anulus fibrosus
b. disc
bulk
b. flow axoplasmic transport
b. graft
bulky hand dressing
bulla, *pl.* **bullae**
hemorrhagic b.

bullae (*pl. of* bulla)
bulldog
b. clamp
b. clamp applier
b. clamp-applying forceps
bullet
b. driver
b. tissue stretching
bullosa
epidermolysis b.
Bullseye femoral guide
bull's eye shoulder
bump
Haglund b.
hip b.
inion b.
pump b.
runner's b.
bumper
axle lock and b.
b. cast
dorsiflexion b.
flexion b.
b. fracture
b. wedge
Buncke
B. microsurgical technique
B. toe to hand transfer
bundle
anterior oblique b.
anteromedial b.
b. bone
cleidoepitrochlear b.
b. dressing
b. function
interdigital nerve b.
intermediate b.
medial neurovascular b.
b. nailing
neurovascular b.
posterolateral b.
posteromedial b.
superior gluteal neurovascular b.
b. suture
bundle-nailing method
Bunge amputation
bungee effect
bunion
b. complex
b. deformity
b. dissector
dorsal b.
Estersohn osteotomy for
tailor's b.
b. formation
juvenile b.
b. pain syndrome
b. shield
tailor's b.

bunionectomy
Akin b.
Austin b.
Austin-Akin b.
b. capsular closure
chevron b.
closing wedge osteotomy b.
DuVries-Mann modified b.
Hauser b.
Hohmann b.
Joplin b.
Juvara b.
juvenile b.
Kalish b.
Kelikian modified Z b.
Keller b.
Kreuscher b.
Lapidus b.
Ludloff b.
Mann b.
Mau b.
Mayo b.
McBride b.
McKeever b.
Mitchell b.
modified Hohmann b.
modified Mau b.
modified McBride b.
modified Z b.
osteotomy b.
Reverdin b.
Reverdin-Green b.
Reverdin-Laird b.
Reverdin-McBride b.
scarf osteotomy b.
scarf Z osteotomy b.
short Z b.
Silver b.
Stone b.
supratubercular wedge
  osteotomy b.
tailor's b.
tricorrectional b.
Wilson b.
Wu b.
Z b.
bunionette
b. deformity
b. excision
b. pain
b. pain syndrome
tailor's b.
**bunionette-hallux valgus-splayfoot
complex**
bunion-hallux valgus complex
bunk
b. bed fracture
b. bed injury
Bunker footpiece

Bunnell
B. active hand and finger
  splint
B. anvil
B. atraumatic technique
B. bone drill
B. crisscross suture
B. digital exertion measurer
B. dissecting probe
B. dressing
B. figure-of-8 suture
B. finger extension splint
B. finger loop
B. forwarding probe
B. gutter splint
B. hand drill
B. knuckle bender
B. modification
B. modification of Steindler
  flexorplasty
B. opponensplasty
B. outrigger splint
B. posterior tibial tendon transfer
  operation
B. pullout nonabsorbable suture
B. pullout wire
B. reverse knuckle-bender splint
B. safety-pin splint
B. solution
B. technique of pulley
  reconstruction
B. tendon needle
B. tendon passer
B. tendon repair
B. tendon repair stitch
B. tendon stripper
B. tendon suturing technique
B. tendon transfer technique
B. wire pullout suture
B. zigzag fashion
Bunnell-Littler wrist contracture test
bunny
B. boot
B. boot foot splint
bupivacaine
lidocaine and b.
Buprenex
buprenorphine
bupropion
bur, burr
acorn-tipped b.
Adson b.
Adson enlarging b.
Adson perforating b.
air-driven b.
Albee olive-shaped b.
arthroplasty b.
Bailey b.
ball b.

bur (*continued*)
    barrel b.
    bone b.
    Borchardt olive-shaped b.
    carbide b.
    coarse carbide cone b.
    coarse olive b.
    cone b.
    conical b.
    crosscut b.
    Cushing b.
    cutting b.
    cylindrical b.
    decortication b.
    dental b.
    D'Errico enlarging drill b.
    D'Errico perforating drill b.
    diamond b.
    Doyen cylindrical b.
    Doyen spherical b.
    b. drill
    Dyonics arthroplasty b.
    enlarging b.
    Fantastic Burr nail b.
    fine olive b.
    finish b.
    fissure b.
    flame-tip b.
    Hall b.
    Happy podiatric b.
    high-speed b.
    high-torque b.
    b. hole
    Hudson b.
    Hudson bone b.
    Hudson brace with b.
    3-in-1 diamond b.
    large-nail spicule b.
    Lindemann b.
    long coarse b.
    long-stemmed powered b.
    McKenzie enlarging b.
    medium carbide cone b.
    medium fine b.
    Midas Rex b.
    motorized b.
    nail b.
    new happy b.
    old smoothie b.
    olive-shaped b.
    orthopaedic b.
    paronychia b.
    pear b.
    perforating b.
    pilot b.
    podiatric b.
    Podi-Burr nail b.
    power b.
    right ankle b.

    Rosen b.
    Rotablator rotating b.
    rotary b.
    rotating b.
    round b.
    short coarse b.
    short fine b.
    side-cutting b.
    small nail spicule b.
    smoothie junior b.
    spherical b.
    Stille b.
    water-cooled power b.
    Zimmer rotary b.
Burch-Schneider antiprotrusio cage
bur-down technique
Burford-Finochietto rib spreader
Burford rib spreader
burgdorferi
    Borrelia b.
Burgess
    B. below-knee amputation
    B. transtibial amputation technique
buried
    b. K-wire fixation
    b. K-wire fixation in digital fusion
Burke
    B. Bariatric bed
    B. test
Burkhalter
    B. modification of Stiles-Bunnell technique
    B. transfer technique
Burkhalter-Reyes
    B.-R. fixation method for phalangeal fracture
    B.-R. method
burn
    B. bench malingering test
    b. boutonnière deformity
    b. contracture
    b. dressing
    irrigation b.
    plaster cast application b.
    b. syndactyly
burner
    b. injury
    B. phenomenon
    b. syndrome
Burnet clonal selection theory
Burnham
    B. finger splint
    B. thumb splint
burning
    b. foot
    b. pain
    paroxysmal b.
burning-feet syndrome
burn-related pigmentation change

Burns
- B. disease
- B. ligament
- B. plate

Burns-Haney incision

Burow
- B. skin flap technique
- B. triangle

burr (*var. of* bur)

Burroughs solution

Burrows distal ulna shortening osteotomy technique

bursa, *pl.* **bursae**
- Achilles tendon b.
- adventitious b.
- anserine b.
- Brodie b.
- calcaneal b.
- deltoid b.
- Fleischmann b.
- infrapatellar b.
- intermetatarsal b.
- intermetatarsophalangeal b.
- ischiogluteal b.
- Luschka b.
- Monro b.
- no-name, no-fame b.
- olecranon b.
- patellar b.
- pisiform b.
- pre-Achilles b.
- prepatellar b.
- radial b.
- radiohumeral b.
- retro-Achilles b.
- retrocalcaneal b.
- rider's b.
- sacral b.
- scapulohumeral b.
- subacromial b.
- subacromiodeltoid b.
- subcutaneous calcaneal b.
- subcutaneous infrapatellar b.
- subcutaneous patellar b.
- subcutaneous synovial b.
- subcutaneous trochanteric b.
- subdeltoid b.
- subtendinous iliac b.
- subtendinous prepatellar b.
- synovial b.
- trochanteric b.
- ulnar b.
- Voshell medial collateral ligament b.

bursae (*pl. of* bursa)

bursal
- b. abscess
- b. cyst
- b. débridement
- b. flap
- b. fluid
- b. inflammation
- b. projection
- b. sac
- b. synovitis
- b. tissue

bursata
- exostosis b.

bursectomy

bursitis
- Achilles b.
- Achilles tendon b.
- anserine b.
- bicipital b.
- calcaneal b.
- calcific b.
- cervicothoracic interspinous b.
- chronic retrocalcaneal b.
- cubital b.
- Duplay b.
- gastrocnemius b.
- gluteal b.
- hip b.
- iliopectinate b.
- iliopectineal b.
- iliopsoas b.
- iliotibial band b.
- infracalcaneal b.
- infrapatellar b.
- intermetatarsal b.
- intermetatarsophalangeal b.
- intertubercular b.
- ischial b.
- ischiogluteal b.
- lateral premalleolar b.
- medial gastrocnemius b.
- olecranon b.
- patellar b.
- pelvic region b.
- pes anserine b.
- pigmented villonodular b.
- popliteal b.
- postcalcaneal b.
- pre-Achilles b.
- premalleolar b.
- prepatellar b.
- psoas b.
- pyogenic b.
- radiohumeral b.
- retrocalcaneal b.
- scapulothoracic b.
- semimembranosus b.
- septic b.
- subacromial b.
- subcalcaneal b.
- subcoracoid b.
- subdeltoid b. (SDB)
- subgluteal b.
- subscapularis b.

B

bursitis (*continued*)
    suprapatellar b.
    tarsal navicular b.
    tibial collateral ligament b.
    trochanteric b.
    tuberculous trochanteric b.
bursocentesis
bursography
    Mikasa subacromial b.
    subacromial b.
bursolith
bursopathy
bursotomy
burst
    b. fracture
    b. injury
    b. resistance fitness ball
bursting dislocation
burst-type laceration
Burton-Pellegrini excision of trapezium
Burton sign
Burwell-Scott
    B.-S. modification
    B.-S. modification of Watson-Jones incision
Busenkell posterior hip retractor
bushing
    guide b.
    Uniflex drill b.
buspirone
Busquet disease
butabarbital sodium
Butalan
butalbital compound and codeine
Butazolidin
butenafine
Buticaps
Butisol Sodium
Butler
    B. fifth toe operation
    B. procedure to correct overlapping toes
butorphanol
butterfly
    B. cushion
    B. cushion with strap
    b. flap
    b. fracture
    b. fracture fragment
    b. vertebra

butterfly-shaped monoblock vertebral plate
buttocks
    heart-shaped b.
    b. pad
button
    b. abscess
    belly b. (BB)
    Biomet b.
    Charnley suture b.
    collared b.
    Drummond b.
    Hewson ligament b.
    b. hook
    ligament b.
    padded b.
    patellar b.
    periosteal b.
    polyethylene b.
    pull-out b.
    b. sequestrum
    silastic b.
    B. Spacer
    subdural b.
    b. suture
    b. toe amputation
    Wisconsin b.
buttonhole
    b. deformity
    b. fracture
    b. rupture
buttress
    b. and button anchor
    b. pad
    b. pie plate
    b. pin
    pretibial b. (PTB)
    rotator cuff b. (RCB)
    b. thread screw
buttressed hook
buttressing
    b. in internal fixation
    b. procedure
buttress-type plate
butyrophenone
BVP
    blood volume pulse
BWO
    base wedge osteotomy
Byars mandibular prosthesis
bypass

C

    C angle
    C knife
    C sign
    C washer

C-2

    C-2 hip system
    C-2 OsteoCap hip prosthesis

CA

    congenital anomaly

Ca

    calcium

cable

    antirotation c. (ARC)
    cerclage c.
    c. cerclage method
    chrome-cobalt c.
    Dall-Miles c.
    Dwyer scoliosis c.
    fiberoptic c.
    Flex Ranger stretch c.
    FlexStrand c.
    Gallie fusion using
     titanium c.
    Howmedica cerclage c.
    interspinous c.
    liquid c.
    c. nerve graft
    scoliosis correction with
     Dwyer c.
    Songer c.
    stretch c.
    c. suspension system
    c. tensioner
    titanium c.
    twister c.

**cable-hook compression
instrumentation**
Cable-Ready cable grip system
cable-twister

    c.-t. brace
    c.-t. orthosis

cable/wire hole
Cabot

    C. leg splint
    C. posterior splint

cacomelia
CAD

    coronary artery disease

cadaver

    c. bone
    c. bone graft

cadaveric

    c. knee
    c. specimen

CAD/CAM

    computer-aided design/computer-aided
     manufacturing
    CAD/CAM prosthesis

caddie (*var. of* caddy)
caddy, caddie

    SwingAlong walker c.

cadence of gait
Cadenza

    C. panty
    C. surgical support girdle

CA-5000 drill-guide isometer
CAECS

    chronic anterior exertional
     compartment syndrome

café au lait spot
caffeine

    acetaminophen, aspirin, c.
    orphenadrine, aspirin, and c.

Caffey

    C. disease
    C. hyperostosis
    C. syndrome

Caffey-Kenny disease
Caffey-Silverman syndrome
Caffinière trapeziometacarpal prosthesis
cage

    antiprotrusio c.
    Bagby and Kuslich lumbar
     fusion c.
    BAK fusion c.
    BAK lumbar fusion c.
    Brantigan interbody fusion c.
    Burch-Schneider antiprotrusio c.
    carbon fiber-composite c.
    carbon fiber-reinforced c.
    carbon fiber-reinforced polymer c.
    CFRP c.
    elastic knee c.
    fusion c.
    Harms c.
    Inter Fix RP threaded spinal
     fusion c.
    Inter Fix titanium threaded spinal
     fusion c.
    lumbar intersomatic fusion
     expandable c. (LIFEC)
    MC+ cervical interbody c.
    Moss c.
    Motech titanium spinal repair c.
    Novus LC threaded interbody
     fusion c.
    Novus LT titanium threaded
     interbody fusion c.
    ogival interbody c. (O.I.C.)

C

cage (*continued*)
    osseocartilaginous thoracic c.
    protrusio c.
    Pyramesh c.
    rib c.
    SL c.
    stereolithography spinal c.
    Swedish knee c.
    threaded fusion c. (TFC)
    threaded spinal fusion c.
cage-back brace
CAH
    camber axis hinge
CAI
    chronic ankle instability
Cairns hemostatic forceps
CAJSA
    computer-aided joint space analysis
CAL
    coracoacromial ligament
Calandriello orthopedic procedure
Calandruccio
    C. cemented hip prosthesis
    C. clamp
    C. external fixation system
    C. fixation
    C. II compression device
    C. impaction screw-plate
    C. nail
    C. side plate
    C. technique
    C. triangular compression apparatus
    C. triangular compression fixation
    device
Calcanea calcaneal fracture plate
calcaneal, calcanean
    c. apophysitis
    c. avulsion fracture
    c. axial view
    c. bone
    c. bone graft
    c. bone plug
    c. branch
    c. bursa
    c. bursitis
    c. compartment pressure
    measurement
    c. displaced fracture
    c. distraction
    c. facet
    c. fat pad
    c. fracture
    c. fracture (I-III)
    c. fracture reduction
    c. gait
    c. gait pattern
    c. inclination angle (CIA)
    c. L osteotomy
    c. malunion

    c. neck lengthening
    c. nerve
    c. pin
    c. pin traction
    c. pitch
    c. pitch angle (CPA)
    c. pseudocyst
    c. region
    c. resection
    c. sliding corrective osteotomy
    c. spreader
    c. spur
    c. spur cookie orthosis
    c. spur pad in shoe
    c. spur syndrome
    c. stance
    c. sulcus
    c. tendon
    c. tenodesis
    c. tuberosity
    c. tumor
    c. tumor
    c. valgus
    c. varus
    c. Y plate
calcaneal-second metatarsal angle
calcanean (*var. of* calcaneal)
calcanectomy
calcanei (*gen. and pl. of* calcaneus)
    sulcus c.
calcaneoapophysitis
calcaneoastragaloid ligament
calcaneocavovarus deformity
calcaneocavus
    c. deformity
    c. foot
    talipes c.
calcaneoclavicular ligament
calcaneocuboid (CC)
    c. articulation
    c. bone
    c. coalition
    c. distraction arthrodesis
    (CCDA)
    dorsal c. (DCC)
    c. joint (CCJ)
    c. joint arthritis
    c. joint nutcracker injury
    lateral c. (LCC)
    c. ligament (CCL)
    short c. (SCC)
    c. subluxation
calcaneocuboideum
    ligamentum c.
calcaneodynia
calcaneofibular
    c. abutment
    c. ligament (CFL)
    c. sprain

calcaneonavicular
    c. articulation
    c. bar
    c. bar resection
    c. bar section
    c. coalition
    inferior c. (ICN)
    c. joint
    c. joint arthroscopy
    c. ligament
    c. ligament-tibialis posterior tendon
      advancement
calcaneopelvic arthrodesis
calcaneoplantar angle
calcaneoscaphoid
calcaneotibial
    c. angle
    c. arthrodesis
    c. fusion
    c. ligament
calcaneovalgocavus
calcaneovalgus
    c. deformity
    c. flatfoot
    c. foot
    talipes c.
calcaneovarus
    c. deformity
    talipes c.
calcaneum (*var. of* calcaneus)
calcaneus, calcaneum, *gen.* and *pl.*
  calcanei
    accessory ossification center of c.
    c. alignment
    c. allograft
    anterior advancement of tendo c.
    c. apophysis
    c. deformity
    displaced intraarticular c.
    distal c.
    c. excursion
    pes c.
    talipes c.
    tendo c.
    thalamic fracture of
      calcaneum
    c. tongue fracture
    tongue fracture of c.
    tuberosity of c.
calcanodynia
calcar
    c. collar
    c. femorale development
    c. pedis
    c. pivot
    pivot of c.
    c. planer
    c. reamer
    c. replacement

    c. replacement femoral prosthesis
    c. replacement stem
Cal Carb-HD
calcareous deposit
Calcichew
Calciday-667
calcidiol test
calcifediol
Calciferol
    C. Injection
    C. Oral
calcific
    c. bursitis
    c. density
    c. deposit
    c. mass
    c. spur
    c. tendinitis
    c. tendinosis
calcificans
    chondrodystrophia c.
calcification
    Achilles tendon enthesis c.
    central c.
    dystrophic c.
    eggshell-like c.
    falx c.
    flocculent focus of c.
    focal c.
    heterotopic c.
    juvenile intervertebral disc c. (JIDC)
    c. of falx
    paraarticular c.
    paraspinal c.
    periarticular c.
    provisional c.
    soft tissue c.
    supraspinatus c.
calcified
    c. cartilage
    c. osteoid
calcify
calcifying aponeurotic fibroma
Calcijex
Calcimar Injection
Calci-Mix
calcinosis
    c. circumscripta
    c. intervertebralis
    c., Raynaud, esophageal motility
      disorders, sclerodactyly,
      telangiectasia (CREST)
    tumoral c.
calciphylaxis
Calcitite
    C. graft
    C. graft material
calcitonin-salmon
calcitriol

C

calcium (Ca)
  c. alginate dressing
  c. carbonate
  c. carbonate bone replacement
    graft
  c. carbonate graft material
  c. channel blocker
  c. deposit
  fenoprofen c.
  c. glubionate
  c. gout
  c. hydroxyapatite (CHA)
  c. hydroxyapatite crystal
  c. hydroxyapatite crystal deposition
    disease
  c. hydroxyapatite pellet
  c. lactate
  c. oxalate deposition
  c. phosphate
  c. phosphate ceramic
  c. phosphate, dibasic (DCP)
  c. pyrophosphate dihydrate
    deposition (CPDD)
  c. pyrophosphate dihydrate
    deposition disease (CPDD, CPPD)
  serum c.
  c. sulfate bone graft barrier
  c. sulfate ceramic
calcodynia
calculation
  Gaines and Ford tendo Achillis
    length c.
calculi (*gen.* and *pl. of* calculus)
calculus, *gen.* and *pl.* **calculi**
  branched c.
  hemic c.
Caldani ligament
Calderol
Caldesene Topical
Caldwell hanging cast
calf, *pl.* **calves**
  c. band
  c. bone dowel
  c. circumference
  football c.
  gnome's c.
  c. hypertension
  c. raise back exercise
  c. shell
  c. squeeze test
calibrated
  c. clubfoot splint
  c. guidepin
  c. guide wire
  c. monofilament
  c. pin
  c. pin guide
  c. probe
calibration curve

calibrator
  screw depth c.
California
  C. soft spinal system
  C. welt construction
Caligamed
  C. ankle orthosis
  C. brace
caliper
  anthropometric c.
  blunt c.
  c. brace
  Digimatic c.
  digital c.
  Harpenden c.
  Lafayette skinfold c.
  Lange skinfold c.
  Mitutoyo digital c.
  c. orthosis
  Redler small bone caliper Redler
    small bone c.
  c. rib movement
  skinfold c.
  Thomas walking c.
  Townley femur c.
  vernier c.
  weight-relieving c.
Callahan
  C. and Scuderi femur neck fracture
    repair approach
  C. method
  C. posterior spinal fusion technique
Callander knee disarticulation
  amputation
Callaway shoulder dislocation test
Calleja exercise
Callender
  C. derotational brace
  C. technique hip prosthesis
callosal lesion
Callos calcium phosphate cement
callosity
  metatarsal c.
  plantar c.
  shearing c.
callotasis
callous
  c. bone union
  c. formation
callus
  bone c.
  bridging c.
  central c.
  definitive c.
  c. distraction
  c. distraction procedure
  elephant-foot c.
  ensheathing c.
  florid c.

fracture c.
horse's foot c.
hyperplastic c.
intermediate c.
irritation c.
c. massage
medullary c.
myelogenous c.
nail groove c.
permanent c.
pinch c.
provisional c.
shearing c.
temporary c.
c. weld
Calmette-Guérin
bacille C.-G. (BCG)
Calnan-Nicolle
C.-N. finger implant
C.-N. finger prosthesis
C.-N. metatarsophalangeal prosthesis
C.-N. synthetic joint prosthesis
calor
Cal-Plus
Caltrate
C. 600
C. Jr.
calvarial
c. free bone
c. free bone graft
Calvé disease
Calvé-Legg-Perthes syndrome
Calvé-Perthes disease
calves (*pl. of* calf)
Calypso lift
CAM
Cognitive Assessment of Minnesota
complementary and alternative
medicine
computer-assisted myelography
controlled ankle motion
cam
c. impingement
C. lock knee joint
C. Walker ankle brace
C. Walker ankle walker
C. Walker II
C. Walker leg brace
Cama Arthritis Pain Reliever
camber axis hinge (CAH)
cambium layer
Cambria thoracolumbar fusion interbody VBR
camelback sign
camera, *pl.* **camerae**
DyoCam 550 arthroscopic video c.
DyoCam arthroscopic view c.
Endius spinal endoscopic c.
gamma c.

Saticon tube c.
Sony CCD/RGB DXC-151 color video c.
Stryker c.
camerae (*pl. of* camera)
Cameron
C. femoral component removal
C. fracture apparatus
C. fracture device
Camino catheter technique
Camitz
C. opponensplasty
C. palmaris longus tendon reconstruction technique
C. palmaris longus tendon transfer
camouflage prosthesis
camp
C. brace
C. corset
C. Diversity arthritis program
Campbell
C. ankle operation
C. ankle procedure
C. cannulated screw
C. corset
C. elbow approach
C. gouge
C. interpositional arthroplasty
C. ligament
C. nerve root retractor
C. onlay bone graft
C. opening-wedge thoracostomy technique
C. osteotome
C. periosteal elevator
C. posterior arthrodesis
C. posterior bone block
C. posterior shoulder approach
C. posterolateral approach
C. reamer
C. resection arthroplasty
C. rongeur
C. screw fixation
C. tibial osteotomy
C. traction splint
C. transfer
C. triceps reflection
Campbell-Akbarnia arthrodesis
Campbell-Rinehard-Kalenak ankle arthrodesis
camper
C. chiasma
C. fascia
Campho-Phenique
camphor and phenol
camplodactyly
camptocormia
camptodactylia (*var. of* camptodactyly)
camptodactylism (*var. of* camptodactyly)

C

**camptodactyly, camptodactylia,
camptodactylism, streblodactyly**
    tendon release in c.
camptomelia
camptomelic dwarfism
camptospasm
CamStar
    C. exercise machine
    C. power leg press
Camurati-Engelmann disease
Canadian
    C. Academy of Sports Medicine
      emergency kit
    Australian and C. (AUSCAN)
    C. crutch
    C. hip disarticulation prosthesis
    C. Knee Orthosis
    C. Occupational Performance
      Measure (COPM)
Canakis beaded hip pin
canal
    Alcock c.
    bony semicircular c.
    carpal c.
    cartilage c.
    central c.
    cerebrospinal c.
    cervical c.
    Civinini c.
    cortical bone primary c.
    Dorello c.
    Dupuytren c.
    endoneural c.
    femoral c.
    femoral medullary c.
    c. finder
    Guyon c.
    haversian c.
    humeral c.
    Hunter c.
    hydrops c.
    iliac c.
    c. innominate osteotomy
    intersacral c.
    intramedullary c.
    lumbar c.
    marrow c.
    medullary c.
    narrowing of spinal c.
    Richet tibial-astragalocalcaneal c.
    sacral c.
    spinal c.
    spinal cord c.
    talar c.
    tarsal c.
    tibial medullary c.
    tight spinal canal trefoil c.
    vertebral c.
    Volkmann c.

Canale
    C. distal humerus fracture pinning
      technique
    C. osteotomy
    C. talus view
Canale-Kelly
    C.-K. talar neck fracture
    C.-K. talar neck fracture
      classification
    C.-K. talar neck view
canaliculi (*pl. of* canaliculus)
canaliculus, *pl.* **canaliculi**
canal-to-calcar-isthmus ratio
Can Am brace
Canavan disease
**Canavan-van Bogaert-Bertrand
disease**
cancellated bone
cancellectomy
cancellous
    c. bone carrier
    c. bone screw
    c. bone surface
    c. chip
    c. chip bone graft
    c. insert
    c. insert graft
    c. morselized bone graft
    c. non-load-bearing bone fracture
    c. pin
    c. screw thread
    c. versus cortical bone
cancer
    American Joint Commission on C.
    c. treatment-related lymphedema
Candela SPTL laser
Candida **onychomycosis**
candle
    c. wax appearance
    c. wax appearance of bone
Can-Do exercise band
cane
    adjustable c.
    broad-based c.
    Double Duty c.
    English c.
    glider c.
    MAFO c.
    offset c.
    quad c.
    single-point c.
    small-base quad c.
    Thera C.
    tripod c.
Canfield shoe
canister
    Autovac autotransfusion c.
**Cannon Law of Denervation
Supersensitivity**

cannula, *pl.* **cannulas, cannulae**
    Acufex double-lumen arthroscopic c.
    arthroscopic c.
    Bergstrom c.
    biopsy c.
    blunt arthroscopic c.
    Bucy-Frazier suction c.
    Concept c.
    Dyonics c.
    Endotrac c.
    Eriksson muscle biopsy c.
    inflow c.
    large-bore inflow c.
    large egress c.
    McCain TMJ c.
    microirrigating c.
    outflow c.
    self-sealing c.
    small egress c.
    suction c.
    suprapatellar c.
    c. system
    Teflon c.
    zone-specific c.
cannulae (*pl. of* cannula)
cannulas (*pl. of* cannula)
cannulated
    c. bolt
    c. bone screw
    c. cancellous lag screw
    c. cortical step drill
    c. drill
    c. drill bit
    c. drill point
    c. expulsion piston
    c. guided hip screw system
    c. Henderson reamer
    c. hip screw
    c. nail
    C. Plus screw system
    c. reaming technique
    c. screwdriver
    c. wrench
cannulation, cannulization
    unilateral pedicle c.
cannulization (*var. of* cannulation)
canted finger hook
Cantharone
cantilever
    c. bending
    c. external fixator
canvas brace
CAOS
    computer-assisted orthopaedic surgery
caoutchouc pelvis
cap
    acetabular c.
    Carnation corn c.'s
    cartilaginous c.

    Cloward drill guard c.
    Compoz Gel c.'s
    digit c.
    egg-shaped c.
    Feverall Sprinkle C.'s
    flexor c.
    nerve c.
    offset c.
    plaster toe c.
    plastic end c.
    Silipos mesh c.
    c. splint
    toe c.
    Zang metatarsal c.
    Zimmer tibial nail c.
capacitive
    c. coupling
    c. sensor
capacity
    aerobic c. (VO_2, VO_2max)
    exercise c.
    forced vital c.
    physical work c. (PWC)
cap-and-anchor plate
Caparosa wire crimper
CAPE
    Children's Assessment of Participation
    and Enjoyment
    Clifton Assessment Procedures for the
    Elderly
    continuous anatomical passive exerciser
capeline bandage
Capello
    C. acetabular reconstruction
    technique
    C. press-fit prosthesis
    C. slim-line abduction pillow
    C. total hip replacement
Capener
    C. brace
    C. coil splint
    C. finger splint
    C. gouge
    C. lateral rhachotomy
capillary
    c. filling time (CFT)
    c. fracture
    c. hemangioma
    c. ischemia
    c. refill
    c. refill, sensation, motor function,
    temperature (CSMT)
    c. refill time (CRT)
capital
    C. and Codeine
    c. crescentic shelf osteotomy
    c. epiphysial angle
    c. epiphysis
    c. femoral epiphysis

C

capital (*continued*)
    c. fragment
    c. ligament
capitate bone
capitate-hamate joint
capitate-lunate
    c.-l. instability
    c.-l. joint
capitellar
    c. fracture
    c. osteochondritis
capitellocondylar
    c. total elbow arthroplasty
    c. unconstrained elbow prosthesis
capitellum
    Hahn-Steinthal fracture of c.
    Kocher-Lorenz fracture of c.
capitolunate angle
capitula (*pl. of* capitulum)
capitular
    c. epiphysis
    c. process
capitulum, *pl.* **capitula**
    c. fracture
    c. humeri
    c. of humerus
Caplan
    C. Indented Paragraph Reading
    Test
    C. syndrome
caplet
    Miles Nervine c.
Capner gouge
capped elbow
caprenin
caprolactam suture
Caprosyn suture
capsaicin topical cream
Capset calcium sulfate bone graft barrier
Capsin
capsular
    c. adhesion
    c. ankylosis
    c. attachment
    c. deficiency
    c. flap
    c. imbrication
    c. imbrication procedure
    c. incision
    c. interposition arthroplasty
    c. layer
    c. length insufficiency
    c. ligament
    c. plication
    c. reconstruction
    c. reefing
    c. release
    c. shift

    c. shift procedure
    c. strap
    c. support tissue
capsular-ligamentous tension
capsular-shift reconstruction
capsulatum
    Histoplasma c.
capsule (cap)
    anterior c.
    anterolateral c.
    anteromedial c.
    apophysial joint c.
    articular c.
    dorsal c.
    elbow c.
    facet c.
    fibrous c.
    c. formation
    Gerota c.
    hip joint c.
    joint c.
    Kadian C.
    medial talonavicular c.
    meniscofemoral c.
    meniscotibial c.
    metatarsophalangeal joint c.
    midlateral c.
    midmedial c.
    peripheral c.
    plantar c.
    posterior c.
    posterolateral c.
    posteromedial c.
    c. repair
    talonavicular c.
    trapeziometacarpal c.
    volar c.
    wrist c.
capsulectomy
    anterior c.
    circumferential c.
    silhouette c.
capsulitis
    adhesive c.
    dorsal carpal c.
    glenohumeral adhesive c.
capsulodesis
    Berger dorsal wrist c.
    Blatt c.
    bleb c.
    dorsal c.
    intercarpal ligament c.
    Zancolli flexion c.
capsulolabral
    c. complex
    c. repair
capsuloligamentous
    c. complex
    c. mechanism

c. system
c. tissue
capsuloperiosteal
c. envelope
c. flap
capsuloplasty
Zancolli c.
capsulorrhaphy
Boyd-Sisk posterior c.
electrothermally assisted c.
(ETAC)
laser-assisted c.
medial c.
open-staple c.
pants-over-vest c.
posterior c.
Rockwood posterior c.
Roux-duToit staple c.
c. staple
staple c.
thermal c.
Tibone posterior shoulder c.
capsulotomy
anterior c.
Curtis PIP joint c.
dorsal transverse c.
dorsolateral and medial c.
dorsoplantar c.
hourglass c.
linear c.
L-shaped c.
medial V-Y c.
metatarsophalangeal c.
posterior c.
stereotaxic anterior c.
subtalar c.
talonavicular c.
transmetatarsal c.
transverse c.
T-shaped c.
V c.
vertical c.
captured interlocking screw
Caput transversum
Capzasin-P
CAQ
Clinical Analysis Questionnaire
car
c. hand control
outdoor emergency c. (OEC)
Carabelt
C. lower back support
C. therapeutic belt
Cara Klenz cleansing agent
carbamate
chlorphenesin c.
carbamazepine
carbapenem
carbenicillin

Carb-HD
Cal Carb-HD
carbide bur
carbidopa-levodopa
Carbocaine
CarboFlex odor-control dressing
carbohydrate oxidation
CarboJet
C. CO_2 lavage system
C. lavage
carbol-fuchsin solution
carbolic acid
carbon
C. Copy high performance foot
prosthesis
C. Copy HP foot prosthesis
C. Copy II foot prosthesis
C. Copy II Light Foot
C. Copy II Light prosthesis
c. dioxide (CO_2)
c. dioxide laser
c. fiber-composite cage
c. fiber fixator
c. fiber graft
c. fiber half ring
c. fiber lamination braid
(CFLB)
c. fiber-reinforced cage
c. fiber-reinforced plate
c. fiber-reinforced polyethylene
c. fiber-reinforced polymer
(CFRP)
c. fiber-reinforced polymer cage
c. implant
c. Monotube long bone fracture
external fixation system
pyrolytic c.
c. steel drill point
carbonate
calcium c.
carbon-based biomaterial
carbon-tungsten rasp
CarbonX active heel
Carboplast
C. II composite
C. II sheeting
C. II sheet orthotic material
carborundum grinding wheel
carcinoembryonic antigen (CEA)
carcinogen
chemical c.
carcinoma, *pl.* **carcinomas,**
carcinomata
clear cell c.
joint verrucous c.
carcinomas (*pl. of* carcinoma)
carcinomata (*pl. of* carcinoma)
carcinomatous myopathy
Carden amputation

cardiac
- c. output
- c. precautions

cardinal axes (X, Y, Z)
cardioboxing
CardioKarate
CardioKickboxing
cardiomyopathy
- dilated c.
- hypertrophic c.
- nonspecific c.
- right ventricular c.

Cardona keratoprosthesis prosthesis
care
- corrective spinal c.
- Miami Acute C. (MAC)
- palliative c.
- postoperative wound c.
- rehabilitation c.

Caregiver Strain Index (CSI)
Carex ambulatory aid
caries (*pl. of* caries)
- c. sicca

carinatum
- pectus c.

carisoprodol
- c. and aspirin
- carisoprodol, aspirin, and codeine

Carl P. Jones traction splint
C-arm
- C-a. fluoroscope
- C-a. fluoroscopy
- C-a. fluoroscopy unit
- C-a. image intensifier
- XiScan portable fluoroscopic C-a.

Carman meniscus sign
Carmody-Batson operation
Carmody perforator drill
Carnation corn caps
Carnesale
- C. acetabular extensile approach
- C. extremity amputation technique
- C. hip approach
- C. hip approach operation

Carnesale-Stewart-Barnes hip dislocation classification
Carolina rocker
Carolon AFO sock
carotid
- c. artery
- c. artery compression
- c. sheath
- c. vein

carpal
- c. arc
- c. arch
- c. articulation
- c. bone
- c. bone fracture ankylosis
- c. bone stress fracture
- c. boss
- c. canal
- C. Care carpal tunnel exerciser
- C. Care exercise
- C. Care rehabilitative program
- c. coalition
- c. compression test
- c. dislocation
- c. height ratio
- c. instability
- c. instability dissociative (CID)
- c. instability nondissociative (CIND)
- c. ligament
- C. Lock cock-up splint
- C. Lock CTS brace
- C. Lock wrist brace
- C. Lock wrist splint
- c. lunate implant prosthesis
- c. navicular fracture
- c. pedal spasm
- c. row
- c. scaphoid
- c. scaphoid bone fracture
- c. scaphoid implant prosthesis
- c. scaphoid screw
- c. sulcus
- c. synovectomy
- C. Trac traction
- C. Trac traction device
- c. tunnel (CT)
- c. tunnel decompression (CTD)
- c. tunnel glove
- c. tunnel release (CTR)
- c. tunnel stretch
- C. Tunnel Stretch exerciser
- c. tunnel surgery relief kit
- c. tunnel syndrome (CTS)
- c. tunnel syndrome injection therapy
- c. tunnel view

carpal-intercarpal joint
Carpal-Lock wrist support
carpal-metacarpal
carpectomy
- distal row c.
- Omer-Capen c.
- proximal row c.

carpenter's
- c. brace
- c. knee

Carpenter syndrome
carpet layer's knee
carpi (*gen.* and *pl. of* carpus)
carpometacarpal
- c. arthroplasty
- c. articulation
- c. boss
- c. fracture-dislocation
- c. joint

c. joint dislocation
c. joint fracture
c. joint radiography
c. ligament
carpometcarpal splint
carpophalangeal joint
carporadial articulation
carposcope
carprofen
carpus, *gen.* and *pl.* **carpi**
complex instability of c. (CIC)
c. curvus
Carrel
C. method
C. patch
C. suture
C. treatment
Carrell
C. distal fibula resection
C. fibular substitution
C. fibular substitution technique
Carrell-Girard screw
Carrie car seat
carrier
cancellous bone c.
clamp c.
double-headed stereotactic c.
Finochietto clamp c.
ligature c.
Miya hook ligature c.
Yasargil ligature c.
Carrington Dermal wound gel
Carroll
C. and Taber arthroplasty
C. arthrodesis
C. bone-holding forceps
C. clubfoot approach
C. dressing forceps
C. hand retractor
C. periosteal elevator
C. skin hook
C. tendon-pulling forceps
C. tendon retriever
C. test
C. tissue forceps
Carroll-Bennett retractor
Carroll-Bunnell drill
Carroll-Legg periosteal elevator
Carr-Purcell-Meiboom-Gill sequence
Carr-Purcell sequence
carrying
c. angle
c. angle of forearm
Carstan reverse wedge osteotomy
cart
Harloff c.
Cartam-Treander reverse wedge osteotomy

Carter
C. elevation pillow
C. foam pillow
C. immobilization cushion
C. mycetoma
C. Rowe awl
C. Rowe shoulder score
C. Rowe shoulder view
C. splint
Carter-Wilkinson criteria for hypermobility syndrome
Carticel
C. autologous cultured chondrocyte
C. cartilage-cell culturing service
C. implant procedure
cartilage
c. ablation
c. abrader
accessory c.
alar c.
anular c.
arthrodial c.
articular c.
arytenoid c.
c. autograft
basilar c.
calcified c.
c. canal
c. cell
c. change
circumferential c.
c. clamp
condylar c.
connecting c.
costal c.
cricoid c.
cryopreserved c.
degenerated c.
diarthrodial c.
eburnation of c.
elastic c.
c. elastic pullover kneecap splint
ensiform c.
falciform c.
fibroelastic c.
fibrous c.
floating c.
c. forceps
free flap of c.
glenoid c.
c. graft
c. healing
hyaline c.
c. hypertrophy
c. implant
interarticular c.
interosseous c.
intervertebral c.
c. knife

C

cartilage (*continued*)
   c. lacuna
   loose c.
   nonossified tarsal navicular c.
   c. oligomeric matrix protein
    (COMP)
   patellofemoral groove c.
   physial c.
   pitted c.
   quadrangular c.
   roughened c.
   c. scissors
   scored c.
   semilunar c.
   c. shaver blade
   shelling off of c.
   slipping rib c.
   c. space
   c. stripper
   c. synovium
   tendon c.
   thyroid c.
   triradial c.
   triradiate c.
   c. volume
   Wrisberg c.
   xiphoid c.
   yellow c.
cartilage-hair hypoplasia (CHH)
cartilaginous
   c. anlage
   c. bar
   c. cap
   c. cap of phalangeal head
   c. coalition
   c. degeneration
   c. disc
   c. fragment
   c. glenoid labrum
   c. growth plate
   c. hallux limitus
   c. hamartoma
   c. hypertrophy
   c. joint
   c. lesion
   c. loose body
   c. metaplasia
   c. navicular
   c. ossification
   c. ring
   c. spur
   c. tissue
   c. tumor
cartwheel fracture
Cartwright implant
casanthranol
cascade
   clotting c.
   C. Up and About system

Casey pelvic clamp
CASH
   cruciform anterior spinal
   hyperextension
    CASH brace
    CASH thoracolumbosacral orthosis
    CASH TLSO
CASP
   Child and Adolescent Social
   Perception Measure
   contoured anterior spinal plate
Caspar
   C. alligator forceps
   C. anterior cervical plating
    technique
   C. anterior instrumentation
   C. blade
   C. cervical plate
   C. cervical screw
   C. retractor
Caspari
   C. arthroscopic portal
   C. shuttle
   C. suture punch
   C. transglenoid repair
CA-6000 spine motion analyzer
Casselberry suture punch
casserian muscle
Casser perforated muscle
cast
   above-elbow c.
   accessory navicular c.
   airplane c.
   c. application
   arm cylinder c.
   banjo c.
   Batchelor plaster hip spica c.
   below-knee walking c. (BKWC)
   c. belt
   c. bender
   bent-knee c.
   Bermuda spica c.
   bivalved c.
   bivalved cylinder c.
   c. blade
   Body Armor walker c.
   body jacket c.
   Böhler skintight c.
   c. boot
   C. Boot polypropylene hip
    abduction brace
   Boston bivalved c.
   c. brace
   c. bracing
   c. breaker
   broomstick c.
   bumper c.
   Caldwell hanging c.
   circular c.

Comfort C.
corrective c.
Cotrel scoliosis c.
cotton c.
c. cover
C. Cozy
C. Cozy toe covering
c. cushion
Cutter c.
c. cutter
cylinder walking c.
double hip spica c.
EDF scoliosis c.
elbow c.
elongation, derotation, flexion
  scoliosis c.
Equalizer short leg walking c.
c. equipped with rubber pedestal
extension body c.
fiberglass c.
figure-of-8 c.
3-finger spica c.
flexion body c.
full thumb spica c.
gaiter c.
C. Gard cast protector
gauntlet c.
gel c.
Gelocast c.
gravity equinus c.
groin-to-ankle c.
gutter c.
Gypsona c.
halo c.
hand c.
handshake c.
hanging arm c.
hinged cylinder c.
hip spica c.
hyperextension c.
c. immobilization
c. immobilizer
inhibitive c.
intermediate c.
intern's triangle in hip spica c.
Jones compression c.
Kite clubfoot c.
Kite metatarsal c.
c. knife
leg walking c.
light c.
c. liner
localizer c.
long arm c. (LAC)
long arm finger c.
long bent-knee leg c.
long leg c. (LLC)
long leg walking c. (LLWC)
long leg weightbearing c. (LLWBC)

Lorenz c.
Lovell clubfoot c.
medial malleolus c.
3M fiberglass c.
Minerva c.
modified Cotrel c.
Moe modified Cotrel c.
Mooney c.
Munster c.
negative impression c.
Neufeld c.
nonwalking c.
O'Donoghue cotton c.
one and one-half spica c.
one-half spica c.
onlay bone graft c.
Orfizip knee c.
Orfizip wrist c.
Orthoplast slipper c.
outrigger c.
c. padding
pancake c.
pantaloon spica c.
pantaloon walking c.
patellar dislocation c.
patellar tendon bearing c.
patellar tendon weightbearing c.
petaling the c.
Petrie spica c.
plaster c.
plaster of Paris c.
plastic c.
3-point pressure c.
polyurethane c.
pontoon spica c.
POP c.
PTB c.
quadriceps femoris muscle c.
Quengel c.
removable c.
c. removal
rigid below-knee c.
Risser localizer scoliosis c.
Risser turnbuckle c.
Sarmiento short leg patellar
  tendon-bearing c.
Sbarbaro spica c.
Schmeisser spica c.
scoliosis c.
semirigid fiberglass c. (SRF)
serial wedge c.
c. shoe
short arm c. (SAC)
short arm fiberglass c.
short arm gauntlet c.
short arm navicular c. (SANC)
short leg c. (SLC)
short leg plaster c.
short leg walking c. (SLWC)

cast (*continued*)
 short walking c.
 shoulder spica c.
 single-leg spica c.
 skin-tight c.
 slipper c.
 c. sock
 spica c.
 SP Walker c.
 sugar-tong c.
 c. syndrome
 c. table
 c. tape
 thumb spica c.
 toe spica c.
 toe-to-groin c.
 toe-to-midthigh c.
 tone-inhibiting leg c.
 total contact c. (TCC)
 traction c.
 turnbuckle c.
 underarm c.
 univalve c.
 Unna boot c.
 unremovable plaster c.
 Velpeau c.
 c. walker
 walking boot c.
 warm and form c.
 c. wedge
 wedging c.
 well-leg c.
 c. window
 windowed c.
 c. with dorsal toe plate extension
 c. with volar toe plate extension
 zipper c.
castaway
 C. ankle walker
 C. leg brace
 C. leg walker
Castech extremity support
Castellani paint
Castiglia ankle brace
casting
 foam c.
 intermittent c.
 negative c.
 postoperative c.
 c. process
 serial c.
 total contact c. (TCC)
Castle femoral resection procedure
Castle-Schneider resection interposition arthroplasty
Castroviejo
 C. bladebreaker knife
 C. needle holder
 C. trephine

CAT
 computerized axial tomography
Cataflam Oral
Catagni criteria
Catalyn vitamin
Catalyst anterior instrument set
cat and camel exercise
catapophysis
Catapres
catarrhalis
 Branhamella c.
catastrophic deterioration
cat-back
 rachitic c.-b.
CAT-CAM
 contoured adduction
 trochanteric-controlled alignment
 method
catch and clunk test
catching sensation
catch-up
 c.-u. clunk
 c.-u. phenomenon
category
 functional ambulation c. (FAC)
 Rehabilitation Impairment C.
 (RIC)
 Risser c.
Catera suture anchor
Cateye
 C. Ergociser
 C. T220 treadmill
Cathcart Orthocentric hip prosthesis
cathepsin
catheter
 condom c.
 c. entrapment
 c. kinking
 Mentor Self-Cath soft c.
 On-Q Soaker c.
 Simpson arthrectomy c.
 tracer c.
 wicking c.
cathode
catlin, catling
 c. amputating knife
catling (*var. of* catlin)
Caton method
cat's
 c. eye injury
 C. Paw exerciser
Catterall
 C. hip score
 C. 4-part (I-IV) Perthes disease
 classification
cauda, *pl.* **caudae**
 c. equina
 c. equina compression
 c. equina syndrome

caudad anterior mold
caudae (*pl. of* cauda)
caudal
    c. compensatory curve
    c. lamina resection
    c. retinaculum
    c. spinal agenesis
    c. translation
    c. vertebra
caudalward
caudocephalad
caudocranial
causal association
causalgia
causalgic pain
cause
    pathoanatomic c.
cauterisation (*var. of* cauterization)
cauterization, cauterisation
    alcohol c.
    bipolar c.
    Bovie c.
    phenol c.
    unipolar c.
cautery
    Aesculap bipolar c.
    BICAP c.
    bipolar c.
    bipolar circumactive probe c.
    Bovie c.
    chemical c.
    Concept handheld c.
    Hotsy C.
    intraarticular c.
    Mira c.
    monopolar c.
    slow c.
    unipolar c.
cava
    inferior vena c. (IVC)
    manus c.
    superior vena c.
    vena c.
cavalry bone
cavalryman's osteoma
cave
    C. hip approach
    C. knee approach
    C. operation
cavern chordoma
cavernous
    c. hemangioma
    c. lymphangioma
Cavin osteotome
cavitary
    c. defect
    c. deficiency
    glenoid c.

cavitation
    joint c.
    manual c.
Cavitron ultrasonic surgical aspirator (CUSA)
cavity
    absorption c.
    bone c.
    cotyloid c.
    glenoid c.
    idiopathic bone c.
    joint c.
    marrow c.
    Meckel c.
    medullary c.
    saclike c.
    synovial c.
    syrinx c.
cavoequinovarus
cavovalgus
    pes c.
    talipes c.
cavovarus
    c. deformity
    c. foot
    pes c.
    talipes c.
cavus
    anterior c.
    anterior pes c.
    combined c.
    combined anterior c.
    c. foot
    c. foot deformity
    c. foot support
    forefoot c.
    global c.
    hindfoot c.
    lesser tarsus c.
    local c.
    midfoot c.
    pes c.
    posttraumatic c.
    c. posture
    pronated pes c.
    rigid foot c.
    talipes c.
CAWO
    closing abductory-wedge osteotomy
CB
    contrast bath
C-bar orthosis
CBCL
    Child Behavior Checklist
CBI
    Child Behaviors Inventory
CBP
    chiropractic biophysics
        CBP technique

C

CBWO
closed base wedge osteotomy
CC
calcaneocuboid
condylocephalic
Adalat CC
CC joint
CC ligament
C1-C7
cervical spine nerves 1-7
cervical spine vertebrae 1-7
CCA
common carotid artery
CCD
cleidocranial dysplasia
CCD angle
CCDA
calcaneocuboid distraction arthrodesis
CCF
compound comminuted fracture
C-Chews
CCJ
calcaneocuboid joint
CCL
calcaneocuboid ligament
costoclavicular ligament
C-clamp
Fukushima C-c.
CCN
cervical cord neurapraxia
C-collar
cervical collar
CCPQ
Children's Comprehensive Pain
Questionnaire
CCS
chronic compartment syndrome
costoclavicular syndrome
CCTA
coronal computed tomographic
arthrography
CCW
counterclockwise
C-D
Cotrel-Dubousset
C-D fixation device
C-D hook
C-D instrumentation
C-D instrumentation device
C-D instrumentation fixation
strength
C-D instrumentation rigidity
C-D rod insertion
C-D screw modification
CD
CD Horizon M8 multiaxial screw
CD Horizon Sextant rod insertion
system
CD Horizon Sextant System

CDH
congenital dysplasia of hip
CDH cup inserter
CDH Precoat Plus hip prosthesis
CdLS
Cornelia de Lange syndrome
CDP
computerized dynamic posturography
CDS
controlled disc stimulation
CDS system
CE
center of femoral head and external
acetabular roof
CE angle
CEA
carcinoembryonic antigen
CEB
cotton elastic bandage
Cebotome
C. bone drill
C. osteotome
CECS
chronic exertional compartment
syndrome
Cedell
C. fracture
C. posterior process of talus
fracture
cefadroxil
Cefadyl
cefamandole
cefazolin
c. assay
c. clearance
c. sodium
cefepime
Cefizox
cefmetazole
Cefobid
cefonicid
cefoperazone
Cefotan
cefotaxime
cefotetan
ceftazidime
Ceftin Oral
ceftizoxime
ceftriaxone
cefuroxime
Celebrex
celecoxib
Celestone Soluspan
Celexa
cell
anterior horn c.
cartilage c.
chondrosarcoma c.
c. cushion

dorsal horn c.
endothelial c.
LE c.
lupus erythematosus c.
Merkel c.
mesenchymal c.
mesenchymal stem c.
osteoclastic giant c.
osteogenic c.
osteoprogenitor c.
osteoprogenitor stem c.
Schwann c.
squamous c.
synovial stromal c.
c. therapy
cell-mediated immunity (CMI), cellular immunity
cellona
cellular
c. level response
c. periosteal osteocartilaginous mass
c. response to implant material
c. schwannoma
cellulitis
aerobic c.
anaerobic c.
celluloid implant material
cellulose
c. hemostatic agent
Oxycel oxidized c.
CEM
central extensor mechanism
cement
acrylic bone c.
antibiotic-impregnated c.
antibiotic-loaded acrylic c.
arthroplasty c.
BA bone c.
bioactive bone c.
biodegradable calcium phosphate c.
bone c.
Boneloc c.
BoneSource hydroxyapatite c.
Callos calcium phosphate c.
c. centralizer
centrifugation of c.
CMW bone c.
c. compactor
c. curette
DePuy CMW 1 bone c.
c. disease
doughy c.
DP-Pour acrylic bone c.
Duall 88 c.
c. eater
Endurance bone c.
excess c.
c. extravasation
Gateway vertebroplastic c.

Howmedica c.
hydroxyapatite c.
hydroxyapatite-coated porous alumni c.
Implast bone c.
c. injection gun
c. interface
Ketac c.
key the c.
KyphX HV-R bone c.
c. leakage
c. line
low-viscosity bone c.
c. mantle
c. mantle grade classification
c. mass
master c.
medium-viscosity c.
methyl methacrylate c.
Norian SRS c.
Orthocomp c.
orthopaedic c.
Orthoset radiopaque bone c.
Osteobond copolymer bone c.
Palacos bone c.
Palacos radiopaque bone c.
Palacos R bone c.
c. patty
c. plug
PMMA bone c.
polymerization of bone c.
polymethyl methacrylate bone c.
pressurized c.
Pronto c.
prosthesis of antibiotic-loaded acrylic c. (PROSTALAC)
Protoplast c.
c. pump
radiopaque bone c.
c. removal
removal of excess c.
residual c.
c. restrictor
c. restrictor inserter
Simplex P bone c.
c. spacer inserter
c. spatula
SRS injectable c.
surface c.
Surgical Simplex P radiopaque c.
Surgical Simplex P radiopaque bone c.
c. syringe
VersaBond medium-viscosity bone c.
vertebroplastic c.
c. viscosity
Zimmer bone c.
Zimmer low-viscosity c.

C

cemental fracture
cementation
cement-bone interface
cemented
    c. broach
    c. component
    c. hip prosthesis
    c. total hip arthroplasty
cementing fibroma
cementless
    c. broach
    c. disease
    c. femoral component
    c. fixation
    c. prosthesis
    c. Spotorno (CLS)
    c. surface replacement arthroplasty
    (CSRA)
    c. technique
    c. total hip arthroplasty
    c. total hip replacement
cementome
    Anspach c.
cementophyte
cement-removal hand chisel
cement-wedge sign
Cemex system
cenesthopathy
Centec Formfit ankle brace
center
    accessory ossification c.
    Arizona Health Science C.
    (AHSC)
    central micturition c.
    C. for Independent Living (CIL)
    growth c.
    Louisiana State University Medical
    C. (LSUMC)
    Midwest Regional Spinal Cord
    Injury C.
    National Aging Information C.
    National Consumer Supporter
    Technical Assistance C.
    National Empowerment C.
    National Rehabilitation
    Information C.
    c. of axial rotation
    c. of femoral head and external
    acetabular roof (CE)
    c. of gravity (COG)
    c. of mass
    ossification primary c.
    ossification secondary c.
    primary c.
    Rancho Los Amigos National
    Rehabilitation C.
    secondary c.
    Veterans Administration Prosthetic
    C. (VAPC)

center-edge
    c.-e. angle
    c.-e. angle of Wiberg
centering
    c. drill
    c. hole
Centinela supraspinatus shoulder test
central
    c. amputation
    c. bone
    c. calcification
    c. callus
    c. canal
    c. canal stenosis
    c. collodiaphysial
    c. collodiaphysial angle
    c. column
    c. cord
    c. cord syndrome
    c. core disease
    c. deficiency
    c. disc protrusion
    c. dislocation
    c. electromyography
    c. extensor mechanism
    (CEM)
    c. fiber-region
    c. heel pad syndrome
    c. herniation
    c. herniation syndrome
    c. horn
    c. meniscal flap
    c. micturition center
    c. modulation
    c. necrosis
    c. nervous system (CNS)
    c. neural blockade
    c. physiolysis
    c. polydactyly
    c. posterior-anterior pressure
    c. ray
    c. ray amputation
    c. segment
    c. semi suture-loop meniscal repair
    technique
    c. slip
    c. slip-sparing technique
    c. spine spondylosis
    c. splitting technique
    c. talus fracture
    c. transpatellar tendon portal
Centralign precoat hip prosthesis
centralization
    Bayne-Klug c.
    Bora c.
    Manske-McCarroll-Swanson c.
    c. of radius operation
    tendon c.

centralizer
    cement c.
    PMMA c.
centralizing rod
centre
    Musculoskeletal Research C.
    (MRC)
centrifugation of cement
centrifuged methyl methacrylate
centromedullary
    c. nail
    c. nailing
centronuclear myopathy
centrosclerosis
cephalad
    c. anterior mold
    c. translation
cephalexin
cephalic
    c. angulation
    c. artery
    c. vein
cephalocaudad (*var. of* cephalocaudal)
cephalocaudal, cephalocaudad
    cephalocaudad direction
cephalomedullary nail fracture
cephaloscapular projection
cephalosporin
Cephalosporium **nail infection**
cephalothin
cephazolin
cephradine
Ceptaz
ceramic
    c. acetabular cup
    alumina c.
    c. bearing
    c. biomaterial
    calcium phosphate c.
    calcium sulfate c.
    c. femoral head
      prosthesis
    c. implant
    c. ossicular prosthesis
    resorbable c.
    c. vertebral spacer
ceramic-on-ceramic
    c.-o.-c. bearing surface
    c.-o.-c. coupling
Ceramion prosthesis
Cerasorb resorbable synthetic bone void filler
cerclage
    c. cable
    Dall-Miles cable c.
    c. fibreux
    Howmedica c.
    c. technique
    c. wire

    c. wire fixation
    c. wire inserter
    c. wire twister
cerclaged component
cerea flexibilitas
cerebella (*pl. of* cerebellum)
cerebellar
    c. ataxia
    c. function test
    c. gait
    c. retractor
cerebellopontine angle tumor
cerebellum, *pl.* **cerebella,** *pl.* **cerebellums**
cerebellums (*pl. of* cerebellum)
cerebral
    c. palsy
    c. palsy-related dystonia
cerebroside reticulocytosis
cerebrospinal (CS)
    c. canal
    c. fluid (CSF)
    c. fluid analysis
cerebrovascular accident (CVA)
Ceres' Secret aloe vera gel
Cerva Crane halter
cervical
    c. acceleration/deceleration syndrome
    c. AOA halo traction
    c. approach
    c. arch
    c. artery
    c. arthritis
    c. arthrodesis
    c. canal
    c. chair
    c. collar (C-collar)
    c. collar brace
    c. compaction test
    c. cord injury
    c. cord neurapraxia (CCN)
    c. corpectomy
    c. cushion
    c. Derefield procedure
      electromyocardiography
    c. disc
    c. disc disease
    c. discectomy
    c. disc excision
    c. discography
    c. discopathy
    c. disc surgery
    c. dorsal glide
    c. dorsal outlet syndrome
    c. drill
    c. epidural steroid injection
    c. extension
    c. extension osteotomy
    c. extension strength
    c. fascia

C

cervical (*continued*)
- c. flexion deformity
- c. fracture tongs
- c. general rotation
- c. halter traction
- c. hypolordosis
- c. interbody fusion
- c. joint
- c. laminaplasty
- c. laminectomy punch
- c. ligament of tarsal sinus
- c. lordosis
- c. mallet
- c. manual traction
- c. microtrauma
- c. midline disc herniation
- c. mover ligament
- c. myelopathy
- c. myelopathy anterior floating procedure
- c. myofascial pain
- c. nerve root encroachment
- c. nerve root injection
- c. nerve root injury
- c. oblique facet wiring
- c. orthosis
- c. ortrochanteric displaced hip fracture
- c. ortrochanteric hip fracture
- c. osteotomy
- c. outlet
- c. pin loosening
- c. plate
- c. plexus
- c. punch forceps
- c. radiculitis
- c. radiculopathy
- c. range of motion (CROM)
- c. range of motion device
- c. region
- c. rib
- c. rib syndrome
- c. roll
- c. rongeur
- c. root
- c. rotation in extension
- c. saddle
- c. sagittal alignment
- c. screw insertion technique
- c. sidegliding test
- c. sleep pillow
- c. specific rotation
- c. specific rotation in flexion
- c. spinal cord
- c. spinal injury
- c. spine (C-spine)
- c. spine decompression
- c. spine extension injury
- c. spine internal fixation

- c. spine kyphotic deformity
- c. spine laminectomy
- c. spine nerves 1-7 (C1-C7)
- c. spine posterior fusion
- c. spine posterior ligament disruption
- c. spine screw-plate fixation
- c. spine stabilization
- c. spine trauma
- c. spine vertebrae 1-7 (C1-C7)
- c. spondylolysis
- c. spondylosis
- c. spondylotic myelopathy (CSM)
- c. spondylotic myelopathy fusion technique
- c. spondylotic myelopathy laminar door technique
- c. spondylotic myelopathy vertebrectomy
- c. stairstep
- c. stenosis
- c. stress line
- c. support
- c. support pillow
- c. sympathectomy
- c. sympathetic chain
- c. sympathetic chain location
- c. synostosis
- c. tension myositis
- c. thoracic orthosis
- c. traction pillow
- c. triangle
- c. vertebral bone
- c. vertebrectomy

cervicalgia
cervical/lumbar hammer
Cervical-Stim noninvasive cervical spine bone growth stimulator
cervicitis
cervicoaxillary
cervicobrachial
cervicobrachialgia
cervicocranial
cervicodorsal
cervicoencephalic syndrome
cervicogenic
- c. dorsalgia
- c. headache
- c. syndrome

cervicomedullary junction
cervicooccipital fusion
cervicoplasty
cervicoscapular
cervicothoracic (CT)
- c. curve
- c. interspinous bursitis
- c. jacket
- c. junction
- c. junction stabilization

c. junction surgery
c. orthosis (CTO)
c. pathology
c. pedicle anatomy
c. pedicle angle
c. transition
cervicothoracolumbosacral orthosis (CTLSO)
cervicotrochanteric
Cervifix system
Cervitrak device
CES
cranial electrical stimulation
Cestan-Chenais syndrome
Cetaphil
cetirizine
CFL
calcaneofibular ligament
CFLB
carbon fiber lamination braid
CFLB prosthesis
C-Flex supine cervical traction
CFRP
carbon fiber-reinforced polymer
CFRP cage
CFS hip prosthesis
CFT
capillary filling time
C-guide
screw placement C-g.
CH
coracohumeral
CH ligament
CHA
calcium hydroxyapatite
CHA crystal
CHA crystal deposition disease
chaddock
C. reflex
c. sign
C. test
CHAG
coralline hydroxyapatite *Goniopora*
CHAG bone graft substitute material
chain
cervical sympathetic c.
closed kinematic c.
closed kinetic c. (CKC)
kinematic c.
kinetic c.
open kinematic c.
paravertebral sympathetic c.
pelvic kinematic c.
c. reaction exercise
sympathetic c.
wheelchair c.
chair
BodyBilt c.
Boyd podiatry c.

cervical c.
dynamic integrated stabilization c. (DISC)
ergonomic c.
ergonomically correct c.
EZ Rider support c.
Gardner c.
Hogg c.
Invacare padded shower c.
Kaleidoscope c.
Orthokinetics travel c.
Pogon c.
Portal Pro 2 treatment c.
sit/stand c.
STC 900-series travel c.
chairback
c. brace
c. lumbosacral orthosis
ChairCiser adjustable exerciser
Chalet frame
chalk-stick fracture
chalky bone
chamber
monoplace hyperbaric c.
multiplace hyperbaric c.
Portable Topical Hyperbaric Oxygen Extremity C.
Chamberlain
C. line
C. method
Chambers
C. osteotomy
C. procedure
chamfer
c. cut
c. cut jig
c. reamer
chamfered cylinder acetabular component
champ
C. elastic bandage
C. Insulated Propac II
champagne bottle leg
champion
C. Power Sox
C. trauma score (CTS)
Championniére bone drill
chance
C. fracture thoracolumbar spine
C. vertebral fracture
Chandler
C. arthrodesis
C. bone elevator
C. disease
C. felt collar splint
C. hip fusion
C. knee retractor
C. patellar advancement
C. procedure

C

Chandler (*continued*)
    C. spinal perforating forceps
    C. tendon transfer
    C. unreamed interlocking tibial
       nail
change
    age-associated degenerative c.
    arthritic talonavicular c.
    burn-related pigmentation c.
    cartilage c.
    Charcot c.
    curvature c.
    degenerative arthritic c.
    diurnal c.
    Fairbanks c.
    global rating of c. (GROC)
    Iowa degenerative c.
    kinematic gait pattern c.
    macroscopic c.
    neuromuscular gait pattern c.
    sarcomatous c.
    spondylolisthetic c.
    therapeutic lifestyle c. (TLC)
    trophic c.
Chang-Miltner incision
Chang pin clamp
channel
    interosseous anastomosing c.
    tibial c.
channel-and-core biopsy
Chapchal knee arthrodesis
Chapman point treatment
Chaput
    C. fracture
    C. fragment
    C. method
    C. tibial tubercle
characteristic
    biocompatibility c.
    electrooptical c. (EOC)
    receiver operating c. (ROC)
Charcot
    C. arthritis
    C. arthropathy
    C. arthroplasty
    C. arthrosis
    C. change
    C. chondroma
    C. collapse
    C. deformity
    C. degeneration
    C. disruption
    C. foot
    C. gait
    C. hip arthrodesis
    C. joint
    C. joint disease
    C. neuroarthropathy
    C. restraint orthotic walker (CROW)

    C. spine
    C. syndrome
    C. triad
Charcot-Marie atrophy
Charcot-Marie-Tooth (CMT)
    C.-M.-T. atrophy
    C.-M.-T. disease
    C.-M.-T. Evaluation
Charité artificial disc
Charleston
    C. nighttime bending brace
    C. scoliosis brace
charley horse
Charlie Chaplin gait
Charlin syndrome
Charnley
    C. acetabular cup
    C. acetabular cup prosthesis
    C. ankle arthrodesis
    C. ankle fusion procedure
    C. arthrodesis clamp
    C. bone clamp
    C. bone curette
    C. brace
    C. brace handle
    C. cemented prosthesis
    C. centering apparatus
    C. centering drill
    C. centering ring
    C. classification of function
    C. compression
    C. compression apparatus
    C. compression arthrodesis
    C. compression clamp
    C. compression-type knee fusion
    C. deepening reamer
    C. expanding reamer
    C. external fixation clamp
    C. external fixation device
    C. femoral broach
    C. femoral condyle drill
    C. femoral condyle radius gauge
    C. femoral inlay aligner
    C. femoral inlay guillotine
    C. femoral prosthesis neck punch
    C. femoral prosthesis pusher
    C. flat-back femoral component
    C. foam suture pad
    C. functional classification
    C. hip score
    C. horizontal retractor
    C. implant
    C. incision
    C. initial incision retractor
    C. introducer
    C. knee retractor
    C. laminar flow room
    C. low-friction arthroplasty
    C. low-friction hip prosthesis

C. narrow-stem component
C. offset-bore cup
C. pain and function grading scale
C. pilot drill
C. pin
C. pin clamp
C. pin retractor
C. rasp
C. self-retaining retractor
C. socket gauge
C. standard-stem component
C. starting drill
C. suction drain
C. suture button
C. taper reamer
C. template
C. tibial onlay jig
C. total hip arthroplasty
C. total hip prosthesis
C. total hip replacement
C. total hip system
C. towel
C. trochanter holder
C. trochanter reamer
C. wire-holding forceps
C. wire passer
C. wire tightener
Charnley-Hastings prosthesis
Charnley-Howorth Exflow system
Charnley-Merle
C.-M. d'Aubigné disability grading scale
C.-M. d'Aubigné disability grading system
Charnley-Müller
C.-M. arthroplasty
C.-M. hip prosthesis
C.-M. lateral hip approach
Charpy impact test
Charriere
C. amputation saw
C. bone saw
CHART
Craig Handicap Assessment and Reporting Technique
chart
body mechanics examination c.
Reality Orientation C.
sclerotome pain c.
Chassaignac
C. axillary muscle
C. 6th cervical vertebra tubercle
Chattanooga
C. balance system
C. traction
C. traction device
Chatzidakis hinged Vitallium implant prosthesis

Chaves
C. pectoralis major transfer
C. pectoralis minor muscle transfer
Chaves-Rapp paralysis
CHD
congenital hip dysplasia
CHD prosthesis
check
Derefield pelvic leg c.
head c.
shoulder-to-head c.
c. socket
Checkerboard wheelchair cushion
checkers
cone c.
checklist
Body Mechanics Evaluation C.
Child Behavior C. (CBCL)
Feasibility Evaluation C. (FEC)
Low Back Pain Symptom C.
McGill pain c.
Mother-Child Interaction c.
role c. (RC)
Ways of Coping c.
checkrein
c. deformity
c. ligament
c. procedure
cheese-grater hemispherical reamer
Cheetah ankle brace
cheilectomy, chilectomy
arthroscopic c.
dorsal c.
first MTP c.
Garceau c.
Mann-Coughlin-DuVries c.
Sage arthroscopic foot joint c.
Sage-Clark foot joint c.
cheilotomy, chilotomy
cheiralgia paresthetica
cheirarthritis
cheiroarthropathy
cheirobrachialgia, chirobrachialgia
cheirognostic, chirognostic
cheiromegaly, chiromegaly
cheiroplasty, chiroplasty
cheiropodalgia, chiropodalgia
cheirospasm, chirospasm
chelation therapy
chelonei
Mycobacterium c.
chemical
AXT-blocking c.
c. carcinogen
c. cautery
c. matricectomy
c. nail avulsion
c. neurolysis

chemical (*continued*)
    c. shift selective suppression
    (CHESS)
    c. sympathectomy (CS)
chemocautery
chemonucleolysis
    chymopapain c.
    double-needle c.
chemosterilized graft
chemosurgery
    phenol c.
chemotactic peptide
chemotherapy
    adjuvant c.
    neoadjuvant c.
chemotherapy-related neuropathy
Cherf
    C. cast stand
    C. legholder
cherry
    C. drill
    C. laminectomy retractor
    C. osteotome
    C. screw extractor
Cherry-Austin drill
CHES
    Children's Handwriting Evaluation
    Scale
CHES-M
    Children's Handwriting Evaluation
    Scale for Manuscript Writing
CHESS
    chemical shift selective suppression
    CHESS MRI technique
chest
    alar c.
    barrel c.
    cobbler's c.
    c. contusion
    c. expansion chest and spine
    arthritis test
    flat c.
    foveated c.
    funnel c.
    keeled c.
    paralytic c.
    phthinoid c.
    pigeon c.
    pterygoid c.
    c. roll
    c. tube (CT)
chest-band transmitter
Chester-Erdheim disease
chevron
    c. bone
    c. bunionectomy
    c. fusion
    c. hallux valgus correction
    c. incision

    c. laceration
    c. modification
    c. modification of Mitchell
    osteotomy
    c. osteotomy
    c. osteotomy with rigid screw
    fixation
    c. procedure
    c. technique
chevron-Akin double osteotomy
CHF
    congestive heart failure
CHH
    cartilage-hair hypoplasia
chi
    tai c.
Chiari
    C. formation
    C. innominate osteotomy
    C. malformation
    C. pelvis osteotomy technique
    C. shelf procedure
chiasma, *pl.* **chiasmata**
    Camper c.
    c. tendinum
chiasmata (*pl. of* chiasma)
Chiba spinal system
chick
    C. CLT operating frame
    C. CLT operating table
    C. fracture table
    C. nail
chicken breast
Chick-Foster orthopaedic bed
Chick-Langren orthopaedic table
Chiene line bilateral greater trochanter test
chilblain
child, *pl.* **children**
    c. amputee
    C. and Adolescent Social Perception
    Measure (CASP)
    Assessment Battery for Children
    (ABC)
    Behavior Assessment System for
    Children (BASC)
    C. Behavior Checklist (CBCL)
    C. Behaviors Inventory (CBI)
    Choosing Outcomes and
    Accommodations for Children
    (COACH)
    C. Development Inventory
    Functional Independence Measure
    for Children (WeeFIM)
    Movement Assessment Battery for
    Children
    sized orthotics for children (SOCS)
    Test of Everyday Attention for
    Children (TEA-Ch)

children (*pl. of* child)
Children's
    C. Advil oral suspension
    C. Assessment of Participation and
      Enjoyment (CAPE)
    C. Comprehensive Pain
      Questionnaire (CCPQ)
    C. Dynafed Jr.
    C. Handwriting Evaluation Scale
      (CHES)
    C. Handwriting Evaluation Scale for
      Manuscript Writing (CHES-M)
    C. Hospital hand drill
    C. Hospital screwdriver
    C. Motrin oral suspension
    C. Paced Auditory Serial Addition
      Test (CHIPASAT)
    C. Silapap
Childress
    C. ankle fixation
    C. ankle fixation technique
    C. duck waddle knee test
child's flatfoot correction
chilectomy (*var. of* cheilectomy)
chilotomy (*var. of* cheilotomy)
Chinese
    C. fingertrap
    C. fingertrap suture
    C. fingertrap tube
    C. medicine
    C. radial forearm flap
    C. red line sign
chin-to-chest test
ChinUpps cervicofacial support
chip
    autologous bone c.
    bone c.
    cancellous c.
    c. fracture
    c. graft
CHIPASAT
    Children's Paced Auditory Serial
    Addition Test
Chippaux-Smirak arch index
chipped-tooth broach
chirarthritis
chirobrachialgia (*var. of* cheirobrachialgia)
Chirocaine
Chiroflow
    C. adjustable back support
    C. back rest
chirognostic (*var. of* cheirognostic)
Chiro-Klenz tea
Chiro-Manis chiropractic table
chiromegaly (*var. of* cheiromegaly)
chiroplasty (*var. of* cheiroplasty)
chiropodalgia
chiropodical
chiropodist

chiropody
chiropractic
    c. adjustment procedure
    c. analysis
    c. biophysics (CBP)
    c. joint manipulation
    c. laser nonsurgical facelift
    c. lesion
    c. management
    c. manipulative reflex technique
      (CMRT)
    c. manipulative therapy
      (CMT)
    c. manual manipulation
    c. manual manipulation of
      spine
    c. mattress
    c. spinal adjustment
    sports c.
    C. Strength Flexall 454
    c. thermography
    c. x-ray film
chiropractor
chiropraxis
chirospasm
Chirotech x-ray system
chisel
    acetabular round c.
    Adson laminectomy c.
    Alexander c.
    ASIF c.
    Association for the Study of
      Internal Fixation C.
    Austin Moore c.
    Ballenger-Hajek c.
    beveled c.
    Biomet cement-removal hand c.
    Bishop c.
    c. blade
    Blair c.
    bone c.
    Bowen c.
    box c.
    Brittain c.
    Bruening c.
    Buckley c.
    cement-removal hand c.
    Cloward spinal fusion c.
    cold c.
    Converse c.
    Cottle c.
    Dautrey c.
    D'Errico lamina c.
    c. elevator
    Fomon c.
    c. fracture
    Freer c.
    Hajek c.
    Harmon c.

C

chisel (*continued*)
    Hibbs c.
    hollow c.
    Kerrison c.
    Lambert-Lowman c.
    laminectomy c.
    Lexer c.
    Lowman c.
    Lowman-Hoglund c.
    Lucas c.
    Magnum c.
    Martin cartilage c.
    meniscotomy c.
    Metzenbaum c.
    Meyerding c.
    Miles bone c.
    Moore prosthesis-mortising c.
    mortising c.
    Oratec c.
    orthopaedic c.
    Partsch c.
    Passow c.
    Pick c.
    Puka c.
    Schwartze c.
    seating c.
    Sheehan c.
    Simmons c.
    Smillie cartilage c.
    Smillie meniscectomy c.
    Smith-Petersen c.
    Sorrells posterior
      condylar c.
    square-hollow c.
    Stille bone c.
    straight c.
    swan-neck c.
    U.S. Army bone c.
    West bone c.
    White c.
chisel-edge elevator
chisel-tip wire
chloral hydrate
chlorambucil
chloramphenicol osteomyelitis
chlordiazepoxide
chlorhexidine gluconate
chloride
    antimicrobial benzalkonium c.
    benzalkonium c.
    ethyl c.
    polyvinyl c. (PVC)
chloroprocaine
chloroquine phosphate
chlorotrianisene
chlorphenesin carbamate
chlorpromazine
chlorprothixene
chlorzoxazone

Cho
    C. anterior cruciate ligament
      reconstruction
    C. tendon technique
choke
    c. hold
    c. syndrome
cholesterol
Cholestin
choline
    c. magnesium trisalicylate
    c. salicylate
cholinergic vagal function
cholinesterase inhibitor
chondral
    c. fracture
    c. fragment
chondralgia
chondrectomy
chondrification
chondritis
chondroblast
chondroblastic sarcoma
chondroblastoma
    benign c.
    humeral c.
chondrocalcinosis
chondroclast
chondrocyte
    c. apoptosis
    autologous cultured c.
    Carticel autologous
      cultured c.
    hypertrophic c.
chondrodiastasis
chondrodynia
chondrodysplasia
    genotypic c.
    hereditary deforming c.
    hyperplastic c.
    McKusick-type metaphysial c.
    metaphysial c.
    c. punctata (CP)
    rhizomelic-type c.
chondrodystrophia (*var. of*
  chondrodystrophy)
chondrodystrophy, chondrodystrophia
    chondrodystrophia calcificans
chondroepiphysis
chondroepiphysitis
chondrofibroma
chondrogenesis
chondrography
chondroid syringoma
chondroitin
chondroitin/glucosamine sulfate
  complex
chondrolipoma
chondrolysis

chondroma
- Charcot c.
- extraskeletal c.
- joint c.
- juxtacortical c.
- periosteal c.
- synovial c.

chondromalacia
- c. patellae
- patellar c.

chondromalacic

chondromatosis
- Henderson-Jones c.
- synovial c. (SCM)

chondromatous hamartoma

chondrometaplasia

chondromyofibroma

chondromyoma

chondromyxofibroma

chondromyxoid fibroma, chondromyxoma

chondromyxoma (*var. of* chondromyxoid fibroma)

chondromyxosarcoma

chondronecrosis

chondroosseous
- c. growth
- c. spur

chondroosteodystrophy

chondropathology

chondropathy

chondrophyte

chondroplastic
- c. dwarfism
- c. myotonia

chondroplasty
- abrasion c.
- arthroscopic abrasion c.
- c. knife

chondroporosis

chondroprotective agent

chondrosarcoma
- c. cell
- clear cell c.
- dedifferentiated c.
- differentiated c.
- extracortical c.
- extraskeletal c.
- juxtacortical c.
- mesenchymal c.
- myxoid c.
- parosteal c.
- periosteal c.
- pseudocapsule c.

chondrosarcomatosis

chondrosis

chondrosteoma

chondrosternal articulation

chondrosternoplasty

chondrotomy

chondrotrophic

chondroxiphoid

chonechondrosternon

Chonstruct chondral repair system

Choosing Outcomes and Accommodations for Children (COACH)

Chooz

Chopart
- C. amputation with tendon balancing
- C. ankle dislocation
- C. articulation
- C. brace
- C. hindfoot amputation
- C. joint line
- C. midtarsal joint
- C. operation
- C. osseous joint injury
- C. partial foot prosthesis

Cho-Pat
- C.-P. Achilles tendon strap
- C.-P. Dual Action Knee Strap
- C.-P. elbow strap
- C.-P. ITB Strap
- C.-P. knitted compression support

Chopin sacral block

chordoblastoma

chordocarcinoma

chordoma
- cavern c.
- sacrococcygeal c.

chordosarcoma

chordotomy

choreatic gait

choreic abasia

choreiform, choreoid

choreoid (*var. of* choreiform)

choristoma

chow
- C. endoscopic carpal tunnel release
- C. transbursal carpal tunnel release technique

Choyce MK II keratoprosthesis prosthesis

CHPS
- chronic heel pain syndrome

Chrisman-Snook
- C.-S. ankle ligament reconstruction
- C.-S. ankle technique
- C.-S. ankle tenodesis
- C.-S. correction
- C.-S. correction of ankle instability
- C.-S. reconstruction of ankle ligament
- C.-S. technique modification
- C.-S. weave procedure

Christensen interlocking nail

Christiani maneuver

Christiansen hip prosthesis

Christian syndrome

Christmas
    C. tree adapter
    C. tree reamer
chromatinolysis (*var. of* chromatolysis)
chromatography
    high-performance liquid c.
chromatolysis, chromatinolysis
chrome
    cobalt c.
chrome-cobalt
    c.-c. cable
    c.-c. screw
chromium (Cr)
    c. implant
chromium-cobalt
    c.-c. alloy implant
    c.-c. mesh
chromomycosis
chronaxia (*var. of* chronaxie)
chronaxie, chronaxia, chronaxy, chronaxis
chronaxis (*var. of* chronaxie)
chronaxy (*var. of* chronaxie)
chronic
    c. absorptive arthritis
    c. Achilles tendinitis
    c. ankle instability (CAI)
    c. ankle sprain
    c. anterior exertional compartment syndrome (CAECS)
    c. compartment syndrome (CCS)
    c. exertional compartment syndrome (CECS)
    c. foot sprain
    c. functional instability
    c. heel pain syndrome (CHPS)
    c. heel wound
    c. hemorrhagic villous synovitis
    c. intractable benign pain syndrome (CIBPS)
    c. lateral ankle instability
    c. low back pain (CLBP)
    c. microtraumatic soft tissue injury
    c. musculoskeletal pain syndrome (CMPS)
    c. noninsertional tendo calcaneus tendinitis
    c. paroxysmal hemicrania
    c. periostalgia
    c. purulent synovitis
    c. recurrent ankle joint dislocation
    c. retrocalcaneal bursitis
    c. rheumatism
    c. sclerosing osteomyelitis of Garré
    c. subtalar joint pain
    c. tophaceous disease
    c. tophaceous gout
    c. traumatic encephalopathy (CTE)

    c. villous arthritis (CVA)
    c. whiplash
chronotropic impairment
CHSD
    congenital hyperphosphatasemic skeletal dysplasia
chuck
    c. adapter
    c. drill
    gold-handled c.
    hand c.
    Jacobs c.
    3-jaw c.
    pin c.
    Steinmann pin with pin c.
    T-handle Zimmer c.
    Zimmer c.
Chuinard autogenous bone graft
Chukka boot
chylothorax
chylous
    c. arthritis
    c. leakage
Chymodiactin
chymopapain
    c. blocking agent
    c. chemonucleolysis
    c. injection
chymotrypsin
    alpha c.
CI
    combined instability
        CI functional knee brace
CIA
    calcaneal inclination angle
    common iliac artery
Cibacalcin Injection
CIBPS
    chronic intractable benign pain syndrome
CIC
    complex instability of carpus
Cica-Care wound dressing
cicatrices (*pl. of* cicatrix)
cicatricial scoliosis
cicatrix, *pl.* **cicatrices**
cicatrization
Cicherelli bone rongeur
ciclopirox
CID
    carpal instability dissociative
Cierny-Mader osteomyelitis staging (type I-V)
ciguatera
CIL
    Center for Independent Living
cilastatin
    imipenem and c.
ciliospinal center of Budge

cimetidine
cinch
>joint c.
>C. Lock CTS brace
>C. suction sleeve for BK prosthetic
>>socket

Cincinnati
>C. ACL brace
>C. incision
>C. Knee Rating System
>C. knee scoring questionnaire
>C. pelvic osteotomy technique

CIND
>carpal instability nondissociative

cine
>c. magnetic resonance imaging
>>(cine-MRI)
>c. memory
>c. view

cinearthrography
>triple-injection c.

cinefluoroscopy
Cinelli osteotome
cinematic amputation
cinematographic gait study
cine-MRI
>cine magnetic resonance imaging

cineplastic amputation, cineplastics
cineplastics (*var. of* cineplastic amputation)
cineradiography, cineroentgenography
cineroentgenography (*var. of*
cineradiography)

Cintor
>C. bone rongeur
>C. knee prosthesis

Cipro
>C. Injection
>C. Oral

ciprofloxacin
CIQ
>Community Integration Questionnaire

circadian oscillator
CircAid elastic stockings
circle
>c. bed
>c. draw test
>perfect c.

CircOlectric
>C. bed
>C. frame

CircPlus bandage/wrap system
Circul'Air shoe process system
circular
>c. bandage
>c. cast
>c. fine-wire external fixator
>c. fixation
>c. fixation device
>c. laminar hook with offset top

c. open amputation
c. saw
c. supracondylar amputation
c. wire
c. wire fixator

circulation
>collateral c.
>extraosseous c.
>femoral c.
>intraosseous c.
>perichondral c.

Circulator boot system
circulatory embarrassment
Circulon dressing
circumduction maneuver
circumductor table
circumference
>calf c.
>pelvic c.

circumferential
>c. capsulectomy
>c. cartilage
>c. dedicated knee coil
>c. dressing
>c. fracture
>c. grommet
>c. lamella
>c. ligamentous sleeve
>c. pelvic antishock sheeting
>c. release
>c. release of clubfoot
>c. wire
>c. wire-loop fixation
>c. wiring

circumflex
>c. iliac artery
>c. scapular artery

circumscribed
circumscribing incision
circumscripta
>calcinosis c.

Cirrus
>C. composite prosthetic foot
>C. foot prosthesis
>C. foot prosthetic

cirsoid angioma
citalopram hydrobromide
Citanest
>C. Forte
>C. Plain

Citelli
>C. punch forceps
>C. sinodural angle

citrate
>orphenadrine c.
>sufentanil c.

Citscope disposable arthroscope
Civinini
>C. canal

Civinini (*continued*)
    C. ligament
    C. process
    C. spine
CIVRA
    continuous intravenous regional anesthesia
C-Jaws
    C-J. cervical compressive mini frame
    C-J. cervical compressive staple
CKC
    closed kinetic chain
CKCE
    closed kinetic chain exercise
CKS
    Continuum knee system
    CKS implant
    CKS knee system
Claforan
Claiborne external fixator
clamp
    Acland microvascular c.
    Aesculap c.
    Allen-Kocher c.
    Allis c.
    angled DeBakey c.
    angled Lowman-type bone c.
    angular hinge c.
    Ann Arbor double towel c.
    appendage c.
    c. approximator
    baby Kocher c.
    baby Satinsky c.
    Backhaus towel c.
    Bahnson appendage c.
    Balfour c.
    Ballantine c.
    Bard c.
    bar-to-bar c.
    Berke c.
    Bernhard c.
    Bircher bone-holding c.
    Bircher cartilage c.
    Bishop bone c.
    Blalock c.
    Böhler c.
    bone extension c.
    bone-holding c.
    Bonney c.
    bulldog c.
    Calandruccio c.
    c. carrier
    cartilage c.
    Casey pelvic c.
    Chang pin c.
    Charnley arthrodesis c.
    Charnley bone c.
    Charnley compression c.

Charnley external fixation c.
Charnley pin c.
Clevis c.
Cooley graft c.
Cooley iliac c.
Cooley multipurpose angled c.
Cooley multipurpose curved c.
Dandy c.
Davidson muscle c.
Diethrich bulldog c.
Dingman bone and cartilage c.
disposable muscle biopsy c.
dissecting c.
distraction c.
Doctor Collins fracture c.
double c.
Edna towel c.
exclusion c.
extension bone c.
femoral c.
Ferguson bone c.
c. fixator
c. forceps
Freeman c.
full-curved c.
Gerster bone c.
Goodwin bone c.
Greenberg c.
Halifax interlaminar c.
Harrington hook c.
Harrington rod c.
hemostat c.
hemostatic thoracic c.
Hex-Fix Universal swivel c.
Hey Groves c.
Hoen c.
Hoffmann ligament c.
c. holder
hook c.
iliac c.
c. insert
interlaminar c.
Jackson bone c.
Jackson bone-extension c.
Jackson bone-holding c.
Jacobson bulldog c.
Jameson muscle c.
Jarit anterior resection c.
Jarit cartilage c.
Jarit meniscal c.
Jarit small bone-holding c.
Johns Hopkins bulldog c.
Jones thoracic c.
Jones towel c.
Kantrowitz thoracic c.
Kelly c.
Kern bone-holding c.
Kocher c.
Lahey c.

Lalonde oblique fracture large bone c.
Lalonde oblique fracture medium
  bone c.
Lalonde oblique metacarpal fracture
  bone c.
Lalonde small bone c.
Lambert-Lowman bone c.
Lambotte bone-holding c.
Lamis patellar c.
Lane bone-holding c.
Lewin bone-holding c.
ligament c.
lobster-type c.
Locke bone c.
locking c.
Lowman bone-holding c.
Lowman-Gerster bone c.
Lowman-Hoglund c.
Malis hinge c.
Martin cartilage c.
Martin meniscal c.
Martin muscular c.
Masterson curved c.
Masterson pelvic c.
Masterson straight c.
Mastin muscular c.
Matthew cross-leg c.
Mayo c.
medial malleolar/small bone
  fragment c.
meniscal c.
metal c.
microvascular c.
miniature multipurpose c.
mini-Ullrich bone c.
Mixter ligature-carrier c.
Mixter right-angle c.
mosquito c.
Moynihan towel c.
multipurpose angled c.
multipurpose curved c.
muscle biopsy c.
muscular c.
Naraghi-DeCoster reduction c.
O'Brien bone c.
osteoplastic flap c.
padded c.
Parham-Martin bone-holding c.
patellar cement c.
patellar reduction c.
Pean c.
pedicle c.
pelvic C c.
Pemberton spur-crushing c.
phalangeal c.
pin c.
pin-to-bar c.
point-of-reduction c.
Price muscular biopsy c.

ratchet c.
Rayport muscular biopsy c.
reamer c.
Richards bone c.
rod c.
rubber shod c.
Rumel myocardial c.
Rumel rubber c.
Rumel thoracic c.
Rush bone c.
saddle c.
Satinsky c.
Schlein c.
Seidel bone-holding c.
self-retaining c.
Semb bone-holding c.
sesamoid c.
single c.
Slocum meniscal c.
Smith bone c.
Southwick c.
speed-lock c.
sponge c.
spur-crushing c.
stainless steel c.
Steinhauser bone c.
Steri-Clamp c.
swivel c.
towel c.
trochanter-holding c.
Ulrich bone-holding c.
universal wire c.
Verbrugge bone c.
Vermont spinal fixator c.
vessel c.
Walton cartilage c.
Walton meniscal c.
West Shur cartilage c.
wire-tightening c.
Wylie lumbar bulldog c.
X c.
Zimmer cartilage c.

clamping mechanism
clamshell
  c. AFO boot
  c. brace
  c. prosthesis
Clancy
  C. cruciate ligament reconstruction
  C. lateral compartment
  C. ligament technique
  C. patellar tendon graft
Clancy-Andrews reconstruction
Clanton
  C. turf toe
  C. turf toe grading system
Clark
  C. classification
  C. classification of melanoma

Clark (*continued*)
    C. pectoralis major transfer
    C. sign
    C. transfer technique
Clarke
    C. arch angle
    C. knee grind sign
    C. patellar compression test
Clarus SpineScope
CLASP
    compression locking anchor with
      secondary purchase
clasp
    Arrow pin c.
    Epi-Sport epicondylitis c.
clasped
    c. thumb
    c. thumb deformity
classification
    AAOS acetabular abnormality c.
    ACR juvenile arthritis c.
    acromioclavicular injury c.
    ACR osteoarthritis of hand c.
    ACR osteoarthritis of hip c.
    ACR Reiter syndrome c.
    ACR rheumatic diseases c.
    Ahlbäck grade c. (1–5)
    Aitken epiphysial fracture c.
    Allman acromioclavicular injury c.
      (1-3)
    Allman-Tossy acromioclavicular
      injury c. (1–3)
    American College of
      Rheumatology c.
    American Research Circulation
      Osseous Osteonecrosis c.
    American Rheumatism Association
      rheumatoid arthritis c.
    American Spinal Cord Injury
      Association c.
    Anderson-D'Alonzo odontoid
      fracture c.
    Anderson modification of
      Berndt-Harty osteochondral talar
      lesion c.
    Anderson tibial pseudarthrosis c.
    ankle fracture c.
    AO and Danis-Weber ankle
      fracture c.
    AO ankle fracture c.
    ARCO osteonecrosis c.
    Arthritis Impact Measurement
      Scale c.
    Ashhurst-Bromer ankle fracture c.
    Ashhurst transcondylar humeral
      fracture c. (I, II)
    Bado Monteggia fracture c.
    Bauer-Jackson traumatic chondral
      lesion c.

Bayne radial agenesis c. (I-IV)
Bayne ulnar ray deficiency c.
    (I-IV)
Bennett thumb fracture c.
Berndt-Harty osteochondral fracture
    c. (I-IV)
Bishop c.
Blauth thumb hypoplasia c. (I-V)
Bleck metatarsus adductus c.
Boyd c.
Boyd and Griffin subtrochanteric
    proximal femur fracture c. (I-IV)
Breslow melanoma c.
Breslow melanoma thickness c.
Brooker heterotopic bone formation
    c. (I-IV)
Bryan-Morrey capitellar fracture c.
    (I-IV)
Canale-Kelly talar neck fracture c.
Carnesale-Stewart-Barnes hip
    dislocation c.
Catterall 4-part (I-IV) Perthes
    disease c.
cement mantle grade c.
Charnley functional c.
Clark c.
Codman c.
Colonna hip fracture c.
3 color concept of wound c.
Colton olecranon fracture c.
Copeland-Kavat metatarsophalangeal
    dislocation c.
Crowe congenital hip dysplasia c.
Daltons dens fracture c. (I–III)
Danis-Weber fracture c.
d'Antonio acetabular c.
Darrow pain c.
David-Chaussé articular arthritis c.
Deknatel suture c.
DeLee pediatric fracture c.
Denis Browne spinal fracture c.
    (1–3)
Denis compression fracture c.
Denis sacral fracture c.
Denis seat-belt injury c.
Devas stress fracture c.
Dorr bone c.
Durie-Salmon c.
Dyck-Lambert c.
Edwards and Lee tibiofibular
    diastasis and syndesmotic injury c.
Ellis tooth fracture c.
Enneking benign tumor c.
Epstein hip dislocation c.
Essex-Lopresti calcaneal fracture c.
Evans intertrochanteric fracture c.
femoral fracture following total hip
    replacement c.
Ficat avascular necrosis c.

Ficat femoral head osteonecrosis c. (stage I-IV)
Fielding femoral fracture c.
Flatt upper extremity congenital anomaly c.
floating knee fracture c.
Foucher distal digital amputation c.
Foucher metacarpal synostosis c. fracture c.
Fränkel neurologic deficit c.
Freeman calcaneal fracture c.
Fries rheumatoid arthritis c.
Frykman distal radius fracture c.
Frykman wrist fracture c.
Garden femoral neck fracture c.
Gartland humeral supracondylar fracture c.
Gartland supracondylar fracture c.
Gartland Universal radial fracture c.
Gertzbein seat-belt injury c.
Graf c.
Grantham femur fracture c.
Greenfield spinocerebellar ataxia c.
Gumley seat beat injury c.
Gustilo-Anderson open fracture c.
Gustilo-Anderson tibial plafond fracture c.
Gustilo puncture wound c.
Gustilo tibial fracture c.
Hahn-Steinthal capitellum fracture c.
Hannover chronic rejection c.
Hansen fracture c.
Hardcastle c.
Hawkins talar fracture c.
Henderson functional results c.
Herbert scaphoid bone fracture c.
Herndon hip c.
Herring lateral pillar Perthes disease (A, B, C) c.
Herring lateral pillar radiographic c.
Heyman hip c.
hip dislocation c.
Hohl-Luck tibial plateau fracture c.
Hohl tibial condylar fracture c.
Holdsworth spinal fracture c.
Hughston Clinic injury c.
Ideberg glenoid fracture c.
Insall patellar injury c.
Jahss ankle dislocation c.
Jahss metatarsophalangeal joint dislocation c.
Janis tibialis posterior tendon dysfunction c.
Jeffery radial fracture c.
Johansson fracture c.
Johnson and Strom tibialis posterior tendon dysfunction c.
Jones congenital tibial deficiency c.
Jones diaphysial fracture c.

Judet epiphysial fracture c.
Kalamchi avascular necrosis c.
Kelikian nail deformity c.
Kilfoyle humeral medial condylar fracture c.
King thoracic scoliosis c.
Kocher humerus fracture c.
Kocher-Lorenz capitellum fracture c. (I-II)
Komori herniated nucleus pulposus migration c.
Kostuik-Errico spinal stability c.
Kuwada Achilles tendon injury c.
Kyle fracture c.
Langenskiöld c. (stage I–VI)
lateral condylar fracture c.
Lauge-Hansen ankle fracture c.
Lauge-Hansen fracture c.
Lenke c.
Lenke and King adolescent idiopathic scoliosis c.
Letournel-Judet acetabular fracture c.
Letournel pelvic ring injury c.
Leung thumb loss c.
Lichtman aseptic necrosis c.
Lindell blanisotropic media c.
load-sharing c.
Louisiana State University Medical Center c.
LSUMC c.
Macewen c.
MacNicol-Voutsinas posterior tibial tear c.
Mason radial head fracture c.
Mathews olecranon fracture c.
Mayo carpal instability c.
Mayo elbow fracture c.
Mazur ankle elevation c.
McDermott radiological c.
Melone distal radius fracture c.
Merland perimedullary arteriovenous fistula c.
Meyers-McKeever tibial fracture c.
Milch elbow fracture c. (I, II)
Milch fracture c. (I, II)
Milch medial condylar of elbow fracture c. (I, II)
modified Bauth thumb hypoplasia c. (I–V)
modified Fränkel c.
modified Sillence c.
modified Stahl c. (stage I-V)
Moore tibial plateau fracture c.
MRC muscle function c.
Mueller femoral supracondylar fracture c.
Mueller humerus fracture c.
Mueller tibial fracture c.
Neer femur fracture c.

classification (*continued*)

Neer-Horowitz humerus fracture c.
Neer humerus fracture c.
Neer shoulder fracture c.
Neviaser frozen shoulder c.
Newman radial neck and head fracture c.
New York diagnostic criteria c.
Nicoll spinal fracture c.
Nurick spondylosis c.
O'Brien radial fracture c.
Oden peroneal tendon subluxation c.
5 c.'s of spondylolisthesis
Ogden epiphysial fracture c.
Ogden knee dislocation c.
Olerud and Molander fracture c.
O'Rahilly limb deficiency c.
ordinal c.
Orthopaedic Trauma Association c.
Orthopaedic Trauma Association fracture c.
osteoarthritis grading c.
OTA fracture c.
Outerbridge chondral knee lesion c.
Ovadia-Beals tibial plafond fracture c.
Paley fibular hemimelia c.
Palmer triangular fibrocartilage complex lesion c.
Papavasiliou olecranon fracture c.
Pauwels femoral neck fracture c.
Pennal pelvic fracture c.
peripheral nerve tumor c.
pilon fracture c.
Pipkin posterior hip dislocation c.
Pipkin subclassification of Epstein-Thomas c.
Poland epiphysial fracture c.
pressure ulcer c.
Pritsch talar osteochondroma c.
Prosthetic Problem Inventory Scale c.
Quénu-Küss tarsometatarsal injury c.
Quinby pelvic fracture c.
Ranawat neurologic deficit (I, II, IIIA, IIIB) c.
Ranawat pneumatoid spondylitis c.
Ratliff avascular necrosis c.
red, yellow, blue wound color c.
Regnaud rigidus c. (I-III)
Regnauld hallux rigidus c.
Riordan clubhand c.
Riseborough-Radin intercondylar fracture c.
Risser c.
Rockwood c.
Rockwood acromioclavicular injury c. (I-VI)

Rosenthal c.
Rowe calcaneal fracture c. (type 1a, 1b, 1c, 2a, 2b, 3-5)
Ruedi-Allgower pilon fracture c.
Russe c.
Russell-Taylor c.
Rüter c.
RYB wound color c.
Salter-Harris-Rang epiphysial fracture c. (1a, b, c, 2a, b, c, 3a, b, 4a, b, 5-9)
Salter-Thomson Perthes disease (A, B) c.
Sanders calcaneal fracture (I-IV) c.
Sanders CT C.
Sangeorzan navicular fracture c. (1–4)
scalar c.
Schatzker tibial plateau fracture c. (I-VI)
Seddon nerve injury c.
Seinsheimer subtrochanteric fracture c. (I-VI)
Severin radiographic residual hip dysplasia c.
Shapiro c.
Shelton femoral fracture c.
Sillence osteogenesis imperfecta c.
simple fifth metatarsal fracture c.
Singh osteoporosis c.
Sorbie calcaneal fracture c.
Speed radial head fracture c.
Stahl Kienbock disease c.
Stahl lunatomalacia c. (I-V)
Steinbrocker rheumatoid arthritis c.
Steinert epiphysial fracture c.
Stewart fifth metatarsal fracture c. (I-V)
Stewart-Milford traumatic pediatric hip dislocation c. (I-IV)
Stulberg hip c.
Sunderland nerve injury first- through fifth-degree c.
Swanson congenital limb anomalies c.
Tachdjian pediatric ankle fracture c.
talar neck injury c. (I–III)
talocalcaneal index c.
Thomas c.
Thompson-Epstein posterior hip fracture dislocation c. (I-V)
tibial tuberosity fractures in children c.
Tile acetabular fracture c.
Tile pelvic injury c.
Torg fifth metatarsal fracture c. (I-III)
Toronto pelvic fracture c.

C

clear
    c. cell acanthoma
    c. cell carcinoma
    c. cell chondrosarcoma
    c. cell sarcoma
    c. space measurement
clearance
    cefazolin c.
    radioactive xenon c.
    spinal c.
Clearfix screw
clearinghouse
    National Accessible
      Apartment C.
    National Maternal and Child
      Health C.
    National Mental Health Consumers'
      Self-Help C.
Clearpro suction socket
cleavage
    c. fracture
    horizontal c.
    c. lesion
    c. line
    c. tear
Cleeman sign
cleft
    c. closure
    c. foot
    c. foot deformity
    c. formation
    gluteal c.
    Hahn c.
    c. hand
    c. hand deformity
    intergluteal c.
    interinnominoabdominal c.
    c. of Hahn
    retropharyngeal fascial c.
    c. spine
    c. spinous process
    venous c.
    c. vertebra
    vertebral column c.
clefting of meniscus
C-Leg
    C-L. lower limb prosthesis
    C-L. microprocessor-controlled
      hydraulic knee
    C-L. prosthesis
    C-L. System artificial leg
cleidagra
cleidal
cleidarthritis
cleidocostal
cleidocranial, clidocranial
    c. dysostosis
    c. dysplasia (CCD)

cleidoepitrochlear bundle
cleidomastoid
Cleland ligament
clenched
    c. fist syndrome
    c. fist view
Cleocin
    C. HCl
    C. Pediatric
    C. Phosphate
Cleveland
    C. bone-cutting forceps
    C. bone rongeur
Clevis clamp
Clevisphere ankle joint
CLI
    critical limb ischemia
click
    hip c.
    Mulder c.
    Ortolani c.
    c. sign
clicker
    compression c.
clidocranial (*var. of* cleidocranial)
Clifton Assessment Procedures for the Elderly (CAPE)
Climara Transdermal
climber
    Fitstep II stair c.
    Sprint C.
clinarthrosis
clindamycin
clinic
    Dickson-Diveley c.
clinical
    C. Analysis Questionnaire (CAQ)
    c. bone sonometer
    c. diagnosis
    c. examination
    c. parameter
    C. Test of Sensory Integration and
      Balance (CTSIB)
    c. trial
Clinisert mattress
Clinitron air bed
clinodactyly
clinoid process
clinometrics
Clinoril
clinotherapy
ClinsWound wound cleanser
clioquinol
clip
    c. applier
    c. gauge
    Indiana tome c.
    Michel c.

palmar c.
towel c.
Weck c.

clip-applying forceps
clip-bending forceps
clip-cutting forceps
clip-introducing forceps
clivi (*pl. of* clivus)
clivus, *pl.* **clivi**
cloacae

Enterobacter c.

clock

c. balance test
shoulder c.

clog

Hollander c.
Markell Mobility Health C.'s
wooden postoperative c.

clomipramine
Clomycin
clonazepam
clonus

ankle c.
3-beat c.
drawn ankle c.
patellar c.
persistent c.
sustained ankle c.
transient c.
unsustained c.

clorazepate dipotassium
Clorpactin WCS-90
closed

c. ankle fracture
c. base wedge osteotomy (CBWO)
c. body
c. core needle biopsy
c. Cotrel-Dubousset hook
c. dislocation
c. drainage system
c. femoral diaphysial shortening
c. flap amputation
c. indirect fracture
c. intramedullary osteotomy
c. irrigation
c. kinematic chain
c. kinetic chain (CKC)
c. kinetic chain exercise (CKCE)
c. kinetic chain injury
c. kinetic chain progressive-
  resistance exercise
c. Küntscher nail
c. Küntscher nailing
c. loop EndoButton
c. manipulation
c. manipulative maneuver
c. medullary nailing
c. pinning

c. pseudarthrosis
c. reduction
c. reduction of fracture
c. rupture
c. soft tissue injury
c. suction irrigation
c. surgery
c. transverse process TSRH hook
c. treatment
c. unlocked nail
c. wedge dorsal osteotomy
c. wedge osteotomy/bunionectomy
c. wound

closed-chain

c.-c. exercise
c.-c. functional assessment

closed-form bar theory
Close Encounter nut
close-packed position
Closer stapler
closing

c. abductory-wedge osteotomy
  (CAWO)
c. base wedge
c. base-wedge osteotomy
voluntary c.
c. wedge arthrodesis
c. wedge greenstick dorsal proximal
  metatarsal osteotomy
c. wedge high tibial osteotomy
  (CWHTO)
c. wedge manipulation
c. wedge manipulation and
  reapplication of plaster
c. wedge osteotomy bunionectomy

clostridial

c. infection
c. myonecrosis
c. myositis

Clostridium

C. difficile (C Diff)
C. perfringens

closure

Barsky cleft hand c.
bunionectomy capsular c.
cleft c.
delayed c.
delayed primary c. (DPC)
epiphysial c.
lace c.
myofascial c.
physial c.
premature c.
primary c.
rotator interval capsule c.
secondary c.
skin c.
Steri-Strip skin c.

C

149

closure (*continued*)
    SureClosure c.
    tissue c.
    vacuum-assisted c. (VAC)
    Velcro c.
    visual c.
    wound c.

clot
    exogenous fibrin c.
    fibrin c.

cloth
    c. binder
    c. tape occlusion method of Litt

clotheslining

clothespin spinal fusion graft

clotrimazole
    betamethasone and c.

clotting
    c. cascade
    c. disorder

Cloutier unconstrained knee prosthesis

cloven-hoof
    c.-h. fracture
    c.-h. fracture of finger

cloverleaf
    c. condylar plate fixation
    c. deformity
    c. Küntscher nail
    c. met foot pad
    c. pattern
    c. pin
    c. pin extractor
    c. plate

Cloward
    C. anterior cervical discectomy and fusion technique
    C. anterior spinal fusion
    C. back fusion
    C. blade retractor
    C. bone graft impactor
    C. cervical arthrodesis
    C. cervical disc approach
    C. cervical drill
    C. cervical drill guard
    C. cervical drill tip
    C. cervical spine fusion operation
    C. depth gauge
    C. dowel cutter
    C. dowel ejector
    C. drill guard cap
    C. drill guide
    C. drill shaft
    C. fusion discography
    C. hammer
    C. intervertebral disc rongeur
    C. osteophyte elevator
    C. periosteal elevator
    C. spinal fusion chisel
    C. spinal fusion osteotome

    C. spreader
    C. surgical saddle

cloxacillin

CLS
    cementless Spotorno
    CLS hip system

club
    c. foot
    c. hand

clubbed
    c. finger
    c. nail
    c. toe

clubfoot, club foot
    acquired c.
    arthrogrypotic c.
    circumferential release of c.
    c. deformity
    extrinsic c.
    intrinsic c.
    posteromedial release of c.
    c. release
    resistant c.
    c. splint

clubhand, club hand
    c. deformity
    radial c.
    ulnar c.

clumsy
    c. gait
    c. hand dysarthria
    c. hand syndrome

cluneal nerve

clunk
    catch-up c.
    c. shoulder test
    spontaneous wrist c.

Clutton joint

Clyburn
    C. Colles fracture fixator
    C. external fixator

Clyde Mood scale

CMAP
    compound muscle action potential
    compound muscle-motor action potential

CM-Band
    CM-B. 505N brace
    CM-B. silicone rubber brace

CMC
    CMC fusion
    CMC joint
    CMC splint

CME-MRI
    contrast medium-enhanced magnetic resonance imaging

CMI
    cell-mediated immunity

CMPS
    chronic musculoskeletal pain syndrome

CMRT
    chiropractic manipulative reflex
      technique
CMT
    Charcot-Marie-Tooth
    chiropractic manipulative therapy
    Contextual Memory Test
      CMT disease
      CMT Evaluation
CMW
      CMW bone cement
      CMW cement gun
C-nail flexible pediatric nail
cnemial
cnemis
cnemitis
CNS
    central nervous system
CO2
    carbon dioxide
    CO_2 powered gun system
COACH
    Choosing Outcomes and
      Accommodations for Children
coach's finger
coagulated plasma
coagulating forceps
coagulation
    c. disorder
    disseminated intravascular c.
      (DIC)
    c. factor
    c. necrosis
coagulative necrosis
coagulator
    ASSI c.
    bipolar c.
    Concept bipolar c.
    Malis CMC-II bipolar c.
    Polar-Mate c.
coalescence
coalition
    acquired tarsal c.
    bilateral talocalcaneal c.
    calcaneocuboid c.
    calcaneonavicular c.
    carpal c.
    cartilaginous c.
    complete c.
    congenital complete subtalar c.
    cubonavicular c.
    fibrous talocalcaneal c.
    c. formation
    incomplete c.
    interphalangeal c.
    lunatotriquetral c.
    Minaar classification of c.
    multiple tarsal c.'s
    naviculocuneiform c.

nonosseous tarsal c.
    c. of bone
    osseous c.
    subtalar c.
    talocalcaneal c.
    tarsal c.
    c. view
coapt
coaptation
    c. plate
    c. splint
coarse
    c. carbide cone bur
    c. olive bur
coast
    c. of California (smooth)
      border
    c. of Maine (irregular) border
coated
    c. implant
    c. prosthesis
coating
    aluminum oxide ceramic c.
    Biolox ceramic c.
    bone fixation surface c.
    cobalt-chrome powder c.
    DePuy total hip system with
      porous c.
    Porocoat porous c.
    porous c.
    sintering of cobalt-chrome powder c.
coat-sleeve amputation
coaxial needle electrode
Coballoy
    C. implant metal
    C. implant metal prosthesis
    C. twist drill
cobalt
    c. chrome
    c. implant
cobalt-based alloy
cobalt-chrome
    c.-c. alloy and polyethylene
      implant
    c.-c. powder coating
    c.-c. power sintering
cobalt-chromium
    c.-c. alloy
    c.-c. alloy prosthesis
    c.-c. head
    c.-c. implant
    ion-bombarded c.-c.
    smooth c.-c.
cobalt-chromium-molybdenum (Co-Cr-Mo)
cobalt-chromium-tungsten-nickel
  (Co-Cr-W-Ni)
Coban
    C. elastic dressing
    C. elastic wrap

Cobb
C. attachment for Albee-Compere fracture table
C. curette
C. gauge
C. method
C. osteotome
C. periosteal elevator
C. scoliosis measuring technique
C. scoliosis spinal curve angle
C. spinal gouge
C. syndrome
technique of C.
C. tibialis posterior tendon dysfunction procedure
cobbler's chest
Cobb-Webb
C.-W. angle of scoliosis
C.-W. method for measuring degree of curve in scoliosis
Coblation spinal surgery system
cobra
C. Master
c. retractor
cobra-design femoral component
cobra-head plate
Coccidioides immitis
coccidioidomycosis
coccyalgia, coccydynia, coccygodynia, coccyodynia
coccydynia (*var. of* coccyalgia)
coccygeal
c. bone
c. joint
c. sinus
c. spine
c. vertebra
coccygectomy
coccygerector
coccygodynia (*var. of* coccyalgia)
coccygotomy
coccyodynia (*var. of* coccyalgia)
coccyx fracture
cockade
c. image
c. image sign
cocked-half flap
Cocke maxillectomy
Cockett communicating perforating veins
cocking injury
Cocklin toe operation
cock-robin head tilt
cock-up
c.-u. arm splint
c.-u. deformity
c.-u. deformity of toe
c.-u. hand splint
c.-u. splint orthosis

c.-u. wrist splint
c.-u. wrist support
co-contraction
active muscle c.-c.
c.-c. exercise
Co-Cr-Mo
cobalt-chromium-molybdenum
Co-Cr-Mo alloy implant metal
Co-Cr-Mo alloy prosthesis
Co-Cr-Mo pin
Co-Cr-W-Ni
cobalt-chromium-tungsten-nickel
Co-Cr-W-Ni alloy implant metal
Co-Cr-W-Ni alloy prosthesis
codeine
acetaminophen and c.
aspirin and c.
butalbital compound and c.
Capital and C.
carisoprodol, aspirin, and c.
Empirin With C.
Fiorinal with C.
Phenaphen With C.
Tylenol With C.
codfish
c. deformity
c. vertebra
Codivilla
C. extension
C. operation
C. tendon lengthening
C. tendon lengthening technique
Codman
C. ACP system
C. anterior cervical plating system
C. bone tumor
C. classification
C. exercise
C. osteosarcoma radiological angle
C. saber-cut shoulder approach
C. sign
C. Ti-frame posterior fixation system
C. tumor-normal bone triangle
C. wire-passing drill
Codman-Kerrison laminectomy rongeur
Codoxy
coefficient of friction (COF)
Coe-pak
C.-p. paste
C.-p. paste adhesive
COF
coefficient of friction
Coffin-Lowry syndrome
Cofield
C. rotator cuff reconstruction technique
C. shoulder prosthesis
C. total shoulder system

CoFilm dressing
Co-Flex
  C.-F. dressing
  C.-F. self-adherent wrap
COG
  center of gravity
cogent
  C. light
  C. LightWear headlight
  C. XL illuminator
Co-Gesic
Cognex
cognitive
  C. Assessment of Minnesota (CAM)
  C. Performance Test (CPT)
cogwheel
  c. gait
  c. rigidity
  c. sign
Cohen
  C. periosteal elevator
  C. rongeur
cohesion
  glenohumeral joint c.
cohort
  C. anterior plate system
  C. bone brush
  C. bone screw
  C. spinal impactor
  c. study
COI
  combination of isotonics
coil
  circumferential dedicated knee c.
  multichannel pelvic phased-array c.
coin
  fracture en c.
Coker-Arnold collar
ColBenemid
colchicine and probenecid
Colclough laminectomy rongeur
cold
  c. abscess
  c. application
  c. chisel
  c. compressive dressing
  c. injury
  c. intolerance
  c. laser
  c. laser treatment
  c. pad
  c. pressor test
  c. rolled rod
  c. therapy
  c. weld
  wind c.

cold-curing polymer
Coldflo
  C. cold therapy
  C. cold therapy and sequential compression
Coldhot pack
cold-mold prosthesis
cold-weld
  c.-w. femoral ball
  c.-w. femoral prosthesis
Cole
  C. fracture frame
  C. hyperextension brace
  C. hyperextension frame
  C. operation
  C. orthopaedic surgical technique
  C. osteotomy
  C. osteotomy for midfoot deformity
  C. procedure
  C. tendon fixation
Coleman
  C. flatfoot technique
  C. lateral block test
  C. plasty
coli
  Escherichia c. (E. coli)
colinear alignment
colistin
collagen
  Avitene microfibrillar c.
  Bio-Oss c.
  bovine c.
  c. fiber
  microcrystalline c.
  c. scaffold
  c. skin dressing
  c. vascular disease (CVD)
collagenase
  Cordase injectable c.
collagen-based biomaterial
collagenous schwannoma
Collagraft bone graft matrix
collapse
  bone graft c.
  Charcot c.
  exercise-associated c.
  exercise-induced c.
  foot c.
  hindfoot-midfoot c.
  hyperthermic exercise-associated c.
  neuropathic c.
  scapholunate advanced c. (SLAC)
  scapholunate arthritis c. (SLAC)
  vertebral body c.
collapsible
  c. internal fixation device
  c. pin
collapsing pes planovalgus

C

collar
- c. and crown scissors
- c. and cuff
- Aspen cervical c.
- c. bone
- c. brace
- Bremer Halo Crown cervical c.
- calcar c.
- cervical c. (C-collar)
- Coker-Arnold c.
- Cowboy C.
- dynamization c.
- Exo-Static cervical c.
- Exo-Static neck c.
- foam c.
- Forrester-Brown c.
- Georgiade visor cervical c.
- hard c.
- Headmaster c.
- Houston halo traction cervical c.
- implant c.
- Lerman-Minerva c.
- Lewin c.
- MAC cervical c.
- Marlin cervical c.
- Mayo rigid cervical c.
- Mayo-Thomas c.
- Miami Acute cervical c.
- Miami J cervical c.
- molded Thomas c.
- myocervical c.
- periosteal bone c.
- Philadelphia cervical c.
- Philadelphia rigid c.
- pillow c.
- Plastazote cervical c.
- plastic c.
- Pneu-trac cervical c.
- 2 + 2 Rehab C.
- rigid c.
- Schanz c.
- serpentine foam c.
- soft c.
- Thomas c.
- Thomas rigid c.
- Tuxedo c.
- wire frame c.

collar-and-cuff sling

collar-button abscess

collar-calcar support femoral prosthesis

collared
- c. button
- c. femoral head
- c. press-fit femoral stem implantation

collarless
- collarless, polished, tapered (CPT)
- c. stem

collateral
- c. artery
- c. circulation
- c. fibular ligament
- c. ligament instability
- c. ligament laxity
- c. ligament rupture
- c. radial ligament
- c. tibial ligament
- c. ulnar ligament

collection
- epidural fluid c.
- multiloculated fluid c.

collectomy
- shortening c.

college
- C. Park TruStep foot
- C. Park TruStep foot prosthesis

Colles
- C. fascia
- C. fracture
- C. ligament
- C. splint

collet
- c. screwdriver adapter
- tibial c.

colli
- fibromatosis c.
- pterygium c.

collicular fracture

colliculi (*pl. of* colliculus)

colliculus, *pl.* **colliculi**
- posterior c.

Collier sign

collimation

collimator
- multileaf c.
- c. plugging pattern

Collin
- C. amputating knife
- C. osteoclast

Collins
- C. dynamometer
- C. rib shears

Collis
- C. broken femoral stem technique
- C. horizontal reaction
- C. horizontal suspension
- C. retractor
- C. TDR instrument
- C. vertical suspension

Collis-Dubrul femoral stem removal

collison
- C. body drill
- C. cannulated hand drill
- C. plate
- C. screw
- C. screwdriver
- C. tap drill

Collis-Taylor retractor
collodiaphysial
    c. angle
    central c.
collodion dressing
colloid solution
Colonna
    C. hip fracture classification
    C. shelf operation
    C. trochanteric arthroplasty
Colonna-Ralston
    C.-R. incision
    C.-R. medial ankle approach
color
    3 c. concept of wound classification
    digital c.
    c. duplex imaging
Colorado internal fixation system
color-coded therapy putty
colored antiseptic
Colpac
Colpacs pack
Coltart
    C. calcaneotibial fusion
    C. fracture
    C. fracture technique
Colton olecranon fracture classification
Columbia
    University of British C. (UBC)
Columbus
    C. McKinnon assist for lifting or transfer
    C. McKinnon Hugger device
3-column
    3-c. cervical spine injury
    3-c. concept
    3-c. spine
    3-c. spine theory
column
    anterior c.
    c. balance
    central c.
    contrast c.
    radial c.
    resistive weighed c.
    spinal c.
    ulnar c.
    vertebral c.
2-column cervical spine injury
comb
    toe c.
Combat Task Test
CombiDERM nonadhesive absorbent dressing
Combi Multi-Traction System
combination
    film-screen c.
    Isola spinal implant system plate-rod c.

jab, hook, punch, injury mechanism c.
    c. of isotonics (COI)
    c. of isotonics therapeutic exercise technique
combined
    c. ankle and knee motion gait determinant
    c. anterior and posterior approach
    c. anterior cavus
    c. cavus
    c. cavus deformity
    c. curve
    c. fixation device
    c. flexion-distraction injury and burst fracture
    c. flexion phenomenon
    C. Instabilities functional knee brace
    c. instability (CI)
    c. low cervical and transthoracic approach
    c. magnetic field system
    c. mechanical
    c. nerve palsy
    penicillin g benzathine and procaine c.
    c. radial-ulnar-humeral fractures
    c. resection arthroplasty and arthrodesis
    c. scintigraphy
    c. stenosis
Combunox
Comed postoperative shoe
Comet fragment
ComfAlign spinal support
Comfeel Ulcus occlusive dressing
Comforfoam splint
comfort
    C. Ag prosthetic sock
    C. Cast
    C. Cast stirrup
    C. Club tub pillow
    C. Cool neoprene support
    c. level
    C. n' Care Seamfree socks
    C. Rite footwear
    C. Take-Along wheelchair cushion
    C. wrist immobilizer
comforter
    C. Splint
    Thermo hand c.
    Thermo knee c.
Comf-Orthotic
    C.-O. 3/4-length insole
    C.-O. sports replacement insole
    C.-O. wool felt insole
Comfortseat
    Flo-Fit C.
Comfort-U total body pillow

ComfortWalk
 C. foot system
 C. prosthetic foot
comfy
 C. Elbow Orthosis
 C. elbow splint
 C. knee orthosis
 C. toilet lift seat
 C. walker
command
 C. hip instrumentation system
 C. instrument system surgical instrument
 C. joint replacement instrument system
comma sign
commemorative sign
comminuted
 c. burst fracture
 c. fracture
 c. intraarticular fracture
 c. pilon fracture
 c. teardrop fracture
comminution
 interposed c.
commissural myelorrhaphy
commissure
 anterior commissure-posterior c. (AC-PC)
committee
 Fitness Safety Standards C.
 International Knee Documentation C. (IKDC)
common
 c. carotid artery (CCA)
 c. digital nerve
 c. dural sac
 c. extensor tendon
 c. fibular nerve injury
 c. iliac artery (CIA)
 c. iliac vein
 c. peroneal nerve
 c. peroneal nerve block
 c. peroneal nerve paralysis
 c. peroneal nerve syndrome
commotio cordis
communicans, *pl.* **communicantes**
 gray ramus c.
communicantes (*pl. of* communicans)
communicating hydrosyringomyelia
communication
 asyndetic c.
communis
 extensor digitorum c. (EDC)
 flexor digitorum c. (FDC)
community
 C. Integration Questionnaire (CIQ)
 c. rehabilitation
Comolli sign

COMP
 cartilage oligomeric matrix protein
compact
 c. bone
 c. osteoma
compaction
 c. pliers
 vertical sacral c.
compactor
 acetabular cement c.
 cement c.
company
 Haynes Stellite C.
 3M C.
 Orthopedic Equipment C. (OEC)
 United States Manufacturing C. (USMC)
comparative radiographic examination
comparison
 Achilles tendon rupture repair c.
compartment
 anterior c.
 Clancy lateral c.
 deep posterior c.
 dorsal c.
 fascial c.
 c. fasciotomy
 interosseous c.
 lateral c.
 medial c.
 Mueller lateral c.
 osteofascial c.
 patellofemoral c.
 plantar c.
 posterior c.
 posterolateral c.
 posteromedial c.
 superficial posterior c.
 c. syndrome
compartmental
 C. II knee prosthesis
 c. pressure
4-compartment fasciotomy
compass
 C. hinge
 C. Hinge external fixator
 C. stereotactic system
Compazine
Compeed protective dressing
compensable accident
compensated
 c. metatarsus adductus
 c. talipes equinus
compensation reaction
compensatory
 c. basilar osteotomy
 c. behavior
 c. curve
 c. deformity

c. hypermobility
c. lordosis
c. movement
c. scoliosis
c. structural subluxation
c. wedge

Compere
C. fixation wire
C. lengthening
C. operation
C. osteotome
C. threaded pin

Compere-Thompson arthrodesis
Comperm tubular elastic bandage
competence, competency
mechanism of reflex immunologic c.
reflex immunologic c.

competency (*var. of* competence)
complement
complementary and alternative medicine
(CAM)
complete
c. amelia
c. amputation
c. aphalangia
c. coalition
c. dislocation
c. fracture
c. paraxial hemimelia
c. phocomelia
c. subtalar release (CSR)
c. syndactyly

complex
c. acetabular reconstruction
ankle joint c. (AJC)
apophysial c.
arcuate c.
atlantoaxial c.
atlas-axis c.
atlas vertebral subluxation c.
borotannic c.
Buford c.
bunion c.
bunionette-hallux valgus-splayfoot c.
bunion-hallux valgus c.
capsulolabral c.
capsuloligamentous c.
chondroitin/glucosamine sulfate c.
Edinger-Westphal c.
epiphysial c.
fabellofibular and arcuate
ligament c.
femur button graft c.
femur, fibula, ulna c.
FFU c.
fibrocartilage c.
foot-ankle c.
forearm c.
c. fracture

c. fracture dislocation
gastrocnemius-soleus c.
Ghon-Sachs c.
hallux valgus-metatarsus primus
varus c.
hindfoot joint c.
c. instability of carpus (CIC)
3-joint c.
knee c.
lateral quadruple c.
ligament-bone c.
ligamentous c.
Lisfranc joint c.
lumbopelvic c.
lymphedema c.
medial quadruple c.
c. meniscal tear
c. motor unit action potential
occipital-atlantoaxial c.
occipitoatlantoaxial joint c.
plantar capsuloligamentous c.
posterior ligamentous c. (PLC)
postural c.
quadruple c.
radial collateral ligament c.
(RCLC)
c. regional pain syndrome (CRPS)
c. regional pain syndrome 2
(CRPS 2)
c. regional pain syndrome (type I)
c. repetitive discharge
semimembranous c.
sensory nerve action potential
receptor c.
shoulder c.
c. skewfoot
SNARE c.
soleus c.
spinal cord-meningeal c.
spring ligament c.
c. syndactyly
talocalcaneonavicular c.
tibiocalcaneal joint c.
trialkylphosphine gold c.
triangular fibrocartilage c.
ulnar collateral ligament c.
(UCLC)
vertebral subluxation c. (VSC)
zygomatic-malar c. (ZMC)

compliant prestress system (CPS)
complicated
c. complex syndactyly
c. dislocation
c. fracture

complication
iatrogenic c.
intraoperative c.
neurologic c.
neurovascular c.

complication (*continued*)
    postoperative c.
    pulmonary c.
    urologic c.

component
    acetabular c.
    AcuMatch A, L, M Series
      acetabular c.
    AcuMatch L Series cemented
      femoral stem c.
    AML trial hip c.
    Amstutz femoral c.
    anatomically graduated c. (AGC)
    anatomic porous replacement
      hemispheric acetabular c.
    Aufranc-Turner femoral c.
    Bechtol acetabular c.
    Biomet MARS acetabular c.
    Biomet revision acetabular c.
    Biomet shoulder c.
    bipolar femoral c.
    bipolar hip arthroplasty c.
    Black Max mid size knee c.
    Bombelli-Morscher femoral c.
    cemented c.
    cementless femoral c.
    cerclaged c.
    chamfered cylinder acetabular c.
    Charnley flat-back femoral c.
    Charnley narrow-stem c.
    Charnley standard-stem c.
    cobra-design femoral c.
    custom-designed swan-neck
      femoral c.
    Definition PM femoral implant c.
    DePuy trispiked acetabular c.
    Duramer polyethylene c.
    Durasul prosthetic c.
    energy conservation walking c.
    failed acetabular c.
    femoral c.
    fluid controlled c.
    glenoid c.
    Gustilo-Kyle femoral c.
    Harris-Galante hip replacement
      acetabular c.
    Harris-Galante I porous-coated
      acetabular c.
    head-neck c.
    Healey revision acetabular c.
    Hoffmann II compact external
      fixation c.
    humeral c.
    hybrid fixation of hip
      replacement c.
    Infinity femoral c.
    internal rotary component of
      force c.
    keel of glenoid c.

    kinesiopathologic c.
    large-head humeral c.
    Lubinus acetabular c.
    MARS c.
    Meridian ST femoral implant c.
    metal-backed acetabular c.
    Metasul hip joint c.
    modular acetabular revision system
      acetabular c.
    modular hip implant c.
    modular large-head c.
    monoblock femoral c.
    Morse taper lock of modular hip
      implant c.
    neck c.
    Neer II humeral c.
    neuromuscular c.
    NexGen c.
    OEC lag screw c.
    c. of gait
    Ogee acetabular c.
    Osteolock acetabular c.
    Osteolock HA femoral c.
    Osteonics Omnifit-HA c.
    performance c.
    polyethylene liner implant c.
    porous cementless c.
    porous-coated c.
    posterior c.
    postural c.
    press-fit femoral c.
    Profix porous femoral c.
    progression walking c.
    prosthesis c.
    quadrant sparing acetabular c.
      (QSAC)
    Reliance CM femoral implant c.
    roof-reinforcement ring hip
      arthroplasty c.
    sensory c.
    short-range elastic c.
    Smith & Nephew reflection
      acetabular cup implant c.
    SPH contact acetabular c.
    Springlite G foot c.
    Springlite II foot c.
    S-ROM modular femoral c.
    standing stability walking c.
    stem c.
    sternal attachment c.
    Stockholm HAVS sensorineural c.
      (0SN, 1SN, 2SN, 3SN)
    straight stem femoral c.
    structural c.
    c. subsidence
    sympathetic c.
    Taperloc femoral c.
    tharies femoral resurfacing c.
    tharies hip c.

thoracic extension c.
Ti-Bac acetabular c.
tibial c.
c. trial
trial femoral c.
Tricon c.
Tricon-M c.
Ultima C femoral c.
uncemented femoral c.
universal radial c.
V40 femoral head implant c.
Vitalock cluster acetabular c.
Vitalock solid-back acetabular c.
wheel chair seating c.
Zimmer NexGen LPS knee
  femoral c.

composite
Carboplast II c.
c. defect
E-A-R Specialty C.'s
c. fracture
c. free tissue transfer
c. groin fascial free flap
c. joint
c. knee score
c. material
c. prosthetic foot
c. rib graft
c. skin graft
c. spring elastic splint
void metal c. (VMC)

composition
body c.

compound
c. comminuted fracture (CCF)
dihydrocodeine c.
c. dislocation
Hurler-Scheie c.
c. joint
c. mixed nerve action potential
c. motor nerve action potential
c. muscle action potential (CMAP)
c. muscle-motor action potential
  (CMAP)
c. nevus
OCT c.
Pediplast moldable footcare c.
pentazocine c.
photoactive naphthalimide c.
c. sensory nerve action potential
c. shattered elbow
Soma c.
Talwin c.

Compoz
C. Gel Caps
C. Nighttime Sleep Aid

compression
c. anesthesia
anterior cord c.

anterior-inferior c.
anterior-posterior c. (APC)
AO c.
c. apparatus
c. arthrodesis
axial c.
c. bandage
c. boot
carotid artery c.
cauda equina c.
Charnley c.
c. clicker
Coldflo cold therapy and sequential c.
cord c.
disc c.
discogenic c.
c. dressing
dynamic c.
elastic c.
c. fracture
c. garment
c. glove
c. Harrington instrumentation
Harrington rod instrumentation c.
c. hip screw
c. hook
c. inserter-extractor
c. instrumentation posterior construct
interfragmentary c.
intermittent impulse c.
intermittent pneumatic c.
ischemic c.
c. lag screw
lateral c.
c. load
c. loading
c. locking anchor
c. locking anchor with secondary
  purchase (CLASP)
lower nerve root c.
lower sacral nerve root c. (LSNRC)
median nerve c.
c. molding
napkin ring c.
nerve root c.
neuraxial c.
c. overload
c. paralysis
c. pattern
c. phenomenon
c. plate
c. plate fixation
plate-to-bone c.
c. plating
pneumatic pedal c.
c. pump
c. rod
c. rod treatment
c. screw-plate device

compression (*continued*)
    sequential c.
    c. sideplate
    c. sleeve
    c. sleeve shin splint
    snap-off c. (SOC)
    spinal cord c.
    c. spring
    static c.
    c. stockings
    c. strain
    c. syndrome
    c. technique
    c. test
    c. testing
    c. therapy
    c. ultrasonography
    c. ultrasound
    c. U-rod instrumentation
    vasopneumatic intermittent c.
    venous c.
    vertebral c.
    vertical c.
    c. wire
    c. wiring
compression-molded
    c.-m. ethylene vinyl acetate (CM EVA)
    c.-m. prosthesis
compression-plus-torque cervical injury
compressive
    c. centripetal wrapping
    c. extension
    c. flexion
    c. flexion injury
    c. hyperextension injury
    c. internal fixating device
    c. myelopathy
    c. neuropathy
compressor
    Adair screw c.
    screw c.
Comprifix
    C. active ankle support
    C. ankle splint
compromise
    nerve root c.
    c. osteotomy
    soft tissue c.
Compro Plus Knee support
Compton clavicle pin
Compudriver digital torque-meter
computed tomography (CT)
computer-aided
    c.-a. design/computer-aided manufacturing (CAD/CAM)
    c.-a. joint space analysis (CAJSA)
computer-assisted
    c.-a. carpal tunnel syndrome

    c.-a. design
    c.-a. design/computer-assisted manufacturing prosthesis
    c.-a. fluoroscopy
    c.-a. mechanical instrument adjusting
    c.-a. myelography (CAM)
    c.-a. orthopaedic surgery (CAOS)
    c.-a. percutaneous internal fixation
computerized
    c. adaptive testing
    c. axial tomography (CAT)
    c. dynamic posturography (CDP)
    c. gait analysis
    c. isokinetic dynamometer
    c. musculoskeletal analysis
Conaxial ankle prosthesis
concave
    c. articular surface
    c. loading socket
    c. rod
concave-surface reamer
concavity
    flexural c.
    glenoid c.
concavity-compression effect
concavoconcave
concavoconvex
concealed straight leg raising test
concentrate
    platelet c.
concentric
    c. bilateral isokinetic
    c. contraction
    c. function
    c. hip cup
    c. isokinetic leg press exercise
    c. lamella
    c. loading
    c. muscle action
    c. needle electrode
    c. reduction
    c. tear
    c. work
concept
    C. ablator
    C. arthroscopy power system
    C. beach chair shoulder positioning system
    C. bipolar coagulator
    C. cannula
    3-column c.
    C. CTS Relief Kit
    Eftekhar c.
    C. handheld cautery
    hinge axis c.
    C. II rowing ergometer
    juvenile hinge axis c.
    Klein-Vogelbach functional movement c.

one wound-one scar c.
C. 2-pin passer
C. Precise ACL guide system
C. rotator cuff repair system
C. self-compressing cannulated screw
   system
C. Sterling arthroscopy blade system
conceptual ability
concetric hip cup
concise
C. cementing sculp
C. compression hip screw
C. compression hip screw system
C. side plate
Conco elastic bandage
concomitant
concretion
concurrent force system
concussion
sideline assessment of c.
Standardized Assessment of C.
   (SAC)
concussor
condensing osteitis
condition
assessment for limiting c.
degenerative spine c.
diabetic foot ulcerative c.
dysvascular c.
limiting c.
postsurgical heel c.
sterile c.
tumorous c.
conditioner
Shuttle cardiomuscular c.
conditioning
aerobic c.
musculoskeletal evaluation,
   rehabilitation and c. (MERAC)
work c.
condom catheter
conduction
c. block
c. time
c. velocity
c. velocity test
volume c.
conductive Hydrogel wound dressing
conductor
Adson c.
Bailey c.
Bozzini light c.
light c.
conduit
Neurotube bioabsorbable nerve c.
condylar
c. angle
c. articulation
c. bolt

c. cartilage
c. compression fracture
c. cuff
c. defect
c. femoral fracture
c. implant
c. implant arthroplasty
c. plate
c. plateau angle (CPA)
press-fit c. (PFC)
c. screw fixation
c. split fracture
condyle
bifid c.
c. block
femoral c.
flare of c.
humeral c.
lateral femoral c.
lateral tibial c.
medial femoral c. (MFC)
medial humeral c.
medial/lateral femoral c.
occipital c.
odontoid c.
tibial c.
volar c.
condylectomy
DuVries phalangeal c.
DuVries plantar c.
phalangeal c.
plantar c.
condylocephalic (CC)
c. nail
c. nailing
condyloid
c. joint
c. process
condylotomy
cone
c. and socket bone
c. arthrodesis
c. bone biopsy
c. bur
c. checkers
cutting c.
hand c.
Posey Palm C.
prosthetic c.
C. ring curette
C. splint
stacking c.
C. suction biopsy curette
Cone-Barton skull traction tongs
coned-down view
configuration
activity c.
Cotrel-Dubousset hook claw c.
double cruciate c.

configuration (*continued*)
    spoke-wheel c.
    triangular base transverse bar c.
confinement
    wheelchair c.
confirmatory testing
confluent
confocal microscopy
Conform dressing
Conformer diabetic boot
confrontational test
congenita
    amyoplasia c.
    amyotonia c.
    arthrogryposis multiplex c.
    dyskeratosis c.
    fragilitas ossium c.
    luxatio coxae c.
    myotonia c.
    osteogenesis imperfecta c. (OIC)
    pachyonychia c.
    SED c.
    spondyloepiphysial dysplasia c.
congenital
    c. above-elbow amputation
    c. anomaly (CA)
    c. anular band
    c. aphalangia
    c. atlantoaxial instability
    c. atonic pseudoparalysis
    c. band syndrome
    c. bar
    c. below-elbow amputation
    c. clasped thumb
    c. complete subtalar coalition
    c. convex pes plano valgus
    c. dislocation of hip
    c. dysplasia of hip (CDH)
    c. dystrophy
    c. fibrous band
    c. fracture
    c. general fibromatosis
    c. hemivertebra
    c. hip dislocation
    c. hip dysplasia (CHD)
    c. hip subluxation
    c. hyperphosphatasemic skeletal
      dysplasia (CHSD)
    c. hypotonia
    c. intercalary limb absence
    c. kyphosis (I, II)
    c. laxity
    c. laxity of ligament
    c. limb deficiency
    c. limb disorder
    c. lymphedema
    c. metatarsus adductus
    c. myopathy
    c. myotonia

    c. nevus
    c. osteochondroma
    c. patella dislocation
    c. plexopathy
    c. posteromedial bowing
    c. predisposition
    c. pseudoarthritis
    c. radioulnar synostosis
    c. ring
    c. rocker-bottom flatfoot
    c. scapular elevation
    c. scoliosis
    c. spondylolisthesis
    c. stenosis
    c. talipes equinovarus
    c. terminal limb absence
    c. tibial deficiency
    c. tibial pseudarthrosis
    c. torticollis
    c. trigger digit
    c. trigger finger
    c. ulnar drift
    c. vertical talus (CVT)
    c. vertical talus foot deformity
    c. wry neck
congenitally short limb
congestion
    flap c.
    intraosseous vascular c.
congestive heart failure (CHF)
congruence
    c. angle
    joint c.
    patellofemoral c.
congruent
    c. articulation
    c. metatarsophalangeal joint
    c. reduction
congruity
    ball-and-socket c.
congruous cup-shaped reamer
conical
    c. bur
    c. nut wrench
    c. obturator
    c. reamer
conical-point wire
conjoined
    c. gastrocnemius soleus fascial
      slip
    c. lateral band
    c. tendons
conjugated linoleic acid
conjunct movement
Conley pin
connecting
    c. bolt
    c. cartilage
    c. plate

connection
        Martin-Gruber c.
        neuroendocrine-immune c.
        Riche-Cannieu c.
connective
        c. tissue
        c. tissue disease
        c. tissue massage (CTM)
        c. tissue plasticity
connector
        adjustable pedicle c.
        anchor c.
        domino spinal instrumentation c.
        intrinsic transverse c.
        longitudinal member to anchor c.
        longitudinal member to longitudinal
          member c.
        nonrigid c.
        pedicle c.
        tandem c.
        transverse c.
Conner
        C. Continuous Performance
        Test
        C. CPT
Con-Nex reamer
Connolly
        C. bone regeneration technique
        C. procedure
Conn operation
conoid
        c. ligament
        c. process
        c. tubercle
conoidal ankle prosthesis
conoideum
        ligamentum c.
        tuberculum c.
Conradi disease
Conradi-Hünermann syndrome
consecutive
        c. amputations
        c. dislocations
conservatism
        therapeutic c.
conservative
        c. management
        c. therapy
Conserve hip system
consideration
        return to play c.
consistency
        boggy c.
        doughy c.
console compression garment
consolidated graft
consolidation
        bony c.
        delayed c.

        fracture line c.
        premature c.
constancy
        form c.
constant
        C. and Murley shoulder scoring
          system
        c. direct current stimulator
        c. massive motion
        c. tension splint
constant-friction knee
**Constant-Murley shoulder assessment
  score**
constant-touch perception
ConstaVac
        C. autoreinfusion system
        C. drainage
constellation of clinical findings
constitutional stenosis
constrained
        c. ankle arthroplasty
        c. condylar knee
        c. hinged knee prosthesis
        c. nonhinged knee prosthesis
        c. shoulder arthroplasty
constriction
        c. band
        c. band syndrome
        hourglass c.
        c. ring
constrictive edema
construct
        all-screw c.
        anterior c.
        AO dynamic compression plate c.
        blade-plate c.
        compression instrumentation
          posterior c.
        disease c.
        double-rod c.
        Edwards modular system bridging
          sleeve c.
        Edwards modular system
          compression c.
        Edwards modular system
          distraction-lordosis c.
        Edwards modular system
          kyphoreduction c.
        Edwards modular system
          neutralization c.
        Edwards modular system rod
          sleeve c.
        Edwards modular system scoliosis c.
        Edwards modular system
          spondylar c.
        Edwards modular system standard
          sleeve c.
        Galveston-type rod c.
        hook-to-screw L4-S1 compression c.

construct (*continued*)
    iliosacral and iliac fixation c.
    interbody c.
    Ogden construct Ogden c.
    pedicle screw c.
    posterior c.
    rod-hook c.
    screw-to-screw compression c.
    segmental compression c.
    single-rod c.
    STALIF interbody c.
    translaminar facet screw c.
    triplane c.
    TSRH double-rod c.
    TSRH pedicle screw-laminar claw c.
    upper cervical spine anterior c.
    upper cervical spine posterior c.
    Wiltse system double-rod c.
    Wiltse system H c.
    Wiltse system single-rod c.
construction
    California welt c.
    corticocancellous c.
constructional ability
contact
    C. ArthroProbe
    first foot c. (FFC)
    first metatarsal c. (FMC)
    c. force
    c. healing
    c. laser delivery system
    last foot c. (LFC)
    c. manipulation
    manual c.
    c. point
    Richards maximum c. (RMC)
    c. shield
    C. SPH cups system
    c. splint
    standing knee bend PSIS-sacrum c.
    c. stress
contained
    c. disc herniation
    c. herniated disc
container
    Quickbox c.
containment bag
content
    bone mineral c. (BMC)
context
    performance c.
Contextual Memory Test (CMT)
contiguity
    amputation in c.
    spatial c.
contiguous
    c. articular surfaces
    c. vertebral structure
continua (*pl. of* continuum)

continuity
    amputation in c.
    neuroma in c.
    c. of bone
    synthesis of c.
continuous
    c. anatomical passive exerciser (CAPE)
    c. cryotherapy
    c. intravenous regional anesthesia (CIVRA)
    c. LVG
    c. mechanical traction
    c. passive motion (CPM)
    c. passive motion apparatus
    c. passive motion exerciser
    c. passive motion machine
    c. performance test (CPT)
    c. stimulation
    c. wave arthroscopy pump
continuum, *pl.* **continua**
    C. bipolar acetabular head
    C. elliptical acetabular cup
    C. hip stem
    C. knee system (CKS)
    C. knee system implant
    C. polyethylene acetabular cup
    C. P/S total knee
    C. total knee base plate
    C. unconstrained prosthesis
contour
    C. DF-80 total hip operation
    double hump c.
    C. internal prosthesis
    C. Meniscus Arrow bioresorbable repair system
    patellar c.
    polyethylene proximal brim in quadrilateral c.
    spinal c.
    Wiberg patellar c. (I-III)
contoured
    c. adduction trochanteric-controlled alignment method (CAT-CAM)
    c. anterior spinal plate (CASP)
    c. anterior spinal plate drill guide
    c. anterior spinal plate technique
    c. felt padding
    c. femoral stem
    c. T-plate plate
    c. washer
contract
contracted foot
contractile force curve
contractility
    muscle c.
contraction
    active c.
    concentric c.

detrusor c.
direct c.
eccentric c.
extrafusal fiber c.
c. fasciculation
isometric c.
isotonic c.
lengthening c.
maintained c.
maximal voluntary c. (MVC)
muscular c.
reflex muscular c.
repeated quick stretch superimposed
  upon an existing c. (RQS-SEC)
shortening c.
tetanic c.
c. tremor
c. type
volitional c.
contractor
Bailey-Gibbon rib c.
Bailey rib c.
Lemmon rib c.
rib c.
Sellors rib c.
contract-relax technique
contracture
abduction c.
Achilles tendon c.
acquired thumb flexion c.
acute ischemic c.
adduction c.
axillary c.
burn c.
clawfoot c.
c. deformity
digital c.
Dupuytren c.
equinus c.
established c.
c. exercise
extension c.
external rotation c.
fixed flexion c. (FFC)
flexion, abduction, external
  rotation c.
flexor digitorum longus tendon c.
flexor hallucis tendon c.
forearm c.
gastrocnemius-soleus c.
hip flexor c.
intrinsic c.
ischemic c.
knee c.
lumbrical intrinsic c.
metacarpophysial joint extension c.
muscle c.
opposition c.
paralytic c.

postpoliomyelitic c.
pronation c.
quadriceps c.
rectus femoris c.
retropatellar fat pad c.
rotational c.
shoulder c.
Skoog procedure for release of
  Dupuytren c.
soft tissue c.
spastic intrinsic c.
supination c.
valgus c.
varus c.
Volkmann c.
Volkmann ischemic c.
web c.
wrist c.
contrafissura
contraflexion brace
contraindication
stretching c.
contralateral
c. double vertical fracture
c. foot
c. hypoplastic/agenetic pedicle
c. pain
c. sign
c. spondylolysis
c. straight leg raising
c. straight leg raising test
contrast
c. agent
air c.
c. arthrography
c. bath (CB)
c. column
c. medium-enhanced magnetic
  resonance imaging (CME-MRI)
contrecoup
c. contusion
c. fracture
fracture by c.
c. injury
control
abnormal motor c. (AMC)
biomechanical c.
car hand c.
3D positional c.
Dupaco knee c.
evaluation, prediction, intervention,
  c. (EPIC)
exsanguination tourniquet c.
fluoroscopic c.
habitual c.
hierarchical c.
hip joint aspiration under
  fluoroscopic c.
maximum c.

C

control (*continued*)
    monitored anesthesia c. (MAC)
    motion c. (MC)
    nudge c.
    postural c.
    pronation c.
    pronation/spring c.
    rotary c.
    somatosensory postural c.
    swing-phase c.
    Total Environment C. (TEC)
    tourniquet c.
    trunk c.
    verticality c.
    vestibular balance c.
    vestibular postural c.
    visual postural c.
    voluntary c.
controlled
    c. ankle motion (CAM)
    c. ankle walker
    c. comminuted fracture
    c. disc stimulation (CDS)
    c. force application
    c. position brace (CPB)
    c. range of motion (CRM)
    c. rotational osteotomy
controlled-motion brace
controller
    shoulder c.
    C. shoulder orthosis
contusion
    chest c.
    contrecoup c.
    coup c.
    cuff c.
    hip pointer c.
    muscle c.
    osteochondral c.
    pelvic region c.
    quadriceps c.
    rib c.
    rotator cuff c.
    shoulder strap c.
    spinal c.
conus medullaris syndrome
ConvaDERM Plus dressing
conventional
    c. cutting needle
    c. osteosarcoma
    c. silicone elastomer (CSE)
    c. single-axis knee
      prosthesis
    c. technique
    c. tomography
convergence
    angle of c.
    c. facilitation
    c. projection

converse
    C. chisel
    C. periosteal elevator
    C. splint
conversion
    Tilt-In-Space wheelchair c.
Convery polyarticular disability index
convex
    c. condylar-implant
      arthroplasty
    c. fusion
    c. pes valgus
    c. rasp
    c. rod
    c. saddle frame
convexity
    distal ulnar c.
    left lumbar c.
    c. of spine
    ulnar c.
convoluted bone
convolution
    Broca c.
Conyers technique
cookbook stimulation of acupuncture points
Cook-Gordon mechanism
cookie
    arch c.
    c. cutter
    Gelfoam c.
    metatarsal c.
    navicular shoe c.
    scaphoid shoe c.
    shoe c.
Cooksey-Cawthorne exercise
Cook walking brace
cool
    c. CPB brace
    c. IROM splint
    c. pack
    c. pack cryotherapy
Cool-Aid continuous controlled cold therapy
Cooley
    C. graft clamp
    C. iliac clamp
    C. multipurpose angled clamp
    C. multipurpose curved
      clamp
    C. rib retractor
    C. rib shears
Cooley-Baumgarten wire twister
Cool-Flex A/K suspension belt
cooling machine
CoolSorb absorbent cold transfer dressing
Coombs bone biopsy system

Coonrad
    C. hinged arthroplasty
    C. semiconstrained elbow prosthesis
    C. total elbow arthroplasty
Coonrad-Bugg
    C.-B. posterior tibial tendon trapping
    C.-B. posterior tibial tendon
      trapping and interposition of soft
      tissue
Coonrad-Morrey
    C.-M. hinged elbow implant
    C.-M. sloppy hinge elbow prosthesis
    C.-M. total elbow arthroplasty
Coonse-Adams
    C.-A. knee approach
    C.-A. quadricepsplasty
    C.-A. V-Y quadriceps turndown
      knee technique
Cooper ankle brace
Coopercare Lastrap support wrap
Coopernail sign
Coopervision irrigation/aspiration
  handpiece
Coordinate complete revision knee
  system
coordinated mobility
coordination
    joint c.
    muscular c.
Copeland-Howard
    C.-H. scapulothoracic fusion
    C.-H. shoulder procedure
Copeland humeral resurfacing head
Copeland-Kavat metatarsophalangeal
  dislocation classification
Coping Strategies Questionnaire (CSQ)
coplaning
    arthroscopic c.
COPM
    Canadian Occupational Performance
    Measure
copolymer
    c. ankle-foot orthosis
    c. foam
    LactoSorb resorbable c.
    c. orthotic material
    c. starch copolymer bead
copper
    c. deficiency syndrome
    c. mallet
copropraxia
coracoacromial
    c. arch
    c. ligament (CAL)
    c. ligament transfer
    c. process
coracobrachialis
    biceps, brachialis, c. (BBC)
coracobrachial muscle

coracoclavicular
    c. arthrodesis
    c. articulation
    c. distance
    c. fixation apparatus
    c. joint
    c. ligament
    c. screw
    c. screw fixation
    c. suture fixation
    c. technique
coracohumeral (CH)
    c. ligament
coracoid
    c. fracture
    c. impingement syndrome
    c. notch
    c. process
    c. tip avulsion
    c. tuberosity
coracoiditis
coracoplasty
coracoradialis
Coraderm dressing
Corail
    C. HA-coated stem
    C. HA-coated stem hip implant
    C. hip system
    C. press-fit prosthesis
coral
    madreporic c.
coralline
    c. hydroxyapatite
    c. hydroxyapatite *Goniopora*
      (CHAG)
Corbett bone rongeur
cord
    anterior horn of spinal c.
    central c.
    cervical spinal c.
    c. compression
    digital c.
    heel c.
    lateral c.
    MGHL c.
    middle glenohumeral ligament c.
    natatory c.
    c. portion
    pretendinous c.
    retrovascular c.
    space available for c.
    spinal c.
    tenodesis of heel c.
    tethered spinal c.
    vocal c.
Cordase injectable collagenase
cordate, cordiform
    c. pelvis
cordiform (*var. of* cordate)

C

cordis
    commotio c.
    C. implantable drug reservoir device
cordlike structure
Cordon-Colles fracture splint
cordotomy
cord-traction syndrome
corduroy cloth pattern
core
    c. biopsy obturator
    bone c.
    c. decompression
    c. decompression of femoral head
    c. drilling procedure
    C. Hibak Rest
    C. Lobak Rest
    C. Max-Relax Cushion
    c. needle biopsy
    C. Reflex wrist support
    C. Sitback Rest
    C. Slimrest
    c. suture
    C. Universal elastic knee support
    C. Universal elbow support
    C. Universal rib support
Corfit System 7000 Series Lumbosacral Support
coring
    c. apparatus
    c. device
Corin hip arthroplasty system
cork
    c. borer
    sheet c.
corkscrew
    c. femoral head extractor
    c. lasso device
    C. Parachute
    C. rotator cuff repair system
    C. suture anchor
Cormet hip resurfacing system
corn
    apical c.
    end c.
    hard c.
    interdigital c.
    Lister c.
    neurovascular c.
    plantar c.
    soft c.
    web c.
Cornelia de Lange syndrome (CdLS)
corner
    c. fracture
    c. fragment
    c. of knee
    posteromedial c.
3-cornered bone
4-corner midcarpal fusion

corneum
    stratum c.
cornuate navicular
cornuradicular zone
Cornwall hip fracture study
Coromega dietary supplement
coronal
    c. computed tomographic arthrography (CCTA)
    c. plane
    c. plane correction
    c. plane deformity
    c. plane deformity sagittal translation
    c. split fracture
    c. tilting
    c. T1-weighted sequence
coronary
    c. artery disease (CAD)
    c. ligament
    c. ligament strain
coronoid
    c. fragment
    c. line
    c. osteophyte
    c. process
    c. process fracture
corpectomy
    anterior c.
    cervical c.
    c. model
    vertebral body c.
corporation
    Accurate Surgical and Scientific Instruments C. (ASSI)
corporectomy
corporotransverse
    c. inferior ligament
    c. superior ligament
correction
    adult flatfoot c.
    anterior c.
    Beckenbaugh c.
    chevron hallux valgus c.
    child's flatfoot c.
    Chrisman-Snook c.
    coronal plane c.
    cubitus varus c.
    curvature c.
    frontal plane c.
    hallux varus c.
    hammertoe c.
    King scoliosis curve posterior c. (I-V)
    kyphosis c.
    Lapidus-type c.
    loss of c.
    mechanism of c.
    neuromechanical c.

c. of dislocated second
  metatarsophalangeal joint
c. of peroneal tendon instability
phalangeal malunion c.
rotational c.
Ruiz-Mora c.
scoliosis c.
somatovisceral c.
Steel pelvic c.
translational c.
V-Y plasty c.

corrective
c. cast
c. lengthening osteotomy
c. orthosis
c. shoe
c. soft dressing
c. spinal care
c. therapy

corrodens
Eikenella c.

corrosion
crevice c.
fretting c.
metal implant c.

corrugated reamer
corrugator muscle
corset, corsette
Boston soft c.
Camp c.
Campbell c.
dorsal lumbar c.
elastic ankle c.
c. front
Hoke lumbar c.
Kampe c.
leather ankle c.
lumbodorsal support c.
lumbosacral c.
soft c.
surgical c.
c. suspension
thigh c.
thoracolumbar c.
Warm 'n' Form lumbosacral c.

corsette (*var. of* corset)
Cort
S-T C.
Cortef
cortex, *pl.* **cortices**
adrenal c. (AC)
articular c.
femoral c.
lateral c.
c. screw
vertebral body anterior c.

cortical
c. ASIF screw
c. atrophy

c. bone
c. bone graft
c. bone modeling
c. bone primary canal
c. bone remodeling
c. bone screw
c. breach
c. cancellous allograft
  plug
c. cancellous screw
c. débridement
c. defect
c. desmoid
c. desmoid tumor
c. destruction
c. fibrous dysplasia
c. fracture
c. fragment
c. index
c. lucency
c. perforation
c. pin
c. plasticity
c. plate
c. ring sign
c. step drill
c. strut graft
c. thickening
c. thickness
c. thumb
c. window
c. windowing

corticalization
cortices (*pl. of* cortex)
corticocancellous
c. bone
c. bone graft
c. bone strip
c. chip graft
c. construction
c. plug

corticospinal
c. tract
c. tract cord injury

corticosteroid
depot c.
c. injection
postoperative c.
c. therapy

corticosteroid-induced avascular
necrosis
corticotomy
DeBastiani c.
Ilizarov c.
c. of proximal tibia
percutaneous c.

corticotropin
cortisol
cortisone injection

Cortisporin
    C. topical cream
    C. topical ointment
Cortone Acetate
Cortoss bone void filler
**corundum ceramic implant
  material**
Coryllos rasp
Corynebacterium
Cosmegen
cosmesis
    foot c.
    poor c.
    scarring c.
cosmetically acceptable foot
Cosmolon closure for splint
costal
    c. angle
    c. bone
    c. cartilage
    c. notch
    c. periosteotome
costalgia
costectomy
Costen syndrome
costocentral articulation
costochondral
    c. joint
    c. junction of ribs
costochondritis
costoclavicular
    c. ligament (CCL)
    c. maneuver
    c. space
    c. syndrome (CCS)
    c. syndrome test
costocoracoid
costogenic
costoinferior
costolumbar angle
costophrenic angle
costopleural
costoscapular
costoscapularis
costosternal
    c. angle
    c. articulation
    c. syndrome
costosternoplasty
costotransversarium
costotransverse
    c. joint
    c. ligament
costotransversectomy
    c. approach
    c. for tumor of spine
    Seddon dorsal
      spine c.
    c. technique

costovertebral
    c. angle (CVA)
    c. angle tenderness (CVAT)
    c. articulation
    c. joint
costoxiphoid
cot
    finger c.
Cotrel
    C. pedicle screw
    C. pedicle screw fixation
      strength
    C. pedicle screw rigidity
    C. scoliosis cast
    C. traction
Cotrel-Dubousset (C-D)
    C.-D. derotation operation
    C.-D. dynamic transverse traction
      device
    C.-D. hook
    C.-D. hook claw configuration
    C.-D. hook-rod
    C.-D. pedicle screw instrumentation
    C.-D. rod
    C.-D. rod flexibility
    C.-D. spinal instrument
Cotting ingrown nail procedure
Cottle
    C. chisel
    C. mallet
    C. osteotome
    C. rasp
    C. saw
cotton
    C. ankle fracture
    C. ankle instability test
    c. ball appearance
    c. bolster
    c. cast
    c. cast padding
    c. dressing
    c. elastic bandage (CEB)
    c. elbow reduction
    C. fibular bone hook test
    C. procedure
    C. reduction of elbow dislocation
    c. roll
    c. sheet wadding
    c. suture
cotton-loader position
cottonoid patty
cotton-wool sign
cotyloid
    c. cavity
    c. notch
cotyloplasty technique
cotylosacral
couch
    CyberKnife treatment c.

cough
- c. fracture
- c. test

Coumadin

council
- Medical Research C. (MRC)

counseling, counselling
- rehabilitation c. (RC)

counselling (*var. of* counseling)

count
- instrument, sponge, needle c.
- lymphocyte c.
- platelet c.
- white blood cell c. (WBC)

counter
- extended medial shoe c.
- heel c.
- c. nutation
- c. rotating saw
- C. Rotation System (CRS)
- C. Rotation System brace

counterbalance

counterclockwise (CCW)

counterextension

counterforce strap

counterrotational splint

countersinking osteotomy

countersink screw head

counterstrain technique

countersunk

countertraction splint

counterweight

Count'R-Force arch brace

coup contusion

coupled
- c. discharge
- c. motion

coupler
- Ferrier c.

coupling
- capacitive c.
- ceramic-on-ceramic c.

Couvelaire incision

Covaderm Plus adhesive barrier dressing

Coventry
- C. distal femoral osteotomy
- C. proximal tibial osteotomy
- C. screw
- C. staple
- C. vagal osteotomy

cover
- Accu-Flo polyethylene bur hole c.
- Accu-Flo silicone rubber bur hole c.
- AquaShield orthopaedic cast c.
- AquaShield reusable cast c.
- cast c.
- Overcast cast c.

ShowerSafe waterproof cast and bandage c.
- soft cosmetic c.
- Springlite polyolefin BK c.
- Springlite polyurethane AK, BK conical c.

coverage
- skin c.
- soft tissue c.

covering
- Cast Cozy toe c.
- epineural c.
- fascial sheath c.

Coverlet
- C. adhesive
- C. adhesive surgical dressing
- C. Strips wound dressing

Cover-Roll
- C.-R. adhesive gauze dressing
- C.-R. gauze
- C.-R. gauze adhesive
- C.-R. stretch bandage

Covertell composite secondary dressing

Cowboy Collar

Cowden syndrome

cowhorn brace

Co-Wrap dressing

coxa, *pl.* **coxae**
- c. adducta
- c. magna
- os c.
- c. plana
- c. senilis
- c. valga
- c. vara
- c. vara luxans

coxae (*pl. of* coxa)

coxal bone

coxalgia

coxalgic pelvis

coxankylometer

coxarthria

coxarthritis

coxarthrocace

coxarthropathy
- Postel c.

coxarthrosis
- end-stage c.

Cox flexion-distraction technique

coxitic scoliosis

coxitis

coxodynia

coxofemoral
- c. articulation
- c. joint

coxotomy

coxotuberculosis

C

Cozen
>C. elbow dislocation test
>C. transverse talonavicular fusion approach

Cozen-Brockway Z-plasty
cozy
>Cast C.

CP
>chondrodysplasia punctata

CPA
>calcaneal pitch angle
>condylar plateau angle

CPB
>controlled position brace

CPDD
>calcium pyrophosphate dihydrate deposition
>calcium pyrophosphate dihydrate deposition disease

CP2 inflatable cold pack
CPM
>continuous passive motion
>>AIM CPM
>>CPM apparatus
>>CPM device
>>CPM exerciser machine

CPPD
>calcium pyrophosphate dihydrate deposition disease

CPS
>compliant prestress system

CPT
>Cognitive Performance Test
>collarless, polished, tapered
>continuous performance test
>cutaneous pressure threshold
>>Conner CPT
>>CPT hip system
>>CPT prosthesis

Cr
>chromium

crab gait
crabmeatlike appearance
Cracchiolo
>C. forefoot arthroplasty
>C. hallux limitus implant arthroplasty procedure

Cracchiolo-Sculco implant arthroplasty
crack
>c. fracture
>hairline c.

cracking
>environmental stress c.
>c. of joint
>stress-corrosion c.

cradle
>c. arm sling
>bed c.
>Posey bed c.

Crafoord thoracic scissors
Craig
>C. abduction splint
>C. Handicap Assessment and Reporting Technique (CHART)
>C. hip test
>C. pin
>C. pin remover
>C. vertebral biopsy set

Craig-Scott orthosis
cram
>C. bowstring sign
>c. sciatic nerve root pressure test

Cramer wire splint
cramp
>c. discharge
>heat c.
>muscle c.
>muscular c.
>writer's c. (WC)

cramping
>heat c.

crane
>C. mallet
>C. osteotome
>C. shoulder exercise

cranial, cranialis
>c. bone
>c. compensatory curve
>c. defect
>c. electrical stimulation (CES)
>c. helmet
>c. Jacobs hook
>c. nerve abnormality
>c. remolding
>c. remolding helmet
>c. remolding orthosis
>c. tongs
>c. vault remodeling

cranialis (*var. of* cranial)
cranial-sacral respiratory mechanism (CSRM)
cranioacromial
craniocaudal glide
craniocervical plate
craniofacial
>c. angle
>c. dysjunction fracture

craniomandibular
>c. dysfunction
>c. joint

craniopagus twins
craniosacral
>c. table
>c. theory
>c. therapy (CST)
>c. therapy technique

craniospinal trauma
craniosynostosis

craniotabes
craniovertebral junction
crank
    c. frame retractor
    c. shoulder test
    c. table
crankshaft phenomenon
crash induction of anesthesia
craterization
cravat bandage
Crawford
    C. head frame
    C. incision
    C. low lithotomy crutch
    C. L-shaped osteotomy
Crawford-Adams
    C.-A. acetabular cup
    C.-A. acetabular cup arthroplasty
crawl
    barrel c.
crazy bone
C-reactive protein (CRP)
creaking
    alar c.
    back c.
    distal medial c.
    flexion c.
    infragluteal c.
    metatarsophalangeal c.
    palmar c.
    PIP flexion c.
    popliteal flexion c.
    skin c.
    thenar c.
    ulnar c.
    wrist c.
cream, creme
    AmLactin c.
    BeneJoint analgesic c.
    capsaicin topical c.
    Cortisporin topical c.
    Diapedic foot c.
    DSC Foot C.
    Free-Up massage c.
    ibuprofen c.
    Lamisil C.
    Lotrimin AF c.
    massage c.
    Maximum Strength Desenex
      Antifungal C.
    Naftin c.
    Neosporin C.
    Noritate C.
    Oxistat c.
    Prevacare moisturizing c.
    terbinafine hydrochloride c.
    Thera-Gesic c.
    Ureacin-20 c.
    Vita ADE c.

crease
    alar c.
    back c.
    distal palmar c. (DPC)
    flexor skin c.
    infragluteal c.
    metatarsophalangeal c.
    palmar c.
    popliteal c.
    skin c.
    thenar palmar c. (TPC)
creatine phosphokinase
creation
    kyphosis c.
    lordosis c.
Creative diabetic socks
Credo operation
Creed dissector
creep
    c. test
    transient compressive c.
    viscoelastic c.
    webspace c.
creeping
    c. palsy
    c. substitution
Crego
    C. elevator
    C. femoral osteotomy
    C. hip reduction
    C. periosteal elevator
    C. retractor
    C. tendon transfer technique
cremasteric reflex
creme (*var. of* cream)
    Aloe Grande c.
    Fungoid C.
    Hydrisinol c.
    Lactinol-E c.
    Ureacin-20 c.
crepitans
    peritendinitis c.
    tenalgia c.
    tenosynovitis c.
crepitant
crepitation
    patellofemoral c.
    Rice Krispies c.
crepitus
    articular c.
    bony c.
crescent
    C. Complete Sleeper pillow
    C. memory pillow
    c. sign
crescentic
    c. base wedge osteotomy
    c. base wedge
      osteotomy/bunionectomy

C

crescentic (*continued*)
    c. basilar first metatarsal osteotomy
    c. calcaneal osteotomy
    c. rupture
    c. saw
    c. shelf osteotomy (CSO)
Crescent-Pillo pillow
crescent-shaped
    c.-s. fibrocartilaginous disc
    c.-s. osteotomy
CREST
    calcinosis, Raynaud, esophageal
    motility disorders, sclerodactyly,
    telangiectasia
    CREST syndrome
crest
    c. buttress pad
    iliac c.
    Maquet elevation of tibial c.
    neural c.
    palpation of iliac c.
    c. sign
    c. sign side
    tibial c.
    toe c.
cretinism
crevice corrosion
crick in neck
cricoid
    c. cartilage
    c. ring
cricopharyngeal sphincter muscle
cricothyroid membrane
Crile
    C. forceps
    C. gasserian ganglion knife and
    dissector
    C. head traction
    C. hemostat
    C. knife
Crile-Wood needle holder
crimped Dacron prosthesis
crimper
    Caparosa wire c.
    pin c.
    Simmons c.
    washer c.
    wire c.
crippled
crisis
    bone c.
crispation
criteria (*pl. of* criterion)
criterion, *pl.* **criteria**
Criticaid lotion
critical
    c. limb ischemia (CLI)
    c. load
    c. pathway

CRM
    controlled range of motion
    CRM cup
    CRM rehab brace
    CRM stem
    CRM system
crochet
    main en c.
crocodile forceps
CROM
    cervical range of motion
Crosby calcaneal fracture
  reduction
cross
    c. bar
    c. friction
    c. leg pain
cross-arm flap
CrossBar thoracolumbar fusion posterior
  fixation link
cross-bracing, crossbracing
    spinal rod c.-b.
crossbracing (*var. of* cross-bracing)
crosscut
    c. bur
    c. saw
crossed
    c. adductor reflex
    c. extensor reflex
    c. flexor reflex
    c. intrinsic transfer
    c. Kirschner wire
    c. straight leg raise
    c. straight leg raise test
    c. straight leg raising
    (CSLR)
crossed-leg pike down stretch
cross-extremity flap
cross-finger flap
cross-friction massage
crosshead displacement
crossing
    nerve c.
    c. screws
cross-leg (*var. of* crossleg)
crossleg, cross-leg
    c. flap
    c. Patrick maneuver
cross-legged gait
crosslink
    Edwards modular system rod c.
    free pyridinium c.
    Galveston fixation with TSRH c.
    c. plate
    c. plate size
    pyridinium collagen c. (PYD)
    TSRH c.
crosslinked EVA copolymer foam
cross-locking screw

crossover
c. impingement of shoulder test
c. second toe
c. syndrome
crossover-toe deformity
cross-screw fixation
cross-sectional anatomy
cross-slot screwdriver
cross-table
c.-t. lateral radiograph
c.-t. lateral view (CTLV)
crossunion
crotch strap
crouch gait
Crouzon syndrome
CROW
Charcot restraint orthotic walker
crowded carpal sign
Crowe
C. congenital hip dysplasia classification
C. congenital hip dysplasia classification system
C. congenital hip dysplasia (I-IV)
C. hip scale
C. pilot point
C. pilot point on Steinmann pin
C. subluxation
C. tip pin
crown
Adaptic c.
c. and collar scissors
c. drill
c. drill screw
Unitek steel c.
CRP
C-reactive protein
CRPS
complex regional pain syndrome
CRS
Counter Rotation System
CRS brace
CRS Tibial Torsion System
CRT
capillary refill time
crucial angle of Gissane
cruciate
anterior c.
c. condylar knee system
c. condylar unconstrained prosthesis
c. fashion
c. head bone screw
c. incision
c. ligament
c. ligament laxity
c. ligament reconstruction
c. ligament rupture
c. paralysis
posterior c.

c. pulley
c. punch
cruciate-retaining prosthesis
cruciate-sacrificing prosthesis
cruciform
c. anterior spinal hyperextension (CASH)
c. anterior spinal hyperextension orthosis
c. head bone screw
c. screwdriver
c. tibial base plate
cruiser
c. buggy
C. hip abduction
C. hip abduction brace
C. OA brace
crunch
Grafton DBM C.
crural fascia
cruris
angina c.
tinea c.
crush
c. fracture
c. injury
c. syndrome
crushed eggshell fracture
crushing osteochondritis
crutch
c. ambulation
c. and belt femoral closed nail
c. and belt femoral closed nailing
axillary c.
Canadian c.
Crawford low lithotomy c.
EuroCuff forearm c.
hands-free c.
Hardy aluminum c.
iWALKfree hands-free c.
Lofstrand c.
c. palsy
c. paralysis
platform c.
c. walking
weightbearing c.
Crutchfield
C. bone drill
C. drill point
C. hand drill
C. operation
C. pin
C. skeletal tong traction
Crutchfield-Raney
C.-R. cervical traction tongs
C.-R. drill
Cruveilhier
C. atrophy
C. disease

C

Cruveilhier (*continued*)
  C. joint
  C. ligament
  C. paralysis
cryoanalgesia
Cryo/Cuff
  Aircast C./C.
  C./C. ankle dressing
  C./C. boot
  C./C. compression support
  C./C. Knee Compression Dressing
  System
Cryocup ice massager
cryogenic
  c. denervation
  c. neuroablation
cryokinetics
cryopreserved cartilage
cryosurgery
cryotherapy
  continuous c.
  cool pack c.
  liquid nitrogen c.
  c. rehabilitation
  verruca c.
cryptococcal infection
cryptococcosis
Cryptococcus neoformans
cryptopodia
cryptotic medial border
cry reflex
crystal
  C. adjusting table
  calcium hydroxyapatite c.
  CHA c.
  c. deposition
  monosodium urate c. (MSU)
  C. polymer gel
  uric acid c.
crystal-induced
  c.-i. arthritis
  c.-i. arthropathy
  c.-i. arthrosis
  c.-i. synovitis
crystalloid solution
crystal-related
  c.-r. arthropathy
  c.-r. joint disease
CS
  cerebrospinal
  chemical sympathectomy
CSE
  conventional silicone
  elastomer
CSF
  cerebrospinal fluid
C-shaped
  C-s. foot
  C-s. plate

CSI
  Caregiver Strain Index
CSLR
  crossed straight leg raising
CSM
  cervical spondylotic myelopathy
CSMT
  capillary refill, sensation, motor
  function, temperature
CSO
  crescentic shelf osteotomy
C-spine
  cervical spine
CSQ
  Coping Strategies Questionnaire
CSR
  complete subtalar release
  McKay-Simons CSR
CSRA
  cementless surface replacement
  arthroplasty
CSRM
  cranial-sacral respiratory
  mechanism
CST
  craniosacral therapy
CT
  carpal tunnel
  cervicothoracic
  chest tube
  computed tomography
  CT bone densitometer
  CT scan
  spiral CT
CTA
  cuff tear arthropathy
**CT-based CAD/CAM revision femoral
  implant**
CTD
  carpal tunnel decompression
  cumulative trauma disorder
CTE
  chronic traumatic encephalopathy
C-Tek anterior cervical plate system
C-telopeptide
**CT-guided percutaneous screw placement
  for sacroiliac joint**
CTi brace
CTi2 knee brace
CTLSO
  cervicothoracolumbosacral
  orthosis
CTLV
  cross-table lateral view
CTM
  connective tissue massage
CTO
  cervicothoracic orthosis
  Aspen CTO

CTR
    carpal tunnel release
CTS
    carpal tunnel syndrome
    Champion trauma score
        CTS gauge
        CTS Gripfit splint
CTSIB
    Clinical Test of Sensory Integration and Balance
Cubbins
    C. arthroplasty
    C. bone screwdriver
    C. incision
    C. open shoulder reduction
    C. operation
    C. screw
    C. shoulder approach
    C. shoulder dislocation technique
cube
    Temper Foam c.
CUBEx multifunctional step
cubital
    c. bursitis
    c. fossa syndrome
    c. joint
    c. nerve
    c. process
    c. tunnel
    c. tunnel splint
    c. tunnel syndrome
cubiti (*gen.* and *pl. of* cubitus)
cubitocarpal
cubitoradial
cubitus, *gen.* and *pl.* **cubiti**
    patella c.
    c. recurvatum
    c. valgus
    c. varus
    c. varus correction
cuboid, cuboidal
    c. abduction angle
    c. bone
    c. decancellation
    c. declination angle
    c. fracture
    c. fusion
    c. notch
    c. sulcus
    c. syndrome
    c. wedge osteotomy
cuboidal (*var. of* cuboid)
    c. tuberosity
cuboid-calcaneal osteotomy
cuboideonavicular ligament
cubonavicular
    c. coalition
    c. joint

Cuda shaver
cuff
    arm c.
    collar and c.
    condylar c.
    c. contusion
    hand c.
    joint distraction c.
    leather c.
    C. Link orthopaedic device
    musculotendinous c.
    c. of fascia
    pneumatic tourniquet c.
    push c.
    Push-Ease Quad C.
    c. resection
    rotator c.
    shoulder c.
    Steri-Cuff disposable tourniquet c.
    supracondylar c.
    suprapatellar c.
    c. suspension
    c. tear arthropathy (CTA)
    c. tear arthroplasty
    thigh c.
    Western Ontario Rotator C. (WORC)
cuing strategy
cul-de-sac of Bruger
Culler hook
Culley ulnar splint
culture
    bacterial c.
    blood c.
    DTM c.
    urine c.
    wound c.
Cummins procedure
cumulative trauma disorder (CTD)
cuneiform
    atavistic c.
    c. bone
    c. fracture
    c. injury
    c. joint
    c. joint arthrodesis
    c. mortise
    c. osteotomy
cuneiform-first metatarsal exostosis
cuneocuboid
cuneometatarsal joint
cuneonavicular
    c. joint
    c. ligament
cuneoscaphoid
Cuniard and Campell technique
cuniculatum
    epithelioma c.
Cunningham brace

cup

AccuPressure heel c.
acetabular c.
c. and cone method
Anti-Shox heel c.
c. arthroplasty
Arthropor acetabular c.
Aufranc modification of
  Smith-Petersen c.
Aufranc-Turner acetabular c.
Bauerfeind SofSpot Heel C.
Bicon-Plus C.
Biomet acetabular c.
bipolar acetabular c.
bipolar prosthetic c.
Buchholz acetabular c.
ceramic acetabular c.
Charnley acetabular c.
Charnley offset-bore c.
concentric hip c.
concetric hip c.
Continuum elliptical acetabular c.
Continuum polyethylene
  acetabular c.
Crawford-Adams acetabular c.
CRM c.
custom-made acetabular c.
DePuy bipolar c.
DePuy Tri-Lock interlocking
  acetabular c.
ESKA UHMWPE acteabular c.
Essential Energy C.
Flo-Trol drinking c.
Ganz c.
Gap c.
Gemini c.
Harris-Galante acetabular c.
Hedrocel c.
heel c.
hip c.
c. holder
c. holder handle
Integrity acetabular c.
interlocking acetabular c.
Interseal acetabular c.
jumbo acetabular c.
Kennedy spillproof c.
Laing concentric hip c.
Lineage acetabular c.
Lord c.
low-profile c.
Luck hip c.
McKee-Farrar acetabular c.
metal-backed acetabular c.
migration of acetabular c.
monolithic A1203 c.
Mueller c.
multipolar bipolar c.
NEB acetabular c.
New England Baptist acetabular c.
oblong polyethylene acetabular c.
Opti-Fix II acetabular c.
Osteonics acetabular c.
patella c.
plastic heel c.
Polysorb heel c.
porous-coated acetabular c.
c. positioner
PQ premium heel c.
press-fit c.
prosthesis c.
c. reamer
Reflection I, V, FSO acetabular c.
Restoration GAP acetabular c.
retroversion of acetabular c.
Riecken PQ premium heel c.
rubber held c.
screw-in ceramic acetabular c.
Silipos Silicone Wonder C.
Smith-Petersen c.
Sorbothane II heel c.
S-ROM acetabular c.
S-ROM Super C.
trial acetabular c.
TTAP-ST acetabular c.
TuliGel heel c.
Tuli Pro heel c.
Tuli rubber heel c.
University of California
  Biomechanics Laboratory heel c.
Viscolas Blue Dot heel c.
Viscolas standard heel c.
Wonder-Cup heel c.
Wonder-Spur heel c.
ZTT acetabular c.
ZTT (I, II) c.
cup-and-ball osteotomy
cup-cement interface
Cupid's
C. bow
C. bow contour sign
C. bow sign
cup-on-cup arthroplasty of hip
cupped
c. curette
c. grasping forceps
Cuprimine
curative
c. soft tissue procedure
c. surgery
curbstone fracture
curb tenotomy
Curdy blade
curet (*var. of* curette)
curettage, curettement
excision and c.

curette, curet
    Acufex c.
    angled Scoville c.
    bone c.
    bowl c.
    box c.
    Bruns bone c.
    Buck bone c.
    cement c.
    Charnley bone c.
    Cobb c.
    Cone ring c.
    Cone suction biopsy c.
    cupped c.
    curved c.
    Daubenspeck bone c.
    Epstein c.
    Faulkner c.
    fine-angled c.
    fine bone c.
    Gillquist suction c.
    Halle bone c.
    Hardy hypophysial c.
    Hatfield bone c.
    hex handle c.
    Hibbs c.
    hypophysial c.
    Innomed bone c.
    Jansen bone c.
    Kerpel bone c.
    Kerrison c.
    Kevorkian c.
    Latitude c.
    Lempert bone c.
    long c.
    Magnum c.
    Malis c.
    Martini bone c.
    mastoid c.
    McCain TMJ c.
    McElroy c.
    meniscal c.
    Meyhoeffer bone c.
    Microsect c.
    Moe bone c.
    orthopaedic c.
    oval curved-cup c.
    Piffard c.
    ring c.
    Schede bone c.
    Scoville c.
    short c.
    Spratt bone c.
    Spratt mastoid c.
    Statak c.
    stout-neck c.
    straight c.
    T-handle c.

    Volkmann bone c.
    Walker ruptured disc c.
    Whitney single-use plastic c.
    Williger bone c.

curettement (*var. of* curettage)

curl
    dynamic trunk c.
    neutral wrist c.
    preacher c.
    reverse wrist c.
    seated hamstring c.
    trunk c.
    wrist c.

curl-up
    broomstick c.-u.

curly
    c. toe
    c. toe deformity

current
    action c.
    amplitude-summation interferential c.
    cutting c.
    direct c.
    interferential c. (IFC)
    low-frequency alternating c. (LFAC)

Currey bone anisotropy model

Curry
    C. hip nail
    C. walking splint

Curschmann-Steinert disease

Curtin
    C. incision
    C. plantar fibromatosis excision

Curtis
    C. flexion contracture release technique
    C. PIP joint capsulotomy

curvatura, *pl.* **curvaturae**

curvaturae (*pl. of* curvatura)

curvature
    angular c.
    anterior c.
    backward c.
    c. change
    c. correction
    dorsal kyphotic c.
    humpbacked spinal c.
    lateral c.
    posterior c.
    Pott spinal c.
    radius of c.
    spinal c.

curve
    Barnes c.
    Blix contractile force c.
    calibration c.
    caudal compensatory c.
    cervicothoracic c.

C

curve (*continued*)
　combined c.
　compensatory c.
　contractile force c.
　cranial compensatory c.
　displacement c.
　double major spinal c.
　double thoracic c.
　flattening of normal lordotic c.
　fractional c.
　full c.
　King thoracic and lumbar c.
　　(I–IV)
　kyphotic c.
　length-tension c.
　load-deflection c.
　load-deformation c.
　load-displacement c.
　lordotic c.
　low single thoracic c.
　lumbar lordotic c.
　c. magnitude
　major c.
　c. measurement
　minor c.
　nonstructural c.
　normal lordotic c.
　c. pattern of scoliosis
　primary c.
　c. progression
　c. progression in scoliosis
　c. progression velocity
　right thoracic c.
　rigid c.
　scoliotic c.
　secondary c.
　segmental c.
　severe rigid thoracic c.
　single overhand thoracic c.
　specific c.
　standardized growth c.
　strain-stress c.
　strength c.
　strength-duration c.
　stress-strain c.
　structural c.
　tension c.
　thoracic c.
　thoracolumbar c.
　torque c.

curved
　c. awl
　c. basket forceps
　c. bone rongeur
　c. curette
　c. gouge
　c. incision
　c. Küntscher nail system
　c. L approach

　c. Mayo scissors
　c. meniscotome
　c. meniscotome blade
　c. osteotome
　c. osteotomy
　c. passer
　c. periosteal elevator
　c. retractor

curvilinear
　c. area
　c. chin implant
　c. incision

CurvTek
　C. drill bone anchor
　C. TSR bone drill

curvus
　carpus c.

CUSA
　Cavitron ultrasonic surgical
　aspirator

Cushing
　C. bur
　C. disc rongeur
　C. dural hook
　C. flat drill
　C. Little Joker elevator
　C. perforator drill
　C. periosteal elevator
　C. retractor
　C. saw guide
　C. syndrome

Cushing-Gigli saw guide

Cushing-Hopkins periosteal elevator

cushion
　abduction c.
　alarm c.
　amputee c.
　Anti-Shox foot c.
　arch c.
　Back Bull lumbar support c.
　Back-Huggar lumbar support c.
　breakaway lap c.
　Butterfly c.
　Carter immobilization c.
　cast c.
　cell c.
　cervical c.
　Checkerboard wheelchair c.
　Comfort Take-Along wheelchair c.
　Core Max-Relax C.
　Disc-O-Sit Jr. c.
　Dry Flotation wheelchair c.
　Easy Up c.
　EcstaSeat seat c.
　enhancer c.
　foam c.
　foot c.
　gel c.
　Gel Foam Ultra-Wedge c.

Geo-Matt contour c.
C. Grip Flatware
Healthier seating c.
c. heel
heel c.
Hudson Hydrofloat C.
hydrofloat c.
Invacare Comfort-Mate
extra c.
invalid c.
Isch-Dish Plus c.
J2 c.
Jay basic c.
Jay Combi c.
Jay Rave c.
Jay Triad c.
Jay Xtreme c.
laptop c.
latex c.
lumbar support c.
MaxiFloat wheelchair c.
Pediplast c.
pommel c.
Postura wheelchair c.
Posture Curve lumbar c.
Posture Wedge seat c.
pressure c.
pressure-relief c.
Prop'R Toes hammertoe c.
Quadtro c.
ring c.
Roho Pack-It c.
saddle c.
Sat-A-Lite contoured wedge
seat c.
seat c.
seating c.
Shockmaster heel c.
c. shoe liner
Sit-Straight wheelchair c.
Skil-Care c.
Sorbothane heel c.
Temper Foam c.
T-Foam c.
T-Gel c.
trilaminate c.
Vac-Lok immobilization c.
Viscoheel K heel c.
Viscoheel N c.
Viscoheel SofSpot viscoelastic
heel c.
Viscolas heel spur c.
ViscoSpot heel c.
wheelchair c.
cushioned shoe insert
cushioning
Abzorb c.
cushion-throat wire cutter
Custodis implant

custom
c. halo
c. implant
c. prosthesis
c. rasp
custom-designed swan-neck femoral component
custom-fitted brace
custom-made
c.-m. acetabular cup
c.-m. insert
c.-m. shoe
custom-molded
c.-m. orthotic
c.-m. shoe
custom-threaded prosthesis
cut
chamfer c.
freehand c.
horizontal gantry c.
jack upper c.
notch c.
Z-step c.
cutaneous
c. amputation
c. axon reflex
c. distribution
c. flap
c. fold
c. graft
c. horn
c. icing
c. maceration
c. nerve
c. neuroma
c. pressure threshold (CPT)
cut-back zone
Cutinova
C. cavity dressing
C. foam dressing
C. thin dressing
cutout
c. knee support
c. patellar brace
c. shoe
c. table
cutter
bolt c.
bone plug c.
Breck pin c.
C. cast
cast c.
Cloward dowel c.
cookie c.
cushion-throat wire c.
diamond pin c.
diamond wire c.
double-action c.
dowel c.

C

cutter (*continued*)
    end c.
    c. guide
    Hefty-bite pin c.
    Horsley bone c.
    Howmedica Microfixation System
      plate c.
    C. implant
    Jarit pin c.
    Kalish Duredge wire c.
    Kirschner wire c.
    Kleinert-Kutz bone c.
    Leibinger Micro System plate c.
    Luhr Microfixation System plate c.
    Martin diamond wire c.
    meniscal c.
    Midas Rex bone c.
    milling c.
    motorized meniscal c.
    M-Pact cast c.
    multiaction pin c.
    multiple action c.
    pin c.
    plate c.
    plug c.
    Redi-Vac cast c.
    rib c.
    Rochester harvest bone c.
    Rochester recipient bone c.
    Roos rib c.
    side c.
    side-cut pin c.
    Sklar pin c.
    Spartan jaw wire c.
    Storz Microsystems plate c.
    Synthes Microsystems plate c.
    toothed c.
    wire c.

cutting
    c. block
    c. bur
    c. cone
    c. current
    c. current knife
    c. forceps
    c. jig
    c. needle
    c. shaver
    c. weight

CVA
    cerebrovascular accident
    chronic villous arthritis
    costovertebral angle
    CVA Sling
    CVA tenderness

CVAT
    costovertebral angle tenderness

CVD
    collagen vascular disease

CVT
    congenital vertical talus
C-Walk foot 1C40 prosthetic foot
CWHTO
    closing wedge high tibial
      osteotomy
C-wire inserter
cyanoacrylate
    c. adhesive
    c. glue
cyanocobalamin
cyanosis
CyberKnife
    C. image-guided surgery
    C. treatment
    C. treatment couch
cybernetics
Cybertech 1000 back support
Cybex
    C. back rehabilitation equipment
    C. cycle ergometer
    C. device
    C. I, II, II+ isokinetic exercise
      system
    C. II isokinetic dynamometer
    C. 340 isokinetic rehabilitation and
      testing system
    C. isokinetic test
    C. machine
    C. tester
    C. testing
    C. Torso Rotation Testing and
      Rehabilitation Unit
    C. training system
    C. Trunk Extension Flexion unit
cycle
    Ergociser exercise c.
    c. ergometer
    Exer-Pedic c.
    gait c.
    c. per second
    Power Trainer c.
    recumbent c.
    Saratoga exercise c.
    Schwinn bi-directional Windjammer
      upper body c.
    c. time
    upper body c.
    walking c.
cycled stimulation
cyclic
    c. loading
    c. mechanical stress
cycling
    studio c.
cyclist's palsy
cyclobenzaprine HCl
cyclooxygenase product
cyclophosphamide

cyclops
>c. formation
>c. lesion
>c. syndrome

cyclosporine

cyclothymia

cylinder
>air c.
>Arthrotek calibrated c.
>Feldenkrais c.
>c. walking cast

cylindrical
>c. autologous dowel graft
>c. bur
>c. dowel
>c. grasp
>c. osteotomy
>c. sleeve

cyma line

cyproheptadine

Cyriax
>C. diagnosis of soft tissue lesions technique
>C. soft tissue injury evaluation

cyst
>c. ablation
>acetabular c.
>acromioclavicular c.
>adventitious c.
>aneurysmal bone c. (ABC)
>Baker c.
>bone c.
>bone aneurysmal c.
>bursal c.
>digital mucoid c.
>expansile c.
>ganglion c.

>giant popliteal synovial c.
>inclusion c.
>c. index
>juxtaarticular bone c.
>lipid inclusion c.
>meniscal c.
>mucous c.
>myxoid c.
>perimeniscal c.
>porencephalic c.
>postfracture c.
>rheumatoid c.
>sacral c.
>simple bone c.
>solitary bone c.
>subarticular c.
>subchondral bone c.
>synovial c.
>Tarlov c.
>tibiofibular c.
>traumatic bone c.
>unicameral bone c.

cystic
>c. arthrosis
>c. bone lesion
>c. defect
>c. disease
>c. hygroma
>c. osteomyelitis
>c. rheumatoid arthritis
>c. tumor

cytoarchitectonic abnormality

cytokine

cytotoxic drug

Cytoxan
>C. injection
>C. Oral

C

3D

3-dimensional
3D fracture walker brace
3D plate
3D positional adjustability
3D positional control
StealthStation with Iso-C 3D

D

25-hydroxyvitamin D

D/3

distal third

1D35

Dynamic Motion Foot 1D35

DA

degenerative arthritis
diagnostic arthroscopy

d'accoucheur

main d.

Dacron

D. batting
D. graft
D. polyester
D. prosthesis
D. stent
D. suture
D. synthetic ligament material

Dacron-impregnated silicone rod
dactinomycin
dactylalgia
dactylitis

blistering distal d. (BDD)
tuberculous d.

dactylocampsis
dactylocampsodynia
dactylodynia
dactylogryposis
dactylospasm
DAF

dynamic axial fixator

Dafilon suture
Dagrofil suture
daily

d. adjusted progressive resistance exercise (DAPRE)
d. adjusted progressive resistance exercise strength training

Dakin

D. solution
D. tubing

Dalalone
Dalco Astro ankle brace
Dale

D. abdominal binder
D. first rib rongeur

Dalgan

Dallas grading system
Dall-Miles

D.-M. cable
D.-M. cable cerclage
D.-M. cable/crimp cerclage system
D.-M. cable grip system
D.-M. cerclage wire

Dalmane
dalteparin
Daltons dens fracture classification (I–III)
DALY

disability adjusted life year

damage

off-axis bone d.
physial d.

damage-control orthopaedics
Damason-P
d'Ambrosia test
damp heat
DANA

designed after natural anatomy
DANA shoulder prosthesis

danaparoid
danazol
dance

high-impact aerobic d. (HIAD)
low-impact aerobic d. (LIAD)
d. medicine

dancer's

d. foot
d. pad
d. 5th metatarsal fracture

dancing

d. bear gait
d. bear syndrome

dandy

D. cerebrospinal fluid leak maneuver
D. clamp

Dandy-Walker deformity
dangling foot
Daniel iliac bone graft
Danis-Weber

D.-W. classification of ankle injury
D.-W. classification of malleolar fracture
D.-W. fracture classification

Danniflex CPM exerciser
Danocrine
Dansko shoe
d'Antonio acetabular classification
Dantrium
dantrolene

DAPRE
>daily adjusted progressive resistance exercise
>DAPRE strength training

Darco
>D. back brace
>D. Body Armor Hi
>D. Body Armor Lo
>D. Body Armor short leg walker
>D. foot splint
>D. Medical-Surgical shoe
>D. Medical-Surgical shoe and toe alignment splint
>D. moldable insole
>D. OrthoWedge healing shoe
>D. Podospray
>D. Softie shoe
>D. surgical shoe
>D. Wedge shoe

DarcoGel ankle brace
Darier-White disease
Darrach
>D. distal ulna resection
>D. extensor carpi ulnaris tendesis procedure
>D. periosteal elevator
>D. retractor
>D. ulnar tenodesis

Darrow pain classification
dart
>Arthrex meniscal d.

Darvocet-N 100
Darvon Compound-65 Pulvules
Darvon-N
Das
>D. Gupta scapular excision
>D. Gupta scapulectomy
>D. Gupta transbronchial needle aspiration procedure

DASA
>distal articular set angle

Dasco Pro angle finder
Daseler-Anson classification of plantaris muscle anatomy
DASH
>Disabilities of Arm, Shoulder, and Hand
>DASH questionnaire
>DASH scale

dashboard
>d. dislocation
>d. fracture
>d. knee injury

dashpot
database
>Joint Theater Trauma Registry military d.
>JTTR military d.

DataHand system

DATT
>deep anterior tibiotalar
>DATT ligament

Daubenspeck bone curette
d'Aubigné
>d. femoral prosthesis
>d. hip status system
>d. patellar transplant

Dautrey
>D. chisel
>D. osteotome

David-Chaussé articular arthritis classification
David drainage
Davidenkow scapuloperoneal syndrome
Davidson muscle clamp
Davidson-Sauerbruch-Doyen periosteal elevator
Davies-Colley operation
Davis
>D. arthrodesis
>D. drainage technique
>D. dura dissector
>D. fusion
>D. law
>D. metacarpal splint
>D. muscle-pedicle graft
>D. percussion hammer
>D. pin
>D. saw guide
>D. series

Dawbarn sign
Dawson-Yuhl
>D.-Y. impactor
>D.-Y. periosteal elevator
>D.-Y. rongeur forceps
>D.-Y. suction tube

Dawson-Yuhl-Kerrison rongeur forceps
Dawson-Yuhl-Key elevator
Dawson-Yuhl-Leksell rongeur forceps
day
>D. fixation device
>D. fixation pin
>D. fixation staple
>d. treatment rehabilitation

Daypro
DayTimer carpal tunnel support
Daytona cervical orthosis
DBM
>demineralized bone matrix
>Grafton DBM

DBS
>deep bonding system
>Denis Browne splint

DCB
>distal communicating branch

DCC
>dorsal calcaneocuboid
>DCC ligament

D-Core support pillow
DCP
    calcium phosphate, dibasic
    dynamic compression plate
DCS
    dorsal column stimulator
    Dynamic condylar screw
        DCS pin
DDA
    dorsal digital artery
DDD
    degenerative disc disease
DDH
    developmental dislocation of hip
    developmental dysplasia of hip
        DDH orthosis
DDP
    dual drop pelvis
        DDP table
DDX
    differential diagnosis
de
    d. Andrade and MacNab anterior
      occipitocervical fusion approach
    d. Barsy syndrome
    d. Kleyn position
    d. Kleyn test
    d. La Caffinière trapeziometacarpal
      prosthesis
    d. Lange syndrome
    D. Lorme boot
    D. Mayo hip positioner
    d. Morgan spot
    d. novo scoliosis
    d. Quervain disease
    d. Quervain fracture
    d. Quervain injury
    d. Quervain stenosing
      tenosynovitis
    d. Quervain synovitis
    d. Quervain tendinitis
dead
    d. arm syndrome
    d. ball exercises
    d. bone
    d. lift
    d. space
deafferentation pain
deafness
    lentigines, electrocardiographic
    abnormalities, ocular hypertelorism,
    pulmonary stenosis, abnormalities
    of genitalia, retardation of growth,
    d. (sensorineural) (LEOPARD)
    d., onychoosteodystrophy, mental
      retardation (DOOR)
dean
    D. bone rongeur
    D. scissors

Deane unconstrained knee prosthesis
death
    exercise-induced sudden d.
    quadrant of d.
Deaver retractor
DeBakey prosthesis
DeBastiani
    D. corticotomy
    D. distractor
    D. external fixator
    D. femoral lengthening
    D. fixation
    D. technique
deBoer lateral knee approach
debonded femoral stem prosthesis
debonding
débridement
    Ahern trochanteric d.
    arthroscopic d.
    bursal d.
    cortical d.
    diagnostic arthroscopy and d.
    enzymatic d.
    exploration and d.
    irrigation and d.
    Magnuson d.
    patella d.
debris
    bone d.
    fibrin d.
    fibrofatty d.
    joint d.
    loose d.
    metallic d.
    particulate wear d.
    polyethylene d.
    polymeric d.
    pulvinar fibrofatty d.
    tissue d.
    wear d.
Debrisan
debris-incited osteolysis
debris-induced osteolysis
debris-retaining reamer
Debrunner kyphometer
debulking
    d. procedure
    Tsuge macrodactyly d.
deburring
Decadron-LA
Decadron Phosphate
Decaject
Decaject-LA
decalcification
decancellation
    cuboid d.
dechondrification
deciduous
Decker rongeur

D

deck plate
declination
  d. angle
  angle of d.
decompression
  anterior d.
  anterior retroperitoneal d.
  anterolateral d.
  bone graft d.
  carpal tunnel d. (CTD)
  cervical spine d.
  core d.
  d. equipment
  extensive posterior d.
  d. fasciotomy
  foot d.
  foramen magnum d.
  fracture d.
  indirect d.
  lateral d.
  leg d.
  lumbar spine d.
  microscopic d.
  nerve root d.
  posterior nerve d.
  posterolateral d.
  retroperitoneal d.
  d. rhachotomy
  sacral spine d.
  spinal d.
  subacromial d.
  d. technique
  thoracic spine d.
  thoracolumbar spine d.
  vertebral axial d.
    (VAX-D)
  vertebral body d.
decompressive
  d. acromioplasty
  d. laminectomy
  d. osteotomy
  d. procedure
deconditioned foot
deconditioning
  bed rest-related d.
  stroke-related d.
  d. syndrome
decorticate posture
decortication
  d. bur
  d. technique
decremental response
DeCube mattress
Decubitene oxygenated oil
decubitus
  d. position
  d. ulcer
decussation
dedifferentiated chondrosarcoma

Dee
  D. elbow hinge
  D. totally constrained elbow
    prosthesis
deep
  d. anterior tibiotalar (DATT)
  d. anterior tibiotalar ligament
  d. arch
  d. bonding system (DBS)
  d. circumflex iliac artery
  d. collateral ligament
  d. delayed infection
  d. fascia
  d. friction massage (DFM)
  d. heat modality
  d. iliac dissection
  d. intracompartmental soft tissue
    sarcoma
  d. knee bend (DKB)
  d. lateral femoral notch sign
  d. muscle therapy
  d. peroneal nerve (DPN)
  d. posterior compartment
  d. posterior sacrococcygeal ligament
  d. posterior tibiotalar (DPTT)
  d. posterior tibiotalar ligament
  D. Relief
  d. retractor
  d. stroking
  d. stroking and kneading massage
  d. tendon reflex (DTR)
  d. transverse carpal ligament
  d. transverse intermetatarsal ligament
  d. transverse metacarpal ligament
  d. transverse metatarsal ligament
  d. venous thrombosis (DVT)
  d. venous thrombosis prophylaxis
  d. wound infection
deepening reamer
de-epithelialized
  d.-e. rectus abdominis muscle
    (DRAM)
  d.-e. rectus abdominis muscle flap
deep-shelled acetabulum
deer tick disease
defect
  acetabular d.
  anteromedial humeral head d.
  Arthropor oblong cup for
    acetabular d.
  articular d.
  barlike ventral d.
  benign cortical d.
  bone d.
  bridging of d.
  cavitary d.
  composite d.
  condylar d.
  cortical d.

cranial d.
cystic d.
developmental d.
diaphysial d.
femoral condylar d.
fibrous cortical d.
fibrous metaphysial d.
fusiform d.
Hill-Sachs d.
impression d.
Klippel-Feil segmentation d.
mapping the d.
metaphysial fibrous cortical d.
neural tube d.
nonsubperiosteal cortical d.
d. nonunion
osseous d.
osteoarticular d.
osteochondral d.
pars d.
posterior superior humeral head d.
radial ray d.
reverse Hill-Sachs d.
segmental bone d.
segmentation d.
skeletal d.
step d.
subcortical d.
subperiosteal cortical d.
tibial d.
triangular d.
trochlear d.
unremodeled d.
defervesce
Defiance functional knee brace
deficiency
acetabular d.
Aitken femoral d.
American Academy of Orthopaedic
  Surgeons classification of
  acetabular d.
biomechanical d.
capsular d.
cavitary d.
central d.
congenital limb d.
congenital tibial d.
factor (VIII, IX) d.
focal d.
Jones classification of congenital
  tibial d.
long bone d.
longitudinal d.
magnesium d.
proximal femoral focal d. (PFFD)
proximal focal femoral d. (PFFD)
radial d.
segmental d.
skeletal limb d.

tibial longitudinal d.
transverse d.
vitamin C, D, K d.
deficient
d. knee
d. spinous process
deficit
executive function d.
glenohumeral internal rotation d.
  (GIRD)
motor d.
motor function d.
neurologic d.
perception d.
proprioceptive d.
sensorimotor d.
sensory d.
somatosensory d.
**Definition PM femoral implant
  component**
definitive
d. callus
d. cerclage wire
d. stabilization
deformability
deformans
arthritis d.
arthrosis d.
dystonia musculorum d.
hyperostosis corticalis d.
malum d.
osteitis d.
osteoarthritis d.
osteochondrodystrophia d.
Paget osteitis d.
spondylitis d.
spondylosis d.
deformation
elastic d.
plastic d.
stem d.
deformational plagiocephaly
deformity
abduction d.
acetabular protrusion d.
adduction d.
adductovarus d.
adult-acquired flatfoot d.
d. analysis
angulation d.
ape hand d.
ape thumb d.
apex plantar d.
Arnold-Chiari d.
arthrosis d.
back-knee d.
Bankart d.
biconcave d.
bifid thumb d.

D

deformity (*continued*)
   bishop's hand d.
   bony d.
   boutonnière d.
   bowing d.
   bowleg d.
   bunion d.
   bunionette d.
   burn boutonnière d.
   buttonhole d.
   calcaneocavovarus d.
   calcaneocavus d.
   calcaneovalgus d.
   calcaneovarus d.
   calcaneus d.
   cavovarus d.
   cavus foot d.
   cervical flexion d.
   cervical spine kyphotic d.
   Charcot d.
   checkrein d.
   clasped thumb d.
   claw toe d.
   cleft foot d.
   cleft hand d.
   cloverleaf d.
   clubfoot d.
   clubhand d.
   cock-up d.
   codfish d.
   Cole osteotomy for midfoot d.
   combined cavus d.
   compensatory d.
   congenital vertical talus foot d.
   contracture d.
   coronal plane d.
   crossover-toe d.
   curly toe d.
   Dandy-Walker d.
   digital d.
   digitus flexus d.
   dinner fork d.
   DISI d.
   dorsal intercalated segment
     instability d.
   double corn d.
   drop wrist d.
   dynamic digital d.
   early-onset spinal d.
   elevatus d.
   equinocavovarus d.
   equinovalgus d.
   equinovarus hindfoot d.
   equinus d.
   Erlenmeyer flask d.
   eversion-external rotation d.
   extension d.
   femoral head d.
   finger d.

fishtail d.
fixed d.
fixed flexion d.
fixed lumbosacral d.
flat back d.
flatfoot d.
flexible clawtoe d.
flexible hammertoe d.
flexion-internal rotational d.
flexion valgus d.
foot d.
forefoot abduction d.
fracture d.
garden spade d.
genu valgum d.
genu varum d.
gibbous d.
gull-wing d.
gunstock d.
Haglund foot d.
hallux limitus d.
hallux valgus d.
hallux varus d.
hammertoe d.
hatchet-head d.
Hibbs extensor tendon transfer
  cavus d.
Hill-Sachs d.
hindfoot d.
hollow foot clawfoot d.
hook-nail d.
hourglass d.
humpback d.
hyperextension d.
Ilfeld-Holder d.
internal rotation d.
intrinsic minus d.
intrinsic plus d.
J-hook d.
joint d.
Kelikian classification of nail d.
Kirner d.
knock-knee d.
kyphotic d.
lobster-claw d.
lumbar spine kyphotic d.
Madelung d.
mallet finger d.
mallet toe d.
medial ray adduction d.
metatarsus adductus d.
metatarsus primus varus d.
metatarsus varus d.
midfoot d.
multiplanar d.
nail d.
neuropathic foot d.
oblique osteotomy for tibial d.
pannus d.

pencil and cup d.
pes arcuatus clawfoot d.
pes cavus clawfoot d.
pes planovalgus d.
pes planus d.
1-plane d.
2-plane d.
3-plane d.
planovalgus d.
plantarflexion-inversion d.
postnatal skeletal growth d.
posttraumatic spinal d.
procurvatum d.
protrusio d.
pseudoboutonnière d.
pseudo-Hurler d.
pump bump d.
rearfoot d.
recurvatum angulation d.
reduction d.
rheumatoid d.
rigid equinovarus d.
rigid flatfoot d.
rockerbottom d.
rotational d.
round shoulder d.
saber shin d.
sagittal d.
scaphoid humpback d.
seal-fin d.
shepherd's crook d.
shoulder d.
silver-fork d.
skeletal d.
skewfoot d.
spastic hindfoot valgus d.
spastic thumb-in-palm d.
spinal coronal plane d.
spine d.
splayfoot d.
split-hand d.
split-nail d.
Sprengel high-grade dislocation of
  scapula d.
S-shaped d.
static foot d.
subcondylar d.
supination d.
swan-neck finger d.
talipes cavus d.
talus foot d.
thoracic spine kyphotic d.
thoracic spine scoliotic d.
thumb d.
thumb-in-palm d.
tibial d.
torsional d.
triphalangeal thumb d.
turned-up pulp d.

ulnar deviation d.
ulnar drift d.
valgus heel d.
varus hindfoot d.
Velpeau d.
vertical talus foot d.
volar angulation d.
Volkmann clawhand d.
windblown d.
windswept d.
wrist d.
Zancolli procedure for clawhand d.
Z foot d.
zigzag compensatory d.
deformity/instability
Defourmentel bone rongeur
DeGangi-Berk Test of Sensory
  Integration
Dega pelvic osteotomy
degenerated cartilage
degeneration
adjacent segment d. (ASD)
axonal d.
cartilaginous d.
Charcot d.
disc d.
endoneurial d.
fascicular d.
fibrinoid d.
immobilization d.
joint d.
Kirkaldy-Willis 3 phases of spinal
  d.
meniscal d.
mucoid d.
osteoarthritic d.
Regnauld great toe d.
retrograde d.
rotator cuff d.
Sandoz 4-phase model of spinal d.
spinal d.
spinocerebellar d.
wallerian d.
wear-and-tear d.
Zenker d.
degenerative
d. arthritic change
d. arthritis (DA)
d. arthrosis
d. disc disease (DDD)
d. disorder
d. joint disease (DJD)
d. lumbar scoliosis
d. lumbar spine
d. lumbar spine fusion
d. meniscal tear
d. meniscus
d. olisthesis
d. osteoarthritis

D

degenerative (*continued*)
    d. spine condition
    d. spondylolisthesis
    d. spondylosis
    d. spondylosis decompression and fusion
    d. spur
    d. spurring
    d. stenosis
    d. vertebral arthropathy
degloving
    d. injury
    internal d.
    phalangeal d.
    d. procedure
degradable polyglycolide rod
degradation
    anulus d.
degree
    d. of freedom
    d.'s of freedom joint motion
    d. of separation
    6 d.'s of freedom electrogoniometer
    d.'s of valgus angulation
    d.'s of varus angulation
dehiscence
    prosthesis d.
    wound d.
    Zuckerkandl d.
dehydration
    nucleus d.
Dejerine
    D. disease
    D. percussion hammer
    D. sign
Dejerine-Davis percussion hammer
Dejerine-Sottas disease
Deknatel
    D. orthopaedic autotransfusion system
    D. suture classification
delamination
DeLaura knee prosthesis
DeLaura-Verner knee prosthesis
delay
    electromechanical d. (EMD)
    sensory d.
delayed
    d. apoplexy
    d. bone imaging
    d. bone maturation
    d. closure
    d. consolidation
    d. femoral osteotomy
    d. fracture union
    d. graft
    d. healing bone fracture
    d. onset
    d. open reduction

    d. primary closure (DPC)
    d. primary repair
    d. reflex
    d. response
delayed-onset muscle soreness (DOMS)
Delbet splint
DeLee
    D. pediatric fracture classification
    D. radiographic analysis
Dellon ulnar nerve transposition
Del-Mycin Topical
DeLorme exercise
Delrin
    D. acetal resin
    D. prosthesis
Delrin-handle bone saw
delta
    d. brush
    D. femoral nail
    d. frame
    d. phalanx
    d. receptor
    D. Recon nail
    D. Recon proximal drill guide
    d. rod
    D. tibial nail
    D. walker
Delta-Cortef Oral
Deltafit Keel
Delta-Lite
    D.-L. casting tape
    D.-L. FlashCast
Deltaloc
    D. Reveal anterior cervical plate
    D. Reveal anterior cervical plating system
Delta-Rol cast padding
Deltasone
deltoid
    d. artery
    d. bursa
    d. fascia
    d. flap
    d. insertion
    d. ligament
    d. ligament sprain
    d. ligament tear
    d. muscle
    d. origin
    d. reflex
    d. region
    d. sprain
Deltoid-Aid arm support
deltoid-splitting
    d.-s. incision
    d.-s. shoulder approach
deltopectoral
    d. approach
    d. flap

d. groove
d. interval
deltotrapezius fascial ligament
deluxe
d. FIN pin
d. FIN pin inserter
demand
motion d.
specific adaptation to imposed d.
(SAID)
demarcation
line of d.
Demariniff protractor
DeMartel wire saw
DeMartel-Wolfson clamp holder
DeMayo suture passer
dementia
Demerol
Demianoff sign
demigauntlet bandage
demineralization
bony d.
demineralized
d. bone
d. bone graft
d. bone matrix (DBM)
demi-pointe position ankle pain
demyelination, demyelinization
demyelinization (*var. of* demyelination)
denatured alcohol
dendritic synovitis
denervation
cryogenic d.
d. disease
d. potential
d. procedure
d. supersensitivity
Denham
D. external fixation
D. external fixation device
D. pin
Denis
D. Browne bar
D. Browne bar foot orthosis
D. Browne bucket
D. Browne clubfoot splint
D. Browne 3-column model
D. Browne 3-column spine theory
D. Browne hip splint
D. Browne sacral fracture
classification
D. Browne spinal fracture
classification (1–3)
D. Browne splint (DBS)
D. Browne talipes hobble splint
D. Browne tray
D. compression fracture classification
D. seat-belt injury classification
Dennison cervical brace

**Dennyson-Fulford extraarticular subtalar
arthrodesis**
DENS
direct electrical nerve stimulation
dens
d. anterior screw fixation
d. fracture
d. x-ray view
dense
d. bone
d. cancellous allograft
densities (*pl. of* density)
densitometer
accuDEXA bone d.
Achilles Plus Ultrasound bone d.
Apollo DXA bone d.
bone d.
CT bone d.
Discovery bone d.
DPX d.
Lunar DPX d.
Lunar Expert d.
Lunar Prodigy bone d.
Norland bone d.
OsteoGram 2000 d.
OsteoView digital bone d.
pDEXA peripheral bone d.
QDR-1500, -2000 d.
QDR-2000 bone d.
Sahara portable bone d.
densitometry
bone d.
dual photon d. (DPD)
fracture site nonunion Norland
bone d.
Norland bone d.
photon d.
scanning d.
video d. (VD)
density, *pl.* **densities**
bone d.
bone mineral d. (BMD)
calcific d.
fiber d.
lumbosacral junction bone d.
proton d.
T-score of bone mineral d.
Z-score of bone mineral d.
dental
d. bur
d. drill
d. mirror
d. pick
dentate
d. fracture
d. ligament
dentinogenesis imperfecta (DGI, DI)
Denucé
quadrate ligament of D.

D

193

denudation
denude
deodorant
    DeoShoes d.
DeoShoes deodorant
deossification band
deoxypyridinoline crosslinks urine assay
DEPA
    depth of ulcer, extent of bacterial colonization, phase of ulcer, associated etiology
        DEPA diabetic foot ulcer scoring system
Depakote
DePalma
    D. hip prosthesis
    D. modified patellar technique
    D. staple
    D. staple procedure
Depen
dependent edema
depletion
    T-cell d.
depMedalone Injection
DepoDur
Depogen Injection
Depoject injection
depolarization block
depolymerisation (*var. of* depolymerization)
depolymerization, depolymerisation
    increased d.
    unbalanced d.
Depo-Medrol injection
Depopred Injection
deposit
    calcareous d.
    calcific d.
    calcium d.
    gouty tophaceous d.
    rotator cuff calcified d.
    tophaceous d.
deposition
    beta-2-microglobulin d.
    bone d.
    calcium oxalate d.
    calcium pyrophosphate dihydrate d. (CPDD)
    crystal d.
    hemosiderin d.
    pseudotumorous mucin d.
depot corticosteroid
depressed
    d. fracture
    d. reflex
depression
    bone d.
    Hamilton Rating Scale for D.

National Alliance for Research on Schizophrenia and D.
d. of fragment
postactivation d.
depth
    acetabular d.
    d. caliper-meter stick method
    d. gauge
    d. inlay shoe
    d. of ulcer, extent of bacterial colonization, phase of ulcer, associated etiology (DEPA)
    d. orthopaedic shoe
    wire penetration d.
depth-check drill
DePuy
    D. acetabular liner
    D. acetabular lining
    D. aeroplane splint
    D. AML hip
    D. AML Porocoat stem prosthesis
    D. any-angle splint
    D. awl
    D. bipolar cup
    D. bolt
    D. calcar grinder
    D. CMW 1 bone cement
    D. coaptation splint
    D. drill
    D. femoral acetabular overlay guide
    D. fracture brace
    D. Global Advantage shoulder eccentric humeral head
    D. Global shoulder glenoid component with fin
    D. graft preparation table
    D. halter
    D. hip prosthesis
    D. hip prosthesis with Scuderi head
    D. interference screw
    D. LCS mobile-bearing knee
    D. open-spindle splint
    D. open-thimble splint
    D. orthopaedic implant
    D. pin
    D. plate
    D. rainbow frame
    D. rasp
    D. reamer
    D. reducing frame
    D. rocking leg splint
    D. rod bender
    D. rolled Colles splint
    D. screwdriver
    D. support
    D. total hip system with porous coating

D. Tri-Lock interlocking acetabular cup

D. trispiked acetabular component

DePuy-Pott splint

derangement

Hey internal d.

internal d.

joint internal d.

structural d.

d. syndrome

vertebral d.

derby

d. hat fracture

D. nail

Derefield

D. leg length test

D. pelvic leg check

Derefield-Thompson leg length test

derivative

DermaBond

dermabrader

Dermacentor

D. andersoni

D. variabilis

DermaFlex Gel

DermaFreeze topical anesthetic

Dermagraft

Dermagran

D. hydrophilic gauze dressing

D. ointment

D. ointment wound dressing

D. spray

D. wound cleanser with zinc

dermal

d. bone

d. fasciectomy

d. fibromatosis

d. interposition splint

d. sinus

d. substitute

DermaMend

D. foam wound dressing

D. Hydrogel dressing

DermaSite dressing

DermAssist wound-filling material

Dermatell hydrocolloid dressing material

DermaTemp infrared thermographic sensor

dermatica

zona d.

dermatitides (*pl. of* dermatitis)

dermatitidis

Blastomyces d.

dermatitis, *pl.* **dermatitides**

atopic d.

shoe d.

venous stasis d.

dermatoarthritis

Dermatobia hominis

dermatocele

dermatofibroma

dermatofibrosarcoma protuberans (DFSP)

dermatogenic torticollis

dermatolymphangitis

dermatomal

d. pain

d. pattern

dermatome

anterior tibial nerve d.

Brown d.

electric d.

d. mapping

mechanical d.

Padgett electric d.

Reese d.

sacral d.

Stryker d.

Zimmer d.

dermatomyositis (DM, DMS)

dermatophyte test medium (DTM)

dermatosensory evoked potential

dermatoses (*pl. of* dermatosis)

dermatosis, *pl.* **dermatoses**

juvenile plantar d.

plantar d.

Derma-Wand germicidal lamp

Dermiflex dressing

dermis

dermodesis

resection d.

dermographia, dermographism

dermographism (*var. of* dermographia)

dermometer

dermomyotome

Dero hole-in-1 prosthetic sock

derotate

derotation

d. boot

d. brace

oblique osteotomy with d.

derotational

d. brace

d. osteotomy

d. pin

d. reflex

derotator

d. bar

d. splint

DeRoyal LMB finger splint

D'Errico

D. enlarging drill bur

D. lamina chisel

D. perforating drill

D. perforating drill bur

D. retractor

deSanctis-Cacchione syndrome

Desault
- D. fracture
- D. sign
- D. wrist bandage
- D. wrist dislocation

descending lymphedema
Deschamps needle
Descot fracture
Desenex
- Prescription Strength D.

design
- ball-and-socket d.
- barrel bur d.
- Blucher d.
- computer-assisted d.
- graft d.
- Harris d.
- hook hollow-ground connection d.
- hook V-groove connection d.
- mechanical plate d.
- metal-on-metal d.
- modular d.
- pedicle screw linkage d.
- prosthetic d.
- prototype d.
- screw d.
- spinal implant d.
- transpedicular fixation system d.
- V-groove hollow-ground connection d.

designation
- ASTM d.

designed after natural anatomy (DANA)
DesignLine orthotic
desipramine
desirudin
desk
- Posture-Rite lap d.

Desk-rest arm support
desktop therapy portal
desmalgia
desmectasis
desmitis
desmocytoma
desmodynia
desmoid
- cortical d.
- d. fibroma
- d. lesion
- periosteal d.
- d. tumor

desmoma
desmopathy
desmoplasia
desmoplastic fibroma
desmorrhexis
desmosis
desmotomy
Desoxyn

desoxyribonuclease
- fibrinolysin and d.

despotic nevus
desquamation
Destot pelvic fracture sign
destroyer
- Doctor Scholl's Maximum Strength Odor D.

destruction
- arthritic d.
- bony element d.
- bony necrosis and d.
- cortical d.
- geographic d.
- localized bone d.
- moth-eaten d.
- pantalocrural arthritic d.
- pantalocrural osteoarthritic d.
- peridiscal bone d.

destructive
- d. articular lesion
- d. bone disease
- d. joint disease
- d. spondyloarthropathy

desyndactylization
- Weinstock d.

detachable extender
detector
- analogous signal d.
- Isometer bone graft placement site d.

deterioration
- arthritic d.
- catastrophic d.
- neurologic d.

determinant
- combined ankle and knee motion gait d.
- knee flexion during stance phase motion gait d.
- pelvic rotation motion gait d.
- pelvic shift motion gait d.
- pelvic tilt motion gait d.

determination
- anteversion d.
- Budin-Chandler anteversion d.
- fusion limit d.
- leg length d.
- skin blood flow d.
- transcutaneous oxygen tension d.
- Whitesides tissue pressure d.

detritus
- d. bone
- hyaline cartilage d.

detrusor
- d. areflexia
- d. contraction
- d. hyperreflexia

detrusor-sphincter synergia
Deune knee prosthesis
Deutschländer disease
Devas stress fracture classification
development

asymmetric subtalar joint d.
Bayley Scales of Infant D.
bone d.
calcar femorale d.
motor d.
National Institute for Child Health
and Human D. (NICHD)
postural d.
reflex d.
D. Test of Visual Perception, 2nd
Edition (DTVP-2)

developmental

d. anatomy
d. coxa vara
d. defect
d. dislocated hip orthosis
d. dislocation of hip (DDH)
d. dyscalculia
d. dysplasia of hip (DDH)
d. hip dysplasia

deviation

angular d.
gait d.
lateral d.
medial d.
d. of atlas on axis
proximal set angle d.
radial d.
rotary d.
standard d.
ulnar d.

device

Acapella chest physical therapy d.
acetabular reinforcement d.
Ace Unifix fixation d.
acrylic orthotic d.
Acufex bioabsorbable fixation d.
AcuSpark piezoelectric d.
adjustable aiming d.
adjustable 2-point caliper sensory
assessment d.
Agee 4-pin fixation d.
AlloAnchor RC allograft d.
Anderson fixation d.
Anderson leg-lengthening d.
ankle disc d.
Antense antitension d.
anterior internal fixation d.
antirotation d.
application of traction d.
Archxerciser foot exercise d.
Arrow absorbable meniscal repair d.
ArtAssist arterial assist d.
Arthrex Bird-Beak d.

arthroscopic Bankart repair using
absorbable fixation d.
ArthroSew arthroscopic suturing d.
Arthrotek tibial fixation d.
ArthroWand d.
articular motion d. (AMD)
articulated tension d.
Artscan 200 arthroscopic cartilage
stiffness testing d.
assistive d.
assistive technology d. (ATD)
Automator d.
A-V Impulse System foot pump
DVT prophylaxis d.
A-V Impulse System foot wrap
DVT prophylaxis d.
Axer compression d.
axis-altering arthroereisis d.
Backbar d.
BackCycler continuous passive
motion d.
back range of motion d.
4-bar external fixation d.
Bassett electrical stimulation d.
Becker orthopaedic spinal system
orthotic d.
biodegradable fixation d.
Biofeedback 5DX d.
BioStinger low-profile fixation d.
Blanchard traction d.
body-powered prosthetic d.
BOING arm exercise d.
bollard d.
Bone-Lok d.
Book Butler book-grip d.
Bovie electrocautery d.
Brannock Foot Measuring D.
Buck convoluted traction d.
Calandruccio II compression d.
Calandruccio triangular compression
fixation d.
Cameron fracture d.
Carpal Trac traction d.
C-D fixation d.
C-D instrumentation d.
cervical range of motion d.
Cervitrak d.
Charnley external fixation d.
Chattanooga traction d.
circular fixation d.
Cleanwheel presterilized
disposable d.
collapsible internal fixation d.
Columbus McKinnon Hugger d.
combined fixation d.
compression screw-plate d.
compressive internal fixating d.
Cordis implantable drug reservoir d.
coring d.

D

device (*continued*)
  corkscrew lasso d.
  Cotrel-Dubousset dynamic transverse
    traction d.
  CPM d.
  Cuff Link orthopaedic d.
  Cybex d.
  Day fixation d.
  Denham external fixation d.
  Deyerle femoral neck fixation d.
  Deyo d.
  Digit-grip d.
  discography d.
  Disk-Criminator nerve stimulation
    measuring d.
  distal targeting d.
  Doctor Grip writing d.
  DressFlex orthotic d.
  Dunn fracture d.
  Dwyer d.
  dynamic transverse traction d.
  Easy-Pull sock aide d.
  EBI d.
  Econo-Cerv traction d.
  Edwards modular system sacral
    fixation d.
  Elbow-Up Protector elbow
    suspension d.
  electronics electrical stimulation d.
  electrotherapy d.
  Encore Orthopedics d.
  EndoPearl bioabsorbable d.
  EndoPearl fixation d.
  Endo-Ring minimal access
    surgery d.
  Endoskeleton TA interbody spinal
    fusion d.
  Epos Ultra extracorporeal shock
    wave therapy d.
  Epos Ultra orthopaedic shock wave
    therapy d.
  Evershears surgical instrument d.
  Exeter intramedullary bone plug d.
  EX-FI-RE d.
  Exogen 2000 noninvasive,
    low-intensity, pulsed ultrasound d.
  E-Z Flex jaw exercising d.
  EZ-Trac orthopaedic suspension d.
  FastOut d.
  fixation d.
  fixation with intramedullary d.
  FootFlex performance stretching d.
  forearm lift assist adjustable
    spring-loaded d.
  d. for transverse traction (DTT)
  d. for transverse traction system
  Fox internal fixation d.
  fracture fixation d.
  Fromm triangle orthopaedic d.

  geometric d.
  Georgiade fixation d.
  Giliberty d.
  Golgi d.
  Graftmaster d.
  Grip-Ease d.
  halo-gravity traction d.
  halo vest d.
  Hare splint d.
  Harrington fixation d.
  Harrington-Kostuik distraction d.
  Harrington rod instrumentation
    distraction outrigger d.
  Harris-Aufranc d.
  Heyer-Schulte antisiphon d.
  hipGRIP body positioning d.
  Hoffmann mini-lengthening
    fixation d.
  Hoffmann-Vidal external fixation d.
  hot/ice cold therapy cooler
    therapy d.
  humeral d.
  Ikuta fixation d.
  Ilizarov d.
  implantable bone anchor d.
  inductive coupling d.
  InFuse bone graft/LT-Cage lumbar
    tapered fusion d.
  Innovasive d.
  Insta-Nerve d.
  Intelect laser system d.
  Inter Fix RP threaded spinal fusion
    cage d.
  Inter Fix threaded spinal fusion
    cage d.
  intraarticular cautery d.
  Intracell mechanical muscle d.
  Intracell myofascial trigger-point d.
  InvertaChair traction d.
  isometric d.
  Jace W550 CPM d.
  JAS EZ elbow d.
  Kaneda distraction d.
  Kendrick extrication d. (KED)
  Kennedy ligament augmenting d.
  Kerboull acetabular reinforcement d.
  Kessler fixation d.
  Kin-Con d.
  kinematic d.
  kinetic rehab d. (KRD)
  Kirschner d.
  Knott rod distraction d.
  KRD L2000 rehab d.
  Kronner external fixation d.
  Kuhlman cervical traction d.
  Küntscher traction d.
  Lawrence d.
  Legasus support CPM d.
  legGRIP body positioning d.

leg-holding d.
leg-lengthening d.
Leinbach d.
Leksell adapter to Mayfield d.
LifeGait partial weightbearing
  therapy d.
ligament augmentation d. (LAD)
Link Orthopaedics d.
LiteGait partial weightbearing gait
  therapy d.
LT-Cage lumbar tapered fusion d.
lumbar tapered-cage lumbar tapered
  fusion d.
Luque fixation d.
Mayfield d.
Mayo elbow distraction d.
McAtee compression screw d.
McKeever patellar resurfacing d.
McLaughlin osteosynthesis d.
MediRule II measuring d.
Merry Walker ambulation d.
metal-on-metal d.
metal-on-polymer d.
MicroFET2 muscle testing d.
Mobilimb CPM d.
Mueller fixation d.
muscle and neurological stimulation
  electrotherapy d.
MyoTrac d.
nail-bending d.
nail-mounted compression d.
nail plate d.
Nauth traction d.
Necktrac traction d.
Nervoscope d.
Neufeld d.
Neuro-Aide testing d.
newer-generation d.
notcher d.
NuPulse d.
Ogden Anchor soft tissue d.
Ommaya reservoir d.
Omni-Flexor d.
Oppociser exercise d.
Orateck d.
Original Jacknobber II
  muscle-massage d.
Orthofix external fixation d.
Orthofix ISKD d.
Ortholav irrigation and suction d.
orthotic d.
OssaTron noninvasive extracorporeal
  shock wave therapy d.
OssaTron Orthotripter d.
OsteoAnalyzer d.
osteosynthesis d.
OsteoView x-ray d.
Oxford uncompartmental d.
Parham-Martin fracture d.

passive motion d.
passive positioning d.
passive thermal d.
PDN d.
peg d.
pegboard lateral positioning d.
Percuss-O-Matic jackhammer d.
Peri-Loc periarticular locked
  plating d.
Pivot Pole walking d.
Plastazote orthotic d.
PlexiPulse intermittent pneumatic
  compression d.
PLM d.
pneumatic external compression d.
pneumatic peripheral circulation
  improvement d. (PPCID)
PodoFlex reflexology d.
Polar Care 500 cryotherapy d.
posterior reduction d. (PORD)
PPT orthotic d.
Pressure-Specified Sensory D.
PRO Balance Master ADL
  evaluation d.
pronation spring-control d.
Pronex patient controlled pneumatic
  traction d.
prosthetic disc nucleus d.
ProTrac measurement d.
pulsatile pneumatic
  plantar-compression d.
pyrolytic carbon d.
Quartzo d.
Quengel d.
Rancho Los Amigos ankle foot
  control d.
recreational terminal d.
Redi-Trac traction d.
Reichert-Mundinger stereotactic d.
Rezaian external fixation d.
Rezaian interbody d.
Richards lag screw d.
RMC knee replacement d.
Rochester bone trephine d.
rod distraction d.
rod-mounted targeting d.
Roeder manipulative aptitude test d.
Roger Anderson compression d.
Roger Anderson external fixation d.
Roger Anderson stabilization d.
RollerBack self-massage d.
Rolz d.
rope stretching d.
rotation d.
Safe-T mate anti-rollback d.
SAFHS ultrasound d.
screw-rod d.
Scully Hip S'port hip d.
sequential compression d. (SCD)

D

device (*continued*)
    sequential foot compression d. (SFCD)
    Servox d.
    Sgarlato d.
    shear-off d.
    sighting d.
    single-use d.
    Sleeper Gripper prosthetic d.
    sliding fixation d.
    sliding nail d.
    Slot distraction d.
    snap-fit d.
    Sock-Assist d.
    Sofamor spinal d.
    SofPulse d.
    SOLEutions custom orthotic d.
    SOLEutions prefab orthotic d.
    Sorbothane orthotic d.
    Southwick pin-holding d.
    Spenco orthotic d.
    spinal fusion d.
    Sport-Rite Olympian d.
    Sport-Rite Runner d.
    sports terminal d.
    SporTX stimulation d.
    StairClimber assist d.
    Statak soft tissue attachment d.
    Stellbrink fixation d.
    Stone clamp-locking d.
    Stress-Ray varus-valgus d.
    Stryker knee joint laxity d.
    STx lumbar traction d.
    STx Saunders lumbar disc d.
    Sukhtian-Hughes fixation d.
    SuperQuad assistive d.
    SureClosure d.
    Suretac bioabsorbable shoulder fixation d.
    Sutter d.
    Sutter-CPM knee d.
    Suture Saver d.
    SynFix-LR stand alone anterior interbody fusion d.
    Tacticon peripheral neuropathy screening d.
    Tekscan in-shoe monitoring d.
    Telectronics electrical stimulation d.
    telescoping tubular d.
    Tenderlett d.
    Teno Fix tendon repair d.
    terminal d.
    T-Fix absorbable meniscal repair d.
    ThermaStim muscle warming d.
    thermocouple skin temperature d.
    The Rope stretch-and-traction d.
    The Rope stretching d.
    Thumper d.
    titanium geometric d.
    toe-straight d.
    totally implantable lengthening d.
    traction d.
    Trans Fix ACL fixation d.
    transpedicularly implanted anterior spinal support d.
    transverse loading d.
    triangular compression d.
    Trigen Peri-Loc periarticular locked plating d.
    TriggerWheel muscle therapy d.
    TSRH corkscrew d.
    TSRH mini-corkscrew d.
    Valenti arthroereisis d.
    Vapr coagulation and cautery d.
    VariFix spinal implant d.
    VariGrip spinal implant d.
    Vectra Genisys laser system d.
    vibrotactile d.
    Vidal-Adrey modified Hoffmann external fixation d.
    Viladot arthroereisis d.
    visor halo fixation d.
    Volkov-Oganesian elbow distraction d.
    Volkov-Oganesian external fixation d.
    voluntary closing terminal d.
    voluntary opening terminal d.
    Wagner distraction d.
    Wagner external fixation d.
    Wagner-Schanz screw d.
    Walk-Rite d.
    Wallis interspinous process stabilization d.
    WasherLoc d.
    Wasserstein external fixation d.
    wood probe reflexology d.
    Wrightlock posterior spinal fixation d.
    Xercise Band exercise d.
    X Stop interspinous process decompression d.
    Zickel supracondylar d.
    Zielke distraction d.
    Zimmer orthopaedic d.

devitalized
    d. bone graft
    d. portion
    d. tissue

DeWald
    D. spinal apparatus
    D. spinal appliance

Dewar
    D. posterior cervical fixation procedure
    D. posterior cervical fusion
    D. posterior cervical fusion technique

Dewar-Barrington
D.-B. arthroplasty
D.-B. clavicular dislocation
technique
Dewar-Harris
D.-H. paralysis
D.-H. shoulder technique
DEXA
dual-energy x-ray absorptiometry
DEXA scan
dexamethasone
neomycin and d.
Dexasone L.A.
Dexatrim
Dexon suture
dexterity
finger d.
dextranomer
dextran prophylaxis
dextromethorphan
acetaminophen and d.
dextropropoxyphene
dextrorotary scoliosis
dextrorotoscoliosis
dextroscoliosis
dextrose
d. solution
tetracaine and d.
Deyerle
D. drill
D. femoral fracture technique
D. femoral neck fixation apparatus
D. femoral neck fixation device
D. interlocking screw
D. plate
D. punch
D. sciatic tension test
Deyo device
dezocine
DFA
dorsiflexion angle
DFM
deep friction massage
D-Foam
DFS
distractive-flexion stage
DFSP
dermatofibrosarcoma protuberans
DGI
dentinogenesis imperfecta
DHC Plus
DH pressure relief walker
DHS
dynamic hip screw
DI
dentinogenesis imperfecta
Diab-A-Foot
D.-A-F. protection system
D.-A-F. rocker insole

Diab-A-Pad insole
Diab-A-Sheet
Diab-A-Sole
D.-A-S. flat insole
D.-A-S. molded insole
Diab-A-Thotics orthotic
diabetes mellitus
diabetic
d. amyotrophy
d. arthropathy
d. Charcot foot
D. Diagnostic insole
D. D-Sole foot orthosis
d. femoral mononeuropathy
d. foot
d. foot ulcerative condition
d. limb salvage
d. neuropathy
d. neurotrophic ulcer
d. orthosis kit
d. plantar hallux ulcer
d. polyneuropathy
d. polyradiculopathy
d. pressure relief shoe
D. Quality of Life
Questionnaire
d. sock
diaclasia (*var. of* diaclasis)
diaclasis, diaclasia
diaclastic amputation
diacondylar fracture
diadochocinesia (*var. of* diadochokinesia)
diadochokinesia, diadochokinesis,
diadochocinesia
diadochokinesis (*var. of* diadochokinesia)
diagnosis
clinical d.
differential d. (DDX)
palpatory d.
diagnostic
d. and operative arthroscopy
(DOA)
d. arthroscopy (DA)
d. arthroscopy and débridement
d. arthroscopy, operative arthroscopy,
possible operative arthrotomy
(AAA)
d. imaging
d. strategy
diagonal stretch
diagram
free body d.
dial
d. pelvic osteotomy
d. periacetabular osteotomy
d. test
dial-lock
d.-l. brace
d.-l. orthosis

D

diameter
>horizontal pedicle d.
>lumbar spine pedicle d.
>neck d.
>orthonormal d.
>pedicle d.
>sagittal pedicle d.
>sagittal spinal canal d.
>thoracic spine pedicle d.
>transpedicular fixation effective
> pedicle d.
>transverse pedicle d.
>vertical pedicle d.

diametral
diametric pelvic fracture
diamond
>D. biomechanical table
>d. bur
>d. fraise
>d. high-speed drill
>d. inlay bone graft
>D. nail
>d. pin cutter
>d. point needle
>d. rasp
>d. tip wire
>d. wire cutter

Diamondback
>D. 1100 recumbent stepper
>D. 1100 self-generated stepper
>D. 100 upright stepper

Diamond-Gould syndactyly operation
diamond-point wire double-strand wire
diamond-shaped medullary nail
diapedesis
Diapedic foot cream
diaphragm
>Bucky d.
>pelvic d.
>urogenital d.

diaphyseal (*var. of* diaphysial)
diaphysectomy
diaphyses (*pl. of* diaphysis)
diaphysial, diaphyseal
>d. aclasis
>d. defect
>d. dysplasia
>d. forearm fracture Nancy nailing
>d. fracture
>d. osteotomy
>d. plating
>d. region
>d. sclerosis
>d. tuberculosis

diaphysial-epiphysial fusion
diaphysis, *pl.* **diaphyses**
>femoral d.
>humeral d.

diaplasis
diaplastic
diarthrodial
>d. cartilage
>d. joint

diarthroses (*pl. of* diarthrosis)
diarthrosis, *pl.* **diarthroses**
diastasis
>ankle mortise d.
>d. fibula
>frank d.
>interosseous d.
>latent d.
>pubic d.
>symphysis pubis d.
>syndesmotic d.
>tibiofibular d.
>tibiotalar d.

diastatic fracture
diastematomyelia
diastrophic
>d. dwarfism
>d. dysplasia

diathermy
>Magnatherm SSP pulse shortwave d.
>microwave d. (MWD)
>pulsed d.
>shortwave d. (SWD)

diatheses (*pl. of* diathesis)
diathesis, *pl.* **diatheses**
>Dupuytren d.

Diaz disease
diazepam
dibasic
>calcium phosphate, d. (DCP)

Dibenzyline
DIC
>disseminated intravascular
> coagulation

Dicarbosil
**dichlorodifluoromethane and
trichloromonofluoromethane**
dichlorotetrafluoroethane
>ethyl chloride and d.

Dick AO fixateur interne
Dickinson
>D. acetabular approach
>D. calcaneal bursitis technique

Dickson
>D. geometric osteotomy
>D. operation
>D. paraffin bath
>D. paralysis
>D. transplant technique
>D. vascularized bone transfer

Dickson-Diveley
>D.-D. clinic
>D.-D. clinic foot operation

D.-D. total joint replacement
procedure
diclofenac sodium and misoprostol
dicloxacillin
dicondylar fracture
Didiee shoulder view
Didronel
Dieffenbach
  D. amputation
  D. operation
die punch fracture
diet
  Gerson d.
  gouty d.
  tea-and-toast d.
  d. therapy
  training d.
dietary
  d. modification
  d. protein
  d. reference intake (DRI)
Diethrich bulldog clamp
Diet-Phen
Diff
difference
differential
  d. diagnosis (DDX)
  d. spinal block
  temperature d.
  d. variable reluctance transducer
  (DVRT)
differentiated chondrosarcoma
differentiation failure
difficile
  Clostridium d. (C Diff)
diffuse
  d. angiokeratoma
  d. axonal injury
  d. fasciitis
  d. idiopathic skeletal hyperostosis
  (DISH)
  d. idiopathic skeletal hyperostosis
  syndrome
  d. infantile fibromatosis
  d. pigmented villonodular synovitis
  (DPVNS)
diflunisal
digastric muscle
DiGeorge syndrome
Digi-Flex
  D.-F. finger exerciser
  D.-F. hand exerciser
Digikit finger tourniquet
Digimatic caliper
Digi Sleeve stockinette dressing
digit
  accessory d.
  arthrodesed d.

d. cap
congenital trigger d.
flail d.
infantile trigger d.
multiple d.'s
replantation of amputated d.
sausage d.
d. splint
supernumerary d.
trigger d.
d. tube
d. wrap
Digit-Aide fifth toe splint
digital
  d. Allen test
  d. amputation
  d. aponeurosis
  d. artery
  d. artery of foot
  d. artery protection
  D. Biofeedback System
  d. block
  d. block anesthesia
  d. blood perfusion
  d. branch
  d. branch of plantar nerve
  d. caliper
  D. Care kit
  d. color
  d. contracture
  d. cord
  d. deformity
  d. edge-detection
  d. extensor mechanism
  d. extensor tendon
  d. flexor tendinitis
  d. flexor tendon
  d. flexor tendon sheath
  d. formula
  d. fusion
  d. impaction
  d. implant
  d. inclinometry
  d. joint
  d. mucoid cyst
  d. nail
  d. nerve block
  D. OsteoView 2000
  d. pad
  d. palpation
  d. photoplethysmography
  d. plethysmography
  d. prosthesis
  d. reflex
  d. response test
  d. self-retaining retractor
  d. shortening
  d. subtraction angiography (DSA)

D

digital (*continued*)
    d. theca
    d. tourniquet
    d. vibrogram
Digit-grip device
digiti (*pl. of* digitus)
digitizer
    Amfit d.
    Metrecom d.
digitorum
    d. brevis avulsion
    d. communis tendon
    extensor d. (ED)
    flexor d. (FD)
digitus, *pl.* **digiti**
    d. adductus
    d. anularis
    d. flexus deformity
    d. medius
    d. pedis minimus
    d. primus
    digiti quinti proprius
      tendon
    d. valgus
    d. varus
Di Guglielmo disease
dihydrocodeine compound
dihydroergotamine
dihydroergotamine-heparin
dihydrostreptomycin
dihydrotachysterol
diisocyanate
    methylene bisphenyl d.
Dilantin
dilatator (*var. of* dilator)
dilated cardiomyopathy
dilation
    flow-mediated d. (FMD)
dilator, dilatator
    Eder-Puestow metal olive
      d.
    incision d.
    lacrimal duct d.
    vessel d.
Dilaudid
Dilaudid-5
Dilaudid-HP
Dillwyn-Evans
    D.-E. osteotomy
    D.-E. relapsed club foot
      resection
Dilocaine
dilutional pseudoanemia
dimelia
    ulnar d.
dimenhydrinate
dimension
    D. hip prosthesis
    D. hip system

3-dimensional (3D)
    3-d. analysis
Dimension-C femoral stem prosthesis
dimethyl sulfoxide (DMSO)
dimidiatum
    Scytalidium d.
diminished sensation
Dimon-Hughston
    D.-H. hip fracture fixation
    D.-H. intertrochanteric medial
      displacement osteotomy
    D.-H. medial displacement
      osteotomy hip fracture
      technique
Dimon osteotomy
dimple
    pilonidal d.
    d. sign
    d. the bone
ding foot
Dingman
    D. bone and cartilage clamp
    D. bone-holding forceps
    D. mouth gag
    D. osteotome
dinner
    d. fork deformity
    d. pad
diode
    infrared light-emitting d.
    d. laser
diorthosis
Dioval Injection
dioxide
    carbon d. (CO_2)
DIP
    distal interphalangeal
    DIP articulation
    DIP fusion
    DIP joint
dipalmitoyl phosphatidylcholine
diparesis
    spastic d.
diphasic
Diphenhist
diphenhydramine
    acetaminophen and d.
diphenylhydantoin
diphosphonate
    aminohydroxypropylidene d.
    methylene d. (MPD)
    technetium labeled methylene
      d.
diplegia
    spastic d.
diplegic foot
Diplococcus pneumoniae
diplomyelia
diploscope

dipotassium
: clorazepate d.

dipropionate
: betamethasone d.

dipyridamole
: d. handgrip test
: d. thallium imaging

direct
: d. contraction
: d. current
: d. current electrotherapy
: d. electrical nerve stimulation (DENS)
: d. fracture
: d. injury elbow dislocation
: d. lateral portal
: d. vertex impact

direct-impact prosthesis

direction
: cephalocaudad d.

director
: grooved d.

direct-vision carpal tunnel release

disability
: d. adjusted life year (DALY)
: atlantooccipital d.
: box and block test of arm d.
: functional d.
: Models of Media Representation of D.
: National Council on D.
: National Information Center for Children and Youth with Disabilities
: Disabilities of Arm, Shoulder, and Hand (DASH)
: Disabilities of Arm, Shoulder, and Hand questionnaire
: Disabilities of Arm, Shoulder, and Hand scale
: Oswestry Low Back Pain D.
: permanent d.
: permanent and total d. (PTD)
: permanent partial d. (PPD)
: reversible ischemic neurologic d. (RIND)
: d. scale
: d. screening questionnaire
: secondary d.
: tapping test of arm d.

Disalcid

disappearing bone disease

disarticulation
: d. amputation
: ankle d.
: Batch-Spittler-McFaddin knee d.
: Boyd hip d.
: elbow d.
: joint d.

Lisfranc d.
Mazet knee d.
metatarsophalangeal joint d.
sacroiliac d.
shoulder d.
toe d.
wrist d.

disassociation (*var. of* dissociation)

DISC
: dynamic integrated stabilization chair

disc, disk
: Acro-Flex artificial d.
: acromioclavicular d.
: amphiarthrodial d.
: articular d.
: Bardeen primitive d.
: Bowman d.
: d. bulge
: bulging d.
: cartilaginous d.
: cervical d.
: Charité artificial d.
: d. compression
: contained herniated d.
: crescent-shaped fibrocartilaginous d.
: d. degeneration
: d. disruption
: Engelmann d.
: d. excision
: excision of intervertebral d.
: extruded d.
: d. extrusion
: fibrocartilaginous d.
: fixation d.
: d. forceps
: d. fragment
: frayed d.
: d. grabber
: hard d.
: herniated d.
: herniated intervertebral d.
: d. herniation
: I d.
: interarticular d.
: intermediate d.
: interpubic d.
: intervertebral d.
: intraarticular d.
: isotropic d.
: J d.
: d. lesion
: locking d.
: lumbar d.
: massive herniated d.
: Mobi-C artificial cervical d.
: Mobidisc artificial lumbar d.
: noncontained d.
: d. of ankle
: d. plication

D

disc (*continued*)
    d. pressure
    d. prolapse
    protruded d.
    protruding d.
    d. protrusion
    Q d.
    Ranvier d.
    d. rongeur
    ruptured d.
    sequestered d.
    sequestrated d.
    slipped d.
    d. space
    d. space infection
    d. space saline acceptance test
    sternoclavicular d.
    swollen d.
    d. syndrome
    thin d.
    transverse d.
    vacuum d.
    Z d.

discectomy, diskectomy
    anterior cervical d.
    automated percutaneous d. (APD)
    automated percutaneous lumbar d.
    (APLD)
    cervical d.
    fluoroscopic d.
    laminotomy and d.
    lumbar d.
    microendoscopic d. (MED)
    microlumbar d. (MLD)
    microsurgical d. (MSD)
    noninstrumented anterior cervical d.
    partial d.
    PercScope percutaneous d.
    percutaneous lumbar d.
    Robinson anterior cervical d.
    SMALL fluoroscopic d.
    Smith-Robinson anterior cervical d.
    Williams d.
    Wiltse d.
    d. with Cloward fusion

discharge
    bizarre high-frequency d.
    bizarre repetitive d.
    complex repetitive d.
    coupled d.
    cramp d.
    double d.
    d. frequency
    grouped d.
    high-frequency d.
    multiple d.
    myokymic d.
    myotonic d.
    neuromyotonic d.

    paired d.
    pseudomyotonic d.
    repetitive d.
    triple d.
    waning d.
disci (*pl. of* discus)
discission knife
discitis, diskitis
    iatrogenic d.
    juvenile d.
    pyogenic d.
    septic d.
disclination
discogenic, diskogenic
    d. compression
    d. neck pain
    d. sciatica
    d. spinal instability
    d. vertebral sclerosis
discogram, diskogram
    d. needle
discography, diskography
    cervical d.
    Cloward fusion d.
    d. device
    functional anesthetic d. (FAD)
    low-pressure positive d.
    lumbar d.
    microlumbar d.
    thoracic d.
    Williams d.
discoid
    d. lateral meniscus
    d. meniscus saucerization
discoligamentous injury
discometry, diskometry
discontinuity
    pelvic d.
discopathogenic
discopathy
    cervical d.
    traumatic cervical d.
Disc-O-Sit Jr. cushion
discotome, diskotome
    Pheasant d.
discovery
    D. bone densitometer
    D. elbow system
discrepancy
    leg length d. (LLD)
    limb length d.
discrete activity
discrimination
    2-point d.
    right/left d.
    sharp/dull d.
    tactile d.
    Weber static 2-point d.
discus, *pl.* **disci**

disease

Albers-Schönberg d.
Albert d.
Albright d.
allograft coronary artery d.
anarthritic rheumatoid d.
Aran-Duchenne d.
Assmann d.
Atton d.
Baastrup d.
Bamberger-Marie d.
basic calcium phosphate crystal
  deposition d.
Bekhterev d.
Blount-Barber d.
Blount pediatric bone
  development d.
bone d.
Bourneville d.
Bowen d.
Brailsford d.
brittle bone d.
Brodie d.
Bruck d.
Buchanan d.
Burns d.
Busquet d.
Caffey d.
Caffey-Kenny d.
calcium hydroxyapatite crystal
  deposition d.
calcium pyrophosphate dihydrate
  deposition d. (CPDD, CPPD)
Calvé d.
Calvé-Perthes d.
Camurati-Engelmann d.
Canavan d.
Canavan-van Bogaert-Bertrand d.
cement d.
cementless d.
central core d.
cervical disc d.
CHA crystal deposition d.
Chandler d.
Charcot joint d.
Charcot-Marie-Tooth d.
Chester-Erdheim d.
chronic tophaceous d.
CMT d.
collagen vascular d. (CVD)
connective tissue d.
Conradi d.
d. construct
coronary artery d. (CAD)
Cruveilhier d.
crystal-related joint d.
Curschmann-Steinert d.
cystic d.
Darier-White d.

deer tick d.
degenerative disc d. (DDD)
degenerative joint d. (DJD)
Dejerine d.
Dejerine-Sottas d.
denervation d.
de Quervain d.
destructive bone d.
destructive joint d.
Deutschländer d.
Diaz d.
Di Guglielmo d.
disappearing bone d.
double Charcot d.
Duchenne d.
Duchenne-Aran d.
Duplay d.
Dupuytren d.
Eddowes d.
Ehlers-Danlos d.
Engelmann d.
Engel-Recklinghausen d.
Erb-Landouzy d.
Erdheim-Chester d.
Erichsen d.
facet joint d. (FJD)
fascioscapulohumeral muscle
  atrophy d.
Felix d.
fibromuscular d. (FMD)
Forestier d.
Freiberg d.
Freiberg-Kohler d.
Friedreich d.
Garré d.
Garrod d.
Gaucher d.
glenohumeral joint d.
Gorham d.
Gorham-Stout d.
Grisel d.
Gumboro d.
Haas d.
Haglund d.
handcuff d.
Hand-Schüller-Christian d.
Hansen d.
Heberden d.
Henderson-Jones d.
hereditary neuropathic d.
Hoffa d.
Hoffa-Kastert d.
Hospital for Joint D. (HJD)
Hurler d.
hydroxyapatite deposition d.
hypophosphatemic bone d.
ischemic leg d.
ischemic limb d. (ILD)
Iselin d.

D

disease (*continued*)

Jaffe d.
Jansen d.
Jansky-Bielschowsky d.
joint d.
Jüngling d.
juvenile Paget d.
Kashin-Bek d.
Kienböck d.
Köhler d.
Köhler-Pellegrini-Stieda d.
Kugelberg-Welander d.
Kümmell d.
Kümmell-Verneuil d.
Lance d.
Larsen d.
Larsen-Johansson d.
Ledderhose d.
Legg-Calvé-Perthes d.
  (LCPD)
Legg-Calvé-Waldenström d.
Legg-Perthes d.
Léri d.
Léri-Weill d.
Letterer-Siwe d.
Lichtman d.
Lichtman radiographic classification
  of Kienböck d. (stages I, II, IIIa,
  IIIb, IV)
Little d.
Lobstein d.
Lyme d.
MacLean-Maxwell d.
Maffucci d.
Marie-Bamberger d.
Marie-Charcot-Tooth d.
Marie-Strümpell d.
Maroteaux-Lamy d.
marrow d.
Martin d.
Mauclaire d.
McArdle d.
metabolic bone d.
metastatic d.
Meyer-Betz d.
milk-alkali d.
mini-core d.
mixed connective tissue d.
modified Kienböck d.
modified Stahl classification of
  Kienböck d. (stage I-V)
Moeller-Barlow d.
Morquio d.
Morquio-Ullrich d.
Morton d.
motor neuron d.
Mouchet d.
Munchmeyer d.
Nakamura d.

National Institute of Arthritis and
  Musculoskeletal and Skin D.'s
  (NIAMS)
Neftel d.
neurogenic d.
neuromuscular d.
neuropathic joint d.
Niemann-Pick d.
noninflammatory degenerative joint
  d. (NIDJD)
oligoarticular d.
Ollier d.
Oppenheim d.
Osgood-Schlatter d.
Otto d.
Otto-Chrobak hip d.
Paas d.
Paget d.
Panner d.
Parkinson d.
Pauzat d.
Pellegrini-Stieda knee ligament
  ossification d.
peripheral arterial occlusive d.
  (PAOD)
peripheral vascular d. (PVD)
peripheral vascular obstructive d.
Perrin-Ferraton d.
Perthes d.
Poncet d.
posttraumatic degenerative d.
Pott d.
Poulet d.
Preiser d.
pseudo-Pott d.
Pyle d.
Quervain d.
quiet hip d.
Raynaud d.
Refsum d.
Reiter d.
rheumatoid d.
Ribbing d.
Roussy-Lévy d.
Rust d.
sacroiliac joint d.
Schanz d.
Schlatter d.
Schlatter-Osgood d.
Schmid d.
Schmorl nucleus pulposus d.
senile hip d.
Sever heel pain d.
Silfverskiöld
  osteochondrodystrophy d.
Sinding-Larsen-Johansson patellar
  tendinitis d.
skeletal hypoplasia d.
spotted bone d.

Steinert d.
steroid-induced bone d.
Still d.
Strümpell d.
Strümpell-Marie d.
Sudeck d.
Swediauer d.
symptomatic cervical disc d.
  (SCDD)
synovial d.
Talma d.
Taratynov d.
Thiemann d.
Thomsen d.
thromboembolic d. (TED)
tophaceous d.
Trevor d.
Trevor-Fairbank d.
Truswell-Hansen d.
upper motor neuron d.
van Buchem d.
van der Hoeve d.
Van Neck d.
venous thromboembolic d. (VTED)
von Recklinghausen
  neurofibromatosis d.
Voorhoeve d.
Vrolik d.
Wegner d.
Werdnig-Hoffmann d.
Wilson d.
Wohlfart-Kugelberg-Welander d.
Woringer-Kolopp d.
Worth d.
Ziehen-Oppenheim d.
disease-modifying antirheumatologic drug
(DMARD)
disfigured foot
DISH
  diffuse idiopathic skeletal hyperostosis
  DISH syndrome
dishpan fracture
DISI
  dorsal intercalated segment instability
  DISI collapse pattern
  DISI deformity
disimpaction
disinfectant
  high-level d.
  intermediate d.
disk (*var. of* disc)
Diskard head halter
Disk-Criminator
  D.-C. nerve stimulation measuring
    device
  D.-C. sensory testing
diskectomy (*var. of* discectomy)
diskitis (*var. of* discitis)
diskogenic (*var. of* discogenic)

diskogram (*var. of* discogram)
diskography (*var. of* discography)
diskometry (*var. of* discometry)
diskotome (*var. of* discotome)
dislocated
  d. knee
  d. patella
dislocating arthropathy
dislocatio erecta
dislocation
  acromioclavicular joint d.
  ankle d.
  antenatal d.
  anterior hip d.
  anterior-inferior d.
  anterior shoulder d.
  anterolateral d.
  arytenoid d.
  atlantoaxial d. (AAD)
  atlantooccipital d.
  atlantooccipital joint d.
  atypical d.
  Bankart shoulder d.
  bayonet d.
  Bell-Dally atlas d.
  Bell-Dally first cervical d.
  bilateral interfacetal d. (BID)
  boutonnière hand d.
  bursting d.
  carpal d.
  carpometacarpal joint d.
  central d.
  Chopart ankle d.
  chronic recurrent ankle joint d.
  closed d.
  complete d.
  complex fracture d.
  complicated d.
  compound d.
  congenital hip d.
  congenital patella d.
  consecutive d.'s
  d. contour abnormality
  Cotton reduction of elbow d.
  dashboard d.
  Desault wrist d.
  direct injury elbow d.
  divergent elbow d.
  dorsal perilunate d.
  dorsal transscaphoid perilunar d.
  elbow d.
  facet d.
  d. factor
  d. fracture
  fracture d.
  frank d.
  gamekeeper's thumb d.
  glenohumeral joint d.
  habitual d.

D

dislocation (*continued*)
    Hill-Sachs shoulder d.
    hip d.
    incomplete d.
    interfacetal d.
    interphalangeal joint d.
    intraarticular d.
    irreducible anterior atlantoaxial d. (IAAD)
    irreducible fracture d.
    isolated d.
    joint d.
    Kienböck d.
    knee d.
    Kocher reduction of shoulder d.
    ligamentous anterior d. (LAD)
    Lisfranc d.
    lumbosacral d.
    lunate d.
    luxatio erecta shoulder d.
    medial swivel d.
    metacarpophalangeal d.
    metatarsophalangeal joint d.
    Meyn reduction of elbow d.
    milkmaid's elbow d.
    Monteggia d.
    Nélaton ankle d.
    neuropathic joint d.
    occipitoatlantal d.
    d. of articular process
    old unreduced d.
    open d.
    Osborne-Cotterill elbow d.
    Otto pelvis d.
    Palmer transscaphoid perilunar d.
    panclavicular d.
    panclavicular fracture d.
    parachute jumper's d.
    partial d.
    patellar intraarticular d.
    pathologic d.
    perilunar transscaphoid d.
    perilunate carpal d.
    peroneal d.
    phalangeal d.
    posterior facet d.
    posterior hip d.
    posterior shoulder d.
    posteromedial d.
    prenatal d.
    primitive d.
    proximal tibiofibular joint d.
    radial head d. (RHD)
    radiocarpal d.
    radioulnar d.
    recent d.
    recurrent patellar d.
    retrosternal d.
    sacroiliac d.

    shoulder d.
    simple d.
    Smith d.
    spontaneous hyperemic d.
    sternoclavicular joint d.
    subastragalar d.
    subcoracoid shoulder d.
    subglenoid shoulder d.
    subspinous d.
    subtalar joint d.
    superior d.
    swivel d.
    talar d.
    talonavicular d.
    tarsal d.
    tarsometatarsal d.
    temporomandibular joint d.
    teratologic d.
    tibialis posterior d.
    tibiofibular joint d.
    transscaphoid perilunate d.
    traumatic d.
    triquetrolunate d.
    unilateral interfacetal d. (UID)
    unreduced d.
    volar semilunar wrist d.

dislodgement (*var. of* dislodgment)

dislodgment, dislodgement
    hook d.

dismember

disodium
    etidronate d.
    tiludronate d.

disorder
    adjustment d.
    adrenal d.
    ARS d.
    clotting d.
    coagulation d.
    congenital limb d.
    cumulative trauma d. (CTD)
    degenerative d.
    fluoroquinolone-associated Achilles tendon d.
    gait d.
    mixed connective tissue d.
    motor speech d.
    movement d.
    muscle d.
    myeloproliferative d.
    National Organization for Rare D.'s (NORD)
    neurocompressive d.
    neurogenic d.
    neurologic d.
    neuromuscular junction d.
    nontotal-contact d.
    occupation-related d.
    patellofemoral d.

peripheral neurocompressive d.
progressive neurologic d.
recurrent d.
repetitive strain d.
repetitive stress d.
repetitive trauma d. (RTD)
retrocalcaneal d.
rheumatoid d.
rheumatologic d.
segmental spinal cord d.
spastic d.
temporomandibular d.
tendon d.
trophic joint d.
vasomotor d.
whiplash-associated d.
work-related musculoskeletal d.
(WMSD)
disorganized bone
disparity
limb length d.
dispenser
Jet Vac cement d.
dispersion
temporal d.
displaced
d. intraarticular calcaneus
d. intraarticular fracture
d. pilon fracture
d. vertebra
displacement
angular d.
d. anterior cavus V osteotomy
atlantoaxial rotary d.
axial d.
crosshead d.
d. curve
Ellis Jones peroneal tendon d.
fracture fragment d.
interregional d.
lateral patella d.
lateral rotary d.
Laurin lateral patella d.
left-right leg d.
load-to-grip d.
medial d.
oblique d.
patella d.
peroneal tendon d.
posterior facet d.
rotary d.
sagittal plane d.
tendon d.
translational d.
traumatic d.
Y-axis translatory d.
display
head-mounted d. (HMD)
high-definition video d.

disposable
d. arthroscope
d. muscle biopsy clamp
d. 1-piece osteotome
Disposatrode disposable electrode
disproportionate dwarfism
disrelationship
persistent occiput/atlas d.
disruption
anterior column d.
cervical spine posterior ligament d.
Charcot d.
disc d.
end-stage d.
facet capsule d.
fibular joint d.
forefoot d.
glenolabral articular d. (GLAD)
interosseous ligament d.
joint d.
lateral compartment d.
ligamentous d.
medial compartment d.
pedicle cortex d.
pelvic ring d.
physial d.
sesamoid d.
skeletal d.
talocalcaneal ligament d.
dissecans
Guhl classification of
osteochondritis d.
osteochondritis d. (OCD)
dissecting
d. clamp
d. probe
d. scissors
dissection
blunt d.
bone d.
deep iliac d.
extracapsular d.
field of d.
fingertip d.
Pack-Ehrlich deep iliac d.
sharp d.
subligamentous d.
subperiosteal d.
dissector
Angell James d.
angled d.
ball d.
blunt hook d.
bunion d.
Creed d.
Crile gasserian ganglion knife
and d.
Davis dura d.
dura d.

D

dissector (*continued*)
    Freer d.
    golf-stick d.
    grooved d.
    Hajek-Ballenger d.
    hand d.
    hockey-stick d.
    joker d.
    Kidner d.
    Kocher d.
    Lewin bunion d.
    McDonald d.
    Penfield 4 d.
    sesamoidectomy d.
    transsphenoidal d.
    West hand d.

disseminated
    d. intravascular coagulation (DIC)
    d. pigmented villonodular
      synovitis

dissociation, disassociation
    hypnotic d.
    lumbopelvic d.
    lunotriquetral d.
    d. movement
    radioulnar d.
    scapholunate d.
    scapulothoracic d.

dissociative
    d. anesthesia
    carpal instability d. (CID)

distal
    d. Akin phalangeal osteotomy
    d. articular set angle (DASA)
    d. biceps brachii tendon rupture
    d. bone end
    d. calcaneus
    d. clavicle
    d. clavicular excision
    d. communicating branch (DCB)
    d. compression test
    d. concave articular surface
    d. dystrophy
    d. femoral cutting guide
    d. femoral epiphysial fracture
    d. femoral resection
    d. femur
    d. fibula
    d. fibulotalar arthrodesis
    d. first metatarsal osteotomy
    d. forearm
    d. fragment
    d. humeral epiphysis
    d. humeral fracture
    d. humerus
    d. interlocking
    d. interphalangeal (DIP)
    d. interphalangeal articulation
    d. interphalangeal joint

    d. interphalangeal joint approach
    d. intrinsic release
    d. junctional kyphosis
    d. latency
    d. locking
    d. locking screw
    d. L osteotomy
    d. medial creaking
    d. metaphysis
    d. metatarsal articular angle
    d. neurolysis
    d. oblique sliding osteotomy
    d. palmar crease (DPC)
    d. parabola toe length
    d. phalanx (DP)
    d. phocomelia
    d. radial fracture
    d. radioulnar (DRU)
    d. radioulnar joint (DRUJ)
    d. radioulnar joint prosthesis
    d. radioulnar joint stabilization
    d. radius
    d. realignment
    d. reference axis (DRA)
    d. row carpectomy
    d. rupture of biceps tendon
    d. segment weight
    d. soft tissue release (DSTR)
    d. star pad
    d. targeting
    d. targeting device
    d. thigh amputation
    d. thigh band
    d. third (D/3, distal/3)
    d. third of shaft
    d. tibia
    d. tibial epiphysial injury
    d. tibial physis
    d. tibiofibular fusion
    d. tibiofibular joint
    d. transfer
    d. tuberosity
    d. tuberosity of finger
    d. tuberosity of toe
    d. tuft
    d. ulna
    d. ulnar convexity
    d. Wagner femoral metaphysial
      shortening

distal/3
    distal third

distalward

distance
    coracoclavicular d.
    focal film d.
    fulcrum d.
    interpediculate d.
    protrusion d.

distension (*var. of* distention)

distention, distension
distoclusal, distoocclusal
distolateral
distoocclusal (*var. of* distoclusal)
distortion
    multisegmental spinal d.
    sacral base d.
    structural intersegmental d.
distracted straight-leg raising
  test
distraction
    apical d.
    d. arthroplasty
    d. bar
    d. bone block arthrodesis
    calcaneal d.
    callus d.
    d. clamp
    fixed d.
    flexion d.
    d. force
    fracture fragment d.
    Guhl d.
    halo-cast d.
    halo-femoral d.
    halo-pelvic d.
    d. histogenesis
    d. hook
    d. injury
    d. instrumentation
    d. instrumentation biomechanics
    joint d.
    d. laminaplasty
    d. lengthening
    longitudinal d.
    manipulation with d.
    Monticelli-Spinelli d.
    d. of fracture
    d. osteogenesis
    d. osteogenesis technique
    physial d.
    d. pin
    d. rod
    d. screw
    slow d.
    small step d.
    spinal d.
    d. subtalar arthrodesis
    d. technique
    d. test
distraction-compression
    d.-c. bone graft arthrodesis
    d.-c. scoliosis treatment
distractive
    d. extension
    d. flexion
    d. force
    d. motion
distractive-flexion stage (DFS)

distractor
    Acufex ankle d.
    Anderson d.
    AO femoral d.
    Bliskunov implantable femoral d.
    DeBastiani d.
    femoral d.
    hook d.
    Ilizarov d.
    intramedullary skeletal kinetic d.
     (ISKD)
    joint d.
    Kessler metacarpal d.
    Mark II distal femur d.
    McCarthy hip d.
    Monticelli-Spinelli d.
    Mueller d.
    Orthofix M-100 d.
    Pinto d.
    Santa Casa d.
    tang d.
    turnbuckle d.
    Wagner d.
distribution
    cutaneous d.
    Moe-Kettleson d.
    stocking-glove d.
    stress d.
disturbance
    articulation d.
    bowel d.
    gait d.
    pain-related sleep d.
    urologic d.
disuse
    d. arthropathy
    d. atrophy
    d. osteoporosis
diurnal
    d. change
    d. variation in straight leg raising
divergence
    angle of d.
    anteroposterior talocalcaneal d.
divergent elbow dislocation
diversified
    d. chiropractic manipulative therapy
    d. manipulation
diversified-type force application
diversional activity
divided navicular
division
    Swafford-Lichtman median nerve d.
divisionary line
divot sign
DJD
    degenerative joint disease
DKB
    deep knee bend

D

D-L internal fixator
DM
  dermatomyositis
  dystrophia myotonica
  myotonic dystrophy
DMARD
  disease-modifying antirheumatologic
    drug
D-Med Injection
DMI
  Duro-Med Industries
    DMI orthopaedic bed
DMP wire twister
dMRI
  dynamic magnetic resonance imaging
DMS
  dermatomyositis
DMSO
  dimethyl sulfoxide
DOA
  diagnostic and operative arthroscopy
Doane knee retractor
Doan's
  Extra Strength D.
dobutamine echocardiography
doctor
  D. Collins fracture clamp
  D. Grip writing device
  D. Joseph's diabetic foot kit
  D. Joseph's Original Footbrush
  D. of Podiatric Medicine (DPM)
  D. Scholl's Athlete's Foot
  D. Scholl's Maximum Strength
    Odor Destroyer
documented pseudarthrosis
Dodd perforator
doffing
  donning and d.
  d. prosthesis
Dogbone ACFS
dog-ear repair
dogleg fracture
Dolacet
Dolene
dolichostenomelia
doll
  D. trochanteric reattachment
  D. trochanteric reattachment
    technique
dollar
  silver d.
  x-ray sign silver d.
dollop
  bone d.
doll's eye sign
Dolobid
Dolophine
Dolorac
dolorimeter

dolorosus
  hallux d.
dome
  d. fracture
  d. knee ArthroWand
  d. plunger
  d. proximal tibial osteotomy
  shoulder d.
  talar d.
  weightbearing acetabular d.
Domeboro
dome-shaped
  d.-s. osteotomy
  d.-s. sacrum
dominance
  hand d.
  left-hand d.
  right-hand d.
dominant
  left-hand d.
  right-hand d.
domino spinal instrumentation connector
DOMS
  delayed-onset muscle soreness
Donaghy angled suture needle holder
Donati vertical mattress suture
DonJoy
  D. ALP brace
  D. Gold Point knee brace
  D. knee splint
  D. OA adjuster
  D. Opal knee brace
  D. 4-point Super Sport knee brace
  D. Quadrant shoulder brace
  D. Ultrasling shoulder immobilizer
  D. Universal ankle brace
  D. wrist splint
donning
  d. and doffing
  d. prosthesis
donning-doffing skill
donor
  d. site
  d. team
donut (*var. of* doughnut)
DOOR
  deafness, onychoosteodystrophy, mental
    retardation
    DOOR syndrome
door
  laminar d.
Doppler
  D. ankle systolic pressure
  D. pulse evaluation
  D. scope
  D. study
  D. technique
  D. ultrasound
  D. ultrasound flowmeter

Doral
Dorello canal
Dormarex 2 Oral
Dormin Oral
Dorr
    D. bone classification
    D. ratio
Dorrance
    D. hand prosthesis
    D. hook
    D. push-back cleft palate procedure
dorsa (*pl. of* dorsum)
dorsal
    d. arch of wrist
    d. aspect
    d. bunion
    d. calcaneocuboid (DCC)
    d. calcaneocuboid ligament
    d. calcaneonavicular ligament
    d. capsule
    d. capsulodesis
    d. carpal capsulitis
    d. carpal ligament
    d. carpometacarpal ligament
    d. cheilectomy
    d. closing wedge osteotomy
    d. closing wedge proximal
      phalangeal osteotomy
    d. columella implant
    d. column stimulator (DCS)
    d. column stimulator implant
    d. compartment
    d. cross-finger flap
    d. cuboideonavicular ligament
    d. cuneocuboid ligament
    d. cuneonavicular ligament
    d. cutaneous nerve
    d. digital artery (DDA)
    d. drainage
    d. drawer test
    d. extension block splint
    d. finger approach
    d. glide
    d. hood
    d. horn cell
    d. intercalated segment instability
      (DISI)
    d. intercalated segment instability
      collapse pattern
    d. intercalated segment instability
      deformity
    d. intercarpal ligament
    d. intercuneiform ligament
    d. interosseous muscle
    d. kyphotic curvature
    d. linear incision
    d. lithotomy position
    d. longitudinal incision
    d. lordosis

    d. lumbar corset
    d. malalignment
    d. metacarpal ligament
    d. metatarsal artery
    d. metatarsal ligament
    d. midline approach
    d. neuroma
    d. pedal pulse
    d. perilunate dislocation
    d. planar x-ray
    d. plate
    d. plate extender
    d. point
    d. proximal metatarsal osteotomy
    d. radial slope
    d. radiocarpal (DRC)
    d. ramus
    d. recumbent position
    d. reflex
    d. ridge
    d. root entry zone (DREZ)
    d. root entry zone lesion
    d. root ganglion (DRG)
    d. root ganglionectomy
    d. scapular nerve
    d. skin
    d. subcutaneous nerve transposition
    d. synovectomy
    d. talonavicular ligament
    d. tarsometatarsal ligament
    d. tenosynovectomy
    d. toe plate extension
    d. T-plate
    d. translation
    d. transscaphoid perilunar dislocation
    d. transverse capsulotomy
    d. transverse incision
    d. ulnar cutaneous branch
    d. venous arch
    d. venous arch of hand
    d. vertebra
    d. V osteotomy
    d. wing
    d. wing fracture
    d. wire-loop fixation
    d. wrist splint
    d. wrist splint with outrigger
dorsalgia
    cervicogenic d.
dorsalia
    ligamenta carpometacarpaliad d.
dorsalis
    d. pedis (DP)
    d. pedis artery anatomy
    d. pedis fasciocutaneous flap
    d. pedis pulse
    tabes d.
dorsalward approach
Dorsey screw-holding screwdriver

D

dorsi
>elastofibroma d.
>latissimus d.
>osteochondritis deformans
>>juvenilis d.

dorsiflexed metatarsal
dorsiflexion
>active d.
>d. angle (DFA)
>d. assist ankle joint ankle-foot
>>orthosis
>d. bumper
>d. flexion
>d. foot splint
>d. metatarsal osteotomy
>passive d.
>resisted d.
>d. stop brace
>d. stress ankle x-ray
>d. view

dorsiflexion-eversion test
dorsiflexion-plantar flexion position
dorsiflexor gait
dorsiflexory wedge osteotomy
Dorsiwedge night splint
dorsodynia
dorsolateral and medial capsulotomy
dorsolumbar area
dorsomedial
>d. approach
>d. cutaneous nerve
>d. incision

dorsoplantar
>d. approach
>d. capsulotomy
>d. projection
>d. radiograph
>d. radiographic view
>d. talometatarsal angle
>d. talonavicular angle

dorsoradial
>d. approach
>d. ligament (DRL)

dorsoulnar approach
dorsovolar approach
dorsum, *pl.* **dorsa**
>d. of hand

Dosepak
>Medrol D.

double
>d. arthrodesis
>d. Becker ankle brace
>d. bent Hohmann acetabular
>>retractor
>d. binocular operating microscope
>d. camelback sign
>d. Charcot disease
>d. clamp
>d. cobra plate

>d. contrast arthrotomography of
>>shoulder
>d. contrast shoulder
>>arthrotomography
>d. corn deformity
>d. cruciate configuration
>d. crush syndrome
>d. discharge
>d. drape
>D. Duty cane
>D. Duty cane reacher
>d. flexion wave
>d. fracture
>d. hemiplegia
>d. hip spica cast
>d. hump contour
>d. incision
>d. inflow cannula system
>d. jointed
>d. leg raise test
>d. limb support
>d. major curve pattern
>d. major curve scoliosis
>d. major spinal curve
>d. osteotomy
>d. PCL sign
>d. pearl-face hip joint
>d. portal technique
>d. posterior collateral ligament sign
>d. right-angle suture
>d. simultaneous sensory stimulation
>d. sugar-tong splint
>d. support time
>d. tendon transfer
>d. thoracic curve
>d. thoracic curve scoliosis
>d. tourniquet
>d. Zielke instrumentation

double-action
>d.-a. ankle joint
>d.-a. bone-cutting forceps
>d.-a. cutter
>d.-a. rongeur

double-arc sign
double-cannula system
double-clamp approximator
double-contrast
>d.-c. arthrogram
>d.-c. arthrography
>d.-c. study

double-ended
>d.-e. nail
>d.-e. right-angle retractor

double-flap amputation
double-flexion knee motion
double-headed stereotactic carrier
double-hollow nail
double-hook Lovejoy retractor
double-H plate

double-incision fasciotomy
double-leg
    d.-l. stance
    d.-l. stance phase
    d.-l. stance phase of gait
double-looped
    d.-l. cerclage wire
    d.-l. gracilis graft
    d.-l. semitendinous and gracilis
      hamstring graft knee reconstruction
      technique
double-L spinal rod
double-needle chemonucleolysis
double-occlusal splint
double-open hook
double-opposing Z-plasty
double-pendulum action
double-pronged skin hook
double-ring frame
double-rod
    d.-r. construct
    d.-r. technique
double-sharp forceps
double-slot screwdriver
double-stem
    d.-s. silicone implant
    d.-s. silicone lesser MP joint
double-step gait
double-stranded wire double-twisted wire
doublet
double-tap gait
double-threaded Herbert screw
double-thumb thrust
double-tunnel PCL reconstruction
double-upright short leg brace
double-Z rhombic skin flap
doughnut, donut
    d. headrest
    d. ring
    d. support brace
doughy
    d. cement
    d. consistency
Douglas skin graft
Dow
    D. Corning titanium hemiimplant
    D. Corning Wright finger joint
      prosthesis
dowager's hump
dowel
    d. arthrodesis
    bone d.
    d. bone graft
    calf bone d.
    d. cutter
    cylindrical d.
    graft d.
    Graftech structural allograft
      cervical d.

    d. graft technique
    d. grip
    iliac crest d.
    d. spinal fusion
    threaded cortical d.
doweled
doweling
    d. spondylolisthesis
    d. spondylolisthesis technique
down
    D. epiphysial knife
    D. syndrome
down-angle hook
downbiting rongeur
Downey
    D. fingertip texture discrimination
      test
    D. hemilaminectomy retractor
    D. modification
    D. modification of Fowler-Philip
      retrocalcaneal exostosis approach
Downey-McGlamery procedure
Downey-Rubin overlapping toe repair
  procedure
downgoing toes
Downing
    D. cartilage knife
    D. staple
downsized circular laminar hook
doxepin
doxorubicin
Doyan periosteal elevator
Doyen
    D. bone mallet
    D. costal rasp
    D. cylindrical bur
    D. cylindrical drill
    D. rib elevator
    D. rib rasp
    D. spherical bur
Dozier radiolucent Bennett
  retractor
DP
    distal phalanx
    dorsalis pedis
      DP pulse
      Springlite Advantage DP
DPA
    dual-photon absorptiometry
DPB
    dynamic pedobarography
DPC
    delayed primary closure
    distal palmar crease
DPD
    dual photon densitometry
d-penicillamine
DPM
    Doctor of Podiatric Medicine

D

DPN
 deep peroneal nerve
DP-Pour acrylic bone cement
DPSI
 dynamic postural stability index
DPTT
 deep posterior tibiotalar
 DPTT ligament
DPVNS
 diffuse pigmented villonodular synovitis
DPX
 dual-photon absorptiometry
 DPX densitometer
DRA
 distal reference axis
drafting
 overlay d.
Dragstedt skin graft
drag-to gait
drain
 Charnley suction d.
 Elutia antimicrobial coated closed
  surgical wound d.
 fishmouth d.
 Hemovac Hydrocoat d.
 Heyer-Schulte wound d.
 Jackson-Pratt d.
 Nélaton rubber tube d.
 open fracture wound d.
 Penrose d.
 polyethylene d.
 PVC d.
 rubber d.
 Shirley d.
 silastic d.
 subcutaneous d.
 Surgivac d.
 Wound-Evac d.
drainage
 anterior d.
 anterolateral d.
 anteromedial d.
 ConstaVac d.
 David d.
 dorsal d.
 ilium d.
 incision and d. (I&D)
 infusion-aspiration d.
 Klein d.
 lateral d.
 medial d.
 Ober posterior d.
 open d.
 pelvic d.
 posterior d.
 posterolateral d.
 posteromedial d.
 suction d.
draining infected nonunion

DRAM
 de-epithelialized rectus abdominis
 muscle
 DRAM flap
drape
 adhesive d.
 double d.
 fenestrated d.
 foot d.
 incise d.
 isolation d.
 lint-free d.
 Loban adhesive d.
 3M skin d.
 NeuroDrape surgical d.
 Opmi microscopic d.
 Opraflex d.
draped out
drawer
 d. sign
 d. test
drawing
 pain d.
 preoperative d.
 Ransford Pain D.
drawn ankle clonus
DRC
 dorsal radiocarpal
 DRC ligament
dream
 D. Pillow
 D. Ride car seat
Drennan
 D. hip adductor posterior transfer
 D. metaphysial-epiphysial angle
DressFlex
 D. orthotic
 D. orthotic device
Dressinet netting bandage
dressing
 abdominal d.
 absorptive d.
 ACU-derm wound d.
 Adaptic d.
 adhesive d.
 Aeroplast d.
 alginate d.
 AlgiSite alginate wound d.
 Allevyn island d.
 Allevyn wound d.
 d. apraxia
 Aquaphor gauze d.
 Aquasorb Hydrogel wound d.
 Arglaes antimicrobial silver film d.
 Arthrosol d.
 Avitene flour d.
 Betadine d.
 Bioclusive select transparent film d.
 biologic d.

blister film d.
bulky hand d.
bundle d.
Bunnell d.
burn d.
calcium alginate d.
CarboFlex odor-control d.
Cica-Care wound d.
Circulon d.
circumferential d.
Coban elastic d.
CoFilm d.
Co-Flex d.
cold compressive d.
collagen skin d.
collodion d.
CombiDERM nonadhesive
  absorbent d.
Comfeel Ulcus occlusive d.
Compeed protective d.
compression d.
conductive Hydrogel wound d.
Conform d.
ConvaDERM Plus d.
CoolSorb absorbent cold transfer d.
Coraderm d.
corrective soft d.
cotton d.
Covaderm Plus adhesive barrier d.
Coverlet adhesive surgical d.
Coverlet Strips wound d.
Cover-Roll adhesive gauze d.
Covertell composite secondary d.
Co-Wrap d.
Cryo/Cuff ankle d.
Cutinova cavity d.
Cutinova foam d.
Cutinova thin d.
Dermagran hydrophilic gauze d.
Dermagran ointment wound d.
DermaMend foam wound d.
DermaMend Hydrogel d.
DermaSite d.
Dermiflex d.
Digi Sleeve stockinette d.
dry sterile d. (DSD)
DuoDerm d.
Eakin cohesive seal d.
elastic d.
Elastikon d.
Elastomull d.
Elastoplast d.
Ensure-It d.
Epigard d.
Esmarch d.
Exu-Dry wound d.
Fabco gauze d.
felt d.
figure-of-8 d.

film blister d.
fixed d.
Flexderm wound d.
flexible burn d.
Flexigrid d.
Flexinet d.
Flexzan foam wound d.
fluff d.
foam wound d.
Fuller shield d.
Furacin gauze d.
FyBron d.
gauze d.
Geliperm d.
Gelocast Unna boot compression d.
Glasscock ear d.
Granuflex d.
hydrocolloid occlusive d.
Hydrocol wound d.
Hydrogel wound d.
hydrophilic d.
Inerpan flexible burn d.
intact d.
Integra bilayer matrix wound d.
IntraSite d.
J&J ulcer d.
Jones d.
Kaltostat d.
Kelikian foot d.
Kerlix d.
Kling adhesive d.
Koch-Mason d.
Kollagen d.
LYOfoam C d.
LYOfoam wound d.
Medi-Rip d.
Microfoam d.
Mills d.
modified Robert Jones d.
moleskin strip d.
Mother Jones d.
neoprene d.
nonadherent gauze d.
N-Terface d.
Nu Gauze d.
NutraFill hydrophilic d.
NutraStat wound d.
Oasis wound d.
occlusive d.
O'Donoghue d.
Omniderm d.
Opraflex d.
OpSite wound d.
Orthoflex d.
Orthoplast d.
OsmoCyte island wound-care d.
Owen gauze d.
palm-to-axilla d.
Panogauze Hydrogel wound d.

D

dressing (*continued*)

    patch d.
    petroleum gauze d.
    pledget d.
    Polyderm hydrophilic polyurethane foam d.
    PolyMem wound care d.
    polymeric d.
    Polyskin d.
    polyurethane foam d. (PFD)
    PolyWic d.
    postoperative d.
    pressure ulcer d.
    Primaderm d.
    Primapore wound d.
    ProCyte transparent d.
    Profore wound d.
    Promogran matrix wound d.
    PVD d.
    RepliCare wound d.
    Reston d.
    Restore CalciCare d.
    rigid d.
    Robert Jones d.
    Schanz d.
    semirigid postoperative d.
    Setopress d.
    SignaDRESS hydrocolloid d.
    silastic gel d.
    silk mesh gauze d.
    SkinTemp collagen skin d.
    sling d.
    Sof-Rol d.
    soft d.
    soft bulky d.
    Sof-Wick d.
    Spenco Second Skin d.
    Spherisorb d.
    stent d.
    sterile dry d. (SDD)
    d. stick
    Stimson figure-of-8 d.
    SuperSkin thin film d.
    Surgilast tubular elastic d.
    Suture-Self d.
    Synthaderm d.
    Tegaderm d.
    Telfa gauze d.
    THINSite d.
    Toe-Aid d.
    toe-to-groin modified Jones d.
    transparent adhesive d.
    Tricodur Epi compression d.
    Tricodur Omos compression d.
    Tricodur Talus compression d.
    Tubex gauze d.
    Tubigrip d.
    ulcer d.
    Ultec thin d.

    Uniflex d.
    V.A.C. GranuFoam heel d.
    Velpeau d.
    Vi-Drape d.
    Vigilon d.
    Webril d.
    wet-to-dry d.
    wide-mesh petroleum gauze d.
    wound d.
    Xeroform gauze d.

Dreyfus

    D. prosthesis forceps
    D. prosthesis placement instrument

DREZ

    dorsal root entry zone
    DREZ lesion
    DREZ lesioning procedure

Drez

    D. modification of Eriksson ankle joint arthroscopy technique

DRG

    dorsal root ganglion

DRI

    dietary reference intake

Driessen hinged plate

drift

    arm d.
    congenital ulnar d.
    leg d.
    osseous d.
    pronator d.
    radial d.
    ulnar d.

drill

    ACL d.
    Acra-Cut wire pass d.
    Acufex d.
    Adson-Rogers perforating d.
    Adson spiral d.
    Adson twist d.
    Aesculap d.
    agility d.
    air d.
    air-powered cutting d.
    Albee d.
    Amico d.
    Anspach power d.
    anticavitation d.
    Archimedean d.
    ASIF twist d.
    ASSI wire-pass d.
    autotome d.
    Bailey d.
    bar d.
    battery-driven hand d.
    biflanged d.
    d. bit
    bit d.
    d. bit fracture

Björk rib d.
bone hand d.
Bosworth crown d.
Bowen suture d.
brace d.
Brunswick-Mack rotating d.
Bunnell bone d.
Bunnell hand d.
bur d.
cannulated d.
cannulated cortical step d.
Carmody perforator d.
Carroll-Bunnell d.
Cebotome bone d.
centering d.
cervical d.
Championniére bone d.
Charnley centering d.
Charnley femoral condyle d.
Charnley pilot d.
Charnley starting d.
Cherry d.
Cherry-Austin d.
Children's Hospital hand d.
chuck d.
Cloward cervical d.
Coballoy twist d.
Codman wire-passing d.
Collison body d.
Collison cannulated hand d.
Collison tap d.
cortical step d.
crown d.
Crutchfield bone d.
Crutchfield hand d.
Crutchfield-Raney d.
CurvTek TSR bone d.
Cushing flat d.
Cushing perforator d.
dental d.
depth-check d.
DePuy d.
D'Errico perforating d.
Deyerle d.
diamond high-speed d.
Doyen cylindrical d.
driver nail d.
Elan d.
Elan-E power d.
extractor nail d.
fingernail d.
Fisch d.
flat d.
Galt hand d.
Gates-Glidden d.
glenoid d.
Gray bone d.
d. guard
d. guide

d. guide forceps
Hall air d.
Hall-Dundar d.
Hall Micro-Aire d.
Hall power d.
Hall stepdown d.
Hall Versipower d.
hand d.
hand-operated d.
Harold Crowe d.
Harris-Smith anterior interbody d.
Hewson d.
high-speed twist d.
hip fracture compaction d.
d. hole
hollow mill d.
Hudson bone d.
Hudson brace d.
initiator d.
intramedullary d.
Jacobs chuck d.
Kerr electro-torque d.
Kerr hand d.
Kirschner bone d.
Kirschner wire d.
Kodex d.
Küntscher d.
Loth-Kirschner d.
Luck bone d.
Lusskin bone d.
Macewen d.
Magnuson twist d.
Mathews hand d.
Mathews load d.
McKenzie bone d.
McKenzie perforating twist d.
Michelson-Sequoia air d.
Micro-Aire d.
Midas Rex d.
mini-Stryker power d.
Minos air d.
Mira d.
Modny d.
Moore bone d.
nail d.
Neurain d.
Neurairtome d.
nipper nail d.
Orthairtome II d.
Osseodent surgical d.
Osteone air d.
Patrick d.
pencil-tip d.
penetrating d.
Penn finger d.
perforating twist d.
perforator d.
pilot d.
d. pin

D

drill (*continued*)
pistol-grip hand d.
Podospray podiatry d.
d. point
Portmann d.
power d.
pronator d.
Ralks bone d.
Ralks fingernail d.
Raney bone d.
Raney perforator d.
retention d.
rib d.
Rica bone d.
Richards Lovejoy bone d.
Richards pistol-grip d.
Richmond subarachnoid
 twist d.
Richter bone d.
right-angle dental d.
Romano curved surgical d.
rotating d.
scissors nail d.
Shea d.
Sherman-Stille d.
Sklar bone d.
d. sleeve
Smedberg hand d.
Smedberg twist d.
Smith automatic perforated d.
spiral d.
Spirec d.
step d.
step-down d.
Stille bone d.
Stille hand d.
Stille-Sherman bone d.
Stiwer hand d.
Stryker d.
Suretac d.
Surgairtome air d.
surgical orthopaedic d.
suture hole d.
Synthes d.
tap d.
Toti trephine d.
trephine d.
Trinkle bone d.
Trinkle power d.
Trinkle Super-Cut twist d.
twist d.
Ullrich d.
Uniflex calibrated step d.
union broach retention d.
universal 2-speed hand d.
wire d.
Wolferman d.
Xomed d.
Zimmer hand d.

Zimmer-Kirschner hand d.
Zimmer universal d.
drill-guide
Acufex d.-g.
drilling
arthroscopic d.
d. broach
excision, curettage, d.
 (ECD)
d. jig
percutaneous transmalleolar d.
retrograde d.
d. technique
transmalleolar d.
drill-tipped guidewire
D-ring strap
drip-suck irrigation
Drisdol Oral
drive
Jacobs chuck d.
drive-extractor
driver
blade-plate d.
bullet d.
femoral head d.
Flatt d.
graft d.
Hall d.
Harrington hook d.
Jewett d.
Ken d.
Kirschner wire d.
Küntscher nail d.
K wire d.
Linvatec d.
Lloyd nail d.
Massie d.
Maxi-Driver d.
McReynolds d.
Micro Series wire d.
Moore d.
nail d.
d. nail drill
Orthairtome wire d.
ParaMax angled d.
plate d.
polyethylene-faced d.
prosthesis d.
Pugh d.
Rush d.
Schneider nail d.
staple d.
supine position d.
surgical pin d.
Teflon-coated d.
tibial d.
trial d.
d. tunnel locator apparatus
wire d.

driver-bender-extractor
    Rush d.-b.-e.
driver-extractor
    Hansen-Street d.-e.
    Ken d.-e.
    McReynolds d.-e.
    Sage d.-e.
    Schneider d.-e.
drivethrough sign
DRL
    dorsoradial ligament
dromedary gait
drooping shoulder sign
droopy shoulder syndrome
drop
    d. arm rotator cuff test
    d. attack
    d. finger
    d. foot
    d. shoulder
    toe d.
    d. vertical jump
    wrist d.
    d. wrist deformity
    d. wrist splint
drop-arm sign
drop-entry closed body hook
droperidol and fentanyl
dropfoot, drop foot
    d. brace
    d. gait
    d. redression stockings
    d. splint
drop-lock
    d.-l. knee brace
    d.-l. ring
dropped hallux
DRU
    distal radioulnar
    DRU joint
drug
    antituberculosis d.
    cytotoxic d.
    disease-modifying antirheumatologic
     d. (DMARD)
    National Collegiate Athletic
     Association prohibited d.
    nonsteroidal antiinflammatory d.
     (NSAID)
    slow-acting antirheumatic d.
     (SAARD)
drug-induced myotonia
drug-infusion fever
drug-related fetal hydantoin
 syndrome
DRUJ
    distal radioulnar joint
    DRUJ instability
    DRUJ prosthesis

drummer-boy palsy
Drummond
    D. and Hastings cuboid extrusion
     injury
    D. button
    D. hook
    D. hook holder
    D. interspinous wiring
     technique
    D. scoliosis repair
    D. segmental wire fixation through
     spinous process
    D. spinal instrumentation
    D. wire
drumstick finger
drunken sailor gait
dry
    d. amputation
    D. Flotation wheelchair cushion
    d. gangrene
    d. heat therapy
    d. hydrotherapy
    d. infected nonunion
    d. joint
    d. necrosis
    d. sterile dressing (DSD)
    d. synovitis
Drysol
Drytex RocketSoc ankle brace
DS
    Anaprox DS
    Tolectin DS
DSA
    digital subtraction angiography
DSC
    DSC Foot Cream
    Parafon Forte DSC
DSD
    dry sterile dressing
DSIS
    dynamic stabilizing innersole system
    DSIS orthotic
D-Soles
    D-S. insole
    D-S. orthotic
DSTR
    distal soft tissue release
DTM
    dermatophyte test medium
    DTM culture
DTR
    deep tendon reflex
DTT
    device for transverse traction
    DTT implant
    DTT system
DTVP-2
    Development Test of Visual
    Perception, 2nd Edition

D

dual
  D. AFO Boot orthotic
  d. compression scoliosis treatment
  d. drop pelvis (DDP)
  d. nerve root suction retractor
  d. onlay cortical bone graft
  d. photon densitometry (DPD)
  d. photon densitometry test
  d. photon densitometry test for osteoporosis
  d. pin redresser
  d. plate
  D. Range Limiter System
  d. square-ended Harrington rod
dual-energy x-ray absorptiometry (DEXA, DXA)
Dualer Plus inclinometer
Duall 88 cement
dual-lock
  d.-l. ankle brace
  d.-l. total hip prosthesis
  d.-l. total hip replacement system
dual-photon
  d.-p. absorptiometry (DPA, DPX)
  d.-p. electrospinal orthosis
dual-threaded screw
Dubreuilh
  melanosis circumscripta praeblastomatosa D.
Duchenne
  D. disease
  D. lower extremity test
  D. muscular atrophy
  D. muscular dystrophy
Duchenne-Aran disease
Duchenne-Erb palsy
duck
  d. waddle
  d. waddle gait
  d. waddle test
duckbill
  d. elevator
  d. rongeur
duct
  thoracic d.
ductile failure
ductility
duction
Dugas dislocated shoulder test
Duhot line
dull aching pain
dumbbell
  d. tumor
  d. wagon
Dumon-Gilliard prosthesis introducer
Duncan
  D. loop

  D. prone rectus femoris dysfunction test
  D. shoulder brace
Dunlop traction
Dunn
  D. acromioclavicular joint technique
  D. biopsy
  D. fracture device
  D. hip operation
  D. multiple comparison test
  D. osteotomy
  D. triple arthrodesis
Dunn-Brittain triple arthrodesis
Duocentric prosthesis
DuoCet
Duo-Cline dual support contoured bed wedge
Duocondylar knee prosthesis
DuoDerm dressing
Duo-Drive screw
Duofilm Solution
Duo-Lock hip prosthesis
duopatellar unconstrained prosthesis
Dupaco
  D. knee control
  D. knee prosthesis
Dupel blue iontophoresis electrode
Duplay
  D. bursitis
  D. disease
  D. periarthritis syndrome
duplex
  d. Doppler ultrasonography
  d. ultrasound
duplicate
  d. sternum
  d. thumb
duplicated metacarpal
duplication
  Marks-Bayne technique for thumb d.
  symmetric thumb d.
  thumb d.
  Wassel thumb d. (I-VI)
Dupont
  D. Bunion Rating Score
  D. distal humeral plate system
Dupré muscle
Dupuytren
  D. amputation
  D. canal
  D. contracture
  D. contracture release
  D. diathesis
  D. disease
  D. exostosis
  D. fascia
  D. fasciitis
  D. fibromatosis

D. fracture
D. hydrocele
D. operation
D. sign
D. splint
D. suture
dura
d. dissector
d. hook
d. mater
d. mater graft
DuraBoot orthosis
Duracon
D. knee implant
D. prosthesis
Duract
Dura-Flex back brace
DuraGen Plus adhesion barrier matrix
Duragesic Transdermal
Dura-Kold reusable compression ice wrap
dural
d. ectasia
d. elevator
d. ligament
d. repair
d. tear
Duraleve custom molded foot orthotic
Durallium implant
Duraloc
D. acetabular cup system
D. acetabular liner
D. prosthesis
Duralone Injection
duralumin
Duramer polyethylene component
Duramorph injection
Duranest
Duran-Houser wrist splint
Duran passive mobilization
Durapatite
D. bone replacement implant
D. bone replacement material
DuraPrep
Dura-Soft soft-compression reusable ice or heat wrap
Dura-Stick adhesive electrode
Durasul
D. head system
D. polyethylene
D. polyethylene, high wear resistant acetabular insert
D. prosthetic component
Duraval hook & loop strap material
Durham
D. flatfoot operation
D. plasty
D. procedure
D. procedure for flatfoot

Durie-Salmon classification
Durkan
D. carpal compression test
D. CTS gauge
Duro-Med Industries (DMI)
durometer
durum
heloma d. (HD)
osteoma d.
dust
nail d.
Dutchman's roll
duToit shoulder staple
Duval elevator
Duverney fracture
DuVries
D. arthroplasty
D. deltoid ligament reconstruction technique
D. hammertoe repair
D. incision
D. metatarsal head resection
D. modified McBride hallux valgus operation
D. phalangeal condylectomy
D. plantar condylectomy
D. plantar fasciotomy approach
D. procedure
D. technique for overlapping fifth toe
DuVries-Mann modified bunionectomy
Dvorak flexion-rotation test
DVR anatomic wrist fracture plate
DVRT
differential variable reluctance transducer
DVT
deep venous thrombosis
Flowtron DVT
DVT prophylaxis
dwarfism
achondroplastic d.
acromelic d.
acromesomelic d.
ateliotic d.
autosomal dominant mild short limb d.
camptomelic d.
chondroplastic d.
diastrophic d.
disproportionate d.
Hunter-Thompson d.
Langer mesomelic d.
Laron d.
metatropic d.
micromelic d.
phocomelic d.
Pott d.
proportionate d.

D

dwarfism (*continued*)
    Russell-Silver d.
    short-limb d.
dwarf pelvis
Dwyer
    D. anterior endoscopic correction of scoliosis
    D. calcaneal osteotomy
    D. clawfoot operation
    D. device
    D. incision
    D. instrumentation biomechanics
    D. orthopaedic procedure
    D. osteotomy
    D. scoliosis cable
    D. spinal instrumentation
    D. spinal mechanical stapler
    D. spinal screw
    D. tensioner
Dwyer-Hall plate
Dwyer-Wickham electrical stimulation system
5DX
    Biofeedback 5DX
DXA
    dual-energy x-ray absorptiometry
    DXA scan
Dycal base
Dycem roll matting
Dycill
Dyck-Lambert classification
Dycor
    D. Geriatric ADL single axis foot prosthesis
    D. prosthetic foot
dye
    d. extravasation
    methylene blue d.
Dyggve-Melchior-Clausen syndrome
dying bug exercise
Dyke-Davidoff-Masson syndrome
Dyna-Disc
    Exertools D.-D.
    D.-D. gymball
DYNAfabric material
Dynafed IB
Dynafill graft biomedium
DynaFix external fixation system
DynaFlex
    D. Gyro exerciser
    D. multilayer compression system
DynaGraft implant
Dynagrip
    D. blade handle
    D. handle of blade
DynaHeat hot pack
Dyna-Hex Topical
Dyna knee splint

Dyna-Lok
    D.-L. pedicle screw system
    D.-L. plating system
Dynalok classic minimal access surgery system
dynametric testing
dynamic
    d. abduction brace
    d. alignment
    d. axial fixator (DAF)
    d. balance
    d. bracing
    d. canal glide
    d. compression
    d. compression plate (DCP)
    d. compression plate fixation
    d. compression plate instrumentation
    D. condylar screw (DCS)
    d. condylar screw fixation
    d. condylar screw tap
    d. digital deformity
    D. digit extensor tube
    d. double tendon replacement
    D. Edge rehabilitation equipment
    D. elbow orthosis
    d. electromyography
    d. external fixation
    d. fault
    D. foot orthosis
    d. footprint
    D. foot stabilizer
    d. friction
    d. gait
    d. gait index
    d. hallux varus
    d. hammertoe
    d. hinge elbow fracture brace
    d. hip screw (DHS)
    d. integrated stabilization chair (DISC)
    d. joint force
    D. knee orthosis
    d. listing
    d. listing nomenclature
    d. loading
    d. locking nail
    d. lumbar stabilization
    d. magnetic resonance imaging (dMRI)
    d. metatarsus adductus
    d. mobility screen
    D. Motion Foot 1D35
    d. motion x-ray
    d. movement
    d. MRI
    d. muscle transfer
    d. pedobarography (DPB)
    d. pedodynographic finding
    d. postural stability index (DPSI)

d. repair
d. splint
d. splinting
d. stability index
d. stabilization trainer
d. stabilizing innersole system (DSIS)
d. standing balance
d. stress x-ray view
d. stump exercise
d. traction method
d. transverse traction device
d. trunk curl
D. wound closure system
D. wrist orthosis

dynamics
foot d.

dynamization collar

dynamometer
Baseline d.
Biodex isokinetic d.
bulb d.
Collins d.
computerized isokinetic d.
Cybex II isokinetic d.
electromechanical d.
hand grip d.
handheld d.
Harpenden d.
isokinetic d.
Isostation B–200 triaxial lumbar d.
Jamar hydraulic hand d.
Lido isokinetic d.
Micro-FET hand held d.
orthopaedic d.
Smedley d.
Spark handheld d.
squeeze d.

dynamometry
isokinetic d.
tip-pinch d.

DynaPak electrode kit
Dynapen
Dynaphor iontophoresis
Dynaplex knee prosthesis
DynaPrene splinting thermoplastic
Dynaslipper night shoe
Dynasplint
D. knee extension
D. knee extension unit
D. shoulder system

DynaSport athletic tape
Dynatron
D. 50, 125, 525 electrotherapy
D. Mini 2000 electrotherapy
D. 2000 muscle test
D. TX 900 electrotherapy

Dynesys dynamic stabilization of spinal segments system

DyoCam
D. 550 arthroscopic video camera
D. arthroscopic view camera

Dyonics
D. arthroplasty bur
D. arthroscope
D. arthroscopic blade
D. cannula
D. Golden Retriever magnet
D. shaver

dysaesthesia (*var. of* dysesthesia)
dysarthria
clumsy hand d.
spinal d.

dysarthrosis
patellofemoral d.

dysbaric
d. osteonecrosis
d. oxygen

dysbasia, dysbasis
d. angiosclerotica
d. lordotica progressiva

dysbasis (*var. of* dysbasia)
dyscalculia
developmental d.

dyschondroplasia
Ollier d.

dyschondrosteosis
dyscinesia (*var. of* dyskinesia)
dyscollagenosis
dyscrasia
plasma cell d.

dyscrasic fracture
dysdiadochocinesia (*var. of* dysdiadochokinesia)
dysdiadochokinesia, dysdiadochocinesia
dysesthesia, dysaesthesia
dysfunction
anterior-inferior capsular ligament d.
bladder d.
craniomandibular d.
endothelial d.
erectile d.
extensor mechanism d.
facet joint d.
FHL d.
fixation d.
iliacus d.
intervertebral d.
joint d.
mechanical d.
motor d.
neuroarticular d.
organic d.
painful minor intervertebral d. (PMID)
patellofemoral d. (PFD)
pelvic ring d.
pilomotor d.

D

dystrophia (*var. of* dystrophy)
dystrophic
    d. calcification
    d. gait
    d. nail
    d. spondylosis
    d. toenail
dystrophica
    myotonia d.
dystrophinopathy
dystrophy, dystrophia
    adult pseudohypertrophic muscular d.
    Barnes d.
    Becker muscular d. (BMD)
    Becker variant of Duchenne d.
    congenital d.
    distal d.
    Duchenne muscular d.
    Emery-Dreifuss muscular d.
    (EDMD)
    Erb muscular d.
    facioscapulohumeral muscular d.
    (FSHD, FSHMD, FSMD)
    fascioscapulohumeral d.
    fascioscapulohumeral muscular d.

    Fröhlich adiposogenital d.
    Gowers muscular d.
    humeroperoneal muscular d.
    juvenile muscular d.
    Kiloh-Nevin ocular form of
    progressive muscular d.
    Landouzy-Dejerine d.
    Leyden-Möbius muscular d.
    limb-girdle muscular d.
    muscular d. (MD)
    myotonic d. (DM, MD)
    dystrophia myotonica (DM)
    myotonic muscular d.
    neurovascular d.
    osseous d.
    pelvofemoral muscular d.
    posttraumatic d.
    progressive muscular d. (PMD)
    pseudohypertrophic d.
    reflex neurovascular d.
    reflex sympathetic d. (RSD)
    sex-linked muscular d.
    sympathetic reflex d.
    tardive muscular d.
dysvascular condition

D

E-2
    E-2 foot prosthesis
    E-2 hydrocollator heating unit
EACS
    exertional anterior compartment
    syndrome
EADL
    electronic aid for daily living
    extended activities of daily living
eagle
    E. arthroscope
    e. beak bone-cutting forceps
    E. rigid anterior cervical plate
    system
    E. straight-ahead arthroscope
    E. syndrome
Eagle-Barrett syndrome
Eakin cohesive seal dressing
Earle sign
EARLY
    ergonomic assessment of risk and
    liability
Early Fit night splint
early-onset spinal deformity
E-A-R Specialty Composites
EAS
    endoskeletal alignment system
Easprin
EAST
    elevated arm stress test
    external rotation-abduction stress
    test
Easton cock-up splint
East-West retractor
Eastwood anesthesia technique
easy
    E. Access foot splint
    E. Lok ankle brace
    E. Up cushion
EasyAnchor
EasyLiner
    ALPS E.
Easy-On elbow brace
Easy-Pull sock aide device
Easyslide sliding mat
Easyspine
    E. pedicle screw and rod system
    E. posterior fixation system
EasyStand 6000 glider
EasyStep pressure relief walker
eater
    cement e.
Eaton
    E. and Glickel carpometacarpal joint
    arthrosis (stage I–IV)

    E. closed carpometacarpal joint
    reduction
    E. implant arthroplasty
    E. splint
    E. trapezium finger joint
    replacement prosthesis
    E. volar plate arthroplasty
Eaton-Lambert syndrome
Eaton-Littler
    E.-L. carpometacarpal thumb repair
    technique
    E.-L. ligament reconstruction
Eberle
    E. contracture release
    E. contracture release technique
EBGS
    electrical bone-growth stimulation
    electrical bone-growth stimulator
EBI
    electronic bone stimulation
    EBI device
    EBI Medical Array spinal system
    EBI Medical SpinalPak II spine
    fusion stimulator
EBL
    estimated blood loss
EBM
    evidence-based medicine
ebonation
eburnate
eburnated
    e. bone
    e. bone surface
eburnation
    bony e.
    e. of cartilage
eburneum
    osteoma e.
eccentric
    e. access
    e. amputation
    e. axis of ankle rotation
    e. contraction
    e. drill guide
    e. dynamic compression plate
    (EDCP)
    e. exercise
    e. function
    e. loading
    e. muscle action
    e. muscle training
    e. wear
    e. work
eccentro-osteochondrodysplasia
ecchondroma, ecchondrosis

E

ecchondrosis (*var. of* ecchondroma)
ecchondrotome
ecchymosis
eccrine
    e. poroma
    e. sweat gland
ECD
    excision, curettage, drilling
echinococciasis (*var. of* echinococcosis)
echinococcosis, echinococciasis
Echlin
    E. bone rongeur
    E. duckbill rongeur
    E. rongeur forceps
Echlin-Luer rongeur
echo
    e. time
    e. train length (ETL)
echocardiography (echo)
    dobutamine e.
echography
eclipse
    E. Gel ankle brace
    E. Gel elbow strap
    E. TENS unit
EC-Naprosyn
EcoNail nail lacquer
econazole
Econo
    E. 90 lumbar home traction
    E. 90 traction unit
Econo-Cerv
    E.-C. supine cervical traction
    E.-C. traction device
economic self-sufficiency WHO Handicap Scale
economy ROM brace
EconoSoc ankle brace
Econo-Strap
Ecotrin Low Adult Strength
ECRB
    extensor carpi radialis brevis
    ECRB muscle
    ECRB tendon
ECRL
    extensor carpi radialis longus
    ECRL muscle
    ECRL tendon
EcstaSeat seat cushion
ECT
    European compression technique
    extended code therapy
    ECT bone screw
    ECT internal fracture fixation
    ECT internal fracture fixation system
ectasia, ectasis
    dural e.
ectasis (*var. of* ectasia)

ectomesomorphic physique
ectomorph
ectomorphic physique
ectopic
    e. bone
    e. bone growth
    e. ossification
ECTR
    endoscopic carpal tunnel release
ectrodactylia (*var. of* ectrodactyly)
ectrodactylism (*var. of* ectrodactyly)
ectrodactyly, ectrodactylia, ectrodactylism
ectromelia
ECU
    extensor carpi ulnaris
    ECU muscle
    ECU tendon
ED
    extensor digitorum
EDB
    extensor digitorum brevis
    EDB muscle
    EDB tendon
EDC
    extensor digitorum communis
EDCP
    eccentric dynamic compression plate
Eddowes
    E. brittle bones syndrome
    E. disease
edema
    bone marrow e.
    constrictive e.
    dependent e.
    endoneurial e.
    goose-egg e.
    e. heat therapy
    intracompartmental e.
    leg e.
    marrow e.
    mushy e.
    nonpitting e.
    pitting e.
    posttraumatic e.
    pretibial e. (PTE)
    rheumatismal e.
    e. sock
    stump e.
    swimming-induced pulmonary e. (SIPE)
    transient bone marrow e.
edematous
Eden-Hybbinette
    E.-H. anterior glenoid bone block procedure
    E.-H. arthroplasty
    E.-H. operation
Eden-Lange trapezius procedure
Eden thoracic outlet test

Eder-Puestow metal olive dilator
EDF
elongation, derotation, flexion
EDF scoliosis cast
EDG
electrodynogram
EDG system
Edgarton-Grand thumb adduction
edge
Acufex E.
E. knee brace
patellar e.
3-edge cutting forceps
edge-detection
digital e.-d.
Edinburgh
E. method
E. Rehabilitation Status Scale
(ERSS)
Edinger-Westphal complex
Edintrak II system
edition
Development Test of Visual
Perception, 2nd E. (DTVP-2)
EDL
extensor digitorum longus
EDM
extensor digiti minimi
EDMD
Emery-Dreifuss muscular dystrophy
Edna towel clamp
EDPA
Erhardt Developmental Prehension
Assessment
EDPCS
exertional deep posterior compartment
syndrome
EDQ
extensor digiti quinti
EDS
Ehlers-Danlos syndrome
EDSS
Expanded Disability Status Scale
education
lifestyle e. (LSE)
posture e.
EDVA
Erhardt Developmental Vision
Assessment
Edwards
E. and Lee tibiofibular diastasis and
syndesmotic injury classification
E. D-L modular fixator
E. D-L modular screw rod
E. hook
E. instrumentation
E. modular system
E. modular system bridging sleeve
construct

E. modular system compression
construct
E. modular system construct
selection
E. modular system
distraction-lordosis construct
E. modular system dynamic loading
E. modular system kyphoreduction
construct
E. modular system load sharing
E. modular system neutralization
construct
E. modular system rod crosslink
E. modular system rod sleeve
construct
E. modular system sacral fixation
device
E. modular system scoliosis
construct
E. modular system spinal/sacral
screw
E. modular system spinal sleeve
E. modular system spondylar
construct
E. modular system standard sleeve
construct
E. modular system Universal rod
E. polyethylene sleeve
E. seamless prosthesis
E. syndrome
E. transposing atrial septum
procedure
Edwards-Levine
E.-L. hook
E.-L. rod
E.-L. sleeve
Edwin Smith papyrus
EDX, EDx
electrodiagnosis
effect
bungee e.
concavity-compression e.
Hick e.
Ilizarov tension-stress e.
magic angle e.
neurophysiologic e.
rake-handle e.
scarring e.
spindle e.
steal e.
Steindler elbow flexion e.
tenodesis e.
tethering e.
vasodilatory e.
windshield wiper e.
effective foot length
efferent nerve impulse
Effler-Groves hook
effleurage massage

E

effluent
    pelvic e.
effort
    brief maximal e. (BME)
    maximum voluntary e. (MVE)
    e. thrombosis
effort-induced thrombosis
effusion
    ankle e.
    bloody e.
    joint e.
    knee joint e.
    shoulder joint e.
Eftekhar
    E. broken femoral stem technique
    E. concept
    E. long-stem prosthesis
Eftekhar-Charnley hip prosthesis
Egawa sign
eggcrate mattress
Eggers
    E. biceps femoris tendon transfer
    E. bone plate
    E. contact splint
    E. neurectomy
    E. operation
    E. screw
    E. spastic quadriplegia crouch gait
      repair tenodesis
    E. tendon transfer technique
Eggsercizer
    E. CTS exerciser
    E. resistive hand exerciser
egg-shaped cap
eggshell
    e. fracture
    e. procedure
eggshell-like calcification
egress of arthroscopic fluid
EGT
    exuberant granulation tissue
Egyptian foot
EHL
    extensor hallucis longus
    EHL tendon
Ehlers-Danlos
    E.-D. disease
    E.-D. syndrome (EDS)
EI
    external ilium
EIA
    exercise-induced asthma
Eichenholz Classification of Charcot arthropathy of foot (stage 1-3)
Eicher
    E. femoral prosthesis
    E. hip prosthesis
eicosanoid
Eikenella corrodens

Eilers-Armstrong unicompartmental knee prosthesis
EIP
    extensor indicis proprius
    EIP muscle
    EIP tendon
ejector
    Cloward dowel e.
Ekbom restless leg syndrome
Ekman brittle bones syndrome
elaiopathia (*var. of* eleopathy)
Elan drill
Elan-E power drill
Elase-Chloromycetin
    E.-C. ointment
    E.-C. Topical
Elase Topical
Elastafit tubing kit
ElastaTrac
    E. home lumbar traction system
    E. home lumbar traction unit
    E. lumbar traction
elastic
    e. ankle corset
    e. bandage
    e. barrier
    e. cartilage
    e. compression
    e. deformation
    e. dressing
    e. fixation
    e. foam bandage
    e. knee cage
    e. knee cage orthosis
    e. knee cage with medial and
      lateral contoured knee joints
    e. knee sleeve brace
    e. limit
    e. plaster of Paris
    e. property
    e. recoil
    e. stable intramedullary nailing
    (ESIN)
    e. stockings
    e. strain
    e. strap
    e. stretch
    e. traction
    e. tubing
    e. twister orthosis
    e. wristlet
    e. zone
elastic-hinge knee brace
elasticity
    modulus of e.
Elastikon
    E. dressing
    E. elastic tape
elastofibroma dorsi

Elasto-Gel
  E.-G. hot/cold therapy wrap
  E.-G. shoulder therapy wrap
elastoidosis
Elasto-Link joint wrap
elastoma
elastomer
  conventional silicone e. (CSE)
  high performance silicone e.
  polyolefin e.
  e. skin molding
  thermoplastic e. (TPE)
Elastomull
  E. dressing
  E. elastic gauze bandage
  E. splint
Elastoplast
  E. bandage
  E. dressing
elastosis
Elavil
elbow
  above e. (AE)
  e. arthrodesis
  e. arthroplasty
  axilla, shoulder, e. (ASE)
  baseball pitcher's e.
  below e. (BE)
  e. bone
  boxer's e.
  capped e.
  e. capsule
  e. cast
  compound shattered e.
  e. disarticulation
  e. dislocation
  epicondylitis of e.
  e. extension splint
  e. extensor tendon
  e. fat-pad
  fat pad of e.
  e. fat-pad sign
  e. flexion splint
  e. flexion test
  floating e.
  e. fracture
  Frohse arcade of e.
  golfer's e.
  e. hinge
  e. injury
  E. Injury Management Kit
  javelin thrower's e.
  e. jerk
  e. jerk reflex test
  e. joint
  Little League e. (LLE)
  e. magnet
  milkmaid's e.
  miner's e.

  nursemaid's e.
  NYU-Hosmer electric e.
  e. orthosis
  e. pad
  e. prosthesis
  pulled e.
  e. radiography
  e. reflex
  e. region
  e. replacement
  reverse tennis e.
  e. sleeve
  slipped e.
  Sorbie-Questor e.
  e. stability
  student's e.
  supermarket e.
  temper tantrum e.
  tennis e.
  thrower's e.
  transverse divergent dislocation of e.
  varus-valgus stress of e.
  Wilson procedure for extraarticular
    fusion of e.
  wrestler's e.
**Elbow-Up Protector elbow suspension
  device**
elbow-wrist-hand orthosis (EWHO)
elderly
  Clifton Assessment Procedures for
    the E. (CAPE)
  e. onset rheumatoid arthritis
electric
  e. artifact
  e. cast saw
  e. dermatome
  e. differential therapy
  e. joint fluoroscopy
  e. wheelchair
electrical
  e. bone-growth stimulation (EBGS)
  e. bone-growth stimulator (EBGS)
  e. implant
  e. inactivity
  e. injury
  e. modality
  e. nerve stimulation
  e. potential
  e. silence
  e. stimulation rehabilitation
  e. stimulation therapy
  e. stimulator waveform
  e. surface stimulation
  e. surface stimulation treatment for
    scoliosis
Electri-Cool
  E.-C. cold therapy system
  E.-C. continuous controlled cold
    therapy

E

electroacupuncture
    Acu-Treat e.
    Electro-Acuscope e.
Electro-Acuscope
    E.-A. electroacupuncture
    E.-A. 85 stimulator
electrocardiography
electrocautery
    e. apparatus
    Aspen e.
electrocoagulation
electrode
    active e.
    ArthroCare e.
    bifilar needle recording e.
    BioKnit garment e.
    bipolar needle recording e.
    bipolar stimulating e.
    coaxial needle e.
    concentric needle e.
    Disposatrode disposable e.
    Dupel blue iontophoresis e.
    Dura-Stick adhesive e.
    Electro-Mesh e.
    Excel Plus e.
    exploring e.
    e. glove
    e. grid
    ground e.
    indifferent e.
    LSI Easy Stims self-adhesive e.
    LSI silver self-adhesive
      disposable e.
    macro-EMG needle e.
    microcurrent e.
    monopolar needle recording e.
    multilead e.
    needle e.
    e. paste
    e. placement
    Polystim e.
    prizm Electro-Mesh Sock e.
    recording e.
    reference e.
    Silver-Thera stocking e.
    single-fiber needle e.
    e. sock
    Sportstim muscle stimulation e.
    stigmatic e.
    stimulating e.
    surface e.
    Teq-Trode e.
    Ultra Stim silver e.
    unipolar needle e.
    Versa-Stim self-adhering e.
electrodesiccated bleeding point
electrodesiccation
electrodiagnosis (EDx, EDX)
    mononeuropathy e.

Electro-Diagnostic Instruments Model 720 bilateral tetrapolar impedance plethysmograph
electrodiagnostic medicine
electrodynogram (EDG)
electrogoniometer
    ankle-foot e.
    6 degrees of freedom e.
    parallelogram e.
electrokinetic potential
Electro-Link joint wrap
electrolyte
    e. balance
    e. replacement
electromagnet
    spring-mounted e.
electromagnetic field
electromassage
electromechanical
    e. delay (EMD)
    e. dynamometer
Electro-Mesh
    E.-M. electrode
    E.-M. sleeve
electromyocardiography
    cervical Derefield procedure e.
electromyogram (EMG)
    integrated rectified e. (IEMG)
    ulnar nerve motor/sensory e.
electromyographic activation
electromyography (EMG)
    central e.
    dynamic e.
    integrated e.
    e. retrainer biofeedback unit
    single-fiber e. (SFEMG)
    surface e. (SEMG, sEMG)
electron-beam therapy
electroneuromyography (ENMG)
electroneurophysiologic
electronic
    e. aid for daily living
      (EADL)
    e. bone stimulation (EBI)
    e. bone stimulation apparatus
    e. goniometer
    e. muscle stimulator (EMS)
electronics
    American Medical E. (AME)
    e. electrical stimulation device
electronystagmography
electrooptical characteristic (EOC)
electrophysiologic study
electrosurgical
    e. generator
    e. instrument
    e. pencil
electrotherapeutic point stimulation (ETPS)

electrotherapy
    e. device
    direct current e.
    Dynatron 50, 125, 525 e.
    Dynatron Mini 2000 e.
    Dynatron TX 900 e.
    Mettler e.
    PET e.
    e. system
    ultrasound e.
electrothermal arthroscopy
electrothermally assisted capsulorrhaphy
    (ETAC)
Elekta stereotactic head frame
element
    neural e.
    posterior e.
elementary fracture
eleopathy, elaiopathia
elephant-ear clavicular splint
elephant-foot
    e.-f. callus
    e.-f. fracture
    e.-f. fracture nonunion
elevata
    scapula e.
elevated
    e. arm stress test (EAST)
    e. rim acetabular liner
    e. scapula
elevating osteotomy
elevation
    e. angle
    congenital scapular e.
    e. exercise
    ice, compression, e. (ICE)
    intracranial pressure e.
    Maquet e.
    e. of extremity
    periosteal e.
    e. pillow
    protection, restricted activity, ice,
        compression, e. (PRICE)
    rest, ice, compression, e. (RICE)
    scapular e.
    E.'s shoe buildup
elevator
    Adson periosteal e.
    Alexander periosteal e.
    angular e.
    APC proximal femoral e.
    Aufranc periosteal e.
    Bennett e.
    Bethune periosteal e.
    biceps e.
    Blair e.
    bone e.
    Bowen periosteal e.
    Bristow periosteal e.

Brophy periosteal e.
Buck periosteal e.
Campbell periosteal e.
Carroll-Legg periosteal e.
Carroll periosteal e.
Chandler bone e.
chisel e.
chisel-edge e.
Cloward osteophyte e.
Cloward periosteal e.
Cobb periosteal e.
Cohen periosteal e.
Converse periosteal e.
Crego e.
Crego periosteal e.
curved periosteal e.
Cushing-Hopkins periosteal e.
Cushing Little Joker e.
Cushing periosteal e.
Darrach periosteal e.
Davidson-Sauerbruch-Doyen
    periosteal e.
Dawson-Yuhl-Key e.
Dawson-Yuhl periosteal e.
Doyan periosteal e.
Doyen rib e.
duckbill e.
dural e.
Duval e.
Endotrac e.
extra-leverage proximal femoral e.
Farabeuf periosteal e.
Fomon periosteal e.
fracture reducing e.
Frazier e.
Freer periosteal e.
Freer septal e.
Gardner e.
hand e.
Harrington spinal e.
Heel Minder foot e.
Herczel rib e.
Hibbs chisel e.
Hoen periosteal e.
Iowa University periosteal e.
Jannetta duckbill e.
joker periosteal e.
Joseph periosteal e.
J-periosteal e.
Kennerdell-Maroon e.
Key e.
Key periosteal e.
Kleinert-Kutz periosteal e.
Kocher e.
Lambotte e.
lamina e.
Lane periosteal e.
Langenbeck periosteal e.
Lempert periosteal e.

E

elevator (*continued*)
Lewis periosteal e.
liberator e.
Locke e.
Love-Adson periosteal e.
lumbosacral fusion e.
Malis e.
Matson-Alexander rib e.
Matson periosteal e.
Matson rib e.
McGlamry e.
Mead periosteal e.
modified Darrach-type e.
Molt periosteal e.
Moore bone e.
e. muscle
narrow proximal femoral e.
nasal e.
orthopaedic shoulder e.
OSI extremity e.
osteophyte e.
Penfield periosteal e.
periosteal e.
e. periosteotome
Phemister e.
posterior glenoid e.
proximal femoral e.
Rhoton e.
rib e.
Rochester lamina e.
Rochester spinal e.
Rolyan arm e.
Rosen e.
round-tapped e.
Sauerbruch rib e.
Sayre e.
Sebileau periosteal e.
Sedillot periosteal e.
Sheffield hand e.
Sisson fracture reducing e.
spiked Darrach-type e.
staphylorrhaphy e.
straight periosteal e.
Sunday staphylorrhaphy e.
Swanson e.
Tenzel e.
T-handle e.
Thornhill offset proximal femoral e.
Tiemann nail e.
Tronzo e.
von Langenbeck periosteal e.
Ward periosteal e.
Wiberg periosteal e.
wide periosteal e.
Williger periosteal e.
Woodson e.
Yasargil e.
elevator-dissector
Freer e.-d.

elevator-periosteotome
elevatus
e. deformity
extrinsic metatarsus primus e.
hallux e.
iatrogenic e.
intrinsic metatarsus primus e.
metatarsus primus e.
Eligoy metal alloy
Eliminator ArthroWand
elite
E. Farley retractor
E. hip system
E. knee brace
E. Plus motion analyzer
E. posterior adjustable stop
E. posterior spring assist
E. Power Station gym
Elithorn perceptual maze test
Elizabethtown osteotomy
Elliott femoral condyle blade plate
ellipsoidal
e. articulation
e. joint
ellipsoid joint
elliptical
e. amputation
e. incision
e. machine
e. overlap shadow
Ellis
E. Jones
E. Jones peroneal tendon
displacement
E. Jones peroneal tendon operation
E. Jones peroneal tendon technique
E. skin traction technique
E. technique for Barton fracture
E. tooth fracture classification
Ellison
E. fixation staple
E. iliotibial band tenodesis
E. iliotibial band transfer for ACL
repair technique
E. lateral knee reconstruction
Ellis-van Creveld syndrome
Elmslie
E. peroneal tendon operation
E. peroneal tendon procedure
E. reconstruction
E. triple arthrodesis
E. weave procedure
Elmslie-Cholmeley
E.-C. foot operation
E.-C. procedure
Elmslie-Trillat
E.-T. knee extensor realignment
E.-T. osteotomy
E.-T. patellar operation

E.-T. patellar procedure
E.-T. patellar realignment method
E.-T. total tendon transplant
elongation
e., derotation, flexion (EDF)
e., derotation, flexion scoliosis
cast
ligament e.
peroneus brevis e.
e. property
repeated quick stretch from e.
(RQS-E)
tissue e.
Elson middle slip finger test
Elutia antimicrobial coated closed
surgical wound drain
Elvarex
E. compression garment
E. support garment
Ely heel-to-buttock test
Emagrin
emanate
Embarc bone repair material
embarrassment
circulatory e.
emboli (*pl. of* embolus)
embolic mononeuropathy
embolism
air e.
arterial gas e.
bone marrow e.
fat e.
pulmonary e.
embolization
Gelfoam e.
embolotherapy
embolus, *pl.* **emboli**
bone marrow e.
embryonal rhabdomyosarcoma
EMD
electromechanical delay
emedullate
emergency
e. closed manipulative measure
e. muscle
Emery-Dreifuss muscular dystrophy
(EDMD)
EMG
electromyogram
electromyography
EMG biofeedback system
fine wire EMG
EMG retrainer biofeedback unit
scanning EMG
single-channel surface EMG
single-fiber EMG
Emgel Topical
eminence
hypothenar e.

medial e.
thenar e.
tibial e.
eminentia, *pl.* **eminentiae**
eminentiae (*pl. of* eminentia)
emission tomography
EMLA
eutectic mixture of local anesthetics
Emmon osteotomy
emollient
vitamin E e.
EMP
extramedullary plasmacytoma
Empirin With Codeine
empty
e. beer can shoulder test
e. can exercise
e. can position
e. can syndrome
e. vertebral body
empyema, *pl.* **empyemata**
empyemata (*pl. of* empyema)
empyemic scoliosis
E-MRI
extremity magnetic resonance
imaging
EMS
electronic muscle stimulator
eosinophilia-myalgia syndrome
EMS 2000 neuromuscular stimulator
en
e. bloc
e. bloc advancement
e. bloc laminectomy
e. bloc resection
enarthrodial joint
Enbrel
encapsulation
encased screw
encephalitides (*pl. of* encephalitis)
encephalitis, *pl.* **encephalitides**
encephalocele
encephalopathia (*var. of* encephalopathy)
encephalopathy, encephalopathia
chronic traumatic e. (CTE)
encerclage
enchondral
e. bone
e. ossification
enchondroma, endochondroma, *pl.*
enchondromata
multiple e.
e. of bone
e. of hand
e. protuberans
solitary e.
enchondromata (*pl. of* enchondroma)
enchondromatosis
multiple e.

E

239

enchondromatous myxoma
encircling wire
enclavement
enclosure
    air-flow e.
encore
    E. Orthopaedics
    E. Orthopedics device
encroachment
    bony e.
    cervical nerve root e.
    foraminal osteophyte e.
    osseous foraminal e.
end
    articulating bone e.
    bone e.
    bony distal e.
    e. corn
    e. cutter
    distal bone e.
    e. feel
    lateral e.
    medial e.
    e. plate
    e. play
    e. point
    e. range of motion
    e. vertebra
endarteritis
    e. deformans
    e. obliterans
    e. proliferans
end-bearing amputation
end-biting forceps
end-cutting
    e.-c. reamer
    e.-c. reciprocating saw
endemic
    e. hypertrophy
    e. osteoarthritis
endemica
    osteoarthritis deformans e.
Ender
    E. awl
    E. elastic condylar nail fracture
    fixation
    E. femoral fracture technique
    E. flexible medullary nail
    E. nail fixation
    E. nailing
    E. pin
    E. rod
    E. rod fixation
    E. rod fixation of fracture
    E. round elastic condylar nail
    E. trochanteric fracture fixation
end-feel
    joint e.-f.
    e.-f. palpation

ending
    flower-spray e.
    nerve e.
Endius
    E. bipolar sheath
    E. endoscopic access system
    E. spinal endoscope/camera
    E. spinal endoscopic camera
    E. TriFix thoracolumbar pedicle
    screw system
Endless Pool physical therapy pool
Endo
    E. Multi-Mode stimulator
    E. rotating knee joint
    prosthesis
endoabdominal fascia
EndoAvitene
EndoButton
    closed loop E.
endochondral
    e. bone
    e. ossification
    e. osteogenesis
endochondroma (*var. of* enchondroma)
endochondromatosis
endocrine fracture
Endo-Fix
    E.-F. bioabsorbable interference
    screw
    E.-F. L screw
Endoflex endoscopic lumbar discectomy
  scope
endogenous pain
Endolite
    E. prosthesis
    E. transtibial system
Endo-Model
    E.-M. hinged knee prosthesis
    E.-M. rotating knee joint prosthesis
    E.-M. sled prosthesis
endomorph
endomysial
endomysium
endoneural
    e. canal
    e. tube
endoneurial
    e. degeneration
    e. edema
    e. fibrosis
endoneurolysis
EndoPearl
    E. bioabsorbable device
    E. fixation device
endoplasmic reticulum (ER)
endoprostheses (*pl. of* endoprosthesis)
endoprosthesis, *pl.* endoprostheses
    acetabular e.
    Atkinson e.

Bio-Moore e.
femoral e.
F.R. Thompson e.
nonporous-coated e.
smooth e.
tibial e.
TPP hip e.
tumor-replacement e.
endoprosthetic flange
end-organ
Endo-Ring minimal access surgery device
endorphin
endorthesis
endorthosis
endoscope
endoscope/camera
Endius spinal e./c.
endoscopic
e. anterior cruciate ligament reconstruction
e. approach
e. carpal tunnel instrumentation
e. carpal tunnel release (ECTR)
e. carpal tunnel release system
e. correction of scoliosis
e. gastrocnemius recession
e. plantar fasciotomy (EPF)
endoscopy
fiberoptic intraosseous e.
laser-assisted spinal e. (LASE)
lumbar epidural e.
percutaneous transcaudal epidural e.
tendon sheath e.
endoskeletal
e. alignment system (EAS)
e. socket
solid ankle flexible e. (SAFE)
stationary attachment flexible e. (SAFE)
Endoskeleton TA interbody spinal fusion device
endosteal
e. hypertrophy
e. lamella
e. revascularization
e. scalloping
e. surface
e. vessel
endosteum
endotenon
endothelia (*pl. of* endothelium)
endothelial
e. cell
e. dysfunction
endothelium, *pl.* **endothelia**
vascular e.
endothoracic fascia

Endotrac
E. blade system
E. cannula
E. carpal tunnel release system
E. elevator
E. endoscopic carpal tunnel release
E. rasp
endotracheal intubation
endovaginal lipoma
end-plate (*var. of* endplate)
endplate, end-plate
e. activity
e. fragmentation
e. invagination
e. noise
e. ossification
posterior e.
e. potential (EPP)
e. sclerosis
e. spike
superior e.
vertebral body e.
e. zone
endpoint of orthopaedic test
end-stage, endstage
e.-s. arthrosis
e.-s. coxarthrosis
e.-s. disruption
endstage (*var. of* end-stage)
end-to-end
e.-t.-e. suture
e.-t.-e. tendon repair
end-to-side repair
EnduraFIX tape
endurance
E. bone cement
e. event
e. exercise
e. limit
e. training
Enduron acetabular liner
energetics
Apex E.
energy
e. absorption
e. conservation walking component
e. expenditure
e. intake
kinetic e.
e. metabolism
muscle e.
E. Plus shoe insert
e. storage
e. storing foot prosthesis
strain e.
thermal e.
enflurane

E

Engebretsen procedure
Engel
    E. hand x-ray angle
    E. plaster saw
Engelmann
    E. disc
    E. disease
    E. thigh splint
Engel-Recklinghausen disease
Engen
    E. extension orthosis
    E. palmar finger orthosis
    E. palmar wrist splint
Engh
    E. porous metal hip prosthesis
    E. total hip replacement
Engh-Glassman femoral stem
engine
    Acrotorque hand e.
engineering
    functional tissue e. (FTE)
Englehardt femoral prosthesis
English
    E. anvil nail nipper
    E. brace
    E. cane
    E. cane board
English-McNab shoulder prosthesis
engulfment abnormality
enhancement
    peridiscal rim e.
enhancer cushion
enjoyment
    Children's Assessment of
      Participation and E.
      (CAPE)
enkephalin
enlarged frontal horn
enlargement
    tibial tunnel e.
enlarging bur
ENMG
    electroneuromyography
Enneking
    E. benign tumor classification
    E. disease stage
    E. knee arthrodesis
    E. malignant bone tumor staging
    E. principle
    E. question
    E. resection arthrodesis
    E. rod
    E. staging (IA, IB, IIA, IIB, III)
      of malignant bone and soft tissue
      tumors
enostosis
enoxacin
enoxaparin
ensheathing callus

ensiform
    e. cartilage
    e. process
Ensolite padded transfer bench
Ensure-It dressing
entacapone
Entegra prosthesis
Enterobacter
    E. agglomerans
    E. cloacae
Enterococcus
enterocutaneous fistula
enteropathic arthritis
enthesis
    Achilles tendon e.
enthesitis
enthesopathic
enthesopathy
enthetic
entrapment
    anterior cutaneous nerve e.
    anular ligament e.
    catheter e.
    ilioinguinal nerve e.
    lateral canal e.
    median nerve e.
    meniscoid e.
    nerve root e.
    e. neuropathy
    peripheral nerve e.
    peroneal nerve e.
    popliteal fossa e.
    posterior interosseous nerve e.
    posterior tibial nerve e.
    suprascapular nerve e.
    e. syndrome
    ulnar nerve e.
entrapped plantar bone
Entrex small joint arthroscopy
  instrument set
entry point
entubulation, entubulization
    nerve e.
entubulization (*var. of* entubulation)
enucleate
enucleation
enucleator
    Rhoton e.
envelope
    e. arm sling
    capsuloperiosteal e.
    soft tissue e.
environment
    Home Observation and Measurement
      of the E. (HOME)
environmental
    e. assessment
    e. stress cracking
Envision anterior cervical plate system

enzymatic, enzymic
    e. débridement
    e. débriding agent
enzyme-based lactic acid blood testing
enzyme-linked immunosorbent assay
enzymic (*var. of* enzymatic)
EOC
    electrooptical characteristic
    EOC goniometer
eosinophilia-myalgia syndrome (EMS)
eosinophilic
    e. granuloma
    e. granuloma of bone
epactal bone
EPB
    extensor pollicis brevis
ependymoma
EPF
    endoscopic plantar fasciotomy
epiarticular osteochondromatous
  dysplasia
EPIC
    evaluation, prediction, intervention,
    control
      EPIC functional evaluation
        system
epicondylalgia
    e. externa
    radial e.
epicondylar
    e. avulsion fracture
    e. resection and anconeus muscle
      transfer
    e. ridge
epicondyle
    femoral e.
    humeral e.
    lateral e.
    medial e.
epicondylectomy
    medial e.
epicondylitis
    external humeral e.
    humeral e.
    lateral humeral e.
    medial e.
    e. of elbow
    radiohumeral e.
epicritic
    e. pain
    e. receptor
    e. sensation
    e. sensation erythrasma
Epic wheelchair
epidermal cell tumor
epidermides (*pl. of* epidermis)
epidermidis
    Staphylococcus e.
epidermis, *pl.* **epidermides**

epidermodysplasia verruciformis
epidermolysis
    e. bullosa
    e. bullosa dermal type
    e. bullosa epidermal type
    e. bullosa junctional type
epidermolytic acanthoma
epidermophytid reaction
Epidermophyton floccosum
epidural
    e. abscess
    e. abscess evacuation
    e. anesthesia
    e. cortisone injection technique
    e. dye flow
    e. fluid collection
    e. neurolysis
    e. space
    e. space infection
    e. steroid
    e. steroid injection (ESI)
    e. tumor evacuation
    e. venography
epidurogram
epidurography
epifascicular epineurotomy
Epigard dressing
epilepsia (*var. of* epilepsy)
epilepsy, epilepsia
    jacksonian e.
    myoclonic e.
    posttraumatic e. (PTE)
epileptic myoclonus
Epi-Lock elbow support
epiloia
epimeric muscle
epimysiotomy
epimysium externum
epinephrine
    admixed e.
    lidocaine and e.
    Marcaine with e.
    Xylocaine with e.
epineural
    e. covering
    e. repair
    e. scarring
epineurectomy
    interfascicular e.
epineurial
    e. neuropathy
    e. neurorrhaphy
epineurial-perineurial neuropathy
epineurium
epineurolysis
    volar e.
epineurotomy
    anterior e.
    epifascicular e.

E

epineurotomy (*continued*)
    interfascicular e.
    local e.
epiphyseal (*var. of* epiphysial)
epiphysealis
    dysplasia e.
epiphyseolysis (*var. of* epiphysiolysis)
epiphyses (*pl. of* epiphysis)
epiphysial, epiphyseal
    e. angle
    e. arrest
    e. artery
    e. aseptic necrosis
    atavistic e.
    e. bar resection
    e. chondromatous giant cell
      tumor
    e. closure
    e. complex
    e. dysgenesis
    e. dysplasia
    e. exostosis
    e. growth plate
    e. growth plate fracture
    e. hyperplasia
    e. injury
    e. ischemic necrosis
    e. line
    e. osteochondritis
    e. osteochondroma
    e. oxygen
    e. ring
    e. slip fracture
    e. staple
    e. stapling
    e. tibial fracture
epiphysial-metaphysial osteotomy
epiphysiodesis
    Abbott-Gill e.
    Blount e.
    bone peg e.
    greater trochanteric e.
    Heyman-Herndon e.
    medial tibial e.
    open bone graft e.
    percutaneous e.
    proximal phalangeal e.
    screw e.
    spontaneous postfracture e.
    White e.
epiphysiolysis, epiphyseolysis
    femoral e.
    proximal femoral e.
epiphysiopathy
epiphysis, *pl.* **epiphyses**
    accessory e.
    capital e.
    capital femoral e.
    capitular e.

    clavicular e.
    distal humeral e.
    femoral e.
    humeral e.
    iliac e.
    Morrissy percutaneous fixation of
      slipped e.
    Perthes e.
    pressure e.
    screw epiphysiodesis for
      hemiepiphysiodesis of distal
      tibial e.
    slipped capital femoral e.
      (SCFE)
    slipped under femoral e. (SUFE)
    stippled e.
    tibial e.
    traction e.
epiphysitis
    transient e.
Epipoint elbow support
epipteric bone
Epi-Sport epicondylitis clasp
epitendineum, epitenon
    epitenon suture
epitenon (*var. of* epitendineum)
epithelialization, epithelization
epithelioid
    e. hemangioepithelioma
    e. sarcoma
epithelioma cuniculatum
epithelioserosa
    zona e.
epithelization (*var. of* epithelialization)
epithesis
Epitrain
    E. active elbow support
    E. knitted elbow support
    E. Viscoped support
epitrochlea
epitrochlear
epitrochlearis
    anconeus e.
epitrochleoanconeus muscle
Epker osteotome
EPL
    extensor pollicis longus
EPO
    erythropoietin
Epoch femoral stem
eponychia
eponychium
Epos
    E. Ultra extracorporeal shock wave
      therapy device
    E. Ultra orthopaedic shock wave
      therapy device
EPP
    endplate potential

Eppright dial osteotomy
epsilon receptor
Epsom salts soak
Epstein
 E. bone rasp
 E. curette
 E. hip dislocation classification
 E. neurological hammer
EPTFE
 expanded polytetrafluoroethylene
 EPTFE graft prosthesis
epX suspension sleeve
Equagesic
equalizer
 E. air walker
 E. cast brace
 E. Pro massager
 E. short leg walking cast
equation
 Bloch e.
 Jackson-Pollock skinfold e.
Equilet
equilibratory ataxia
equilibrium
 intrinsic e.
 e. reaction
 e. reflex
equina
 cauda e.
equine gait
equinocavovarus deformity
equinocavus foot
equinovalgus
 e. deformity
 e. foot
 pes e.
 spastic e.
 talipes e.
equinovarus
 congenital talipes e.
 e. foot
 e. hindfoot deformity
 pes e.
 e. posturing
 psychogenic e.
 talipes e. (TEV)
 Turco repair of talipes e.
equinus
 ankle e.
 anterior e.
 compensated talipes e.
 e. contracture
 e. deformity
 e. foot
 forefoot e.
 gastrocnemius e.
 gastrosoleal e.
 global e.
 global metatarsus e.

 heel e.
 osseous e.
 pes e.
 e. position
 residual heel e.
 residual hindfoot e.
 spastic e.
 e. step
 talipes e.
equipment
 accommodative e.
 adaptive e.
 adjustment e.
 AquaMED dry hydrotherapy e.
 Austin Medical E. (AME)
 Baltimore Therapeutic E. (BTE)
 Body-Solid exercise e.
 Cybex back rehabilitation e.
 decompression e.
 Dynamic Edge rehabilitation e.
 home medical e.
 insertion e.
 Invertrac e.
 National Operating Committee on
  Standards for Athletic E.
  (NOCSAE)
 OsteoStat single-use power
  surgical e.
 personal protective e. (PPE)
 Reflex exercise and rehabilitation e.
 Response rehabilitation and
  fitness e.
 stainless steel e.
EquiTest CDP testing system
equivalent
 human skin e.
ER
 endoplasmic reticulum
E-R
 Indochron E-R
Erb
 E. atrophy
 E. muscular dystrophy
 E. palsy
 E. point
Erb-Duchenne palsy
Erb-Goldflam syndrome
Erb-Landouzy disease
Erdheim-Chester disease
Erdheim syndrome
ERE
 external rotation in extension
erect
 e. position
 e. view
erecta
 dislocatio e.
 luxatio e.
erectile dysfunction

E

erector spinae
ERF
    external rotation in flexion
Ergo
    E. Cush back support
    E. style flexion table
ergocalciferol
Ergociser
    Cateye E.
    E. exercise cycle
Ergoflex Premiere back support
ergogenic aid
ergograph
    Mosso e.
ErgoLogic keyboard
ergolytic
ergometer
    bicycle e.
    Biodex cycle e.
    Concept II rowing e.
    Cybex cycle e.
    cycle e.
    handgrip e.
    upper body e. (UBE)
ergometry
    bicycle e.
ergonomic
    e. assessment
    e. assessment of risk and liability
    (EARLY)
    e. chair
    e. factor
    e. injury
    e. risk
    e. safety
ergonomically
    e. correct chair
    e. designed transducer
ergoreceptor
ergostat
Ergos work simulator
ergotherapy
Erhardt
    E. Developmental Prehension
    Assessment (EDPA)
    E. Developmental Vision Assessment
    (EDVA)
Erichsen
    E. disease
    E. sign
Erich splint
erigentes
    nervi e.
Eriksson
    E. brachial block technique
    E. cruciate ligament reconstruction
    E. knee prosthesis
    E. ligament technique
    E. muscle biopsy cannula

ER:IR
    external rotation-to-internal rotation
    ratio
Erlenmeyer
    E. flask deformity
    E. flask shape
ERLP
    exercise-related leg
    pain
erosion
    bony e.
    e. of articular surface
    osteoclastic e.
    pedicle e.
erosive
    e. arthritides
    e. osteoarthritis
ERSS
    Edinburgh Rehabilitation Status
    Scale
EryDerm Topical
Erygel Topical
Erymax Topical
erythema of joint
erythematosus
    lupus e. (LE)
    systemic lupus e. (SLE)
erythralgia
erythrasma
    epicritic sensation e.
erythrocyte sedimentation rate
(ESR)
erythromelalgia
    idiopathic e.
    secondary e.
erythromycin
erythropoietin (EPO)
    recombinant human e.
    (rHuEPO)
ES
    extra strength
    Forte ES
    Vicodin ES
eschar
escharotic
escharotomy
Escherichia coli **(E. coli)**
Esclim Transdermal
E-Series hip system
ESI
    epidural steroid injection
ESIN
    elastic stable intramedullary nailing
    ESIN pediatric fracture fixation
Eska
    E. Implant artificial joint
    replacement
    E. modular hip system
    E. UHMWPE acetabular cup

Esmarch
> E. bandage
> E. dressing
> E. plaster knife
> E. plaster shears
> E. tourniquet
> E. tube

E-Solve-2 Topical
ESR
> erythrocyte sedimentation rate

essential
> E. Energy Cup
> E. Energy Water
> e. fatty acid
> e. tremor

Esser skin graft
Essex-Lopresti
> E.-L. axial fixation technique
> E.-L. calcaneal fracture
> classification
> E.-L. calcaneal fracture technique
> E.-L. calcaneal injury
> E.-L. fixation
> E.-L. fixation of calcaneal fracture
> E.-L. joint depression-type calcaneal
> fracture
> E.-L. lesion
> E.-L. method
> E.-L. open radial head fracture
> reduction
> E.-L. tongue type calcaneal fracture

ESSF
> external spinal skeletal fixator

Essiac
ESSKA
> European Society of Sports
> Traumotology, Knee Surgery, and
> Arthroscopy

established contracture
estazolam
Esterom solution
Estersohn
> E. osteotomy
> E. osteotomy for tailor's bunion

esthesia, aesthesia
esthesiometry, aesthesiometry
> Semmes-Weinstein monofilament
> pressure e.

estimated blood loss (EBL)
estimation
> Simple Calculated Osteoporosis Risk
> E. (SCORE)

Estinyl
estradiol
Estratab
Estring
ETAC
> electrothermally assisted capsulorrhaphy

etanercept

Ethafoam
ethambutol
ethanol
> anhydrous e.

ethchlorvynol
Ethibond suture
Ethicon suture
Ethiflex suture
Ethilon suture
ethmoid forceps
ethyl
> e. chloride
> e. chloride and
> dichlorotetrafluoroethane

ethylene
> e. oxide
> e. oxide sterilization
> e. vinyl acetate (EVA)

etidocaine
etidronate
> e. disodium
> sodium e.

etiology
> depth of ulcer, extent of bacterial
> colonization, phase of ulcer,
> associated e. (DEPA)
> e. undetermined
> e. unknown

ETL
> echo train length

etodolac
ETPS
> electrotherapeutic point stimulation
> ETPS therapy

ETS-2% Topical
Eucalyptamint arthritis pain ointment
eukinesia
Euler
> E. angle
> E. angle of wrist motion
> E. load

eulerian angle
eumelanin
eumycetoma
EuroCuff forearm crutch
Euroglide MKII slide board
European
> E. Chiropractic Union
> E. compression technique (ECT)
> E. Society of Sports Traumotology,
> Knee Surgery, and Arthroscopy
> (ESSKA)

European-style screwdriver
Eurotaper 12/14 taper
Eurotech
> E. Diamond table
> E. Emerald table
> E. Platinum table
> E. Sapphire table

E

eutectic mixture of local anesthetics (EMLA)
EVA
    ethylene vinyl acetate
evacuation
    epidural abscess e.
    epidural tumor e.
    nail bed hematoma e.
evaluation
    Acute Physiology and Chronic Health E. (APACHE)
    Arnadottir OT-ADL Neurobehavioral E. (A-ONE)
    baseline capacity e.
    Bay Area Functional Performance E. (BaFPE)
    Charcot-Marie-Tooth E.
    CMT E.
    Cyriax soft tissue injury e.
    Doppler pulse e.
    Evans tenodesis e.
    Evolution hip prosthesis e.
    Fugl-Meyer e.
    functional capacity e. (FCE)
    Hughston knee e.
    isokinetic e.
    job capacity e. (JCE)
    Mazur ankle e.
    motion analysis e.
    orthopaedic e.
    physical capacity e. (PCE)
    e., prediction, intervention, control (EPIC)
    preoperative e.
    Smith physical capacities e.
    static e.
    Toddler and Infant Motor E. (TIME)
    E. Tool of Children's Handwriting
    uniaxial balance e. (UBE)
    vocational e. (VE)
evaluation-revised
    Rabideau Kitchen E.-R. (RKE-R)
evaluator
    Touch-Test sensory e.
Evans
    E. ankle instability procedure
    E. ankle joint instability operation
    E. ankle reconstruction technique
    E. ankle tenodesis
    E. anterior opening wedge calcaneal osteotomy
    E. calcaneal lengthening
    E. calcaneal lengthening osteotomy site
    E. calcaneal reconstruction
    E. fracture classification system

    E. intertrochanteric fracture classification
    E. lateral ankle reconstruction
    E. tenodesis evaluation
Evans-Burkhalter protocol
Evazote
    E. cushioning material
    E. foam
Eve
    E. reconstruction of gliding tissue defects procedure
    E. vascularized seventh rib fascia cartilage and serratus muscle
event
    endurance e.
eventration
Ever-Flex insole
Evershears surgical instrument device
eversion
    ankle e.
    heel e.
    e. injury
    e. osteotomy
    e. stress test
eversion-external rotation deformity
evertor
    e. force
    e. tendon
evidence-based
    e.-b. medicine (EBM)
    e.-b. orthopaedics
Evista
Evithrom
evoked
    e. compound muscle action potential
    e. potential study
    e. response
Evolis femoral cutting guide
evolution
    E. hip prosthesis
    E. hip prosthesis evaluation
Ewald
    E. capitellocondylar total elbow arthroplasty
    E. elbow arthroplasty rating system
    E. total elbow replacement
    E. unconstrained elbow prosthesis
Ewald-Walker
    E.-W. kinematic knee arthroplasty
    E.-W. knee implant
EWHO
    elbow-wrist-hand orthosis
Ewing
    E. family of tumors
    E. sarcoma
E.X.
    Extra Strength Dynafed E.X.

exacerbation
Exactech Ziramic femoral head
Exact-Fit ATH hip replacement system
exaggeration reaction
examination
    Apley e.
    ARM method of physical e.
    arthroscopic e.
    BB to MM e.
    belly button to medial malleolus e.
    bench e.
    Boston Diagnostic Aphasia e.
    Broden subtalar instability stress e.
    clinical e.
    comparative radiographic e.
    full spine radiographic e.
    lateral full-spine radiographic e.
    Mini Mental State E. (MMSE)
    motor e.
    neurologic e.
    neurological nerve conduction
      velocity e.
    palpatory e.
    pedodynographic e.
    physical e.
    radiographic e.
    reflex e.
    sensory e.
    stress e.
    tender point e.
    thermographic e.
exarteritis
exarticulation
Ex-Balls medicine ball
excavatum
    pectus e.
Excedrin
    Extra Strength E.
    E. P.M.
Excel Plus electrode
excentric amputation
excess cement
excessive
    e. joint play
    e. laxity test
    e. sweating
    e. thoracic slumping
exchange
    isolated modular tibial
      insert e.
    e. nailing
excision
    e. and curettage
    e. and implantation
    e. arthroplasty
    bar e.
    Bartlett nail fold e.
    bone cyst e.
    Bose nail fold e.

    bunionette e.
    cervical disc e.
    clavicle e.
    e., curettage, drilling
      (ECD)
    Curtin plantar fibromatosis e.
    Das Gupta scapular e.
    disc e.
    distal clavicular e.
    Ferciot e.
    Ferciot-Thompson knee ossicle e.
    Flatt e.
    funicular e.
    hemivertebral e.
    intracapsular e.
    intralesional e.
    marginal e.
    McKeever-Buck fragment e.
    meniscal e.
    microlumbar disc e.
    e. of dorsal wrist ganglion
    e. of intervertebral disc
    e. of osteochondroma
    e. of volar wrist ganglion
    radical compartmental e.
    retropulsed bone e.
    ruptured disc e.
    split-thickness skin e. (STSE)
    Stewart distal clavicular e.
    ulnar head e.
    wide e.
    Williams microlumbar disc e.
excisional
    e. arthrodesis
    e. biopsy
excision-curettage technique
excitatory postsynaptic potential
exclusion clamp
excoriation
excrescence
    bony e.
excretory function
excursion
    e. amplifier sleeve
    calcaneus e.
    hindfoot e.
    insertional e.
    range of e.
    tendon e.
executive function deficit
Exelderm Topical
Exerball kit
Exerband
    E. Pak bilateral tube
    E. Pak unilateral tube
    E. therapy band
    E. tubing
Exerboard
    Velcro Hand E.

E

exercise

active-assisted range of motion e.
active-assistive e. (AAE)
active back e.
active range of motion e.
aerobic e.
anaerobic e.
ankle-pump e.
aquatic e.
back e.
Back Revolution Stick e.
back stretch on ball e.
e. band
e. board
e. bone
Brügger relief position e.
Buerger-Allen circulation of feet e.
calf raise back e.
Calleja e.
e. capacity
Carpal Care e.
cat and camel e.
chain reaction e.
closed-chain e.
closed kinetic chain e. (CKCE)
closed kinetic chain
  progressive-resistance e.
co-contraction e.
Codman e.
concentric isokinetic leg press e.
contracture e.
Cooksey-Cawthorne e.
Crane shoulder e.
daily adjusted progressive resistance
  e. (DAPRE)
dead ball e.'s
DeLorme e.
dying bug e.
dynamic stump e.
eccentric e.
elevation e.
empty can e.
endurance e.
explosive e.
external rotation e.
FITT e.
flexibility e.
flexion-extension e.
forearm ischemic e.
Frenkel e.'s
frequency, intensity, type, time e.
gastrocnemius resistive e.
e. grab bar
gripping e.'s
hamstring-setting e.
handgrip e.
heel cord stretching e.
heel raise e.
heel rock e.

hip abductor strengthening e.
hip extension e.
hook-lying pectoral stretch e.
horizontal shoulder abduction e.
increment after e.
internal rotation e.
e. intolerance
inversion-eversion e.
e. ischemia
isokinetic e.
isometric e. (IME)
isotonic e.
kinesthetic e.
knee extension e.
knee pump e.
Kolár wall slide with arm
  elevation e.
e. log
low-stress aerobic e.
McKenzie extension e.
muscle-setting e.
muscle-strengthening e.
e. myopathy
open-chain e.
open kinetic chain e.
orthokinetic e.
6-pack hand e.
parallel squat e.
passive assistance e.
passive range of motion e.
passive resistive e.
passive stretch e.
pelvic floor e.
pendulum e.
peroneal strengthening e.
e. physiology
Pilates method e.
plyometric e.
pneumatic resistance e.
PNF e.
e. program
progressive-resistance e. (PRE)
progressive-resistive e. (PRE)
prone scapular retraction e.
proprioceptive e.
proprioceptive neuromuscular
  facilitation e.
pulley e.
e. putty
quadriceps-setting e.
quadriceps strengthening e.
race-pace e.
range of motion e.
regeneration flexion e.
rehabilitation flexibility e.
remedial e.
repetitive e.
resistive e.
rotation e.

E. Sandal
e. science
seated scapular retraction e.
e. self-efficacy
E. Self-Efficacy Scale
Seradge hand e.'s
single-row e.
sports anemia e.
stair-climbing e.
step e.
straight leg raising e.
Superman back e.
Super-Seven e.
supported extension e.
tai chi chuan e.
e. testing
Thera-Band Max resistive e.
therapeutic e.
toe gripping e.
toe raise e.
towel e.
unrestricted closed and open chain
  knee extension e.
vastus medialis obliquus e.
VMO e.
volitional e.
wall-slide e.
Williams flexion e. (WFE)
work hardening e.
wrist stretch e.

exercise-associated
e.-a. collapse
e.-a. hyponatremia

exercise-induced
e.-i. amenorrhea
e.-i. anaphylaxis
e.-i. asthma (EIA)
e.-i. breast pain
e.-i. collapse
e.-i. compartment syndrome
e.-i. myokymia
e.-i. sudden death

exerciser
AccessTrainer e.
animal beanbag e.
Ankle Isolator foot and ankle e.
axial resistance e.
bicycle e.
Builder Grip hand e.
Carpal Care carpal tunnel e.
Carpal Tunnel Stretch e.
Cat's Paw e.
ChairCiser adjustable e.
continuous anatomical passive e.
  (CAPE)
continuous passive motion e.
Danniflex CPM e.
Digi-Flex finger e.
Digi-Flex hand e.

DynaFlex Gyro e.
Eggsercizer CTS e.
Eggsercizer resistive hand e.
Exer-Cor e.
ExtendaFLEX e.
finger e.
Finger Helper hand e.
Finger Platter hand e.
Flextender Plus hand e.
Grahamizer I e.
Gripp squeeze ball hand e.
Gyro-Flex upper extremity e.
hand e.
Hand Helper hand e.
isokinetic Unex III e.
Iso-Quadron e.
Jace shoulder e.
jaw e.
Jux-A-Cisor e.
Knead-A-Ball e.
microcomputer upper limb e.
  (MULE)
MiniMedBall hand e.
Morpho E.
Motivator FTR2000 e.
Nelson finger e.
NordiCare Enabler e.
NordiCare Strider e.
NordicTrack ski e.
NuStep e.
Omni-Flexor wrist e.
Oppociser hand e.
Orthotron e.
pedal e.
Plyo-Sled e.
Powerflex CMP e.
Power Pogo stationary e.
Power Web hand e.
Power Web Jr. e.
Preston Traveler CPM e.
ProStretch e.
Pul-Ez e.
resistive e.
rickshaw rehabilitation e.
rocky boat e.
Rotaflex e.
Roylan ergonomic hand e.
Seated Cable Row e.
soft touch hand e.
squeeze e.
strengthening e.
Stronghands hand e.
Stryker CPM e.
Stryker leg e.
Swanson Grip-X hand e.
Thera-Band Assist e.
Thera-Band hand e.
Thera-Band resistive e.
Thera Cane shoulder e.

E

exerciser (*continued*)
    Theraflex wrist e.
    Ther-A-Hoop e.
    Thera-Loop e.
    Thera-Putty CTS e.
    Toronto Medical CPM e.
    Tuf Nex neck e.
    Tunturi hand e.
    Versa-Trainer e.
    Walk-'n-Tone e.
    Wristiciser e.
    Zimmer continuous anatomical
      passive e.

exercise-related
    e.-r. headache
    e.-r. leg pain (ERLP)

Exer-Cor exerciser
Exercycle
ExerFlex ball
Exer-Pedic cycle
Exerstrider walking pole
exertion
    Borg Scale of Rating
      Perceived E.
    rated perceived e. (RPE)
    rating of perceived e. (RPE)

exertional
    e. anterior compartment syndrome
      (EACS)
    e. deep posterior compartment
      syndrome (EDPCS)
    e. hypotension
    e. rhabdomyolysis

Exertools
    E. Dyna-Disc
    E. gymball

Exeter
    E. cemented hip prosthesis
    E. intramedullary bone plug
      device
    E. Plug
    E. stem
    E. total hip system

Exeter-Femora press fit prosthesis
EX-FI-RE
    external fixation reduction
    EX-FI-RE device
    EX-FI-RE system

exhaustion
    postactivation e.
    posttetanic e.

Exidine Scrub
Exo-Bed traction unit
exoccipital bone
Exogen
    E. bone healing system
    E. 2000 noninvasive, low-intensity,
      pulsed ultrasound device
    E. 2000+ noninvasive ultrasound

    E. 2000+ noninvasive ultrasound
      therapy
    E. 2000 sonic accelerated fracture
      healing system

exogenous
    e. fibrin clot
    e. reconstruction

Exo-Overhead traction unit
Exo-Static
    E.-S. cervical collar
    E.-S. neck collar
    E.-S. traction

exostectomy, exostosectomy
    lateral e.
    medial e.

exostosectomy
exostoses (*pl. of* exostosis)
exostosis, *pl.* **exostoses**
    blocker's e.
    bony e.
    e. bursata
    cuneiform-first metatarsal e.
    Dupuytren e.
    epiphysial e.
    Haglund e.
    hereditary multiple e.
    hypertrophic e.
    impinging e.
    marginal e.
    metatarsal cuneiform e.
    metatarsocuneiform joint e.
    multiple hereditary osteochondral e.
      (MHOCE)
    osteocartilaginous e.
    pump bump e.
    retrocalcaneal e.
    subungual e.
    tackler's e.
    talar neck e.
    talotibial e.
    thrower's e.
    traction e.
    turret e.

Exotec brace
expanded
    E. Disability Status Scale
      (EDSS)
    e. polytetrafluoroethylene (EPTFE)

expander
    AccuSpan tissue e.
    acetabular e.
    Mentor tissue e.
    skin e.
    tissue e.

expanding reamer
Expandover athletic tape
expansile
    e. cyst
    e. lesion

expansion
    e. bolt
    lateral extensor e.
    medial extensor e.
    e. screw
expansive laminaplasty
Expedium anterior spine system
expenditure
    energy e.
experimental threshold
exploration
    e. and débridement
    e. and revision
exploratory incision
exploring electrode
explosion
    e. fracture
    front kick e.
    e. injury
explosive exercise
exposure
    Abbott-Gill epiphysial plate e.
    anterior surgical e.
    bone-tendon e.
    extrapharyngeal e.
    Henry posterior interosseous nerve
      e.
    Kocher-Langenbeck e.
    Smith-Petersen anterior hip surgical
      e.
    subperiosteal e.
    surgical e.
    thoracolumbar junction surgical
      e.
    thoracolumbar spine anterior e.
    transperitoneal e.
    upper cervical spine anterior e.
    vertebral e.
expulsion
    graft e.
exsanguinate
exsanguination tourniquet control
extend
    E. stem
    E. total hip system
ExtendaFLEX exerciser
extended
    e. activities of daily living
      (EADL)
    e. ADLs
    e. care facility
    e. code therapy (ECT)
    e. iliofemoral approach
    e. maxillotomy
    e. medial shoe counter
    e. slide trochanteric osteotomy
    e. steel shank
    e. steel-shank shoe
extended-counter shoe

extender
    bone graft e.
    detachable e.
    dorsal plate e.
    nail e.
    Rousek e.
    Rush e.
    Superstabilizer cemented stem e.
    Superstabilizer press-fit stem e.
Extend-It finger splint
extensibility
extensible
extensile
    e. anterior approach
    e. lateral approach
extension
    active knee e. (AKE)
    e. aid
    angle of greatest e. (AGE)
    Bardenheuer e.
    basal e.
    e. block splint
    e. block splinting method
    e. body cast
    e. bone clamp
    e. bow
    brachioradialis transfer for wrist e.
    brake lever e.
    Buck e.
    cast with dorsal toe plate e.
    cast with volar toe plate e.
    cervical e.
    cervical rotation in e.
    Codivilla e.
    compressive e.
    e. contracture
    e. deformity
    distractive e.
    dorsal toe plate e.
    Dynasplint knee e.
    external rotation in e. (ERE)
    femoral trunk e.
    flexion, abduction, external rotation,
      e. (fabere)
    flexion, adduction, internal rotation,
      e. (fadire)
    flexion and e.
    e. gap
    headrest e.
    hip e.
    Hittenberger halo e.
    e. injury posterior atlantoaxial
      arthrodesis
    e. instability
    internal rotation in e. (IRE)
    isokinetic knee e.
    joint e.
    Legg-Perthes shoe e.
    lumbar e.

E

extension (*continued*)
    e. malposition
    e. maneuver
    Maquet table e.
    e. nail
    nail e.
    NexGen offset stem e.
    e. osteotomy
    range of e.
    e. restriction
    shoe e.
    sitting knee e.
    skeletal e.
    Telos fracture table e.
    terminal knee e.
    toe plate e.
    volitional resisted flexion
     and e.
    wrist e.

extensive
    e. posterior approach
    e. posterior decompression

extensometer
    strain-gauge e.

extensor
    apparatus e.
    e. brevis arthroplasty
    e. carpi radialis brevis (ECRB)
    e. carpi radialis brevis muscle
    e. carpi radialis brevis tendon
    e. carpi radialis longus (ECRL)
    e. carpi radialis longus muscle
    e. carpi radialis longus tendon
    e. carpi ulnaris (ECU)
    e. carpi ulnaris muscle
    e. carpi ulnaris tendinitis
    e. carpi ulnaris tendon
    e. communis muscle
    e. digiti minimi (EDM)
    e. digiti minimi muscle
    e. digiti minimi tendon
    e. digiti quinti (EDQ)
    e. digiti quinti muscle
    e. digiti quinti tendon
    e. digitorum (ED)
    e. digitorum brevis (EDB)
    e. digitorum brevis flap
    e. digitorum brevis muscle
    e. digitorum brevis tendon
    e. digitorum communis (EDC)
    e. digitorum communis muscle
    e. digitorum communis tendon
    e. digitorum longus (EDL)
    e. digitorum longus muscle
    e. digitorum longus tendon
    e. digitorum transfer
    e. hallucis
    e. hallucis brevis muscle
    e. hallucis longus (EHL)

    e. hallucis longus muscle
    e. hallucis longus strength
    e. hallucis longus tendon
    e. hallucis longus tenodesis
    e. hallucis longus transfer
    e. hood
    e. hood mechanism
    e. hood release
    e. indicis muscle
    e. indicis proprius (EIP)
    e. indicis proprius tendon
    knee e.
    long e.
    e. mechanism dysfunction
    e. pollicis brevis (EPB)
    e. pollicis brevis muscle
    e. pollicis brevis tendon
    e. pollicis longus (EPL)
    e. pollicis longus muscle
    e. pollicis longus tendon
    e. quinti tendon
    radial wrist e.
    e. retinaculum
    e. substitution
    e. tendon blockage
    e. tendon injury
    e. tendon lengthening
    e. tendon repair
    e. tendon transfer
    e. tenotomy
    e. thrust reflex
    toe e.
    ulnar e.
    e. wad of 3 muscles
    e. wand
    wrist e.

extensus
    hallux e.

exteriorization

externa
    epicondylalgia e.

external
    e. band
    e. elastic strap
    e. fixation reduction (EX-FI-RE)
    e. fixator
    e. fixator frame
    e. hamstring reflex
    e. humeral epicondylitis
    e. ilium (EI)
    e. ilium movement
    e. immobilization
    e. immobilizer
    e. intercostal muscle
    e. malleolus
    e. neurolysis
    e. oblique muscle
    e. oblique reflex
    posteroinferior e. (PIEX)

e. prehallux
e. recurvatum knee test
e. ring fixation
e. rotation
e. rotation-abduction stress test
  (EAST)
e. rotation contracture
e. rotation exercise
e. rotation in extension (ERE)
e. rotation in flexion (ERF)
e. rotation recurvatum knee test
e. rotation stress test
e. rotation-to-internal rotation ratio
  (ER:IR)
e. rotator
e. sequential pneumatic compression
  boot
e. skeletal fixation apparatus
e. spinal fixation
e. spinal skeletal fixator (ESSF)
e. support
e. tibial torsion
e. traction
e. version
external-alignment compression jig
external-coil electrical stimulation
externally
e. powered tenodesis orthosis
e. rotated
externum
epimysium e.
perimysium e.
externus
malleolus e.
exteroceptive sensation
exteroceptor
postural e.
extirpation
surgical e.
extorsion
extra
Aspercin E.
Buffinol E.
e. strength (ES)
E. Strength Adprin-B
E. Strength Bayer Enteric 500
  Aspirin
E. Strength Bayer Plus
E. Strength Deep Relief
E. Strength Doan's
E. Strength Dynafed E.X.
E. Strength Excedrin
e. toe
Valorin E.
extraabdominal desmoid tumor
extraarticular
e. ankylosis
e. arthrodesis
e. arthroscopy

e. augmentation
e. fracture
e. graft
e. Grice procedure
e. hip fusion
e. knee ligament
e. pain syndrome
e. pigmented villonodular synovitis
e. pseudarthrosis
e. reconstruction
e. resection
e. structure
e. subtalar fusion
e. subtalar joint
e. technique
e. tuberculosis
extrabursal approach
extracapsular
e. ankylosis
e. arterial ring
e. dissection
e. fracture
e. ligament
e. rupture
extracompartmental
e. lesion
e. soft tissue sarcoma
extracorporeal shock wave therapy
extracortical chondrosarcoma
extract
feverfew e.
extracting forceps
extraction
e. of broken femoral antegrade
  nail
e. of unbroken antegrade femoral
  nail
e. pliers
extractor
Austin Moore e.
ball e.
Bilos pin e.
bone plug e.
broach e.
Cherry screw e.
cloverleaf pin e.
corkscrew femoral head e.
femoral head e.
femoral trial e.
FIN e.
Intraflex intramedullary pin e.
Jewett e.
Kalish Duredge wire e.
Küntscher e.
Mark II femoral component e.
Mark II tibial component e.
Massie e.
metatarsal head e.
Moore prosthesis e.

E

extractor (*continued*)
    Moreland femoral component e.
    e. nail drill
    Nicoll e.
    Rousek e.
    Snap Lock wire/pin e.
    Southwick screw e.
    staple e.
    stem e.
    Sven-Johansson e.
    Take-Out E.
    Universal modular femoral hip
      component e.
    Zimmer e.
extractor-driver
extractor-impactor
    Fox e.-i.
extra-depth
    e.-d. posterior acetabular
      retractor
    e.-d. shoe
extradural
    e. anastomosis
    e. granulation
extrafascial nerve injection
extrafusal fiber contraction
extra-large hip retractor
**extra-leverage proximal femoral
elevator**
extramedullary
    e. alignment
    e. alignment guide
    e. fixation
    e. nail extraction by proximal
      stacked wire technique
    e. plasmacytoma (EMP)
    e. tibial alignment jig
extraoctave fracture
extraosseous
    e. circulation
    e. factor
    e. leakage
extraperitoneal approach
extrapharyngeal
    e. approach
    e. exposure
extrapyramidal gait
extraskeletal
    e. chondroma
    e. chondrosarcoma
    e. osteosarcoma
extravasation
    cement e.
    dye e.
    e. extremity
    e. extrusion
    e. injury
    e. irrigation solution
    transcortical contrast e.

Extreme foot orthotic
extremitas (*var. of* extremity)
extremity, extremitas
    both lower extremities
      (BLE)
    both upper extremities
      (BUE)
    elevation of e.
    extravasation e.
    left lower e. (LLE)
    left upper e. (LUE, LUX)
    lower e. (L ext)
    e. magnetic resonance imaging
      (E-MRI)
    e. mobilization strap
    e. mobilization technique
    e. pump
    right lower e. (RLE)
    right upper e. (RUE)
    scanogram of lower e.
    upper e. (UE)
extrinsic
    e. clubfoot
    e. entrapment test
    e. ligament
    e. metatarsus primus elevatus
    e. muscle
    e. muscle strength
    e. rearfoot post
    e. tightness test
    e. toe flexor
extrinsics
    finger e.
extruded
    e. bar polyethylene
    e. disc
extruding-type herniation
extrusion
    bone graft e.
    disc e.
    extravasation e.
extubation
    postoperative e.
exuberant
    e. granulation tissue (EGT)
    e. synovium
exudate
exude
Exu-Dry wound dressing
eye sign
Eyler flexorplasty
Eyre-Brook epiphysial index
EZ
    EZ Bend sponge
    EZ hand pump
    EZ Rider support chair
    EZ ROM postoperative knee
      brace
    EZ T orthopaedic shirt

E-Z
    E-Z arm abduction orthosis
    E-Z Flex jaw exercising device
    E-Z Reacher
Ezeform splint

EZ-Trac orthopaedic suspension device
EZ-Up inversion table
Ezy
    E. Wrap lumbosacral support
    E. Wrap shoulder immobilizer

E

F
French scale
F wave latency
FA
femoral anteversion
Fabco
F. gauze bandage
F. gauze dressing
fabella syndrome
fabellofibular
f. and arcuate ligament complex
f. ligament
faber
flexion, abduction, external rotation
faber test
fabere
flexion, abduction, external rotation, extension
fabere sign
fabere test
Fabian screw
fabric
neoprene f.
Staph-Chek Synergy f.
fabrication
solid freeform f.
FAC
functional ambulation category
face
f. validity
f. validity of rehabilitation testing
face-bow (*var. of* facebow)
facebow, face-bow
Ortho-Yomy f.
face-lift (*var. of* facelift)
facelift, face-lift
chiropractic laser nonsurgical f.
facet, facette
f. angle
f. anomaly
f. apposition
articular f.
calcaneal f.
f. capsule
f. capsule disruption
f. degenerative arthropathy
f. dislocation
f. excision technique
fibular f.
f. fracture
f. fracture stabilization wiring
f. fusion
fusion f.
f. hypertrophy
inferior f.

f. injection
f. joint
f. joint block
f. joint disease (FJD)
f. joint dysfunction
f. joint irritation
f. joint preparation
f. joint syndrome
f. joint vacuum
lateral patellar f.
locked f.
malleolar f.
oblique wiring f.
f. plane
posterior f.
proximal fibular f.
f. replacement
f. screw system
f. subluxation
f. subluxation stabilization wiring
f. surface
f. synovial impingement
f. tropism
facetectomy
O'Donoghue f.
facette (*var. of* facet)
facial
f. artery
f. grading system
facies
acromegalic f.
f. articularis malleolus medialis tibiae
facilitated
f. spinal system
f. subluxation
facilitation
convergence f.
Law of F.
neuromuscular f.
f. pattern
postactivation f.
posttetanic f.
proprioceptive neuromuscular f. (PNF)
facilitatory technique
facility
adult congregate living f.
extended care f.
health-related f.
intermediate care f. (ICF)
skilled nursing f. (SNF)
Xtra Depth University pedorthic educational f.
facioauriculovertebral (FAV)
f. syndrome

F

faciodigitogenital dysplasia
facioscapulohumeral (FSH)
f. muscular dystrophy (FSHD, FSHMD, FSMD)
factitious
f. injury
f. lymphedema
factor
analog neurotrophic f.
atrial natriuretic f. (ANF)
autologous growth f. (AGF)
biomechanical f.
coagulation f.
dislocation f.
ergonomic f.
extraosseous f.
FFC gait-related risk f.
FFF gait-related risk f.
FMC gait-related risk f.
high-risk f.
HO gait-related risk f.
insulin-like growth f. (IGF)
insulin-like growth f. I
leg protection f. (LPF)
LFC gait-related risk f.
nerve growth f.
neurotrophic f.
platelet-derived growth f. (PDGF)
prognostic f.
RA f.
rheumatoid arthritis f. (RAF)
skeletal growth f.
transforming growth f. (TGF)
f. (VIII, IX) deficiency
FAD
functional anesthetic discography
fadir
flexion, adduction, internal rotation
fadir sign
fadir test
fadire
flexion, adduction, internal rotation, extension
fadire test
fad therapy
faecalis
Streptococcus f.
Fahey
F. hip approach
F. pin
F. retractor
F. technique
failed
f. acetabular component
f. back surgery syndrome (FBSS)
f. back syndrome (FBS)
f. back syndrome with documented pseudarthrosis
f. femoral osteotomy

f. flatfoot surgery
f. implant arthroplasty
f. joint replacement
f. procedure
f. surgery syndrome
f. triple arthrodesis
fail-safe mechanism
failure
brittle bone f.
congestive heart f. (CHF)
differentiation f.
ductile f.
fatigue f.
Harrington rod instrumentation f.
heart f.
implant f.
instrumentation f.
metal f.
f. of conservative management
spinal implant load to f.
stem f.
Fairbanks
F. change
F. sign
F. technique with Sever modification
F. uvulopalatopharyngoplasty technique
Fairbanks-Sever brachial plexus repair procedure
Fajersztajn crossed sciatic sign
FAL
functional and anatomic loading
falces (*pl. of* falx)
falciform
f. cartilage
f. ligament
falciparum
Plasmodium f.
Fallat-Buckholz method
fallen
f. arch
f. fragment sign
fallen-leaf sign
fall reduction
false
f. acetabulum
f. aneurysm
f. ankylosis
f. articulation
f. coxa vara
f. joint
f. ligament
f. neuroma
f. pelvis
f. profile view
f. rib
f. vertebra
false-negative result

falx, *pl.* **falces**
    f. calcification
    calcification of f.
FAM
    functional assessment measure
familial
    f. expansile osteolysis
    f. idiopathic scoliosis (FIS)
    f. lymphedema
    f. myoglobinuria
    f. osteoectasia
    f. periodic paralysis
    f. shape
    f. spinal muscular atrophy
family management model
fan
    Schmitt f.
    f. sign
Fanconi
    F. anemia
    F. syndrome
Fanconi-Albertini-Zellweger syndrome
Fantastic Burr nail bur
Farabeuf
    F. amputation
    F. bone-holding forceps
    F. bone rasp
    F. periosteal elevator
Farabeuf-Lambotte
    F.-L. bone-holding forceps
    F.-L. rasp
far fashion
far-field potential
farmer
    F. in utero myelomeningocele repair
     operation
    F. technique
far-near
    f.-n. near-far suture technique
    f.-n. suture
far-out L5 nerve root compression syndrome
Farrior wire-crimping forceps
fartlek training
fascia, *pl.* **fasciae,** *pl.* **fascias**
    Abernethy f.
    antebrachial f.
    anterior cervical f.
    Buck f.
    Camper f.
    cervical f.
    clavipectoral f.
    Colles f.
    crural f.
    cuff of f.
    deep f.
    deltoid f.
    Dupuytren f.
    endoabdominal f.

endothoracic f.
gluteal f.
hypothenar f.
infraspinous f.
investing f.
f. lata
f. lata freeze-thawed graft
lumbar f.
lumbodorsal f. (LDF)
medial geniculate f.
f. of quadratus lumborum
  muscle
Osborne f.
palmar f.
plantar f.
popliteal f.
pubic f.
quadratus femoris f.
retrosacral f.
Scarpa f.
f. sheath
Sibson f.
thenar f.
transversalis f.
vertebral f.
fasciae (*pl. of* fascia)
fascial
    f. arthroplasty
    f. band
    f. bridge
    f. compartment
    f. fibromatosis
    f. flap augmentation
    f. graft
    f. plane
    f. plexus
    f. release
    f. sarcoma
    f. septum
    f. sheath covering
    f. space
    f. space infection
    f. subcutaneous turn-down flap
    f. suture
fascial-muscle interface
fasciaplasty, fascioplasty
fascias (*pl. of* fascia)
fascia-splitting incision
fascicle
    anterior tibiotalar f. (ATTF)
    motor f.
    muscle f.
    popliteomeniscal f.
    sensory f.
    silent f.
fascicular
    f. degeneration
    f. neuropathy
    f. repair

F

fasciculation
  benign f.
  contraction f.
  malignant f.
  f. potential
fasciculi (*pl. of* fasciculus)
fasciculus, *pl.* **fasciculi**
  arcuate f. (AF)
fasciectomy
  dermal f.
  limited f.
  partial f.
  radical palmar f.
  subtotal plantar f.
fasciitis, fascitis
  diffuse f.
  Dupuytren f.
  iliotibial band f.
  ITB f.
  necrotizing f.
  nodular f.
  plantar f.
  proliferative f.
  pseudosarcomatous f.
   (PSF)
  recalcitrant plantar f.
fasciocutaneous
  f. axial pattern flap
  f. island flap
fasciodesis
fascio-fat graft
fasciogram
fascioplasty (*var. of* fasciaplasty)
fasciorrhaphy
fascioscapulohumeral
  f. dystrophy
  f. muscle atrophy disease
  f. muscular atrophy
  f. muscular dystrophy
fasciotome
  intercompartment f.
  Masson f.
  Moseley f.
fasciotomy
  4-compartment f.
  compartment f.
  decompression f.
  double-incision f.
  endoscopic plantar f. (EPF)
  minimal incision plantar f.
  palmar f.
  percutaneous plantar f. (PPF)
  plantar f.
  prophylactic f.
  single-incision f.
  subcutaneous palmar f.
  uniportal plantar f.
  Yount f.
fascitis (*var. of* fasciitis)

fashion
  aseptic f.
  barber-pole f.
  Bunnell zigzag f.
  cruciate f.
  far f.
  near-far f.
FASS
  foot and ankle severity scale
FAST
  Functional Assessment Staging
fast
  f. axoplasmic transport
  f. imaging with steady procession
   (FISP)
  f. low-angle shot (FLASH)
  f. muscle
FASTak
  F. suture anchor
  F. suture anchor system
fastener
  Intrafix ACL tibial f.
**Fastex proprioceptive and agility
 test**
Fastin
  F. suture anchor
  F. threaded anchor
FAST1 intraosseous infusion system
Fastlok implantable staple
FastOut device
Fas-Trac strip
fast-twitch muscle fiber
FAT
  female athlete triad
fat
  f. and fat-free mass (FFM)
  aspirated f.
  autogenous f.
  f. embolism
  f. embolism syndrome (FES)
  f. graft
  f. loading
  f. oxidation
  f. pad
  f. pad atrophy
  f. pad of elbow
  f. pad retractor
  f. pad syndrome
  f. saturation
fat-blood
  f.-b. interface (FBI)
  f.-b. interface sign
fat-fluid level
fatigue
  f. failure
  f. fracture
  implant f.
  metal f.
  static f.

f. strength
f. stress
f. tolerance
volitional f.
fatigued bone graft
fat-pad
elbow f.-p.
foveal f.-p.
heel f.-p.
Hoffa f.-p.
patellar f.-p.
pre-Achilles f.-p.
scalene f.-p.
f.-p. sign
fat-suppressed turbo spin-echo T2-weighted sequence
fatty
f. tissue
f. tissue tumor
Faulkner curette
fault
dynamic f.
faulty union
FAV
facioauriculovertebral
FAV syndrome
Fazio-Londe
F.-L. atrophy
F.-L. syndrome
FBI
fat-blood interface
FBI sign
FBS
failed back syndrome
FBSS
failed back surgery syndrome
FCE
functional capacity evaluation
FCER
Foundation for Chiropractic Education and Research
FCL
fibular collateral ligament
FCR
flexor carpi radialis
FCS
fluorescence correlation spectroscopy
full cervical spine
FCS view
FCS x-ray
FCU
flexor carpi ulnaris
FD
flexor digitorum
FDB
flexor digitorum brevis
FDC
flexor digitorum communis

FDICT
frequency-difference interferential current therapy
FDL
flexor digitorum longus
FDMA
first dorsal metatarsal artery
FDP
flexor digitorum profundus
FDQB
flexor digitorum quinti brevis
FDS
flexor digitorum sublimis
flexor digitorum superficialis
Feagin shoulder dislocation test
feasibility
F. Evaluation Checklist (FEC)
vocational f.
febricitans
pes f.
FEC
Feasibility Evaluation Checklist
feedback
force f.
vibrotactile f.
feeder
offset suspension f.
suspension f.
Tumble Forms f.
feel
end f.
initiation f.
through-range f.
feet (*pl. of* foot)
Feiss
F. line
F. medial malleolus to plantar first MTP joint line
Feldene
Feldenkrais
F. cylinder
F. foam roll
F. method
Felix disease
fell
f. on outstretched hand (FOOSH)
f. on outstretched hand injury
felon
aseptic f.
f. infection
felt
f. apron Bowden cable suspension system
f. brace
f. collar splint
f. dressing
orthopaedic f.
f. padding
f. patch

F

felt (*continued*)
    rolled f.
    F. shears
female
    f. athlete triad (FAT)
    f. reamer
    f. washer
Femizol-M
femora (*pl. of* femur)
femoral
    f. aligner
    f. alignment jig
    f. antetorsion
    f. anteversion (FA)
    f. approach
    f. arteriography
    f. attachment
    f. bone
    f. Buck plug procedure
    f. canal
    f. canal restrictor
    f. circulation
    f. circumflex artery
    f. clamp
    f. component
    f. component pusher
    f. component removal
    f. condylar defect
    f. condylar shaving
    f. condylar template
    f. condyle
    f. cortex
    f. cortical index
    f. cortical perforation
    f. cortical ring allograft
    f. cortical window
    f. cutaneous nerve
    f. derotation osteotomy
    f. diaphysial allograft
    f. diaphysis
    f. distractor
    f. drill bit
    f. drill tunnel
    f. endoprosthesis
    f. epicondyle
    f. epiphysiolysis
    f. epiphysis
    f. footprint
    f. fossa
    f. fracture following total hip
     replacement classification
    f. fracture Ogden construct repair
    f. groove
    f. guide pin
    f. guidepin
    f. head
    f. head amputation
    f. head and neck
    f. head bone removal reamer

    f. head cork screw
    f. head deformity
    f. head driver
    f. head dysplasia
    f. head extractor
    f. head line (FHL)
    f. head-neck anteversion
    f. head-neck junction
    f. head osteonecrosis
    f. head-to-neck ratio
    f. head vascularity
    f. impactor
    f. intramedullary guide
    f. intratrochanteric fracture
    f. lengthening
    f. medullary canal
    f. metaphysial shortening
    f. metaphysis
    f. muscle
    f. nailing
    f. neck fracture (FNF)
    f. neck fracture reduction
    f. neck nail
    f. neck prosthesis
    f. neck version
    f. nerve block (FNB)
    f. nerve paralysis
    f. nerve stretch test (FNST)
    f. nerve traction hip test
    f. neuropathy
    f. notch guide
    f. offset
    f. osteolysis
    f. osteomyelitis
    f. osteoporosis
    f. plate
    f. plug
    f. prosthesis broach
    f. prosthesis fixation
    f. rasp
    f. reflex
    f. region
    f. resection
    f. resector
    f. retrotorsion
    f. retroversion
    f. rollback
    f. sarcoma
    self-articulating f. (SAF)
    f. shaft
    f. shaft axis
    f. shaft fracture
    f. shaft malunion
    f. sheath
    f. stem removal
    f. stress fracture
    f. supracondylar fracture
    f. torsion
    f. trial extractor

f. trunk angle
f. trunk extension
f. trunk flexion
f. tuberosity
f. tunnel
f. vein injury
femoris (*gen. of* femur)
femoroacetabular impingement
femoroiliac thrombophlebitis
femoroischial transplant
femoropatellar joint
femorotibial
f. angle (FTA)
f. joint
f. ligament tenodesis
f. torsion
femur, *pl.* **femora,** *gen.* **femoris**
adductor tubercle of f.
biceps femoris
f. button graft complex
distal f.
f., fibula, ulna (FFU)
f., fibula, ulna complex
F. Finder instrument
fovea capitis femoris
fovea centralis of f.
f. graft
f. length
f. length-to-abdominal circumference ratio (FL:AC)
proximal f.
quadratus femoris (QF)
rectus femoris
resection of distal f.
spiral line of f.
swashbuckler approach to distal f.
Universal Proximal F. (UPF)
fenamic acid
fence splint
fender fracture
fenestrated
f. drape
f. reamer
f. stem
f. tenotomy
fenestration
Fenlin total shoulder system
fenoprofen calcium
fentanyl
droperidol and f.
F. Oralet
Fenton tibial bolt
Ferciot
F. excision
F. tiptoe splint
Ferciot-Thompson knee ossicle excision
Ferguson
F. bone clamp
F. bone holder

F. bone-holding forceps
F. hip reduction
F. method for measuring spinal curvature scoliosis
F. sacral base angle
F. sacroiliac view
F. scoliosis measuring method
Ferguson-Frazier suction tube
Fergusson forceps
Ferkel
F. bipolar muscular torticollis release
F. C guide
F. torticollis technique
Fernandez
F. extensile anterior knee approach
F. osteotomy
F. point-score wrist assessment system
F. scale posttraumatic wrist assessment system
Ferno
F. AquaCiser underwater treadmill system
F. custom therapy pool
Ferran awl
ferric subsulfate
Ferrier coupler
Ferris-Smith
F.-S. bone-biting forceps
F.-S. rongeur
F.-S. rongeur forceps
F.-S. tissue forceps
Ferris-Smith-Kerrison
F.-S.-K. forceps
F.-S.-K. laminectomy rongeur
Ferris-Smith-Spurling disc rongeur
ferromagnetic
f. metal plate
f. relaxation
ferrous sulfate
ferumoxide injectable solution
FES
fat embolism syndrome
functional electrical stimulation
FES exercise bicycle
festinating gait, festination
festination (*var. of* festinating gait)
fetal
f. alcohol syndrome
f. substantia nigra graft
fetalis
myodystrophia f.
fever
drug-infusion f.
fracture f.
f. of undetermined origin (FUO)
rheumatic f.

F

Feverall
    Infants F.
    F. Sprinkle Caps
feverfew extract
FFC
    first foot contact
    fixed flexion contracture
    FFC gait-related risk factor
FFF
    forefoot flat
    FFF gait-related risk factor
FFI
    foot function index
FFM
    fat and fat-free mass
FFU
    femur, fibula, ulna
    FFU complex
F3 hand, foot, wrist fracture fragment plating system
FHB
    flexor hallucis brevis
FHL
    femoral head line
    flexor hallucis longus
    FHL dysfunction
    FHL release technique
    FHL tendon transfer/augmentation
FI
    Functional Integration
fiber, fibre, *pl.* **fibrae**
    A-delta f.
    afferent f.
    f. analysis
    anular f.
    collagen f.
    f. density
    fast-twitch muscle f.
    intrafusal f.
    f. metal taper
    ragged red f.
    Sharpey f.
    skeletal muscle f.
    tendinous f.
fiberglass
    f. bandage
    f. cast
    f. splint
fiberglass-free cast tape
fiber-metal peg
fiberoptic
    f. arthroscope
    f. cable
    f. intraosseous endoscopy
    f. light source
fiber-region
    anterior f.-r.
    central f.-r.
fiber-splitting incision

fibra, *pl.* **fibrae**
fibrae (*pl. of* fiber, *pl. of* fibra)
fibre (*var. of* fiber)
fibreux
    cerclage f.
fibrillar absorbable hemostat material
fibrillation
    muscle f.
    f. potential
    synchronized f.
fibrin
    f. clot
    f. debris
    f. glue adhesive
    f. island
fibrinogen
    iodine-labeled f.
    radioactive iodine-labeled f.
fibrinoid degeneration, fibrinous degeneration
fibrinolysin and desoxyribonuclease
fibrinolysis
fibrinolytic agent
fibrinous degeneration
fibroadipose tissue
fibroblast
    regenerated f.
fibroblastic
    f. phase
    f. proliferation
    f. sarcoma
    f. tumor
fibrocartilage
    f. complex
    triangular f. (TFC)
fibrocartilaginous
    f. disc
    f. joint
    f. pad
    f. plate
    f. tissue
fibrochondrocyte
fibroconnective tissue
fibrodysplasia ossificans progressiva
fibroelastic cartilage
fibroepithelial polyp
fibroepithelioma of Pinkus
fibroepitheliomatous
fibrofatty
    f. debris
    f. infiltrate
    f. tissue
fibroid tumor
fibrokeratoma
    acquired digital f.
    acral digital f.
fibrolipoma
    massive f.

fibrolipomatosis
  macrodactylia f.
fibroma
  aponeurotic f.
  calcifying aponeurotic f.
  cementing f.
  chondromyxoid f.
  desmoid f.
  desmoplastic f.
  juvenile aponeurotic f.
  Koenen periungual f.
  f. molle
  nonossifying f. (NOF)
  nonosteogenic f.
  ossifying f.
  osteogenic f.
  perineural f. (PNR)
  periosteal f.
  periungual f.
  soft f.
  subungual f.
fibromatosis
  aggressive infantile f.
  f. colli
  congenital general f.
  dermal f.
  diffuse infantile f.
  Dupuytren f.
  fascial f.
  Garrod f.
  generalized f.
  infantile dermal f.
  irradiation f.
  juvenile hyaline f.
  palmar f.
  plantar f.
  pseudosarcomatous f.
  solitary f.
  sternocleidomastoid muscle f.
  subcutaneous pseudosarcomatous f.
fibromuscular disease (FMD)
fibromyalgia syndrome (FMS)
fibromyalgic pain
fibromyositis
fibromyxoma
fibronectin
fibroosseous
  f. pulley
  f. ring
  f. ring of Lacroix
  f. sheath
  f. tunnel
fibropathic abnormality
fibroplasia
fibrosa (*var. of* fibrous)
fibrosarcoma
fibrosis
  anular f.
  endoneurial f.

intraneural f.
perineural f.
retroperitoneal f.
fibrositis
  f. ossificans progressiva
  periarticular f.
fibrosus
  anulus f.
  bulging anulus f.
  lacertus f.
fibrotic strut
fibrous, fibrosa
  f. adhesion
  f. ankylosis
  f. attachment
  f. band
  f. capsule
  f. cartilage
  f. cortical defect
  f. dysplasia
  f. dysplasia ossificans progressiva
  f. hamartoma
  f. histiocytoma
  f. hyperplasia
  f. joint
  f. lesion
  f. loose body
  f. metaphysial defect
  f. metaplasia
  myositis fibrosa
  progressive myositis fibrosa
  f. scar tissue
  f. spur
  f. talocalcaneal coalition
  f. tissue implant
  f. transformation
  f. tumor
  f. union
  f. xanthoma
fibrovascular connective tissue stroma
fibroxanthoma
fibula, *pl.* **fibulae, fibulas**
  diastasis f.
  distal f.
  dysplastic f.
  head of f.
  f. protibial synostosis
  proximal f.
  short f.
  f. shortening
fibulae (*pl. of* fibula)
fibular
  f. anlage
  f. bone
  f. bone hook test
  f. collateral ligament (FCL)
  f. collateral sprain
  f. compression test
  f. diaphysial fracture

F

fibular (*continued*)
    f. facet
    f. groove
    f. head
    f. head resection
    f. hemimelia
    f. joint disruption
    f. malleolus
    f. margin
    f. metaphysis
    f. muscle
    f. neck
    f. onlay-inlay graft
    f. ostectomy
    f. osteotomy
    f. peg
    f. plantar marginal artery
    f. pseudarthrosis
    f. ring allograft
    f. sesamoid
    f. sesamoidal ligament
    f. sesamoidectomy
    f. shortening
    f. strut graft
    f. transfer
    f. transplant
fibulas (*pl. of* fibula)
fibulectomy
    partial f.
fibulocalcaneal
    f. ligament
    f. ligament strain
    f. pain syndrome
fibulotalar
    f. arthrodesis
    f. ligament
fibulotalocalcaneal (FTC)
    f. ligament
Ficat
    F. and Arlet classification of major joint osteonecrosis
    F. and Arlet radiographic classification of humeral head osteonecrosis (stage I-IV)
    F. avascular necrosis classification
    F. femoral head osteonecrosis classification (stage I-IV)
    F. radiographic classification of femoral head osteonecrosis (stage I-IV)
    F. view
Fick method
fiducial
field
    F. blade
    f. block
    f. block anesthesia
    bloodless f.
    electromagnetic f.

    ionized gas f.
    f. of dissection
    peripheral nerve cutaneous f.
    pulsating electromagnetic f. (PEMF)
    pulsed electromagnetic f. (PEMF)
    QRS pulsating magnetic f.
field focusing nuclear magnetic resonance (FONAR)
Fielding
    F. femoral fracture classification
    F. modification of Gallie atlantoaxial instability spine fusion technique
fifth
    f. finger
    f. metacarpal
fighter's fracture
figure-of-4
    f.-o.-4 position
    f.-o.-4 test
figure-of-8
    f.-o.-8 adjustment
    f.-o.-8 bandage
    f.-o.-8 brace
    f.-o.-8 cast
    f.-o.-8 dressing
    f.-o.-8 harness
    f.-o.-8 suture
    f.-o.-8 taping
    f.-o.-8 test
    f.-o.-8 thoracic orthosis
    f.-o.-8 wire
    f.-o.-8 wire loop
    f.-o.-8 wiring
filarial
    f. arthritis
    f. synovitis
file
    bone f.
    orthopaedic bone f.
    orthopaedic surgical f.
filgrastim
filiform
fill
    fit and f.
Fillauer
    F. bar
    F. bar foot orthosis
    F. dorsiflexion assist ankle joint
    F. endoskeletal alignment system
    F. modular shuttle lock system
    F. night splint
    F. PDC ankle joint
    F. prosthesis liner
    F. Scottish Rite orthosis kit
    F. silicone suction liner
    F. silicone suspension liner
filler
    BF+ bone void f.
    f. block

BonePlast bone void f.
Cerasorb resorbable synthetic bone
    void f.
Cortoss bone void f.
nonosteoconductive bone void f.
OsteoSet bone f.
Plexur P bone void f.
ProOsteon implant 500 coralline
    hydroxyapatite bone void f.
shoe f.
Springlite toe f.
synthetic cancellous bone void f.
synthetic cortical bone void f.
TheriLok bone void f.
Vitoss Scaffold synthetic cancellous
    bone void f.

filleted graft
fillet local flap graft
filling pattern
film
    f. blister dressing
    chiropractic x-ray f.
    lateral cervical spine f.
    scout f.
    spot f.
    stress f.
    working orthopaedic surgery f.
film-screen combination
filmy adhesion
filtration system
filum terminale syndrome
FIM
    functional independence measure
FIN
    flexible intramedullary nail
    FIN extractor
    FIN pin guide
    FIN system
fin
    DePuy Global shoulder glenoid
        component with f.
    F. & Flipper exercise log
    f. of the implant
    prosthetic stem lateral f.
finder
    angle f.
    canal f.
    Dasco Pro angle f.
    gravity-driven angle f.
    Leisure Activities F. (LAF)
    pedicle f.
finding
    bone in bone f.
    constellation of clinical f.'s
    dynamic pedodynographic f.
    thermographic f.
fine
    f. bone curette
    f. manipulation

f. olive bur
f. osteotome
f. wire EMG
fine-angled curette
fine-tooth electric saw
finger
    adduction stress to f.
    f. agnosia
    f. amputation
    f. angle
    baseball f.
    base of f.
    F. Blocking Tree
    f. bolster
    claw f.
    cloven-hoof fracture of f.
    clubbed f.
    coach's f.
    congenital trigger f.
    f. cot
    f. cot splint
    f. deformity
    f. dexterity
    distal tuberosity of f.
    drop f.
    drumstick f.
    f. exerciser
    f. extension bow
    f. extension clockspring splint
    f. extension test
    f. extrinsics
    fifth f.
    F. Fitness Spring Ball
    f. flap
    f. flexion glove
    f. flexion splint
    f. flexor muscle
    football f.
    f. gauge
    f. goniometer
    hammer f.
    F. Helper hand exerciser
    hippocratic f.
    f. hook
    hypoplastic f.
    f. in balloon sign
    index f.
    f. intrinsics
    jammed f.
    jerk f.
    jersey f.
    f. joint
    f. joint arthroplasty
    f. joint implant
    f. joint implant prosthesis
    f. ladder
    little f.
    lock f.
    long f.

F

finger (*continued*)
    f. loop
    lumbrical plus f.
    lumbrical syndrome f.
    mallet f.
    middle f.
    multiple f.'s
    f. opposition
    f. pad
    paradoxical lumbrical-plus f.
    F. Platter hand exerciser
    prosthetic f.
    f. pulp
    f. ray
    release of trigger f.
    replantation of f.
    ring f.
    rugby jersey f.
    sausage f.
    f. separator
    Silastic HP-100 prosthetic f.
    f. sled splint
    f. sling
    snap f.
    spade f.
    spider f.
    f. splint (type 501, 502, 504, 602)
    spring f.
    stuck f.
    syndactylized f.
    f. technique
    f. tourniquet
    f. trap
    f. trap suspension
    f. trap suture
    f. trap traction
    f. trap tube
    trigger f.
    f. tuft
    f. web
    webbed f.
fingerbreadth
Finger-Hugger splint
fingernail
    base of f.
    f. drill
    parrot beak f.
3-finger spica cast
finger-thumb reflex
fingertip
    f. amputation
    f. cold intolerance
    f. dissection
    f. guard
    f. pad
fingertips-to-floor test
finger-to-finger test
finger-to-nose test (FNT)

fingertrap
    Chinese f.
finish bur
finisher
    Küntscher f.
Finkelstein
    F. maneuver
    F. sign
    F. tendonitis of wrist test
    F. test for synovitis
Finn
    F. hinged knee prosthesis
    F. knee system
Finney-Flexirod prosthesis
Finney prosthesis
Finochietto
    F. clamp carrier
    F. rib retractor
Fiorinal with Codeine
FIQ
    Functional Index Questionnaire
firearm injury
firing
    f. pattern
    f. rate
Firm D-Ring wrist support splint
FirmFlex
    F. custom orthosis
    F. custom orthotic
first
    f. carpometacarpal joint fracture
    f. cervical vertebra
    f. cuneiform joint arthrodesis
    f. cuneiform-navicular joint arthrodesis
    f. dorsal interosseous assist
    f. dorsal metacarpal artery
    f. dorsal metatarsal artery (FDMA)
    f. foot contact (FFC)
    f. intention
    f. intermetacarpal ligament
    f. metacarpal
    f. metatarsal contact (FMC)
    f. metatarsal-first cuneiform arthrodesis
    f. metatarsus rise test
    f. MTP cheilectomy
    f. plantar metatarsal artery (FPMA)
    f. ray surgery
    f. rib rasp
    f. rib resection
    f. toe Jones repair
    f. web space
    wrist f.
first–fifth intermetatarsal angle
first–second intermetatarsal angle
FirstSTEP Developmental Screening Test

FIS
    familial idiopathic scoliosis
Fisch
    F. bone drill irrigator
    F. bone rongeur
    F. drill
Fischer
    F. pressure threshold meter
    F. ring
    F. tendon stripper
    F. transfixing pin
fish
    F. cuneiform osteotomy
    F. cuneiform osteotomy
     technique
    f. vertebra
    f. vertebra sign
Fisher
    F. advancement flap
    F. brace
    F. guide
    F. half pin
    F. rasp
fishmouth
    f. amputation
    f. anastomosis
    f. drain
    f. end-to-end suture
    f. incision
fishtail
    f. deformity
    f. sign
Fiskars scissors
Fisk-Fernandez volar wedge bone
  graft
FISP
    fast imaging with steady procession
fissure bur
fissured
    f. fracture
    f. nail
fist-edge-palm test
fist-palm-side test
fist position
fist-ring test
fistula, *pl.* **fistulae, fistulas**
    arteriovenous f. (AVF)
    enterocutaneous f.
    perilymphatic f. (PLF)
    synovial f.
fistulae (*pl. of* fistula)
fistulas (*pl. of* fistula)
fistulography
FIT
    Footwear Integration Technology
    Fracture Intervention Trial
    functional integrated training
fit
    f. and fill

    interference f.
    press f.
    snap f.
    trial f.
Fit-Lastic
    F.-L. therapy band
    F.-L. therapy tubing
fitness
    F. Ball
    F. Safety Standards
     Committee
Fitnet joint testing system
Fits-All
    F.-A. sling
    F.-A. support
Fitstep
    F. II stair climber
    Universal F.
FITT
    frequency, intensity, time, type
    FITT exercise
fitting
    immediate postsurgical f.
     (IPSF)
    prosthetic f.
    temporary prosthetic f.
    Velcro f.
Fitzgerald rating
fixateur
    f. interne fixation system
    f. interne rod
    f. interne screw
fixating apparatus
fixation
    abnormal f.
    Ace-Colles f.
    Ace-Fischer f.
    Ace Unifix f.
    adjunctive screw f.
    Allen-Ferguson Galveston
     pelvic f.
    Ambi f.
    AMS intramedullary f.
    Anderson pin f.
    angled blade-plate f.
    anterior cervical f.
    anterior internal f.
    anterior metallic f.
    anterior odontoid f.
    anterior plate f.
    anterior screw f.
    anterior spinal f.
    AO external f.
    AO screw f.
    AO spinal internal f.
    APR cement f.
    Arbeitsgemeinschaft für
     Osteosynthesefragen-Association for
     Internal F. (AO-ASIF)

F

fixation (*continued*)

Arbeitsgemeinschaft für Osteosynthesefragen-Association for the Study of Internal F. (AO-ASIF)
arthroscopic screw f.
Association for the Study of Internal F. (ASIF)
atlantoaxial rotatory f. (AARF)
Austin chevron osteotomy f.
axial f.
bar bolt f.
Barbour cervical f.
4-bar external f.
Barr open reduction and internal f.
Barr tibial fracture f.
biaxial compression plate f.
bicortical screw f.
Biofix absorbable f.
biologic f.
blade-plate f.
f. bolt
bolt f.
bone-ingrowth f.
bone suture f.
bridge plate f.
buried K-wire f.
buttressing in internal f.
Calandruccio f.
Campbell screw f.
cementless f.
cerclage wire f.
cervical spine internal f.
cervical spine screw-plate f.
chevron osteotomy with rigid screw f.
Childress ankle f.
circular f.
circumferential wire-loop f.
cloverleaf condylar plate f.
Cole tendon f.
compression plate f.
computer-assisted percutaneous internal f.
condylar screw f.
coracoclavicular screw f.
coracoclavicular suture f.
cross-screw f.
DeBastiani f.
Denham external f.
dens anterior screw f.
f. device
Dimon-Hughston hip fracture f.
f. disc
dorsal wire-loop f.
dynamic compression plate f.
dynamic condylar screw f.
dynamic external f.
f. dysfunction

f. dysfunction of lumbar spine
ECT internal fracture f.
elastic f.
Ender elastic condylar nail fracture f.
Ender nail f.
Ender rod f.
Ender trochanteric fracture f.
ESIN pediatric fracture f.
Essex-Lopresti f.
external ring f.
external spinal f.
extramedullary f.
femoral prosthesis f.
fracture f.
Gallie subtalar f.
Galveston pelvic f.
Ganz f.
Georgiade visor halo f.
Gouffon pin f.
graft f.
greenstick f.
Hackethal intramedullary bouquet f.
half-pin f.
Halifax clamp posterior cervical f.
Hammer external f.
Harrington rod f.
Herbert bone screw f.
Hex-Fix external f.
Hoffmann external f.
3-hole suture tendon f.
hook-pin f.
hook-plate f.
Hughes f.
hybrid f.
Ikuta f.
iliac f.
Ilizarov external f.
f. imaging
ingrowth f.
Innovasive f.
interference fit f.
internal f. (IF)
internal fracture f.
internal spinal f.
interosseous wire f.
intersegmental f.
Intrafix f.
intramedullary bouquet f.
intramedullary rod f.
intraosseous f.
intrapedicular f.
intrapelvic f.
f. jig
Kavanaugh-Brower-Mann f.
Kempf internal screw f.
Kirschner pin f.
Kirschner wire f.
Kristiansen-Kofoed external f.

Kronner external f.
Kronner ring f.
K wire f.
Kyle internal f.
lag screw f.
long-bone f.
loop f.
LPPS hydroxyapatite f.
lumbar pedicle f.
lumbar spine segmental f.
lumbar spine transpedicular f.
Luque-Galveston f.
Luque loop f.
Luque rod f.
Luque segmental f.
Magerl posterior cervical screw f.
Magerl transarticular screw f.
Matta-Saucedo f.
McKeever medullary clavicle f.
mechanical f.
medial malleolus f.
medullary nail f.
Meniscus Arrow f.
Minerva f.
minifragment plate f.
Modulock posterior spinal f.
monofilament wire f.
Monticelli-Spinelli leg f.
Morrissy percutaneous slipped
  epiphysis f.
multiple-point sacral f.
Murray f.
nail plate f.
neutralization plate f.
nonloop f.
Obwegeser-Dalpont internal screw f.
occipitocervical f.
odontoid fracture internal f.
Olerud transpedicular f.
open condylar plate f.
open reduction and internal f.
  (ORIF)
OrthoSorb pin f.
os calcis pin f.
pedicle screw f.
pedicular f.
f. peg
pelvic f.
percutaneous f.
phalangeal fracture f.
Phemister acromioclavicular pin f.
pin f.
f. pin
pin-and-plaster f.
plate f.
plate-screw f.
4-point f.
porous ingrowth f.
posterior cervical f.

posterior screw f.
posterior segmental f.
Precision Osteolock f.
press-fit f.
prophylactic skeletal f.
provisional f.
radial neck fracture f.
reduction f.
ReUnite hand f.
Rezaian spinal f.
rib f.
rigid internal f.
rod sleeve f.
Roger Anderson f.
Rogozinski spinal f.
Roy-Camille posterior screw plate f.
sacral fusion screw f.
sacral pedicle screw f.
sacral spine f.
sacroiliac extension f.
sacroiliac flexion f.
sacropelvic f.
Sangeorzan foot and ankle
  internal f.
Schneider f.
Schuind external f.
scoliosis f.
scoliotic curve f.
screw f.
f. screw
screw-and-keel f.
screw-and-plate f.
screw-and-wire f.
screw-plate f.
segmental f.
Seidel intramedullary f.
Shepherd internal screw f.
short-segment posterior f.
short-segment transpedicular f.
  (SSTF)
Slatis pelvic f.
SmartTack f.
spinal f.
spinopelvic transiliac f. (STIF)
spondylolisthesis reduction f.
spring f.
Stableloc II external f.
staple f.
static f.
Steinmann pin f.
f. strength
strut plate f.
sublaminar f.
f. subluxation
Sukhtian-Hughes f.
supraacetabular compression
  external f.
suprasyndesmotic screw f.
Suretac shoulder f.

F

fixation (*continued*)
    surgical f.
    suture f.
    Syracuse anterior spinal f.
    table-skeletal f.
    f. technique
    temporary external transpedicular f.
    tendon f.
    tension band f.
    thin pin f.
    TiMesh implantable hardware f.
    transarticular screw f.
    transarticular wire f.
    transcapitellar wire f.
    TransFix ACL system f.
    transiliac rod f.
    transpedicular f.
    transsyndesmotic screw f.
    transverse f.
    triangular external ankle f.
    TSRH rod f.
    tunnel-and-sling f.
    Turvy internal screw f.
    Versa-Fx femoral f.
    Vidal-Adrey modified Hoffmann f.
    Volkov-Oganesian external f.
    VSP f.
    Wagner f.
    Webb f.
    wedge f.
    Wilson-Jacobs tibial f.
    wire loop f.
    Wisconsin wire f.
    f. with intramedullary device
    Zickel nail f.
    Zickel subtrochanteric
      fracture f.

fixator
    Ace-Colles external f.
    Ace-Fischer external f.
    Agee-WristJack external f.
    AO internal f.
    articulated external f.
    1-bar external f.
    biplanar f.
    Block f.
    cantilever external f.
    carbon fiber f.
    circular fine-wire external f.
    circular wire f.
    Claiborne external f.
    clamp f.
    Clyburn Colles fracture f.
    Clyburn external f.
    Compass Hinge external f.
    DeBastiani external f.
    D-L internal f.
    dynamic axial f. (DAF)
    Edwards D-L modular f.

external f.
external spinal skeletal f. (ESSF)
f. frame
Ganz antishock pelvic f.
half-pin external f.
Herbert screw f.
Hex-Fix monolateral external f.
high tibial osteotomy f.
hinged articulated f.
hinged elbow external f.
Hoffmann C-series external f.
Hoffmann dynamic external f.
Hoffmann-Vidal external f.
HTO f.
hybrid external f.
Ilizarov circular external f.
Ilizarov external ring f.
Ilizarov hybrid f.
Jacquet f.
Kessler external f.
L-frame f.
Lima external f.
Manuflex external f.
mini-Hoffmann external f.
mini-Kessler external f.
mini-Orthofix f.
modified Hoffmann quadrilateral
  external f.
Monofixateur external f.
Monticelli-Spinelli f.
f. muscle
Olerud internal f.
Orthofix monolateral femoral
  external f.
Oxford f.
Pennig dynamic wrist f.
pin external f.
1-plane bilateral external f.
2-plane bilateral external f.
1-plane unilateral external f.
2-plane unilateral external f.
preoperative planning under pin f.'s
Rezaian spinal f.
Richards Colles external f.
ring external f.
Roger Anderson external f.
Sheffield Ring F.
spanning external f.
Stableloc Colles fracture
  external f.
temporary external f.
thin-wire Ilizarov f.
Thomas f.
True/LOK external f.
Vermont spinal f. (VSF)
Wagner f.
Wagner device external f.
Wiltse f.

fixator-augmented nailing

fixed
- f. anatomic patellar implant
- f. bearing knee implant
- f. deformity
- f. distraction
- f. dressing
- f. femoral head prosthesis
- f. flexion contracture (FFC)
- f. flexion deformity
- f. hammertoe
- f. hammertoe deformity repair
- f. inversion
- f. lumbosacral deformity
- f. sagittal imbalance
- f. torticollis

fixed-angle AO blade-plate
fixed-offset guide
Fixion
- F. intramedullary humeral nail
- F. proximal femoral nail

Fix-Sil silicone adhesive
FJD
- facet joint disease

FL:AC
- femur length-to-abdominal circumference ratio

flaccid
- f. cerebral palsy
- f. flatfoot
- f. gait
- f. leg
- f. paralysis

flaccidity
flag
- f. flap
- f. sign

Flagg fiberglass knee brace
Flagyl
flail
- f. arm
- f. digit
- f. foot
- f. implant
- f. joint
- f. knee
- f. shoulder
- f. toe

flail-elbow hinge
FLAIR
- fluid attenuation inversion recovery

flake hamate fracture
flame-tip bur
Flanagan-Burem apposing hemicylindric graft
flange
- endoprosthetic f.

4-flanged nail
flanged revision prosthesis
flank bone

flap
- abdominal f.
- abductor hallucis longus f.
- adductor magnus adductor f.
- adipofascial f.
- advancement f.
- f. amputation
- anterior myocutaneous f.
- anterior tibial fasciocutaneous f.
- arm f.
- arterial f.
- Atasoy-Kleinert hand advancement f.
- Atasoy triangular advancement f.
- Atasoy volar V-Y f.
- axial pattern f.
- axillary f.
- biaxial f.
- bilateral V-Y Kutler f.
- bilobed digital neurovascular island f.
- bilobed skin f.
- bipedicle dorsal f.
- brachioradialis f.
- buccinator myomucosal f.
- bursal f.
- butterfly f.
- capsular f.
- capsuloperiosteal f.
- central meniscal f.
- Chinese radial forearm f.
- cocked-half f.
- composite groin fascial free f.
- f. congestion
- cross-arm f.
- cross-extremity f.
- cross-finger f.
- crossleg f.
- cutaneous f.
- de-epithelialized rectus abdominis muscle f.
- deltoid f.
- deltopectoral f.
- dorsal cross-finger f.
- dorsalis pedis fasciocutaneous f.
- double-Z rhombic skin f.
- DRAM f.
- extensor digitorum brevis f.
- fascial subcutaneous turn-down f.
- fasciocutaneous axial pattern f.
- fasciocutaneous island f.
- finger f.
- Fisher advancement f.
- flag f.
- flexor hallucis brevis f.
- foot first-web f.
- forearm f.
- free fasciocutaneous f.

F

flap (*continued*)

free latissimus dorsi f.
free microsurgical f.
free scapular f.
free skin f.
gastrocnemius f.
Gilbert scapular f.
gluteus maximus f.
gracilis f.
f. graft
groin f.
hemipulp f.
horseshoe-shaped f.
hypogastric f.
iliac osteocutaneous f.
iliofemoral pedicle f.
intercostal f.
inverted skin f.
island adipofascial f.
island skin f.
Kutler double lateral advancement f.
Kutler V-Y f.
lateral arm f.
lateral thigh f.
lateral thoracic f.
latissimus dorsi f.
lazy-V de-epithelialized turn-over
  fasciocutaneous f.
Limberg pilonidal disease f.
local f.
long posterior f.
medialis pedis f.
medial plantar fasciocutaneous f.
f. meniscal tear
microvascular free muscle f.
Moberg advancement f.
Morrison neurovascular free f.
multistaged carrier f.
muscle f.
musculocutaneous free f.
musculotendinous f.
myocutaneous f.
neurocutaneous hand f.
neurovascular free f.
nutrient f.
omental f.
f. operation
osteocutaneous free f.
osteomusculocutaneous f.
osteoperiosteal f.
palmar advancement f.
palmar cross-finger f.
parascapular f.
pectoralis major f.
pedicle groin f.
peroneal island f.
plantar artery f.
plantar V-Y advancement f.
f. plasty

posterior f.
pulp f.
radial-based f.
radial forearm f.
random pattern f.
rectus abdominis f.
rectus femoris f.
remote pedicle f.
reverse cross-finger f.
reverse-flow f.
reverse forearm island f.
rhomboid f.
rotational f.
saphenous f.
scapular f.
Schrudde rotational f.
serratus anterior f.
single-lobed skin f.
skew f.
skin f.
sliding f.
soft tissue f.
Steichen digital neurovascular
  free f.
supramalleolar f.
sural island f.
temporalis fascia f.
tensor fasciae latae muscle f.
thenar f.
thoracoepigastric f.
TRAM f.
transposition f.
transverse rectus abdominis
  muscle f.
triangular advancement f.
turn-down tendon f.
Urbaniak neurovascular free f.
Urbaniak scapular f.
vascularized free f.
V-Y advancement f.
V-Y Kutler fingertip f.
webspace f.
wraparound neurovascular
  free f.

flapless amputation
4-flap Z-plasty
flare

foot f.
medial tibial f.
f. of condyle

flared spinal rod
FLASH

fast low-angle shot

FlashCast

Delta-Lite F.

flat

f. back deformity
f. bone
f. bone graft

f. chest
f. drill
f. flexible foot
f. foot
F. Foot insole
forefoot f. (FFF)
f. hand
f. metatarsal head
f. palpation
f. plate
f. plate radiography
f. retractor
f. splint
flat-back (*var. of* flatback)
flatback, flat-back
f. syndrome
flat-bottomed Kerrison rongeur
flat-cut
f.-c. arthrodesis
f.-c. technique
flat-foot (*var. of* flatfoot)
flatfoot, flat-foot
acquired f.
adult acquired f.
calcaneovalgus f.
congenital rocker-bottom f.
f. deformity
Durham procedure for f.
flaccid f.
f. gait
hypermobile f.
Kidner f.
neonatal f.
pediatric f.
peroneal spastic f.
physiologic f.
posttraumatic f.
pronated straight f.
rigid f.
rockerbottom f.
spastic f.
flat-hand (*var. of* flathand)
flathand, flat-hand
f. test
Flatt
F. driver
F. excision
F. finger-joint prosthesis
F. finger-thumb prosthesis
F. hand surgery technique
F. implant
F. recess
F. self-retaining screwdriver
F. tendon transfer
F. upper extremity congenital
anomaly classification
flattening of normal lordotic curve
F&L attenuating glove
flattop talus

flatware
Cushion Grip F.
Melaware f.
flava
flaval ligament
flavectomy
flavum
hypertrophied ligamentum f.
ligamentum f.
Flaxedil
fleck
f. fracture
f. sign
Fleischmann bursa
flesh
proud f.
flex
f. against gravity
F. Foam brace
F. Foam orthosis
Grafton DBM F.
F. H/A total ossicular prosthesis
F. Ranger stretch cable
F. Ranger stretch cable with
pulley
Flexall
Chiropractic Strength F. 454
F. gel
Flexaphen
Flexderm wound dressing
flexed position
Flexeril
Flex-Foam bandage
Flex-Foot Modular III prosthesis
flexibilitas
cerea f.
flexibility
f. conditioning program
Cotrel-Dubousset rod f.
f. exercise
f. training
flexible
f. bandage
f. burn dressing
f. clawtoe deformity
f. digital implant
f. hammertoe
f. hammertoe deformity
f. hinge implant
f. hinge suspension
f. intramedullary nail (FIN)
f. intramedullary nail guide
f. medullary nail
f. medullary reamer
f. nailing of the femoral
shaft
f. orthosis
f. pes planus
f. pes valgus

F

flexible (*continued*)
    f. socket
    f. sound
    f. talipes
Flexicair bed
Flexigrid dressing
Flexi-Grip exercise putty
Flexilite conforming elastic bandage
fleximeter
Flexinet dressing
flexing
flexion
    f., abduction, external rotation
      (faber)
    f., abduction, external rotation
      contracture
    f., abduction, external rotation,
      extension (fabere)
    f., abduction, external rotation,
      extension test
    f., abduction, internal rotation
      test
    active f.
    f., adduction, internal rotation (fadir)
    f., adduction, internal rotation,
      extension (fadire)
    f., adduction, internal rotation
      test
    f. and extension
    f. angle
    angle of greatest f. (AGF)
    f. axis
    back f.
    f. body cast
    f. body jacket
    f. bumper
    f. burst fracture
    cervical specific rotation in f.
    f. compression spine injury
     stabilization
    compressive f.
    f. creaking
    f. distraction
    distractive f.
    dorsiflexion f.
    elongation, derotation, f. (EDF)
    external rotation in f. (ERF)
    femoral trunk f.
    forced passive full forward f.
    forced plantar f.
    forward f.
    full fist f.
    further f.
    f. gap
    f. glove
    hip f.
    f. injury
    f. instability
    internal rotation in f. (IRF)

    knee f.
    lateral f.
    left lateral f.
    lumbar lateral f.
    lumbosacral f.
    f. malposition
    f. osteotomy
    palmar f.
    plantar f. (PF)
    resisted active f.
    f. restriction
    right lateral f.
    Riordan finger f.
    Schober test of lumbar f.
    shelf f.
    sitting f.
    f. spinal radiography test
    spine f.
    standing f.
    f. teardrop fracture
    toe f.
    transverse axis knee f.
    uninhibited f.
    f. valgus deformity
    volar f.
    volitional resisted f.
flexion-adduction
flexion-compression fracture
flexion-distraction
    f.-d. chiropractic table
    f.-d. fracture
    f.-d. injury
    f.-d. therapy
flexion-extension
    f.-e. arc
    f.-e. axis
    f.-e. control cervical orthosis
    f.-e. exercise
    f.-e. gap
    hip f.-e.
    f.-e. injury
    knee f.-e.
    f.-e. maneuver
    f.-e. MRI
    f.-e. plane
    f.-e. radiography
flexion-internal rotational deformity
flexion-rotation-compression
  maneuver
flexion-rotation-drawer (FRD)
    f.-r.-d. knee instability test
    f.-r.-d. test
Flexisplint flexed arm board
FlexiSport orthotic
FlexiTherm
    F. diabetic diagnostic insole
    F. Thermographic System
FlexLite hinged knee support
Flex-Master bandage

flexometer
    Moeltgen f.
flexor
    anterior long toe f.
    f. cap
    f. carpi radialis (FCR)
    f. carpi radialis muscle
    f. carpi radialis tendon
    f. carpi ulnaris (FCU)
    f. carpi ulnaris muscle
    f. carpi ulnaris syndrome
    f. carpi ulnaris tendinitis
    f. carpi ulnaris tendon
    f. digiti quinti muscle
    f. digitorum (FD)
    f. digitorum brevis (FDB)
    f. digitorum communis (FDC)
    f. digitorum communis tendon
    f. digitorum longus (FDL)
    f. digitorum longus muscle
    f. digitorum longus tendon
    f. digitorum longus tendon contracture
    f. digitorum longus tendon transfer
    f. digitorum profundus (FDP)
    f. digitorum profundus muscle
    f. digitorum profundus tendon
    f. digitorum quinti brevis (FDQB)
    f. digitorum slip
    f. digitorum sublimis (FDS)
    f. digitorum sublimis muscle
    f. digitorum sublimis tendon
    f. digitorum superficialis (FDS)
    f. digitorum superficialis muscle
    f. digitorum superficialis tendon
    extrinsic toe f.
    f. glove
    f. groove
    f. hallucis brevis (FHB)
    f. hallucis brevis flap
    f. hallucis brevis muscle
    f. hallucis brevis tendon
    f. hallucis longus (FHL)
    f. hallucis longus muscle
    f. hallucis longus release technique
    f. hallucis longus tendon
    f. hallucis longus tendon release
    f. hallucis longus tenosynovitis
    f. hallucis tendon contracture
    f. hinge hand-splint brace
    f. hinge orthosis
    f. hinge splint
    long toe f.
    f. mechanism
    f. origin syndrome
    f. phase
    f. plate
    f. plate release
    f. pollicis brevis (FPB)
    f. pollicis brevis muscle
    f. pollicis brevis tendon
    f. pollicis longus (FPL)
    f. pollicis longus abductorplasty
    f. pollicis longus muscle
    f. pollicis longus tendon
    f. profundus tendon
    f. pronator slide
    f. pronator syndrome test
    f. retinaculum
    f. retinaculum of hand
    f. skin crease
    snapping thumb f.
    f. sublimis tendon
    f. tendon anastomosis
    f. tendon graft
    f. tendon laceration
    f. tendon repair
    f. tendon rupture
    f. tendon sheath
    f. tenolysis
    f. tenosynovectomy
    f. tenotomy
    toe f.
    f. wad
    f. wad of 5 muscles
    f. withdrawal reflex
flexorplasty
    Bunnell modification of Steindler f.
    Eyler f.
    Steindler elbow f.
flexor-pronator
    f.-p. origin
    f.-p. origin release
flexor-to-extensor tendon transfer
FlexPosure endoscopic retractor
Flex-Sprint prosthesis
FlexStrand cable
FlexTech knee brace
Flextender Plus hand exerciser
flexural concavity
flexure
    perineal f.
flexus
    hallux f.
Flex-Walk
    F.-W. II prosthesis
    F.-W. II prosthetic foot
    F.-W. prosthesis
Flexzan foam wound dressing
Flip-Flop pillow
flipped meniscus sign
flipper hand
flip test
F2L Multineck femoral stem
Floam ankle stirrup brace

F

floating
- f. arch fracture
- f. cartilage
- f. clavicle
- f. elbow
- f. gait
- f. knee
- f. knee fracture classification
- f. ligament
- f. patella
- f. rib
- f. shoulder
- f. thumb
- f. time
- f. toe
- f. traction

floccosum
- *Epidermophyton f.*

flocculent
- f. focus
- f. focus of calcification

Flo-Fit Comfortseat
floor
- f. mat
- f. of acetabulum
- f. sitter

floor-reaction ankle-foot orthosis
floppy
- f. infant
- f. infant syndrome
- f. toe

flora
- bacterial f.

Floralax
Florical
florid
- f. callus
- f. reactive periostitis
- f. rickets
- f. synovitis

Florida
- F. back brace
- F. cervical brace
- F. contraflexion brace
- F. extension brace
- F. hyperextension brace
- F. J-24, J-35, J-45, J-55 brace
- F. post-fusion brace
- F. spinal brace

Flo-Tech prosthetic socket
Flo-Trol drinking cup
flottant
- pouce f.

flounce
- meniscal f.

flow
- blood f.
- epidural dye f.
- f. meter

flower-spray ending
flowing hyperostosis
flow-mediated
- f.-m. dilation (FMD)
- f.-m. vasodilation (FMV)

flowmeter, flow meter
- Doppler ultrasound f.

flowmetry
- laser Doppler f. (LDF)

Flowtron
- F. DVT
- F. pneumatic compression system
- BioCryo system

FLP
- Functional Limitation Profile

fluctuation test
flucytosine
fluff dressing
Fluftex gauze roll
fluid
- f. absorption ability
- f. attenuation inversion recovery (FLAIR)
- f. balance
- f. barrier boot
- bursal f.
- cerebrospinal f. (CSF)
- f. controlled component
- egress of arthroscopic f.
- f. homeostasis
- hypotonic f.
- interstitial f.
- f. overhydration
- f. prosthesis
- f. sign
- synovial f.

FluidAir bed
fluid-fluid
- f.-f. level
- f.-f. level sign

Fluidotherapy sterile dry heat modality
fluocinolone acetonide
fluorescein
- f. perfusion monitoring
- f. study

fluorescence correlation spectroscopy (FCS)
Fluori-Methane topical spray
fluormethane
fluorometholone
FluoroNav
- StealthStation with F.
- F. virtual fluoroscopy system

fluoroquinolone
fluoroquinolone-associated Achilles tendon disorder
FluoroScan imaging system

fluoroscope
  C-arm f.
  Siremobil Iso-C3D f.
  XiScan f.
fluoroscopic
  f. control
  f. discectomy
  f. table
fluoroscopy
  C-arm f.
  computer-assisted f.
  electric joint f.
  intraoperative f.
  2-plane f.
  portable C-arm image intensifier f.
  spinal f.
  XiScan f.
flurazepam
flurbiprofen
flush
  heparinized saline f.
  peroxide f.
fluted
  f. medullary rod
  f. reamer
  f. Sampson nail
  f. titanium nail
flute of cannulated screw
Flutex Topical
Flynn
  F. femoral neck fracture reduction
  F. technique
FMC
  first metatarsal contact
  FMC gait-related risk factor
FMD
  fibromuscular disease
  flow-mediated dilation
FMH
  1st metatarsal head
FMP acetabular system
fMRI
  functional magnetic resonance imaging
FMS
  fibromyalgia syndrome
  FMS Intracell stick
FMV
  flow-mediated vasodilation
FNB
  femoral nerve block
FNF
  femoral neck fracture
FNS
  functional neuromuscular stimulation
FNST
  femoral nerve stretch test
FNT
  finger-to-nose test

foam
  f. casting
  f. collar
  f. compression molded ethylene vinyl acetate foam
  copolymer f.
  crosslinked EVA copolymer f.
  f. cushion
  Evazote f.
  gelatin f.
  high-density f.
  Neoplush f.
  f. pad
  Pedilen polyurethane f.
  f. pillow
  Plastazote f.
  polyethylene f.
  prosthetic f.
  f. ring
  f. slant
  soft copolymer f.
  f. tape
  Temper F.
  tube f.
  f. tubing
  f. wound dressing
Foamart foot impression system
FoamWrap
  F. BuddyWrap
  F. Final Flexion wrap
  F. finger sling
  F. finger trapper
  F. ThumDuction strap
  F. ThumWrap
focal
  f. back pain
  f. calcification
  f. deficiency
  f. dystonia
  f. fibrocartilaginous dysplasia
  f. film distance
  f. nodular myositis
  f. pigmented villonodular synovitis
  f. scleroderma
foci (*pl. of* focus)
focus, *pl.* **foci**
  flocculent f.
Foerster forceps
fold
  asymmetric skin f.
  Bartlett nail f.
  cutaneous f.
  nail f.
  synovial f.
folding
  f. fracture
  f. frame wheelchair
fold-over finger splint
Folex PFS

F

folic acid
folliculitis
fomentation therapy
Fomon
    F. chisel
    F. periosteal elevator
    F. periosteotome
    F. rasp
FONAR
    field focusing nuclear magnetic
    resonance
    FONAR Stand-Up MRI
fondaparinux sodium
Fontan
    F. operation
    F. physiology
Fontan-type procedure
FOOSH
    fell on outstretched hand
    FOOSH injury
foot, *pl.* feet
    adolescent rigid f.
    Aftate for Athlete's F.
    f. alignment
    f. and ankle severity scale
    (FASS)
    f. anesthetic
    f. angle
    f. architecture
    arch of f.
    articulation of f.
    artificial f.
    atavistic f.
    athlete's f.
    ball of f.
    basketball f.
    Beachcomber prosthetic f.
    bifid f.
    broad f.
    burning f.
    calcaneocavus f.
    calcaneovalgus f.
    Carbon Copy II Light F.
    cavovarus f.
    cavus f.
    f. central compartment pressure
    measurement
    Charcot f.
    Cirrus composite prosthetic f.
    clavus f.
    claw f.
    cleft f.
    f. collapse
    College Park TruStep f.
    ComfortWalk prosthetic f.
    composite prosthetic f.
    contracted f.
    contralateral f.
    f. cosmesis

cosmetically acceptable f.
C-shaped f.
f. cushion
C-Walk foot 1C40 prosthetic f.
dancer's f.
dangling f.
f. decompression
deconditioned f.
f. deformity
diabetic f.
diabetic Charcot f.
digital artery of f.
ding f.
diplegic f.
disfigured f.
Doctor Scholl's Athlete's F.
f. drape
drop f.
f. drop strap
Dycor prosthetic f.
f. dynamics
f. dysplasia
Egyptian f.
Eichenholz Classification of Charcot
    arthropathy of f. (stage 1-3)
equinocavus f.
equinovalgus f.
equinovarus f.
equinus f.
f. first-web flap
flail f.
f. flare
flat f.
flat flexible f.
Flex-Walk II prosthetic f.
forced f.
Friedreich f.
functional disability of f.
f. function index (FFI)
F. Function Index questionnaire
Greek f.
Hardy-Clapham classification of
    sesamoid bones of f.
F. Health Status Questionnaire
hemiplegic f.
hollow f.
hooked f.
F. Hugger foot support
hypermobile f.
hypoflexibility of f.
immersion f.
f. imprinter
inferior extensor of f.
insensate f.
f. ischemia
ischemic f.
Kingsley Steplite f.
lateral spring ligament of f.
F. Levelers custom orthotic

F. Levelers orthosis
F. Levelers sandalthotics
f. lift-off
lobster-claw f.
Lo Rider prosthetic f.
low-arch f.
Madura f.
f. magnet
malodorous f.
march f.
f. model
Morand f.
Morton f.
mossy f.
multiaxis f.
neuroarthropathic f.
neuropathic f.
f. orthosis
f. orthotic management
Otto Bock 1A30 Greissinger
 Plus f.
Otto Bock 1D25 Dynamic Plus f.
paralytic f.
parrot f.
Pathfinder prosthetic f.
Persian slipper f.
f. pillow
f. placement test
planovalgus f.
plantar f.
plantigrade f.
f. plate
polydactylous cleft f.
f. progression angle (FPA)
pronated f.
pronation of f.
f. prosthesis
prosthetic f.
f. puncture wound
Quantum f.
reel f.
Re-Flex VSP artificial f.
f. rest
rheumatoid f.
rigid f.
rockerbottom f.
f. rotation
SACH f.
SAFE f.
F. screw system
serpentine f.
shortened f.
single-axis Syme Dycor f.
skew f.
f. slap
f. sling
sole of f.
solid ankle cushioned heel f.
spatula f.

split f.
f. sprain
spread f.
S-shaped f.
f. stabilization
f. stabilizer
f. stagnation
stairclimber's f.
stationary ankle flexible
 endoskeleton f.
f. stool
f. strain
f. stump
superior extensor retinaculum
 of f.
supination of f.
Sure-Flex III prosthetic f.
Syme Dycor prosthetic f.
tabetic f.
taut f.
trench f.
tripod f.
Trowbridge Terra-Round
 accessory f.
f. type
valgus f.
Vari-Flex prosthetic f.
f. volumeter
weak f.
Z f.
foot-ankle
 f.-a. assembly
 f.-a. brace
 f.-a. complex
football
 f. calf
 f. finger
 f. player's shoulders
footballer's
 f. ankle
 f. groin
 f. hernia
footbed
 Velocor f.
Footbrush
 Doctor Joseph's Original F.
footdrop
 f. brace
 f. gait
 f. night splint
Foot-Fitter
FootFlex performance stretching device
footgear
Footmaster orthotic
footpiece
 Bunker f.
 traction f.
foot-plate (*var. of* footplate)
footplate, foot-plate, foot plate

F

footprint
    f. analysis
    dynamic f.
    femoral f.
    Harris-Beath f.
    f. index
    f. mat
    static f.
    tibial f.
footrest
Foot-Station 3-D foot imaging system
foot-strike
    f.-s. hemolysis
    f.-s. hemolysis anemia
    f.-s. phase
    f.-s. phase of gait
foot-thigh axis
footwear
    Ambulator biomechanical f.
    Ambulator conform f.
    AquaRunners resistance f.
    Aravon f.
    Comfort Rite f.
    F. Integration Technology (FIT)
    Milano Shoethotic f.
    Mobils Professionals pedorthic f.
forage
    f. biopsy
    f. core decompression biopsy
      procedure
foramen, *pl.* **foramina**
    arcuate f.
    Hartigan f.
    intravertebral f.
    ischiopubic f.
    f. magnum
    f. magnum decompression
    neural f.
    open exit f.
    sciatic f.
    f. transversarium
    Weitbrecht f.
foramina (*pl. of* foramen)
foraminal
    f. compression test
    f. encroachment subluxation
    f. osteophyte encroachment
    f. stenosis
foraminoplasty
    laminaplasty with extended f.
foraminotomy
    microsurgical anterior cervical f.
    neural f.
Forbes
    F. modification of Phemister graft
      technique
    F. onlay bone graft
force
    activation f.

    f. application
    contact f.
    distraction f.
    distractive f.
    dynamic joint f.
    evertor f.
    f. feedback
    forefoot f.
    f. gauge
    gravity ground reaction f.
    ground reaction f.
    hamstring f.
    invertor f.
    isometric f.
    joint f.
    knee f.
    lateral compression f.
    moment of f.
    muscle f.
    Newton f.
    f. nucleus
    patellofemoral joint reaction f.
    f. plate
    f. plate foot analysis
    f. platform
    prehension f.
    reaction f.
    shearing f.
    subthreshold f.
    tensile f.
    tension f.
    torque f.
    f. transducer
    translatory f.
    vertical ground reaction f. (VGRF)
    weightbearing ground reaction f.
forcé
    brisement f.
    redressement f.
force-couple splint reduction
forced
    f. adduction test
    f. flexion injury
    f. foot
    f. passive full forward flexion
    f. passive internal rotation
    f. plantar flexion
    f. vital capacity
forceps
    Acland clamp-applying f.
    Acufex curved basket f.
    Acufex rotary biting basket f.
    Adson clip-introducing f.
    Adson drill guide f.
    Adson hypophysial f.
    adventitial f.
    Aesculap bipolar cautery f.
    alligator bone-reduction f.
    alligator grasping f.

Allis tissue f.
Angell James hypophysectomy f.
angled-down f.
angled-up f.
anterior f.
AO reduction f.
arthroscopy basket f.
arthroscopy grasping f.
Asch f.
atraumatic f.
Babcock f.
baby Lane f.
Backhaus towel f.
Baer bone-cutting f.
Bane rongeur f.
Bardeleben bone-holding f.
basket f.
bearing-seating f.
Beasley-Babcock f.
biarticular bone-cutting f.
biopsy f.
bipolar f.
Bircher-Ganske cartilage f.
blunt f.
Boies f.
bone-biting f.
bone-breaking f.
bone-cutting f.
bone-grasping f.
bone-holding f.
bone punch f.
bone-splitting f.
Brand tendon-holding f.
Brand tendon-passing f.
Brown-Adson f.
Brown-Cushing f.
Brown tissue f.
bulldog clamp-applying f.
Cairns hemostatic f.
Carroll bone-holding f.
Carroll dressing f.
Carroll tendon-pulling f.
Carroll tissue f.
cartilage f.
Caspar alligator f.
cervical punch f.
Chandler spinal perforating f.
Charnley wire-holding f.
Citelli punch f.
clamp f.
Cleveland bone-cutting f.
clip-applying f.
clip-bending f.
clip-cutting f.
clip-introducing f.
coagulating f.
Crile f.
crocodile f.
cupped grasping f.

curved basket f.
cutting f.
Dawson-Yuhl-Kerrison rongeur f.
Dawson-Yuhl-Leksell rongeur f.
Dawson-Yuhl rongeur f.
Dingman bone-holding f.
disc f.
double-action bone-cutting f.
double-sharp f.
Dreyfus prosthesis f.
drill guide f.
eagle beak bone-cutting f.
Echlin rongeur f.
3-edge cutting f.
end-biting f.
ethmoid f.
extracting f.
Farabeuf bone-holding f.
Farabeuf-Lambotte bone-holding f.
Farrior wire-crimping f.
Ferguson bone-holding f.
Fergusson f.
Ferris-Smith bone-biting f.
Ferris-Smith-Kerrison f.
Ferris-Smith rongeur f.
Ferris-Smith tissue f.
Foerster f.
Friedman rongeur f.
gall duct f.
Gardner bone f.
glenoid-reaming f.
grasping f.
Greene f.
Gunderson bone f.
Gunderson muscle f.
Hajek-Koffler bone punch f.
Halsted f.
Harrington clamp f.
Harrison bone-holding f.
Hartmann mosquito f.
Heermann alligator f.
hemostatic f.
Hibbs bone-cutting f.
Hinderer cartilage f.
Hirsch hypophysis punch f.
Hoen f.
Horsley bone-cutting f.
Horsley-Stille bone-cutting f.
Horsley-Stille rib shears f.
Howmedica Microfixation System f.
Hudson f.
Hurd bone-cutting f.
implant f.
Jackson broad-blade staple f.
Jackson dressing f.
Jackson tendon-seizing f.
Jacobson mosquito f.
James wound f.
Jansen monopolar f.

F

forceps (*continued*)
    Jarell f.
    Jarit tendon-pulling f.
    jeweler's f.
    Juers-Lempert rongeur f.
    Kelly f.
    Kern bone-holding f.
    Kern-Lane bone f.
    King wound f.
    Kleinert-Kutz bone-cutting f.
    Kleinert-Kutz rongeur f.
    Kleinert-Kutz tendon f.
    Knight bone-cutting f.
    knotting f.
    Kocher f.
    Lalonde hook f.
    Lambotte bone-holding f.
    Landolt spreading f.
    Lane bone-holding f.
    Lane screw-holding f.
    Lane self-retaining bone-holding f.
    Langenbeck bone-holding f.
    Larsen tendon-holding f.
    Leibinger Micro System
      plate-holding f.
    Leksell rongeur f.
    Lempert rongeur f.
    LeRoy clip-applying f.
    Lester muscle f.
    Lewin f.
    Lewin bone-holding f.
    Lewin spinal perforating f.
    lion f.
    lion-jaw f.
    Liston bone-cutting f.
    Liston-Key bone-cutting f.
    Liston-Littauer bone-cutting f.
    Liston-Stille bone-cutting f.
    Littauer-Liston bone-cutting f.
    Llorente dissecting f.
    long-jaw basket f.
    Lore suction tube and tip-holding f.
    Love-Gruenwald alligator f.
    Love-Kerrison rongeur f.
    Lowman bone-holding f.
    Luer rongeur f.
    Luer-Whiting rongeur f.
    Luhr Microfixation System
      plate-holding f.
    Malis-Jensen microbipolar f.
    Malis jeweler bipolar f.
    Mantis retrograde f.
    Markwalder rib f.
    Martin cartilage f.
    Mayfield f.
    McGee-Priest wire f.
    McGee wire-crimping f.
    McIndoe rongeur f.
    meniscus f.

    MicroBite f.
    Micro-One dissecting f.
    Micro-Two f.
    Mixter f.
    mosquito f.
    mosquito-tip grasping f.
    nail-pulling f.
    Nicola f.
    Niro bone-cutting f.
    Niro wire-twisting f.
    Olivecrona clip-applying and
      removing f.
    orthopaedic f.
    Overholt clip-applying f.
    perforating f.
    Perman cartilage f.
    pick-up f.
    pin-seating f.
    plain tissue f.
    plate-holding f.
    Poppen f.
    Potts-Smith dressing f.
    Preston ligamentum flavum f.
    punch f.
    Raimondi hemostatic f.
    rat-tooth f.
    reduction f.
    rib f.
    Riches artery f.
    ring f.
    Rochester-Carmalt f.
    Rochester-Ochsner f.
    Rochester-Pean f.
    rongeur f.
    rotary basket f.
    Rowe disimpaction f.
    Rowe glenoid-reaming f.
    Rowe-Harrison bone-holding f.
    Rowe modified-Harrison f.
    Ruskin bone-cutting f.
    Ruskin bone-splitting f.
    Ruskin-Liston bone-cutting f.
    Ruskin rongeur f.
    Ruskin-Rowland bone-cutting f.
    Russian f.
    Samuels f.
    Sauerbruch rib f.
    Schlesinger cervical punch f.
    Schlesinger rongeur f.
    Schwartz clip-applying f.
    Schwartz temporary
      clamp-applying f.
    screw-holding f.
    Seaber f.
    seizing f.
    self-centering bone-holding f.
    self-retaining bone-holding f.
    Selverstone rongeur f.
    Semb bone f.

Semb rib f.
septal f.
sequestrum f.
Shutt Mantis retrograde f.
side-cutting basket f.
small plate f.
Smithwick clip-applying f.
smooth-tipped jeweler's f.
spatula f.
Spence rongeur f.
sponge-holding f.
spreading f.
Spurling-Kerrison rongeur f.
Steinmann tendon f.
Stille-Horsley bone f.
Stille-Horsley rib f.
Stille-Liston bone-cutting f.
Stille-Luer rongeur f.
Stiwer bone-holding f.
straight basket f.
Synthes Microsystems
  plate-holding f.
tack-and-pin f.
Take-apart f.
taper-jaw f.
tenaculum-reducing f.
tendon f.
tendon-braiding f.
tendon-holding f.
tendon-passing f.
tendon-pulling f.
tendon-retrieving f.
tendon-seizing f.
tendon-tunneling f.
Thompson hip prosthesis f.
thumb f.
tissue f.
titanium microsurgical bipolar f.
Toennis tumor f.
toothed tissue f.
Tudor-Edwards bone-cutting f.
tumor-grasping f.
tying f.
Ulrich bone-holding f.
Ulrich-St. Gallen f.
universal bone grafting/impacting f.
upbiting basket f.
upcurved punch f.
Utrata f.
van Buren sequestrum f.
vascular f.
Verbrugge bone-holding f.
Walton-Liston f.
Walton wire-pulling f.
Weller cartilage f.
Wiet cup f.
Wilde ethmoid f.
Wilde rongeur f.
wire-cutting f.

wire-extracting f.
wire-holding f.
wire prosthesis-crimping f.
wire-pulling f.
wire-tightening f.
wire-twisting f.
X-long cement f.
Zimmer-Hoen f.
Zimmer-Schlesinger f.

force-time integral
Ford triangulation technique
forearm
  f. amputation
  balanced f.
  1-bone f.
  3-bone f.
  carrying angle of f.
  f. compartment syndrome
  f. complex
  f. contracture
  distal f.
  f. flap
  f. fracture
  f. ischemic exercise
  f. lift assist adjustable spring-loaded
    device
  f. lift assist prosthesis
  f. splint
  f. stabilizer
  f. supination test
  f. tourniquet
forefoot
  f. abduction deformity
  f. abductus
  f. adduction correction test
  f. adductovarus
  f. adductus
  f. angulation
  f. arthroplasty
  f. block test
  f. cavus
  f. compression sleeve
  f. digital amputation
  f. disruption
  f. equinus
  f. flat (FFF)
  f. force
  f. FPA
  hooked f.
  Larmon f.
  narrowing of f.
  f. nerve block
  f. peak pressure
  f. sleeve
  f. splaying
  f. striker
  f. valgus
  f. varus
forefoot-to-rearfoot striker

F

foreign
    f. body
    f. body granuloma
    f. body of synovitis
    f. body reaction
    f. body response
    f. body screw
forequarter amputation
Forestier
    F. bowstring sign
    F. disease
forged cobalt-chromium alloy prosthesis
fork
    f. strap
    f. strap prosthetic support
form
    f. constancy
    IKDC f.
    International Knee Documentation
      Committee f.
    International Knee Documentation
      Committee Subjective Knee F.
    Jettmobile positioning and tumble f.
    warm and f.
formal hemipelvectomy
formation
    adhesion f.
    beaklike osteophyte f.
    bone f.
    bunion f.
    callous f.
    capsule f.
    Chiari f.
    clavus f.
    cleft f.
    coalition f.
    cyclops f.
    gouty tophus f.
    intramembranous f.
    lappet f.
    new bone f.
    osteomyelitic cloaca f.
    osteophyte f.
    periosteal new bone f.
    Pfitzner theory of coalition f.
    pincer nail f.
    procallus f.
    reactive bone f.
    rouleaux f.
    scar f.
    spur f.
    subperiosteal new bone f.
    tophus f.
    trellis f.
Formatray mandibular splint
forme
    f. fruste
    f. of neurofibromatosis
formes (*pl. of* forme)

formula, *pl.* **formulae, formulas**
    Arth-Aid Joint F.
    Arth-Support F.
    Bayer Select Pain Relief F.
    Bjure spinal deformity f.
    Boyd f.
    digital f.
    pediatric nutritional f.
    Resistance Support F.
    vertebral f.
formulae (*pl. of* formula)
formulas (*pl. of* formula)
Forrester
    F. cervical collar brace
    F. splint
Forrester-Brown collar
Fortaz
Forte
    Aristocort F.
    Citanest F.
    F. ES
    F. harness
    Intenzyme F.
    Norgesic F.
    Parafon F.
    Triam F.
Fortin finger low back pain test
fortitude
    F. Ti titanium spinal fixation
      product
    F. Vue titanium spinal fixation
      product
fortuitum
    Mycobacterium f.
forward
    f. bending
    f. flexion
    f. flexion posture
    f. head posture
forward-cutting knife
FOS
    fructooligosaccharides
Fosamax
Fosnaugh nail biopsy
fossa, *pl.* **fossae**
    acetabular f.
    antecubital f.
    bony f.
    femoral f.
    glenoid f.
    intercondylar f.
    ischiorectal f.
    Jobert f.
    lower f. active, lateral knee pain,
      long leg on side ipsilateral to
      weak f. (LLL)
    Mohrenheim f.
    olecranon f.
    patellar f.

popliteal f.
sphenoid f.
supinator f.
supraclavicular f.
upper f. active, medial knee pain, and short leg on side ipsilateral to weak f. (UMS)

fossae (*pl. of* fossa)
Foster
F. bed
F. splint
F. turning frame

Foster-Kennedy
F.-K. frame
F.-K. maneuver

Foucher
F. classification of digital amputation
F. distal digital amputation classification
F. metacarpal synostosis classification

fouet
foulage
foundation
Arthritis F.
F. for Chiropractic Education and Research (FCER)
level f.
Musculoskeletal Transplant F. (MTF)
National Headache F.
National Osteoporosis F.
Osteogenesis Imperfecta F. (OIF)
F. total knee and hip system

fourchée
main f.

Fourier transform infrared spectroscopy
fourth
f. metacarpal
f. metatarsophalangeal joint
f. turbinated bone

fovea, *pl.* **foveae**
f. capitis femoris
f. centralis of bone
f. centralis of femur

foveae (*pl. of* fovea)
foveal fat-pad
foveate, foveated
foveated (*var. of* foveate)
f. chest

foveation
Fowler
F. central slip tenotomy
F. dynamic hand tenodesis
F. foot arch prosthesis test
F. knee system
F. maneuver
F. osteotomy
F. position

F. procedure
F. spread
F. technique
F. tendon transfer

Fowler-Philip
F.-P. back of heel angle
F.-P. incision
F.-P. retrocalcaneal exostosis approach

Fowles
F. dislocation technique
F. open elbow reduction

fox
F. clavicular splint
F. extractor-impactor
F. impactor-extractor
F. internal fixation apparatus
F. internal fixation device
F. wrench

FPA
foot progression angle
forefoot FPA
hindfoot FPA

FPB
flexor pollicis brevis

FPL
flexor pollicis longus

FPMA
first plantar metatarsal artery

FP5000 pump system
F.R.
F.R. Thompson endoprosthesis
F.R. Thompson femoral prosthesis

fraction
linear f.
motor unit f.

fractional
f. curve
f. lengthening

fractionation
Fractomed splint
fracture
abduction-external rotation f.
accessory navicular f.
accessory ossicle f.
acetabular posterior wall f.
acetabular rim f.
acute avulsion f.
adduction f.
agenetic f.
AIIS avulsion f.
Aitken classification of epiphysial f.
Allen open reduction of calcaneal f.
alveolar bone f.
anatomic neck f.
Anderson-Hutchins unstable tibial shaft f.
angulated f.
ankle mortise f.

F

fracture (*continued*)
    anterior calcaneal process f.
    anterior column f.
    anterior wedge compression f.
    anterolateral compression f.
    AO classification of ankle f.
    apical non-load-bearing bone f.
    apophysial f.
    arch f.
    articular mass separation f.
    articular pillar f.
    Atkin epiphysial f.
    atlas f.
    atraumatic f.
    atrophic f.
    avulsion chip f.
    avulsion stress f.
    axial load teardrop f.
    backfire f.
    Bankart f.
    Barton f.
    basal neck f.
    baseball finger f.
    basilar femoral neck f.
    basocervical f.
    bayonet position of f.
    beak f.
    f. bed
    bedroom f.
    bend f.
    bending f.
    Bennett f.
    Berndt-Harty classification of
      transchondral f.
    bicolumn f.
    bicondylar T-shaped f.
    bicondylar Y-shaped f.
    bicycle spoke f.
    bimalleolar ankle f.'s
    bipartite f.
    birth f.
    f. blister
    blow-in f.
    blow-out f.
    bone shaft f.
    f. boot
    boot-top f.
    Bosworth f.
    both-bone f.
    both-column f.
    bowing f.
    f. box
    boxer's f.
    f. bracing
    Broberg-Morrey f.
    bucket-handle f.
    buckle f.
    bumper f.
    bunk bed f.

    Burkhalter-Reyes fixation method for
      phalangeal f.
    burst f.
    butterfly f.
    buttonhole f.
    f. by contrecoup
    calcaneal f.
    calcaneal avulsion f.
    calcaneal displaced f.
    calcaneal f. (I-III)
    calcaneus tongue f.
    f. callus
    f. callus loading
    Canale-Kelly talar neck f.
    cancellous non-load-bearing bone f.
    capillary f.
    capitellar f.
    capitulum f.
    carpal bone stress f.
    carpal navicular f.
    carpal scaphoid bone f.
    carpometacarpal joint f.
    cartwheel f.
    Cedell f.
    Cedell posterior process of talus f.
    cemental f.
    central talus f.
    cephalomedullary nail f.
    cervical ortrochanteric displaced
      hip f.
    cervical ortrochanteric hip f.
    chalk-stick f.
    Chance vertebral f.
    Chaput f.
    chip f.
    chisel f.
    chondral f.
    circumferential f.
    f. classification
    clavicular birth f.
    clay shoveler's f.
    cleavage f.
    closed ankle f.
    closed indirect f.
    closed reduction of f.
    cloven-hoof f.
    coccyx f.
    Colles f.
    collicular f.
    Coltart f.
    combined flexion-distraction injury
      and burst f.
    combined radial-ulnar-humeral f.'s
    comminuted f.
    comminuted burst f.
    comminuted intraarticular f.
    comminuted pilon f.
    comminuted teardrop f.
    complete f.

complex f.
complicated f.
composite f.
compound comminuted f. (CCF)
compression f.
condylar compression f.
condylar femoral f.
condylar split f.
congenital f.
contralateral double vertical f.
contrecoup f.
controlled comminuted f.
coracoid f.
corner f.
coronal split f.
coronoid process f.
cortical f.
Cotton ankle f.
cough f.
crack f.
craniofacial dysjunction f.
crush f.
crushed eggshell f.
cuboid f.
cuneiform f.
curbstone f.
dancer's 5th metatarsal f.
Danis-Weber classification of
  malleolar f.
dashboard f.
f. decompression
f. deformity
delayed healing bone f.
dens f.
dentate f.
depressed f.
de Quervain f.
derby hat f.
Desault f.
Descot f.
diacondylar f.
diametric pelvic f.
diaphysial f.
diastatic f.
dicondylar f.
die punch f.
direct f.
dishpan f.
dislocation f.
f. dislocation
displaced intraarticular f.
displaced pilon f.
distal femoral epiphysial f.
distal humeral f.
distal radial f.
distraction of f.
dogleg f.
dome f.
dorsal wing f.

double f.
drill bit f.
Dupuytren f.
Duverney f.
dyscrasic f.
eggshell f.
elbow f.
elementary f.
elephant-foot f.
Ellis technique for Barton f.
f. en coin
Ender rod fixation of f.
endocrine f.
f. en rave
epicondylar avulsion f.
epiphysial growth plate f.
epiphysial slip f.
epiphysial tibial f.
Essex-Lopresti fixation of
  calcaneal f.
Essex-Lopresti joint depression-type
  calcaneal f.
Essex-Lopresti tongue type
  calcaneal f.
explosion f.
extraarticular f.
extracapsular f.
extraoctave f.
facet f.
fatigue f.
femoral intratrochanteric f.
femoral neck f. (FNF)
femoral shaft f.
femoral stress f.
femoral supracondylar f.
fender f.
f. fever
fibular diaphysial f.
fighter's f.
first carpometacarpal joint f.
fissured f.
f. fixation
f. fixation device
flake hamate f.
fleck f.
flexion burst f.
flexion-compression f.
flexion-distraction f.
flexion teardrop f.
floating arch f.
folding f.
forearm f.
fragility f.
f. fragment
f. fragment displacement
f. fragment distraction
f. fragment nonunion
f. fragment separation
f. frame

F

fracture (*continued*)

Freiberg f.
fresh f.
Frykman radial f.
fulcrum f.
Gaenslen f.
Gaenslen spike fixation of fresh neck of femur f.
Galeazzi f.
f. gap
Garden femoral neck f.
glenoid f.
glenoid rim f.
Gosselin f.
graft f.
greater trochanteric femoral f.
greenstick f.
grenade thrower's f.
gross f.
growing f.
growth plate f.
Guérin f.
gunshot f.
Gustilo-Anderson open clavicular f.
Gustilo open femur f. (GI, GII, GIIIA, GIIIB, GIIIC)
Gustilo tibial f.
Hahn-Steinthal f.
hairline f.
hamate tail f.
hangman's f.
Hansen-Winquest femoral diaphysial f. (1–4)
Hawkins talus f. (I-IV)
head f.
head-splitting humeral f.
healed f.
f. healing
heat f.
hemicondylar f.
Henderson f.
Herbert scaphoid bone f.
Hermodsson f.
hickory-stick f.
high-energy f.
high-energy metaphysial distal tibia f.
Hill-Sachs f.
hip avulsion f.
hockey-stick f.
Hoffa intercondylar femoral f.
Holstein-Lewis f.
hoop stress f.
horizontal f.
humeral head-splitting f.
humeral physial f.
humeral shaft f.
humeral supracondylar f.

Hutchinson f.
hyperextension teardrop f.
hyperflexion teardrop f.
ice skater's f.
idiopathic f.
impacted articular f.
impacted valgus f.
impaction f.
implant f.
impression f.
incomplete f.
indirect f.
inflammatory f.
infraction f.
infratectal transverse f.
insufficiency f.
interarticular f.
intercondylar femoral f.
intercondylar humeral f.
intercondylar tibial f.
internally fixed f.
interperiosteal f.
intertrochanteric f. (ITFx)
intertrochanteric femoral f.
intertrochanteric 4-part f.
F. Intervention Trial (FIT)
intraarticular calcaneal f.
intraarticular proximal tibial f.
intracapsular f.
intraoperative f.
intraperiosteal f.
inverted-Y f.
ipsilateral femoral neck f.
ipsilateral femoral shaft f.
irreducible f.
ischioacetabular f.
Jefferson cervical burst f.
Jeffrey radial head f. (type I–II)
joint depression f.
Jones f.
junctional f.
juvenile Tillaux f.
juxtaarticular f.
juxtacortical f.
juxtatectal transverse f.
Kapandji f.
knee f.
Kocher f.
Kocher-Lorenz capitellum f.
Köhler f.
laminar f.
lap seatbelt f.
lateral column calcaneal f.
lateral humeral condyle f.
laterally displaced f.
lateral malleolus f.
lateral mass f.
lateral talar process f.
lateral tibial plateau f.

lateral wedge f.
Lauge-Hansen stage II
  supination-eversion f.
Laugier f.
lead-pipe f.
Le Fort fibular f.
Le Fort (I-III) f.
Le Fort mandible f.
Le Fort-Wagstaffe f.
lesser trochanter f.
f. line
linear f.
f. line consolidation
Lisfranc f.
Lloyd-Roberts f.
local compression f.
local decompression f.
long-bone f.
longitudinal f.
long oblique f.
loose f.
Looser zone in insufficiency f.
lorry driver's f.
low-energy f.
low lumbar spine f.
low T humerus f.
lumbar spine burst f.
lumbosacral junction f.
lunate f.
Maisonneuve fibular f.
malar f.
Malgaigne pelvic f.
malleolar chip f.
mallet f.
f. malreduction
malunited calcaneus f.
malunited forearm f.
malunited radial f.
f. management
mandibular f.
march f.
marginal f.
Marmor-Lynn f.
Mason f.
maxillary f.
f. mechanics
f. mechanism
medial column calcaneal f.
medial epicondyle humeral f.
medial malleolar f.
medial wall f.
metacarpal neck f.
metaphysial tibial f.
metatarsal f.
middle tibial shaft f.
midface f.
midfacial f.
midfoot f.
midnight f.

midshaft f.
minimally displaced f.
mini-pilon f.
missed f.
monomalleolar ankle f.
Monteggia forearm f.
Montercaux f.
Moore f.
Mouchet f.
multangular ridge f.
multilevel f.
multipartite f.
multiple f.'s
multiray f.
nasoethmoid f.
navicular dorsal lip f.
navicular tuberosity f.
naviculocapitate f.
neck f.
Neer-Horowitz classification of
  humeral f.
neoplastic f.
neurogenic f.
neuropathic f.
neurotrophic f.
Newman radial f.
nightstick f.
night-walker f.
nonarticular distal radial f.
noncontiguous f.
nondisplaced f.
nonloadbearing bone f.
nonphysial f.
nonrotational burst f.
nonunion horse-hoof f.
nonunion long-bone f.
nonunion torsion wedge f.
nonunited f.
nutcracker f.
oblique f.
obliquity f.
obturator avulsion f.
occipital condyle f.
occult f.
occult sacral f.
odontoid condyle f.
f. of fifth metacarpal
f. of necessity
old f.
olecranon tip f.
open f.
open-book f.
open-break f.
open f. (I, II, III, IIIA, IIIB,
  IIIC)
open reduction of f.
ossification-associated f.
osteochondral non-load-bearing
  bone f.

F

fracture (*continued*)
osteochondral nonunion articular f.
osteochrondral slice f.
osteoporotic ankle f.
os trigonum f.
Pais f.
Palmer primary f.
paranasal sinus f.
paratrooper's f.
parry f.
pars interarticularis f.
1-, 2-, 3-, 4-part f.
patellar f.
patellar sleeve f.
pathologic f.
f. pattern
Pauwels f.
pedicle f.
pelvic avulsion f.
pelvic rim f.
pelvic ring f.
pelvic straddle f.
penetrating f.
percutaneous pinning of f.
perforating f.
periarticular f.
PER (I-IV) f.
periprosthetic f.
peritrochanteric f.
pertrochanteric f.
phalangeal diaphysial f.
physial plate f.
physis f.
Piedmont f.
pillow f.
pilon f.
ping-pong f.
pin placement for treatment of
pelvic f.
Pipkin-type femoral head f.
plafond f.
plastic bowing f.
plateau f.
pond f.
Posada f.
posterior arch f.
posterior column f.
posterior element f.
posterior process f.
posterior talar process f.
posterior wall f.
postirradiation f.
postmortem f.
postoperative f.
Pott ankle f.
Pouteau wrist f.
pressure f.
Prevent Recurrence of Osteoporotic
F.'s (PROOF)

profundus artery f.
pronation-abduction f.
pronation-eversion f.
pronation-eversion-external rotation
f.
pronation-external rotation (I-IV)
f.
proximal end tibia f.
proximal femoral f.
proximal humeral f.
proximal tibial metaphysial f.
pseudo-Bennett f.
pseudo-Jones f.
puncture f.
pyramidal f.
quadruped f.
radial head f.
radial neck f.
radial styloid f.
f. reducing elevator
f. reduction
reduction of f.
f. repair
f. repair with intramedullary
nailing
resecting f.
retrodisplaced f.
reverse Barton f.
reverse Colles f.
reverse Monteggia f.
reverse obliquity f.
rib f.
ring f.
f. risk
Rolando f.
rotational burst f.
Ruedi f.
Ruedi-Allgower tibial plafond f.
sacral f.
sacroiliac f.
Salter epiphysis f.
Salter-Harris distal tibial-fibular
physis f.
Salter-Harris epiphysial f. (I-VI)
sandbagging long bone f.
Sanders calcaneal f.
Sanders calcaneal f. (type I-IV)
Sanders highly comminuted
calcaneal f.
Sanders nondisplaced calcaneal f.
Sanders 3-part calcaneal f.
Sanders 4-part calcaneal f.
Sanders split calcaneal f.
scaphoid f.
scapular f.
Schatzker tibial plateau f.
secondary f.
segmental f.
Segond tibial avulsion f.

Séguin f.
senile subcapital f.
sentinel f.
SER (I-IV) f.
sesamoid f.
shaft f.
shear f.
Shepherd posterior process of talus f.
short oblique f.
sideswipe elbow f.
silver-fork f.
simple f.
single-column f.
sinus f.
f. site
f. site nonunion Norland bone densitometry
skier's f.
Skillern radius f.
sleeve f.
small f.
Smith ankle f.
Sneppen talar f.
snowboarder's f.
sourcil f.
spinal f.
spinous process f.
spiral f.
spiral oblique f.
f. splint
splintered f.
split f.
split-depression f.
split heel f.
spontaneous f.
sprain f.
sprinter's f.
f. stabilization
stable burst f.
stairstep f.
stellate f.
step-off of f.
sternum f.
Stieda medial femoral condyle avulsion f.
straddle f.
strain f.
stress f.
styloid f.
subcapital f.
subcutaneous f.
subperiosteal f.
subtrochanteric femoral f.
supination-adduction f.
supination-eversion f.
supination-external rotation (I-IV) f.
supracondylar humeral f.
supracondylar Y-shaped f.

suprasyndesmotic f.
supratectal transverse f.
surgical neck f.
sustentaculum tali f.
synchondritic f.
T f.
f. table
talar avulsion f.
talar neck f.
talar osteochondral f.
talus body f.
tarsal bone f.
T condylar f.
teacup f.
teardrop f.
teardrop-shaped flexion-compression f.
temporal bone f.
tennis f.
tension f.
thalamic fragment of calcaneal f.
thoracic spine f.
thoracolumbar burst f.
through-and-through f.
thrower's f.
Thurston-Holland fragment f.
tibial plafond f.
tibial plateau f.
tibial stress f.
tibiofibular f.
Tillaux anterolateral tibial epiphysis f.
Tillaux-Chaput anterolateral tibial epiphysis f.
toddler's f.
torsion f.
torsional f.
torus f.
total talus f.
f. toughness
traction f.
transcapitate f.
transcervical femoral f.
transchondral f.
transcondylar f.
transepiphysial f.
transhamate f.
transiliac f.
transsacral f.
transscaphoid dislocation f.
transtriquetral f.
transverse process f.
trapezium f.
trimalleolar f.
trimalleolar ankle f.
triplane tibial f.
triquetral f.
trophic f.
Tscherne closed femur f. (0-III)

F

fracture (*continued*)
 T-shaped f.
 tuberosity avulsion f.
 tuft f.
 ulnar styloid f.
 unciform f.
 uncinate process f.
 undisplaced f.
 unicondylar f.
 unstable f.
 ununited f.
 vertebral body f.
 vertebral [body] compression f.
  (VCF)
 vertebral body wedge f.
 vertebral compression f.
 vertebral plana f.
 vertebral stable burst f.
 vertebral wedge compression f.
 vertical shear f.
 volar shear f.
 Volkmann posterior tibia f.
 Vostal radial head f.
 V-shaped f.
 wagon wheel f.
 Wagstaffe f.
 Wagstaffe-Le Fort f.
 waist f.
 Walther hip f.
 Watson-Jones navicular f.
 Weber (A, B, C) f.
 wedge compression f.
 wedge flexion-compression f.
 wedge-shaped uncomminuted tibial
  plateau f.
 willow f.
 Wilson f.
 Winquist-Hansen classification (0–IV)
  of femoral f.
 f. with scoliosis
 wrist f.
 Y f.
 Y-T f.
 Zickel f.
 ZMC f.
 f. zone
fractured
 f. bone
 f. bone mobility
 f. vertebra
fracture-dislocation
 atlantoaxial f.-d.
 carpometacarpal f.-d.
 Galeazzi f.-d.
 intermediate cuneiform f.-d.
 Lisfranc f.-d.
 Monteggia f.-d.
 perilunate f.-d. (PLFD)
 posterior f.-d.

 f.-d. reduction
 tarsometatarsal f.-d.
 thoracolumbar spine f.-d.
 tibial plateau f.-d.
 transcapitate f.-d.
 transhamate f.-d.
 transtriquetral f.-d.
 unstable f.-d.
 f.-d. with anterior ligament
fragile X syndrome
fragilitas
 f. ossium
 f. ossium congenita
fragility fracture
Fragmatome tip
fragment
 alignment of fracture f.'s
 anterolateral f.
 articular f.
 avascular f.
 avulsion f.
 bone f.
 bucket-handle f.
 butterfly fracture f.
 capital f.
 cartilaginous f.
 Chaput f.
 chondral f.
 Comet f.
 corner f.
 coronoid f.
 cortical f.
 depression of f.
 disc f.
 distal f.
 fracture f.
 free f.
 free-floating cartilaginous f.
 hinged f.
 hypervascular f.
 intraarticular f.
 loose f.
 major fracture f.
 osteochondral f.
 retrolisthesed f.
 retropulsed bony f.
 step-off between bone
  fracture f.'s
 superomedial f.
 sustentacular f.
 Thurston-Holland f.
 tuberosity f.
 wedge-shaped uncomminuted f.
fragmental bone
fragmentation
 endplate f.
 graft f.
fragment-in-notch sign
Fragmin

fraise
    diamond f.
frame
    Ace-Colles fracture f.
    Ace-Fischer fracture f.
    Ace-Fischer ring f.
    Alexian Brothers overhead f.
    Anderson f.
    Andrews spinal surgery f.
    anterior quadrilateral triplane f.
    f. application
    Balkan fracture f.
    basic Ilizarov-type f. (I-IV)
    bilateral f.
    Böhler-Braun f.
    Böhler fracture f.
    Böhler reducing f.
    Bradford fracture f.
    Braun f.
    Brooker f.
    Brown-Roberts-Wells stereotactic f.
    Chalet f.
    Chick CLT operating f.
    CircOlectric f.
    C-Jaws cervical compressive mini f.
    claw-type basic f.
    Cole fracture f.
    Cole hyperextension f.
    convex saddle f.
    Crawford head f.
    delta f.
    DePuy rainbow f.
    DePuy reducing f.
    double-ring f.
    Elekta stereotactic head f.
    external fixator f.
    fixator f.
    Foster-Kennedy f.
    Foster turning f.
    fracture f.
    fusion f.
    GaitMaster low-profile f.
    Gardner-Wells fixation f.
    Goldthwait f.
    Granberry f.
    Hastings f.
    Herzmark f.
    Hibbs f.
    Hitchcock stereotactic
      immobilization f.
    Hoffmann f.
    Hoffmann-Vidal double f.
    Ilizarov f.
    Jones abduction f.
    Jordan f.
    Kessler traction f.
    laminectomy f.
    Malcolm-Lynn C-RXF cervical
      retractor f.

    Mayfield fixation f.
    Monticelli-Spinelli f.
    f. of reduction
    f. of reference
    pelvic fracture f.
    phantom f.
    Pittsburgh pelvic f.
    1-plane bilateral f.
    2-plane bilateral f.
    1-plane unilateral f.
    2-plane unilateral f.
    4-poster f.
    quadrilateral f.
    rectangular f.
    Relton-Hall f.
    Risser f.
    scoliosis operating f.
    Slatis pelvic fracture f.
    sling f.
    spinal turning f.
    spine f.
    Stealth f.
    Stryker fracture f.
    Stryker turning f.
    table-skeletal fixation f.
    Taylor spinal f.
    tent f.
    Thomas f.
    Thompson f.
    triangular ankle fusion f.
    triangulate triple f.
    triple f.
    Wagner f.
    Watson-Jones f.
    Whitman f.
    Wilson convex f.
    Zimmer fracture f.
    Zimmer laminectomy f.
Framer
    F. finger extension bow
    F. splint
    F. tendon passer
    F. tendon-passing needle
frank
    F. and Johnson modification
    F. and Johnson modification of
      Heyman procedure
    f. diastasis
    f. dislocation
Fränkel
    F. neurologic deficit classification
    F. sign
    F. white line
Frankfort horizontal plane
frayed
    f. disc
    f. meniscus
fraying of meniscus
Frazer carpal tunnel wrist brace

F

Frazier
    F. elevator
    F. suction tip
FRD
    flexion-rotation-drawer
    FRD test
free
    f. body diagram
    f. fasciocutaneous flap
    f. fat graft
    f. flap of cartilage
    f. flap transfer
    f. fragment
    f. gracilis muscle transfer
    f. latissimus dorsi flap
    f. microsurgical flap
    f. phalangeal bone autograft
    f. pyridinium crosslink
    f. revascularized autograft
    f. scapular flap
    f. skin flap
    f. skin graft
    f. tie
    f. tissue transfer
    f. toe transfer
    f. vascularized bone graft (FVBG)
    f. vascularized bone transplant
    f. vascularized fibula graft
    f. weight rehabilitation
Freebody
    F. pin
    F. stay-retractor
freedom
    F. accommodator arch support
    F. arthritis support
    F. back support
    degree of f.
    F. elastic long wrist support
    F. Micro Pro stimulator
    F. neutral position splint
    f. of movement
    F. Omni Progressive splint
    F. Palm Guard
    F. Progressive Resting splint
    F. SportsFit splint
    F. thumbkeeper
    f. thumb spica
    f. thumb stabilizer
    F. ultimate grip splint
    F. USA wristlet
free-floating
    f.-f. cartilaginous fragment
    f.-f. osteotomy
Free-Flow system prosthesis
freehand
    f. CT-guided biopsy
    f. cut
    f. prosthesis system
    f. suturing technique

freely movable joint
Freeman
    F. calcaneal fracture classification
    F. clamp
    F. modular total hip prosthesis
Freeman-high neck press fit
  prosthesis
Freeman-Samuelson knee prosthesis
Freeman-Sheldon syndrome
Freeman-Swanson
    F.-S. knee prosthesis
    F.-S. knee system
Freer
    F. chisel
    F. dissector
    F. elevator-dissector
    F. periosteal elevator
    F. septal elevator
free-spinning probe
free-swinging knee gait
Free-Up massage cream
free-walking velocity
freeze-dried
    f.-d. bone
    f.-d. bone pin
    f.-d. cancellous allograft
    f.-d. cortical bone
    f.-d. graft
freeze-thawed graft
Freiberg
    F. cartilage knife
    F. disease
    F. fracture
    F. infarction
    F. meniscectomy knife
    F. traction
Freiberg-Kohler disease
Frejka
    F. jacket
    F. pillow
    F. pillow orthosis
    F. pillow splint
    F. traction
fremitus
frena (*pl. of* frenum)
French
    F. adapter
    F. fracture technique
    F. lateral closing-wedge osteotomy
    F. rod bender
    F. scale (F)
    F. supracondylar fracture operation
frenectomy
Frenkel
    F. exercises
    F. movement
    F. track
frenula (*pl. of* frenulum)
frenulum, *pl.* **frenula**

frenum, *pl.* **frena,** *pl.* **frenums**
frenums (*pl. of* frenum)
frequency
    f. analysis
    discharge f.
    f., intensity, time, type
      (FITT)
    f., intensity, type, time
      exercise
    onset f.
    recruitment f.
frequency-difference interferential current
  therapy (FDICT)
freshening of bone
freshen the surface
fresh fracture
fresh-frozen
    f.-f. graft
    f.-f. nonirradiated bone-patellar
      tendon-bone allograft
Fresnel prism
fretting corrosion
friable
Friatec manual arthroscopy instrument
fricative
friction
    f. artifact
    coefficient of f. (COF)
    cross f.
    dynamic f.
    f. lock pin
    f. massage
    patient-on-table f.
    f. rub
frictional torque
friction-reduced
    f.-r. examination table
    f.-r. segmented table
Fried-Hendel procedure
Friedman
    F. bone rongeur
    F. brace
    F. rongeur forceps
    F. splint
    F. support
Friedreich
    F. ataxia
    F. disease
    F. foot
Fries
    F. rheumatoid arthritis classification
    F. rheumatoid arthritis score
fringe
    f. joint
    f. of osteophyte
    synovial f.
frog-leg
    f.-l. lateral radiograph
    f.-l. lateral view

    f.-l. position
    f.-l. splint
Fröhlich adiposogenital dystrophy
Frohse
    arcade of F.
    F. arcade of elbow
    arch of F.
    F. ligamentous arcade
Froimson
    F. bicipital groove keyhole
      technique
    F. splint
    F. tendon interposition thumb
      procedure
Froimson-Oh
    F.-O. arm procedure
    F.-O. upper limb tendon
      interposition repair
frôlement
FROM
    full range of motion
Froment
    F. nerve palsy sign
    F. paper sign
    F. ulnar nerve function test
Fromm triangle orthopaedic device
frond
    synovial f.
front
    corset f.
    f. kick explosion
frontal
    f. bone
    f. bossing
    f. motion
    f. plane
    f. plane correction
    f. plane growth abnormality
    f. plane XY
    f. plane Z-plasty
    f. plate
front-entry guide
fronting of velar
frontoorbital advancement
front-opening orthosis
frontside snowboard stance
frost
    F. foot operation
    F. foot procedure
    F. H-block
    F. partial matricectomy
    F. posterior tibialis technique
    F. posterior tibialis tendon
      lengthening
frostbite
    f. acroosteolysis
    f. injury
    f. of hand
frottage

F

frozen
    f. pelvis
    f. shoulder
    f. shoulder syndrome
FRS
    fusion and reconstruction system
    FRS screw
fructooligosaccharides (FOS)
fruste, *pl.* **frustes**
    forme f.
frustes (*pl. of* fruste)
Frykman
    F. distal radius fracture
      classification
    F. radial fracture
    F. wrist fracture classification
F-Scan
    F-S. foot force and gait analysis
      system
    F-S. foot pressure analysis
    F-S. in-shoe system
    F-S. pressure measurement system
FSH
    facioscapulohumeral
FSHD
    facioscapulohumeral muscular dystrophy
FSHMD
    facioscapulohumeral muscular dystrophy
FSI
    Functional Status Index
FSMD
    facioscapulohumeral muscular dystrophy
FSQ
    Functional Status Questionnaire
FSU
    functional spinal unit
FTA
    femorotibial angle
FTC
    fibulotalocalcaneal
    FTC ligament
FT03C transducer
FTE
    functional tissue engineering
F-tool
FTSG
    full-thickness skin graft
fuel
    Ripped F.
Fugl-Meyer
    F.-M. evaluation
    F.-M. Evaluation of Physical
      Performance
Fukuda humeral head retractor
Fukushima C-clamp
fulcra (*pl. of* fulcrum)
fulcrum, *pl.* **fulcra, fulcrums**
    f. distance
    f. fracture

    joint f.
    f. test
fulcruming
fulcrums (*pl. of* fulcrum)
Fulford subtalar arthrodesis procedure
fulgurate
Fulkerson
    F. functional knee score
    F. oblique tibial tubercle osteotomy
full
    f. cervical spine (FCS)
    f. cervical spine view
    f. cervical spine x-ray
    f. curve
    f. fist flexion
    f. interference pattern
    f. lateral position
    f. range of motion (FROM)
    f. spine radiographic examination
    f. thumb spica cast
    f. weightbearing (FWB)
full-circle goniometer
full-curved clamp
Fuller shield dressing
full-hand splint
full-occlusal splint
full-radius
    f.-r. resector
    f.-r. resector knife
full-thickness
    f.-t. cuff tear
    f.-t. skin graft (FTSG)
fully constrained tricompartmental knee
  prosthesis
fulminans
    purpura f.
fulminate
Fulvicin
    F. P/G
    F. U/F
fumigatus
    Aspergillus f.
function
    adrenergic vagal f.
    ambulatory f.
    bundle f.
    Charnley classification of f.
    cholinergic vagal f.
    concentric f.
    eccentric f.
    hand f.
    intrinsic f.
    Jebsen assessment of hand f.
    LSUMC classification of motor and
     sensory f.
    motor f.
    neurologic f.
    passive f.
    perverted f.

physical condition, upper limb
function, lower limb function,
sensory component, excretory
function, support f. (PULSES)
position of f.
Quadriplegia Index of F. (QIF)
reflex f.
rotator cuff f.
sensory f.
splinted in position of f.
subtalar joint f. (SJF)
sudomotor f.
throwing f.
tibialis posterior f.
functional
    f. activity
    f. ambulation
    f. ambulation category (FAC)
    f. and anatomic loading (FAL)
    f. anesthetic discography (FAD)
    f. assessment measure (FAM)
    F. Assessment Staging (FAST)
    f. axial rotation
    f. back pain
    f. capacity assessment
    f. capacity evaluation (FCE)
    f. capacity measurement
    f. cross-sectional area
    f. disability
    f. disability of foot
    f. electrical stimulation (FES)
    f. fracture brace
    f. grip pushup block
    f. independence measure (FIM)
    F. Independence Measure for
    Children (WeeFIM)
    F. Index Questionnaire (FIQ)
    f. instability
    f. integrated training (FIT)
    F. Integration (FI)
    f. intermetatarsal angle
    f. knee brace
    f. leg length inequality
    F. Limitation Profile (FLP)
    f. loss
    f. magnetic resonance imaging
    (fMRI)
    f. neuromuscular stimulation (FNS)
    f. orthotic
    f. outcome
    f. performance
    f. phase rehabilitation
    f. rating score
    f. recovery
    f. refractory period
    f. restoration
    f. scoliosis
    f. short leg
    f. spinal unit (FSU)

    f. splint
    f. squats back exercise technique
    F. Status Index (FSI)
    F. Status Questionnaire (FSQ)
    f. subluxation
    f. tissue engineering (FTE)
    f. training
functionally debilitating symptom
functioning
    Assessment of Occupational F.
    (AOF)
    Self-Assessment of Occupational F.
    (SAOF)
fungal, fungous
    f. arthritis
    fungous infection
    fungous synovitis
Fungi-Nail antifungal solution
fungoid
    F. AF Topical Solution
    F. Creme
fungous (*var. of* fungal)
funicular excision
funiculi (*pl. of* funiculus)
funiculitis
funiculus, *pl.* **funiculi**
Funk tibialis posterior tendon
  dysfunction syndrome
funnel
    f. breast
    f. chest
    f. technique
funnelization of metaphysis
funny bone
Funsten supination splint
FUO
    fever of undetermined origin
Furacin gauze dressing
furniture brace
furrowing
    scarring and f.
further flexion
furunculosis
Fusarium solani
fused
    f. ankle
    f. arthrodesis
    f. hip
    f. vertebra
fusiform
    f. defect
    f. periosteal new bone
    f. soft tissue swelling
fusimotor
    f. neuron
    f. system
fusion
    Adkins spinal f.
    Albee lumbar spinal f.

F

fusion (*continued*)
  Anderson ankle f.
  f. and reconstruction system (FRS)
  ankle f.
  anterior and posterior f.
  anterior cervical f. (ACF)
  anterior cervical body f.
  anterior cervical discectomy and f.
   (ACDF)
  anterior-inferior f.
  anterior lumbar interbody f. (ALIF)
  anterior lumbar vertebral
   interbody f.
  anterior spinal f.
  AP f.
  atlantoaxial f.
  atlantooccipital f.
  Bailey-Badgley cervical spine f.
  balloon-assisted endoscopic
   retroperitoneal anterior lumbar
   interbody f.
  f. bed
  BERG anterior lumbar interbody f.
  bilateral lateral f.
  Blair ankle f.
  Bohlman triple-wire f.
  bone block f.
  Bosworth lumbar spinal f.
  Bradford f.
  Brooks cervical f.
  Brooks-Gallie cervical f.
  Brooks-Jenkins atlantoaxial f.
  Brooks-Jenkins cervical f.
  Brooks-type f.
  buried K-wire fixation in digital f.
  f. cage
  calcaneotibial f.
  cervical interbody f.
  cervical spine posterior f.
  cervicooccipital f.
  Chandler hip f.
  Charnley compression-type knee f.
  chevron f.
  Cloward anterior spinal f.
  Cloward back f.
  CMC f.
  Coltart calcaneotibial f.
  convex f.
  Copeland-Howard scapulothoracic f.
  4-corner midcarpal f.
  cuboid f.
  Davis f.
  degenerative lumbar spine f.
  degenerative spondylosis
   decompression and f.
  Dewar posterior cervical f.
  diaphysial-epiphysial f.
  digital f.
  DIP f.

discectomy with Cloward f.
distal tibiofibular f.
dowel spinal f.
extraarticular hip f.
extraarticular subtalar f.
facet f.
f. facet
f. frame
Gallie atlantoaxial f.
Gallie cervical f.
Gallie subtalar ankle f.
Gallie wire f.
Gissane ankle f.
Goldstein spinal f.
f. graft
Hall facet f.
hammertoe correction with
  interphalangeal f.
H-graft f.
Hibbs spinal f.
Horwitz-Adams ankle f.
Horwitz ankle f.
hyperostotic bony f.
instrumented spinal f.
interbody spinal f.
interdigital bone f.
interfacet wiring and f.
interphalangeal f.
intersegmental f.
interspinal process f.
intertransverse f.
intraarticular hip f.
intraarticular knee f.
joint f.
Kellogg-Speed lumbar spinal f.
Kennedy modification of Gallie
  ankle f.
King intraarticular hip f.
knee f.
Langenskiöld f.
lateral f.
f. limit determination
long segment spinal f.
lower cervical spine f.
lumbar spine f.
lumbar vertebral interbody f.
lumbosacral f.
lunotriquetral f.
f. mass
McKeever metatarsophalangeal f.
metatarsocuneiform joint f.
metatarsophalangeal joint f.
minimally invasive lumbar interbody
  f. (MiLIF)
Müller intraarticular shoulder f.
multilevel f.
naviculocuneiform f.
f. nonunion rate
occipitoatlantoaxial f.

occipitocervical f.
osteotomy and f.
pantalar ankle f.
f. plate
posterior cervical f.
posterior lumbar interbody f. (PLIF)
posterior spinal f. (PSF)
posterolateral f. (PLF)
posterolateral interbody f.
posterolateral lumbosacral f.
posterolateral spine f.
radiolunate f.
radioscaphoid f.
Robinson anterior cervical f.
Robinson cervical spine f.
Robinson-Southwick f.
Robins-Riley spinal f.
Rowe f.
sacral spine f.
sacroiliac joint f.
salvage f.
scaphocapitate f.
scapulothoracic f.
scoliosis spinal f.
screw f.
selective thoracic spine f.
short segment spinal f.
Simmons cervical spine f.
single-level spinal f.
Smith-Petersen sacroiliac joint f.
Smith-Robinson anterior f.
Smith-Robinson cervical interbody f.
Soren ankle f.
spinal f.
2-stage hip f.
Stamm procedure for intraarticular
hip f.
stand alone lumbar intervertebral f.
(STALIF)
f. stiffness
subastragalar f.
subaxial posterior cervical spinal f.
subtalar distraction bone block f.
symmetric vertebral f.
talar body f.
talocalcaneal f.
talocrural f.

talonavicular f.
f. technique
Thermo F.
thoracic facet f.
thoracic spinal f.
thoracolumbar f.
tibiocalcaneal f.
tibiofibular f.
tibiotalar f.
tibiotalocalcaneal ankle f.
transfibular f.
transpedal multiplanar wedge f.
trapeziometacarpal f.
triple tarsal f.
triple-wire f.
triscaphe f.
upper cervical spine f.
vertebral f.
Watkins spinal f.
Watson scaphotrapeziotrapezoidal f.
White posterior ankle f.
Wilson ankle f.
Wiltse bilateral lateral f.
Winter hemivertebrae convex f.
Zielke instrumentation for scoliosis
spinal f.
fusionless
f. scoliosis surgery
f. surgery
Fusobacterium nucleatum
fustigation
Futrex body fat analyzer
Futura
F. conical subtalar implant
F. flexible digital implant
F. metal hemi-toe implant
Future implant
Futuro
F. splint
F. wrist brace
F. wrist support
FVBG
free vascularized bone graft
F-wave response
FWB
full weightbearing
FyBron dressing

F

G

penicillin G
G suit

G5

G5 Fleximatic massage/percussion
unit
G5 Fleximatic massager/percussor
massager
G5 Porta-Plus muscle stimulator
G5 Vibracare massager/percussor
G5 Vibramatic massage/percussion
unit

gabapentin
gadolinium-diethylenetriamine pentaacetic
acid (gadolinium-DTPA)
gadolinium-DTPA

gadolinium-diethylenetriamine
pentaacetic acid

gadolinium-enhanced MRI
gadolinium-labeled diethylenetriamine
pentaacetic acid
gadopentetate-dimeglumine-enhanced
magnetic resonance imaging
GADS

gas atomized dispersion strengthened
GADS vitallium alloy

Gaenslen

G. fracture
G. osteomyelitis
G. sacroiliac joint and lumbar
vertebrae inflammation test
G. sign
G. spike fixation of fresh neck of
femur fracture
G. split-heel incision
G. split-heel technique

Gaffney

G. ankle prosthesis
G. joint

gag

Dingman mouth g.

Gage

G. distal rectus femoris
transfer
G. sign

gain

Body Oscillation Integrates
Neuromuscular G.
(BOING)
heat g.

Gaines and Ford tendo Achillis length
calculation
GAIT

great toe arthroplasty implant
technique

gait

abductor lurch g.
G. Abnormality Rating Scale
(GARS)
adult g.
g. analysis
g. and mobility
g. and station
angle of g.
antalgic g.
apraxic g.
apropulsive g.
g., arms, legs, and spine (GALS)
g., arms, legs, spine screening
arthrogenic g.
g. assessment
astasia-abasia g.
ataxic g.
avoidance g.
base of g.
batrachian g.
g. belt
biomechanical evaluation of foot
function during stance phase of g.
g. biomechanics
broad-based g.
cadence of g.
calcaneal g.
cerebellar g.
Charcot g.
Charlie Chaplin g.
choreatic g.
clumsy g.
cogwheel g.
component of g.
crab g.
cross-legged g.
crouch g.
g. cycle
dancing bear g.
g. deviation
g. disorder
g. disorder, autoantibody, late-age
onset, polyneuropathy (GALOP)
g. disturbance
dorsiflexor g.
double-leg stance phase of g.
double-step g.
double-tap g.
drag-to g.
dromedary g.
dropfoot g.
drunken sailor g.
duck waddle g.
dynamic g.

G

gait (*continued*)
dystrophic g.
equine g.
extrapyramidal g.
festinating g.
flaccid g.
flatfoot g.
floating g.
footdrop g.
foot-strike phase of g.
free-swinging knee g.
gastrocnemius-soleus g.
glue-footed g.
gluteal g.
gluteus maximus g.
gluteus medius g.
heel-and-toe g.
heel-contact phase of g.
heel-off phase of g.
heel-strike phase of g.
heel-toe g.
helicopod g.
hemiparetic g.
hemiplegic g.
high-steppage g.
hip extensor g.
hobbling g.
hyperextended knee g.
hysterical g.
instability g.
intermittent double-step g.
internal rotational g.
intoeing g.
jerky g.
kinematic g.
g. laboratory
g. line
listing g.
g. lock splint (GLS)
g. lock splint brace
lurching g.
marche à petits pas g.
midstance period of g.
myopathic g.
narrow-base g.
Oppenheim g.
opposite foot-strike phase of g.
opposite toe-off phase of g.
out-toeing g.
painful g.
paraparetic g.
parkinsonian g.
g. pathomechanics
g. pattern
penguin g.
petit pas g.
Petren g.
pigeon-toeing g.
g. plate

2-point g.
3-point g.
4-point g.
pronatory g.
propulsion g.
push-off phase of g.
reeling g.
retropulsion of g.
reversal of fore-aft shear phase of g.
rigid g.
scissors g.
scissors-leg g.
scraping toe g.
short leg g.
shuffling g.
skater's g.
slap foot g.
slapping g.
spastic g.
spastic equinus g.
stable g.
staggering g.
stamping g.
stance phase of g.
star g.
station and g.
steppage g.
stiff g.
stiff-knee g.
stiff-legged g.
stride length of g.
strike phase of g.
stuttering of g.
swaying g.
swing phase of g.
swing-through g.
swing-to g.
tabetic g.
tandem g.
tiptoe g.
Todd g.
toe g.
toe-heel g.
toeing-in g.
toeing-out g.
toe-off phase of g.
toe-toe g.
toe-walking g.
tottering g.
g. training
Trendelenburg g.
tripoding g.
uncoordinated g.
unsteady g.
waddling g.
wide-based g.
gaiter cast
GaitKeeper cast shoe

GaitMaster low-profile frame
GAITRite mat
Galante hip prosthesis
Galant sign
galaxy
    G. 900HS adjusting table
    G. McManis hylo table
Galeazzi
    G. fracture
    G. fracture-dislocation
    G. hip dislocation sign
    G. patella realignment
    G. patellar operation
    G. pediatric hip dysplasia test
Galen scoliosis
Gallagher rasp
gallamine triethiodide
Gallannaugh plate
gall duct forceps
Gallie
    G. ankle arthrodesis
    G. atlantoaxial arthrodesis
    G. atlantoaxial fusion
    G. atlantoaxial fusion technique
    G. atlantoaxial wiring
    G. cervical fusion
    G. fusion using titanium cable
    G. needle
    G. procedure
    G. subtalar ankle fusion
    G. subtalar bone block arthrodesis
     approach
    G. subtalar fixation
    G. wire fixation technique
    G. wire fusion
    G. wiring technique
gallium citrate scan
gallium-67 scan
Gallo traction
Gallows splint
GALOP
    gait disorder, autoantibody, late-age
    onset, polyneuropathy
    GALOP syndrome
GALS
    gait, arms, legs, and spine
    GALS screening
Galt hand drill
galvanic
    g. bath
    g. electrode stimulator
    high-voltage pulsed g.
    g. skin response
    g. stimulation
galvanism
    high-voltage g.
    low-voltage g. (LVG)
    medical g.
    surgical g.

Galveston
    G. fixation with TSRH crosslink
    G. intrasacral post
    G. metacarpal brace
    G. Orientation and Amnesia Test
    (GOAT)
    G. pelvic fixation
    G. plate
    G. reconstruction
    G. spinopelvic reconstruction
    technique
    G. splint
Galveston-type rod construct
gambiense
    Trypanosoma g.
game
    g. knee
    g. leg
gamekeeper's
    g. injury
    g. thumb
    g. thumb dislocation
gamma
    g. aminobutyric acid
    g. camera
    g. camera imaging
    G. locking nail
    G. trochanteric locking nail
gamma-aminobutyric acid agonist
gammopathy
    monoclonal g.
ganciclovir
ganglia (*pl. of* ganglion)
ganglion, *pl.* **ganglia, ganglions**
    Acrel g.
    arthroscopic resection of dorsal
    wrist g.
    g. block
    g. cyst
    dorsal root g. (DRG)
    excision of dorsal wrist g.
    excision of volar wrist g.
    intraosseous g.
    metatarsophalangeal joint g.
    periosteal g.
    radiocapitellar joint g.
ganglionectomy
    dorsal root g.
ganglioneuroma
ganglionic block
ganglionostomy
ganglions (*pl. of* ganglion)
gangrene
    dry g.
    gas g.
    ischemic g.
    Meleney synergistic g.
    peripheral g.
    postnatal g.

G

gangrene (*continued*)
    Pott g.
    Raynaud g.
    synergistic g.
    vascular g.
    wet g.
gangrenosum
gangrenous necrosis
Ganley
    G. extensor hallucis brevis
      transfer
    G. forefoot osseous reconstruction
      technique
    G. modification of Keller
      arthroplasty
    G. splint
Gant
    G. hip arthrodesis
    G. operation
    G. osteotomy
gantry
    scanner g.
Ganz
    G. antishock pelvic fixator
    G. cup
    G. fixation
    G. periacetabular osteotomy
gap
    g. arthroplasty
    G. cup
    extension g.
    flexion g.
    flexion-extension g.
    fracture g.
    g. healing
    g. nonunion
    scapholunate g.
Garamycin Topical
Garceau
    G. cheilectomy
    G. tendon technique
Garceau-Brahms arthrodesis
Garcia wrist laxity criteria
garden
    G. alignment index
    G. femoral neck fracture
    G. femoral neck fracture
      angle
    G. femoral neck fracture
      classification
    G. screw
    g. spade deformity
Gardner
    G. bone forceps
    G. chair
    G. elevator
    G. operation
    G. syndrome
Gardner-Diamond syndrome

Gardner-Wells
    G.-W. fixation frame
    G.-W. tongs
    G.-W. tong traction
garment
    antishock g.
    compression g.
    console compression g.
    Elvarex compression g.
    Elvarex support g.
    g. hook
    pneumatic g.
    pneumatic antishock g. (PASG)
    support g.
Garré
    chronic sclerosing osteomyelitis of
      G.
    G. disease
    G. osteitis
    G. sclerosing osteomyelitis
Garrick popliteus tendon test
Garrod
    G. disease
    G. fibromatosis
GARS
    Gait Abnormality Rating Scale
GARS-M
    Modified Gait Abnormality Rating
      Scale
garter strapping
Garth shoulder view
Gartland
    G. forefoot reconstruction procedure
    G. humeral supracondylar fracture
      classification
    G. supracondylar fracture
      classification
    G. Universal radial fracture
      classification
GAS
    general adaption syndrome
gas
    g. atomized dispersion strengthened
      (GADS)
    g. gangrene
    ionized g.
    g. sterilization
gasless
    balloon-assisted endoscopic
      retroperitoneal g. (BERG)
gas-producing streptococcal infection
gastrocnemius
    g. angle
    Baker tongue in groove slide
      lengthening of g.
    Baumann and Koch intramuscular
      lengthening of g.
    g. bursitis
    g. equinus

g. flap
lateral head of g.
g. lengthening
g. muscle
g. recession
g. resistive exercise
g. rupture
g. soleus
g. tendon
g. tendon transfer

gastrocnemius-soleus
g.-s. complex
g.-s. contracture
g.-s. fascial strip
g.-s. gait
g.-s. junction
g.-s. muscle
g.-s. muscle group
g.-s. recession
g.-s. stretching
g.-s. tendon

gastrointestinal
g. anastomosis (GIA)
g. tract

gastrosoleal equinus
Gatch bed
gate control theory of pain
Gatellier-Chastang
G.-C. ankle approach
G.-C. incision

Gates-Glidden drill
gateway
G. Expedium anterior spine system
G. thoracolumbar system
G. vertebroplastic cement

Gator
G. gait trainer
G. Grip
G. plastic orthosis

Gaucher disease
gauge
acetabular g.
aneroid g.
B&L pinch g.
bone screw depth g.
bone screw ruler g.
Charnley femoral condyle radius g.
Charnley socket g.
clip g.
Cloward depth g.
Cobb g.
CTS g.
depth g.
Durkan CTS g.
finger g.
force g.
isometric strain g.
Jamar hydraulic pinch g.
measuring g.

5.07 monofilament g.
orthopaedic depth g.
pain threshold g.
Philips toe force g.
pinch g.
Preston pinch g.
Rocabado posture g.
Rosette strain g.
screw depth g.
socket g.
spanner g.
strain g.
tourniquet g.
uniaxial strain g.
vernier caliber g.

gauntlet
AFG ankle/foot g.
g. anesthesia
g. atrophy
g. bandage
g. cast
Jobst g.
leather lacer g.
wrist g.

gauze
Adaptic g.
Cover-Roll g.
g. dressing
iodoform g.
Kerlix g.
g. packing
petrolatum g.
plain g.
pledget of g.
Safe-Wrap g.
g. sponge
Surgitube tubular g.
Telfa g.
g. wrap

Gaynor-Hart
G.-H. carpal tunnel view
G.-H. position

GC
gonococcal
GCS
Glasgow coma scale
GCT
giant cell tumor
GDLH posterior spinal system
GD Regainer System
gear
shoe g.
gearshift
g. probe
thoracic g.
gear-stick sign
GEIN
gradual elongation intramedullary
nailing

Geissling rating scale
gel
- Adcon adhesive control g.
- Adcon-L anti-adhesion barrier g.
- Aquasonic Transmission G.
- atelocollagen g.
- Biofreeze topical analgesic g.
- G. Care self-adhesive gel
- Carrington Dermal wound g.
- g. cast
- Ceres' Secret aloe vera g.
- Crystal polymer g.
- g. cushion
- DermaFlex G.
- Flexall g.
- G. Foam Ultra-Wedge cushion
- Grafton DBM g.
- H.P. Acthar G.
- hydrisalic g.
- Iamin hydrating g.
- Keralyt G.
- Lam IPM Wound G.
- Mederma topical g.
- Naftin g.
- osteoinductive enhanced-graft g.
- Oxiplex/SP g.
- g. pack
- 0.01% Regranex G.
- silicone g.
- Silipos g.
- Silosheath g.
- sodium hyaluronate wound g.
- g. stump sock
- g. suspension sleeve
- g. tubing
- Uni-Patch electrode g.
- g. warmer
- wound g.
- g. wrap

gelatin
- g. compression boot
- g. foam

gelatinous
gelatin-resorcin-formalin glue
GelBand arm band
Gel-Bank patellar strap
Gel-Care
Gelfoam
- G. cookie
- G. embolization
- G. pack
- G. pledget
- G. stamp
- thrombin-soaked G.

Geliperm dressing
gelling phenomenon
Gelman
- G. foot operation
- G. foot procedure

Gelocast
- G. cast
- G. Unna boot compression dressing
- G. Unna boot compression wrap

Gelpi retractor
Gelpirin
GelPort hand access laparoscopy
GELS
- gravity extension locking system

Gel-Sole shoe insert
gemellus
Gemini
- G. chiropractic table
- G. cup
- G. hip system prosthesis
- G. MKII mobile-bearing knee implant

Gem total knee system
GEN
- gradual elongation nailing

Genahist Oral
Genapap
Genaspor
Gencalc 600
Gendron bariatric wheelchair
general
- g. ability
- g. adaption syndrome (GAS)
- g. adjustment
- g. capsular stretch
- g. endotracheal anesthesia
- g. thrust manipulation

generalized fibromatosis
generation
- G. II 3DX brace
- G. II KAFO
- G. II knee brace
- G. II Unloader ADJ knee brace
- G. II Unloader Select knee brace

generator
- electrosurgical g.

Genesis
- G. arthroplasty hardware
- G. II foot/ankle system
- G. II foot system
- G. II mobile-bearing knee implant
- G. II total knee system
- G. knee prosthesis
- G. unicompartmental knee

genetic scoliosis
genicula (*pl. of* geniculum)
genicular
- g. artery
- medial g.

geniculate neuralgia
geniculum, *pl.* **genicula**
genital system
genitofemoral nerve

Gennari band
genotypic chondrodysplasia
Genpril
gentamicin
    g. bead
    g. implant
gentle
    G. Threads interference screw
    g. traction
GentleStep shoe
genu, *pl.* **genua**
    g. recurvatum
    g. valgum
    g. valgum deformity
    g. varum
    g. varum deformity
genua (*pl. of* genu)
Genucentric knee hinge
Genucom
    G. ACL laxity analysis system
    G. arthrometer
    G. knee flexion analysis system
Genutrain
    G. knee brace
    G. PE patellar realignment
    G. P3 knee support
Genzyme Tissue Repair
GeoFlex
    G. knee
    G. knee prosthesis
geographic destruction
Geo-Matt contour cushion
Geo-Mattress bariatric mattress
Geomedic
    G. system
    G. total knee prosthesis
geometric
    g. device
    g. supracondylar extension
    osteotomy
    g. total knee prosthesis
Geo Rectangles spinal implant
George
    G. line
    G. vertebrobasilar insufficiency test
Georgiade
    G. fixation device
    G. visor cervical collar
    G. visor cervical traction
    G. visor halo fixation
    G. visor halo fixation apparatus
Gerard
    G. prosthesis
    G. resurfacing procedure
Gerber subscapularis test
Gerbert osteotomy
Gerdy
    G. ligament
    G. tibial tubercle

geriatric
    g. chair trunk support
    g. physical therapy
    g. trauma
germicidal lamp
germinal matrix
germinative matrix
Gerota capsule
Gerson diet
Gerster
    G. bone clamp
    G. traction bar
Ger technique
Gertie ball
Gertzbein
    G. classification of seat-belt injury
    G. seat-belt injury classification
Gerzog bone mallet
GET
    graded exposures training
Get-A-Grip grip
Ghajar guide
GHE Eska femoral stem
GHL
    glenohumeral ligament
Ghon-Sachs complex
GIA
    gastrointestinal anastomosis
    GIA staple
    GIA stapler
Giannestras
    G. modification of Lapidus hallux
    valgus technique
    G. oblique metatarsal osteotomy
    G. step-down modified osteotomy
giant
    g. bone island
    g. cell reaction
    g. cell reparative granuloma
    g. cell sarcoma
    g. cell tumor (GCT)
    g. cell tumor of tendon sheath
    g. motor unit action potential
    g. osteoid osteoma
    g. popliteal synovial cyst
giantism (*var. of* gigantism)
Gianturco
    G. macrocoil
    G. prosthesis
gibbosity
gibbous
    g. deformity
    g. deformity of spine
gibbus
Gibney
    G. boot
    G. fixation bandage
    G. perispondylitis
    G. taping

G

Gibson
  G. bandage
  G. posterior hip approach
  G. splint
Gibson-Piggott osteotomy
Giebel blade-plate
Giertz rib shears
Giertz-Shoemaker rib shears
Giertz-Stille scissors
Gifford mastoid retractor
gigantism, giantism
  hyperpituitary g.
  pituitary g.
gigas
  pes g.
Gigli
  G. saw
  G. saw blade
  G. saw guide
  G. saw osteotomy
Gilbert
  G. harvesting
  G. procedure
  G. scapular flap
Gilchrist
  G. splint
  G. test
Gilfillan humeral prosthesis
Giliberty
  G. acetabular prosthesis
  G. apparatus
  G. bipolar femoral head
  G. device
  G. femoral neck prosthesis
  G. hip prosthesis
gill
  G. arthrodesis
  G. lumbar spondylolisthesis
    decompression laminectomy
  G. massive sliding graft
  G. posterior bone block
  G. shelf procedure
  G. sliding graft technique
Gillet marching sacroiliac joint motion test
Gillette
  G. brace
  G. double-flexure ankle joint
  G. double-flexure ankle joint system
  G. joint orthosis
  G. joint prosthesis
  G. modification
  G. modification of ankle-foot
    orthosis
Gilliat-Summer nerve-damaged hand
Gillies
  G. bone graft
  G. bone hook
  G. pollicization

  G. prosthesis
  G. suture
Gillies-Dingman hook
Gill-Manning-White surgical treatment of spondylolisthesis
Gillquist
  G. procedure
  G. suction curette
  G. suction tube
Gill-Stein arthrodesis
Gilmer splint
Gilmore groin
Gimbel glove
gimpy
  g. knee
  g. leg
ginglymoarthrodial
ginglymoid joint
ginglymus
Ginkgo biloba
Girard keratoprosthesis prosthesis
GIRD
  glenohumeral internal rotation
    deficit
girdle
  Cadenza surgical support g.
  limb g.
  pectoral g.
  pelvic g.
  shoulder g.
Girdlestone
  G. flexor to extensor tendon
    transfer
  G. hip resection
  G. operation
  G. orthopedic procedure
  G. pseudarthrosis
  G. resection arthroplasty
Girdlestone-Taylor muscle transfer clawtoe repair procedure
Gissane
  G. ankle fusion
  G. arthrodesis
  G. calcaneal x-ray angle
  crucial angle of G.
  G. spike
give-way
  g.-w. phenomenon
  g.-w. weakness
giving
  g. way
  g. way of ankle
  g. way of knee
glabella
glabellar rasp
glacier
  G. ceramic 4-in-1 cutting guide
  G. ceramic knee cutting guide
  G. Pack

GLAD
glenolabral articular disruption
GLAD lesion
gladiatorum
herpes g.
tinea g.
gland
eccrine sweat g.
haversian g.
parathyroid g.
thyroid g.
Glasgow
G. coma scale (GCS)
G. screw
Glasscock ear dressing
Glassman-Engh-Bobyn trochanteric slide
glatiramer acetate
Gleich
G. osteotomy
G. osteotomy for pes valgo planus
G-lengthening of semitendinosus tendon
glenohumeral
g. adhesive capsulitis
g. arthrodesis
g. dislocation repair
g. glide
g. instability
g. internal rotation deficit
 (GIRD)
g. joint
g. joint cohesion
g. joint disease
g. joint dislocation
g. joint stability
g. joint subluxation
g. ligament (GHL)
g. pain
g. shift
glenoid
g. alignment peg
g. cartilage
g. cavitary
g. cavity
g. component
g. concavity
g. drill
g. drill guide
g. fixation screw
g. fossa
g. fossa of scapula
g. fracture
g. implant base impactor
g. labrum
lip of g.
g. metal tray
g. neck
g. osteotomy
g. point
g. rim

g. rim fracture
g. slot
glenoid-reaming forceps
glenolabral
g. articular disruption (GLAD)
g. articular disruption lesion
g. ovoid mass (GLOM)
g. ovoid mass lesion
g. ovoid mass sign
glenoplasty
posterior g.
Scott posterior g.
Gliadel implant
glide
anterior g.
anterior-inferior g.
anterior-posterior g.
cervical dorsal g.
craniocaudal g.
dorsal g.
dynamic canal g.
glenohumeral g.
g. hole
g. hole for screw placement
g. hook
inferior g.
mushroom walker g.
natural apophysial g. (NAG)
patellar g.
posterior g.
posterior-anterior g.
self-sustained natural apophysial g.'s
superior g.
sustained natural apophysial g.'s
 (SNAGS)
volar g.
glider
g. cane
g. cane board
EasyStand 6000 g.
G. II patient transfer system
gliding
g. hinge joint
g. hole
g. hole first technique
g. layer
g. mechanism
g. principle
glioma
gliosis
Glisson sling
global
g. cavus
g. equinus
G. Fx shoulder fracture system
g. kyphosis
g. metatarsus equinus
g. rating of change (GROC)
G. total shoulder arthroplasty

G

global (*continued*)
G. total shoulder arthroplasty system
g. total shoulder implant
G. total shoulder implant
globose
globulin
immune g.
tetanus immune g.
Globus Pivot spinal implant
GLOM
glenolabral ovoid mass
GLOM lesion
GLOM sign
glomangiosarcoma
glomus
g. tumor
g. tumor of hand
glossopharyngeal neuralgia
glove
g. anesthesia
antivibration g.
Biobrane g.
Bio-Form g.
carpal tunnel g.
compression g.
electrode g.
finger flexion g.
F&L attenuating g.
flexion g.
flexor g.
Gimbel g.
Handeze fingerless g.
impact g.
Isotoner g.
Jobst g.
Kevlar g.
Life Liner stick and cut-resistant g.
Maxxus orthopaedic latex
  surgical g.
Medak g.
Medarmor puncture-resistant g.
Necelon surgical g.
peripheral nerve g.
pressure g.
Push-Ease wheelchair g.
radial nerve g.
SoftFlex computer g.
Sorbothane antivibration g.
surgical g.
TheraKnit electrode g.
Tubigrip g.
vibration g.
weighted g.
WHECS g.
glove-and-stocking anesthesia
GLS
gait lock splint
GLS brace
GLS suture anchor

glubionate
calcium g.
Gluck rib shears
glucocerebroside
glucocorticoid
gluconate
chlorhexidine g.
glucosamine sulfate
glucosteroid
glue
cyanoacrylate g.
gelatin-resorcin-formalin g.
Histoacryl g.
skin g.
Tisseel fibrin g.
glued-to-the-floor phenomenon
glue-footed gait
glutamic-oxaloacetic
  transaminase
glutamic-pyruvic transaminase
  (GPT)
glutaraldehyde
gluteal
g. artery
g. bonnet
g. bursitis
g. cleft
g. fascia
g. gait
g. lurch
g. nerve
g. reflex
g. region
g. sulcus
gluteal/hamstring raise back exercise
  technique
glutethimide
gluteus
g. maximus flap
g. maximus gait
g. maximus muscle
g. maximus pain syndrome
g. maximus tensing test
g. medius gait
g. medius limp
g. medius muscle
g. medius pain syndrome
g. medius paralysis
g. minimus muscle
glycation
nonenzymatic connective
  tissue g.
glycocalyx
glycogen sparing
glycol
salicylic acid and propylene g.
glycosaminoglycan
GMFM
Gross Motor Function Measure

G-myticin Topical
gnathodynamics
gnathodynamometer
gnathologic, gnathological
gnathological (*var. of* gnathologic)
gnome's calf
goal
    rehabilitation g.
GOAT
    Galveston Orientation and Amnesia
    Test
goblet incision
Goethe bone
Gohil-Cavolo method
Golaski graft
gold (Au)
    g. probe
    g. salt
    g. sodium thiomalate
    g. therapy
    g. weight and wire spring implant
      material
Goldberg clavicle fracture repair
  technique
golden
    G. closing wedge osteotomy
    G. Comfort orthotic
    G. Fitness orthotic
    G. mean testing system
Goldenberg footplate shoe
GoldenEye arthroscope
Goldenhar syndrome
gold-handled chuck
Goldman-Fristoe
    G.-F. articulation test
    G.-F. Test of Articulation
Goldmar opponensplasty
Goldner
    G. spinal arthrodesis
    G. thumb reconstruction
Goldner-Clippinger multangular bone
  excision technique
GoldPoint
    G. ACL functional knee brace
    G. hinged knee brace
    G. PCL functional knee brace
Goldstein
    G. spinal fusion
    G. spinal fusion technique
Goldthwait
    G. brace
    G. frame
    G. sign
golfer
    Thera-Band Exercise System for
      G.'s
golfer's
    g. elbow
    g. elbow test

    g. nails
    g. wrist
Golf Exercise System
golf-stick dissector
Golgi
    G. apparatus
    G. device
    G. tendon
    G. tendon organ
gonadotrophin (*var. of* gonadotropin)
gonadotropic hormone
gonadotropin, gonadotrophin
    human chorionic g.
gonalgia
gonarthritis
gonarthromeningitis
gonarthrosis
gonarthrotomy
gonatagra
gonatocele
gonial angle
goniometer
    2-arm g.
    electronic g.
    EOC g.
    finger g.
    full-circle g.
    O'Brien g.
    orthopaedic g.
    Polk finger g.
    Sammons biplane g.
    universal full-circle
      manual g.
    Zimmer g.
goniometric
goniometry
Goniopora
    coralline hydroxyapatite *G.*
    (CHAG)
gonitis
gonococcal (GC)
    g. arthropathy
    g. septic arthritis
gonococcic tenosynovitis
gonorrheal, gonorrhoeal
    g. heel
    g. tenosynovitis
gonorrhoeae
    Neisseria g.
gonorrhoeal (*var. of* gonorrheal)
Gonstead
    G. pelvic marking system
    G. technique
gonycampsis
good
    G. Grips utensil
    G. 'N Bed wedge
    G. rasp
Goode wrap

G

Goodman orthopaedic bed
Goodwin bone clamp
Goody's Headache Powders
goose-egg edema
gooseneck gouge
Go-Ped motorized scooter
Gordon
    G. calf squeeze test
    G. hip approach
    G. joint injection technique
    G. knee phenomenon
    G. reflex
    G. reflex sign
    G. splint
gordonae
    Mycobacterium g.
Gordon-Broström single-contrast
  arthrogram
Gordon-Taylor hindquarter
  amputation
Gore
    G. bit
    G. smoother
    G. smoother crucial tool
Gore-Tex
    G.-T. anterior cruciate ligament
    G.-T. interpositional
      arthroplasty
    G.-T. knee prosthesis
    G.-T. nonabsorbable suture
    G.-T. waterproof cast liner
Gorham
    G. disease
    G. massive osteolysis
    G. syndrome
Gorham-Stout
    G.-S. disease
    G.-S. syndrome
gorilloid
Gosselin fracture
Gotfried percutaneous compression
  plating
Gottron
    G. papule
    G. sign
Gouffon pin fixation
gouge
    Abbott g.
    Acufex g.
    Alexander g.
    Andrews g.
    Army bone g.
    arthroplasty g.
    Aufranc g.
    Bishop g.
    bone g.
    Buck-Gramcko g.
    Campbell g.
    Capener g.

    Capner g.
    Cobb spinal g.
    curved g.
    gooseneck g.
    Guy g.
    Hibbs g.
    Hoen g.
    Jewett g.
    Killian g.
    Lexer g.
    Lucas g.
    Metzenbaum g.
    Meyerding g.
    Moe g.
    Murphy g.
    orthopaedic g.
    oscillating g.
    Partsch g.
    Read g.
    Rubin g.
    Sheehan g.
    Smith-Petersen curved g.
    Smith-Petersen gooseneck g.
    Smith-Petersen straight g.
    Stagnara g.
    Stille bone g.
    straight g.
    swan-neck g.
    tendon g.
    U.S. Army g.
    Watson-Jones bone g.
    West bone g.
    Zielke g.
    Zimmer g.
Gould ankle procedure
gout
    acute g.
    articular g.
    calcium g.
    chronic tophaceous g.
    latent stage of g.
    tophaceous g.
gouty
    g. arthritis
    g. diet
    g. node
    g. pain
    g. tophaceous deposit
    g. tophus
    g. tophus formation
Gowers
    G. maneuver
    G. muscular dystrophy
    G. phenomenon
    G. sign
Gowers-Welander musclar dystrophy
  syndrome
GPS
    gravitational platelet separation

GPT
glutamic-pyruvic transaminase
grab
g. bar
g. sign
grabber
arthroscopic g.
disc g.
Tab G.
tendon g.
grace
G. method
G. method of metatarsal length ratio
G. plate 4-hole adapter
gracilis
g. flap
g. muscle
g. muscle graft
g. procedure
g. syndrome
g. tendon
g. test
graciloplasty
grade
g. (A, B, C1, C2, D) cement mantle
Boyer degenerative joint disease g. (0–4)
g. (I, II) oscillation
Kellgren and Lawrence osteoarthritis g. (0–4)
Kendall muscle g. (1–5)
g. (1–5) of mobilization
Risser g.
Tachdjian flatfoot g.
Wagner diabetic foot ulcer g.
Zachary sensory g.
graded
g. exposures training (GET)
g. Gore-Tex tape
g. spinal anesthesia
gradient-recalled acquisition in steady state (GRASS)
grading
activity g.
g. of manipulation
osteoarthritis radiographic g.
gradual
g. elongation intramedullary nailing (GEIN)
g. elongation nailing (GEN)
graduated
g. spinal block (GSB)
g. tenotomy
graduated-height block
Graf
G. classification
G. stabilization system

Graflex material
graft
AAA bone g.
acetabular augmentation g.
ACL g.
advancement flap g.
Albee bone g.
allogenic bone g.
allograft bone g.
alloplastic g.
antebrachial fascial g.
anterior sliding tibial g.
anterosuperior iliac spine g.
autochthonous g.
autogenous cancellous bone g.
autogenous fibular g.
autogenous patellar ligament g.
autogenous quadrupled hamstring tendon g.
autogenous semitendinosus-gracilis g.
autologous cancellous bone g.
autologous reverse g.
autolyzed antigen-extracted allogenic bone g.
autoplastic g.
banked bone g.
barber-pole vein g.
bicondylar g.
bicortical iliac bone g.
bicortical ilial strip g.
bifid g.
biopolymeric g.
Blair-Brown skin g.
bone g. (BG)
bone autogenous g.
bone block g.
bone chip g.
bone marrow g.
bone peg g.
bone replacement g.
bone-tendon g.
bone-tendon-bone g.
bone-to-bone g.
Bonfiglio bone g.
bovine collagen g.
Boyd dual-onlay bone g.
BPB autologous g.
BPTB g.
Braun skin g.
bridge g.
bulk g.
cable nerve g.
cadaver bone g.
calcaneal bone g.
Calcitite g.
calcium carbonate bone replacement g.
calvarial free bone g.
Campbell onlay bone g.

G

graft (*continued*)

cancellous chip bone g.
cancellous insert g.
cancellous morselized bone g.
carbon fiber g.
cartilage g.
chemosterilized g.
chip g.
Chuinard autogenous bone g.
Clancy patellar tendon g.
clothespin spinal fusion g.
composite rib g.
composite skin g.
consolidated g.
g. containment system
cortical bone g.
cortical strut g.
corticocancellous bone g.
corticocancellous chip g.
cutaneous g.
cylindrical autologous dowel g.
Dacron g.
Daniel iliac bone g.
Davis muscle-pedicle g.
delayed g.
demineralized bone g.
g. design
devitalized bone g.
diamond inlay bone g.
double-looped gracilis g.
Douglas skin g.
g. dowel
dowel bone g.
Dragstedt skin g.
g. driver
dual onlay cortical bone g.
dura mater g.
Esser skin g.
g. expulsion
extraarticular g.
fascial g.
fascia lata freeze-thawed g.
fascio-fat g.
fat g.
fatigued bone g.
femur g.
fetal substantia nigra g.
fibular onlay-inlay g.
fibular strut g.
filleted g.
fillet local flap g.
Fisk-Fernandez volar wedge bone g.
g. fixation
Flanagan-Burem apposing
  hemicylindric g.
flap g.
flat bone g.
flexor tendon g.
Forbes onlay bone g.

g. fracture
g. fragmentation
free fat g.
free skin g.
free vascularized bone g. (FVBG)
free vascularized fibula g.
freeze-dried g.
freeze-thawed g.
fresh-frozen g.
full-thickness skin g. (FTSG)
fusion g.
Gillies bone g.
Gill massive sliding g.
Golaski g.
gracilis muscle g.
Haldeman bone g.
hamstring g.
Harris superior acetabular g.
g. harvest
Hemashield enhanced g.
hemicondylar g.
hemicylindrical bone g.
Henderson onlay bone g.
Henry bone g.
heterodermic g.
heterogeneous g.
heterogenous g.
H-graft bone g.
Hoaglund bone g.
homogeneous g.
homologous g.
homoplastic g.
H-shaped g.
Huntington bone g.
iliac bone g. (IBG)
iliac crest bone g. (ICBG)
iliac crest bone free g.
iliac crest-inlay g.
iliac slot g.
iliac strut bone g.
iliotibial band g.
g. impingement
Inclan bone g.
Infuse bone g.
inlay bone g.
insert g.
interbody g.
intercalary g.
interpositional tricortical g.
interposition bone g.
intramedullary bone g.
ipsilateral slide g.
irradiation sterilized g.
island g.
isologous g.
Isotec patellar tendon g.
Judet vascularized bone g.
jump g.
keystone g.

Krause-Wolfe skin g.
Kutler V-Y flap g.
LAD composite g.
Langenskiöld bone g.
lateral patellar autologous g.
Lee anterosuperior iliac spine g.
Lee bone g.
ligamentous anterior dislocation
  composite g.
load-bearing g.
lyophilized bone g.
Massie sliding g.
massive sliding g.
matchstick g.
g. material
g. material alternative
Matti-Russe bone g.
McFarland bone g.
McMaster bone g.
medullary bone g.
meniscus g.
mesh g.
Meyers quadratus muscle-pedicle
  bone g.
Millesi nerve g.
Moberg dowel g.
morcellized bone g.
morcellized cancellous g.
Mueller patellar tendon g.
multiple cancellous chip g.
muscle pedicle bone g.
nail bed g.
nerve g.
neurovascular island g.
Nicoll cancellous bone g.
Nicoll cancellous insert g.
nonisometric g.
nontubed closed distant flap g.
nontubed open distant flap g.
OATS g.
Ollier thick split free g.
Ollier-Thiersch skin g.
onlay bone g.
onlay cancellous iliac g.
OP-1 implant/bone g.
Opteform 100HT bone g.
osteoarticular g.
osteocartilaginous g.
osteochondral g.
osteochondral autograft transfer
  system g.
osteogenic protein-1 bone g.
osteoperiosteal bone g.
Overton dowel g.
Papineau g.
particulate cancellous bone g.
patellar tendon g.
pedicle bone g.
pedicle fat g.

peg bone g.
percutaneous autogenous dowel
  bone g.
peroneus brevis g.
Phemister onlay bone g.
pie-crusting skin g.
g. placement
plantaris tendon g.
polytetrafluoroethylene g.
porous polyethylene g.
posterior bone g.
posterior cruciate ligament g.
posterolateral bone g.
powdered bone g.
g. preparation
prophylactic bone g.
prosthetic femorodistal g.
PTFE g.
QSGT g.
quadriceps tendon g.
quadruple semitendinosus and
  gracilis tendons g.
rectus femoris g.
revascularization of g.
Reverdin epidermal free g.
rib g.
Russe bone g.
Ryerson bone g.
sandwiched iliac bone g.
scapular g.
segmental tendon g.
semitendinosus-gracilis g.
semitendinous g.
single-condylar g.
single-onlay cortical bone g.
single-stage tendon g.
skin g.
sliding bone g.
soft tissue g.
Soto-Hall bone g.
split calvarial bone g.
split-thickness skin g. (STSG)
Stark bone g.
Stark iliac bone to mandibular
  body g.
g. strength
structural bone g.
g. structure
strut bone g.
subclavius tendon g.
Tait vascular g.
temporal fascia g.
tendon g.
g. tension
tension-free Millesi nerve g.
textured allograft bone g.
Thiersch medium split free g.
Thiersch thin split free g.
Thomas extrapolated bar g.

G

319

graft (*continued*)
tibial bone g.
tricortical iliac crest bone g.
tricortical ilial strip g.
tube flap g.
tubularization of g.
tumbler g.
vascularized bone g. (VBG)
vascularized fibular g.
vascularized osteoseptocutaneous
  fibular autogenous g.
vascularized rib strut g.
VertiGraft textured allograft bone g.
wedge g.
Weiland iliac crest bone g.
Whitecloud-LaRocca fibular strut g.
Wilson bone g.
Wolfe hand surgery g.
Wolf full-thickness free g.
wraparound flap bone g.
Z-plasty local flap g.
graft-bony tunnel wall abrasion
GraftCage TLX spinal implant
Graftech
G. structural allograft anterior ramp
G. structural allograft cervical dowel
G. structural allograft cervical spacer
G. structural allograft posterior ramp
grafted
g. bone
g. material
grafting vein
**GraftJacket regenerative tissue repair
  matrix**
Graftmaster device
Grafton
G. bone matrix and marrow
G. DBM
G. DBM Crunch
G. DBM Flex
G. DBM gel
G. DBM Matrix plug
G. DBM putty
G. demineralized bone matrix
  putty
G. Plus DBM paste
Graham
G. ankle arthrodesis
G. muscle hook
G. nerve hook
G. traction
Grahamizer I exerciser
gram-negative
gram-positive
Gram stain
Granberg cervical traction system
Granberry
G. frame
G. traction

Grand Stand support stand
Grantham femur fracture classification
Grant, Surrall, and Lehman procedure
Granuflex dressing
granular
g. cell myoblastoma
g. histiocytosis
granulation
extradural g.
healing by g.
g. phase
g. tissue
granule
ProOsteon Implant 500 g.'s
Granulex
granuloma, *pl.* **granulomas,** *pl.*
  granulomata
eosinophilic g.
foreign body g.
giant cell reparative g.
Mignon eosinophilic g.
pyogenic g.
g. pyogenicum
reparative g.
rheumatic g.
subperiosteal giant cell reparative g.
subungual g.
swimming pool g.
tubercular g.
granulomas (*pl. of* granuloma)
granulomata (*pl. of* granuloma)
granulomatosis
Langerhans cell g.
Wegener g.
granulomatous
g. fungal infection
g. mass
g. myositis
g. tenosynovitis
graph
Moseley bone age g.
Moseley straight line g.
Graphic Rating Scale (GRS)
graphospasm
Grashey shoulder view
grasp
cylindrical g.
hook g.
pinch g.
prehension g.
g. reflex
thumb-pinch g.
grasper
Acufex g.
Ideal suture g.
loose body g.
pituitary g.
grasper-cutter
Questus leading edge g.-c.

grasping
    g. forceps
    g. power
    g. suture
GRASS
    gradient-recalled acquisition in steady
    state
grasshopper
    g. patella
    G. positioner
Grass neurostimulator
Graston soft tissue technique
grater reamer
Graves scapula
gravis
    myasthenia g.
    Tensilon test for myasthenia g.
gravitational
    g. insecurity
    g. line
    g. platelet separation (GPS)
    g. platelet separation system
    g. proprioception
gravity
    center of g. (COG)
    g. drawer knee test
    g. equinus cast
    g. extension locking system
    (GELS)
    flex against g.
    g. ground reaction force
    g. inflow irrigation
    line of g.
    g. method
    g. method of Stimson
    g. plumb line
    g. stress test
gravity-driven angle finder
gray
    G. bone drill
    g. matter
    periaqueductal g.
    g. ramus communicans
    G. reamer
    G. revision instrument
    system
Grayson
    G. ligament
    G. ligament in hand
grease gun injury
great
    g. sciatic nerve
    g. toe
    g. toe amputation
    g. toe arthroplasty implant technique
    (GAIT)
    g. toe bone
    g. toe implant
    g. toe implant prosthesis

    g. toe push-off
    g. toe reflex
    g. vessel
greater
    g. multangular
    g. multangular bone
    g. multangular ridge
    g. pelvis
    g. rhomboid muscle
    g. trochanter
    g. trochanteric apophysial arrest
    g. trochanteric epiphysiodesis
    g. trochanteric femoral fracture
    g. tuberosity
    g. tuberosity osteotomy
Greek foot
green
    G. and McDermott gastrocnemius
    lengthening
    G. and OBrien wrist function
    score
    G. arthroplasty
    G. muscle hook
    G. procedure
    G. tendon transfer
Green-Anderson growth table
Green-Banks technique
Greenberg clamp
Greene forceps
Greenfield
    G. osteotomy
    G. spinocerebellar ataxia
    classification
Green-Grice procedure
Green-Laird
    G.-L. modification
    G.-L. modification of Reverdin
    osteotomy
Green-O'Brien evaluation system
Green-Reverdin osteotomy
Green-Seligson-Henry (GSH)
    G.-S.-H. nail
Greenspan scoliosis assessment
method
greenstick
    g. dorsal proximal metatarsal
    osteotomy
    g. fixation
    g. fracture
Green-Watermann osteotomy
Greifer prosthesis
Greissinger
    G. foot prosthesis
    G. Multiaxis joint
grelot
    image en g.
grenade
    g. thrower's arm
    g. thrower's fracture

G

Greulich-Pyle
  G.-P. bone age
  G.-P. skeletal age estimation
    technique
  G.-P. skeletal maturation stage
Grice
  G. extraarticular subtalar arthrodesis
  G. incision
  G. procedure
Grice-Green
  G.-G. extraarticular subtalar
    arthrodesis
  G.-G. operation
  G.-G. subtalar extraarticular
    arthrodesis technique
grid
  electrode g.
  g. maze board
  g. maze set
  radiographic g.
  Shar-Tek foot positioning g.
Grierson meniscal shaver
griffe
  main en g.
Griffith incision
Grifulvin V
grimace test
grinder
  DePuy calcar g.
grind shoulder test
grip
  dowel g.
  Gator G.
  Get-A-Grip g.
  key g.
  g. lock
  pencil g.
  Posey g.
  Skil-Care cushion g.
  g. strength
  g. strength test
  syringe g.
  g. tester
  ulnar side g.
Grip-Ease device
Gripp
  G. squeeze ball
  G. squeeze ball hand exerciser
Gripper acetabular cup prosthesis
gripping exercises
GripTrack Commander strength tester
Grisactin Ultra
Grisel
  G. disease
  G. syndrome
griseofulvin
Gris-PEG
Gristina-Webb total shoulder
  arthroplasty

Griswold distraction machine
grit-blasted prosthesis
Gritti
  G. amputation
  G. operation
Gritti-Stokes
  G.-S. amputation
  G.-S. distal thigh
    procedure
  G.-S. knee prosthesis
Grix-Blankenship-Peterson
  syndrome
GROC
  global rating of change
groin
  g. flap
  footballer's g.
  Gilmore g.
  g. pain
  sportsman's g.
groin-to-ankle cast
grommet
  g. bone liner
  circumferential g.
  press-fit circumferential g.
  titanium circumferential g.
groove
  anular g.
  bicipital g.
  deltopectoral g.
  g. distal tibia
  femoral g.
  fibular g.
  flexor g.
  intercollicular g.
  intercondylar g.
  intertubercular g.
  nail g.
  g. of Ranvier
  parasagittal g.
  patellar g.
  patellofemoral g.
  peroneal g.
  spiral humeral g.
  trochlear g.
grooved
  g. director
  g. dissector
  G. Pegboard Test
  g. protector
grooving
  g. osteotome
  g. reamer
gross
  g. fracture
  g. manipulation
  G. Motor Function Measure
    (GMFM)
  g. motor skills

Grosse-Kempf
    G.-K. interlocking medullary nail
    G.-K. interlocking medullary nailing
    G.-K. locking nail
    G.-K. tibial locked nailing technique

ground
    g. electrode
    g. lamella
    purchase and press the g.
    g. reaction
    g. reaction force

group
    activity g.
    adductor muscle g.
    ancillary muscle g.
    AO g.
    g. fascicular repair
    gastrocnemius-soleus muscle g.
    International Clubfoot Study G.
    levator ani g.
    muscle g. (MG)
    Prevent Recurrence of Osteoporotic
      Fractures G.
    PROOF g.
    quadriceps muscle g.

grouped discharge
Grover
    G. meniscotome
    G. meniscus knife

Groves opponensplasty
growing
    g. fracture
    g. pain

growth
    anchorage-dependent g.
    appositional g.
    g. arrest
    g. arrest line
    asymmetrical g.
    bone g.
    g. center
    g. center of bone
    chondroosseous g.
    ectopic bone g.
    g. hormone
    g. hormone hypersecretion
    g. hormone resistance
    latitudinal g.
    physial g.
    g. plate
    g. plate abscess
    g. plate fracture
    g. plate injury
    g. prediction
    g. retardation
    unsynchronous g.
    g. zone

GRS
    Graphic Rating Scale

Gruca lower leg procedure
Gruca-Weiss spring
Gruen
    G. mode
    G. zone

gryphotic toenail
GSB
    graduated spinal block
    GSB elbow prosthesis
    GSB expanded version for knee
      prosthesis

GSH
    Green-Seligson-Henry
    GSH nail

GSW
    gunshot wound

guard
    ankle g.
    Brain Pad mouth g.
    Cloward cervical drill g.
    drill g.
    fingertip g.
    Freedom Palm G.
    McDavid ankle g.
    McDavid hinged knee g.
    McDavid Knee G. (MKG)
    Omed vented instrument g.
    PAL-Guard postamputation limb g.
    palm g.
    pin g.
    Pro-Designed wrist g.
    Progressive palm g.
    Ullrich drill g.

guarded osteotome
guardian
    G. limb salvage system
    G. Red Dot walker

guarding
    muscle g.

Guardsman femoral interference
screw
Gubler wrist tumor
Gudas
    G. scarf Z-plasty
    G. scarf Z-plasty osteotomy

Guepar hinged knee prosthesis
Guérin fracture
Guhl
    G. ankle arthroscopy technique
    G. classification of osteochondritis
      dissecans
    G. distraction

guide
    Accu-Cut osteotomy g.
    Accu-Line g.
    acetabular cup peg drill g.
    Achillon instrument g.
    ACL drill g.
    acrylate drill g.

G

guide (*continued*)
Acufex alignment g.
Acufex tibial g.
Adapteur multifunctional drill g.
adjustable angle g.
Adson drill g.
Adson saw g.
aiming g.
alignment g.
apical axis g.
Arthrex Adapteur C-ring
  drill g.
Arthrex femoral g.
Arthrex subcoracoid drill g.
Arthrex tibial g.
axis g.
Bailey-Gigli saw g.
Bailey saw g.
ball-tipped Küntscher g.
barrel g.
g. barrel
Blair saw g.
bone wire g.
Bow & Arrow cannulated drill g.
Bullseye femoral g.
g. bushing
calibrated pin g.
Cloward drill g.
contoured anterior spinal plate
  drill g.
Cushing-Gigli saw g.
Cushing saw g.
cutter g.
Davis saw g.
Delta Recon proximal drill g.
DePuy femoral acetabular overlay g.
distal femoral cutting g.
drill g.
eccentric drill g.
Evolis femoral cutting g.
extramedullary alignment g.
femoral intramedullary g.
femoral notch g.
Ferkel C g.
FIN pin g.
Fisher g.
fixed-offset g.
flexible intramedullary nail g.
front-entry g.
Ghajar g.
Gigli saw g.
Glacier ceramic 4-in-1 cutting g.
Glacier ceramic knee cutting g.
glenoid drill g.
handheld drill g.
Hewson cruciate g.
Hewson ligament drill g.
Hoffmann pin g.
g. hole

Howell tibial g.
humeral cutting g.
intercondylar drill g.
intramedullary g.
Lebsche saw g.
Levin drill g.
ligature g.
Lipscomb-Anderson
  drill g.
long axial alignment g.
long nail-mounted drill g.
nail-driving g.
nail rotational g.
neutral drill g.
notch cutting g.
nut alignment g.
patellar drill g.
patellar reamer g.
patellar resection g.
PCA cutting g.
PCA medullary g.
picket fence g.
pin g.
g. pin
Poppen Gigli saw g.
porous-coated anatomic g.
ProTrac alignment g.
Puddu drill g.
Raney saw g.
reamer g.
rear-entry ACL drill g.
Reece osteotomy g.
Richards angle g.
Richards drill g.
g. rod
saw g.
scaphoid screw g.
Scott RCE osteotomy g.
screw angle g.
Stader pin g.
stationary angle g.
Synthes wire g.
targeting drill g.
T-Bar g.
telescopic view g.
tibial cutting g.
tibial drill g.
tissue anchor g. (TAG)
Todd-Wells stereotactic
  arc g.
tube g.
tunnel drill g.
tunnel locator g.
Tworek screw g.
Uslenghi drill g.
g. wire
wire and drill g.
wound measuring g.
Yasargil ligature g.

guideline
- AHRQ g.'s
- Böhler g.
- Hartel g.
- Letournel g.

guidepin, guide pin
- AO g.
- ball g.
- ball-point g.
- ball-tip g.
- beaded reamer g.
- calibrated g.
- femoral g.
- lateral g.
- nonbeaded g.
- precurved ball-tipped g.
- Rica wire g.
- Synthes g.
- threaded g.
- tibial g.
- Watson-Jones g.

guidewire, guide wire
- beaded g.
- drill-tipped g.
- Suretac g.

Guilford cervical brace
Guilford-Wright prosthesis
Guillain-Barré syndrome
Guilland sign
guillotine
- g. amputation
- Charnley femoral inlay g.

Guldmann Overhead Trac System
Guleke bone rongeur
Gulick II tape
Guller sigmoid resection
gull-wing deformity
Gumboro disease
Gumley seat beat injury classification
gummatous
- g. abscess
- g. necrosis

gum rubber Martin bandage
gun
- Arthrex meniscal dart g.
- g. barrel sign
- Biofix arrow g.
- cement injection g.
- CMW cement g.
- Harris cement g.
- heat g.
- Reflex G.
- rivet g.
- staple g.
- Sterivap cement g.

Gunderson
- G. bone forceps
- G. muscle forceps

Gunning splint
Gunn jaw winking
gunshot
- g. fracture
- g. wound (GSW)

GunSlinger shoulder orthosis
gunstock deformity
Gunston
- G. arthroplasty
- G. polycentric knee prosthesis

Gunston-Hult knee prosthesis
Gurd
- G. distal clavicle open resection procedure
- G. distal clavicle resection

Gustilo
- G. classification of puncture wound
- G. hip prosthesis
- G. knee prosthesis
- G. open femur fracture (GI, GII, GIIIA, GIIIB, GIIIC)
- G. puncture wound classification
- G. tibial fracture
- G. tibial fracture classification
- G. unconstrained prosthesis

Gustilo-Anderson
- G.-A. open clavicular fracture
- G.-A. open fracture classification
- G.-A. tibial plafond fracture classification

Gustilo-Kyle
- G.-K. cementless total hip arthroplasty
- G.-K. femoral component

gutter
- g. cast
- g. splint

Guttmann
- G. subtalar arthrodesis
- G. technique

guy
- G. gouge
- g. suture

Guyon
- G. amputation
- G. canal
- G. canal syndrome
- G. operation
- G. tunnel release
- G. tunnel syndrome

G/W Heel Lift, Inc. orthosis
gym
- g. ball
- Elite Power Station g.
- hand g.
- limb g.
- Total G.
- Zuni g.

G

gymball
    Dyna-Disc g.
    Exertools g.
Gymmy exercise unit
gymnastics
    pommel horse g.
    Swedish g.
Gymnastik ball
gymnast's wrist

Gymnic Plus exercise ball
Gyne-Lotrimin
Gynogen L.A. Injection
Gypsona
    G. cast
    G. cast material
Gyro-Flex upper extremity exerciser
Gyroscan superconducting MRI

H
hydrogen
H buttress support patellofemoral brace
Kenalog H
Margesic H
H reflex
H region
H vertebra sign
H wave
HA
hydroxyapatite
Proplast HA
Haas
H. disease
H. operation
H. osteotomy
H. paralysis
H. trapezius muscle transfer
habit scoliosis
habitual
h. control
h. dislocation
h. patella luxation
habituation
habitus
varus h.
Hackethal
H. intramedullary bouquet fixation
H. nail
H. stacked nailing humeral shaft technique
hacking
hacksaw
HA-coated hip implant
Haddad metatarsal osteotomy
Hadfield hand board
Hadley S-curve
haemangioendothelioma (*var. of* hemangioendothelioma)
haemangioma (*var. of* hemangioma)
haemangiomatosis (*var. of* hemangiomatosis)
haemangiopericytoma (*var. of* hemangiopericytoma)
haemangiosarcoma (*var. of* hemangiosarcoma)
haemarthrosis (*var. of* hemarthrosis)
haemastatic (*var. of* hemostatic)
haematoma (*var. of* hematoma)
haematomyelia (*var. of* hematomyelia)
haematorrhachis (*var. of* hematorrhachis)
haematosteon (*var. of* hematosteon)
haematothorax (*var. of* hemothorax)

haemochromatosis (*var. of* hemochromatosis)
haemogenesis (*var. of* hemogenesis)
haemolysis (*var. of* hemolysis)
haemophilic (*var. of* hemophilic)
Haemophilus
H. influenzae
H. parainfluenzae
haemorrhage (*var. of* hemorrhage)
haemorrhagic (*var. of* hemorrhagic)
haemostasis (*var. of* hemostasis)
haemostat (*var. of* hemostat)
haemostatic (*var. of* hemostatic)
haemothorax (*var. of* hemothorax)
Hafnia alvei
Hagie
H. hip pin
H. pin nail
H. sliding nail plate
HAGL
humeral avulsion of glenohumeral ligament
HAGL lesion
Haglund
H. bump
H. disease
H. exostosis
H. foot deformity
H. syndrome
Haglund-Stille plaster spreader
Hahn
H. bone nail
H. cleft
cleft of H.
H. screw
Hahn-Steinthal
H.-S. capitellum fracture classification
H.-S. fracture
H.-S. fracture of capitellum
Haid
H. cervical plate
H. UBP system
H. Universal bone plate
hairline
h. crack
h. fracture
hair-on-end sign
hairpin
h. knot
h. splint
Hajdu-Cheney syndrome
Hajdu staging system

H

Hajek
  H. chisel
  H. mallet
Hajek-Ballenger dissector
Hajek-Koffler bone punch forceps
halazepam
Halcion
Haldeman bone graft
Halder locking nail
Haldol
Haldrone
half
  h. ring
  h. ring leg splint
  h. stitch knot
half-and-half nail
half-circle plate
half-hitch arthroscopic knot
half-moon sign
half-pin
  h.-p. external fixator
  h.-p. fixation
Halfprin 81
half-shell splint
half-shoe
Halifax
  H. clamp posterior cervical
    fixation
  H. interlaminar clamp
  H. interlaminar clamp kit
halisteresis phenomenon
hall
  H. air drill
  H. air-driven oscillating saw
  H. bur
  H. double-hole spinal stapler
  H. driver
  H. facet fusion
  H. Kalamchi shelf procedure
  H. mandibular implant system
  H. Micro-Aire drill
  H. Micro E power instrument
  H. modular acetabular reamer
    system
  H. Neurairtome
  H. power drill
  H. preformed metal crown technique
  H. sagittal saw
  H. screwdriver
  H. series 4 large bone instrument
  H. spinal screw
  H. stepdown drill
  H. Versipower drill
  H. Versipower oscillating saw
  H. Versipower reamer
  H. Versipower reciprocating saw
Hall-Dundar drill
Halle bone curette
Hall-effect strain transducer

Hallpike maneuver
hallucal sesamoid
hallucination
  stump h.
hallucis
  accessory abductor h.
  h. brevis tenodesis
  extensor h.
  hyperdynamic abductor h.
  h. longus laceration
hallus (*var. of* hallux)
hallux, hallus
  h. abductovalgus (HAV)
  clawed h.
  h. dolorosus
  dropped h.
  h. elevatus
  h. extensus
  h. flexus
  hammer h.
  h. interphalangeal abductus
  h. interphalangeal joint
    arthrodesis
  intrinsic minus h.
  h. IP joint
  h. limitus
  h. limitus deformity
  h. malleus
  h. metatarsophalangeal
    interphalangeal scale (HMIS)
  h. migration
  h. nail
  rectus h.
  h. rigidus
  h. rigidus arthrodesis
  h. sesamoid
  h. valgus (HV)
  h. valgus angle (HVA)
  h. valgus deformity
  h. valgus interphalangeus angle
  h. valgus-metatarsus primus varus
    complex
  h. valgus night splint
  h. valgus orthosis
  h. valgus procedure
  h. varus
  h. varus correction
  h. varus deformity
Hall-Zimmer power instrument
halo
  h. body jacket
  h. brace
  BRW head ring h.
  h. cast
  h. cast/vest immobilization
  h. cervical orthosis
  h. cervical traction
  h. cervical traction system
  custom h.

h. extension orthosis
h. immobilization
Lerman noninvasive h.
h. nevus
noninvasive h.
h. pedestal
pericellular h.
Perry-Nickel cranial h.
h. pin
h. ring
h. sign
h. traction jacket
h. traction orthosis
Twin Cities Lo-Profile h.
h. vest
h. vest apparatus
h. vest device
halo-cast distraction
halo-dependent traction
halo-femoral
h.-f. distraction
h.-f. traction
halogen lamp
halo-gravity traction device
halo-Ilizarov distraction instrumentation
halo-pelvic
h.-p. distraction
h.-p. traction
haloprogin
Halotex
halo-vest orthosis
halo-wheelchair traction
Halsey
H. nail scissors
H. needle holder
Halsted
H. forceps
H. thoracic outlet maneuver
halter
Cerva Crane h.
DePuy h.
Diskard head h.
head h.
Repro head h.
h. traction
Upper 7 head h.
Zimfoam head h.
Zimmer head h.
Haltran
hamartoma
cartilaginous h.
chondromatous h.
fibrous h.
leiomyomatous h.
lipofibromatous h.
neuromuscular h.
polymorphic h.
hamartomatous lesion

Hamas
H. endoscopic facial rejuvenation technique
H. upper limb prosthesis
hamate
h. bone
h. hook
h. hook nonunion
hook of h.
h. ligament
h. tail fracture
hamate-lunate joint
hamatometacarpal ligament
Hamilton
H. apparatus
H. jaw bandage
H. pelvic traction screw tractor
H. Rating Scale for Depression
H. ruler test
H. screw
H. traction
Hamilton-Russell traction
hammer
Babinski percussion h.
Berliner percussion h.
Buck neurological h.
Buck percussion h.
cervical/lumbar h.
Cloward h.
Davis percussion h.
Dejerine-Davis percussion h.
Dejerine percussion h.
h. digit syndrome
Epstein neurological h.
H. external fixation
h. finger
h. hallux
hypothenar h.
Küntscher h.
orthopaedic h.
OrthoVise with slap h.
percussion h.
reflex h.
slap h.
sliding h.
Taylor percussion h.
h. toe pain syndrome
h. toe syndrome (HTS)
Trömner percussion h.
hammertoe, hammer toe
h. correction
h. correction with interphalangeal fusion
h. deformity
dynamic h.
fixed h.
flexible h.
h. repair

H

329

Hammon
    H. foot operation
    H. foot procedure
Hammond splint
hamstring
    anterior cruciate ligament
      reconstruction using h.'s
    h. fixation technique
    h. force
    h. graft
    lateral h.
    h. lengthening
    h. ligament augmentation
    medial h.
    h. muscle
    h. reflex
    h. release
    h. stretcher
    h. syndrome
    h. tendinitis
    h. tendon
    h. tightness
hamstring-setting exercise
hamstrung knee
hamulus
    sphenoid h.
Hancock amputation
hand
    accoucheur h.
    American Society for Surgery of
      the H. (ASSH)
    h. amputation
    h. anomaly
    ape h.
    apelike h.
    artificial h.
    baseball fracture of h.
    bear's paw h.
    h. block
    h. board
    h. brace
    h. cast
    h. chuck
    claw h.
    cleft h.
    h. cock-up splint
    h. cone
    h. cuff
    Disabilities of Arm, Shoulder, and
      H. (DASH)
    h. dissector
    h. dominance
    dorsal venous arch of h.
    dorsum of h.
    h. drill
    h. elevator
    enchondroma of h.
    h. evaluation set
    h. exercise ball

    h. exerciser
    fell on outstretched h. (FOOSH)
    flat h.
    flexor retinaculum of h.
    flipper h.
    frostbite of h.
    h. function
    H. Functional Index (HFI)
    h. function test
    Gilliat-Summer nerve-damaged h.
    glomus tumor of h.
    h. grasp strength
    Grayson ligament in h.
    h. grip dynamometer
    h. grip strength
    h. gym
    H. Helper
    H. Helper hand exerciser
    hemiplegic h.
    hypoplastic h.
    intrinsic minus h.
    intrinsic plus h.
    h. intrinsics
    Krukenberg h.
    lobster-claw h.
    mirror h.
    mitten h.
    monkey fist h.
    Myobock artificial h.
    myopathy h.
    no man's land of h.
    oath h.
    obstetric h.
    obstetrician's h.
    opera-glass h.
    h. orthosis
    Otto Bock system electric h.
    outstretched h.
    pancake h.
    h. paralysis
    h. placement
    pretendinous band of h.
    proprioception of h.
    h. prosthesis
    h. reconstruction
    h. rest
    h. saw
    skeleton h.
    spade h.
    spastic h.
    split h.
    spread h.
    tangential h.
    trident h.
    vaginal ligament of h.
    h. volumeter
    web area of h.
    web border of h.
    writing h.

**hand-arm vibration syndrome
(HAVS)**
handbag muscle
handball
    team h.
handbreadth
HandClens ultra antiseptic spray
handcuff disease
1-handed kitchen tool
handedness
Handeze fingerless glove
hand-foot syndrome
hand-foot-uterus syndrome
hand-glove prosthesis
handgrip
    h. ergometer
    h. exercise
handheld
    h. drill guide
    h. dynamometer
    h. retractor
    h. weight (HHW)
**hand-honed reverse cutting
needle**
handicap
    International Classification of
    Impairments, Disabilities, H.'s
    (ICIDH)
    visual analog scale of h.
handle
    Bard-Parker h.
    Barton traction h.
    Beaver blade h.
    Charnley brace h.
    cup holder h.
    Dynagrip blade h.
    multisided blade h.
    Ortho-Grip silicone rubber h.
    stone basket screw mounted h.
    surgical knife h.
    Thera-Band h.
    Therap-Loop door h.
    T-pin h.
    traction h.
    Transfer Handle support h.
handlebar palsy
handle-type reamer
hand-operated drill
handpiece
    Coopervision irrigation/aspiration h.
    Max 3 electric h.
    reciprocating power h.
Hand-Schüller-Christian disease
hands-free crutch
handshake cast
handwriting
    Evaluation Tool of Children's H.
Handy-Buck traction
Hanger ComfortFlex knee prosthesis

hanging
    h. arm cast
    h. cast sling
    h. heel sign
    h. hip
    h. hip operation
    h. of limb
    h. toe operation
hangman's fracture
Hang Ups gravity boot
Hankin
    H. lung volume reduction
    H. posterior elbow reduction
Hanna night splint
Hannover
    H. chronic rejection classification
    H. scoring system
Hansen
    H. disease
    H. fracture classification
    H. pin
Hansen-Street
    H.-S. driver-extractor
    H.-S. nail
**Hansen-Winquest femoral diaphysial
fracture (1–4)**
Hanslik patellar prosthesis
Hansson
    Lars Ingvar H. (LIH)
Hapad
    H. felt insert
    H. heel pad
    H. heel wedge
    H. longitudinal metatarsal arch pad
    H. medial arch pad
    H. metatarsal arch
    H. metatarsal insole
    H. prefabricated wool felt pad
    H. scaphoid arch
    H. shoe insert
Happy podiatric bur
Hapset hydroxyapatite bone graft plaster
haptic
HAQ
    Headache Assessment Questionnaire
    HAQ Index
Hara infiltration block
hard
    h. callus stage
    h. collar
    h. corn
    h. disc
    h. socket
Hardcastle
    H. classification
    H. classification of tarsometatarsal
    joint injury
hardening
    work h.

H

Hardinge
    H. expansion bolt
    H. femoral hip approach
    H. hip prosthesis measurement
      technique
    H. lateral hip approach
    H. vastus lateralis procedure
hardware
    Genesis arthroplasty h.
    orthopaedic h.
    h. photopenia
hardy
    H. aluminum crutch
    H. hypophysial curette
**Hardy-Clapham classification of sesamoid
bones of foot**
hare
    H. apparatus
    H. compact traction splint
    H. pin
    H. splint device
    H. traction
hark
    H. foot operation
    H. pes planus procedure
Harken prosthesis
Harloff cart
Harlow plate
Harmon
    H. cervical approach
    H. chisel
    H. hip reconstruction
    H. modified posterolateral approach
    H. procedure
    H. shoulder approach
    H. tendon transfer
    H. transfer technique
harmonic imaging
Harmony PLIF instrument set
Harms
    H. anterior scoliosis technique
    H. cage
    H. posterior cervical plate
    H. thoracic spine fracture repair
      technique
**Harms-Moss anterior thoracic
instrumentation**
harness
    figure-of-8 h.
    Forte h.
    Kicker Pavlik h.
    Pavlik h.
    weight-relieving Forte h.
    Wheaton Pavlik h.
    Zuni h.
Harold Crowe drill
Harpenden
    H. caliper
    H. dynamometer

Harpoon suture anchor
Harriluque technique
Harrington
    H. clamp forceps
    H. compression rod
    H. distraction instrumentation
    H. distraction outrigger
    H. distraction rod
    H. fixation device
    H. flat wrench
    H. hook clamp
    H. hook driver
    H. nail
    H. outrigger splint
    H. pedicle (bifid) hook
    H. rod and hook system
    H. rod clamp
    H. rod distraction instrumentation
    H. rod fixation
    H. rod instrumentation
    H. rod instrumentation compression
    H. rod instrumentation distraction
      outrigger device
    H. rod instrumentation failure
    H. rod instrumentation force
      application
    H. spinal elevator
    H. spreader
    H. total hip arthroplasty
Harrington-Kostuik
    H.-K. distraction device
    H.-K. instrumentation
Harrington-Luque technique
Harris
    H. anterolateral ankle approach
    H. axial heel view
    H. bolt
    H. brace-type reamer
    H. broach
    H. cemented hip prosthesis
    H. cement gun
    H. center-cutting acetabular reamer
    H. condylocephalic nail
    H. condylocephalic nailing
    H. condylocephalic rod
    H. criteria
    H. criteria for implant loosening
    H. design
    H. Design femoral prosthesis
    H. Design-2 implant
    H. femoral component removal
    H. footprint mat
    H. growth arrest line
    H. Hemi Arm Sling
    H. hip line
    H. hip nail
    H. hip scale
    H. hip score (HHS)
    H. hip status system

H. Infant Neuromotor Test (HINT)
H. knotter
H. lateral trigeminal neurolytic
approach
H. medullary nail
H. Micromini prosthesis
H. plate
H. scope
H. splint
H. splint sling
H. superior acetabular graft
H. wire tier
H. 4-wire trochanter reattachment
Harris-Aufranc device
Harris-Beath
H.-B. axial calcaneus view
H.-B. axial hindfoot x-ray
H.-B. footprint
H.-B. footprinting mat sign
H.-B. footprint mat
H.-B. projection
Harris-Galante
H.-G. acetabular cup
H.-G. hip replacement acetabular
component
H.-G. I porous-coated acetabular
component
H.-G. porous hip prosthesis
H.-G. stem
Harrison bone-holding forceps
Harrison-Nicolle polypropylene peg
Harris-Smith anterior interbody drill
Hartel guideline
Hart extension finger splint
Hartigan foramen
Hartmann
H. bone rongeur
H. mosquito forceps
Hartshill-Ransford loop
Hartshill rectangle
harvest
graft h.
h. site
harvester
Hermosa bone h.
minimally invasive bone graft h.
QuickDraw bone h.
tendon h.
harvesting
bone h.
Gilbert h.
Weiland h.
Harvey wire-cutting scissors
Hass
H. osteotomy
H. procedure
Hastings
H. bipolar hemiarthroplasty
H. frame

H. hip prosthesis
H. open radius reduction
Hatcher pin
hatchet-head
h.-h. deformity
h.-h. shoulder
Hatfield bone curette
Hauser
H. Achilles lengthening procedure
H. ambulation index
H. bunionectomy
H. heel cord procedure
H. lateral retinacular release
realignment
H. patellar operation
H. patellar realignment technique
H. patellar tendon procedure
Hausmann
H. weight rack
H. Work-Well work hardening
system
Hausted orthopaedic bed
Hautant test
HAV
hallux abductovalgus
haversian
h. bone remodeling
h. canal
h. gland
h. lamella
h. space
h. system
h. vessel
HAVS
hand-arm vibration syndrome
HAVS staging (0–4)
Hawaii Early Learning Profile (HELP)
Hawkeye
H. suture needle
H. suture needle for arthroscopy
Hawkins
H. impingement sign
H. line
H. shoulder procedure
H. talar fracture classification
H. talus fracture (I-IV)
**Hawkins-Kennedy shoulder impingement
test**
Haygarth node
Hay lateral hip approach
Haynes
H. pin
H. Stellite Company
Haynes-Stellite
H.-S. 21 implant metal
H.-S. implant metal prosthesis
Hays hand retractor
hazard
job-related h.

H

H-block
    Frost H-b.
    H-b. nail surgery
H2 blocker
HBO
    hyperbaric oxygen
    HBO therapy
HBr
    hydrobromide
HBS
    headless bone screw
    HBS system
HC
    Bancap HC
HCA
    heel cord advancement
HCl
    hydrochloride
        Cleocin HCl
        cyclobenzaprine HCl
        Isocaine HCl
        tacrine HCl
        terbinafine HCl
        tramadol HCl
HCMI
    Health Care Manufacturing Inc.
    HCMI Chiropractic System
HCT
    helical computed tomography
HCTU
    home cervical traction unit
HD
    heloma durum
HD-2 cemented total hip prosthesis
head
    abductor hallucis oblique h.
    abductor hallucis transverse h.
    Aequalis humeral h.
    avascular necrosis of femoral h.
      (AVNFH)
    BioPro ceramic TARA h.
    h. brace
    cartilaginous cap of phalangeal h.
    h. check
    cobalt-chromium h.
    collared femoral h.
    Continuum bipolar acetabular h.
    Copeland humeral resurfacing h.
    core decompression of femoral h.
    countersink screw h.
    DePuy Global Advantage shoulder
      eccentric humeral h.
    DePuy hip prosthesis with Scuderi h.
    Exactech Ziramic femoral h.
    femoral h.
    fibular h.
    flat metatarsal h.
    h. fracture
    Giliberty bipolar femoral h.

    h. halter
    H. hip arthroplasty
    HIP Vitox femoral h.
    h. holder
    humeral h.
    infrared h.
    ischemic necrosis of femoral h.
      (INFH)
    J-FX bipolar h.
    long h.
    Matroc femoral h.
    metatarsal flat h.
    h. of fibula
    h. of patella
    phalangeal h.
    Phillips screw h.
    pseudometatarsal h.
    radial h.
    h. rest
    screw h.
    1st metatarsal h. (FMH)
    talar h.
    terminal h.
    ulnar h.
    V40 forged femoral h.
    zirconia orthopaedic prosthetic h.
    Zyranox femoral h.
headache
    H. Assessment Questionnaire (HAQ)
    cervicogenic h.
    exercise-related h.
    ice pick h.
    post dural puncture h.
    posttraumatic h.
head-at-risk sign
headed Bio-Corkscrew
head-first slide
head-halter traction
headholder, head holder
    Aesculap h.
headless
    h. bone screw (HBS)
    h. bone screw system
headlight
    Cogent LightWear h.
Headmaster collar
head-mounted display (HMD)
head-neck component
headrest, head rest
    doughnut h.
    h. extension
    Mayfield neurosurgical h.
    McConnell orthopaedic h.
    pin h.
    3-prong h.
head-shaft angle
head-splitting humeral fracture
head-stem offset
healed fracture

Healey revision acetabular component
healing
- bone h.
- bony h.
- h. by first intention
- h. by granulation
- h. by second intention
- cartilage h.
- contact h.
- fracture h.
- gap h.
- organizational phase of tendon h.
- PER primam h.
- plasmatic phase of skin h.
- h. retardation
- h. shoe
- soft tissue h.
- spiritual h.
- tendon h.
- therapeutic ultrasound for tendon h.

Healos
- H. bone graft substitute
- H. synthetic bone grafting material

health
- H. Assessment Questionnaire index
- H. Care Manufacturing Inc. (HCMI)
- H. O Meter Scale

Healthflex orthotic
Healthier seating cushion
health-related
- h.-r. facility
- h.-r. quality of life (HRQOL)

Heal Well night splint
heart
- athlete's h.
- h. failure
- h. rate

heart-and-hand syndrome
heart-shaped buttocks
heat
- h. allodynia
- h. application
- h. cramp
- h. cramping
- damp h.
- h. fracture
- h. gain
- h. gun
- h. injury prevention
- h. injury risk
- h. loss
- moist h.
- h. stress
- h. stroke
- h. syncope
- h. therapy
- wind h.

heat-cured acrylic femoral head
prosthesis

Heath mallet
heat-molded petroplastic ankle-foot orthosis
heavy
- h. cross-slot screwdriver
- h. side plate

heavy-duty
- h.-d. femur plate
- h.-d. 2-tooth retractor

Heberden
- H. arthropathy
- H. disease
- H. node
- H. nodosity
- H. rheumatism

hebosteotomy
hebotomy
Hebra blade
Heck screw
Hector tendon
Hedrocel
- H. cup
- H. proximal tibia augmentation implant
- H. tantalum metal structure
- H. titanium screw

heel
- h. and sole insert
- anterior h.
- black-dot h.
- CarbonX active h.
- h. compression syndrome
- h. cord
- h. cord advancement (HCA)
- h. cord lengthening
- h. cord stretch
- h. cord stretching exercise
- h. counter
- h. cup
- cushion h.
- h. cushion
- h. equinus
- h. eversion
- h. fat-pad
- H. Free splint
- gonorrheal h.
- h. height
- high-prow h.
- H. Hugger therapeutic heel stabilizer
- h. jar
- jogger's h.
- h. lift
- h. lock
- H. Minder foot elevator
- h. pad pathology
- h. pad sign
- h. pad thickening
- painful h.
- h. pain syndrome
- policeman's h.

H

heel (*continued*)
- h. posting
- h. prominence
- prominent h.
- h. raise exercise
- reverse Thomas h.
- h. rock exercise
- rubber walking h.
- h. sleeve
- solid ankle cushioned h. (SACH)
- h. spike
- h. spur
- h. spur/plantar fasciitis syndrome
- H. Spur Special
- h. spur surgery
- h. spur syndrome
- h. stand
- h. strike
- tennis h.
- h. tension
- Thomas h.
- h. valgus
- h. varus
- h. varus sign
- h. walk
- walking h.
- h. wedge
- wedge adjustable cushioned h. (WACH)

heel-and-toe
- h.-a.-t. gait
- h.-a.-t. walk
- h.-a.-t. walking

Heelbo decubitus heel/elbow protector
heel-contact
- h.-c. phase
- h.-c. phase of gait

Heelift
- H. suspension boot
- H. traction boot

heel-off (HO)
- h.-o. phase
- h.-o. phase of gait

heel-palm test
heel-rise test
heel-strike
- h.-s. phase
- h.-s. phase of gait

heel-tap
- h.-t. reflex
- h.-t. test

heel-tap reflex
heel-tip test
heel-toe
- h.-t. gait
- h.-t. pattern
- h.-t. runner

heel-to-knee test
heel-to-shin test

heel-to-toe medial shoe wedge
Heel-Up Boot suspension boot
HeelWedge healing shoe
Heerfordt syndrome
Heermann alligator forceps
Hefty-bite pin cutter
Hegge pin
Heifetz nail matrix excision procedure
height
- heel h.
- intervertebral disc h.

Hein rongeur
Heiple arthrodesis
Heiss soft tissue retractor
Helal
- H. flap arthroplasty
- H. modification
- H. osteotomy

Helbing sign
Helenca
- H. binder
- H. stockinette bandage

Helfet test
helical computed tomography (HCT)
helicopod gait
helicopodia
Heliodorus T bandage
Helistat absorbable collagen hemostatic sponge
helmet
- cranial h.
- cranial remolding h.

heloma
- h. durum (HD)
- h. miliare
- h. molle (HM)
- h. neurovasculare
- h. vasculare

helotomy
HELP
- Hawaii Early Learning Profile

Helparm
- Swedish H.

helper
- Hand H.

hemangiectasia
- Klippel-Trenaunay osteohypertrophic h.

hemangioendothelioma, haemangioendothelioma
hemangioendotheliosarcoma
hemangioepithelioma
- epithelioid h.

hemangioma, haemangioma
- capillary h.
- cavernous h.

hemangiomatosis, haemangiomatosis
hemangiopericytoma, haemangiopericytoma

hemangiosarcoma, haemangiosarcoma
hemarthrosis, haemarthrosis
    acute traumatic h.
    posttraumatic h.
    traumatic h.
Hemashield enhanced graft
hemathorax (*var. of* hemothorax)
hematogenous
    h. infection
    h. osteomyelitis
hematoma, haematoma
    iliopsoas muscle h.
    intramedullary h.
    postoperative drainage-related h.
    pulsating h.
    sciatic nerve palsy h.
    subgluteal h.
    subungual h.
hematomyelia, haematomyelia
hematorrhachis, hemorrhachis, haematorrhachis
hematosteon, haematosteon
hemianopsia
    homonymous h.
hemiarthroplasty
    Austin Moore h.
    Bateman h.
    Hastings bipolar h.
    I-beam hip h.
    large humeral head h.
    Miller-Galante I h.
    Neer h.
    prosthetic h.
    Smith-Petersen h.
hemiballism
hemicallotasis
    arthritic knee h.
hemic calculus
hemicondylar
    h. fracture
    h. graft
hemicord
hemicrania
    chronic paroxysmal h.
hemicylindrical bone graft
hemidystonia
hemiepiphysiodesis
hemigigantism
hemihypertrophy
hemi-implant
    Dow Corning titanium h.
hemi-interpositional implant
hemijoint arthroplasty
hemiknee
hemilaminectomy knife
hemimelia
    complete paraxial h.
    fibular h.

    paraxial h.
    partial h.
    radial h.
    tibial h.
hemimelic progressive osseous heteroplasia
hemiparetic gait
hemipelvectomy
    formal h.
    internal h.
hemipelvis
hemiphalangectomy
    Johnson h.
hemiplegia
    bilateral h.
    double h.
    spastic h.
    traumatic h.
hemiplegic
    h. amyotrophy
    h. foot
    h. gait
    h. hand
hemiprosthesis
    single-stemmed silicone h.
hemipulp flap
hemiresection interposition arthroplasty
hemisection
    triple h.
hemisemilaminotomy
hemisilastic implant
hemispatial neglect
hemispherical
    h. pusher
    h. reamer
hemivertebra, *pl.* **hemivertebrae**
    balanced h.
    congenital h.
    thoracic hemivertebrae
    unbalanced h.
hemivertebrae (*pl. of* hemivertebra)
hemivertebral excision
hemochromatosis, haemochromatosis
hemodialysis-related arthropathy
hemogenesis, haemogenesis
hemolymphangioma
hemolysis, haemolysis
    foot-strike h.
    intravascular h.
hemophilic, haemophilic
    h. arthritis
    h. arthropathy
    h. joint
hemorrhachis (*var. of* hematorrhachis)
hemorrhage, haemorrhage
    intramedullary h.
    retroperitoneal h.
    subacute subperiosteal h.

H

hemorrhagic, haemorrhagic
- h. bulla
- h. osteomyelitis
- h. villous synovitis

hemosiderin deposition
hemostasia (*var. of* hemostasis)
hemostasis, hemostasia, haemostasis
hemostat, haemostat
- blunt nose h.
- h. clamp
- Crile h.
- Kelly h.
- mosquito h.
- Nu-Knit absorbable h.
- orthopaedic h.
- Surgicel fibrillar h.
- Surgicel Nu-Knit absorbable h.

hemostatic, haemastatic, haemostatic
- h. forceps
- h. thoracic clamp
- Thrombostat topical h.

hemothoraces (*pl. of* hemothorax)
hemothorax, hemathorax, haematothorax, haemothorax, *pl.* **hemothoraces**
Hemovac
- H. Hydrocoat drain
- H. suction tube

Hendel guided osteotome
Henderson
- H. arthrodesis
- H. clamp approximator
- H. fracture
- H. functional results classification
- H. lag screw
- H. onlay bone graft
- H. posterolateral tibia approach
- H. posteromedial knee approach
- H. skin incision

Henderson-Jones
- H.-J. chondromatosis
- H.-J. disease

Hendler unitunnel ACL repair technique
Hendren self-retaining retractor
Henle
- H. ligament
- trapezoid bone of H.

Hennessy knee brace
Henning
- H. cast spreader
- H. inside-to-outside meniscal repair technique
- H. instrument set
- H. mallet
- H. meniscal retractor
- H. plaster spreader

Henoch-Schönlein purpura
Henry
- H. acromioclavicular technique
- H. anterior strap approach

- H. anterolateral radial shaft approach
- H. bone graft
- H. extensile approach
- H. femoral neck resection
- H. incision
- H. knot
- knot of H.
- leash of H.
- ligament of H.
- master knot of H.
- H. paralysis
- H. posterior interosseous nerve approach
- H. posterior interosseous nerve exposure
- posterolateral approach of H.
- H. radial approach

Hensen plane
heparin
- reconstituted depolymerized h.

heparinized
- h. Ringer lactate solution
- h. saline flush

hepatotoxicity
herb
- ayurvedic h.

herbal therapy
Herbert
- H. bone screw
- H. bone screw fixation
- H. bone screw system
- H. jig
- H. knee prosthesis
- H. saw
- H. scaphoid bone fracture
- H. scaphoid bone fracture classification
- H. scaphoid screw
- H. screw fixator

Herbert-Whipple bone screw
Hercules
- H. plaster shears
- H. TM drop-adjusting table

Herczel rib elevator
hereditaria
- myotonia h.

hereditary
- h. deforming chondrodysplasia
- h. essential myoclonus
- h. motor sensory neuropathy (HMSN)
- h. multiple exostosis
- h. neuropathic disease
- h. onychoosteodysplasia
- h. osteoonychodysplasia (HOOD)
- h. progressive arthroophthalmopathy
- h. spinocerebellar ataxia

heredopathia atactica polyneuritiformis

Herendeen phenomenon
Heritage hip system
Hermes
    H. Evolution tricompartmental knee
    system
    H. total knee system
Hermodsson
    H. fracture
    H. internal rotation
    H. internal rotation shoulder view
    H. internal rotation technique
    H. tangential shoulder view
Hermosa bone harvester
Hernandez-Ros bone staple
Herndon hip classification
hernia, *pl.* **hernias,** *pl.* **herniae**
    footballer's h.
    muscle h.
    Schmorl h.
    sportsman's h.
    synovial h.
herniae (*pl. of* hernia)
hernias (*pl. of* hernia)
herniated
    h. disc
    h. intervertebral disc
    h. nucleus pulposus (HNP)
herniation
    central h.
    cervical midline disc h.
    contained disc h.
    disc h.
    extruding-type h.
    intervertebral disc h.
    intraspongy nuclear disc h.
    midline disc h.
    migrating-type h.
    noncontained disc h.
    phalangeal h.
    posterolateral h.
    synovial h.
    traumatic cervical disc h.
herpes
    h. gladiatorum
    h. simplex
herpetic whitlow
Herring
    H. lateral pillar Perthes disease (A,
    B, C) classification
    H. lateral pillar radiographic
    classification
Herzenberg bolt
Herzmark frame
Hessco 300, 500 series hydrotherapy
  table
Hessing brace
heterodermic graft
heterogeneous graft
heterogenesis

heterogenous graft
heterograft
heteroplasia
    hemimelic progressive osseous h.
    progressive osseous h.
heterotopic
    h. bone
    h. calcification
    h. ossification
    h. ossification prevention
Heuter-Volkmann law
Hewson
    H. breakaway pin
    H. cruciate guide
    H. drill
    H. ligament button
    H. ligament drill guide
    H. suture passer
    H. suture retriever
hex
    h. handle curette
    h. head bolt
    h. head pin
    h. head screwdriver
    h. screw
    h. wrench
hexachlorophene
Hexadrol Phosphate
hexagonal slot-cap screw
Hexcel
    H. knee prosthesis
    H. total condylar knee system
    H. total condylar prosthesis
Hexcelite
Hex-Fix
    H.-F. Add-A-Clamp
    H.-F. external fixation
    H.-F. monolateral external fixator
    H.-F. Universal swivel clamp
hexhead
Hey
    H. amputation
    H. Groves clamp
    H. Groves fascia lata technique
    H. Groves-Kirk technique
    H. Groves ligament reconstruction
    technique
    H. Groves procedure
    H. internal derangement
    H. operation
Heyer-Schulte
    H.-S. antisiphon device
    H.-S. bur hole valve
    H.-S. wound drain
Heyman
    H. hip classification
    H. operation
    H. procedure
    H. technique

H

Heyman-Herndon
 H.-H. clubfoot operation
 H.-H. epiphysiodesis
 H.-H. procedure
 H.-H. release
Heyman-Herndon-Strong capsular release
HFI
 Hand Functional Index
Hg
 mercury
HG
 HG multilock hip prosthesis
 HG multilock hip stem
hGH
 human growth hormone
HGO
 hip guidance orthosis
H-graft
 H-g. bone graft
 H-g. fusion
H1209 healing shoe
H1215 healing shoe
HHS
 Harris hip score
HHW
 handheld weight
Hi
 Darco Body Armor H.
 H. Speed Pulse lavage
HIAD
 high-impact aerobic dance
hiatal sign
hiatus (*pl. of* hiatus)
 adductor h.
 popliteal h.
 h. totalis sacralis
Hibbs
 H. arthrodesis
 H. blade
 H. bone-cutting forceps
 H. chisel
 H. chisel elevator
 H. curette
 H. curved osteotome
 H. extensor tendon transfer cavus deformity
 H. frame
 H. gouge
 H. lumbar fusion procedure
 H. mallet
 H. metatarsocalcaneal angle
 H. operation
 H. retractor
 H. spinal fusion
 H. straight osteotome
 H. tendosuspension
hibernoma
Hibiclens
 H. scrub

H. solution
H. Topical
Hibistat Topical
Hick effect
hickory-stick fracture
Hicks lugged plate
hidroacanthoma simplex
hierarchial
 h. ADL scale
 h. scale of ADLs
hierarchical control
HIFix skull pin
high
 h. heel shoe
 h. Knight brace
 h. median-high radial palsy
 h. median-high ulnar palsy
 h. molecular weight polyethylene (HMWPE)
 h. muscular resistance bed
 h. performance silicone elastomer
 h. tibial osteotomy (HTO)
 h. tibial osteotomy fixator
 h. toe box
 h. ulnar-high radial palsy
 h. velocity, low amplitude
high-air-loss bed
high-altitude
 h.-a. activity
 h.-a. adaptation
 h.-a. maladaptation
high-assimilation pelvis
high-definition video display
high-density foam
high-dose traction
high-energy
 h.-e. fracture
 h.-e. metaphysial distal tibia fracture
 h.-e. trauma
highest turbinated bone
high-frequency discharge
high-grade
 h.-g. spondylolisthesis
 h.-g. surface osteogenic sarcoma
 h.-g. ulcer
high-impact
 h.-i. activity
 h.-i. aerobic dance (HIAD)
high-level disinfectant
high-performance liquid chromatography
high-power athlete
high-prow heel
high-resolution analysis
high-riding patella
high-risk factor
high-speed
 h.-s. bur
 h.-s. twist drill
high-steppage gait

high-tide walking brace
high-torque bur
high-velocity low-amplitude thrust technique
high-voltage
    h.-v. galvanism
    h.-v. pulsed galvanic
    h.-v. pulsed galvanic stimulation (HVPGS)
    h.-v. pulsed stimulation (HVPS)
    h.-v. therapy (HVT)
hila (*pl. of* hilum)
hilar
Hilgenreiner
    H. acetabular angle
    H. brace
    H. horizontal Y line
Hilgenreiner-Perkins (H-P)
    H.-P. pelvic x-ray line
Hill Air-Drop HA90C table
Hillock arch
Hill-Rom orthopaedic bed
Hill-Sachs
    H.-S. AP shoulder view
    H.-S. defect
    H.-S. deformity
    H.-S. fracture
    H.-S. lesion
    H.-S. shoulder dislocation
    H.-S. sign
hill-shaped ossification
hi-lo table
hilum, *pl.* **hila**
    neurovascular h.
    h. of tendon
Hinderer
    H. cartilage forceps
    H. malar prosthesis
hindfoot
    h. amputation
    h. anatomic variation
    h. arthrodesis
    h. cavus
    h. deformity
    h. excursion
    h. FPA
    h. instability
    h. joint complex
    h. kinematics
    lateral h.
    h. motion
    h. orthosis
    h. pronation
    h. reconstruction
    spastic varus h.
    h. supination
    h. valgus
    varus h.
hindfoot-midfoot collapse

hindquarter amputation
hinge
    h. abduction
    Adjusta-Wrist h.
    AHSC-Volz h.
    Arizona Health Sciences Center-Volz h.
    h. articulation
    h. axis concept
    Bahler h.
    camber axis h. (CAH)
    Compass h.
    Dee elbow h.
    elbow h.
    flail-elbow h.
    Genucentric knee h.
    implant h.
    Kinematic rotation h.
    Kudo h.
    Lacey h.
    medial/plantar h.
    Noiles h.
    offset h.
    Quengel h.
    Rancho Los Amigos swivel h.
    h. rod
    rotating h.
    soft tissue h.
    stabilizing h.
hinged
    h. articulated fixator
    h. constrained knee prosthesis
    h. cylinder cast
    h. cylinder splint
    h. elbow external fixator
    h. fragment
    h. great toe replacement prosthesis
    h. implant
    h. implant prosthesis
    h. joint
    h. knee brace
    h. Thomas splint
    h. total knee prosthesis
hinged-distraction apparatus
hinging
    hip h.
HINT
    Harris Infant Neuromotor Test
HIO
    hole-in-1
    hole-in-1 technique
    HIO technique
hip
    h. abduction
    h. abduction stress test
    h. abductor strengthening exercise
    anthropometric total h. (ATH)
    h. arthroplasty
    h. avulsion fracture

H

hip (*continued*)
  h. axis length
  biologically designed h. (BDH)
  h. bump
  h. bursitis
  h. click
  h. compression screw
  congenital dislocation of h.
  congenital dysplasia of h. (CDH)
  h. cup
  cup-on-cup arthroplasty of h.
  DePuy AML h.
  developmental dislocation of h.
    (DDH)
  developmental dysplasia of h.
    (DDH)
  h. disarticulation prosthesis
  h. disarticulation suspension
  h. dislocation
  h. dislocation classification
  h. dysplasia
  dysplasia of h.
  h. epiphysial injury
  h. extension
  h. extension exercise
  h. extension range of motion
  h. extensor gait
  h. flexion
  h. flexion-extension
  h. flexor contracture
  h. fracture compaction drill
  h. fracture compaction drill bit
  fused h.
  h. guidance orthosis (HGO)
  hanging h.
  h. hemipelvectomy suspension
  h. hinge back exercise technique
  h. hinging
  hockey player's h.
  irritable h.
  ischemic disease of growing h.
    (IDGH)
  h. joint angle (HJA)
  h. joint aspiration under fluoroscopic
    control
  h. joint capsule
  h. joint syndrome
  Kinamed anthropometric total h.
  Link anatomical h.
  Metasul metal-on-metal h.
  h. mobility
  observation h.
  1-stage correction of spastic
    dislocated h.
  h. orthosis
  pillow orthosis for h.
  h. pin
  h. pinning
  h. pocket neuropathy

  h. pointer
  h. pointer contusion
  Precision total h.
  h. quadrant test
  h. reduction
  h. replacement
  h. replacement prosthesis
  h. revision
  revision of total h.
  h. roll
  h. rotation
  h. scouring test
  Senegas transtrochanteric lateral
    approach to h.
  h. skid
  snapping h.
  H. Society
  h. spica
  h. spica cast
  h. subluxation
  tuberculosis of h.
  H. Vitox
  H. Vitox alumina ceramic material
  H. Vitox femoral head
  windblown h.
  windswept h.
  Zimmer MIS 2-incision
    posterior h.
HIPciser abduction splint
hipGRIP body positioning device
hip-knee-ankle (HKA)
  h.-k.-a. angle
hip-knee-ankle-foot orthosis (HKAFO)
Hipokrat bimodular shoulder system
Hippocrates
  H. cap-shaped bandage
  H. manipulation
hippocratic
  h. finger
  h. maneuver
hipRAP
  orthoRAP h.
HipSaver protective underwear
hip-to-ankle
  h.-t.-a. view
  h.-t.-a. x-ray
Hirabayashi
  H. laminaplasty
  H. unilateral open door cervical
    laminaplasty
Hirabayashi-type laminaplasty
Hirayma osteotomy
Hiroshima free muscle transfer
Hirsch
  H. hypophysial punch
  H. hypophysis punch forceps
Hirschberg
  H. reflex
  H. sign

Hirschhorn
    H. compression technique
    H. fracture compression plate
      approach
Hirschtick utility shoulder splint
hirudin
His-Haas procedure
histiocytic tumor
histiocytoma
    angiomatoid malignant fibrous h.
      (AMFH)
    fibrous h.
    malignant fibrous h. (MFH)
    nevoid h.
    pleomorphic fibrous h.
histiocytosis
    granular h.
    Langerhans cell h.
    sinus h.
Histoacryl
    H. glue
    H. glue adhesive
histochemistry
Histofreezer
    H. cryosurgical system
    H. cryosurgical wart treatment
      kit
histogenesis
    distraction h.
histologic, histological
histological (*var. of* histologic)
histomorphometry
histopathology
    synovial h.
Histoplasma capsulatum
histoplasmosis
hitch
    ankle h.
    spinal h.
Hitchcock
    H. arm procedure
    H. biceps tendon technique
    H. stereotactic immobilization
      frame
hitchhiker's thumb
Hi-Top
    H.-T. foot/ankle brace
    H.-T. foot/ankle walker
    H.-T. II adjustable walker
    H.-T. shoe
Hittenberger
    H. halo extension
    H. prosthesis
Hivid
HJA
    hip joint angle
HJD
    Hospital for Joint Disease
    HJD total hip system

HKA
    hip-knee-ankle
    HKA angle
HKAFO
    hip-knee-ankle-foot orthosis
HLA
    human leukocyte antigen
    HLA B27 blood antigen
    HLA B27 related
      spondyloarthropathy syndrome
HLT-405 instrument adjusting table
HM
    heloma molle
HMD
    head-mounted display
HMIS
    hallux metatarsophalangeal
      interphalangeal scale
HMS
    hypermobility syndrome
HMSN
    hereditary motor sensory neuropathy
HMWPE
    high molecular weight polyethylene
HNA
    hypothalamoneurohypophysial axis
HNP
    herniated nucleus pulposus
HO
    heel-off
    HO gait-related risk factor
H₂O2
    hydrogen peroxide
HOA
    hypertrophic osteoarthroscopy
Hoaglund bone graft
hobbling gait
Hobb sternoclavicular joint view
hockey
    ice h.
    h. player's hip
    h. stick incision
hockey-stick
    h.-s. dissector
    h.-s. fracture
Hodgen
    H. hip splint
    H. leg splint
Hodge plane
**Hodgkinson acetabular component
loosening criteria**
Hodgson hypospadias repair technique
Hodor-Dobbs procedure
Hoen
    H. clamp
    H. forceps
    H. gouge
    H. periosteal elevator
    H. retractor

H

Hoen (*continued*)
    H. rongeur
    H. skull plate
Hoffa
    H. disease
    H. fat-pad
    H. fracture
    H. intercondylar femoral fracture
    H. massage
    H. operation
    H. sign
    H. syndrome
    H. tendon shortening
    H. tendon-shortening method
    H. test
Hoffa-Kastert disease
Hoffa-Lorenz operation
Hoffer
    H. ankle procedure
    H. split tendon transfer
Hoffmann
    H. apex fixation pin
    H. approach
    H. C-series external fixator
    H. dynamic external fixator
    H. external fixation
    H. external fixation system
    H. frame
    H. II compact external fixation
      component
    H. ligament clamp
    H. metatarsal operation
    H. metatarsal procedure
    H. mini-lengthening fixation device
    H. muscular atrophy
    H. panmetatarsal head resection
    H. pin guide
    H. reflex
    H. sign
    H. syndrome
    H. transfixion pin
Hoffmann-Vidal
    H.-V. double frame
    H.-V. external fixation apparatus
    H.-V. external fixation device
    H.-V. external fixator
Hogg chair
Hohl-Luck tibial plateau fracture
    classification
Hohl-Moore tibial plateau fracture
    repair technique
Hohl tibial condylar fracture
    classification
Hohmann
    H. bone retractor
    H. bunionectomy
    H. hallux osteotomy procedure
    H. operation
    H. osteotomy

Hohmann-Thomasen metatarsal osteotomy
Hoke
    H. Achilles tendon lengthening
    H. Achilles tendon lengthening
      operation
    H. lumbar brace
    H. lumbar brace/corset
    H. lumbar corset
    H. osteotome
    H. procedure for tibial palsy
    H. tibial palsy procedure
    H. triple arthrodesis
    H. triple-section method
Hoke-Kite arthrodesis technique
Hoke-Martin traction
Hoke-Miller pes planus procedure
hold
    choke h.
holder
    acetabular cup h.
    Alvarado knee h.
    arm h.
    arthroscopic leg h.
    Barraquer needle h.
    Böhler-Steinmann pin h.
    bone h.
    Castroviejo needle h.
    Charnley trochanter h.
    clamp h.
    Crile-Wood needle h.
    cup h.
    DeMartel-Wolfson clamp h.
    Donaghy angled suture needle h.
    Drummond hook h.
    Ferguson bone h.
    Halsey needle h.
    head h.
    hook h.
    hookbar h.
    Jacobson needle h.
    knee h.
    leg h.
    limb h.
    Malis needle h.
    Mayo-Hegar needle h.
    McConnell arm h.
    microneedle h.
    needle h.
    neonatal tracheostomy tube h.
    octopus h.
    operative leg h.
    OSI arthroscopic leg h.
    pin h.
    Rhoton needle h.
    rod h.
    Ryder needle h.
    Sarot needle h.
    Schmidt rod h.
    shoulder h.

staple h.
thigh h.
tibial track h.
trochanter h.
TSRH hook h.
Wangensteen needle h.
washer h.
Watanabe pin h.
Webster needle h.
well-leg h.
Yasargil needle h.

holder/scissors
holding mitt
hold-relax
h.-r. method
h.-r. technique
Holdsworth spinal fracture classification
3-hole
3-h. plate
3-h. suture tendon fixation
4-hole
4-h. Alta straight plate
4-h. side plate
hole
acetabular seating h.
anchor h.
anchoring h.
blind anchorage h.
bone hook with cable/wire h.
bur h.
cable/wire h.
centering h.
drill h.
glide h.
gliding h.
guide h.
lag screw thread h.
offset drill h.
h. preparation method
10-hole blade-plate
hole-in-1 (HIO)
h.-i.-1. technique (HIO)
9-hole peg test
2-hole plate
5-hole plate
6-hole plate
7-hole plate
11-hole plate
17-hole plate
holism
Hollander clog
Hollingshead Index
Hollister Hot/Ice knee blanket
hollow
h. back
h. bone
h. bone trephine
h. chisel

h. foot
h. foot clawfoot deformity
h. mill Asnis cannulated screw
h. mill drill
h. mill instrumentation
h. mill reamer
Hollywood
H. bed
H. bed extension hook set
H. roll technique
H. thoracolumbar fusion interbody VBR
Holmes
H. operation
H. phenomenon
rebound phenomenon of H.
Holmes-Rahe Life Change Index
Holmes-Stewart phenomenon
holmium YAG laser
holorachischisis
Holscher
H. knee retractor
H. root retractor
Holstein fracture of humerus
Holstein-Lewis fracture
Holt
H. bolt
H. nail
H. nail plate
Holter traction
Holt-Oram dysplasia
Holzheimer retractor
Homans
H. sign
H. venous thrombosis of leg test
HOME
Home Observation and Measurement of the Environment
home
h. assessment
h. cervical traction unit (HCTU)
h. exercise program
h. medical equipment
H. Observation and Measurement of the Environment (HOME)
H. Ranger shoulder pulley
h. rehabilitation
h. spinal stabilization program
homeopathy
homeostasis
fluid h.
osseous h.
HomeStretch lumbar traction
HomeTrac
Saunders cervical H.
hominis
Dermatobia h.
homogeneous graft

H

homograft
    h. implant material
    h. prosthesis
homolog
    meniscus h.
homologous graft
homonymous hemianopsia
homoplastic graft
homuncular organization
homunculus
honeycomb pattern
HOOD
    hereditary osteoonychodysplasia
hood
    dorsal h.
    extensor h.
    retinacular h.
hook
    Acufex nerve h.
    anatomic h.
    h. approximator
    APRL prosthetic h.
    Army Prosthetic Research Lab
      prosthetic h.
    Austin Moore h.
    Barr h.
    bifid h.
    h. blade
    h. blocker
    blunt h.
    Bobechko sliding barrel h.
    h. body
    bone h.
    Boyes-Goodfellow h.
    button h.
    buttressed h.
    canted finger h.
    Carroll skin h.
    C-D h.
    h. clamp
    clawed pedicle h.
    closed Cotrel-Dubousset h.
    closed transverse process TSRH h.
    compression h.
    Cotrel-Dubousset h.
    cranial Jacobs h.
    Culler h.
    Cushing dural h.
    h. dislodgment
    distraction h.
    h. distractor
    Dorrance h.
    double-open h.
    double-pronged skin h.
    down-angle h.
    downsized circular laminar h.
    drop-entry closed body h.
    Drummond h.
    dura h.

    Edwards h.
    Edwards-Levine h.
    Effler-Groves h.
    finger h.
    garment h.
    Gillies bone h.
    Gillies-Dingman h.
    glide h.
    Graham muscle h.
    Graham nerve h.
    h. grasp
    Green muscle h.
    hamate h.
    Harrington pedicle (bifid) h.
    H. hemi-harness shoulder
      immobilizer
    h. holder
    h. hollow-ground connection design
    Hosmer Dorrance h.
    h. impactor
    intermediate C-D h.
    Isola spinal implant system h.
    Jameson muscle h.
    Jannetta h.
    jig h.
    Joseph h.
    Keene compression h.
    Kennerdell-Maroon h.
    Kilner h.
    Kirby muscle h.
    Knodt rod and h.
    Küntscher nail-extracting h.
    Lahey Clinic dural h.
    Lambotte bone h.
    laminar C-D h.
    Leatherman h.
    lyre-shaped finger h.
    meniscus h.
    Micro-One h.
    Moe alar h.
    Moss h.
    multispan fracture h.
    nail-extracting h.
    nerve h.
    neutral h.
    O'Brien rib h.
    Oesch h.
    h. of hamate
    h. of hamate bone
    open C-D h.
    Osher irrigating implant h.
    PCL-oriented placement marking h.
    pediatric C-D h.
    pediatric TSRH h.
    pedicle C-D h.
    h. pin
    h. plate
    h. probe system
    prosthetic h.

h. pusher
ribbed h.
right-angle h.
Rogozinski h.
h. rotary scissors
Selby I, II h.
sharp worm h.
side-opening laminar h.
h. site
skin h.
sliding barrel h.
split-finger h.
square-ended h.
T-handled h.
top-entry h.
traction h.
h. trial set screw
TSRH buttressed laminar h.
TSRH circular laminar h.
TSRH pedicle h.
TSRH trial h.
twist h.
up-angle h.
vessel h.
h. V-groove connection design
Vilex Ouchless H.
Volkmann bone h.
Yasargil spring h.
Zielke bifid h.
Zuelzer h.
hookbar holder
hooked
h. acromion
h. bone
h. foot
h. forefoot
h. intramedullary nail
h. knife
h. medullary nail
hook-end intramedullary pin
hookian region
hook-lying pectoral stretch
  exercise
hook-nail deformity
hook-pin fixation
hook-plate fixation
hook-rod
Cotrel-Dubousset h.-r.
Isola h.-r.
TSRH h.-r.
hook-to-screw L4-S1 compression
  construct
hoop stress fracture
Hoover
H. paralyzed leg test
H. sign
hop
h. index
h. test

hope
Planning Alternative Tomorrows with
  H. (PATH)
Hopkins plaster knife
Hoppenfeld lateral knee approach
Hori umbilicus reconstruction
  technique
horizontal
h. cleavage
h. external rotation
h. fracture
h. gantry cut
h. mattress suture
h. meniscal tear
h. osteotomy
h. pedicle diameter
h. plane
h. platform support (HPS)
h. position
h. shoulder abduction exercise
h. suspension
h. suspension response
h. Y line
hormone
adrenocorticotropic h. (ACTH)
growth h.
human growth h. (hGH)
thyrotropin-releasing h.
  (TRH)
horn
anterior h.
bone graft shoe h.
central h.
cutaneous h.
enlarged frontal h.
posterior h.
shoulder h.
horse
charley h.
horseback rider's knee
horse-hoof fracture nonunion
horse's foot callus
horseshoe
h. abscess
h. appearance
h. heel pad
h. patellofemoral brace
h. therapy table
horseshoe-shaped
h.-s. felt pad
h.-s. flap
horse-tail Achilles tendon tear
Horsley
H. bone cutter
H. bone-cutting forceps
H. bone rongeur
H. bone saw
H. bone wax
H. separator

H

Horsley-Stille
    H.-S. bone-cutting forceps
    H.-S. rib shears forceps
Horwitz
    H. ankle fusion
    H. ankle fusion approach
    H. transmalleolar arthrodesis
Horwitz-Adams
    H.-A. ankle fusion
    H.-A. arthrodesis
hose
    TED h.
    Venosan support h.
Hosmer
    H. above-knee rotator
    H. Dorrance hook
    H. Dorrance voluntary control 4-bar
    knee mechanism
    H. Endurance knee
    H. single-axis friction knee
    H. single-axis locking knee
    H. VC 4-bar knee orthosis
    H. WALK prosthesis
    H. weight-activated locking knee
hospital
    H. for Joint Disease (HJD)
    H. for Special Surgery (HSS)
    H. for Special Surgery knee score
    H. for Special Surgery scale
    Imperial College London H.
    (ICLH)
    Texas Scottish Rite H.
    (TSRH)
    H. Trauma Index
host
    h. bone
    h. immune reaction
host-allograft junction
hot
    h. and cold contrast bath
    h. dog technique
    h. fomentation therapy
    h. joint
    h. knife
    h. moist pack
    h. plate
    h. water bath
    h. weld
hot-cross-bun
    h.-c.-b. skull
    h.-c.-b. skull sign
hot/ice
    h. cold therapy cooler therapy
    device
    H. System III
Hotsy Cautery
hourglass
    h. capsulotomy
    h. constriction

    h. deformity
    h. vertebra
    H. vertebral body spacer
House-Dieter malleus nipper
household ambulatory
housemaid's knee
House upper limb reconstruction
Houston
    H. halo cervical support
    H. halo cervical traction
    H. halo traction cervical collar
    H. operation
Howard
    H. bone block
    H. differential ureteral catheterization
    technique
Howell tibial guide
Howmedica
    H. bone anchor
    H. cement
    H. cerclage
    H. cerclage cable
    H. Duracon implant
    H. ICS screw
    H. Kinematic II knee prosthesis
    H. knee instrumentation
    H. knee system
    H. Microfixation System drill bit
    H. Microfixation System forceps
    H. Microfixation System plate
    cutter
    H. Microfixation System pliers
    H. monospherical implant
    H. monotube
    H. monotube external rotator
    H. PCA prosthesis
    H. total ankle system
    H. universal compression screw
    H. Vitallium staple
    H. VSF fixation system
Howmedica-Osteonics instrument
Howorth
    H. approach
    H. hip procedure
    H. prosthesis
Howse
    H. prosthesis
    H. total hip replacement
Howship lacuna
Hoyer
    H. lift
    H. traction
H-P
    Hilgenreiner-Perkins
    H-P pelvic x-ray lines
HP
    Vicodin HP
HP-100
    Silastic HP-100

HPA
  hypothalamic-pituitary-adrenal
    HPA axis
H.P. Acthar Gel
HPS
  horizontal platform support
    HPS II total hip prosthesis
H-reflex
HRQOL
  health-related quality of life
H-shaped
    H-s. capsular incision
    H-s. graft
    H-s. plate
HSS
  Hospital for Special Surgery
    HSS knee ligament rating
    HSS knee score
    HSS total condylar knee
      prosthesis
HTO
  high tibial osteotomy
    HTO fixator
    HTO wedge human donor tissue
      allograft
HTS
  hammer toe syndrome
H-type sacral fracture with associated
  spinopelvic dissociation injury
Hubbard
    H. bolt
    H. physical therapy tank
    H. side plate
hubbed needle
Huber
    H. abductor digiti minimi transfer
    H. adductor digiti quinti
      opponensplasty
    H. transfer of abductor digiti quinti
Hubscher adult flatfoot maneuver
Huckstep
    H. nail
    H. nail arthrodesis
Hudson
    H. bone bur
    H. bone drill
    H. brace drill
    H. brace with bur
    H. bur
    H. chuck adapter
    H. forceps
    H. Hydrofloat Cushion
    H. TLSO brace
Hudson-Jones knee-cage brace
Hueter
    H. bandage
    H. line
    H. sign
Hughes fixation

Hughston
    H. Clinic injury classification
    H. external rotation recurvatum test
    H. hypoplastic dislocation of patella
      realignment
    H. knee evaluation
    H. knee jerk test
    H. knee scope
    H. knee score
    H. lateral compartment
      reconstruction
    H. lateral knee instability procedure
    H. patella view
    H. plica knee test
    H. posterolateral drawer knee test
    H. posteromedial drawer knee test
Hughston-Losee jerk test
human
    h. botfly
    h. cancellous bone
    h. chorionic gonadotropin
    h. cortical bone
    h. growth hormone (hGH)
    h. leukocyte antigen (HLA)
    h. lymphocyte antigen
    h. osteogenic sarcoma
    h. skin equivalent
humanism
Humby knife
humeral
    h. avulsion
    h. avulsion of glenohumeral
      lesion
    h. avulsion of glenohumeral
      ligament (HAGL)
    h. bone
    h. brace
    h. canal
    h. chondroblastoma
    h. circumflex vessel
    h. component
    h. condyle
    h. cutting guide
    h. device
    h. diaphysis
    h. epicondyle
    h. epicondylitis
    h. epiphysis
    h. fracture abduction splint
    h. fracture malunion
    h. head
    h. head retractor
    h. head-splitting fracture
    h. impactor
    h. joint
    h. mechanism
    h. neck
    h. physial fracture
    h. reamer

H

humeral (*continued*)
  h. saw
  h. shaft fracture
  h. supracondylar fracture
humeri (*gen.* and *pl. of* humerus)
humeroperoneal muscular dystrophy
humeroradial
  h. articulation
  h. joint
humerothoracic abduction
humeroulnar
  h. angle
  h. articulation
  h. joint
humerus, *gen.* and *pl.* **humeri**
  articulatio humeri
  capitulum humeri
  capitulum of h.
  distal h.
  Holstein fracture of h.
  medial epicondyle of h.
  periarthrosis humeri
  proximal h.
  pseudocyst of h.
  pseudodislocation of h.
  h. sulcus
humoral immunity
hump
  buffalo h.
  dowager's h.
  rib h.
humpback deformity
humpbacked spinal curvature
Humphry ligament
hunchback
Hungarian grip plate
Hungerford-Krackow-Kenna knee arthroplasty
Hungerford technique
hungry bone syndrome
hung-up knee jerk
hunter
  H. canal
  H. open cord tendon implant
  H. silastic prosthesis
  H. silastic rod
  H. tendon prosthesis
Hunter-Thompson dwarfism
hunting
  h. reaction
  h. response
Huntington
  H. bone graft
  H. sign
  H. tibial technique
Hunt paradoxical phenomenon
Hunt-Thompson pantalar arthrodesis
Hurd bone-cutting forceps

Hurler
  H. disease
  H. polydystrophy
  H. syndrome
Hurler-Scheie
  H.-S. compound
  H.-S. syndrome
Husk bone rongeur
Hutchinson
  H. fracture
  melanotic whitlow of H.
  H. teeth
HV
  hallux valgus
  HV NightSplint splint
  HV SoftSplint splint
HVA
  hallux valgus angle
HVPGS
  high-voltage pulsed galvanic stimulation
HVPS
  high-voltage pulsed stimulation
HVT
  high-voltage therapy
Hyalgan injection
hyaline
  h. cartilage
  h. cartilage detritus
  h. cartilage implant
  h. necrosis
hyalinization
hyalinum
  Scytalidium h.
hyaluronan
hyaluronate
  sodium h.
hyaluronidase
hybrid
  h. external fixator
  h. fixation
  h. fixation of hip replacement component
  h. instrumentation
  h. total hip replacement
HybridFit
  H. total hip system
  H. total knee system
Hycort
hydatidosis
  spinal h.
  vertebral h.
hydatid resonance
Hydra-Cadence
  H.-C. gait-control unit
  H.-C. knee prosthesis
Hydragrip clamp insert
hydrarthrodial

hydrarthrosis
    intermittent h.
hydrate
    chloral h.
hydration status
hydraulic
    h. knee unit
    h. knee unit prosthesis
    h. test system
hydrisalic gel
Hydrisinol
    H. creme
    H. lotion
hydrobromide (HBr)
    citalopram h.
hydrocele
    Dupuytren h.
hydrocephalus, hydrocephaly
hydrocephaly (*var. of* hydrocephalus)
Hydrocet
hydrochloride (HCl)
    alfentanil h.
    amiprilose h.
    naloxone h.
    oxycodone h.
    oxymorphone h.
    pentazocine h.
    phencyclidine h.
    propoxyphene h.
    tramadol h.
hydrocodone
    h. and acetaminophen
    h. and aspirin
    h. and ibuprofen
    h. bitartrate and ibuprofen
hydrocollator
    h. heating unit
    H. pad
    h. steam pack
hydrocolloid occlusive dressing
Hydrocol wound dressing
hydrocortisone
    bacitracin, neomycin, polymyxin B, and h.
    neomycin and h.
    neomycin, polymyxin B, and h.
    h. phonophoresis
Hydrocortone
    H. Acetate
    H. Phosphate
Hydrocort Topical
HydroFlex arthroscopy irrigating system
hydrofloat cushion
Hydrogel
    Lido-Gel topical anesthetic H.
    H. wound dressing
hydrogen (H)
    h. peroxide (H_2O_2, H_2O_2)
    h. washout blood flow method

Hydrogesic
hydroma (*var. of* hygroma)
hydromassage table
hydromelia
hydromorphone
Hydron Burn Bandage
hydrophilia
    Aeromonas h.
hydrophilic dressing
hydropneumogony
hydrops canal
HydroSoothe recliner
hydrostatic pressure
HydroStat IR
hydrosyringomyelia
    communicating h.
hydrotherapy
    AquaMED dry h.
    dry h.
Hydro-Tone Bell
HydroTrack underwater treadmill system
hydroxyapatite (HA), hydroxylapatite
    h. adhesive
    h. bone
    h. bone replacement material
    calcium h. (CHA)
    h. cement
    coralline h.
    h. deposition disease
    h. implant material
    LLPS h.
    PureFix h.
    h. tetra-tri-calcium phosphate
hydroxyapatite-coated
    h.-c. ankle arthroplasty
    h.-c. porous alumni cement
    h.-c. stem
hydroxychloroquine
hydroxylapatite (*var. of* hydroxyapatite)
25-hydroxyvitamin D
hydroxyzine
hygroma, hydroma
    cystic h.
Hylamer
    H. enhanced ultra-high molecular weight polyethylene acetabular liner
    H. orthopaedic bearing polymer
Hyland's Leg Cramps with Quinine
Hylin rasp
hyoid
    h. bone
    h. syndrome
hypaesthesia (*var. of* hypesthesia)
hypalgesia, hypoalgesia, hypalgia
hypalgia (*var. of* hypalgesia)
hyperabduction
    h. maneuver
    h. thoracic outlet test

H

hyperactive
  h. reflex
  h. response
hyperactivity
  physiological h.
hyperaemic (*var. of* hyperemic)
hyperaesthesia (*var. of* hyperesthesia)
hyperaesthetic (*var. of* hyperesthetic)
hyperalgesia, hyperalgia
hyperalgia (*var. of* hyperalgesia)
hyperalimentation
hyperanteflexion sprain
hyperbaric
  h. oxygen (HBO)
  h. oxygen therapy
hypercalcaemia (*var. of* hypercalcemia)
hypercalcemia, hypercalcaemia
hypercortisolism
hyperdorsiflexion
hyperdynamic abductor hallucis
hyperemia
hyperemic, hyperaemic
hyperesthesia, hyperaesthesia
hyperesthetic, hyperaesthetic
hyperextend
hyperextended knee gait
hyperextensibility
  joint h.
  h. of joint
hyperextension
  h. brace
  h. cast
  cruciform anterior spinal h.
    (CASH)
  h. deformity
  h. elbow test
  h. injury
  intraoperative neck h.
  neck h.
  h. orthosis
  rebound h.
  recurrent h.
  rigid neck h.
  segmental h.
  h. stress
  h. teardrop fracture
  h. trauma
hyperextension-hyperflexion injury
Hyperex thoracic orthosis
hyperflexed toe compartment syndrome
hyperflexion
  h. injury
  h. teardrop fracture
  h. trauma
hyperhidrosis, hyperidrosis
hyperidrosis (*var. of* hyperhidrosis)
hyperintense
  h. signal
  h. zone

hyperkeratosis
  Kyrle h.
hyperkeratotic lesion
hyperkyphoscoliosis
  neuropathic h.
hyperkyphosis
  thoracic h.
hyperlordosis
hypermobile
  h. flatfoot
  h. foot
  h. joint
  h. joint syndrome
  h. pes planovalgus
hypermobility
  compensatory h.
  joint h.
  h. syndrome (HMS)
hypermyotrophy
hypernephroma
hyperosmotic
hyperosteoidosis
hyperostosis
  ankylosing spinal h.
  Caffey h.
  h. corticalis deformans
  diffuse idiopathic skeletal h.
    (DISH)
  flowing h.
  h. frontalis interna
  infantile cortical h.
  Morgagni h.
  sesamoid h.
  h. syndrome
hyperostotic
  h. bony fusion
  h. spondylosis
hyperparathyroidism
  brown tumor of h.
  h. tumor
hyperpathia
hyperphalangism
hyperphosphatasemic skeletal dysplasia
hyperphosphatasia
hyperpigmented lesion
hyperpituitary gigantism
hyperplantarflexion injury
hyperplasia
  epiphysial h.
  fibrous h.
hyperplastic
  h. bone
  h. callus
  h. chondrodysplasia
  h. osteoarthritis
hyperplastica
  synovitis h.
hyperpolarization
hyperpronation

hyperpyrexia
    malignant h. (MH)
hyperreflexia
    autonomic h.
    detrusor h.
hypersecretion
    growth hormone h.
hypersensitivity syndrome
hyperspectral near-infrared Raman imaging microscopy
hypertension
    calf h.
hyperthermia
    malignant h. (MH)
hyperthermic exercise-associated collapse
hypertonia, hypertonicity
hypertonicity
hypertonus
    thoracolumbar h.
hypertrophia (*var. of* hypertrophy)
hypertrophic
    h. arthritis
    h. cardiomyopathy
    h. chondrocyte
    h. exostosis
    h. flexor retinaculum
    h. granulation tissue
    h. interstitial neuropathy
    h. ligament
    h. osteoarthritis
    h. osteoarthropathy
    h. osteoarthroscopy (HOA)
    h. pulmonary osteoarthropathy
    h. scar
    h. skin
    h. spondylitis
    h. strength training
    h. synovitis
    h. vital nonunion
    h. zone
hypertrophica
    tenosynovitis h.
hypertrophied ligamentum flavum
hypertrophy, hypertrophia
    bone h.
    cartilage h.
    cartilaginous h.
    endemic h.
    endosteal h.
    facet h.
    ligamentous-muscular h.
    smooth muscle h.
    uncinate h.
hypervagotonia
hypervascular
    h. fragment
    h. nonunion
hypesthesia, hypoesthesia, hypaesthesia
Hy-Phen

hypnoanalgesia
hypnoanesthesia
hypnopedia
hypnotic
    h. dissociation
    h. reinterpretation
    h. replacement
    h. therapy
hypoactive deep tendon reflex
hypoaldosteronism
    hyporeninemic h.
hypoalgesia (*var. of* hypalgesia)
hypobaric
    h. microvalve
    H. transfemoral system
    H. transtibial system
hypochondriac region
hypochondriasis
hypochondroplasia
hypocycloidal ankle tomography
hypoechogenicity
hypoechoic intermetatarsal web space mass
hypoesthesia (*var. of* hypesthesia)
hypofibrinolysis
hypoflexibility of foot
hypogastric
    h. artery
    h. flap
hypoglossal nerve
hypointense signal
hypokinetic aberration
hypokyphosis
    right thoracic curve with h.
    thoracic h.
hypolordosis
    cervical h.
    lumbar h.
hypomelia
hypomobile
hyponatremia
    exercise-associated h.
hyponychium
hypoosmotic
hypophalangism
    pedal h.
hypophosphatemic bone disease
hypophyseal (*var. of* hypophysial)
hypophysial, hypophyseal
    h. curette
hypoplasia
    cartilage-hair h. (CHH)
    odontoid h.
    phalangeal h.
    skeletal h.
hypoplastic
    h. disc space
    h. finger
    h. first rib

H

hypoplastic (*continued*)
    h. hand
    h. thumb
hyporeninemic hypoaldosteronism
hypostatic abscess
hypostosis
hypotension
    exertional h.
    postexercise h.
hypotensive
    h. anesthesia
    h. surgery
hypothalamic-pituitary-adrenal (HPA)
    h.-p.-a. axis
hypothalamoneurohypophysial axis (HNA)
hypothenar
    h. eminence
    h. fascia
    h. hammer
    h. hammertoe syndrome
    h. muscle
    h. reflex
hypothermia

hypothermic
hypotheses (*pl. of* hypothesis)
hypothesis, *pl.* **hypotheses**
    axoplasmic aberration h.
    instability h.
    neuroimmune h.
    somatoautonomic reflex h.
hypotonia, hypotonus
    congenital h.
hypotonic fluid
hypotonicity
hypotonus (*var. of* hypotonia)
hypotrophic arthritis
HyProCure
    H. sinus tarsi implant
    H. sinus tarsi implant block
hysteric (*var. of* hysterical)
    h. joint
hysterical, hysteric
    h. gait
    h. joint
    h. scoliosis
Hytakerol

I
 I disc
IAAD
 irreducible anterior atlantoaxial
 dislocation
IADL
 instrumental activity of daily
 living
Iamin hydrating gel
IAR
 instantaneous axis of
 rotation
IASTM
 instrument-assisted soft tissue
 mobilization
iatrogenic
 i. complication
 i. discitis
 i. dural tear
 i. elevatus
 i. infection
 i. injury
 i. loss
 i. lumbar kyphosis
 i. osteomyelitis
 i. spinal cord injury
IB
 Dynafed IB
 Motrin IB
 Sine-Aid IB
I-beam
 I-b. cement punch
 I-b. hemiarthroplasty hip
 prosthesis
 I-b. hip hemiarthroplasty
 I-b. hip operation
 Jergesen I-b.
IBF
 Insall-Burstein-Freeman
 IBF knee instrument
IBG
 iliac bone graft
IBT
 inflatable bone tamp
 KyphX Elevate IBT
 KyphX Exact IBT
ibuprofen
 i. cream
 hydrocodone and i.
 hydrocodone bitartrate and i.
 pseudoephedrine and i.
ICBG
 iliac crest bone graft
ICE
 ice, compression, elevation

ice
 i. application
 i., compression, elevation (ICE)
 i. hockey
 i. immersion
 Liquid I.
 i. massage
 N'ice Stretch night splint suspension
 system with Sealed I.
 i. pack (IP)
 i. pick headache
 i. skater's fracture
 I. Wedge hot/cold therapy wrap
I.C.E. Down cold pack
Iceflex Endurance suction suspension
sleeve
Iceross Comfort Plus silicone gel liner
Icex socket
ICF
 intermediate care facility
ichnogram
ICIDH
 International Classification of
 Impairments, Disabilities, Handicaps
icing
 cutaneous i.
ICLH
 Imperial College London Hospital
 ICLH ankle prosthesis
 ICLH double cup arthroplasty
 ICLH knee prosthesis
ICN
 inferior calcaneonavicular
 intercostal neuralgia
Icon pylon
ICRS
 International Cartilage Repair Society
 ICRS arthroscopic knee, shoulder,
 and ankle joint staging system
I&D
 incision and drainage
IDCN
 intermediate dorsal cutaneous nerve
ideal
 I. spinal implant
 I. suture grasper
Ideberg glenoid fracture classification
Identifit hip prosthesis
IDET
 intradiscal electrothermal therapy
 intradiscal electrothermal treatment
 IDET procedure
IDGH
 ischemic disease of growing hip
idiomuscular

idiopathic
 i. anterior knee pain
 i. arm pain
 i. avascular necrosis
 i. bone cavity
 i. erythromelalgia
 i. fracture
 i. genu valgum (IGV)
 i. hallux valgus
 i. hypertrophic osteoarthropathy (IHO)
 i. juvenile osteoporosis
 i. osteonecrosis
 i. polymyositis myopathy
 i. scoliosis
 i. skeletal
 i. skeletal hyperostosis syndrome
 i. toe-walker (ITW)
 i. toe walking (ITW)
 i. transient osteoporosis

IDK
 internal derangement of knee

IDN
 interdigital neuroma

IEMG
 integrated rectified electromyogram

IF
 internal fixation

IFC
 interferential current
 IFC stimulation
 IFC stimulator
 IFC therapy

I-Flow nerve block infusion kit

IGF
 insulin-like growth factor
 IGF binding protein

IGHL
 inferior glenohumeral ligament
 IGHL insertion

IGV
 idiopathic genu valgum

IHO
 idiopathic hypertrophic osteoarthropathy

IKDC
 International Knee Documentation Committee
 IKDC form
 IKDC score

Ikuta
 I. clamp approximator
 I. fixation
 I. fixation device
 I. free muscle transfer

ILD
 ischemic limb disease

Ilex
 Biofreeze with I.

Ilfeld
 I. brace
 I. splint
 I. splint orthosis

Ilfeld-Gustafson splint

Ilfeld-Holder deformity

ilia (*pl. of* ilium)

iliac
 i. apophysis
 i. apophysis sign
 i. apophysitis
 i. artery
 i. bone
 i. bone graft (IBG)
 i. buttressing procedure
 i. canal
 i. clamp
 i. compression test
 i. crest
 i. crest bone block
 i. crest bone free graft
 i. crest bone graft (ICBG)
 i. crest bone graft stabilization
 i. crest bridge
 i. crest dowel
 i. crest-inlay graft
 i. crest ossification
 i. epiphysis
 i. fixation
 i. oblique view
 i. osteocutaneous flap
 i. osteotomy
 i. post
 i. region
 i. screw
 i. slot graft
 i. spine
 i. strut bone graft
 i. tuberosity
 i. vein
 i. wing
 i. wing resection

iliacus
 i. dysfunction
 i. muscle
 i. syndrome
 i. test

ilial

ilii (*gen. of* ilium)
 ala ossis i.

iliococcygeus muscle

iliocostalis lumborum syndrome

iliocostal muscle

iliofemoral
 i. approach
 i. flap artery
 i. ligament
 i. pedicle flap

i. thrombosis
i. triangle
iliofemoroplasty
iliohypogastric nerve
ilioinguinal
i. acetabular approach
i. nerve
i. nerve entrapment
i. syndrome
iliolumbar
i. artery
i. ligament
i. vein
iliometer
iliopatellar
i. band
i. ligament
iliopectinate bursitis
iliopectineal
i. bursitis
i. line
iliopelvic
iliopsoas
i. bursitis
i. muscle
i. muscle hematoma
i. recession
Sharrard posterior transfer of i.
i. tendon
i. test
i. transfer
iliopubic
iliosacral (IS)
i. and iliac fixation construct
i. articulation
i. implant
i. screw
iliospinal
iliotibial
i. band (ITB)
i. band bursitis
i. band fasciitis
i. band friction syndrome (ITBFS)
i. band graft
i. band graft augmentation
i. band strap
i. band syndrome (ITBS)
i. band tenodesis
i. band transfer
i. tract (ITT)
iliotrochanteric ligament
ilioxiphopagus
ilium, *pl.* **ilia,** *gen.* **ilii**
anterosuperior i.
anterosuperior external i. (ASEX)
anterosuperior internal i. (ASIN)
AS i.
ASEX i.
ASIN i.

i. drainage
external i. (EI)
INEX i.
OS i.
PIEX i.
PIIN i.
piriform sclerosis of i.
wing of i.
Ilizarov
I. ankle arthrodesis
I. ankle fusion technique
I. apparatus
I. circular external fixator
I. corticotomy
I. device
I. distractor
I. external fixation
I. external ring fixator
I. frame
I. hybrid fixator
I. limb lengthening
I. limb lengthening method
I. limb-lengthening system
I. limb-lengthening technique
I. procedure
I. ring
I. screw
I. technique
I. tension-stress effect
I. wire
ill-fitting shoe
illness
illuminator
Cogent XL i.
IM
intramuscular
IM angle
IM joint
IMA
intermetatarsal angle
image
body i.
cockade i.
i. en grelot
i. intensification
i. intensifier
postinjection i.
Image-I analysis software
imagery
mental i.
imaging
bone-forming sarcoma bone i.
cine magnetic resonance i.
(cine-MRI)
color duplex i.
contrast medium-enhanced magnetic
resonance i. (CME-MRI)
delayed bone i.
diagnostic i.

imaging (*continued*)
    dipyridamole thallium i.
    dynamic magnetic resonance i.
      (dMRI)
    extremity magnetic resonance i.
      (E-MRI)
    fixation i.
    functional magnetic resonance i.
      (fMRI)
    gadopentetate-dimeglumine-enhanced
      magnetic resonance i.
    gamma camera i.
    harmonic i.
    indirect magnetic resonance
      arthrography nuclear bone i.
    magnetic resonance i. (MRI)
    magnetic resonance spectroscopic i.
      (MRSI)
    magnetic source i. (MSI)
    magnetization transfer magnetic
      resonance i. (mtMRI)
    multiplanar virtual fluoroscopic i.
    multiple line-scan i. (MLSI)
    orthopantogram i.
    radionucleotide i.
    Raman spectroscopic i.
    sagittal plane i.
    trapezoidal i.

imbalance
    fixed sagittal i.
    isokinetic torque i.
    muscle i.
    rotator cuff i.
    sagittal i.
    sagittal plane i.

imbrication
    capsular i.
    MacNab line for facet i.
    medial capsular i.

IME
    isometric exercise

imipenem and cilastatin

imipramine

IML
    intermetacarpal ligament

immature
    i. achondroplast
    i. bone
    skeletally i.

immediate
    i. amputation
    i. postoperative prosthesis (IPOP)
    i. postoperative stability (IPS)
    i. postsurgical fitting (IPSF)
    i. release
    i. tibial nailing without reaming

immersion
    i. foot
    ice i.

immitis
    Coccidioides i.

immobilisation (*var. of* immobilization)

immobilization, immobilisation
    cast i.
    i. degeneration
    external i.
    halo i.
    halo cast/vest i.
    i. jacket
    joint i.
    i. method
    postoperative i.
    Rowe-Zarins shoulder i.
    skull-occiput-mandibular i. (SOMI)
    sling i.
    sternal-occipital-mandibular i. (SOMI)
    Velcro i.
    Webril i.

immobilizer
    acromioclavicular i.
    ankle i.
    cast i.
    Comfort wrist i.
    DonJoy Ultrasling shoulder i.
    external i.
    Ezy Wrap shoulder i.
    Hook hemi-harness shoulder i.
    joint i.
    knee i.
    Kuz-Medics disposable knee i.
    long leg i.
    OEC knee i.
    Pedi-Wrap i.
    Plastazote-Kydex cervical i.
    postoperative i.
    QuickCast wrist i.
    Raymond shoulder i.
    sateen knee i.
    shoulder abduction i.
    single-panel knee i.
    sling i.
    Slingshot shoulder i.
    sternal-occipital-manubrial i.
    Tab-Strap knee i.
    thumb-wrist i.
    Trimline knee i.
    tri-panel knee i.
    universal sling and swathe
      shoulder i.
    universal tri-panel knee i.
    Velcro i.
    Velpeau shoulder i.
    Watco knee i.
    Westfield-style acromioclavicular i.
    wrist i.
    Y-strap knee i.
    Zimmer knee i.

immobilizing bandage

immovable
    i. articulation
    i. bandage
    i. joint
immune
    i. globulin
    i. system
immunity
    cell-mediated i. (CMI)
    humoral i.
immunoassay
    Alkphase-B i.
immunocompetence
immunogenicity
Immunomount
immunosuppression (IS)
    tolerogenic i.
immunosuppressive therapy (IST)
IMN
    intramedullary nailing
IMP
    Innovative Medical Products
    intramuscular pressure
    IMP bone screw targeter
    IMP knee positioning triangle
    IMP Steri-Clamp
    IMP surgical leg pedestal
    IMP turnstile casting stand
    IMP universal knee positioner
    IMP universal lateral positioner
impact
    i. biomechanics
    direct vertex i.
    i. glove
    i. index
    i. mitt
    I. modular porous prosthesis
    I. modular total hip system
    I. total hip prosthesis
    I. total hip system
impacted
    i. articular fracture
    i. valgus fracture
impaction
    atlantoaxial i.
    i. cancellous autografting
    digital i.
    i. fracture
impactor
    Austin Moore i.
    bone i.
    Cloward bone graft i.
    Cohort spinal i.
    Dawson-Yuhl i.
    femoral i.
    glenoid implant base i.
    hook i.
    humeral i.
    Küntscher i.

    Moe bone i.
    mushroom i.
    orthopaedic i.
    i. rod
    shell i.
    Smith-Petersen i.
    vertebral body i.
impactor-extractor
    Fox i.-e.
impact-reducing pylon
impact-release binding on ski
impaired competitor policy
impairment
    i. assessment
    BFM i.
    chronotropic i.
    neurovascular i.
    physical i.
    proprioceptive i.
    sensory i.
    visual-spatial ability i.
impedance
    bioelectrical i.
    i. plethysmography
imperfecta
    Adair-Dighton osteogenesis i.
    dentinogenesis i. (DGI, DI)
    luxatio i.
    osteogenesis i. (OI)
Imperial College London Hospital (ICLH)
impingement
    ankle i.
    anterior ankle i.
    anterior cord i.
    anterior joint i.
    anterior soft tissue i.
    cam i.
    facet synovial i.
    femoroacetabular i.
    graft i.
    lateral i.
    i. lesion
    i. of shoulder test
    i. pain
    peroneal tendon i.
    pincer-type i.
    posterior i.
    i. reduction test
    repetitive osseous i.
    i. rod
    roof i.
    rotator cuff i.
    i. sign
    i. spur
    i. syndrome
    tibiotalar i.
    ulnocarpal i.
Impingement-Free Tibial Guide System

impinging exostosis
implant

advanced mobile-bearing knee i.
i. alloy aluminum
AO-ASIF orthopaedic i.
i. arthroplasty
articulated chin i.
artificial joint i.
Ascension MCP finger joint i.
Ascension MCP total joint i.
Avanta total wrist surface
  replacement prosthesis i.
Avanta uHead ulnar head i.
BAK/Proximity interbody fusion i.
Bankart Tack i.
bicompartmental i.
BioAction great toe i.
bioactive i.
i. biocompatibility
BioCuff bioresorbable screw and
  spiked washer i.
BioCuff C bioresorbable cannulated
  screw and spike washer i.
BioCuff C bioresorbable spike
  washer i.
biodegradable i.
Biodel i.
Biofix biodegradable i.
biomechanical failure of i.
Biomet custom i.
bioresorbable i.
BioSphere suture anchor i.
i. blank
bone i.
bovine collagen i.
Calnan-Nicolle finger i.
carbon i.
cartilage i.
Cartwright i.
ceramic i.
Charnley i.
chromium i.
chromium-cobalt alloy i.
CKS i.
coated i.
cobalt i.
cobalt-chrome alloy and
  polyethylene i.
cobalt-chromium i.
i. collar
condylar i.
Continuum knee system i.
Coonrad-Morrey hinged elbow i.
Corail HA-coated stem hip i.
CT-based CAD/CAM revision
  femoral i.
curvilinear chin i.
Custodis i.
custom i.

Cutter i.
DePuy orthopaedic i.
digital i.
dorsal columella i.
dorsal column stimulator i.
double-stem silicone i.
DTT i.
Duracon knee i.
Durallium i.
Durapatite bone replacement i.
DynaGraft i.
electrical i.
Ewald-Walker knee i.
i. failure
i. fatigue
fibrous tissue i.
finger joint i.
fin of the i.
fixed anatomic patellar i.
fixed bearing knee i.
flail i.
Flatt i.
flexible digital i.
flexible hinge i.
i. forceps
i. fracture
Futura conical subtalar i.
Futura flexible digital i.
Futura metal hemi-toe i.
Future i.
Gemini MKII mobile-bearing
  knee i.
Genesis II mobile-bearing knee i.
gentamicin i.
Geo Rectangles spinal i.
Gliadel i.
global total shoulder i.
Global total shoulder i.
Globus Pivot spinal i.
GraftCage TLX spinal i.
great toe i.
HA-coated hip i.
Harris Design-2 i.
Hedrocel proximal tibia
  augmentation i.
hemi-interpositional i.
hemisilastic i.
i. hinge
hinged i.
Howmedica Duracon i.
Howmedica monospherical i.
Hunter open cord tendon i.
hyaline cartilage i.
HyProCure sinus tarsi i.
Ideal spinal i.
iliosacral i.
Insall-Burstein intracondylar
  knee i.
Insall-Burstein total knee i.

Interax Integrated Secure Asymmetric mobile-bearing knee i.
Inter Fix interbody fusion cage i.
Interpore i.
joint i.
Kalix flatfoot i.
Kinetik great toe i. (KGTI)
Kinetikos joint i.
knee i.
Koenig total great toe i.
KPS bipolar vitallium-polyethylene i.
LaPorta great toe i.
Lawrence first metatarsophalangeal joint i.
LCS total knee system i.
i. loosening
lumbar anterior-root stimulator i. (LARSI)
i. material
Maxwell-Brancheau arthroereisis i.
McCutchen hip i.
metacarpophalangeal i.
i. metal
metal-backed acetabular component hip i.
metal-backed patellar i.
metal hemi-toe i.
metallic i.
metal orthopaedic i.
Metasul hip i.
methyl methacrylate bead i.
Microloc knee i.
mobile-bearing knee i.
modular i.
Natural-Knee i.
Neer II total shoulder system i.
NeuFlex metacarpophalangeal joint i.
NexGen knee i.
Nexus i.
Niebauer i.
Niebauer-Cutter i.
nonfusion spine i.
O.I.C. PEEK cage i.
OP-1 putty spinal fusion i.
OP-1 TM bone i.
orthobiologic i.
orthotic attachment i.
OsteoGen resorbable osteogenic bone-filling i.
Osteonics HA femoral i.
oxidized zirconium alloy on i.
Partnership i.
patellar resurfacing i.
pectoralis muscle i.
pedicle i.
percutaneous dorsal column stimulator i.
permanent i.
phalangeal i.

pin i.
plastic ball i.
PLLA i.
PMMA i.
polyglycolide i.
polylactide i.
polymethylmethacrylate i.
Polypin biodegradable pin i.
porous-coated i.
primus i.
Primus flexible great toe i.
processed carbon i.
Prodisc-C cervical artificial disc i.
Prodisc II lumbar i.
Profix mobile-bearing knee i.
ProOsteon I. 500
pyrocarbon i.
Ray cage i.
i. reaction
i. removal
Restore cuff tear i.
Restore orthobiologic soft-tissue i.
rHead Recon i.
ROI intersomatic i.
Rotaglide knee i.
rotating patellar i.
Seeburger first metatarsophalangeal joint i.
self-aligning mobile-bearing knee i.
self-centering i.
self-sealing i.
Septacin i.
Sgarlato toe i.
Shaw-SHIP rod hammertoe i.
silastic finger i.
silastic toe i.
silicone breast i.
silicone elastomer rubber ball i.
silicone MP i.
simple button patellar i.
single-stemmed toe i.
Sinterlock i.
Smart Screw bioabsorbable i.
spike washer i.
spinal i.
i. stage
STA-peg i.
StayFuse i.
i. stem
subtalar MBA i.
supraspinatus i.
Surgibone i.
Surgicel i.
i. survival rate
Sutter i.
Swanson carpal lunate i.
Swanson carpal scaphoid i.
Swanson finger joint i.
Swanson great toe i.

implant (*continued*)
    Swanson metacarpophalangeal i.
    Swanson radial head i.
    Swanson radiocarpal i.
    Swanson small joint i.
    Swanson trapezium i.
    Swanson ulnar head i.
    Swanson wrist joint i.
    Swiss MP joint i.
    symptomatic i.
    synthetic bone i.
    Techmedica i.
    I. Technology LSF prosthesis
    Teflon i.
    Telamon carbon i.
    The Wedge bioresorbable
      interference-fit i.
    Thompson-Parkridge-Richards i.
    TissueTak corkscrew i.
    titanium i.
    tobramycin-impregnated
      PMMA i.
    toe i.
    TOPS i.
    total knee i.
    Trac II knee i.
    trial i.
    tricompartmental i.
    TSRH i.
    UltraFix RC i.
    UltraFix rotator cuff repair i.
    unicompartmental knee i.
    Unilab Surgibone surgical i.
    VerteFill i.
    Viladot i.
    vitallium i.
    Voltz wrist i.
    Volz wrist i.
    Wallis interspinous i.
    Weber hip i.
    Weil i.
    Weil modified Swanson i.
    Weil type Swanson-design
      hammertoe i.
    white band on degenerated i.
    Wright monoblock titanium i.
    Zang metatarsal cap i.
    Zeichner i.
    Zymderm collagen i.
implantable
    i. bone anchor
    i. bone anchor device
    i. internal system
implantation
    autologous chondrocyte i. (ACI)
    collared press-fit femoral stem i.
    excision and i.
    1-level i.
    2-level i.

    3-level i.
    noncollared press-fit femoral
      stem i.
    periosteal i.
    screw i.
    vascular bundle i.
implant-cement interface
implanted bone growth stimulator
Implast
    I. adhesive
    I. bone cement
impressio, *pl.* **impressiones**
impression
    basilar i.
    i. defect
    i. fracture
impressiones (*pl. of* impressio)
imprinter
    foot i.
improvement
    maximal medical i.
impulse
    afferent nerve i.
    efferent nerve i.
    i. inertial exercise trainer
    mobilization with i.
impulse-based nerve transmission
IMSC
    intramedullary supracondylar
      IMSC multihole nail
Imuran
^{111}In
    indium-111
in
    toeing i.
    i. toto
    i. vivo study
4-in-1
    4-i.-1 arthroplasty
    4-i.-1 cutting block
    4-i.-1 positioning block system
5-in-1
    5-i.-1 knee ligament repair
    5-i.-1 knee reconstruction
inactivity
    i. atrophy
    electrical i.
    physical i.
In-Bed AFO boot
Inc.
    incorporated
    Health Care Manufacturing Inc.
      (HCMI)
    National Foundation for Depressive
      Illness Inc.
    Orthopaedic Systems Inc. (OSI)
Inca bone
InCare brace
incarial bone

incarnatus
> unguis i.

Incavo wire passer

incidence
> myelopathy i.
> nonunion i.

incise drape

incised wound

incision
> i. and drainage (I&D)
> anteromedial i.
> Banks-Laufman i.
> Bardenheuer i.
> battledore i.
> bifrontal i.
> Brockman i.
> Brunner modified i.
> Brunner palmar i.
> Bruser skin i.
> Burns-Haney i.
> Burwell-Scott modification of
>   Watson-Jones i.
> capsular i.
> Chang-Miltner i.
> Charnley i.
> chevron i.
> Cincinnati i.
> circumscribing i.
> Colonna-Ralston i.
> Couvelaire i.
> Crawford i.
> cruciate i.
> Cubbins i.
> Curtin i.
> curved i.
> curvilinear i.
> deltoid-splitting i.
> i. dilator
> dorsal linear i.
> dorsal longitudinal i.
> dorsal transverse i.
> dorsomedial i.
> double i.
> DuVries i.
> Dwyer i.
> elliptical i.
> exploratory i.
> fascia-splitting i.
> fiber-splitting i.
> fishmouth i.
> Fowler-Philip i.
> Gaenslen split-heel i.
> Gatellier-Chastang i.
> goblet i.
> Grice i.
> Griffith i.
> Henderson skin i.
> Henry i.
> hockey stick i.

> H-shaped capsular i.
> inverted-L lateral periosteal i.
> inverted-Y i.
> Jergesen i.
> J-shaped skin i.
> Kocher collar i.
> Koenig-Schaefer i.
> Langenbeck i.
> lateral utility i.
> lazy-C i.
> lazy-L i.
> lazy-S skin i.
> L-curved i.
> Loeffler-Ballard i.
> longitudinal i.
> L-shaped capsular i.
> Ludloff i.
> Mayfield i.
> McLaughlin-Ryder i.
> medial parapatellar i.
> midaxillary line i.
> muscle-splitting i.
> Nicola i.
> Ober i.
> oblique i.
> Ollier i.
> palmar i.
> parapatellar i.
> parathenar i.
> Picot i.
> plantar longitudinal i.
> posterior i.
> posterolateral costotransversectomy i.
> Pridie i.
> racquet-shaped i.
> relaxing i.
> relieving i.
> right-sided submandibular
>   transverse i.
> S i.
> saber-cut i.
> Seattle modification of Kocher i.
> serpentine i.
> S-flap i.
> skin i.
> skived i.
> split i.
> split heel i.
> S-shaped i.
> stab i.
> STALIF single i. (360°)
> straight i.
> subfascial i.
> Sutherland-Rowe i.
> tangential i.
> Texas T i.
> thoracoabdominal i.
> transverse i.
> triradial i.

incision (*continued*)
  T-shaped i.
  Turco oblique
    posteromedial i.
  universal i.
  upright-Y i.
  U-shaped i.
  volar midline oblique i.
  volar zigzag finger i.
  V-shaped i.
  Wagner skin i.
  Watson-Jones i.
  webspace i.
  Y i.
  Y-shaped i.
  Y-V plasty i.
  zigzag finger i.
  Z-plasty i.
incisional
  i. biopsy
  i. neuroma
  i. skin-slough
4-incision procedure
5-incision procedure
incisive bone
Incisor arthroscopic
  blade
incisural notch
Inclan
  I. bone graft
  I. modification
  I. modification of Campbell ankle
    operation
  I. modification of Campbell ankle
    procedure
  I. posterior bone block
Inclan-Ober
  I.-O. arthroplasty
  I.-O. procedure
inclination
  i. angle
  angle of thoracic i.
  sacral i.
  thoracic i.
inclinometer
  Baseline Bubble i.
  Dualer Plus i.
1-inclinometer method
2-inclinometer method
inclinometry
  digital i.
inclusion
  i. body myositis
  i. cyst
InCompass
  I. polyaxial screw
  I. spinal fixation system
  I. thoracolumbar spine fixation
    screw

incomplete
  i. amputation
  i. coalition
  i. dislocation
  i. fracture
  i. fracture of bone
  i. luxation
  i. paraplegia
  i. reduction
  i. ring sign
  i. syndactyly
  i. tear
incongruency
  subtalar joint i.
incongruent articulation
incongruity
  angle of i.
incontinence, incontinentia
  oral i.
  incontinentia pigmenti
  urinary i.
incontinentia (*var. of* incontinence)
incoordination
incorporated (Inc.)
incorporation
  bone graft i.
increased
  i. carrying angle
  i. depolymerization
  i. lateral joint space
increment after exercise
incremental
  i. range of motion (IROM)
  i. range of motion splint
  i. response
incubation period
incudomalleolar
  i. articulation
  i. joint
incurvated
incurvatum reflex
independent
  i. exercise program
  i. transfer
Inderal
index, *pl.* indices, indexes,
  gen. indicis
  acetabular i.
  acetabular head i. (AHI)
  acromial spur i. (ASI)
  activities of daily living i.
  ADL i.
  alignment i.
  alpha i.
  ambulation i.
  arch i.
  arch-height i.
  Arthritis Helplessness I. (AHI)
  Australia/Canada osteoarthritis i.

axial acetabular i. (AAI)
Barthel ADL i.
Benink tarsal i.
beta i.
body mass i. (BMI)
Caregiver Strain I. (CSI)
Chippaux-Smirak arch i.
Convery polyarticular disability i.
cortical i.
cyst i.
dynamic gait i.
dynamic postural stability i. (DPSI)
dynamic stability i.
Eyre-Brook epiphysial i.
femoral cortical i.
i. finger
i. finger abduction
foot function i. (FFI)
footprint i.
Functional Status I. (FSI)
Garden alignment i.
Hand Functional I. (HFI)
HAQ I.
Hauser ambulation i.
Health Assessment Questionnaire i.
Hollingshead I.
Holmes-Rahe Life Change I.
hop i.
Hospital Trauma I.
impact i.
Insall-Salvati patellar height i.
Ishihara cervical spine curve i.
Jette Functional Status i.
Katz ADL i.
Keitel i.
Kenny ADL i.
I. Knobber II massage tool
laxity i.
Lequesne Severity of Osteoarthritis I.
Life Satisfaction I. (LSI)
lift-up i.
Lucas and Drucker Motor I.
malleolar i.
McDowell Impairment I. (MII)
McMurtry kinematic i.
i. metacarpophalangeal joint
reconstruction
Motricity I.
neck disability i. (NDI)
Northwick Park I.
notch width i. (NWI)
Nottingham Extended ADL i.
osteoarthritis global i. (OGI)
Oswestry i.
posterior inferior cerebellar artery i.
predictive salvage i. (PSI)
pressure excursion i.
I. prosthesis
Quetelet i.

i. ray amputation
Reimers hip instability i.
Reimers hip position migration i.
Reintegration to Normal Living i.
rib-hump scoliosis i.
right and left ankle indices
Ritchie rheumatoid arthritis i.
Rivermead ADL i.
Rivermead Mobility I. (RMI)
Roland low back pain i.
sciatic function i. (SFI)
Singh osteoporosis i.
Spinal Cord Motor Index and
Sensory Indices
Spotorno i.
Stahl lunate disease i.
Takakura tarsal i.
talocalcaneal i.
toe i.
upper extremity functional i. (UEFI)
Western Ontario and McMaster
University osteoarthritis i.
Western Ontario Instability I.
(WOSI)
Western Ontario Rotator Cuff i.
Wheelchair User's Shoulder Pain I.
(WUSPI)
WOMAC osteoarthritis i.
WORC i.
indexes (*pl. of* index)
3-in-1 diamond bur
Indiana
I. conservative prosthesis
I. reamer
I. tome carpal tunnel syndrome
release system
I. tome clip
I. tome open carpal tunnel release
knife
indices (*pl. of* index)
indicis (*gen. of* index)
indifferent electrode
indirect
i. decompression
i. fracture
i. magnetic resonance arthrography
nuclear bone imaging
i. manipulation
i. reduction
i. triangulation
indium-111 (^{111}In)
i.-111 scintigraphy
individual physiotherapy
Indochron E-R
Indocin
I. I.V.
I. SR
indoleacetic acid
indomethacin

Indong Oh hip prosthesis
indoprofen
induced
    intraorganically i.
induction
    pain i.
inductive coupling device
indurated plantar keratoma
induration
industry
    Duro-Med Industries (DMI)
inelastic
inequality
    anatomic leg length i.
    functional leg length i.
    i. in leg length
    leg length i. (LLI)
Inerpan flexible burn dressing
inertia
INEX
    internal-external
    INEX ilium
    INEX movement
inextensibility
infant
    i. abduction splint
    i. clown cast shoe
    I.'s Feverall
    floppy i.
    Movement Assessment of I.'s
    (MAI)
infantile
    i. cortical hyperostosis
    i. dermal fibromatosis
    i. idiopathic scoliosis
    i. progressive spinal muscular
    atrophy
    i. tibia vara (ITV)
    i. trigger digit
Infants' Silapap
infarct, infarction
    bone i.
infarction
    bone i.
    Freiberg i.
In-Fast bone screw system
infected
    i. bone
    i. nondraining nonunion
infection
    aerobic i.
    anaerobic i.
    aspergillosis i.
    blood-borne i.
    bone i.
    Cephalosporium nail i.
    clostridial i.
    cryptococcal i.
    deep delayed i.

    deep wound i.
    disc space i.
    epidural space i.
    fascial space i.
    felon i.
    fungous i.
    gas-producing streptococcal i.
    granulomatous fungal i.
    hematogenous i.
    iatrogenic i.
    Meleney i.
    musculoskeletal i.
    mycobacterial i.
    nontuberculous mycobacterial i.
    percutaneous bone marrow i.
    pin tract i.
    postoperative i.
    i. prevention
    pyogenic spinal i.
    skeletal i.
    spinal i.
    superficial i.
    suppurative joint i.
    tarsal joint i.
    webspace i.
infectious
    i. arthritis
    i. bulbar necrosis
    i. tenosynovitis
inferential
    i. current stimulation
    i. current stimulator
    i. current therapy
    i. therapy
inferior
    i. angle
    anterior and i. (AI)
    atraumatic multidirectional bilateral
    rehabilitation i. (AMBRI)
    i. band cruciform ligament
    i. calcaneal nerve
    i. calcaneonavicular (ICN)
    i. capsular shift
    i. capsular split technique
    i. costal sulcus
    i. extensor of foot
    i. extensor retinaculum
    i. facet
    i. gemelli muscle
    i. glenohumeral ligament (IGHL)
    i. glenohumeral ligament insertion
    i. glide
    i. ilioischial ligament
    i. laryngeal nerve
    i. leaf
    i. movement
    i. outline
    i. peroneal retinaculum
    i. process

i. radioulnar joint
i. ramus
i. spur
i. spurring
i. thyroid artery
i. tibiofibular joint
i. tibiofibular repair
i. vena cava (IVC)
inferoposterior acetabular capsule retractor
infestation
pressure ulcer-related maggot i.
INFH
ischemic necrosis of femoral head
infiltrate
fibrofatty i.
infiltration
root i.
infinity
I. femoral component
I. hip system
I. modular hip prosthesis
InFix interbody fusion system
inflamed synovial pouch
inflammation
bursal i.
i. management
polyarticular symmetric tophaceous joint i.
prepatellar bursa i.
tendon i.
inflammatory
i. arthropathy
i. bowel disease associated arthritis
i. fracture
i. myositis
i. phase
i. scoliosis
i. spondyloarthropathy
i. synovitis
i. tenovaginitis
inflatable
i. bone tamp (IBT)
i. elbow splint
inflexion point
inflow
i. cannula
vascular i.
influenzae
Haemophilus i.
infracalcaneal bursitis
infraclavicular
i. region
i. triangle
infraction fracture
infracture
infraganglionic injury
infraglenoid tuberosity

infragluteal
i. creaking
i. crease
infraisthmal
infrapatellar
i. bursa
i. bursitis
i. contracture syndrome (IPCS)
i. fat pad
i. ligament
i. plica
i. strap
i. tendinitis
i. tendon
i. tendon rupture
i. view
infrared (IR)
i. applicator
i. head
i. light
i. light-emitting diode
i. therapy
i. thermography
infrascapular region
infraspinatus
i. muscle
i. tendinitis
i. tendon
infraspinous
i. fascia
i. region
infrasternal
infratectal transverse fracture
infratrochlear
Infumorph Injection
infuse
I. bone graft
I. bone graft/LT-Cage lumbar tapered fusion device
Infusible pressure infusion bag
infusion-aspiration drainage
infusion pump
Inge
I. retractor
I. spreader
Ingebrightsen traction
Inglis-Cooper release
Inglis-Pellicci elbow arthroplasty rating system
Inglis triaxial total elbow arthroplasty
Ingram
I. bony bridge resection
I. osteotomy
I. procedure
ingrowing toenail
ingrown
i. nail
i. toenail

ingrowth
- bone i.
- i. fixation

inguinal
- i. approach
- i. ligament
- i. ligament syndrome

inhalant anesthesia

inhalation anesthesia

inherent motion

inhibition test

inhibitive
- i. cast
- i. traction

inhibitor
- aldose reductase i.
- anion transport i.
- cholinesterase i.
- monoamine oxidase-B i.
- shoulder subluxation i. (SSI)
- tissue i.

inhibitory postsynaptic potential

inhomogeneity

iniencephaly

inion bump

initial
- i. contact phase
- i. manifestation
- i. stance

initiation
- i. feel
- rhythmic i.

initiator drill

injection
- Adlone i.
- alcohol i.
- Alfenta i.
- A-methaPred I.
- Articulose-50 I.
- Astramorph PF i.
- Ben-Allergin-50 I.
- Bicillin C-R 900/300 i.
- Botox i.
- Calciferol I.
- Calcimar I.
- cervical epidural steroid i.
- cervical nerve root i.
- chymopapain i.
- Cibacalcin I.
- Cipro I.
- corticosteroid i.
- cortisone i.
- Cytoxan i.
- depMedalone I.
- Depogen I.
- Depoject i.
- Depo-Medrol i.
- Depopred I.
- Dioval I.

- D-Med I.
- Duralone I.
- Duramorph i.
- epidural steroid i. (ESI)
- extrafascial nerve i.
- facet i.
- Gynogen L.A. I.
- Hyalgan i.
- Infumorph I.
- i. injury
- intraarticular i.
- intramuscular i.
- intraosseous i.
- joint i.
- Kefurox I.
- Key-Pred I.
- Lovenox I.
- low-pressure i.
- lumbar facet i.
- lumbar nerve root i.
- lumbar transforaminal epidural i.
- Medralone I.
- Miacalcin i.
- M-Prednisol I.
- Nafcil I.
- Nallpen I.
- Neosar i.
- nerve root i.
- Novocain I.
- Octocaine I.
- Oncovin i.
- osteocalcin i.
- peroneal bupivacaine i.
- peroneal tendon sheath i.
- Pontocaine With Dextrose I.
- Predcor-TBA I.
- Prednisol TBA i.
- i. pressure
- procaine-phenol motor point i.
- Salmonine I.
- Sandimmune i.
- Seconal I.
- selective nerve root i.
- Solu-Medrol i.
- steroid i.
- i. study
- subacromial bursa i.
- Sublimaze i.
- Sufenta i.
- i. technique
- tenosynovial i.
- thecal i.
- i. therapy
- thoracic epidural i.
- Toposar I.
- Toradol i.
- trigger point i.
- Unipen I.
- VePesid I.

Vincasar PFS I.
Zinacef i.
zygapophysial joint i.
injurious energy input spearing
injury
    acceleration i.
    acceleration/deceleration i.
    accessory nerve i.
    acquired brain i. (ABI)
    acromioclavicular joint i.
    acute stretch i.
    i. algorithm
    American Spinal Injury Association
      standard neurological classification
      of spinal cord i.
    ankle i.
    anular i.
    ASIA standard neurological
      classification of spinal cord i.
    i. assessment
    athletic i.
    avulsion i.
    axial compression i.
    axial loading i.
    axillary nerve i.
    axonal i.
    ballistic i.
    barked i.
    bending toward the side of i.
    bicycle i.
    birth i.
    bladder i.
    brachial artery i.
    brachial plexus i.
    brachial plexus traction i. (BPTI)
    Brief Test of Head I. (BTHI)
    bunk bed i.
    burner i.
    burst i.
    calcaneocuboid joint nutcracker i.
    cat's eye i.
    cervical cord i.
    cervical nerve root i.
    cervical spinal i.
    cervical spine extension i.
    Chopart osseous joint i.
    chronic microtraumatic soft tissue i.
    closed kinetic chain i.
    closed soft tissue i.
    cocking i.
    cold i.
    2-column cervical spine i.
    3-column cervical spine i.
    common fibular nerve i.
    compression-plus-torque cervical i.
    compressive flexion i.
    compressive hyperextension i.
    contrecoup i.
    corticospinal tract cord i.

    crush i.
    cuneiform i.
    Danis-Weber classification of
      ankle i.
    dashboard knee i.
    degloving i.
    de Quervain i.
    diffuse axonal i.
    discoligamentous i.
    distal tibial epiphysial i.
    distraction i.
    Drummond and Hastings cuboid
      extrusion i.
    elbow i.
    electrical i.
    epiphysial i.
    ergonomic i.
    Essex-Lopresti calcaneal i.
    eversion i.
    explosion i.
    extensor tendon i.
    extravasation i.
    factitious i.
    fell on outstretched hand i.
    femoral vein i.
    firearm i.
    flexion i.
    flexion-distraction i.
    flexion-extension i.
    FOOSH i.
    forced flexion i.
    frostbite i.
    gamekeeper's i.
    Gertzbein classification of
      seat-belt i.
    grease gun i.
    growth plate i.
    Hardcastle classification of
      tarsometatarsal joint i.
    hip epiphysial i.
    H-type sacral fracture with
      associated spinopelvic
      dissociation i.
    hyperextension i.
    hyperextension-hyperflexion i.
    hyperflexion i.
    hyperplantarflexion i.
    iatrogenic i.
    iatrogenic spinal cord i.
    infraganglionic i.
    injection i.
    internal degloving i.
    interosseous nerve i.
    inversion ankle i.
    ipsilateral foot i.
    Klumpke i.
    knee ligamentous i.
    laryngeal nerve i.
    lateral compartment i.

injury (*continued*)
lateral compression i.
lawn mower i.
ligamentous i.
Lisfranc i.
long thoracic nerve i.
low back i.
lower plexus i.
lumbar plexus i.
lunate facet dye punch i.
MacKinnon nerve i.
mangling i.
marching band i.
matrix i.
medial brachial cutaneous nerve i.
medial compartment i.
median nerve i.
meniscal i.
mesencephalic i.
metatarsophalangeal joint i.
midcarpal i.
middle column i.
missile i.
multiple injuries
muscle-tendon i.
musculocutaneous nerve i.
nail i.
nerve i.
neural i.
neurovascular i.
nutcracker i.
obstetric brachial plexus i. (OBPI)
obturator nerve i.
Ontario Cohort of
  Running-Related I.
open-book pelvic i.
osteochondral i.
overuse i.
paint gun i.
paint thinner i.
paracetamol-induced renal i.
paracetamol-induced renal tubular i.
i. pattern
pelvic i.
PER i.
perihamate i.
peripheral nerve i. (PNI)
peripisiform i.
peritrapezial i.
peritrapezoidal i.
peroneal nerve i.
physial i.
pitching i.
plantarflexion i.
plantar plate i.
pleural i.
pneumatic tire i.
Poland classification of physial i.
posterior ligamentous i.

predictor of i.
pronation i.
pronation-abduction i.
pronation-eversion i.
pronation-eversion-external rotation i.
pronation-external rotation i.
pseudogamekeeper's i.
pudendal nerve i.
Pugil stick i.
radial artery i.
radial nerve i.
radioulnar joint i.
recurrent laryngeal nerve i.
reperfusion i.
repetition strain i. (RSI)
repetitive stress i.
road burn i.
roller i.
Rosenthal classification of nail i.
rotator cuff i.
running-related i.
sacral plexus i.
sacroiliac joint i.
Sage-Salvatore classification I-III of
  acromioclavicular joint i.
sailboarder i.
Salter-Harris classification of
  epiphysial plate i.
Salter-Harris tibial-fibular physis i.
sand toe i.
Scales of Cognitive Ability for
  Traumatic Brain I. (SCATBI)
scaphoid tuberosity i.
scapuloclavicular i.
sciatic nerve i.
seat belt i.
sesamoid i.
I. Severity Score (ISS)
shaken impact i.
shearing i.
shotgun i.
sideswipe i.
skier's i.
snowboarding i.
softball sliding i.
soft tissue i.
spinal accessory nerve i.
spinal cord i. (SCI)
sports i.
stable cervical spine i.
steering wheel i.
sternoclavicular joint i.
stinger i.
straddle i.
strain-sprain i.
stress i.
stretch i.
subaxial i.
subclavian artery i.

subclavian vein i.
subscapular artery i.
subscapular nerve i.
Sunderland classification of nerve i.
  (1st-5th degree)
Sunderland first-degree – fifth-degree
  nerve i.
supination i.
supination-adduction i.
supination-eversion i.
supination-external rotation i.
supination-inversion rotation i.
supination-outward rotation i.
supination-plantarflexion i.
supraganglionic i.
suprascapular nerve i.
synovial i.
tarsometatarsal joint i.
thoracic duct i.
thoracic nerve i.
thoracoabdominal artery i.
thoracodorsal nerve i.
thoracolumbar spinal i.
thoracolumbar spine
  flexion-distraction i.
throwing i.
tibial axial load i.
tibial nerve i.
tornado i.
tracheal i.
trampoline i.
transcutaneous crush i.
translation i.
traumatic brain i. (TBI)
traumatic burn i.
turf toe i.
ulnar artery i.
ulnar collateral ligament i.
ulnar nerve i.
unstable cervical spine i.
vascular i.
vertebrobasilar i.
weightbearing rotation i.
whiplash i.
windup i.
wringer i.

Inland Super Multi-Hite orthopaedic bed
inlay
  i. bone graft
  Sher diabetic shoe i.
inlet view
inner
  i. heel wedge
  I. Lip Plate
  I. Lok ankle brace
  i. malleolus
  i. table
innervation
  muscle i.

parasympathetic i.
reciprocal i.
somatic i.
sympathetic i.
Innoboot splint
Innomed
  I. arthroplasty measuring system
  I. Assistant Free surgical
    instrument
  I. bone curette
innominate
  anterior i.
  i. bone
  i. bone resection
  left i.
  i. movement
  i. osteotomy
  posterior i.
  right posterior i.
  i. tilt
  i. vein
Innovar
innovasive
  I. bone anchor
  I. device
  I. fixation
innovation
  I. Sports bracing product
  I. Sports bracing support
innovative
  I. COR/T implant system
  I. Medical Products (IMP)
  I. Medical Products knee positioning
    triangle
  I. Medical Products Steri-Clamp
inochondritis
inosculation phase
inotropism
Inpatient Rehabilitation Facility Patient
  Assessment Instrument (IRFPAI)
Inro surgical nail
Insall
  I. anterior cruciate ligament
    reconstruction
  I. anterior knee approach
  I. criteria
  I. ligament reconstruction technique
  I. patella alta method
  I. patellar injury classification
  I. patellar instability repair
    procedure
  I. proximal realignment
  I. ratio
Insall-Burstein
  I.-B. II modular total knee system
  I.-B. intracondylar knee implant
  I.-B. semiconstrained
    tricompartmental knee prosthesis
  I.-B. total knee implant

Insall-Burstein-Freeman (IBF)
    I.-B.-F. knee arthroplasty
Insall-Hood reconstruction technique
Insall-Salvati
    I.-S. measurement
    I.-S. patellar height index
    I.-S. ratio
insecurity
    gravitational i.
insensate foot
insert
    AliMed i.
    angled bearing i.
    articular i.
    cancellous i.
    clamp i.
    cushioned shoe i.
    custom-made i.
    Durasul polyethylene, high wear
      resistant acetabular i.
    Energy Plus shoe i.
    Gel-Sole shoe i.
    i. graft
    Hapad felt i.
    Hapad shoe i.
    heel and sole i.
    Hydragrip clamp i.
    Johnson & Johnson PFC
      cruciate-substituting i.
    New York University orthotic i.
    NYU orthosis i.
    Orthex Relievers shoe i.
    orthotic shoe i.
    Osteonics Scorpio i.
    Poly-Dial i.
    polyethylene tibial i.
    polypropylene i.
    POWERPoint orthotic shoe i.
    Profix confirming tibial i.
    retrieved i.
    Roho solid seat i.
    shoe i.
    silicone gel socket i.
    soft socket i.
    sole i.
    Spenco shoe i.
    S-ROM Poly-Dial i.
    thermomoldable i.
    tibial i.
    UCB shoe i.
    viscoelastic heel i.
    warm and form i.
    WonderZorb silicone shoe i.
    Xpanse bone i.
    Xpanse R bone i.
    Xpanse S bone i.
inserter
    Buck femoral cement restrictor i.
    CDH cup i.

    cement restrictor i.
    cement spacer i.
    cerclage wire i.
    C-wire i.
    deluxe FIN pin i.
    Kirschner wire i.
    Massie i.
    prosthesis i.
    Shaffner orthopaedic i.
    spacer i.
    staple i.
    T-shaped i.
    TSRH hook i.
inserter-extractor
    compression i.-e.
insertion
    anatomic i.
    anomalous i.
    Bosworth bone peg i.
    C-D rod i.
    deltoid i.
    i. equipment
    IGHL i.
    inferior glenohumeral ligament i.
    lag screw i.
    ligamentous i.
    oblique screw i.
    pedicle screw i.
    percutaneous pin i.
    Pierrot and Murphy advancement i.
    rerouting i.
    screw i.
    i. tendinopathy
insertional
    i. Achilles tendinosis
    i. activity
    i. excursion
    i. tendo calcaneus tendinitis
in-shoe transducer
inside-out
    i.-o. Bankart shoulder instability
      operation
    i.-o. meniscal repair
    i.-o. technique for establishing ankle
      portal
    i.-o. tissue repair technique
inside-to-outside technique
**Insight knee positioning and alignment
    system**
insole
    Aliplast i.
    Anti-Shox gel i.
    Apex i.
    Bestfoam i.
    Comf-Orthotic 3/4-length i.
    Comf-Orthotic sports replacement i.
    Comf-Orthotic wool felt i.
    Darco moldable i.
    Diab-A-Foot rocker i.

Diab-A-Pad i.
Diab-A-Sole flat i.
Diab-A-Sole molded i.
Diabetic Diagnostic i.
D-Soles i.
Ever-Flex i.
Flat Foot i.
FlexiTherm diabetic diagnostic i.
Hapad metatarsal i.
Kinetic Wedge molded i.
molded postpartum i.
Orthex reliever i.
Plastazote i.
Plexidure i.
Poron 400 i.
PPT flat i.
PPT MXL soft molded i.
PPT Plastizote i.
PPT RX firm molded i.
ProThotics i.
PumpPals i.
Reflex Comfort i.
Sherform silicone i.
silicone i.
Sof Airr i.
SofSole Airr i.
Sorbothane i.
Spenco i.
S-Soles i.
TechnoGel i.
viscoelastic i.
ViscoPed S i.

inspiration and expiration breathing thoracic spine test

instability

AMBRI glenohumeral i.
ankle i.
anterior shoulder i.
anterolateral-anteromedial rotary i.
anterolateral rotary i. (ALRI)
anterolateral rotary knee i.
anteromedial-posteromedial rotary i.
anteromedial rotary i.
articular i.
atlantoaxial i. (AAI)
atraumatic multidirectional i.
axial i.
capitate-lunate i.
carpal i.
Chrisman-Snook correction of ankle i.
chronic ankle i. (CAI)
chronic functional i.
chronic lateral ankle i.
collateral ligament i.
combined i. (CI)
congenital atlantoaxial i.
correction of peroneal tendon i.

discogenic spinal i.
dorsal intercalated segment i. (DISI)
DRUJ i.
extension i.
flexion i.
functional i.
i. gait
glenohumeral i.
hindfoot i.
i. hypothesis
intercalated segment i.
inversion i.
joint i.
knee i.
lateral rotatory ankle i.
lumbar spinal i.
lumbar spine i.
lunotriquetral i.
mechanical i.
medial column i.
membrane i.
midcarpal i. (MCI)
multidirectional i. (MDI)
i. of the ankle
open stabilization of traumatic anterior shoulder i.
osseous i.
patellar i.
pelvic i.
perilunar i.
1-plane i.
posterior shoulder i.
posterolateral rotary i.
posteromedial rotary i.
postural i.
progressive perilunar i.
push-pull i.
radiocarpal i.
repair of forearm malunions with distal radioulnar joint i.
rotary ankle i.
rotational i.
sagittal plane i.
scapholunate i.
shoulder i.
spinal i.
spinal deformity i.
straight lateral i.
subtalar joint i.
thumb i.
tibiofibular joint i.
tibiotalar i.
traumatic anterior i.
traumatic anterior shoulder i.
triquetrolunate i.
valgus i.
varus-valgus i.
vertebral i.

instability (*continued*)
    volar flexed intercalated segment i.
      (VISI)
    volar intercalary wrist i.
    wrist i.
installation
    i. method
    i. of orthosis procedure
Insta-Nerve device
instantaneous axis of rotation (IAR)
instant cold pack
Instat collagen sponge
instill
instillation
    i. of anesthetic
    i. procedure
institute
    Podiatry I.
    Southern California Orthopaedic I.
      (SCOI)
Instratek titanium cannulated small bone
  screw system
Instron machine
instrument
    Accu-Line knee i.
    AccuSharp carpal tunnel release i.
    Achieve computer-assisted i.'s
    activating adjusting i. (AAI)
    Acufex arthroscopic i.
    Acufex MosaicPlasty i.
    American Academy of Orthopaedic
      Surgeons Pediatrics Outcomes I.
    Arthrex arthroscopy i.
    Arthroforce III hand i.
    arthroscopic laser i.
    Atlas orthogonal percussion i.
    AxyaWeld i.
    back range of motion i.
    battery-powered i.
    Collis TDR i.
    Command instrument system surgical i.
    Cotrel-Dubousset spinal i.
    Dreyfus prosthesis placement i.
    electrosurgical i.
    Femur Finder i.
    Friatec manual arthroscopy i.
    Hall Micro E power i.
    Hall series 4 large bone i.
    Hall-Zimmer power i.
    Howmedica-Osteonics i.
    IBF knee i.
    Innomed Assistant Free surgical i.
    Inpatient Rehabilitation Facility
      Patient Assessment I. (IRFPAI)
    Kinetix i.
    Kirschner surgical i.
    laser i.
    I. Makar biodegradable interference
      screw

    microsurgical i.
    Midas Rex pneumatic i.
    i. migration
    Mitek SuperAnchor i.
    Monogram total knee i.
    Nicolet Compass EMG i.
    Ohio Medical I.'s (OMI)
    orthopaedic cutting i.
    OrthoVise orthopaedic i.
    oscilloscope i.
    paraspinal skin temperature
      thermocouple i.
    Partnership i.
    passivation metal i.
    PowerTrack II muscle testing i.
    quadriceps-sparing, minimally
      invasive total knee i.
    Rancho Los Amigos external
      fixation i.
    reciprocal planing i.
    RingLoc i.
    ScoliTron i.
    Shea prosthesis placement i.
    single reference point i.
    instrument, sponge, needle count
    StealthStation Treon plus
      neurosurgical i.
    Steffee i.
    Sulzer Orthopaedics i.
    thermocouple i.
    Ultra-Cut i.
    Universal Minimally Invasive
      Assistant Free hip surgery i.'s
    Wiet graft-measuring i.
instrumental
    i. activity of daily living (IADL)
    i. ADLs
instrument-assisted soft tissue
  mobilization (IASTM)
instrumentation
    Accu-Line knee i.
    Acufex arthroscopic i.
    anterior distraction i.
    anterior Zielke i.
    AO fixateur interne i.
    AO notched i.
    Apofix cervical i.
    Arthrotek Ellipticut hand i.
    biodegradable fixation i.
    bone-holding i.
    cable-hook compression i.
    Caspar anterior i.
    C-D i.
    compression Harrington i.
    compression U-rod i.
    Cotrel-Dubousset pedicle screw i.
    distraction i.
    double Zielke i.
    Drummond spinal i.

Dwyer spinal i.
dynamic compression plate i.
Edwards i.
endoscopic carpal tunnel i.
i. failure
halo-Ilizarov distraction i.
Harms-Moss anterior thoracic i.
Harrington distraction i.
Harrington-Kostuik i.
Harrington rod i.
Harrington rod distraction i.
hollow mill i.
Howmedica knee i.
hybrid i.
interspinous segmental spinal i. (ISSI)
Jacobs locking hook spinal rod i.
Kaneda anterior spinal i.
Kostuik-Harrington spinal i.
locking hook i.
Louis i.
lumbar spine i.
lumbosacral spine transpedicular i.
Luque II segmental spinal i.
Luque semirigid segmental spinal i.
Mayfield i.
McElroy i.
modular i.
Moreland total hip revision i.
Moss i.
Moss-Miami scoliosis i.
Moss-Miami transforaminal interbody
fusion i.
multiple hook assembly C-D i.
Passport i.
posterior cervical spinal i.
posterior distraction i.
posterior hook-rod spinal i.
Putti-Platt i.
rod-sleeve i.
sacral spine modular i.
segmental spinal i. (SSI)
short-segment pedicle screw i. (SSPI)
Sielke i.
skin-contact i.
Smith-Richards i.
spinal i.
Steffee spinal i.
Stryker power i.
i. system
thoracoscopic i.
total knee i.
TSRH i.
universal sacral spine i.
variable screw placement system i.
VSP plate i.
Wisconsin interspinous segmental
spinal i.
Zielke pedicular i.

instrumented spinal fusion
insufficiency
abductor i.
active i.
capsular length i.
i. fracture
ligamentous i.
mechanical i.
muscle i.
passive i.
peripheral vascular i. (PVI)
posterior tibial tendon i.
PTT i.
thoracic i.
transverse plane motion i.
vertebrobasilar i. (VBI)
insufflate
insulin-dependent diabetes
  mellitus
insulin-like
i.-l. growth factor (IGF)
i.-l. growth factor I
insulin-like growth factor I
In-Tac bone-anchoring system
intact
i. dressing
neurologically i.
neurovascularly i.
i. neurovascular status
i. peripheral pulses
i. spinous lamina
i. spinous process
intake
dietary reference i. (DRI)
energy i.
Integra
I. bilayer matrix wound dressing
I. Mozaik osteoconductive scaffold
integral
force-time i.
I. hip system
I. Interlok femoral prosthesis
pressure-time i.
integrated
I. Ankle orthotic ankle joint
i. electromyography
i. rectified electromyogram
  (IEMG)
i. shape and imaging system
I. Shape Imaging System scoliosis
  screening
integration
Beery-Buktenica Developmental Test
  of Visual-Motor I.
body side i.
DeGangi-Berk Test of Sensory I.
Functional I. (FI)
sensory i.
visual-motor i. (VMI)

integrity
  I. acetabular cup
  I. acetabular cup prosthesis
  I. acetabular cup screw
  i. and alignment
  biochemical i.
  biomechanical i.
  bone plate i.
  maintenance of bone plate i.
  soft tissue i.

Intelect
  I. Combo stimulator/ultrasound
  I. electric stimulator
  I. laser system device
  I. Legend stimulator
  I. 600MP microcurrent
    stimulator

InteliJET fluid management system
Intelligent Prosthesis Plus
  prosthesis
IntelliTemp insulation material
intensification
  image i.
intensifier
  C-arm image i.
  image i.
intention
  first i.
  healing by first i.
  healing by second i.
  i. myoclonus
  primary i.
  second i.
  secondary i.
  i. tremor
intentional
  i. movement
  i. rotation
Intenzyme Forte
Inteq small joint suturing system
Inter
  I. Fix interbody fusion cage implant
  I. Fix RP threaded spinal fusion cage
  I. Fix RP threaded spinal fusion
    cage device
  I. Fix threaded spinal fusion cage
    device
  I. Fix titanium threaded spinal
    fusion cage
interaction
  surface shoe i.
  tibiofemoral i.
interarticular
  i. cartilage
  i. disc
  i. fracture
  i. joint
  i. ligament of head of rib
  i. sulcus

interarticularis
  pars i.
Interax
  I. Integrated Secure Asymmetric
    mobile-bearing knee implant
  I. total knee system
interbody
  i. arthrodesis
  i. construct
  i. fusion cage system
  i. graft
  i. rasp
  i. spinal fusion
  i. stabilization
intercalary
  i. allograft procedure
  i. diaphysial allograft
  i. graft
  i. resection
  i. segmental replacement
intercalated segment
  instability
intercarpal
  i. arthrodesis
  i. articulation
  i. joint
  i. ligament
  i. ligament capsulodesis
interchondral joint
interclavicular
  i. ligament
  i. notch
intercollicular groove
intercompartment fasciotome
intercondylar, intercondylic,
  intercondyloid
  i. drill guide
  i. femoral fracture
  i. fossa
  i. groove
  i. humeral fracture
  i. notch
  i. process
  i. roof
  i. space
  i. tibial fracture
intercondylic (*var. of* intercondylar)
intercondyloid (*var. of*
  intercondylar)
intercostal
  i. artery
  i. flap
  i. nerve
  i. nerve block
  i. neuralgia (ICN)
  i. restriction
  i. space
  i. vein
intercostobrachial nerve

intercritical time
intercuneiform joint
interdigital
    i. bone fusion
    i. corn
    i. ligament
    i. neoplasia
    i. nerve
    i. nerve bundle
    i. neuroma (IDN)
    i. neuroma test
    i. webspace
interdischarge interval
interdisciplinary vocational evaluation program
interepicondylar axis
interface
    acetabular prosthetic i.
    bone-cement i.
    bone-implant i.
    bone-peg i.
    bony i.
    cement i.
    cement-bone i.
    cup-cement i.
    fascial-muscle i.
    fat-blood i. (FBI)
    implant-cement i.
    long-term bone-
      instrumentation i.
    paraspinal i.
    patient-table i.
    pin-bone i.
    prosthesis i.
    prosthesis-cement i.
    ShearBan low-friction i.
    shoe-foot i.
    soft tissue i.
interfacet
    i. wiring
    i. wiring and fusion
interfacetal dislocation
interfacial porosity
interfascicular
    i. epineurectomy
    i. epineurotomy
    i. neurolysis
interference
    i. fit
    i. fit fixation
    nerve i.
    i. pattern
    i. screw
    i. screw technique
    vertebrogenic i.
interferential
    i. current (IFC)
    i. electrical
      stimulation

    i. stimulator
    i. therapy
interfragmentary
    i. compression
    i. lag screw
    i. plate
    i. wire
intergluteal cleft
interilioabdominal amputation
interinnominate asymmetry
interinnominoabdominal
    i. amputation
    i. cleft
interlaminar clamp
interleukin-1 beta release
interline
    Lisfranc articular i.
interlocking
    i. acetabular cup
    distal i.
    i. medullary nail
    i. nailing
    proximal i.
    i. screw
intermaxillary bone
intermediary amputation
intermediate
    i. amputation
    i. bundle
    i. callus
    i. care facility (ICF)
    i. cast
    i. C-D hook
    i. cuneiform fracture-dislocation
    i. disc
    i. disinfectant
    i. dorsal cutaneous nerve
      (IDCN)
    i. interference pattern
    i. lamella
    i. phalangectomy
    i. socket
Intermedics
    I. natural hip system
    I. Natural-Knee knee
      prosthesis
intermediolateral nucleus
intermediomedial nucleus
intermedius
    vastus i. (VI)
intermetacarpal
    i. articulation
    i. joint
    i. ligament (IML)
intermetatarsal
    i. angle (IMA)
    i. angle-reducing operation
    i. angle-reducing procedure
    i. artery

intermetatarsal (*continued*)
    i. bursa
    i. bursitis
    i. joint
    i. ligament
    i. nerve
    i. space
    i. vein
intermetatarsophalangeal
    i. bursa
    i. bursitis
intermittens
    dyskinesia i.
    myotonia congenita i.
intermittent
    i. arthralgia
    i. casting
    i. cervical traction
    i. claudication
    i. double-step gait
    i. extremity pump
    i. hydrarthrosis
    i. impulse compression
    i. paresthesia
    i. pneumatic compression
    i. torticollis
intermuscular
    i. neuroma transposition
    i. septum
interna
    hyperostosis frontalis i.
internal
    i. band
    i. carotid artery
    i. degloving
    i. degloving injury
    i. derangement
    i. derangement of knee (IDK)
    i. femoral rotation
    i. fixation (IF)
    i. fixation apparatus
    i. fixation, closed reduction
    i. fixation compression arthrodesis
    i. fixation compression arthrodesis
    of ankle
    i. fixation plate-screw system
    i. fixation spring
    i. fracture fixation
    i. gel pad
    i. hemipelvectomy
    i. iliac artery
    i. iliac vein
    i. jugular vein
    i. malleolus
    i. movement
    i. neurolysis
    i. oblique muscle
    posteroinferior i. (PIIN)
    i. process

    i. rotary component of force
    component
    i. rotational gait
    i. rotation deformity
    i. rotation exercise
    i. rotation in extension (IRE)
    i. rotation in flexion (IRF)
    i. rotator
    i. snapping hip syndrome
    i. spinal fixation
    i. tibial torsion (ITT)
    i. tibial torsion brace
    i. tibiofibular torsion
    i. topography
    i. traction
    i. version
internal-external (INEX)
    i.-e. rotation
internally
    i. fixed fracture
    i. rotated
international
    I. Cartilage Repair Society (ICRS)
    I. Classification for Surgery of the
    Hand in Tetraplegia
    I. Classification of Impairments,
    Disabilities, Handicaps (ICIDH)
    I. Clubfoot Study Group
    I. 10-20 EEG scalp electrode
    placement system
    I. Knee Documentation Committee
    (IKDC)
    I. Knee Documentation Committee
    form
    I. Knee Documentation Committee
    knee scale
    I. Knee Documentation Committee
    Subjective Knee Form
    I. Knee Ligament Standard
    Evaluation questionnaire
    I. Listing System
    I. Society of Arthroscopy, Knee
    Surgery, and Orthopaedic Sports
    Medicine (ISAKOS)
    I. Spine Intervention Society
    (ISIS)
interne
    AO-ASIF fixateur i.
    AO fixateur i.
    Dick AO fixateur i.
internervous plane
intern's
    i. triangle
    i. triangle in hip spica cast
internus
    malleolus i.
    metatarsus i.
interoceptor
    postural i.

Inter-Op
    I.-O. acetabular prosthesis
    I.-O. acetabular shell
    I.-O. hip prosthesis
interossei (*pl. of* interosseus)
interosseous
    i. anastomosing channel
    i. artery
    i. branch
    i. cartilage
    i. compartment
    i. cuneocuboid ligament
    i. cuneometatarsal ligament
    i. diastasis
    i. intercuneiform ligament
    i. ligament disruption
    i. membrane (IOM)
    i. metacarpal ligament
    i. metatarsal ligament
    i. muscle
    i. nerve
    i. nerve injury
    i. nerve syndrome
    i. sacroiliac ligament
    i. talocalcaneal ligament
      (ITCL)
    i. tendon
    i. wire fixation
interosseum
interosseus, *pl.* **interossei**
interparietal bone
interpeak interval
interpedicular (*var. of* interpedicutate)
    i. distance widening joint widening
interpediculate, interpedicular
    i. distance
interpeduncular
    i. notch
    i. space
interpelviabdominal
  amputation
interperiosteal fracture
interphalangeal (IP)
    i. amputation
    i. arthrodesis
    i. arthroplasty
    i. articulation
    i. coalition
    distal i. (DIP)
    i. fusion
    i. joint
    i. joint dislocation
    i. joint space
    i. osteoarthritis
    proximal i. (PIP)
    proximal interphalangeal/distal i.
    i. sesamoid management
    i. tenodesis
interphalangectomy

Interpore
    I. bone
    I. bone replacement material
    I. implant
interposed comminution
interposition
    i. arthroplasty
    i. bone graft
    ligament reconstruction with tendon
      i. (LRTI)
    i. membrane
    soft tissue i.
    tendon i.
interpositional
    i. arthroplasty
    i. tricortical graft
interpotential interval
interpubic disc
interquantile range
interregional displacement
interrupted
    i. LVG
    i. suture
intersacral canal
interscalene block
interscapular
    i. aching
    i. amputation
    i. reflex
interscapulothoracic forequarter
  amputation
Interseal
    I. acetabular cup
    I. Variant (I–IV) prosthesis
intersection syndrome
intersegmental
    i. fixation
    i. fusion
    i. mobility
    i. motion
    i. movement
    i. range of motion palpation
      (IRMP)
    i. rotation
    i. traction chiropractic table
intersesamoidal
intersesamoid ligament
interspace
    atlantoodontoid i.
    I. hip spacer
    I. knee spacer
    wedging of vertebral i.
interspinal
    i. ligament
    i. ligament
    i. process fusion
interspinous
    i. cable
    i. pseudarthrosis

interspinous (*continued*)
    i. segmental spinal instrumentation (ISSI)
    i. wiring
interstice, *pl.* **interstices**
interstices (*pl. of* interstice)
interstitial
    i. fluid
    i. lamella
    i. meniscal tear
    i. myofasciitis
interstitium
    bone i.
Intertan femoral fracture nail
interteardrop line
intertendinous vinculum
intertransverse
    i. fusion
    i. ligament
    i. process arthrodesis
intertrigo
intertrochanteric
    i. femoral fracture
    i. fracture (ITFx)
    i. 4-part fracture
    i. plate
    i. varus osteotomy
Intertron therapy microprocessor
intertubercular
    i. bursitis
    i. groove
    i. plane
    i. sulcus
interval
    acromiohumeral i. (AHI)
    anterior atlantoodontoid i.
    arthroscopic capsulolateral augmentation and rotator i.
    atlantoaxial i.
    atlantodens i. (ADI)
    atlas-dens i.
    biceps i.
    deltopectoral i.
    interdischarge i.
    interpeak i.
    interpotential i.
    Kocher i.
    posterior atlantoodontoid i.
    recruitment i.
    response i.
    scaphocapitate i.
    i. training
    trapeziodeltoid i.
intervening
    i. connective tissue
    i. muscle
intervention
    late i.

    prosthetic i.
    rehabilitation i.
intervertebral
    i. body stapling
    i. cartilage
    i. disc
    i. disc height
    i. disc herniation
    i. disc narrowing
    i. disc nucleus signal
    i. dysfunction
    i. joint
    i. motion
    i. motor unit
    i. notch
    i. space
intervertebralis
    calcinosis i.
interview
    Occupational Performance History I. (OPHI)
    School Setting I. (SSI)
    Worker Role I. (WRI)
intervolar plate ligament
intoe
intoeing gait
intolerance
    cold i.
    exercise i.
    fingertip cold i.
intorsion
intraacetabular
intraarticular
    i. adhesion
    i. arthrodesis
    i. calcaneal fracture
    i. cautery
    i. cautery device
    i. clavicle
    i. disc
    i. disc ligament
    i. dislocation
    i. fragment
    i. hip fusion
    i. injection
    i. jamming
    i. knee fusion
    i. loose body
    i. malunion
    i. osteochondroma
    i. osteoid osteoma
    i. osteotomy
    i. procedure
    i. proximal tibial fracture
    i. reconstruction
    i. structure
intracapsular
    i. ankylosis
    i. excision

i. fracture
i. osteoid osteoma
i. osteotomy
i. rupture
Intracell
  I. massage stick
  I. mechanical muscle device
  I. myofascial trigger-point device
  I. Sprinter stick
  I. trigger point massager
intracellulare
  Mycobacterium i.
intrachondrial bone
intracompartmental
  i. edema
  i. ischemia
  i. pressure
Intracone intramedullary reamer
intracortical
  i. fibrous dysplasia
  i. osteogenic sarcoma
  i. radiolucent lesion
intracranial pressure elevation
intractable plantar keratosis
intracuticular stitch
intradermal suture
intradiscal, intradiskal
  i. electrothermal therapy (IDET)
  i. electrothermal therapy procedure
  i. electrothermal treatment (IDET)
  i. electrothermal treatment procedure
  i. pressure
intradiskal (*var. of* intradiscal)
intradural
  i. anastomosis
  i. dorsal spinal root rhizotomy
  i. tumor surgery
intraepiphysial osteotomy
Intrafix
  I. ACL tibial fastener
  I. fixation
  I. screw
Intraflex
  I. intramedullary pin
  I. intramedullary pin extractor
intrafocal reduction technique
intraforaminal approach
intrafusal fiber
intralesional
  i. excision
  i. resection
  i. vascular resistance
intramedullary
  Ace i. (AIM)
  i. alignment jig
  i. alignment rod
  i. ANK nail
  i. arthrodesis
  i. bar

i. bone graft
i. bouquet fixation
i. canal
i. drill
i. elastic nail
i. fibular allograft
i. guide
i. hematoma
i. hemorrhage
i. lesion
i. nailing (IMN)
i. pin
i. reamer
i. rod fixation
i. saw
i. skeletal kinetic distractor (ISKD)
i. stem
i. supracondylar (IMSC)
i. supracondylar multihole nail
intramembranous
  i. formation
  i. ossification
intramuscular (IM)
  i. injection
  i. lengthening
  i. nerve transposition
  i. pressure (IMP)
  i. recording
intraneural
  i. fibrosis
  i. lipofibroma
intraoperative
  i. Cell Saver
  i. complication
  i. dural tear
  i. fluoroscopy
  i. fracture
  i. neck hyperextension
  i. roentgenography
  i. spinal cord monitoring
  i. stress-relaxation
  i. view
  i. x-ray
intraorganically induced
intraosseous
  i. abscess
  i. circulation
  i. fixation
  i. ganglion
  i. injection
  i. lipoma
  i. lipomatosis
  i. membrane
  i. nerve transposition
  i. osteosarcoma
  i. pneumatocyst
  i. probe
  i. suture anchor
  i. therapy

intraosseous (*continued*)
    i. tibiofibular ligament
    i. tophaceous gouty invasion
    i. tumor
    i. vascular congestion
    i. venography
    i. wire
    90-90 i. wire Nitinol flexible
    wire
    i. wiring
intrapedicular fixation
intrapelvic fixation
intraperiosteal fracture
intraprosthetic
intrapyretic amputation
intrascaphoid angle
IntraSite dressing
intraspinous muscle
intraspongy nuclear disc
  herniation
intratendinous
intrathecal
    i. anesthesia
    Lioresal I.
    i. neurolysis
intrathecally enhanced CT scan
intravascular hemolysis
intravenous
    i. block anesthesia
    i. regional anesthesia (IVRA)
    i. therapy
intravertebral
    i. foramen
    i. vacuum cleft sign
Intrepid functional knee brace
intrinsic
    i. clubfoot
    i. contracture
    i. equilibrium
    i. function
    i. metatarsus primus elevatus
    i. minus deformity
    i. minus hallux
    i. minus hand
    i. minus position
    i. muscle
    i. muscle strength
    i. paralysis
    i. plus deformity
    i. plus hand
    i. restoration
    i. tightness test
    i. transverse connector
    i. transverse connector role
intrinsics
    finger i.
    hand i.
introducer
    Charnley i.

    Dumon-Gilliard prosthesis i.
    staple i.
intubation
    endotracheal i.
Invacare
    I. APM mattress
    I. Comfort-Mate extra cushion
    I. manual wheelchair
    I. padded shower chair
    I. vinyl transfer bench
invagination
    basilar i.
    endplate i.
invalid
    i. cushion
    i. ring
invasion
    intraosseous tophaceous gouty i.
    vascular i.
inventory
    Brief Pain I.
    Child Behaviors I. (CBI)
    Child Development I.
    Mayo-Portland Adaptability I. 3
      (MPAI-3)
    Millon Behavioral Health I.
    Millon Clinical Multiaxial I.
      (MCMI)
    Multidimensional Pain i.
    Neurobehavioral Functioning I. (NFI)
    Pediatric Evaluation of Disability I.
      (PEDI)
    Vanderbilt Pain Management I.
    Westhaven Yale Multidimensional
      Pain I. (WHYMPI)
inversion
    ankle i.
    i. ankle injury
    i. ankle sprain
    i. ankle stress view
    fixed i.
    i. instability
    i. of muscle action
    restricted i.
    i. stress test
inversion-eversion
    ankle i.-e.
    i.-e. exercise
    i.-e. rotation
InvertaChair traction device
inverted
    i. champagne bottle leg
    i. Napoleon hat sign
    i. orthotic
    i. radial reflex
    i. scarf Z-osteotomy
    i. skin flap
    i. smile
inverted-L lateral periosteal incision

inverted-Y
>   i.-Y Achilles tenotomy
>   i.-Y fracture
>   i.-Y incision

inverting knot technique
invertor force
Invertrac equipment
investing fascia
involucra (*pl. of* involucrum)
involucre (*var. of* involucrum)
involucrum, involucre, *pl.* **involucra**
involuntary activity
involvement
>   pantalocrural arthritic i.
>   tumorous i.

inward rotation
Ioban Vi-Drape
Iodex
Iodex-p
iodine
iodine-labeled fibrinogen
iodoform gauze
iodoform-impregnated plastic sheet
iodophor solution
IOM
>   interosseous membrane

Ionact antibacterial protection
ion-bombarded cobalt-chromium
IonGuard orthopaedic surface treatment
ionized
>   i. gas
>   i. gas field

iontophoresis
>   Dynaphor i.

iopamidol myelography
Iowa
>   I. degenerative change
>   I. hip score
>   I. hip status rating system
>   I. implant material
>   I. internal prosthesis
>   I. stem
>   I. total hip prosthesis
>   I. University periosteal elevator

IP
>   ice pack
>   interphalangeal
>   IP joint

IPCS
>   infrapatellar contracture syndrome

I-plate
>   Syracuse I-p.

I-Plus
>   I-P. system humeral fracture brace
>   I-P. system ulnar fracture brace

Ipomax orthosis
IPOP
>   immediate postoperative prosthesis

Ipos
>   I. arch support system
>   I. forefoot relief orthosis
>   I. heel relief orthosis
>   I. heel relief shoe
>   I. postoperative shoe

ipriflavone
>   Pinna-Cal i.

IPS
>   immediate postoperative stability
>   IPS total hip system

IPSF
>   immediate postsurgical fitting

ipsilateral
>   i. approach
>   i. femoral neck fracture
>   i. femoral shaft fracture
>   i. foot injury
>   i. rotation
>   i. side bending
>   i. slide graft
>   i. total elbow arthroplasty
>   i. total shoulder arthroplasty
>   i. vascularized fibula transfer (IVFT)

IR
>   infrared
>   isotonic reversal
>   HydroStat IR

IRE
>   internal rotation in extension

IRF
>   internal rotation in flexion

IRFPAI
>   Inpatient Rehabilitation Facility Patient Assessment Instrument

iris scissors
IRMP
>   intersegmental range of motion palpation

IROM
>   incremental range of motion

Irom
>   I. bilateral splint
>   I. Regal splint
>   I. splint with shells

iron
>   i. deficiency anemia
>   Jewett bending i.

Ironman Triathlon Pro-Power massager
irradiation
>   i. fibromatosis
>   i. sterilized graft

irreducible
>   i. anterior atlantoaxial dislocation (IAAD)
>   i. fracture
>   i. fracture dislocation

irregular
   i. articular surface
   i. bone
   i. potential
irregularity
   tendon i.
irregular-shaped lesion
irrigating solution
irrigation
   i. and débridement
   i. bulb
   i. burn
   closed i.
   closed suction i.
   drip-suck i.
   gravity inflow i.
   Pulsavac i.
   i. solution
   i. suction
   Systec i.
   i. system
   i. tube
   WaterPik i.
   wound i.
irrigator
   Arthro-Flo i.
   Baumrucker clamp i.
   Fisch bone drill i.
   jet i.
   pulse i.
irritability
   nerve root i.
   soft tissue i.
irritable
   i. hip
   i. joint
   i. lesion
   i. symptom
irritation
   i. callus
   facet joint i.
   nerve root i.
   sciatic nerve i.
   spinal cord i.
Irvine
   I. ankle
   I. ankle arthroplasty
   University of California I.
     (UCI)
Irwin osteotomy
IS
   iliosacral
   immunosuppression
Isaac-Merton syndrome
Isaac syndrome, Isaac-Merton syndrome
ISAKOS
   International Society of Arthroscopy,
   Knee Surgery, and Orthopaedic
   Sports Medicine

ischaemia (*var. of* ischemia)
ischaemic (*var. of* ischemic)
Isch-Dish Plus cushion
ischemia, ischaemia
   capillary i.
   critical limb i. (CLI)
   exercise i.
   foot i.
   intracompartmental i.
   muscle i.
   myocardial i.
   myoneural i.
   postural i.
   tourniquet i.
   vasospastic i.
   Volkmann i.
   warm i.
ischemic, ischaemic
   i. compression
   i. contracture
   i. disease of growing hip (IDGH)
   i. foot
   i. forearm exercise test
   i. gangrene
   i. leg disease
   i. lesion
   i. limb
   i. limb disease (ILD)
   i. lumbago
   i. myositis
   i. necrosis
   i. necrosis of femoral head (INFH)
   i. tourniquet technique
   i. ulcer
ischia (*pl. of* ischium)
ischial
   i. bone
   i. bursitis
   i. containment socket
   i. spine
   i. tuberosity (IT)
   i. weightbearing leg brace
   i. weightbearing orthosis
   i. weightbearing prosthesis (IWP)
   i. weightbearing ring
ischial-bearing seat
ischialgia
ischial-gluteal weightbearing socket
ischiatic scoliosis
ischii (*gen. of* ischium)
ischiectomy
ischioacetabular fracture
ischiodynia
ischiofemoral ligament
ischiogluteal
   i. bursa
   i. bursitis
ischiohebotomy
ischionitis

ischiopubic
    i. arch
    i. foramen
    i. ramus
ischiopubiotomy
ischiorectal
    i. abscess
    i. fossa
    i. region
ischium, *pl.* **ischia,** *gen.* **ischii**
Iselin disease
Ishihara cervical spine curve index
Ishizuki unconstrained elbow prosthesis
ISIS
    International Spine Intervention Society
    ISIS scoliosis screening
ISKD
    intramedullary skeletal kinetic distractor
    ISKD system
island
    i. adipofascial flap
    bone i.
    fibrin i.
    giant bone i.
    i. graft
    i. skin flap
Isobaric epidural/spinal anesthesia technique
Isobar LP low profile pedicle screw system
Isocaine HCl
isodynamic
IsoDyn knee brace
isoelastic pelvic prosthesis
isograft
    bone i.
isoinertial
isokinetic
    i. assessment
    concentric bilateral i.
    i. dynamometer
    i. dynamometry
    i. evaluation
    i. exercise
    i. joint apparatus
    i. knee extension
    i. movement
    i. performance
    i. resistance apparatus
    i. strength test maximal
    i. testing
    i. torque imbalance
    i. Unex III exerciser
Isola
    I. fixation system
    I. hook-rod
    I. spinal implant system accessory
    I. spinal implant system anchor
    I. spinal implant system application

    I. spinal implant system eye rod
    I. spinal implant system hook
    I. spinal implant system iliac post
    I. spinal implant system iliac screw
    I. spinal implant system plate-rod combination
    I. spinal instrumentation system
    I. vertebral screw
    I. wire
isolated
    i. avulsion
    i. dislocation
    i. modular tibial insert exchange
    i. paralysis
    i. zone
isolation drape
isolator
    Ankle I.
isologous graft
isometer
    I. bone graft placement site detector
    CA-5000 drill-guide i.
    PCL Protension i.
    tension i.
isometheptene mucate
isometric
    i. cervical extension strength
    i. contraction
    i. device
    i. exercise (IME)
    i. force
    i. motor testing
    i. point
    i. resistance
    i. strain gauge
    i. strength testing
    i. technique
    i. traction
    i. training
isometricity
isometrics
isoniazid
isophendylate
Isoprene plastic splint
isoproterenol
Isoptin
Iso-Quadron exerciser
Isostation B–200 triaxial lumbar dynamometer
Isotechnologies B-200 low back exercise machine
Isotec patellar tendon graft
Isotoner glove
isotonic
    combination of i.'s (COI)
    i. contraction
    i. exercise
    i. machine
    i. motor testing

isotonic (*continued*)
    i. resistance
    i. reversal (IR)
    i. traction
    i. training
isotope
    bone mineralization i.
    i. bone scan
isotropic disc
Isovue myelography
Israel
    I. rasp
    I. retractor
ISS
    Injury Severity Score
ISSI
    interspinous segmental spinal
    instrumentation
**Issys inverted polyaxial pedicle screw
system**
IST
    immunosuppressive therapy
iStep FIT digital scanner
isthmic spondylolisthesis
isthmi (*pl. of* isthmus)
isthmus, *pl.* **isthmi, isthmuses**
isthmuses (*pl. of* isthmus)
isuprel
IT
    ischial tuberosity
ITB
    iliotibial band
        ITB fasciitis
        ITB strap
ITBFS
    iliotibial band friction
    syndrome

ITBS
    iliotibial band syndrome
ITCL
    interosseous talocalcaneal ligament
ITFx
    intertrochanteric fracture
itraconazole
Itrel
    I. II, III spinal cord stimulation
    system
    I. programmed transmitter-receiver
ITT
    iliotibial tract
    internal tibial torsion
ITV
    infantile tibia vara
ITW
    idiopathic toe-walker
    idiopathic toe walking
I.V.
    Indocin I.V.
    Merrem I.V.
Ivalon prosthesis
IVC
    inferior vena cava
IVFT
    ipsilateral vascularized fibula transfer
ivory
    i. bone
    i. osteoma
    i. phalanx sign
    i. vertebra
IVRA
    intravenous regional anesthesia
iWALKfree hands-free crutch
IWP
    ischial weightbearing prosthesis

J

J board
J disc
J pad
J patellofemoral brace
J septum
J sign

JA

juvenile arthritis

jab, hook, punch, injury mechanism combination

Jaboulay amputation

Jaccoud

J. arthritis
J. arthropathy
J. arthroplasty
J. syndrome

Jace

J. hand continuous passive motion unit
J. shoulder exerciser
J. W550 CPM device

jack

J. Frost hot/cold pack
J. test
turnbuckle j.
j. upper cut

jacket

body j.
Boston soft body j.
cervicothoracic j.
flexion body j.
Frejka j.
halo body j.
halo traction j.
immobilization j.
Kydex body j.
Lexan j.
Low Profile plastic body j.
LS^4 custom spinal j.
Minerva cervical j.
Orfizip body j.
Orthoplast j.
plaster cast j.
plastic body j.
Prenyl j.
Royalite body j.
Sayre j.
underarm body j.
Vitrathene j.
von Lackum transection shift j.
Wilmington plastic j.

jackknife

j. position
j. test

Jacknobber

The J. II

Jackson

ankle scoring system of Baird and J.
J. bone clamp
J. bone-extension clamp
J. bone-holding clamp
J. broad-blade staple forceps
J. cerebellar syndrome
J. compression test
J. dressing forceps
J. intervertebral disc rongeur
J. intrasacral bar Jackson intrasacral bar
J. spinal surgery and imaging table
J. tendon-seizing forceps

Jackson-Gorham syndrome

jacksonian epilepsy

Jackson-Pollock skinfold equation

Jackson-Pratt drain

Jacksonville sling

Jackson-Weiss syndrome

Jacobs

J. chuck
J. chuck adapter
J. chuck drill
J. chuck drive
J. distraction rod
J. locking hook spinal rod
J. locking hook spinal rod instrumentation
J. locking hook spinal rod instrumentation modification
J. locking hook spinal rod technique

Jacob shift test

Jacobson

J. bulldog clamp
J. mosquito forceps
J. needle holder
J. resonator
J. suture pusher
J. system

Jacoby

J. bunion splint
J. heel splint

Jacquet fixator

Jadassohn-Lewandowsky syndrome

JAFAR

Juvenile Arthritis Functional Assessment Report

Jaffe
J. disease
J. press-fit prosthesis
J. procedure
Jaffe-Campanacci syndrome
jagged osteophyte
Jahss
J. ankle dislocation classification
J. dorsal wedge osteotomy
procedure
J. metacarpal neck fracture
reduction maneuver
J. metatarsophalangeal joint
dislocation classification
J. 90-90 method
Jakob
J. knee test
J. shoulder test
Jamaica Sandalthotics orthotic
Jamar
J. grip strength test
J. grip tester
J. hydraulic hand
dynamometer
J. hydraulic pinch gauge
James
J. position
J. procedure
J. splint
J. wound forceps
Jameson
J. muscle clamp
J. muscle hook
jammed finger
jamming
intraarticular j.
Jamshidi needle
**Janis tibialis posterior tendon
dysfunction classification**
Jannetta
J. duckbill elevator
J. hook
Jansen
J. bone curette
J. disease
J. metaphysial dysostosis
J. monopolar forceps
J. rasp
J. test
Jansey
J. shoulder arthrodesis technique
J. toenail ablation procedure
Jansky-Bielschowsky disease
Jan van Breemen (JVB)
Japanese
J. Orthopaedic Association
(JOA)
J. Orthopaedic Association
Scale

Japas
J. osteotomy
J. V-osteotomy
jar
heel j.
Jarcho-Levin syndrome
Jarell forceps
Jarit
J. anterior resection clamp
J. cartilage clamp
J. meniscal clamp
J. pin cutter
J. rotator
J. small bone-holding clamp
J. tendon-pulling forceps
JAS
Joint Active Systems
JAS EZ elbow device
Jaszczak phantom
javelin thrower's elbow
jaw
j. claudication
j. exerciser
j. opening reflex (JOR)
3-jaw chuck
Jay
J. basic cushion
J. Combi cushion
J. J2 wheelchair
J. Rave cushion
J. Triad cushion
J. Xtreme cushion
JCE
job capacity evaluation
J-24 cervical orthosis
J-45 contraflexion orthosis
JCS
joint coordinate system
J2 cushion
Jeanie
J. Rub
J. Rub Massager
Jebsen
J. assessment
J. assessment of hand function
J. hand function test
Jebsen-Taylor hand function test
Jefferson cervical burst fracture
Jeffery
J. radial fracture classification
J. technique
Jeffrey radial head fracture (type I–II)
Jendrassik maneuver
Jergesen
J. I-beam
J. I-beam plate
J. incision
J. tapered plate
J. tube

jerk
- Achilles j.
- ankle j.
- elbow j.
- j. finger
- hung-up knee j.
- knee j.
- j. knee test
- patellar j.
- quadriceps j.
- j. sign
- supinator j.
- tendon j.
- triceps j.
- triceps surae j.

jerky gait
jersey finger
jet
- j. irrigator
- j. lavage
- Ortholav j.
- J. Vac cement dispenser

Jet-Air splint
Jeter lag/position screw
jet-pilot position
Jette Functional Status index
Jettmobile positioning and tumble form
jeweler's
- j. forceps
- j. thumb

Jewett
- J. bending iron
- J. contraflexion orthosis
- J. driver
- J. extractor
- J. gouge
- J. hyperextension orthosis
- J. nail
- J. nail overlay plate
- J. operation
- J. pick-up screw
- J. postfusion orthosis
- J. prosthesis
- J. thoracolumbosacral orthosis

Jewett-Benjamin
- J.-B. cervical brace
- J.-B. cervical orthosis

J-FX bipolar head
J-hook deformity
J-35 hyperextension orthosis
JIDC
- juvenile intervertebral disc calcification

jig
- chamfer cut j.
- Charnley tibial onlay j.
- cutting j.
- drilling j.
- external-alignment compression j.
- extramedullary tibial alignment j.

- femoral alignment j.
- fixation j.
- Herbert j.
- j. hook
- intramedullary alignment j.
- Miller-Galante j.
- Osteonics j.
- Plexiglas j.
- precompression j.
- spacer-tensor j.
- tibial j.

J&J
- Johnson & Johnson
- J&J postoperative shoe
- J&J ulcer dressing

JOA
- Japanese Orthopaedic Association
- JOA Scale

job
- j. capacity evaluation (JCE)
- j. redesign
- j. task analysis (JTA)

Jobe relocation shoulder test
Jobert fossa
job-related hazard
Jobst
- J. air band
- J. appliance
- J. athrombotic pump
- J. boot
- J. brassiere
- J. gauntlet
- J. glove
- J. prosthesis
- J. stockings

jockey cap patella
Joerns orthopaedic bed
jogger's
- j. heel
- j. nipples
- j. toe

jogging in place test
Johannesberg staple
Johannson lag screw
Johanson-Blizzard syndrome
Johansson fracture classification
John
- J. Barnes myofascial release
- J. C. Wilson arthrodesis

Johns
- J. Hopkins bulldog clamp
- J. Hopkins National Low Back Pain Study

Johnson
- J. and Strom tibialis posterior tendon dysfunction classification
- J. chevron osteotomy
- J. hemiphalangectomy
- J. & Johnson (J&J)

Johnson (*continued*)
    J. & Johnson PFC
      cruciate-substituting insert
    J. medial meniscal suturing
    J. pelvic fracture technique
    J. procedure
    J. pronator advancement
    J. resection arthroplasty
    J. screwdriver
    J. staple technique
Johnson-Boseker scale
Johnson-Elloy Accord unconstrained
prosthesis
Johnson-Jahss classification of posterior
tibial tendon tear
Johnson-Spiegl procedure
Johnston-Iowa hip prosthesis
joint
    AC j.
    acromioclavicular j. (ACJ)
    J. Active Systems (JAS)
    adjustable dynamic j. (ADJ)
    amphidiarthrodial j.
    ankle j.
    anterior sternoclavicular j.
    apophysial j.
    j. arthrodesis
    j. arthrogram
    j. arthrography
    j. arthrometer
    j. arthropathy
    arthroscopy of subtalar j.
    Ascension MCP total j.
    Ascension PIP total j.
    j. aspiration
    j. assessment
    atlantoaxial j.
    atlantooccipital j.
    atlantoodontoid j.
    bail-lock knee j.
    ball-and-socket j.
    basal j.
    beaking j.
    biaxial j.
    bilocular j.
    j. block
    Budin j.
    calcaneocuboid j. (CCJ)
    calcaneonavicular j.
    Cam lock knee j.
    capitate-hamate j.
    capitate-lunate j.
    j. capsule
    j. capsule mechanoreceptor
    carpal-intercarpal j.
    carpometacarpal j.
    carpophalangeal j.
    cartilaginous j.
    j. cavitation

j. cavity
CC j.
cervical j.
Charcot j.
j. chondroma
Chopart midtarsal j.
j. cinch
Clevisphere ankle j.
Clutton j.
CMC j.
coccygeal j.
composite j.
compound j.
condyloid j.
j. congruence
congruent metatarsophalangeal j.
j. coordinate system (JCS)
j. coordination
coracoclavicular j.
correction of dislocated second
    metatarsophalangeal j.
costochondral j.
costotransverse j.
costovertebral j.
coxofemoral j.
cracking of j.
craniomandibular j.
Cruveilhier j.
CT-guided percutaneous screw
    placement for sacroiliac j.
cubital j.
cubonavicular j.
cuneiform j.
cuneometatarsal j.
cuneonavicular j.
j. debris
j. deformity
j. degeneration
j. depression fracture
diarthrodial j.
digital j.
DIP j.
j. disarticulation
j. disease
j. dislocation
j. disruption
distal interphalangeal j.
distal radioulnar j. (DRUJ)
distal tibiofibular j.
j. distraction
j. distraction cuff
j. distractor
double-action ankle j.
double pearl-face hip j.
double-stem silicone lesser MP j.
DRU j.
dry j.
j. dysfunction
j. effusion

elastic knee cage with medial and
  lateral contoured knee j.'s
elbow j.
ellipsoid j.
ellipsoidal j.
enarthrodial j.
j. end-feel
erythema of j.
j. extension
extraarticular subtalar j.
facet j.
false j.
femoropatellar j.
femorotibial j.
fibrocartilaginous j.
fibrous j.
Fillauer dorsiflexion assist ankle j.
Fillauer PDC ankle j.
finger j.
flail j.
j. force
fourth metatarsophalangeal j.
freely movable j.
fringe j.
j. fulcrum
j. fusion
Gaffney j.
Gillette double-flexure ankle j.
ginglymoid j.
glenohumeral j.
gliding hinge j.
Greissinger Multiaxis j.
hallux IP j.
hamate-lunate j.
hemophilic j.
hinged j.
hot j.
humeral j.
humeroradial j.
humeroulnar j.
j. hyperextensibility
hyperextensibility of j.
hypermobile j.
j. hypermobility
hysteric j.
hysterical j.
IM j.
j. immobilization
j. immobilizer
immovable j.
j. implant
incudomalleolar j.
inferior radioulnar j.
inferior tibiofibular j.
j. injection
j. instability
Integrated Ankle orthotic ankle j.
interarticular j.
intercarpal j.

interchondral j.
intercuneiform j.
intermetacarpal j.
intermetatarsal j.
j. internal derangement
interphalangeal j.
intervertebral j.
IP j.
irritable j.
j. kinematics
knee j.
lap j.
lateral atlantoaxial j.
j. lavage
j. laxity
lesser metatarsophalangeal j.
j. leveling
limited motion metal ankle j.
j. line
j. line pain
j. line tenderness
Lisfranc j.
Lisfranc Charcot j.
locking of j.
LT j.
lumbosacral j.
lunocapitate j.
lunotriquetral j.
Luschka j.
j. manipulation
manubriosternal j.
j. meniscoid
metacarpocapitate j.
metacarpocarpal j.
metacarpohamate j.
metacarpophalangeal j.
  (MPJ)
metacarpophysial j.
metacarpotrapezoid j.
Metasul j.
metatarsal j.
metatarsal-tarsal j.
metatarsocuboid j.
metatarsocuneiform j.
metatarsophalangeal j.
metatarsosesamoid j.
j. mice
midcarpal j.
middle atlantoepistrophic j.
middle carpal j.
midfoot j.
midtarsal j.
j. mobility
j. mobilization
j. model
mortise and tenon j.
j. motion
movable j.
MTP j.

joint (*continued*)
    multiaxial j.
    multiple-axis knee j.
    naviculocuneiform j.
    near-anatomic position of j.
    neuropathic j.
    neurotrophic j.
    noncongruent metatarsophalangeal j.
    nonsubluxated metatarsophalangeal j.
    oblique metatarsocuneiform j.
    occipital-atlantal j.
    occipital-axis j.
    occipitoatlantoaxial j.
    Oklahoma ankle j.
    j. osteoarthritis
    Otto Bock 3R65 children's hydraulic
      knee j.
    Otto Bock 3R45 modular knee j.
    patellofemoral j.
    PIP j.
    pisotriquetral j.
    pivot j.
    plane j.
    plastic limited-motion j.
    j. play
    polyaxial j.
    j. popping
    j. position sense (JPS)
    posterior approach to sacrum and
      sacroiliac j.
    prosthetic replacement for j.
    proximal interphalangeal j.
    proximal radioulnar j.
    proximal tibiofibular j.
    pseudo-Charcot j.
    radiocapitellar j.
    radiocarpal j.
    radiohumeral j.
    radiolunate j.
    radioscaphoid j.
    radioscapholunate j.
    radioulnar j.
    j. reconstruction
    j. release
    j. replacement surgery
    j. rice
    3R80 modular hydraulic knee j.
    rotary j.
    sacrococcygeal j.
    sacroiliac j.
    saddle-shaped j.
    j. salvage procedure
    SC j.
    scaphocapitate j.
    scapholunate j.
    scaphotrapezoid-trapezial j.
    scapuloclavicular j.
    scapulothoracic j. (STJ)
    Scotty stainless ankle j.

Select j.
septic finger j.
sesamoidometatarsal j.
shoulder j.
SI j.
silastic finger j.
Silastic HP-100 prosthetic finger j.
simple j.
single-axis ankle j.
single pearl-face hip j.
single smooth-face hip j.
S-K reconstruction of distal
  radioulnar j.
slip j.
solid ankle j.
j. space
j. spacer
spheroidal j.
spiral j.
j. sprain
stable hinge j.
sternoclavicular j.
sternocostal j.
j. stiffness
stifle j.
STT j.
subcrural j.
subluxated metatarsophalangeal j.
j. subluxation
subtalar j. (STJ)
superior radioulnar j.
superior tibiofibular j.
Sutter silicone
  metacarpophalangeal j.
Swanson finger j.
j. swelling
synarthrodial j.
synovial j.
talocalcaneal j.
talocalcaneonavicular j.
talocrural j.
talofibular j.
talonavicular j.
Tamarack flexure j.
tarsal j.
tarsometatarsal j.
temporomandibular j. (TMJ)
J. Theater Trauma Registry (JTTR)
J. Theater Trauma Registry military
  database
tibiofemoral j.
tibiofibular j.
tibiotalar j.
TN j.
total replacement j.
track-bound j.
transverse tarsal j.
trapeziometacarpal j.
trapeziotrapezoidal j.

triscaphe j.
trochoid j.
ulnocarpal j.
ulnohumeral j.
ulnomeniscotriquetral j.
Ultraflex dynamic j.
uncovertebral j.
uniaxial j.
unilocular j.
unstable j.
j. verrucous carcinoma
Virtual hip j.
von Gies j.
j. warmth
wedge-and-groove j.
weightbearing j.
j. wound
j. wrap
wrist j.
xiphisternal j.
zygapophysial j.
3-joint complex
joint-destructive procedure
jointed
double j.
Joint-Jack finger splint
joint-preservation surgery
joker
j. dissector
j. periosteal elevator
Jolly myasthenic reaction test
Jonas prosthesis
Jonell
J. countertraction finger splint
J. thumb splint
Jones
J. abduction frame
J. and Brackett anterior approach
J. arm splint
J. brace
J. classification of congenital tibial deficiency
J. cock-up toe operation
J. compression cast
J. compression pin
J. compression plate
J. congenital tibial deficiency classification
J. diaphysial fracture classification
J. dressing
J. elbow in flexion view
Ellis J.
J. first toe repair
J. fracture
J. metacarpal splint
J. position
J. resection arthroplasty
J. retinaculum reconstruction procedure

J. scissors
J. screw
J. suspension traction
J. tendon test
J. tendosuspension
J. thoracic clamp
J. towel clamp
J. traction splint
Jones-Ellison ACL reconstruction
Joplin
J. bunionectomy
J. operation
J. toe prosthesis
JOR
jaw opening reflex
Jordan frame
Joseph
J. hook
J. nasal rasp
J. osteotome
J. periosteal elevator
J. periosteotome
J. splint
Journal of Manipulative and Physiological Therapeutics
Jousto dropfoot splint, skid orthosis
JoyBags therapeutic heat pack
J-periosteal elevator
J-55 postfusion orthosis
JPS
joint position sense
Jr.
Caltrate Jr.
Children's Dynafed Jr.
JRA
juvenile rheumatoid arthritis
J.R. Moore procedure
J-shaped skin incision
JSMA
juvenile spinal muscular atrophy
JTA
job task analysis
JTTR
Joint Theater Trauma Registry
JTTR military database
Judet
J. epiphysial fracture classification
J. hip status system
J. oblique acetabulum view
J. press-fit hip prosthesis
J. quadricepsplasty
J. radiograph
J. vascularized bone graft
Juers-Lempert rongeur forceps
jugal
j. bone
j. suture
Julstro Self-Treatment system

jumbo
- j. acetabular cup
- j. uncemented cup acetabular component revision

jump
- drop vertical j.
- j. graft
- j. sign
- squat j.

jumper's
- j. knee
- j. knee position

jumping leg

junction
- allograft-host j.
- atlantooccipital j.
- beaked cervicomedullary j.
- cervicomedullary j.
- cervicothoracic j.
- craniovertebral j.
- femoral head-neck j.
- gastrocnemius-soleus j.
- host-allograft j.
- lumbosacral j.
- meniscocapsular j.
- meniscosynovial j.
- metaphysial-diaphysial j.
- modified anterior approach to cervical thoracic j.
- musculotendinous j.
- myotendinous j.
- occipitocervical j.
- tarsometatarsal j.
- thoracolumbar j.

junctional
- j. fracture
- j. kyphosis
- j. nevus

junctura, *pl.* **juncturae**

juncturae (*pl. of* junctura)

Jüngling disease

Jung muscle

junior
- J. Strength Motrin
- J. Strength Panadol

Junod boot

Jurgan
- J. Fixator Ball
- J. pin
- J. Pin Ball
- J. Pin Ball pin protector
- J. Pin Ball system

jury-rig

Juvara
- J. bunionectomy
- J. closing abudetory wedge for feet procedure
- J. foot operation

juvenile
- j. aponeurotic fibroma
- j. arthritis (JA)
- J. Arthritis Functional Assessment Report (JAFAR)
- j. bunion
- j. bunionectomy
- j. chronic arthritis
- j. discitis
- j. flatfoot pathomechanics
- j. hallux valgus
- j. hinge axis concept
- j. hyaline fibromatosis
- j. idiopathic scoliosis
- j. intervertebral disc calcification (JIDC)
- j. kyphosis
- j. muscular atrophy
- j. muscular dystrophy
- j. osteoporosis
- j. Paget disease
- j. pelvis
- j. plantar dermatosis
- j. polyarthritis
- j. rheumatoid arthritis (JRA)
- j. spinal muscular atrophy (JSMA)
- j. thoracic kyphosis
- j. Tillaux fracture
- j. xanthogranuloma

juvenile-onset
- j.-o. ankylosing spondylitis
- j.-o. rheumatoid arthritis

juvenilis
- osteochondritis j.
- osteochondritis deformans j.

Jux-A-Cisor exerciser

juxtaarticular
- j. bone cyst
- j. fracture
- j. lesion

juxtaarticulation

juxtacortical
- j. chondroma
- j. chondrosarcoma
- j. fracture

juxtacubital reconstruction

juxtaepiphysial

juxtaspinal

juxtatectal transverse fracture

Juzo
- J. brace
- J. Patellaligner brace
- J. support

J-Vac closed drainage system

JVB
- Jan van Breemen
- JVB function questionnaire

K
> kiintscher
> Kirschner
> potassium
> > K blade
> > K nail
> > K needle
> > K rod
> > K wire
> > K wire driver
> > K wire fixation
> > K wire placement

K2
> > K2 hemi toe implant system
> > K2 sensation prosthesis

Kadian Capsule
Kaesar
> scapuloperoneal syndrome type K.

KAFO
> knee-ankle-foot orthosis
> Generation II KAFO
> PRAFO KAFO

Kager
> K. Achilles tendon triangle
> K. fat pad

Kalamchi
> K. avascular necrosis
> classification
> K. osteotomy

Kaleidoscope chair
Kalish
> K. bunionectomy
> K. bunionectomy modification
> K. Duredge wire cutter
> K. Duredge wire extractor
> K. osteotomy

Kalix flatfoot implant
Kallassy
> K. ankle support
> K. brace
> K. orthosis

Kaltenborn joint mobilization system
Kaltostat dressing
Kambin triangular working zone
Kampe corset
kanamycin
Kanavel
> K. cock-up splint
> K. palm triangle
> K. sign

Kaneda
> K. anterior spinal instrumentation
> K. anterior spinal/scoliosis system
> (KASS)

> K. distraction device
> K. plate
> K. rod

kansasii
> *Mycobacterium k.*

Kantrex
Kantrowitz thoracic clamp
Kapandji
> K. fracture
> K. fracture of radius
> K. pinning technique
> K. thumb opposition score

Kapandji-Sauvé
> K.-S. arthrodesis
> K.-S. technique

Kapel
> K. elbow dislocation technique
> K. operation

Kaplan
> K. modification
> K. modification of Ruiz-Mora
> procedure
> K. oblique line
> K. open metacarpophalangeal joint
> reduction
> K. osteotomy
> K. sign
> K. technique

Kaposi sarcoma
kappa receptor
Kaprelian easy-access tweezers (KEAT)
karate
> Shotokan k.

karate-inspired aerobics
Karfoil splint
Karlsson
> K. and Peterson scoring scale
> K. ankle instability correction
> procedure

Karsch-Neugebauer syndrome
KAS
> Kofoed ankle score

Kasdan retractor
Kashin-Bek disease
Kashiwagi
> K. elbow arthroplasty technique
> K. ulnohumeral resection

KASS
> Kaneda anterior spinal/scoliosis
> system

Kast syndrome
KAT
> Kinesthetic Ability Trainer

Kates forefoot arthroplasty

K

Katz
>K. ADL index
>K. index of activities of daily
>living

Kaufer tendon technique
Kaufmann subpial transection technique
Kavanaugh-Brower-Mann fixation
Kawamura
>K. dome osteotomy
>K. pelvic osteotomy

Kay scissors
Kazanjian splint
K-Cap
Keane mobility bed
Kearns-Sayre syndrome
KEAT
>Kaprelian easy-access tweezers

KED
>Kendrick extrication device

keel
>All Poly Deltafit k.
>k. and wing
>k. bone punch
>Deltafit K.
>k. of glenoid component

keeled
>k. chest
>k. prosthesis

Keene
>K. compression hook
>K. obturator

Keen sign
Kefurox Injection
Kefzol
Kehr
>K. procedure
>K. sign

Keitel index
Keithley clamp kit
Keith needle
Kelikian
>K. classification of nail deformity
>K. foot dressing
>K. lateral ankle suture anchor
>procedure
>K. metatarsal push-up test
>K. modified Z bunionectomy
>K. modified Z osteotomy
>K. modified Z
>osteotomy/bunionectomy
>K. nail deformity classification

Keller
>K. arthroplasty
>K. bunionectomy
>K. bunionectomy procedure
>K. bunionectomy with prosthesis
>K. foot operation
>K. hallux valgus operation
>K. resection arthroplasty

Keller-Blake
>K.-B. half-ring splint
>K.-B. leg splint

Keller-Brandes
>K.-B. procedure
>K.-B. resection arthroplasty

Keller-Lelièvre arthroplasty
Keller-Mann resection arthroplasty
Keller-Mayo diabetic foot arthroplasty
Kellgren
>K. and Lawrence osteoarthritis
>grade (0–4)
>K. degenerative disc disease
>criteria
>K. knee scale
>K. sign

Kellgren-Lawrence grading system
Kellogg-Speed
>K.-S. lumbar spinal fusion
>K.-S. operation

Kelly
>K. clamp
>K. forceps
>K. hemostat
>K. peroneal tendon dislocation
>procedure
>K. tendon lengthening osteotomy

Kelly-Keck osteotomy
Kelly-Kelly osteotomy
keloid scar
KELS
>Kohlman Evaluation of Living Skills

Kelsey unloading exercise therapy
Kelvin body
Kempf internal screw fixation
Kempson-Campanacci lesion
Kemp spinal test
Kemron
Ken
>K. driver
>K. driver-extractor
>K. screwdriver
>K. sliding nail

Kenacort
Kenaject-40
Kenalog-10, -40
Kenalog H
Kendall
>K. A-V impulse system
>K. muscle grade (1–5)
>K. muscle grade percent (0–100)

Kendrick
>K. below-knee amputation
>procedure
>K. extrication device (KED)

Kenna Knee Scale
Kennedy
>K. LAD
>K. ligament augmenting device

K. ligament technique
K. modification of Gallie ankle
 fusion
K. spillproof cup
Kennerdell-Maroon
K.-M. elevator
K.-M. hook
Kenny
K. ADL index
K. Self-Care Questionnaire
K. treatment
Kenny-Caffey syndrome
Kenny-Howard
K.-H. shoulder sling
K.-H. splint
Keolar implant material
Keralyt Gel
**Keramos ceramic/ceramic total hip
system**
Kerasal ointment
keratoderma blennorrhagica
keratolysis
pitted k.
keratolytic agent
keratoma
indurated plantar k.
keratome, keratotome
automated disposable k.
k. Beaver blade
keratoprosthesis
keratoses (*pl. of* keratosis)
keratosis, *pl.* **keratoses**
actinic k.
intractable plantar k.
plantar k.
k. punctata
stucco k.
keratotome (*var. of* keratome)
keraunoparalysis
keraunopathology
**Kerboull acetabular reinforcement
device**
Kerlix
K. bandage
K. cast padding
K. dressing
K. gauze
K. wrap
Kern
K. bone-holding clamp
K. bone-holding forceps
Kernig sign
Kern-Lane bone forceps
Kerpel bone curette
Kerr
K. abduction splint
K. electro-torque drill
K. hand drill
K. sign

Kerrison
K. chisel
K. curette
K. downbiting rongeur
K. punch
Kerr-Lagen abdominal support
Kessel-Bonney
K.-B. extension osteotomy
K.-B. hallux osteotomy
 procedure
Kessel plate
Kessler
K. external fixator
K. fixation device
K. grasping suture
K. metacarpal distractor
K. metacarpal lengthening
K. modified Achilles tendon repair
K. posterior tibial tendon transfer
 operation
K. prosthesis
K. 4-strand suture
K. suture technique
K. tendon repair stitch
K. tendon transfer
K. traction
K. traction frame
Kessler-Tajima suture
Ketac cement
ketamine
ketanserin
ketoconazole
ketoprofen
ketorolac tromethamine
Kevlar glove
Kevorkian curette
key
K. elevator
k. grip
K. intraarticular knee arthrodesis
K. periosteal elevator
k. pinch
K. rasp
k. release
k. the cement
K. wrist brace
keyboard
ErgoLogic k.
Kinesis k.
wave k.
keyboarder
key-grip tenodesis
keyhole
k. approach
k. method
k. punch
k. tenodesis
k. tenodesis technique
key-lock wrench

K

Key-Pred Injection
keystone
    k. graft
    k. of the calcar arch
    K. splint
    k. structure
keyway
    OEC lag screw component
    with k.
K-Fix fixator system
KGTI
    Kinetik great toe implant
Khan-Lewis phonological analysis
kicker
    K. Pavlik harness
    K. Pavlik harness hip abduction
    brace
kick-point
Kid-Dee-Lite orthosis
Kidner
    K. dissector
    K. excision of accessory navicular
    bone procedure
    K. flatfoot
    K. foot operation
    K. lesion
kidney rest
Kiel bone
Kienböck
    K. atrophy
    K. disease
    K. dislocation
    K. phenomenon
kiintscher (K)
Kikuchi-MacNob-Moreau anterior cervical disectomy approach
Kilfoyle humeral medial condylar fracture classification
Kilian line
Killian gouge
Kilner hook
Kiloh-Nevin
    K.-N. myopathy
    K.-N. ocular form of progressive
    muscular dystrophy
kilopond (kp)
kilovoltage potential
Kimerle anomaly
kinaesthesia (*var. of* kinesthesia)
kinaesthesiometer (*var. of* kinesthesiometer)
kinaesthetic (*var. of* kinesthetic)
KinAir bed
Kinamed
    K. anthropometric total hip
    K. Exact-Fit ATH system
Kinast indirect multifragmenting femur fracture reduction

Kin-Con
    K.-C. device
    K.-C. isokinetic exercise system
kinematic
    k. chain
    k. device
    K. fully constrained tricompartmental
    knee prosthesis
    k. gait
    k. gait pattern
    k. gait pattern change
    K. II condylar and stabilizer total
    knee system
    K. II rotating hinge knee system
    K. II rotating hinge total knee
    prosthesis
    k. index of McMurtry
    k. linkage
    K. rotation hinge
    k. study
kinematics
    hindfoot k.
    joint k.
    knee k.
    spine k.
Kinemax
    K. modular condylar and stabilizer
    total knee system
    K. Plus knee prosthesis
    K. Plus total knee system
    K. removable fixation peg
    K. spacer
Kinemetric guide system
kineplastic amputation
kineplastics
kinesiatrics
Kinesio elastic therapeutic taping
kinesiology
    applied k.
kinesiopathologic component
kinesiopathology
kinesipathist
kinesipathy
Kinesis keyboard
kinesitherapy
kinesthesia, kinesthesis, kinaesthesia
    knee k.
kinesthesiometer, kinaesthesiometer
kinesthesis (*var. of* kinesthesia)
kinesthetic, kinaesthetic
    K. Ability Trainer (KAT)
    k. awareness
    k. exercise
KineTec
    K. ECT system
    K. hip CPM machine
kinetic
    k. cervical spine
    k. chain

k. energy
k. energy theory
k. foot pain
k. gait analysis
k. rehab device (KRD)
k. splint
K. Wedge molded insole
K. Wedge orthotic
kinetics
Kinetik
K. great toe implant (KGTI)
K. great toe implant system
Kinetikos joint implant
Kinetix
K. instrument
K. instrument for carpal tunnel
release
Kinetron muscle strengthening apparatus
king
K. cervical brace
K. cervical traction
K. contrast venography technique
K. 2-curve classification of scoliosis
(type I-V)
K. intraarticular hip fusion
K. intraarticular hip fusion
procedure
K. maneuver
K. open radial head reduction
K. scoliosis curve posterior
correction (I-V)
K. thoracic and lumbar curve
(I–IV)
K. thoracic scoliosis classification
K. wound forceps
King-Moe
K.-M. classification of scoliosis
K.-M. idiopathic scoliosis
classification system
King-Richards dislocation technique
Kingsley Steplite foot
King-Steelquist hindquarter
amputation
kinking
catheter k.
pedicular k.
Kinsbourne syndrome
Kirby muscle hook
Kirk
K. distal thigh amputation
K. distal thigh operation
K. orthopaedic mallet
Kirkaldy-Willis
K.-W. arthrodesis
K.-W. back pain criteria
K.-W. operation
K.-W. 3 phases of spinal
degeneration
Kirner deformity

Kirschenbaum
K. foot positioner
K. retractor
Kirschner (K)
K. apparatus
K. bone drill
K. device
K. II-C shoulder system
K. integrated shoulder system
K. Medical Dimension hip
replacement
K. Medical Dimension prosthesis
K. pin fixation
K. skeletal traction
K. stem
K. surgical instrument
K. tightener
K. total shoulder prosthesis
K. traction bow nut
K. wire (K wire)
K. wire cutter
K. wire drill
K. wire driver
K. wire fixation
K. wire inserter
K. wire pin
K. wire tensioner
K. wire traction bow
kissing
k. lesions
k. sequestra
k. spines
k. spines syndrome
Kistler force platform
kit
Alpha suction attachment block k.
Arthrex Trim-It drill pin osteotomy
fixation k.
Balcones Sensory Integration
Screening K.
BFO K.
Bio-Dermal Hydrogel k.
bone fixation k.
Canadian Academy of Sports
Medicine emergency k.
carpal tunnel surgery relief k.
Concept CTS Relief K.
diabetic orthosis k.
Digital Care k.
Doctor Joseph's diabetic foot k.
DynaPak electrode k.
Elastafit tubing k.
Elbow Injury Management K.
Exerball k.
Fillauer Scottish Rite orthosis k.
Halifax interlaminar clamp k.
Histofreezer cryosurgical wart
treatment k.
I-Flow nerve block infusion k.

K

kit (*continued*)

    Keithley clamp k.
    Leukotape P combo pack taping k.
    MediCordz rehabilitation k.
    Merit final flexion k.
    nerve block infusion k.
    OsteoSet resorbable bead k.
    Oval-8 k.
    palmar swab k.
    parallel pin k.
    pelvic reconstruction k.
    portable diagnostic k.
    Posey bar k.
    resistive chair exercise k.
    sensory stimulation k.
    Shoulder Therapy K.
    Skin Care k.
    SOS Safe Salon Pedicure K.
    Tacticon peripheral neuropathy k.
    Unna-Flex Plus venous ulcer k.
    VersaFlex tubing k.

Kitaoka clinical rating scale

kite

    K. and Lovell technique
    K. clubfoot cast
    K. measurement
    K. metatarsal cast
    K. slipper
    K. talocalcaneal index angle

kitesurfing

Klebsiella

    K. oxytoca
    K. pneumoniae

Kleiger ankle test

Klein

    K. drainage
    K. technique

Klein-Bell Activities of Daily Living Scale

Kleinert

    K. flexor tendon repair
    K. modification
    K. postoperative traction brace
    K. splint
    K. technique of pulley reconstruction

Kleinert-Kutz

    K.-K. bone cutter
    K.-K. bone-cutting forceps
    K.-K. bone rongeur
    K.-K. clamp approximator
    K.-K. periosteal elevator
    K.-K. rasp
    K.-K. rongeur forceps
    K.-K. synovectomy rongeur
    K.-K. tendon forceps
    K.-K. tendon retriever

Kleinert-Ragnell retractor

Kleinman shear carpal ligament test

Klein-Vogelbach functional movement concept

Klemm nail

Klengall brace

Klenzak

    K. double-upright splint
    K. orthosis
    K. spring brace

Kline line

Kling

    K. adhesive dressing
    K. cervical brace
    K. elastic bandage

Klippel-Feil

    K.-F. malformation
    K.-F. segmentation defect
    K.-F. sign

Klippel-Trenaunay

    K.-T. osteohypertrophic hemangiectasia
    K.-T. syndrome (KTS)

Klippel-Trenaunay-Weber syndrome

Kloehn craniofacial remodeling technique

Klumpke

    K. injury
    K. palsy
    K. plexopathy

KMFTR

    Kotz modular femur and tibia resection

KMnO4

    potassium permanganate

KMP

    KMP femoral stem
    KMP femoral stem prosthesis

Knavel table

Knead-A-Ball exerciser

kneading massage

knee

    above k. (AK)
    acetabular k.
    ACL-deficient k.
    anatomic modular k. (AMK)
    anterior cruciate deficit k.
    k. arthrodesis
    k. arthroplasty
    k. arthroscopy
    Axiom total k.
    barked k.
    below k. (BK)
    bicompartmental replacement of k.
    Biomet Ascent total k.
    k. bolster
    k. brace splint
    breaststroker's k.
    Brodie k.
    cadaveric k.
    k. cage brace

carpenter's k.
carpet layer's k.
C-Leg microprocessor-controlled
  hydraulic k.
k. complex
constant-friction k.
constrained condylar k.
Continuum P/S total k.
k. contracture
corner of k.
deficient k.
DePuy LCS mobile-bearing k.
k. disarticulation amputation
k. disarticulation suspension
dislocated k.
k. dislocation
k. extension assist
k. extension exercise
k. extension orthosis
k. extensor
k. extensor system
flail k.
k. flexion
k. flexion during stance phase
  motion gait determinant
k. flexion-extension
k. flexion reflex
k. flexion stress test
floating k.
k. force
k. fracture
k. fusion
game k.
Genesis unicompartmental k.
GeoFlex k.
gimpy k.
giving way of k.
hamstrung k.
k. holder
horseback rider's k.
Hosmer Endurance k.
Hosmer single-axis friction k.
Hosmer single-axis locking k.
Hosmer weight-activated locking k.
housemaid's k.
k. immobilizer
k. immobilizer splint
k. implant
k. instability
k. instability test
internal derangement of k. (IDK)
k. jerk
k. jerk reflex
k. jerk reflex test
k. joint
k. joint effusion
k. joint position sense
jumper's k.
k. kinematics

k. kinesthesia
k. knob
k. laxity arthrometer
k. laxity test
k. ligament arthrometer
k. ligamentous injury
k. lock
locked k.
k. management orthosis
Mauch Swing and Stance hydraulic
  k.
k. MD brace
Miller-Galante k.
mobile-bearing k.
Most Options system rotating hinge
  revision k.
motorcyclist's k.
moviegoer's k.
neuropathic k.
NexGen LPS Flex-Mobile bearing k.
NexGen LPS-Mobile bearing k.
Noiles posterior stabilized k.
Noiles rotating hinge k.
k. orthosis
k. osteoarthritis
Otto Bock 3R60 EBS k.
Otto Bock 3R80 modular rotary
  hydraulic k.
Otto Bock Safety constant-friction
  k.
Oxford unicompartmental k.
PC Performer k.
K. Pillo
pneumatic 4-bar linkage k.
PolymerFriction total k.
porous-coated anatomic total k.
k. positioner
k. positioning triangle
posterior cruciate ligament of k.
press-fit condylar total k.
ProAdvantage k.
k. prosthesis
k. pump
k. pump exercise
k. retractor
k. rotation
runner's k.
SAL k.
k. saver
Seattle safety k.
self-aligning k.
septic k.
k. signature system
single-axis friction k. (SAFK)
single-axis locking k. (SALK)
k. sleeve
K. Sleeve knee support
k. sling
snowstorm k.

K

knee (*continued*)
  K. Society score
  K. Society Total Knee Arthroplasty
    Roentgenographic Evaluation and
    Scoring System
  k. stability
  k. strike
  surfer's k.
  tension band of k.
  total condylar k.
  Total Knee 2100 prosthetic k.
  total rotating k. (TRK)
  translating and congruent
    mobile-bearing k.
  transverse ligament of k.
  trick k.
  USMC stance locking safety k.
  valgus k.
  varus k.
  k. varus-valgus
  voluntary control 4-bar k.
  weight-activated locking k. (WALK)
  windblown k.
  wrenched k.
knee-ankle-foot orthosis (KAFO)
kneecap stabilizer
knee-chest
  k.-c. push
  k.-c. rocking
  k.-c. table
knee-control orthosis pad
Kneed-It kneeguard
knee-drop test
kneeGRIP
kneeguard
  Kneed-It k.
kneeling
  k. bench test
  k. position
  90-90 k. position
  k. reciprocal back exercise technique
KneeRanger hinged knee brace
kneeRAP
Kniest syndrome
knife, *pl.* **knives**
  acetabular k.
  ACL graft k.
  amputation k.
  arthroscopic k.
  backward-cutting k.
  Ballenger swivel k.
  banana k.
  Bard-Parker k.
  bayonet k.
  Beaver cataract k.
  Beaver-DeBakey k.
  Bircher meniscus k.
  k. blade
  Blair k.

Blount k.
Bovie k.
C k.
cartilage k.
cast k.
Castroviejo bladebreaker k.
catlin amputating k.
chondroplasty k.
Collin amputating k.
Crile k.
cutting current k.
discission k.
Down epiphysial k.
Downing cartilage k.
Esmarch plaster k.
forward-cutting k.
Freiberg cartilage k.
Freiberg meniscectomy k.
full-radius resector k.
Grover meniscus k.
hemilaminectomy k.
hooked k.
Hopkins plaster k.
hot k.
Humby k.
Indiana tome open carpal tunnel
  release k.
Langenbeck flap k.
Langenbeck resection k.
Lindvall-Stille k.
Liston amputating k.
Liston phalangeal k.
Lowe-Breck cartilage k.
Lowe-Breck meniscectomy k.
Maltz cartilage k.
McKeever cartilage k.
meniscectomy k.
meniscus k.
Midas Rex k.
Neff meniscus k.
Oretorp retractable k.
orthopaedic k.
Reiner plaster k.
retrograde-cutting hook-shaped k.
Ridlon plaster k.
rocker k.
Salenius meniscus k.
sculp k.
semilunar cartilage k.
serrated fine-cutting k.
sheathed k.
skiving k.
Smillie-Beaver k.
Smillie cartilage k.
Smillie meniscal k.
Smith cartilage k.
Stryker cartilage k.
tenotomy k.
upward-cutting triangular k.

Weck k.
Yamada myelotomy k.
knight
K. back brace
K. bone-cutting forceps
Knight-Taylor
K.-T. thoracic brace
K.-T. thoracolumbosacral orthosis
Knit-Rite suspension sleeve
knitting
knives (*pl. of* knife)
knob
knee k.
Knobber
Original Index K. II
Knobble massager
knocked-down shoulder
knock-knee
k.-k. brace
k.-k. deformity
Knodt
K. distraction rod
K. rod and hook
knot
arthroscopic k.
hairpin k.
half-hitch arthroscopic k.
half stitch k.
Henry k.
lockable arthroscopic k.
k. of Henry
PDS k.
k. pusher
Revo k.
sliding k.
surfer's k.
wire k.
knotter
Harris k.
knotting forceps
Knott rod distraction device
Knowles
K. hip pin
K. pin nail
K. pinning
Knox
K. Cube Imitation Test
K. Preschool Play Scale
knuckle
k. bone
boxer's k.
k. pad
k. shaped
knuckle-bender splint
KobyGard system
Koby Isogard surgical treatment system
Kocher
K. clamp
K. collar incision

K. curved-L approach
K. dissector
K. elevator
K. forceps
K. fracture
K. humerus fracture classification
K. interval
K. lateral J approach
K. reduction of shoulder dislocation
K. retractor
K. shoulder reduction
Kocher-Debré-Semelaigne syndrome
Kocher-Gibson posterolateral approach
Kocher-Langenbeck
K.-L. exposure
K.-L. posterior approach for
acetabular fracture repair
K.-L. posterior proximal femur and
acetabulum approach
Kocher-Lorenz
K.-L. capitellum fracture
K.-L. capitellum fracture
classification (I-II)
K.-L. fracture of capitellum
Koch-Mason dressing
Kodel knee sling
Kodex drill
Kodros radiolucent awl
Koenen periungual fibroma
Koenig, König
K. metatarsal broach
K. metatarsophalangeal joint
arthroplasty
K. MPJ prosthesis
K. nail-splitting scissors
K. rasp
K. total great toe implant
Koenig-Schaefer incision
Kofoed
K. ankle score (KAS)
K. scoring system
Köhler
K. disease
K. fracture
K. hip protrusion grading scale
K. line
Köhler-Pellegrini-Stieda disease
Kohlman Evaluation of Living Skills
(KELS)
Kohs block
koilonychia
koilosternia
Kolár wall slide with arm elevation
exercise
Kold Wrap
Kollagen dressing
Komori herniated nucleus pulposus
migration classification
Kondoleon operation

K

König (*var. of* Koenig)
Kool Kit cold therapy pack
Korean hand acupuncture
Korex cork sheet
Kortzeborn
    K. hand operation
    K. procedure
Kosair Scoliosis Orthosis (KSO)
Kostuik-Errico spinal stability
  classification
Kostuik-Harrington
    K.-H. distraction system
    K.-H. spinal instrumentation
Kostuik screw
Kotz modular femur and tibia resection
  (KMFTR)
Koutsogiannis
    K. calcaneal displacement osteotomy
    K. sliding calcaneal osteotomy
      procedure
kp
  kilopond
KPS bipolar vitallium-polyethylene implant
Krackow
    K. Achilles tendon repair
    K. HTO blade staple
    K. locking loop technique
    K. locking suture technique
    K. obese patient tourniquet maneuver
    K. point
    K. suture
Krackow-Thomas-Jones technique
Kramer
    K. modification
    K. modification of Hohmann
      osteotomy
Kraske
    K. operation
    K. position
Krause
    K. bone
    suture of K.
    ulnar collateral nerve of K.
Krause-Wolfe skin graft
KRD
  kinetic rehab device
  KRD L2000 rehab device
Kreuscher
    K. bunionectomy
    K. operation
Kristiansen-Kofoed external fixation
K rod
  Kuntscher rod
Kronfeld pin
Kronner
    K. external fixation
    K. external fixation apparatus
    K. external fixation device
    K. ring fixation

Krukenberg
    K. amputation
    K. hand
    K. hand operation
    K. hand reconstruction
    K. reconstruction of BKA procedure
KS 5 ACL brace
K9 Scooter
KSO
  Kosair Scoliosis Orthosis
  KSO brace
KT
  Orudis KT
KT-1000
  KT-1000 foot stabilizer
  KT-1000 joint arthrometer
  KT-1000, 2000 knee ligament
    arthrometer
KT-1000/Jr arthrometer
KTS
  Klippel-Trenaunay syndrome
KT-1000/s surgical arthrometer
kudo
    K. hinge
    K. unconstrained elbow prosthesis
Kugelberg reconstruction
Kugelberg-Welander
    K.-W. disease
    K.-W. juvenile spinal muscle
      atrophy
    K.-W. syndrome
Kuhlman
    K. cervical traction device
    K. traction
Kumar
    K. application
    K. spica cast technique
Kümmell
    K. disease
    K. spondylitis
Kümmell-Verneuil disease
Küntscher
    K. awl
    K. drill
    K. extractor
    K. finisher
    K. hammer
    K. humeral prosthesis
    K. impactor
    K. intramedullary nailing technique
    K. medullary nailing
    K. modified knee arthrodesis
    K. nail (K nail)
    K. nail driver
    K. nail-extracting hook
    K. ossimeter
    K. pin
    K. reamer
    K. rod (K rod)

K. traction apparatus
K. traction device
Küntscher-Hudson brace
Kurosaka interference-fit screw
Kurtzke
K. Expanded Disability scale
K. Expanded Disability Status scale
score
K. functional system
Kuschkin Ace wheelchair
Kuskokwim congenital hip contracture
syndrome
Kuslich
Bagby and K. (BAK)
Kutler
K. double lateral advancement flap
K. V-Y flap
K. V-Y flap graft
Kuwada Achilles tendon injury
classification
Kuz-Medics disposable knee
immobilizer
Kydex
K. body jacket
K. brace
K. chairback orthosis
Kyle
K. fracture classification
K. fracture classification system
K. internal fixation
kyllosis
kyphectomy
Sharrard-type k.
kyphometer
Debrunner k.
kyphoplastic procedure
kyphoplasty
balloon k.
kyphorachitic pelvis
kyphoscoliorachitic pelvis
kyphoscoliosis
neurofibromatosis k.
Scheuermann k.
k. secondary to neurofibromatosis
severe k.
thoracolumbar k.
kyphoscoliotic pelvis
kyphosing scoliosis
kyphosis
acute angular k.
adolescent k.
anterior k.
apprentice k.

k. brace
congenital k. (I, II)
k. correction
k. correction surgery
k. creation
distal junctional k.
global k.
iatrogenic lumbar k.
junctional k.
juvenile k.
juvenile thoracic k.
long-radius k.
lumbar k.
lumbosacral k.
Luque rod fixation for k.
maximum-curve k.
myelodysplastic k.
paralytic k.
postlaminectomy k.
postradiation k.
posttraumatic k.
k. progression
rotational k.
sagittal k.
Scheuermann juvenile k. (SJK)
segmental k.
short-radius k.
thoracic k.
thoracolumbar k.
T4-T8 k.
upper thoracic k.
kyphos resection
kyphotic
k. angle
k. angulation
k. curve
k. decompression syndrome
k. deformity
k. deformity pathomechanics
k. lift
k. pelvis
kyphotone
KyphX
K. Elevate IBT
K. Elevate inflatable bone
tamp
K. Exact IBT
K. Exact inflatable bone tamp
K. HV-R bone cement
K. inflatable bone tamp
K. Xpander inflatable bone tamp
Kyrle hyperkeratosis
kyrtorrhachic

K

L
  lumbar
  L plate
  L rod
L.A.
  L.A. cervical orthosis
  Dexasone L.A.
  Solurex L.A.
lab
  laboratory
laboratory (lab)
  Army Prosthetics Research L.
    (APRL)
  gait l.
  Orthopaedic Casting L. (OCL)
  University of California Berkeley L.
    (UCBL)
labra (*pl. of* labrum)
labral
  l. avulsion
  l. lesion
  l. tear
labrum, *pl.* **labra**
  acetabular l.
  anterior glenoid l. (AGL)
  articular l.
  cartilaginous glenoid l.
  glenoid l.
  posterior glenoid l.
LAC
  long arm cast
lace
  l. closure
  no-tie stretch l.
laced blucher of shoe
lace-lock ankle splint
lace-on brace
laceration
  boot-top l.
  burst-type l.
  chevron l.
  flexor tendon l.
  hallucis longus l.
  stellate nail bed l.
lacertus
  l. fibrosus
  l. medius
  l. syndrome
lace-up RocketSoc ankle brace
Lacey
  L. fully constrained tricompartmental
    knee prosthesis
  L. hinge
  L. hinged knee prosthesis
  L. rotating hinge arthroplasty

Lachman
  L. knee ligamentous instability
    test
  L. knee ligament tear maneuver
  L. sign
lachrymal (*var. of* lacrimal)
Lac-Hydrin lotion
lacing ankle brace
laciniate ligament
lacquer
  EcoNail nail l.
  Penlac Nail L.
lacrimal, lachrymal
  l. bone
  l. duct dilator
Lacroix
  fibroosseous ring of L.
  L. osseous ring
  osseous ring of L.
lacrosse
lactate
  blood l.
  calcium l.
  Ringer l.
  l. threshold
lactic
  l. acid
  l. acidosis
  l. acidosis threshold
Lactinol-E creme
Lactinol lotion
Lactobacillus
LactoSorb
  L. orthopaedic wound material
  L. resorbable copolymer
  L. screw
lacuna, *pl.* **lacunae**
  bone l.
  cartilage l.
  Howship l.
  osseous l.
lacunae (*pl. of* lacuna)
LAD
  ligament augmentation device
  ligamentous anterior dislocation
    LAD composite graft
    Kennedy LAD
ladder
  finger l.
  shoulder l.
  l. splint
laevodopa (*var. of* levodopa)
LAF
  Leisure Activities Finder
Lafayette skinfold caliper

L

lag
   l. screw
   l. screw fixation
   l. screw insertion
   l. screw thread hole
Laguere sacroiliac test
Lahey
   L. clamp
   L. Clinic dural hook
Laing
   L. concentric hip cup
   L. H-beam nail
   L. hip cup prosthesis
Lalonde
   L. hook forceps
   L. oblique fracture large bone
     clamp
   L. oblique fracture medium bone
     clamp
   L. oblique metacarpal fracture bone
     clamp
   L. small bone clamp
   L. tendon approximator
LAM
  limb accurate measurement
Lam
   L. inversion tarsal tunnel test
   L. IPM Wound Gel
lambdoid suture
Lambert cosine law
Lambert-Eaton
   L.-E. myasthenic syndrome
     (LEMS)
   L.-E. syndrome (LES)
Lambert-Lowman
   L.-L. bone clamp
   L.-L. chisel
Lambeth disability screening
questionnaire
Lamb muscle transfer
Lambotte
   L. bone-holding clamp
   L. bone-holding forceps
   L. bone hook
   L. elevator
   L. osteotome
   L. principle
Lambrinudi
   L. dropfoot operation
   L. osteotomy
   L. splint
   L. technique
   L. triple arthrodesis
lamb's
   l. wool
   l. wool pad
lamella, *pl.* **lamellae**
   articular bone l.
   basic l.

   circumferential l.
   concentric l.
   endosteal l.
   ground l.
   haversian l.
   intermediate l.
   interstitial l.
   osseous l.
   periosteal l.
lamellae (*pl. of* lamella)
lamellar
   l. bone
   l. pattern
   l. separation
   l. thickening
lamellated bone
lamellation
lamina, *pl.* **laminae**
   l. elevator
   intact spinous l.
laminae (*pl. of* lamina)
laminagram
laminaplasty, laminoplasty
   cervical l.
   distraction l.
   expansive l.
   Hirabayashi l.
   Hirabayashi-type l.
   Hirabayashi unilateral open door
     cervical l.
   midsagittal splitting l.
   open-door expansive l.
   Tsuji l.
   l. with extended
     foraminoplasty
laminar, laminated
   l. bone
   l. C-D hook
   l. cortex posterior aspect
   l. door
   l. fracture
   l. spreader
laminated (*var. of* laminar)
lamination
laminectomized spine
laminectomy
   cervical spine l.
   l. chisel
   decompressive l.
   en bloc l.
   l. frame
   Gill lumbar spondylolisthesis
     decompression l.
   multilevel l.
   osteoplastic l.
   radial l.
laminoforaminotomy
laminoplasty (*var. of* laminaplasty)
laminotomy and discectomy

Lamisil
> L. Cream
> L. Oral

Lamis patellar clamp

lamp
> l. cord sign
> Derma-Wand germicidal l.
> germicidal l.
> halogen l.

lance
> L. acetabuloplasty
> L. disease
> L. shelf procedure

Lanceford prosthesis

lancinating pain

lancing

Landeez all-terrain wheelchair

Landers-Foulks prosthesis

landmark
> anatomic l.
> bony l.
> pedicle l.

Landolt spreading forceps

Landouzy-Dejerine dystrophy

Landsmeer ligament

lane
> L. bone-holding clamp
> L. bone-holding forceps
> L. bone lever
> L. bone screw
> L. periosteal elevator
> L. plate
> L. procedure
> L. screwdriver
> L. screw-holding forceps
> L. self-retaining bone-holding
> forceps

Lanex screen

Lange
> L. Achilles tendon reconstruction
> L. bone retractor
> L. hip reduction
> L. operation
> L. procedure
> L. skinfold caliper
> L. tendon lengthening
> L. tendon lengthening and repair
> L. tendon-lengthening method

Lange-Hohmann bone retractor

Langenbeck
> L. amputation
> L. anteromedial approach
> L. bone-holding forceps
> L. bone saw
> L. flap knife
> L. hip joint triangle
> L. incision
> L. metacarpal saw
> L. operation

> L. periosteal elevator
> L. rasp
> L. resection knife
> L. retractor

Langenskiöld
> L. bone graft
> L. bony bridge resection
> L. central physeal bar excision
> procedure
> L. classification (stage I–VI)
> L. fusion
> L. grading system
> L. osteotomy

Langer
> L. axillary arch
> L. axillary arch muscle
> L. line
> L. mesomelic dwarfism

Langerhans
> L. cell granulomatosis
> L. cell histiocytosis

Langoria sign

lap
> l. joint
> l. seatbelt fracture

laparoscopic surgeon's thumb

laparoscopy
> GelPort hand access l.

laparotomy
> l. sheet
> l. sponge

Lapidus
> L. alternating air-pressure
> mattress
> L. arthrodesis
> L. bed
> L. bunionectomy
> L. hammertoe technique
> L. modified arthrodesis
> L. operation
> L. procedure

Lapidus-type correction

LaPorta
> L. great toe implant
> L. total toe prosthesis

lappet formation

L'Aprina topical spray

laptop cushion

large
> l. callus Podi-Burr
> l. Cobra retractor
> l. composite allograft
> l. egress cannula
> l. humeral head hemiarthroplasty
> l. nail Podi-Burr

large-bore inflow cannula

large-head humeral component

large-nail spicule bur

Lark scooter

L

Larmon
    L. forefoot
    L. forefoot arthroplasty
    L. forefoot procedure
Laron dwarfism
Larrey
    L. amputation
    L. operation
Larsen
    L. disease
    L. lateral ankle stabilization
      procedure
    L. syndrome
    L. tendon-holding forceps
Larsen-Johansson disease
LARSI
    lumbar anterior-root stimulator implant
Lars Ingvar Hansson (LIH)
Larson
    L. hip score
    L. hip status system
    L. ligament reconstruction
    L. posterolateral instability of knee
      repair technique
laryngeal
    l. nerve
    l. nerve injury
LAS
    local adaptation syndrome
    long arm splint
LASA
    Lisfranc articular set angle
Laschal suture scissors
LASE
    laser-assisted spinal endoscopy
    LASE probe
Lasègue
    L. rebound herniated nucleus
      pulposus test
    L. sign
    L. sitting test
    L. straight leg raising test
laser
    l. acupuncture
    ArthroProbe arthroscopic l.
    l. arthroscopy
    Candela SPTL l.
    carbon dioxide l.
    cold l.
    diode l.
    l. Doppler flowmetry (LDF)
    l. Doppler probe
    holmium YAG l.
    l. image custom arthroplasty (LICA)
    l. instrument
    low-energy l. (LEL)
    low-power l.
    l. nucleotomy
    l. partial matricectomy

    red light neon l.
    SilkTouch CO_2 l.
    Surgilase CO_2 l.
    Trimedyne Omnipulse holmium l.
    VersaPulse holmium l.
laser-assisted
    l.-a. capsular shift
    l.-a. capsulorrhaphy
    same-day microsurgical arthroscopic
      lateral approach l.-a. (SMALL)
    l.-a. spinal endoscopy (LASE)
Laserflo BPM
LaserPen laser therapy
lashing suture
last
    l. foot contact (LFC)
    l. normal vertebra (LNV)
lata, *gen.* and *pl.* **latae**
    fascia l.
latae (*gen.* and *pl. of* lata)
    tensor fasciae l. (TFL)
Latarjet procedure
late
    l. intervention
    l. operative site pain (LOSP)
    l. response
    l. stage
    l. stance
late-age onset
latency
    distal l.
    F wave l.
    motor l.
    muscle reflex l.
    l. of activation
    onset l.
    peak l.
    proximal l.
    residual l.
    sensory peak l.
    terminal l.
latent
    l. diastasis
    l. period
    l. stage of gout
lateral
    l. acetabular shelf operation
    l. acromial border
    l. and anteroposterior rib
      compression thoracic spine test
    l. ankle sprain
    l. antebrachial cutaneous nerve
    l. anterior thoracic nerve
    l. arm flap
    l. aspiration
    l. atlantoaxial joint
    l. atlantooccipital ligament
    l. band
    l. band mobilization

l. bending
l. bending view
l. bicipital sulcus
l. block test
l. bowing
l. buttress support
l. calcaneal artery
l. calcaneocuboid (LCC)
l. canal entrapment
l. capsular release
l. capsular sign
l. cervical spine film
l. closing wedge osteotomy
l. collateral ligament (LCL)
l. collateral sprain
l. column calcaneal fracture
l. column lengthening
l. column lengthening surgery
l. column syndrome
l. common digital nerve
l. compartment
l. compartment disruption
l. compartment injury
l. compartment reconstruction
l. compression
l. compression force
l. compression injury
l. condylar fracture classification
l. cord
l. cortex
l. corticospinal tract
l. costotransverse ligament
l. curvature
l. decompression
l. decubitus position
l. deltoid-splitting approach
l. deviation
l. deviation angle
l. disc protrusion
l. displacement osteotomy
l. distal femoral angle
l. drainage
l. elbow epicondyle test
l. elbow tendinosis
l. electrical surface stimulation
  (LESS)
l. end
l. epicondyle
l. exostectomy
l. extensor expansion
l. extensor release
l. femoral condyle
l. femoral cutaneous nerve
l. femoral notch sign
l. flexion
l. flexion dynamic visual analysis
l. flexion malposition
l. flexion restriction
l. forefoot overload

l. full-spine radiographic examination
l. fusion
l. gap sign
l. guidepin
l. gutter syndrome
l. hamstring
l. head of gastrocnemius
l. hindfoot
l. hip arthroscopy
l. hip rotation
l. humeral condyle fracture
l. humeral epicondylitis
l. hyperpressure syndrome
l. impingement
l. interosseous ligament
l. J approach
l. joint line
l. joint space
l. Kocher approach
l. listhesis
l. lumbar shift
l. lumbosacral ligament
l. malleolus
l. malleolus fracture
l. malleolus muscle
l. mass articulation (LMA)
l. mass fracture
l. meniscectomy
l. meniscus
l. monopodal stance view
l. motion racket sport
l. oblique view
l. Ollier approach
l. opening wedge osteotomy
l. pad
l. parapatellar approach
l. park-bench position
l. patella displacement
l. patellar autologous graft
l. patellar compression syndrome
l. patellar facet
l. patellofemoral angle
l. pivot shift
l. pivot shift knee ligamentous
  instability test
l. plantar artery
l. plantarflexion talar angle
l. plantar metatarsal angle
l. plantar nerve
l. plica
l. premalleolar bursitis
l. process
l. projection
l. quadruple complex
l. recess
l. recess stenosis (LRS)
l. retinaculum release
l. rhachotomy
l. roentgenogram

L

lateral (*continued*)
    l. root pressure
    l. rotary displacement
    l. rotatory ankle instability
    l. sacrococcygeal ligament
    l. scapular slide test (LSST)
    l. sesamoid
    l. sesamoidectomy
    l. shear
    l. shelf
    l. sling procedure
    l. slip
    l. slip angle
    l. spring ligament
    l. spring ligament of foot
    l. spring-loaded lock
    l. squeeze pinch
    l. squeeze test
    l. stability
    l. step-up
    l. superior genicular nerve
    l. sway
    l. talar-first metatarsal angle
    l. talar process fracture
    l. talocalcaneal angle
    l. talocalcaneal ligament (LTC)
    l. tarsometatarsal angle
    l. tear
    l. thigh flap
    l. thoracic flap
    l. tibial condyle
    l. tibial plateau fracture
    l. tibial tubercle
    l. tilt stress ankle view
    l. tilt stress ankle x-ray
    l. to medial screw
    l. transfer
    l. transmalleolar portal
    l. trap suture
    l. trunk shift
    l. tuberosity
    l. utility incision
    l. wedge
    l. wedge fracture
    l. weightbearing radiograph
lateralis
    malleolus l.
    vastus l. (VL)
    vastus medialis obliquus to vastus l.
laterality
    atlas l.
lateralization
laterally displaced fracture
lateral-to-medial thrust
lateroduction
lateropulsion
latex
    l. anaphylaxis
    l. cushion

latissimus
    l. dorsi
    l. dorsi flap
    l. dorsi muscle
Latitude curette
latitudinal growth
latticework
latus
    metatarsus l.
Lauenstein ulnar head resection
  procedure
Lauge-Hansen
    L.-H. ankle fracture classification
    L.-H. fracture classification
    L.-H. stage II supination-eversion
      fracture
Laugier
    L. fracture
    L. sign
Laurence-Biedl syndrome
Laurence-Moon-Biedl
    L.-M.-B. law
    L.-M.-B. syndrome
Laurence-Moon syndrome
Laurin
    L. lateral patella displacement
    L. lateral patellofemoral angle
    L. patella view
    L. tangential patella view
lavage
    bone l.
    CarboJet l.
    Hi Speed Pulse l.
    jet l.
    joint l.
    pulsatile jet l.
    pulsatile pressure l.
    Pulsavac l.
    pulsed l.
    Simpulse pulsing l.
    Simpulse S/I l.
law
    Davis l.
    Heuter-Volkmann l.
    Lambert cosine l.
    Laurence-Moon-Biedl l.
    L. of Facilitation
    Ollier l.
    Palmerian l.
    Sherrington reciprocal
      innervation l.
    sports medicine l.
    von Schwann l.
    Wolff l.
lawn mower injury
Lawrence
    L. device
    L. first metatarsophalangeal joint
      implant

L. lateral proximal humerus view
L. transthoracic lateral humerus
view
Lawrence-Seip syndrome
Lawson-Thornton plate
Lawton procedure
laxity
    ankle l.
    anterior knee l.
    collateral ligament l.
    congenital l.
    cruciate ligament l.
    l. index
    joint l.
    ligamentous l.
    radioscaphocapitate ligament l.
    subtalar l.
    l. to varus stress
    valgus l.
    varus l.
layer
    cambium l.
    capsular l.
    gliding l.
    Ollier l.
    parietal tendon sheath l.
    periosteal cambium l.
    tangential l.
LazerSporin-C solution
lazy-C incision
lazy-L incision
lazy-S skin incision
**lazy-V de-epithelialized turn-over
fasciocutaneous flap**
LB
    loose body
L-bolt
    TSRH L-b.
LBP
    low back pain
LBS
    Leisure Boredom Scale
LBW
    lean body weight
LCC
    lateral calcaneocuboid
        LCC ligament
LCL
    lateral collateral ligament
LCPD
    Legg-Calvé-Perthes disease
LCR
    ligamentous and capsular repair
        LCR system
LCS
    low-contact stress
        LCS meniscal bearing
            semiconstrained prosthesis
        LCS mobile bearing knee system

LCS New Jersey knee prosthesis
LCS rotating platform
    semiconstrained prosthesis
LCS substituting semiconstrained
    prosthesis
LCS total knee system
LCS total knee system
    implant
LCS universal APG
    semiconstrained prosthesis
LCT
    liquid crystal thermography
L-curved incision
LDF
    laser Doppler flowmetry
    lumbodorsal fascia
LE
    lupus erythematosus
    LE cell
Le
    Le Dentu suture
    L. Fort amputation
    L. Fort fibular fracture
    Le Fort (I-III) fracture
    Le Fort (I-III) osteotomy
    Le Fort mandible fracture
    L. Fort-Wagstaffe fracture
LEA
    lower extremity amputation
**Leach-Schepsis-Paul
augmentation**
lead (Pb)
    Axxess spinal cord
        stimulation l.
    l. line
    l. synovitis
Leadbetter
    L. hip manipulation
    L. hip reduction maneuver
    L. technique
leader
    l.'s and trailers
    tendon l.
lead-filled mallet
lead-line scan
lead-pipe fracture
leaf, *pl.* **leaves**
    inferior l.
    l. splint
    superior l.
leaf-spring
    AFO posterior l.-s.
    l.-s. brace
    plastic l.-s. (PLS)
leakage
    bony slurry l.
    cement l.
    chylous l.
    extraosseous l.

lean
> antalgic l.
> l. body weight (LBW)

Leander
> L. chiropractic table
> L. motorized flexion table

leaning hop test

LEAP
> Lewis expandable adjustable prosthesis
> Lower Extremity Amputation Prevention
> LEAP monofilament test
> LEAP program

learning
> spinal l.

leash of Henry

leather
> l. ankle corset
> l. cuff
> l. lacer gauntlet
> l. orthosis

Leatherman hook

leaves (*pl. of* leaf)

Lebsche
> L. rongeur
> L. saw guide
> L. wire saw

LeCocq brace

Ledderhose disease

Ledraplastic exercise ball

Lee
> L. anterosuperior iliac spine graft
> L. bone graft
> L. laryngotracheal stenosis management technique
> L. procedure
> L. reconstruction

leech
> artificial l.
> medicinal l.
> North American l.

Leeds-Keio Dacron mesh replacement

Leeds spinal procedure

Lefferts rib shears

LEFS
> Lower Extremity Functional Scale

left
> l. erector spinae musculature
> l. innominate
> l. lateral flexion
> l. lower extremity (LLE)
> l. lower limb (LLL)
> l. lumbar convexity
> l. rotation
> l. thoracolumbar major curve pattern
> l. upper extremity (LUE, LUX)
> l. upper limb (LUL)

left-hand
> l.-h. dominance
> l.-h. dominant

left-right leg displacement

left-sided
> l.-s. nail
> l.-s. thoracotomy

1-leg
> 1-l. hop for distance test
> 1-l. stance test

leg
> anatomic short l.
> l. axis
> badger l.
> baker's l.
> bayonet l.
> bowed l.
> l. brace
> champagne bottle l.
> C-Leg System artificial l.
> l. compartment release
> l. decompression
> l. drift
> l. edema
> L. Extension Power Rig
> flaccid l.
> functional short l.
> game l.
> gimpy l.
> l. holder
> inverted champagne bottle l.
> jumping l.
> l. length
> l. length determination
> l. length discrepancy (LLD)
> l. lengthening
> l. length inequality (LLI)
> lusty l.
> nonpreferred l.
> paretic l.
> l. positioner
> l. press
> l. protection factor (LPF)
> restless l.
> rider's l.
> scissors l.
> short l.
> l. shortening
> l. sling
> stork l.
> stovepipe l.
> table short l.
> tennis l.
> l. traction
> unilateral spastic l.
> l. walking cast

Legasus support CPM device

leg-curl
> ankle joint l.-c.

legend
  L. ACL functional knee brace
  L. Hy-Lo adjusting table
  L. PCL functional knee brace
  L. stationary adjusting table
leg-foot-toe syndrome
Legg-Calvé-Perthes
  L.-C.-P. disease (LCPD)
  L.-C.-P. syndrome
Legg-Calvé-Waldenström
  L.-C.-W. disease
  L.-C.-W. syndrome
Legg-Perthes
  L.-P. disease
  L.-P. disease orthosis
  L.-P. shoe extension
  L.-P. sling
Legg procedure
legGRIP body positioning device
legholder
  Alvarado l.
  Arthroplasty Products Consultants
    foot and l.
  arthroscopic l.
  Bickel l.
  Cherf l.
  LH1000 arthroscopic l.
  lithotomy l.
  Low Profile l.
  operative l.
  Prep-Assist l.
  Surbaugh l.
  SurgAssist surgical l.
  Zollinger l.
leg-holding
  l.-h. apparatus
  l.-h. device
leg-lengthening device
Legs (*var. of* gait, arms, legs, and spine)
Lehman endoscopic pancreatic
  sphincterotomy technique
Leibinger
  L. Micro System drill bit
  L. Micro System plate cutter
  L. Micro System plate-holding
    forceps
  L. Profyle hand system
Leibolt pantalar arthrodesis technique
Leica model 1600 water-cooled diamond
  saw
Leichtenstern sign
Leinbach
  L. device
  L. femoral prosthesis
  L. hip prosthesis
  L. olecranon screw
  L. osteotome
leiomyomatous hamartoma
leisure

  L. Activities Finder (LAF)
  L. Boredom Scale (LBS)
Leksell
  L. adapter
  L. adapter to Mayfield device
  L. laminectomy rongeur
  L. rongeur forceps
  L. stereotactic arc
Leksell-Stille thoracic rongeur
LEL
  low-energy laser
Lelièvre osteotomy
Lema strap
Lemmon rib contractor
Lempert
  L. bone curette
  L. bone rongeur
  L. periosteal elevator
  L. rongeur forceps
LEMS
  Lambert-Eaton myasthenic
    syndrome
Lengemann wire
length
  distal parabola toe l.
  echo train l. (ETL)
  effective foot l.
  femur l.
  hip axis l.
  inequality in leg l.
  leg l.
  limb l.
  metatarsal l.
  needle cord l.
  l. of stay (LOS)
  pedicle screw cord l.
  pedicle screw path l.
  resting l.
  step l.
  stride l.
lengthening
  Achilles tendon l.
  Anderson tibial l.
  anterior calcaneal lateral
    column l.
  aponeurotic l.
  Armistead ulnar l.
  calcaneal neck l.
  Codivilla tendon l.
  Compere l.
  l. contraction
  DeBastiani femoral l.
  distraction l.
  Evans calcaneal l.
  extensor tendon l.
  femoral l.
  fractional l.
  Frost posterior tibialis tendon l.
  gastrocnemius l.

L

lengthening (*continued*)
    Green and McDermott
      gastrocnemius l.
    hamstring l.
    heel cord l.
    Hoke Achilles tendon l.
    Ilizarov limb l.
    intramuscular l.
    Kessler metacarpal l.
    Lange tendon l.
    lateral column l.
    leg l.
    limb l.
    limb-girdle l.
    metacarpal l.
    l. over nails procedure
    percutaneous heel cord l.
    percutaneous tendo Achillis l.
    posterior tibialis tendon l.
    l. reflex
    reverse undercutting l.
    Silfverskiöld Achilles tendon l.
    Spencer Achilles tendon l.
    step-cut l.
    Strayer l.
    subscapularis capsular l.
    Tachdjian fractional l.
    Tachdjian hamstring l.
    tendo Achillis l. (TAL)
    tendo calcaneus l.
    tendon l.
    tibial l.
    transiliac l.
    ulnar l.
    Vulpius gastrocnemius muscle l.
    Wagner femoral l.
    Wagner tibial l.
    Warren-White open sliding Achilles
      tendon l.
    Wasserstein limb l.
    White tendo calcaneus l.
    Z-slide l.
length-tension curve
Lenke
    L. and King adolescent idiopathic
      scoliosis classification
    L. classification
    L. 3–component classification (I-V)
      of adolescent idiopathic scoliosis
Lenox
    L. bucket
    L. Hill derotational knee brace
    L. Hill knee orthosis
    L. Hill Spectralite knee brace
lens
    Nikon SMZ 2T magnifying l.
lenticular bone
lenticularis
    dystonia l.

lentigines, *pl. of* **lentigo**
lentigo, *pl.* **lentigines**
    lentigines, electrocardiographic
      abnormalities, ocular hypertelorism,
      pulmonary stenosis, abnormalities
      of genitalia, retardation of growth,
      deafness (sensorineural)
      (LEOPARD)
    l. maligna
    l. maligna melanoma
Leo Bathlifter
Leone expansion screw
LEOPARD
    lentigines, electrocardiographic
      abnormalities, ocular hypertelorism,
      pulmonary stenosis, abnormalities of
      genitalia, retardation of growth,
      deafness (sensorineural)
    LEOPARD syndrome
Lepird metatarsus adductus procedure
L'Episcopo
    L. hip reconstruction
    L. obstetric brachial plexus injury
      repair procedure
leptopodia
Lequesne Severity of Osteoarthritis
  Index
Lere bone mill
Léri
    L. disease
    L. pleonosteosis
    L. sign
Leriche syndrome
Léri-Weill
    L.-W. disease
    L.-W. syndrome
Lerman
    L. hinge brace
    L. multiligamentous knee control
      orthosis
    L. noninvasive halo
Lerman-Minerva collar
LeRoy clip-applying forceps
LES
  Lambert-Eaton syndrome
lesion
    acute traumatic l.
    ALPSA l.
    anterior labrum periosteal sleeve
      avulsion l.
    articular cartilage l.
    atlantoaxial l.
    Bankart shoulder l.
    Bennett l.
    Bennett posterior inferior glenoid l.
    BHAGL l.
    biceps interval l. (BIL)
    bone surface l.
    bony l.

bony humeral avulsion of
  glenohumeral ligament l.
Brown-Séquard l.
bubbly bone l.
callosal l.
cartilaginous l.
chiropractic l.
cleavage l.
cyclops l.
cystic bone l.
desmoid l.
destructive articular l.
disc l.
dorsal root entry zone l.
DREZ l.
Essex-Lopresti l.
expansile l.
extracompartmental l.
fibrous l.
GLAD l.
glenolabral articular disruption l.
glenolabral ovoid mass l.
GLOM l.
HAGL l.
hamartomatous l.
Hill-Sachs l.
humeral avulsion of glenohumeral l.
hyperkeratotic l.
hyperpigmented l.
impingement l.
intracortical radiolucent l.
intramedullary l.
irregular-shaped l.
irritable l.
ischemic l.
juxtaarticular l.
Kempson-Campanacci l.
Kidner l.
kissing l.'s
labral l.
lytic l.
lytic bone l.
meniscoid l.
metastatic bone l.
Modic vertebral endplate l. (1–2)
Monteggia equivalent l.
Morel-Lavallée l.
Morel-Lavallée internal degloving l.
morphealike l.
muscular l.
nail bed l.
neoplastic l.
nerve root l.
neuromechanical l.
nonlinear l.
Nora l.
occult talar l.
Osgood-Schlatter l.
osseous l.

osteoblastic l.
osteocartilaginous l.
osteochondral l.
osteopathic l.
paraosseous l.
parosteal l.
pedal hyperpigmented l.
Perthes l.
Perthes-Bankart l.
POLPSA l.
polyostotic bone l.
posterior labrocapsular periosteal
  sleeve avulsion l.
posterior-superior humeral head l.
postfracture l.
pseudoneoplastic l.
radiolucent l.
retroacetabular l.
reverse Bankart l.
reverse Hill-Sachs l.
rim l.
rotator cuff l.
shoulder l.
Sinding-Larsen-Johansson knee
  growth plate l.
SLAP l.
soft tissue l.
Stener gamekeeper's thumb l.
striatal l.
subchondral l.
superior labrum anterior and
  posterior l.
transfer l.
transient l.
traumatic, unidirectional instability
  and Bankart l.
tuberculous l.
uncommitted metaphysial l.
upper motor neuron l.
verrucous l.
vertebral l.
Woofry-Chandler classification of
  Osgood-Schlatter l.
Wrisberg l.

Leslie-Ryan anterior axillary
  approach
LESS
  lateral electrical surface
    stimulation
lesser
  l. metatarsal
  L. Metatarsophalangeal-
    Interphalangeal Scale (LMIS)
  l. metatarsophalangeal joint
  l. multangular
  l. multangular bone
  l. pelvis
  l. rhomboid muscle
  l. tarsal arthrodesis

L

lesser (*continued*)
    l. tarsus cavus
    l. toe
    l. trochanter
    l. trochanter fracture
    l. tuberosity
**less invasive stabilization system
  (LISS)**
Lester muscle forceps
Letournel
    L. guideline
    L. pelvic ring injury classification
    L. plate
Letournel-Judet
    L.-J. acetabular approach
    L.-J. acetabular fracture classification
Letterer-Siwe disease
Leukeran
leukocyte scan
LeukoScan
Leukotape
    L. P combo pack taping
      kit
    L. P stretch bandage
    L. sports tape
Leung thumb loss classification
levator
    l. ani group
    l. scapulae muscle
    l. scapulae syndrome
level
    comfort l.
    fat-fluid l.
    fluid-fluid l.
    l. foundation
    long and short l.
    myoinositol l.
    l. of activity
    parathormone l.
    segmental l.
    sorbitol l.
    spinal l.
    transcutaneous oxygen l.
    vertebral l.
1-level implantation
2-level implantation
3-level implantation
leveling
    joint l.
4-level radiculopathy
level-specific chiropractic adjustment
lever
    l. arm
    Lane bone l.
levering
Levin drill guide
Levine
    L. and Drennan metaphysial to
      diaphysial angle

    L. Orthopaedic Outcomes
      Questionnaire
    L. patellar tendon strap
Levis arm splint
levodopa, laevodopa
Levo-Dromoran
Levoprome
levorphanol tartrate
levoscoliosis scoliosis
Levy & Rappel foot orthosis
Lewin
    L. bone-holding clamp
    L. bone-holding forceps
    L. bunion dissector
    L. collar
    L. finger splint
    L. forceps
    L. punch referred back pain
      test
    L. reverse Lasègue test
    L. snuff disc rupture test
    L. spinal perforating forceps
    L. standing hamstring test
    L. supine ankylosing spinal lesion
      test
Lewin-Gaenslen sacroiliac lesion test
Lewin-Stern
    L.-S. finger splint
    L.-S. thumb splint
Lewis
    L. expandable adjustable prosthesis
      (LEAP)
    L. intercalary resection
    L. nail
    L. periosteal elevator
    L. periosteal rasp
    L. Trapezio prosthesis
**Lewis-Prusik capillary circulation
  test**
Lewit stretch technique
Lexan jacket
Lexer
    L. chisel
    L. gouge
    L. osteotome
Leyden-Möbius muscular dystrophy
Leyla
    L. arm
    L. bar
LFAC
    low-frequency alternating current
LFC
    last foot contact
    LFC gait-related risk factor
LFIT
    low-friction ion treatment
L-frame fixator
LH1000 arthroscopic legholder
Lhermitte sign

liability
>ergonomic assessment of risk and l. (EARLY)

LIAD
>low-impact aerobic dance

liberator elevator

liberty
>L. CMC thumb brace
>L. One splint
>L. spinal system

Librium

LICA
>laser image custom arthroplasty

lichen
>l. nitidus
>l. planus

Lichtblau
>L. osteotomy
>L. tenotomy

Lichtman
>L. aseptic necrosis classification
>L. disease
>L. lunatomalacia staging
>L. midcarpal shift test
>L. modification of stahl technique
>L. radiographic classification of Kienböck disease (stages I, II, IIIa, IIIb, IV)
>L. staging of Kienböck disease technique

Lido
>L. Active Multijoint System
>L. isokinetic dynamometer
>L. lift
>L. lift and work set
>L. Passive Multijoint System
>L. WorkSET work simulator

Lidoback isokinetic dynamometry system

lidocaine
>l. and bupivacaine
>l. and epinephrine
>l. and prilocaine
>bacitracin, neomycin, polymyxin B, and l.
>l. patch

Lidoderm

Lido-Gel
>L.-G. topical anesthetic
>L.-G. topical anesthetic Hydrogel

Liebolt radioulnar technique

life
>health-related quality of l. (HRQOL)
>L. Liner stick and cut-resistant glove
>quality of l.
>L. Satisfaction Index (LSI)

LIFEC
>lumbar intersomatic fusion expandable cage

LifeGait partial weightbearing therapy device

Lifeline Wall Gym 2000 fitness system

Lifestride treadmill

lifestyle
>l. education (LSE)
>sedentary l.

lift
>BTE dynamic l.
>Calypso l.
>dead l.
>heel l.
>Hoyer l.
>kyphotic l.
>Lido l.
>ML l.
>shoe l.
>squat l.
>VuRyser monitor l.

lifting
>static l.

lift-off
>foot l.-o.
>l.-o. of heel in walk
>l.-o. subscapularis test
>tibial l.-o.
>varus-valgus l.-o.

lift-up index

Ligaclip applier

ligament
>accessory atlantoaxial l.
>accessory lateral collateral l.
>acromioclavicular l.
>acromiocoracoid l.
>adipose l.
>alar l.
>allograft reconstruction of fibular collateral l.
>l. anchor
>ankle inferior transverse l.
>anterior collateral l.
>anterior cruciate l. (ACL)
>anterior fibular l.
>anterior longitudinal l. (ALL)
>anterior medial ankle l.
>anterior meniscofemoral l.
>anterior oblique l. (AOL)
>anterior sacrococcygeal l.
>anterior sacroiliac l.
>anterior talofibular l. (ATFL)
>anterior talotibial l.
>anterior tibiofibular l.
>anterior tibiotalar l.
>anteroinferior glenohumeral l.
>anteroinferior tibiofibular l.
>anteromedial glenohumeral l.
>anterosuperior glenohumeral l.
>anular l.
>arcuate popliteal l.

ligament (*continued*)
- artificial l.
- atlantal transverse l.
- atlantoaxial l.
- atlantooccipital l.
- l. augmentation device (LAD)
- avulsed l.
- l. avulsion
- Barkow l.
- beak l.
- Bertin l.
- Bichat l.
- bifurcate l.
- Bigelow l.
- bony humeral avulsion of glenohumeral l. (BHAGL)
- Bourgery l.
- Brodie l.
- Burns l.
- l. button
- calcaneoastragaloid l.
- calcaneoclavicular l.
- calcaneocuboid l. (CCL)
- calcaneofibular l. (CFL)
- calcaneonavicular l.
- calcaneotibial l.
- Caldani l.
- Campbell l.
- capital l.
- capsular l.
- carpal l.
- carpometacarpal l.
- CC l.
- cervical mover l.
- CH l.
- checkrein l.
- Chrisman-Snook reconstruction of ankle l.
- Civinini l.
- l. clamp
- Cleland l.
- collateral fibular l.
- collateral radial l.
- collateral tibial l.
- collateral ulnar l.
- Colles l.
- congenital laxity of l.
- conoid l.
- coracoacromial l. (CAL)
- coracoclavicular l.
- coracohumeral l.
- coronary l.
- corporotransverse inferior l.
- corporotransverse superior l.
- costoclavicular l. (CCL)
- costotransverse l.
- cruciate l.
- Cruveilhier l.
- cuboideonavicular l.

- cuneonavicular l.
- DATT l.
- DCC l.
- deep anterior tibiotalar l.
- deep collateral l.
- deep posterior sacrococcygeal l.
- deep posterior tibiotalar l.
- deep transverse carpal l.
- deep transverse intermetatarsal l.
- deep transverse metacarpal l.
- deep transverse metatarsal l.
- deltoid l.
- deltotrapezius fascial l.
- dentate l.
- dorsal calcaneocuboid l.
- dorsal calcaneonavicular l.
- dorsal carpal l.
- dorsal carpometacarpal l.
- dorsal cuboideonavicular l.
- dorsal cuneocuboid l.
- dorsal cuneonavicular l.
- dorsal intercarpal l.
- dorsal intercuneiform l.
- dorsal metacarpal l.
- dorsal metatarsal l.
- dorsal talonavicular l.
- dorsal tarsometatarsal l.
- dorsoradial l. (DRL)
- DPTT l.
- DRC ligament
- dural l.
- l. elongation
- extraarticular knee l.
- extracapsular l.
- extrinsic l.
- fabellofibular l.
- falciform l.
- false l.
- fibular collateral l. (FCL)
- fibular sesamoidal l.
- fibulocalcaneal l.
- fibulotalar l.
- fibulotalocalcaneal l.
- first intermetacarpal l.
- flaval l.
- floating l.
- fracture-dislocation with anterior l.
- FTC l.
- Gerdy l.
- glenohumeral l. (GHL)
- Gore-Tex anterior cruciate l.
- Grayson l.
- hamate l.
- hamatometacarpal l.
- Henle l.
- humeral avulsion of glenohumeral l. (HAGL)
- Humphry l.
- hypertrophic l.

iliofemoral l.
iliolumbar l.
iliopatellar l.
iliotrochanteric l.
inferior band cruciform l.
inferior glenohumeral l. (IGHL)
inferior ilioischial l.
infrapatellar l.
inguinal l.
intercarpal l.
interclavicular l.
interdigital l.
intermetacarpal l. (IML)
intermetatarsal l.
interosseous cuneocuboid l.
interosseous cuneometatarsal l.
interosseous intercuneiform l.
interosseous metacarpal l.
interosseous metatarsal l.
interosseous sacroiliac l.
interosseous talocalcaneal l. (ITCL)
intersesamoid l.
interspinal l.
interspinal l.
intertransverse l.
intervolar plate l.
intraarticular disc l.
intraosseous tibiofibular l.
ischiofemoral l.
laciniate l.
Landsmeer l.
lateral atlantooccipital l.
lateral collateral l. (LCL)
lateral costotransverse l.
lateral interosseous l.
lateral lumbosacral l.
lateral sacrococcygeal l.
lateral spring l.
lateral talocalcaneal l. (LTC)
LCC l.
limited proteoglycan matrix of l.
Lisfranc l.
long calcaneocuboid l.
longitudinal l.
long plantar l. (LPL)
LRL l.
LT l.
lumbocostal l.
lunotriquetral l.
medial capsular l.
medial collateral l. (MCL)
medial patellofemoral l. (MPFL)
medial sesamoid l.
medial talocalcaneal l.
medial ulnar collateral l. (MUCL)
meniscofemoral l.
meniscotibial l.
metacarpal l.
metacarpoglenoid l.

metacarpophalangeal l.
metatarsal l.
metatarsosesamoid l.
middle glenohumeral l. (MGHL)
midline l.
natatory l.
navicular cuneiform l.
naviculocuneiform l.
nuchal l.
oblique popliteal l.
oblique retinacular l.
l. of Henry
l. of Struthers
l. of tarsus
l. of Wrisberg
olecranon l.
orbicular l.
ossification of posterior longitudinal
   l. (OPLL)
palmar carpal l.
palmar carpometacarpal l.
palmar intercarpal deltoid l.
palmar metacarpal l.
palmar radiocarpal l.
palmar ulnocarpal l.
patellar l.
patellofemoral l.
patellomeniscal l.
patellotibial l.
petroclinoid l.
pisiform metacarpal l.
pisohamate l.
pisometacarpal l.
plantar l.
plantar calcaneocuboid l.
plantar calcaneonavicular l.
plantar cuboideonavicular l.
plantar cuneocuboid l.
plantar cuneonavicular l.
plantar intercuneiform l.
plantar metatarsal l.
plantar spring l.
plantar tarsometatarsal l.
popliteal l.
popliteofibular l.
posterior cruciate l. (PCL)
posterior longitudinal l. (PLL)
posterior meniscofemoral l.
posterior sacroiliac l.
posterior talofibular l. (PTFL)
posterior tibiofibular l.
posterior tibiotalar l.
posteroinferior tibiofibular l.
Poupart inguinal l.
pubocapsular l.
pubofemoral l.
quadrate l.
radial carpal collateral l.
radial collateral l. (RCL)

L

ligament (*continued*)
    radial metacarpal l.
    radiate carpal l.
    radiate sternocostal l.
    radiocapitate l.
    radiocarpal l.
    radiolunotriquetral l.
    radioscaphocapitate l.
    radioscaphoid l.
    radioscapholunate l.
    radiotriquetral l.
    rearfoot l.
    l. reconstruction
    l. reconstruction with tendon
      interposition (LRTI)
    repair of spring l.
    l. replacement
    retinacular l.
    rhomboid l.
    Robert l.
    round l.
    Rouviere l.
    l. rupture sprain
    sacrococcygeal l.
    sacroiliac l.
    sacrospinal l.
    sacrospinous l.
    sacrotuberale l.
    sacrotuberous l.
    scapholunate interosseous l.
    scaphotrapezoid interosseous l.
    scapular l.
    scapulohumeral l.
    SCC l.
    sesamoid l.
    sesamophalangeal l.
    short calcaneocuboid l.
    short plantar l. (SPL)
    short radiolunate l.
    spinal posterior l.
    spinal transverse l.
    spinoglenoid l.
    spiral oblique retinacular l.
    spring l.
    SRL l.
    sternoclavicular l.
    sternocostal l.
    STT l.
    subtalar interosseous l.
    superficial medial l.
    superficial posterior sacrococcygeal l.
    superficial tibiotalar l.
    superficial transverse l.
    superficial transverse metacarpal l.
    superficial transverse metatarsal l.
    superficial TV metacarpal l.
    superficial TV metatarsal l.
    superior costotransverse l.
    superomedial calcaneonavicular l.

    supraspinal l.
    supraspinous l.
    syndesmotic l.
    talocalcaneal l.
    talofibular l.
    talonavicular l.
    tarsometatarsal l.
    tectoral l.
    tendinotrochanteric l.
    tibial collateral l. (TCL)
    tibial sesamoid l.
    tibiocalcaneal l.
    tibiofibular l.
    tibionavicular l.
    tibiospring l.
    torn l.
    transverse acetabular l.
    transverse atlantal l.
    transverse carpal l. (TCL)
    transverse intertarsal l.
    transverse metatarsal l.
    transverse retinacular l.
    transverse scapular l.
    transverse spinal l.
    transverse tibiofibular l.
    trapezoid l.
    traumatized l.
    triangular l.
    ulnar carpal collateral l.
    ulnar collateral l. (UCL)
    ulnocarpal l.
    ulnolunate l.
    ulnotriquetral l.
    vaginal hand l.
    vertebropelvic l.
    volar beak l.
    volar carpal l. (VCL)
    Weitbrecht l.
    Wrisberg l.
    yellow l.
ligament-bone complex
ligamentoplasty
ligamentotaxis
    multiplanar l.
ligamentous
    l. and capsular repair (LCR)
    l. ankylosis
    l. anterior dislocation (LAD)
    l. anterior dislocation composite
      graft
    l. attachment
    l. attrition
    l. bouncing
    l. box
    l. complex
    l. control brace
    l. disruption
    l. injury
    l. insertion

l. instability test
l. insufficiency
l. laxity
l. luxation
l. release
l. stability
l. structure
l. support tissue
l. thickening
l. weave procedure

ligamentous-muscular hypertrophy
ligament-scar matrix
ligamentum

l. bifurcatum
l. calcaneocuboideum
ligamenta carpometacarpaliad dorsalia
l. conoideum
l. flavum
l. radiatum
l. sacrospinale
l. sacrotuberale

ligand adhesive
ligation
ligature

l. carrier
l. guide
l. passer
stick tie l.

light

l. cast
Cogent l.
l. conductor
l. cross-slot screwdriver
infrared l.
l. intensity training
l. microscopy
l. source
therapeutic l.
l. touch sensation
l. touch test
ultraviolet l.
L. V sign

Lightplast athletic tape
LIH

Lars Ingvar Hansson
LIH hook pin

Likert and Borg scale
Lilienthal rib spreader
Lima external fixator
limb

l. absence
l. accurate measurement (LAM)
artificial l.
l. ataxia
l. brace
l. bud
congenitally short l.
l. girdle
l. gym

hanging of l.
l. holder
ischemic l.
left lower l. (LLL)
left upper l. (LUL)
l. length
l. length angulation
l. length discrepancy
l. length disparity
l. lengthening
phantom l.
plantigrade l.
l. position
posture of l.
l. replantation
residual l.
right lower l. (RLL)
right upper l. (RUL)
l. salvage
seal l.
l. synergy
Trowbridge Terra-Round sports l.
Utah artificial l.

Limberg pilonidal disease flap
limb-girdle

l.-g. lengthening
l.-g. muscular dystrophy

limb-girdle-trunk paresis
limbi (*pl. of* limbus)
limb-salvage

l.-s. procedure
l.-s. surgery

limb-sparing operation
limbus, *pl.* **limbi**

l. anulare

4-limb Z-plasty
limit

elastic l.
endurance l.
metal endurance l.
motion l.
l.'s of stability (LOS)
within functional l.'s (WFL)

limitation

motion l.
l. of motion (LOM)
l. of movement (LOM)
protective l.

limited

l. compression-dynamic compression
plate
l. fasciectomy
l. intertarsal arthrodesis
l. joint mobility (LJM)
l. motion metal ankle joint
l. performance measure
l. proteoglycan matrix of ligament

limited-contact dynamic compression
plate

L

limiter
> Becker 655 motion control l.
> motion control l.

limiting condition

limitus
> bony hallux l.
> cartilaginous hallux l.
> hallux l.
> McKeever arthrodesis for hallux l.
> Regnauld free phalangeal base autograft for hallux l.
> Z-slide lengthening in hallux l.

limp
> antalgic l.
> gluteus medius l.
> new-onset l.
> Trendelenburg l.

LINAC
> linear accelerator
> Boston LINAC
> University of Florida LINAC

Linberg restrictive thumb-index tenosynovitis syndrome

Lincoln-Oseretsky Motor Development Scale

Lindell blanisotropic media classification

Lindeman laryngeal diversion procedure

Lindemann bur

Linder sign

Lindgren oblique osteotomy

Lindholm
> L. Achilles lengthening procedure
> L. Achilles tendon rupture repair technique
> L. open surgical tendon repair
> L. tendo calcaneus repair

Lindseth osteotomy

Lindsjö method

Lindvall-Stille knife

line
> acetabular l.
> AC-PC l.
> action l.
> Andren-von Rosen l.
> anterior axillary l. (AAL)
> anterior humeral l.
> anterior spinal l.
> antitension l.
> AxyaWeld product l.
> Beau l.
> bisector l.
> Blumensaat anterior cruciate ligament l.
> Bryant l.
> cement l.
> cervical stress l.
> Chamberlain l.
> Chopart joint l.
> cleavage l.

> coronoid l.
> cyma l.
> divisionary l.
> Duhot l.
> epiphysial l.
> Feiss l.
> Feiss medial malleolus to plantar first MTP joint l.
> femoral head l. (FHL)
> fracture l.
> Fränkel white l.
> gait l.
> George l.
> gravitational l.
> gravity plumb l.
> growth arrest l.
> Harris growth arrest l.
> Harris hip l.
> Hawkins l.
> Hilgenreiner horizontal Y l.
> Hilgenreiner-Perkins pelvic x-ray l.
> horizontal Y l.
> H-P pelvic x-ray l.'s
> Hueter l.
> iliopectineal l.
> interteardrop l.
> joint l.
> Kaplan oblique l.
> Kilian l.
> Kline l.
> Köhler l.
> Langer l.
> lateral joint l.
> lead l.
> Looser l.
> lumbar gravitational l.
> MacNab l.
> Maquet l.
> McGregor l.
> McRae l.
> Meary l.
> medial joint l. (MJL)
> Meyer l.
> Meyerding spondylolisthesis classification l.
> midaxillary l. (MAL)
> midheel l.
> midmalleolar l.
> midsternal l. (MSL)
> Moloney l.
> Moyer l.
> Nélaton l.
> oblique metacarpal l.
> obturator/brim l.
> odontoid perpendicular l.
> l. of demarcation
> l. of gravity
> l. of Zahn
> Ogston l.

parajugular l.
parallel pitch l.'s
Perkins-Ombredanne l.
Perkins vertical l.
physial l.
plumb l.
posterior axillary l. (PAL)
posterior cervical l.
radiocapitellar l.
radiolucent l.
relaxed skin tension l.
Roser l.
Roser-Nélaton l.
sacral arcuate l.
sacral horizontal plane l. (SHPL)
sacroiliac l.
sacroiliac-symphysis l.
Schoemaker congenital hip
  dislocation l.
sclerotic l.
scurvy l.
Shenton l.
Shenton-Ménard l.
Skinner pelvic menstruation l.
skin tension l.
spinolaminar l. (SLL)
superior nuchal l.
Sydney l.
teardrop l.
tibiofibular l.
trapezoid l.
trough l.
Trümmerfeld scurvy l.
Ullmann spondylolisthesis l.
Wegner l.
Whitesides l.
Winberger l.
Y l.
Z l.

linea, *pl.* **lineae**
l. aspera
l. semilunaris
lineae (*pl. of* linea)
Lineage acetabular cup
linear
l. accelerator (LINAC)
l. amputation
l. analog pain scale
l. capsulotomy
l. fraction
l. fracture
L. hip stem
l. osteotomy
l. potentiometer
l. scar
L. total hip system
l. variable differential transducer
linebacker's arm
linen suture

liner
acetabular l.
acetabular prosthetic l.
Alpha cushion l.
ALPS CustomPro custom l.
bone l.
cast l.
cushion shoe l.
DePuy acetabular l.
Duraloc acetabular l.
elevated rim acetabular l.
Enduron acetabular l.
Fillauer prosthesis l.
Fillauer silicone suction l.
Fillauer silicone suspension l.
Gore-Tex waterproof cast l.
grommet bone l.
Hylamer enhanced ultra-high
  molecular weight polyethylene
  acetabular l.
Iceross Comfort Plus silicone
  gel l.
Medium-Plus alpha l.
metal acetabular l.
l. micromotion
OrthoGel l.
Plastazote shoe l.
polyethylene l.
Polysorb l.
polyurethane l.
Reflection l.
RingLoc hip l.
SiloLiner gel l.
Spenco l.
splint l.
TEC l.
USMC luxury l.
line-to-line reaming technique
Ling
L. cemented hip prosthesis
L. method
lingism
lingual
l. artery
l. vein
lining
DePuy acetabular l.
shoe l.
Thermold heat moldable
  shoe l.
link
L. anatomical hip
4-bar l.
CrossBar thoracolumbar fusion
  posterior fixation l.
L. custom partial pelvis replacement
  system
L. Endo-Model rotational knee
  prosthesis

L

link (*continued*)

L. Endo-Model rotational knee system

L. Lubinus SP II hip replacement system

malleable l.

L. MP hip noncemented reconstruction prosthesis

L. MP microporous hip stem

L. MP reconstruction hip stem

musculotendinous-osseous l.

offset l.

L. Orthopaedics device

L. Saddle Prosthesis Endo-Model hip replacement system

L. Stack Split Splint

L. toe splint

linkage

kinematic l.

rod l.

linked potential

lint-free drape

Linton varicose vein procedure

Linvatec

L. absorbable screw

L. arthroscopic infusion pump

L. arthroscopy product

L. bone anchor

L. driver

L. product

lion forceps

lion-jaw forceps

Lioresal Intrathecal

lip

bone l.

l. of acetabulum

l. of glenoid

l. of navicular

l. of tibia

osteophytic bone l.

posterior l.

lipid

l. inclusion cyst

l. tumor

lipoarthritis

lipoblastomatosis

lipocalcinogranulomatosis

lipochondrodystrophy

lipofibroma

intraneural l.

lipofibromatosis

lipofibromatous hamartoma

lipohemarthrosis

lipoma, *pl.* **lipomas**

l. arborescens

endovaginal l.

intraosseous l.

pleomorphic l.

spinal l.

spindle cell l.

lipomas (*pl. of* lipoma)

lipomatosa

macrodystrophia l.

lipomatosis

intraosseous l.

lipomeningocele

liposarcoma

myxoid l.

myxoid-type l.

pleomorphic l.

round cell l.

round cell-type l.

well-differentiated myxoid l.

lipping

Lippman

L. biceps tendinopathy test

L. hip prosthesis

L. screw

Lippman-Cobb

L.-C. classification (I-VII) of curvature in scoliosis

L.-C. technique

Lipscomb

L. metatarsophalangeal arthrodesis

L. modified McKeever arthrodesis

L. procedure

L. technique

Lipscomb-Anderson drill guide

liquid

l. cable

l. crystal thermography (LCT)

L. Ice

Lotrimin AF spray l.

l. nitrogen cryotherapy

Tums Extra Strength L.

Liquiprin

Lisch nodule

Lisfranc

L. amputation

L. arthrodesis

L. articular interline

L. articular set angle (LASA)

L. below-knee prosthesis

L. Charcot joint

L. disarticulation

L. dislocation

L. fracture

L. fracture-dislocation

L. injury

L. joint

L. joint articulation

L. joint complex

L. ligament

L. operation

L. scalene tubercle

LISS
>less invasive stabilization system
>Synthes LISS

Lissauer zone

list
>postural l.

Lister
>L. corn
>L. dorsal radius tubercle
>L. flexor tendon pulley
>reconstruction technique
>L. technique of pulley
>reconstruction

listhesis
>anterior-posterior l.
>lateral l.

listing
>dynamic l.
>l. gait
>static l.

Liston
>L. amputating knife
>L. bone-cutting forceps
>L. bone rongeur
>L. operation
>L. phalangeal knife
>L. shears
>L. splint

Liston-Key bone-cutting forceps
Liston-Key-Horsley rib shears
Liston-Littauer
>L.-L. bone-cutting forceps
>L.-L. rongeur

Liston-Stille bone-cutting forceps
**LiteGait partial weightbearing gait
 therapy device**
LiteNest portable seating system
lithotomy
>l. legholder
>l. position

Litroff test
Litt
>cloth tape occlusion method
>of L.

**Littauer-Liston bone-cutting
 forceps**
litter
>Neal-Robertson l.

Littig strut
little
>L. area
>L. disease
>l. finger
>L. League elbow (LLE)
>L. release
>L. technique

Littler
>L. operation
>L. opponensplasty

>L. pollicization
>L. swanneck deformity repair
>technique
>wing excision of L.

Littler-Cooley
>L.-C. abductor digiti minimi transfer
>L.-C. opponensplasty technique
>L.-C. tendon transfer

livedo reticularis
Liverpool
>L. elbow prosthesis
>L. knee prosthesis

live splint
living
>activity of daily l. (ADL)
>Center for Independent L. (CIL)
>electronic aid for daily l. (EADL)
>extended activities of daily l.
> (EADL)
>instrumental activity of daily l.
> (IADL)
>Katz index of activities of daily l.
>Occupational Therapy Activities of
>Daily L. (OTADL)

Livingstone therapy
Livingston intramedullary bar
Liviscope scope
Livotrit Plus
LJM
>limited joint mobility

L1-L5
>lumbar (spine) nerves 1-5
>lumbar (spine) vertebrae 1-5

LLC
>long leg cast

LLD
>leg length discrepancy

LLE
>left lower extremity
>Little League elbow

LLI
>leg length inequality

LLL
>left lower limb
>lower fossa active, lateral knee pain,
>long leg on side ipsilateral to weak
>fossa

LLO
>lower limb orthosis

Llorente dissecting forceps
Lloyd
>L. adapter
>L. adapter for Smith-Petersen
>nail
>L. chiropractic table
>L. nail driver

Lloyd-Roberts
>L.-R. fracture
>L.-R. fracture technique

L

Lloyd-Roberts-Swann trochanteric advancement
LLP
    lower limb prosthesis
LLPS
    low-load prolonged stretch
    low-pressure plasma spray
       LLPS hydroxyapatite
       LLPS hydroxyapatite
        adhesive
LLWBC
    long leg weightbearing cast
LLWC
    long leg walking cast
LMA
    lateral mass articulation
LMB
       LMB finger splint
       LMB wire-foam economical resting
       splint
LMIS
    Lesser
      Metatarsophalangeal-Interphalangeal
      Scale
LMJA
    longitudinal midtarsal joint
    axis
L'Nard
      L. boot
      L. Multi Podus orthosis
      L. thoracolumbosacral orthosis
LNS
    localized nodular synovitis
LNV
    last normal vertebra
Lo
      L. Bak spinal support
      L. Bak spinal support prosthesis
      Darco Body Armor L.
      L. Rider prosthetic foot
load
    l. and shift shoulder test
    applied l.
    axial compression l.
    l. beam
    bending l.
    compression l.
    critical l.
    Euler l.
    ramp l.
    rotatory l.
    spinal axial l.
    torque l.
    torsional l.
    l. transfer
load-and-shift maneuver
load-bearing graft
load-deflection curve
load-deformation curve

load-displacement
    l.-d. curve
    l.-d. plot
loading
    anatomic l.
    arch l.
    axial l.
    compression l.
    concentric l.
    cyclic l.
    dynamic l.
    eccentric l.
    Edwards modular system
      dynamic l.
    fat l.
    fracture callus l.
    functional and anatomic l. (FAL)
    lumbar spine l.
    l. mode
    musculoskeletal l.
    progressive l.
    repetitive l.
    status l.
    sustained l.
    tension l.
    l. time
    trunk l.
    vertical l.
load-sharing classification
load-to-grip displacement
Loban adhesive drape
Lobstein
      L. brittle bones syndrome
      L. disease
lobster-claw
    l.-c. deformity
    l.-c. foot
    l.-c. hand
lobster-type clamp
local
    l. adaptation syndrome (LAS)
    l. cavus
    l. compression fracture
    l. decompression fracture
    l. epineurotomy
    l. flap
    l. radical resection
    l. standby anesthesia
    l. standby anesthesia technique
Localio procedure
localization
    pedicle l.
localized
    l. bone destruction
    l. nodular synovitis (LNS)
    l. nodular tenosynovitis
    l. thermoregulation
localizer cast
locating pin

location
    cervical sympathetic chain l.
    pedicle l.
locator
    Berman-Moorhead metal l.
    metal l.
locator/stimulator
    Pointer-Plus l./s.
lock
    Ball knee l.
    l. finger
    grip l.
    heel l.
    knee l.
    lateral spring-loaded l.
    Morse taper l.
    physiologic l.
    Ratchet Lock variable flexion
     knee l.
    spring-loaded knee l.
    VariLock socket l.
lockable arthroscopic knot
Locke
    L. bone clamp
    L. elevator
locked
    l. facet
    l. intramedullary osteosynthesis
    l. intramedullary osteosynthesis pin
    l. knee
    l. nailing
    l. scapula
Lockhart toe splint
locking
    anatomic medullary l. (AML)
    l. clamp
    l. compression plate
    l. disc
    distal l.
    l. hook instrumentation
    l. horizontal mattress suture
    l. loop
    medullary l.
    l. nail
    l. nut
    l. of joint
    l. peg
    l. pliers
    l. prosthesis
    proximal l.
    sacroiliac joint l.
    l. screw
    single axis l. (SAL)
locking-head screw
locking-hook spinal rod
locking-position test
locking-suture technique
lock-jaw (*var. of* lockjaw)
lockjaw, lock-jaw

locknut wrench
lockout suture
Locksley occipitocervical fusion technique
locomotion
locomotor
    l. ataxia
    l. mechanism
    l. pattern
    l. system
LoCon-T
    L.-T distal radial plate
    L.-T distal radial plating system
Lodine XL
Loeffler-Ballard incision
Lofstrand crutch
log
    exercise l.
    Fin & Flipper exercise l.
    motor activity l.
Logan traction
logrolling maneuver
Lok-it screwdriver
LOM
    limitation of motion
    limitation of movement
    loss of motion
London unconstrained elbow prosthesis
Lone Star retractor system
long
    l. alignment rod
    l. and short level
    l. arm brace
    l. arm cast (LAC)
    l. arm finger cast
    l. arm splint (LAS)
    l. axial alignment guide
    l. axis
    l. axis of bone
    l. axis traction chiropractic table
    L. Beach pedicle screw
    l. bent-knee leg cast
    l. bone compression test
    l. bone deficiency
    l. bone osteomyelitis
    l. calcaneocuboid ligament
    l. coarse bur
    l. curette
    l. deltopectoral approach
    l. extensor
    l. external rotator
    l. fibular muscle
    l. finger
    l. head
    l. head biceps tendon
    l. head of biceps
    l. leg arthropathy
    l. leg brace
    l. leg cast (LLC)
    l. leg hinged brace

L

long (*continued*)
    l. leg immobilizer
    l. leg orthosis
    l. leg splint
    l. leg stockings
    l. leg walking cast (LLWC)
    l. leg weightbearing cast (LLWBC)
    l. lever low-amplitude type manipulation
    l. nail-mounted drill guide
    l. oblique fracture
    l. opponens orthosis
    l. plantar ligament (LPL)
    l. posterior flap
    l. radiolunate (LRL)
    l. segment spinal fusion
    l. stem
    l. thoracic nerve injury
    l. thoracic nerve injury orthosis
    l. thoracic nerve palsy
    l. toe flexor
    l. tract sign
longa
    vincula l.
long-axis ray
long-bone
    l.-b. fixation
    l.-b. fracture
long-edge medullary nail
Longevity V-Lign hip prosthesis
longissimus colli muscle
longitudinal
    l. arch stress
    l. axis
    l. blood supply
    l. deficiency
    l. displaced complete tear
    l. distraction
    l. epiphysial bracket
    l. fracture
    l. incision
    l. incomplete intrameniscal tear
    l. ligament
    l. ligament rupture
    l. member to anchor connector
    l. member to longitudinal member connector
    l. meniscal tear
    l. midtarsal joint axis (LMJA)
    l. plantar arch
    l. ridge
    l. spinal bar
    l. split tear
    l. tendon split
    l. traction
long-jaw basket forceps
long-latency somatosensory evoked potential

long-radius kyphosis
long-stemmed powered bur
long-term bone-instrumentation interface
longus
    abductor pollicis l. (APL)
    adductor hallucis l.
    l. capitis muscle
    l. cervicis colli muscle
    l. colli muscle
    extensor carpi radialis l. (ECRL)
    extensor digitorum l. (EDL)
    extensor hallucis l. (EHL)
    extensor pollicis l. (EPL)
    flexor digitorum l. (FDL)
    flexor hallucis l. (FHL)
    flexor pollicis l. (FPL)
    palmaris l.
    peroneus l.
loop
    Bunnell finger l.
    l. circumferential wire
    Duncan l.
    figure-of-8 wire l.
    finger l.
    l. fixation
    Hartshill-Ransford l.
    l. & hook strapping
    locking l.
    Ohio Medical Instruments l.
    OMI l.
    perineal l.
    Ransford l.
    l. scissors
    thumb l.
    toe l.
    wire l.
loop-lock cock-up splint
loop-over wrap
loose
    l. body (LB)
    l. body grasper
    l. cartilage
    l. debris
    l. fracture
    l. fragment
    l. joint body
    l. knee procedure
    l. procedure
    l. shoulder
loosening
    acetabular component l.
    aseptic l.
    cervical pin l.
    Harris criteria for implant l.
    implant l.
    prosthetic l.
    screw l.
    sterile l.

loose-packed position
Looser
> L. line
> L. zone
> L. zone in insufficiency
> fracture

Looser-Milkman syndrome
Lo-Por vascular graft prosthesis
Loprox
LOPS
> loss of protective sensation

Lopurin
lorazepam
Lorcet
> L. 10
> L. Plus

Lorcet-HD
lord
> L. cup
> L. press-fit hip prosthesis
> L. total hip arthrodesis
> L. total hip prosthesis

Lordex lumbar spine system
lordoscoliosis
lordosis
> cervical l.
> compensatory l.
> l. creation
> dorsal l.
> lumbar spine l.
> occipitocervical l.
> l. preservation
> reversal of cervical l.
> thoracic spine l.

lordotic
> l. curve
> l. pelvis

lordoticiser
> Posture Pump l.

Lorenz
> L. brace
> L. cast
> L. congenital clubfoot procedure
> L. hip reduction
> L. operation
> L. osteosynthesis system
> L. osteotomy
> L. sign

Lorenzo screw
Lore suction tube and tip-holding forceps
lorgnette
> main en l.

lorry driver's fracture
LOS
> length of stay
> limits of stability

Los
> L. Angeles

Losee
> L. knee instability test
> L. modification of MacIntosh ACL
> repair technique
> L. sling and reef ACL repair
> technique

LOSP
> late operative site pain

loss
> blood l.
> bone l.
> estimated blood l. (EBL)
> functional l.
> heat l.
> iatrogenic l.
> lumbar lordosis iatrogenic l.
> motor l.
> l. of correction
> l. of motion (LOM)
> l. of protective sensation (LOPS)
> periprosthetic bone l.
> postmenopausal bone l.
> segmental bone l.
> sensory l.
> vertebral body height l.

LOTCA
> Löwenstein Occupational Therapy
> Cognitive Assessment

LOTCA-G
> Löwenstein Occupational Therapy
> Cognitive Assessment-Geriatric

Loth-Kirschner drill
lotion
> AmLactin l.
> Biotone Polar l.
> Bromi-Lotion antiperspirant l.
> Criticaid l.
> Hydrisinol l.
> Lac-Hydrin l.
> Lactinol l.
> Lotrimin AF l.
> Myossage l.
> Polysonic ultrasound l.
> Restore AF antifungal l.
> Senuva l.
> Tineacide antifungal l.
> Ultra Mide 25 l.
> Ureacin-10 l.

Lotrimin
> L. AF cream
> L. AF lotion
> L. AF Solution
> L. AF spray liquid
> L. AF spray powder

Lotrisone
Lottes
> L. nailing
> L. pin
> L. triflanged medullary nail

L

lotus
    l. position
    L. unicompartment prosthesis
Loughheed and White procedure
Louis
    L. instrumentation
    L. plate
Louisiana
    L. ankle wrap technique
    L. State University (LSU)
    L. State University Medical Center
    (LSUMC)
    L. State University Medical Center
    classification
loupe
    binocular l.
    l. magnification
    magnifying l.
    surgical l.
love
    L. nerve root retractor
    L. splint
Love-Adson periosteal elevator
Love-Gruenwald alligator forceps
Love-Kerrison rongeur forceps
Lovell clubfoot cast
Lovenox Injection
Lovett
    L. clinical scale of zero-normal
    strength
    L. muscle strength test
    L. spring balance muscle test
Lovibond nail fold and plate angle
loving
    L. Comfort maternity support
    L. Comfort postpartum support
low
    l. back injury
    l. back neurosis
    l. back pain (LBP)
    L. Back Pain Symptom Checklist
    l. bone mass
    l. cervical approach
    l. impedance thermocouple
    l. lumbar spine fracture
    l. median-low ulnar palsy
    L. Profile legholder
    L. Profile plastic body jacket
    l. quarter Blucher shoe
    l. single thoracic curve
    l. T humerus fracture
low-air-loss bed
low-arch foot
low-assimilation pelvis
low-contact
    l.-c. dynamic compression plate
    l.-c. stress (LCS)
    l.-c. stress semiconstrained
    prosthesis

low-dose traction
Low-Dye
    L.-D. strapping
    L.-D. taping
    L.-D. taping technique
Lowe-Breck
    L.-B. cartilage knife
    L.-B. meniscectomy knife
Lowell hip reduction
low-energy
    l.-e. fracture
    l.-e. laser (LEL)
Löwenstein
    L. frog-leg lateral hips view
    L. Occupational Therapy Cognitive
    Assessment (LOTCA)
    L. Occupational Therapy Cognitive
    Assessment-Geriatric (LOTCA-G)
lower
    l. cervical spine
    l. cervical spine fusion
    l. cervical spine posterior
    stabilization
    l. cervical spine procedure
    l. extremity (L ext)
    l. extremity amputation (LEA)
    L. Extremity Amputation Prevention
    (LEAP)
    l. extremity bypass surgery
    L. Extremity Functional Scale
    (LEFS)
    l. extremity noninvasive
    l. extremity prosthesis
    l. fossa active, lateral knee pain,
    long leg on side ipsilateral to
    weak fossa (LLL)
    l. hand retractor
    l. hook trial
    l. limb dysmetria
    l. limb orthosis (LLO)
    l. limb prosthesis (LLP)
    l. lumbar spine
    l. nerve root compression
    l. plexus injury
    l. posterior lumbar spine and
    sacrum surgery
    l. sacral nerve root compression
    (LSNRC)
    l. thoracic pedicle
    l. thoracic spine
low-frequency alternating current
  (LFAC)
low-friction ion treatment (LFIT)
low-grade
    l.-g. central osteosarcoma
    l.-g. ulcer
low-heeled shoe
low-impact aerobic dance (LIAD)
low-load prolonged stretch (LLPS)

Lowman
    L. balance board
    L. bone-holding clamp
    L. bone-holding forceps
    L. chisel
    L. hand retractor
    L. shelf procedure
Lowman-Gerster bone clamp
Lowman-Hoglund
    L.-H. chisel
    L.-H. clamp
low-neck femoral prosthesis
low-power laser
low-pressure
    l.-p. injection
    l.-p. plasma spray (LLPS)
    l.-p. plasma-sprayed (LPPS)
    l.-p. positive discography
low-profile
    l.-p. cup
    l.-p. dorsal plate
    l.-p. femoral prosthesis
    l.-p. halo traction
low-riding patella
low-set thumb
low-stress aerobic exercise
low-surface reactive
low-temperature plastic
low-tide walking brace
low-turnover osteoporosis
low-viscosity bone cement
low-voltage galvanism (LVG)
loxoscelism
loxotomy
LP
    lumbar puncture
LPF
    leg protection factor
LPL
    long plantar ligament
L-plate
    Synthes mini L-p.
LPPS
    low-pressure plasma-sprayed
    LPPS hydroxyapatite
        fixation
LRL
    long radiolunate
    LRL ligament
L-rod
    Luque L-r.
LRS
    lateral recess stenosis
LRTI
    ligament reconstruction with tendon
        interposition
LS
    lumbosacral
LS⁴ custom spinal jacket

LSE
    lifestyle education
L-shaped
    L-s. capsular incision
    L-s. capsulotomy
    L-s. osteotomy
    L-s. pad
    L-s. plate
    L-s. rod
    L-s. rotator cuff tear
LSI
    Life Satisfaction Index
    LSI Easy Stims self-adhesive
        electrode
    LSI silver self-adhesive disposable
        electrode
LSNRC
    lower sacral nerve root compression
LSO
    lumbosacral orthosis
L-spine
    lumbar spine
LSST
    lateral scapular slide test
LSU
    Louisiana State University
    LSU reciprocation-gait orthosis
    LSU reciprocation-gait orthosis brace
    LSU reciprocator
LSUMC
    Louisiana State University Medical
      Center
    LSUMC classification
    LSUMC classification of motor and
      sensory function
LT
    L-tryptophan
    lunotriquetral
    LT joint
    LT ligament
LTC
    lateral talocalcaneal ligament
LT-Cage lumbar tapered fusion device
L-tryptophan (LT)
Lubinus
    L. acetabular component
    L. AP hip system
    L. knee prosthesis
    L. SP II anatomically adapted hip
      system
Lucae bone mallet
Lucas
    L. and Drucker Motor Index
    L. chisel
    L. gouge
lucency
    cortical l.
    subchondral l.
    syndesmosis screw l.

L

lucent
luck
    L. bone drill
    L. hand procedure
    L. hip cup
    L. nail
    L. operation
Luck-Bishop bone saw
Ludington
    L. shoulder test
    L. sign
Ludloff
    L. bunionectomy
    L. congenital hip dislocation repair technique
    L. incision
    L. medial open reduction hip approach
    L. operation
    L. osteotomy
    L. sign
Ludwig
    L. plane
    L. sternal angle
LUE
    left upper extremity
Luer
    L. bone rongeur
    L. rongeur forceps
Luer-Lok needle
Luer-Whiting rongeur forceps
Luhr
    L. fixation system
    L. Microfixation cranial plate
    L. Microfixation System drill bit
    L. Microfixation System plate cutter
    L. Microfixation System plate-holding forceps
    L. Microfixation System pliers
    L. microplate
    L. miniplate
    L. pan plate
    L. screw
LUL
    left upper limb
lumbago
    ischemic l.
lumbago-mechanical instability syndrome
lumbar (L)
    l. abscess
    l. accessory movement technique
    l. agenesis
    l. anesthesia
    l. anterior-root stimulator implant (LARSI)
    l. brace
    l. canal
    l. disc
    l. discectomy

l. discography
l. distraction manipulation
l. epidural endoscopy
l. extension
l. extension test
l. facet injection
l. fascia
l. flat back syndrome
l. gravitational line
l. hypolordosis
l. intersomatic fusion expandable cage (LIFEC)
l. kyphosis
l. lateral flexion
l. lateral flexion test
l. lordosis iatrogenic loss
l. lordosis preservation
l. lordotic curve
l. microtrauma
l. myofascial pain syndrome
l. nerve root injection
l. olisthesis
l. pedicle
l. pedicle fixation
l. pedicle marker
l. pedicle screw
l. plexus injury
l. protective mechanism test
l. puncture (LP)
l. range of motion
l. reflex
l. region
l. rheumatism
l. roll
l. rotation
l. rotation test
l. sagittal mobility
l. scoliosis
l. spinal instability
l. spine (L-spine)
l. spine biopsy
l. spine burst fracture
l. spine decompression
l. spine fusion
l. spine instability
l. spine instrumentation
l. spine kyphotic deformity
l. spine loading
l. spine lordosis
l. spine model
l. (spine) nerves 1-5 (L1-L5)
l. spine pedicle diameter
l. spine rotational stability
l. spine segmental fixation
l. spine transpedicular fixation
l. spine trauma
l. (spine) vertebrae 1-5 (L1-L5)
l. spine vertebral osteosynthesis
l. spondylosis

l. support cushion
l. sympathectomy
l. sympathetic block
l. tapered-cage lumbar tapered fusion device
l. thecoperitoneal shunt syndrome
l. traction
l. transforaminal epidural injection
l. tumor
l. vein
l. vertebra
l. vertebral interbody fusion
lumbarization
lumbocostal ligament
lumbodorsal
l. fascia (LDF)
l. support corset
Lumbo 90 home care traction system
lumbopelvic
l. complex
l. dissociation
l. motion
l. radiograph
lumbosacral (LS)
l. brace
l. cartilaginous system
l. corset
l. dislocation
l. flexion
l. fusion
l. fusion elevator
l. joint
l. joint angle
l. junction
l. junction bone density
l. junction fracture
l. kyphosis
l. mechanical syndrome
l. orthosis (LSO)
l. plexus
l. radiculopathy
l. segmental angle
l. series
l. spine
l. spine transpedicular instrumentation
l. spondylolisthesis
l. traction
l. vertebra
Lumbotrain lumbosacral support
lumbrical
l. bar
l. intrinsic contracture
l. muscle
l. plus
l. plus finger
l. plus phenomenon
l. syndrome finger
l. tendon

Lumex
L. lightweight wheelchair
L. Tub-Guard safety rail
L. walker
lunar
L. DPX densitometer
L. Expert densitometer
L. Prodigy bone densitometer
lunate
l. acrylic cement wrist prosthesis
l. bone
l. dislocation
l. facet dye punch injury
l. fracture
l. sinus
lunatomalacia
lunatotriquetral coalition
Lunceford-Pilliar-Engh hip prosthesis
Lund
L. operation
L. prototype unicompartment prosthesis
Lundholm
L. plate
L. screw
lunocapitate
l. bone
l. joint
lunotriquetral (LT)
l. arthrodesis
l. ballottement test
l. dissociation
l. fusion
l. instability
l. joint
l. ligament
l. shear test
lunula, *pl.* **lunulae**
lunulae (*pl. of* lunula)
Luongo hand retractor
lupus
l. anticoagulant
l. erythematosus (LE)
l. erythematosus cell
Luque
L. cerclage wire
L. fixation device
L. II fixation system
L. II plate
L. II screw
L. II segmental spinal instrumentation
L. instrumentation concave technique
L. instrumentation convex technique
L. loop fixation
L. L-rod
L. pedicle screw
L. rectangle
L. ring
L. rod

L

Luque (*continued*)
    L. rod bender
    L. rod fixation
    L. rod fixation for kyphosis
    L. rod migration
    L. segmental fixation
    L. semirigid segmental spinal
      instrumentation
    L. sublaminar wiring technique
    L. wiring
Luque-Galveston
    L.-G. fixation
    L.-G. post
    L.-G. rod
lurch
    abductor l.
    gluteal l.
    Trendelenburg l.
lurching gait
Luschka
    L. bursa
    L. joint
    L. muscle
Lusskin bone drill
Lust phenomenon
lusty leg
LUX
    left upper extremity
luxans
    coxa vara l.
luxated bone
luxatio
    l. coxae congenita
    l. erecta
    l. erecta shoulder dislocation
    l. imperfecta
    l. perinealis
luxation
    atlantoaxial l.
    habitual patella l.
    incomplete l.
    ligamentous l.
    Malgaigne l.
    palmar l.
    patella l.
LVG
    low-voltage galvanism
    continuous LVG
    interrupted LVG
Lyden real-time cerebral angiography technique
Lyman-Smith traction
Lyme
    L. disease
    L. disease arthritis
lymphadenopathy
lymphangiography
lymphangioma
    cavernous l.

lymphangiosarcoma
LymphaPress traction
lymphatic
lymphedema, lymphoedema
    cancer treatment-related l.
    l. complex
    congenital l.
    descending l.
    factitious l.
    familial l.
    l. sling
lymphocyte count
lymphoedema (*var. of* lymphedema)
lymphoma
    angiotropic l.
    primary l.
lymph vessel
Lynco
    L. biomechanical orthotic system
    L. foot orthosis
Lynn
    L. Achilles lengthening procedure
    L. Achilles tendon repair technique
    L. tendo calcaneus repair
Lynx wrist, hand, finger orthosis arm positioner splint
LYOfoam
    L. C dressing
    L. wound dressing
lyophilization of bone
lyophilized bone graft
Lyphocin
lyre-shaped finger hook
Lyser
    trapezoid bone of L.
Lysholm
    L. knee function scoring scale
    L. knee joint instability scope
    L. knee score (1–5)
    L. knee scoring questionnaire
Lysholm-Gillquist
    L.-G. knee subjective function scale
    L.-G. knee subjective function
      score
lysis
lysosomal absorption
Lyte Fit orthotic
lytic
    l. bone lesion
    l. lesion
    l. spine
Lytle metacarpal splint
3M
    3M Company
    3M fiberglass cast
    3M Maxi Driver blade
    3M preparation
    3M skin drape
    3M staple

M

mitochondria
M band
M wave

M/3

middle third

mA

milliampere

MAC

Miami Acute Care
monitored anesthesia control
MAC cervical collar

MacAusland

M. lumbar brace
M. operation
M. procedure

MacCarthy excision of sacrum procedure

maceration

cutaneous m.

Macewen

M. classification
M. drill
M. osteotomy

Mache electromyogram setting

machine

Accu-SPINA cervical
decompression m.
Accu-Tron microcurrent m.
ankle exercise m.
BackStrong lumbar extension m.
Biodex isokinetic testing m.
Bionx servohydraulic testing m.
borazone blade cutting m.
CamStar exercise m.
continuous passive motion m.
cooling m.
CPM exerciser m.
Cybex m.
elliptical m.
Griswold distraction m.
Instron m.
Isotechnologies B-200 low back
exercise m.
isotonic m.
KineTec hip CPM m.
MB-900 AC m.
Med-Fit Senior Circuit exercise m.
MedX functional testing m.
MedX Mark II lumbar extension m.
MedX stretch m.
Orthion traction m.
Paramount total body
plate-loaded m.
passive motion m.
Pec-Dec m.

PodoFlex m.
SAM spinal analysis m.
Schwinn elliptical full body
exercise m.
m. screw
spinal analysis m. (SAM)
SurgiLav m.
VersaClimber RX exercise m.
Wilkco ankle exercise m.

machine-gunlike pain

MacIntosh

M. extraarticular ruptured anterior
cruciate ligament tenodesis
M. iliotibial band tenodesis
M. laryngoscopy technique
M. lateral pivot shift knee test
M. over-the-top ACL reconstruction
M. over-the-top anterior cruciate
ligament repair
M. tibial plateau prosthesis

Mackenzie amputation

MacKinnon

M. modification
M. modification of Dellon ulnar
nerve transposition
M. nerve injury

Mackinnon-Dellon staging system

Maclaren mobile buggy

MacLean-Maxwell disease

Macleod

M. capsular rheumatism
M. rheumatism

MacNab

M. line
M. line for facet imbrication
M. patella operation
M. shoulder repair

MacNab-English shoulder prosthesis

MacNicol-Voutsinas posterior tibial tear
classification

MacReflex infrared motion analysis
system

macroadhesion

macrobrachia

macrocheiria, macrochiria

macrochiria (*var. of* macrocheiria)

macrocnemia

macrocoil

Gianturco m.

macrodactylia

m. fibrolipomatosis
pedal m.
progressive m.
m. reduction
m. reduction procedure

M

macrodactylism (*var. of* macrodactyly)
macrodactyly, macrodactylism
macrodystrophia lipomatosa
macroelectromyography (macro-EMG)
macro-EMG
    macroelectromyography
      macro-EMG needle electrode
macronutrient
macronychia
MacroPore OS spinal system
macroradiograph
macroscopic change
macrotrauma rehabilitation program
macularis eruptiva perstans
Madajet
    M. XL jet-injection anesthesia
      system
    M. XL local anesthesia
Maddacare child bath seat
Maddacrawler prone support walker
Maddapult Asissto-Seat
Madelung
    M. deformity
    M. subluxation
madreporic
    m. coral
    m. hip prosthesis
Madura foot
maduromycosis
mafenide acetate
Maffucci disease
Maffucci-Kast syndrome
MAFO
    molded ankle-foot orthosis
      MAFO cane
Magerl
    M. hook-plate system
    M. plate-screw system
    M. posterior cervical screw
      fixation
    M. screw placement technique
    M. transarticular screw fixation
    M. translaminar facet screw fixation
      technique
maggot debridement therapy
magic
    m. angle effect
    m. angle phenomenon
    M. Wand vibrator
Magilligan femoral anteversion
  measuring technique
magna
    coxa m.
Magna-FX cannulated screw system
MagnaPod pain relief magnet
MagnaScanner Picker Magnet
Magnassager
    M. massager
    M. massage tool

Magnatherm
    M. SSP electromagnetic therapy unit
    M. SSP pulse shortwave diathermy
Magnathotic orthotic
MagneCore magnetic therapy pad
magnesium (Mg)
    m. deficiency
    m. salicylate
    m. sulfate ($MgSO_4$)
magnet
    ankle m.
    BIOflex medical m.
    Dyonics Golden Retriever m.
    elbow m.
    foot m.
    MagnaPod pain relief m.
    MagnaScanner Picker M.
    m. splint
    Tectonic m.
magnetic
    m. motion transducer
    m. resonance arteriography (MRA)
    m. resonance arthrography (MRAr)
    m. resonance imaging (MRI)
    m. resonance neurography (MRN)
    m. resonance spectroscopic imaging
      (MRSI)
    m. resonance spectroscopy
      (MRS)
    m. resonance venography (MRV)
    m. retriever
    m. sensor
    m. source imaging (MSI)
    m. source imaging mapping
    m. stimulation
    M. Support brace
    m. therapy
magnetization
    m. transfer
    m. transfer magnetic resonance
      imaging (mtMRI)
magnification
    loupe m.
    m. view
magnifying loupe
magnitude
    curve m.
magnum
    M. 800 bed
    M. chisel
    M. curette
    foramen m.
    M. 101 Plus stimulator
    M. 101 Plus table
    M. 100 stimulator
    M. Tiger blade
magnus
    adductor m.
    nucleus raphe m. (NRM)

Magnuson
- M. abduction humeral splint
- M. anterior dislocation of shoulder repair technique
- M. débridement
- M. low back pain site test
- M. operation
- M. twist drill
- M. wire

Magnuson-Stack
- M.-S. arthroplasty
- M.-S. shoulder arthroplasty
- M.-S. shoulder arthrotomy
- M.-S. shoulder procedure

Ma-Griffith
- M.-G. Achilles tendon rupture repair technique
- M.-G. percutaneous Achilles tendon repair
- M.-G. ruptured Achilles tendon repair

Mahan pediatric sedation procedure

MAI
- Movement Assessment of Infants
- *Mycobacterium avium-intracellulare*

Maigne vertebrobasilar insufficiency test

main
- m. d'accoucheur
- m. en crochet
- m. en griffe
- m. en lorgnette
- m. fourchée

maintained contraction

maintenance of bone plate integrity

Maisel congenital hand transverse deficiency suppression theory

Maisonneuve
- M. amputation
- M. fibular fracture
- M. sign

Maitland
- M. manipulation
- M. manual spinal therapy technique
- M. slump neural tissue tension test

Majestro-Ruda-Frost tendon technique

major
- m. amputation
- anterosuperior ilium m.
- m. curve
- m. fracture fragment
- m. injury vector (MIV)
- m. lumbar curve pattern
- posteroinferior ilium m.
- m. thoracic curve pattern

making
- M. Action Plans (MAPs)
- return-to-play sidelines decision m.

MAL
- midaxillary line

malabsorption

maladaptation
- high-altitude m.
- soft tissue m.

maladjustment

malakopathy

malalignment
- dorsal m.
- malicious m.
- radial m.
- rotational m.
- varus m.

malangulation

malar
- m. bone
- m. fracture

Malawer
- M. excision technique
- M. fibula tumor resection (type I, II)

malaxation

Malcolm-Lynn
- M.-L. C-RXF cervical retractor frame
- M.-L. radiolucent spinal retraction system

Malcolm-Rand radiolucent headrest and retraction system

maldevelopment

male
- m. reamer
- m. washer

malformation
- Arnold-Chiari m.
- arteriovenous m.
- Chiari m.
- Klippel-Feil m.
- medullary venous m. (MVM)
- retromedullary arteriovenous m.

Malgaigne
- M. amputation
- M. luxation
- M. pelvic fracture

Malibu
- M. cervical orthosis
- M. Sandalthotics orthotic
- M. thoracolumbar fusion posterior fixation pedicle screw system

malicious malalignment

maligna
- lentigo m.

malignancy
- spinal m.

malignant
- m. acetabular osteolysis
- m. fasciculation
- m. fibrous histiocytoma (MFH)
- m. fibrous xanthoma
- m. hyperpyrexia (MH)
- m. hyperthermia (MH)

M

malignant (*continued*)
    m. melanoma
    m. myeloid sarcoma
    m. osteopetrosis
    m. schwannoma
    m. soft tissue tumor
    m. synovioma
Malis
    M. CMC-II bipolar coagulator
    M. curette
    M. elevator
    M. hinge clamp
    M. jeweler bipolar forceps
    M. ligature passer
    M. needle holder
Malis-Jensen microbipolar forceps
Mallamint
malleable
    m. link
    m. metal finger splint
    structural aluminum m. (SAM)
    m. template
mallei (*pl. of* malleus)
malleolar
    m. chip fracture
    m. facet
    m. gel sleeve
    m. index
    m. osteotomy
    m. screw
    m. sulcus
malleoli (*pl. of* malleolus)
Malleoloc
    M. anatomic ankle arthrosis
    M. ankle orthosis
    M. ankle support
malleolus, *pl.* **malleoli**
    belly button to medial m. (BB to MM)
    external m.
    m. externus
    fibular m.
    inner m.
    internal m.
    m. internus
    lateral m.
    m. lateralis
    medial m. (MM)
    m. medialis
    outer m.
    posterior m.
    radial m.
    m. radialis
    tibial m.
    tip of medial m.
    ulnar m.
    m. ulnaris
Malleo-Med soft ankle support
malleotomy

Malleotrain ankle support
mallet
    Acufex m.
    Bergman m.
    bone m.
    boxwood m.
    cervical m.
    copper m.
    Cottle m.
    Crane m.
    Doyen bone m.
    m. finger
    m. finger deformity
    m. finger orthotic
    m. fracture
    Gerzog bone m.
    Hajek m.
    Heath m.
    Henning m.
    Hibbs m.
    Kirk orthopaedic m.
    lead-filled m.
    Lucae bone m.
    Mead m.
    Meyerding m.
    Miltex m.
    Ombredanne m.
    orthopaedic m.
    polyethylene-faced m.
    Richards m.
    Rush m.
    slotted m.
    Steinbach m.
    Swanson m.
    m. thumb
    m. toe
    m. toe deformity
    Williger bone m.
malleus, *gen.* and *pl.* **mallei**
    hallux m.
Mallory
    M. prosthesis
    M. technique
Mallory-Head
    M.-H. femoral stem
    M.-H. I, II prosthesis
    M.-H. modular calcar system
    M.-H. porous primary femoral prosthesis
    M.-H. rasp
    M.-H. revision operation
    M.-H. total hip prosthesis
    M.-H. total hip revision
Malmö hip splint
malnutrition
    protein m.
malodorous foot
mal perforans ulcer
malposed vertebra

malposition
    extension m.
    flexion m.
    lateral flexion m.
    rotational m.
    screw m.
malreduction
    fracture m.
malrotation
Malteno tube implant material
maltracking patella
Maltz
    M. cartilage knife
    M. rasp
malum
    m. coxae senilis
    m. deformans
malunion
    angulatory m.
    calcaneal m.
    femoral shaft m.
    humeral fracture m.
    intraarticular m.
    talar m.
    varus m.
malunited
    m. acetabulum
    m. calcaneus fracture
    m. forearm fracture
    m. radial fracture
mammillary process
management
    airway m.
    biologic fracture m.
    chiropractic m.
    conservative m.
    failure of conservative m.
    foot orthotic m.
    fracture m.
    inflammation m.
    interphalangeal sesamoid m.
    neuromechanical spinal
     chiropractic m.
    nonoperative orthopaedic m.
    nonsurgical m.
    preoperative m.
    pressure ulcer m.
    reflex tracheostomy m.
Mancini plate
mandible
    m. ossification
    Spiessel internal screw fixation
     of m.
mandibular
    m. angle
    m. fracture
    m. nerve
    m. osteotomy
    m. spine

maneuver, manoeuvre
    Adson thoracic outlet m.
    Allen scalenous anterior
     syndrome m.
    Allis hip dislocation m.
    Apley m.
    Bárány-Nylen vertigo m.
    Bigelow posterior hip dislocation m.
    Bouvier MCP joint flexion m.
    Christiani m.
    circumduction m.
    closed manipulative m.
    costoclavicular m.
    crossleg Patrick m.
    Dandy cerebrospinal fluid leak m.
    extension m.
    Finkelstein m.
    flexion-extension m.
    flexion-rotation-compression m.
    Foster-Kennedy m.
    Fowler m.
    Gowers m.
    Hallpike m.
    Halsted thoracic outlet m.
    hippocratic m.
    Hubscher adult flatfoot m.
    hyperabduction m.
    Jahss metacarpal neck fracture
     reduction m.
    Jendrassik m.
    King m.
    Krackow obese patient tourniquet m.
    Lachman knee ligament tear m.
    Leadbetter hip reduction m.
    load-and-shift m.
    logrolling m.
    manipulative m.
    McElvenny m.
    McKenzie extension m.
    McMurray circumduction m.
    McMurray twist m.
    Mendelsohn m.
    Meyn-Quigley m.
    military m.
    military brace m.
    milking m.
    Ortolani m.
    osteoclasis m.
    Parvin m.
    Patrick cross-leg m.
    Phalen m.
    postural fixation back m.
    Queckenstedt m.
    relative response attributable to m.
     (RRAM)
    reverse Bigelow m.
    rotation-compression m.
    scalene m.
    Schreiber patellar reflex test m.

M

maneuver (*continued*)
    shear m.
    Slocum knee m.
    Slocum knee rotatory instability m.
    Soto-Hall m.
    Spurling cervical foraminal
      compression m.
    Spurling cervical nerve root
      impingement m.
    Stimson posterior hip dislocation
      reduction m.
    twist m.
    Valsalva m.
    Walton acromioclavicular joint pain
      m.
    Watson wrist m.
    Whitman m.
    Wright m.
**Mangled Extremity Severity Score
(MESS)**
mangling injury
manifestation
    initial m.
manipulable subluxation
manipulation
    back m.
    m. board
    chiropractic joint m.
    chiropractic manual m.
    closed m.
    closing wedge m.
    contact m.
    diversified m.
    fine m.
    general thrust m.
    grading of m.
    gross m.
    Hippocrates m.
    indirect m.
    joint m.
    Leadbetter hip m.
    long lever low-amplitude
      type m.
    lumbar distraction m.
    Maitland m.
    medical m.
    myofascial m.
    noncontact m.
    m. of articulation
    opening wedge m.
    osteopathic m.
    passive joint m.
    rotational m.
    soft tissue m.
    specific thrust m.
    spinal m.
    target of m.
    thrust m.
    m. with distraction

manipulative
    m. maneuver
    m. procedure
    m. technique
    m. therapy
Mankin
    M. knee resection
    M. technique
Manktelow
    M. pectoralis major muscle transfer
    M. transfer procedure
Mann
    M. bunionectomy
    M. hallux valgus repair procedure
    M. modified McKeever arthrodesis
    M. protocol
    M. resection arthroplasty
    M. technique
Mann-Coughlin-DuVries cheilectomy
manoeuvre (*var. of* maneuver)
Manske-McCarroll-Swanson centralization
Manske radioulnar osteoclasis technique
Mantis retrograde forceps
mantle
    cement m.
    grade (A, B, C1, C2, D) cement
      m.
manual
    m. adjustment
    m. cavitation
    m. contact
    m. fracture reduction
    m. gun system
    m. locking knee prosthesis
    m. medicine
    m. muscle test (MMT)
    m. muscle testing (MMT)
    m. pressure
    m. push-pull technique
    m. reflex neurotherapy
    m. resistance
    m. resistance technique (MRT)
    m. talar tilt
    m. therapy
    m. traction
    m. treatment
    m. wheelchair
    m. work
manubria (*pl. of* manubrium)
manubriosternal
    m. angle
    m. joint
    m. joint pain
    m. joint pain syndrome
manubrium, *pl.* **manubria**
manufacturing
    computer-aided design/computer-aided
      m. (CAD/CAM)
Manuflex external fixator

ManuTrain active wrist support
Maolate
MAP
> Miller Assessment for Preschoolers
> Multiaxial Assessment of Pain

map
> aquatic m.

Mapap
Maple Leaf hip orthosis
mapping
> behavioral m.
> dermatome m.
> magnetic source imaging m.
> MSI m.
> paraspinal m.
> m. the defect

MAPs
> Making Action Plans

Maquet
> M. dome osteotomy
> M. elevation
> M. elevation of tibial crest
> M. line
> M. patellar realignment procedure
> M. table extension
> M. tibial tuberosity advancement

Maramed
> M. Miami fracture brace system
> M. ThermoFlex

Maranox
marathoner's toe
marathon running
marble
> m. bone
> m. bone pin

Marcaine with epinephrine
marcescens
> Serratia m.

march
> m. foot
> m. fracture

marche
> m. à petits pas
> m. à petits pas gait

marching band injury
Marfan syndrome
Margesic H
margin
> anterior tibial m.
> fibular m.

marginal
> m. excision
> m. exostosis
> m. fracture
> m. osteophyte
> m. resection

margines (*pl. of* margo)
margin-free spondylectomy
margo, *pl.* **margines**

Marie-Bamberger disease
Marie-Charcot-Tooth disease
Marie-Foix sign
Marie-Léri syndrome
Marie-Strümpell
> M.-S. arthritis
> M.-S. disease
> M.-S. spondylitis

marinum
> Mycobacterium m.

Marion screw
mark
> M. II Chandler total knee retractor
> M. II concave total knee retractor
> M. II distal femur distractor
> M. II femoral component extractor
> M. III halo system
> M. II lateral collateral ligament
> retractor
> M. II modular weight retractor
> M. II Sorrells hip arthroplasty
> retractor system
> M. II S total knee retractor
> M. II Stubbs short prong collateral
> ligament retractor
> M. II Stulberg hip positioner
> M. II Stulberg leg positioner
> M. II tibial component extractor
> M. II wide PCL knee retractor
> M. II Wixson hip positioner
> M. II Z knee retractor

Markell
> M. brace boot
> M. Mobility Health Clogs
> M. Mobility Shoes
> M. open-toe boot
> M. open-toe shoe
> M. tarso medius straight shoe
> M. tarso pronator outflare shoe

marker
> BB m.
> biochemical m.
> bone turnover m.
> lumbar pedicle m.
> pedicle m.
> retroreflective m.
> skin m.
> tantalum ball m.
> thoracic pedicle m.
> X-Act podiatric m.

Markham-Meyerding retractor
Markley retention pin
Marks-Bayne
> M.-B. technique
> M.-B. technique for thumb
> duplication

Markwalder
> M. bone rongeur
> M. rib forceps

M

Markwort ankle support
Marlex
    M. and methyl methacrylate
      prosthesis
    M. mesh
Marlin
    M. cervical collar
    M. cervical orthosis
Marmor
    M. modular knee prosthesis
    M. replacement
Marmor-Lynn fracture
maroon spoon
Maroteaux
    spondyloepiphysial dysplasia of M.
Maroteaux-Lamy
    M.-L. disease
    M.-L. syndrome (MLS)
MARP
    Military Amputee Research Program
Marquardt
    M. angulation osteotomy
    M. bone rongeur
Marquet fracture table
marrow
    bone m.
    m. canal
    m. cavity
    m. disease
    m. edema
    Grafton bone matrix and m.
    m. nailing
    red m.
    m. stimulation
    yellow m.
MARS
    Modular Acetabular Revision System
    Multicenter ACL Revision Study
    MARS component
Marshall
    M. anterior cruciate ligament repair
    M. Hall theory of reflex action
    M. knee score
    M. ligament repair technique
    M. patelloquadriceps tendon
      substitution
Marshall-McIntosh ACL repair technique
Martel sign
martensitic stainless steel
Marthritic
Martin
    M. cartilage chisel
    M. cartilage clamp
    M. cartilage forceps
    M. cartilage scissors
    M. diamond wire cutter
    M. disease
    M. loop circumferential wire
    M. meniscal clamp

    M. muscular clamp
    M. osteotomy
    M. patellar wiring technique
    M. screw
    M. sheet rubber bandage
Martin-Gruber
    M.-G. anastomosis
    M.-G. connection
Martini bone curette
Marx osteoradionecrosis protocol
Maryland
    M. foot score
    M. Foot Score Profile
MAS
    modified Ashworth scale
mason
    M. fracture
    M. fracture classification system
    M. radial head fracture classification
    M. splint
Mason-Allen
    M.-A. suture
    M.-A. Universal hand splint
masRAP
MASS
    minimal access spinal surgery
mass
    bone m.
    bony m.
    calcific m.
    cellular periosteal osteocartilaginous
      m.
    cement m.
    center of m.
    fat and fat-free m. (FFM)
    fusion m.
    glenolabral ovoid mass (GLOM)
    granulomatous m.
    hypoechoic intermetatarsal web
      space m.
    low bone m.
    osteocartilaginous m.
    peak bone m.
    plantar-hindfoot-midfoot bony m.
    pre-Achilles m.
    radiodense m.
    masses sign
    soft tissue m.
    tumorous m.
massage
    aqua PT water m.
    m. ball
    Bindegewebsmassage connective
      tissue m.
    callus m.
    connective tissue m. (CTM)
    m. cream
    cross-friction m.
    deep friction m. (DFM)

deep stroking and kneading m.
effleurage m.
friction m.
Hoffa m.
ice m.
kneading m.
m. oil
pneumatic m.
Shiatsu therapeutic m.
Silhouette therapeutic m.
soft tissue m.
stimulating m.
Swedish m.
m. therapy (MT)
M. Time Pro hydromassage table
transverse friction m. (TFM)
vibratory m.

massager
AcuVibe m.
Body Sticks m.
Cryocup ice m.
Equalizer Pro m.
G5 Fleximatic massager/percussor m.
Intracell trigger point m.
Ironman Triathlon Pro-Power m.
Jeanie Rub M.
Knobble m.
Magnassager m.
Medisana M.
Morfam Quality Jeanie Rub m.
Omni Roller m.
Original Backnobber muscle m.
Original Index Knobber II m.
Power Pillow cervical m.
Reach Easy m.
Saso Variable Speed M.
Scrip Muscle Master m.
T-Bar trigger point m.
Thera Cane m.

massager/percussor
G5 Vibracare m.

masseur
masseuse
Massie
M. driver
M. extractor
M. II nail
M. inserter
M. nail assembly
M. plate
M. screwdriver
M. sliding graft
M. sliding nail

massive
m. fibrolipoma
m. herniated disc
m. osteolysis
m. osteoplysis
m. sliding graft

Masson fasciotome
massotherapy
MAST
military antishock trousers
master
Balance M.
m. cement
Cobra M.
m. knot of Henry
NeuroCom Balance M.
Pro Balance M.
M. screwdriver
Smart Balance M.
M. step foot prosthesis
Masterson
M. curved clamp
M. pelvic clamp
M. straight clamp
Master-Stim interferential stimulator
Mastin muscular clamp
Mastisol liquid adhesive
mastocytosis
mastoid
m. curette
m. process
m. rongeur
mat
Airex m.
air flow m.
AliMed sensor floor m.
AquaBodyCiser aquatic m.
Easyslide sliding m.
floor m.
footprint m.
GAITRite m.
Harris-Beath footprint m.
Harris footprint m.
Minislide sliding m.
Scoot-Gard m.
sliding m.
sting m.
m. table
matchstick
m. graft
m. test
match to sample test
mater
dura m.
material
acrylic implant m.
Actifuse bone graft m.
Alisoft splinting m.
allogenic lyophilized bone graft
   implant m.
AlloGro bone graft m.
alloplastic m.
alpha-BSM bone repair m.
aluminum oxide arthroplasty m.

M

material (*continued*)

American Society for Testing and M.'s (ASTM)

amorphous eosinophilic m.

Aquaplast splinting m.

Aquarelle hydrogel nucleus viscoelastic m.

bioabsorbable m.

bioceramic implant m.

bone implant m.

Bone Plast bone replacement m.

bone-tendon graft m.

Calcitite graft m.

calcium carbonate graft m.

Carboplast II sheet orthotic m.

cellular response to implant m.

celluloid implant m.

CHAG bone graft substitute m.

composite m.

copolymer orthotic m.

corundum ceramic implant m.

Dacron synthetic ligament m.

DermAssist wound-filling m.

Dermatell hydrocolloid dressing m.

Durapatite bone replacement m.

Duraval hook & loop strap m.

DYNAfabric m.

Embarc bone repair m.

Evazote cushioning m.

m. failure break point

fibrillar absorbable hemostat m.

gold weight and wire spring implant m.

Graflex m.

graft m.

grafted m.

Gypsona cast m.

Healos synthetic bone grafting m.

HIP Vitox alumina ceramic m.

homograft implant m.

hydroxyapatite bone replacement m.

hydroxyapatite implant m.

implant m.

IntelliTemp insulation m.

Interpore bone replacement m.

Iowa implant m.

Keolar implant m.

LactoSorb orthopaedic wound m.

Malteno tube implant m.

methyl methacrylate implant m.

National Center to Improve Practice through Technology, Media, and M.'s

Nicoll bone replacement m.

NovaBone Bioglass bone grafting m.

Omega splinting m.

Ommaya reservoir implant m.

Opteform bone graft m.

OrthoDyn bone substitute m.

Ortho-Glass synthetic m.

Ortho-Jel impression m.

OsSatura synthetic bone graft substitution m.

Osteogenics BoneSource synthetic bone replacement m.

OsteoSponge osteoinductive bone allograft m.

paraffin implant m.

Pelite thermoplastic crepe m.

PerioGlas bone graft m.

Plasti-Pore prosthetic m.

polyether implant m.

polyethylene implant m.

polyurethane implant m.

polyvinyl alcohol splinting m.

polyvinyl implant m.

porcine graft m.

Porocoat prosthetic m.

porous prosthetic m.

ProOsteon bone graft m.

Proplast I, II porous implant m.

Proplast prosthetic m.

purulent m.

Pyrost bone graft m.

Shearing posterior chamber implant m.

shell implant m.

silicone m.

Silon silicone thermoplastic splinting m.

solid buckling implant m.

solid silicone exoplant implant m.

splinting m.

Stimoceiver implant m.

Synergy flexible splinting m.

synthetic m.

thermomoldable m.

ThermoSKY orthotic m.

tissue mandrel implant m.

titanium implant m.

Trilon multilayered m.

Unigraft bone graft m.

Unilab Surgibone bone replacement m.

Virtullene brace m.

viscoelastic m.

vitallium implant m.

zirconium oxide arthroplasty m.

Zorbacel shock-absorbing m.

Matev sign

mathematical processing test

Mathews

M. drill point

M. hand drill

M. load drill

M. olecranon fracture classification

Mathew scale

Mathieu rasp
Mathys prosthesis
matricectomy, matrixectomy
    chemical m.
    Frost partial m.
    laser partial m.
    partial m.
    phenol m.
    phenol-alcohol m.
    Steindler ungual m.
    total m.
    Winograd partial m.
    Zadik total m.
matrices (*pl. of* matrix)
matrix, *pl.* **matrices**
    Accell 100 m.
    Accell Connexus bone m.
    Accell Evo3 m.
    Accell total bone m.
    bone m.
    Collagraft bone graft m.
    demineralized bone m. (DBM)
    DuraGen Plus adhesion barrier m.
    germinal m.
    germinative m.
    GraftJacket regenerative tissue
      repair m.
    m. Grafton putty
    m. injury
    ligament-scar m.
    nail m.
    proteoglycan m.
    scaffold m.
    m. seating system
    sterile m.
    Surgiflo hemostatic m.
    total bone m. (TBM)
    Trinity multipotential cellular
      bone m.
matrix-bone marrow slurry
matrixectomy (*var. of* matricectomy)
Matroc femoral head
Matrol femoral head prosthesis
Matson
    M. Evaluation of Social Skills in
      Individuals with Severe Retardation
      (MESSIER)
    M. periosteal elevator
    M. procedure
    M. rib elevator
Matson-Alexander rib elevator
Matta-Saucedo fixation
matter
    gray m.
    white m.
Matthew cross-leg clamp
Matthews-Green pin
matting
    Dycem roll m.

Matti-Russe
    M.-R. bone graft
    M.-R. scaphoid nonunion bone graft
      technique
mattress
    Akros extended care m.
    Akros pressure m.
    AkroTech m.
    antidecubitus m.
    chiropractic m.
    Clinisert m.
    DeCube m.
    m. double anchor footprint rotator
      cuff tear repair
    eggcrate m.
    Geo-Mattress bariatric m.
    Invacare APM m.
    Lapidus alternating air-pressure m.
    Nirvana m.
    OptiMax Supreme pressure
      reduction m.
    overlay m.
    PressureGuard m.
    Q Star Voyager pressure
      reduction m.
    Rik fluid m.
    Sofflex m.
    Sof Matt pressure relieving m.
    m. suture
    Tempur-Pedic m.
    Tempur-Pedic pressure relieving
      Swedish m.
    T-Foam m.
    Tri-Float pressure reduction m.
Mattrix spinal cord stimulation system
maturation
    accelerated bone m.
    bone m.
    delayed bone m.
    m. phase
    skeletal m.
    m. zone
maturity
    bone m.
    Oxford method for scoring
      skeletal m.
    skeletal m.
Mau
    M. and Ludloff procedure
    M. bunionectomy
    M. osteotomy
Mauch Swing and Stance hydraulic
  knee
Mauck
    M. knee procedure
    M. operation
Mauclaire disease
Maudsley tennis elbow test
Max 3 electric handpiece

M

Maxi-Driver driver
MaxiFloat wheelchair cushion
maxillary
    m. fracture
    m. process
    m. spine
maxillectomy
    Cocke m.
    subtotal m.
maxillofacial bone screw
maxillomandibular
maxillotomy
    extended m.
Maxima II transcutaneous electrical nerve stimulator
maximal (*var. of* maximum)
    isokinetic strength test m.
    m. medical improvement
    m. oxygen uptake (VO$_2$max)
    m. stimulus
    m. voluntary contraction (MVC)
Maxim Modular Knee System
maximum, maximal
    m. conduction velocity
    m. control
    m. eversion velocity
    m. inversion velocity
    m. oxygen uptake (VO$_2$max)
    m. pressure picture
    m. radial bow
    1-repetition m. (1-RM)
    repetition m. (RM)
    M. Strength Desenex Antifungal Cream
    M. Strength Nytol
    m. voluntary effort (MVE)
    M. Voluntary Efforts Test
maximum-curve kyphosis
Maxon suture
Maxwell body
Maxwell-Brancheau
    M.-B. arthroereisis implant
    M.-B. arthrorisis (MBA)
Maxxus orthopaedic latex surgical glove
May anatomical bone plate
Mayday
    M. distal first metatarsal osteotomy
    M. distal first metatarsal osteotomy for hallux valgus
Mayer
    M. orthotic
    M. reflex
    M. splint
    M. trapezius transfer operation
Mayfield
    M. adapter
    M. device
    M. fixation frame

    M. forceps
    M. head rest
    M. incision
    M. instrumentation
    M. miniature clip applier
    M. neurosurgical headrest
    M. temporary aneurysm clip applier
Mayo
    M. ankle arthroplasty
    M. approach
    M. block anesthesia
    M. bunionectomy
    M. carpal instability classification
    M. clamp
    M. Clinic congruent elbow plate
    M. Clinic congruent elbow plate system
    M. Clinic forefoot score
    M. Clinic Forefoot Scoring System
    M. elbow distraction device
    M. elbow fracture classification
    M. elbow performance score
    M. hallux valgus modified operation
    M. hip score
    M. hip scoring system
    M. metatarsal head resection
    M. nerve block
    M. resection arthroplasty
    M. rigid cervical collar
    M. scissors
    M. semiconstrained elbow prosthesis
    M. total ankle prosthesis
    M. total elbow arthroplasty
Mayo-Collins retractor
Mayo-Hegar needle holder
Mayo-Portland Adaptability Inventory 3 (MPAI-3)
Mayo-Stone-Valenti hallux limitus/rigidus arthroplasty
Mayo-Thomas collar
Mazabraud syndrome
Mazas totally constrained elbow prosthesis
Mazet
    M. knee disarticulation
    M. knee disarticulation technique
Mazur
    M. ankle elevation classification
    M. ankle evaluation
    M. ankle rating
    M. operation
MBA
    Maxwell-Brancheau arthrorisis
MB-900 AC machine
M-Brace knee brace
MBS
    Multi Balance System
    MBS snap-on orthotic

MC
metacarpal
motion control
MC walker brace
MCA
motorcycle accident
McArdle
M. disease
M. syndrome
McAtee compression screw device
McBride
M. bunionectomy
M. bunion hallux valgus operation
M. femoral prosthesis
M. hallux abductovalgus reduction
M. hallux valgus reduction
M. pin
M. plate
M. procedure
M. tripod
M. tripod pin traction
McCain
M. TMJ arthroscopic system
M. TMJ cannula
M. TMJ curette
McCarthy
M. hip distractor
M. hip procedure
M. Scale of Children's Abilities
M. test
McCash
M. hand procedure
M. hand surgery
McCauley foot procedure
MC+ cervical interbody cage
McClintoch brace
McCollough internal tibial torsion brace
McConnell
M. arm holder
M. extensile knee approach
M. median and ulnar nerve approach
M. orthopaedic headrest
M. patellar taping technique
M. patellofemoral treatment plan
M. shoulder positioner
M. taping technique method
McCullough retractor
McCune-Albright syndrome
McCutchen hip implant
McDavid
M. ankle guard
M. hinged knee guard
M. knee brace
M. Knee Guard (MKG)
M. knee guard support
McDermott radiological classification
McDonald dissector

McDowell Impairment Index (MII)
McElroy
M. curette
M. instrumentation
McElvenny
M. foot procedure
M. maneuver
M. orthopaedic technique
McFarland
M. bone graft
M. syndrome
McFarland-Osborne hip joint lateral incision technique
McGee
M. prosthesis needle
M. splint
M. wire-crimping forceps
McGee-Priest wire forceps
McGill
M. pain checklist
M. pain questionnaire (MPQ)
M. pain scale
M. standing overhead arm reach
McGlamry
M. and Feldman modification
M. elevator
M. procedure
McGlamry-Downey forefoot procedure
McGregor line
McGuire
M. ankle score
M. pelvic positioner
M. rating
MCI
midcarpal instability
McIndoe
M. bone rongeur
M. rongeur forceps
M. scissors
McIntire splint
McIvor ENT retractor
McKay
M. hip procedure
M. osteotomy
McKay-Simons
M.-S. complete subtalar release
M.-S. CSR
McKee
M. brace
M. femoral prosthesis
M. totally constrained elbow prosthesis
M. tri-fin nail
McKee-Farrar
M.-F. acetabular cup
M.-F. total hip arthroplasty
M.-F. total hip prosthesis

M

McKeever
   M. arthrodesis for hallux limitus
   M. bunionectomy
   M. cartilage knife
   M. medullary clavicle fixation
   M. metatarsophalangeal
      arthrodesis
   M. metatarsophalangeal fusion
   M. open reduction
   M. operation
   M. patellar cap prosthesis
   M. patellar resurfacing device
   M. procedure
   M. vitallium knee prosthesis
McKeever-Buck fragment excision
McKenzie
   M. back and neck pain treatment
   M. back pain and neck pain
      therapy
   M. bone drill
   M. cervical roll
   M. enlarging bur
   M. extension exercise
   M. extension maneuver
   M. lumbar roll
   M. method
   M. night roll
   M. perforating twist drill
   M. Repex table
McKittrick transmetatarsal amputation
McKusick-type metaphysial
   chondrodysplasia
MCL
   medial collateral ligament
   MCL brace
McLaughlin
   M. acromionectomy
   M. approach
   M. arthroplasty
   M. carpal scaphoid screw
   M. modification of Bunnell pullout
      suture
   M. nail
   M. osteosynthesis apparatus
   M. osteosynthesis device
   M. plate
   M. posterior dislocated shoulder
      repair
   M. posterior shoulder dislocation
      repair procedure
   M. subscapularis tendon
      transfer
McLaughlin-Ryder incision
McLeod padded clavicular splint
McMaster bone graft
McMaster-Toronto Arthritis Patient
   Preference Disability Questionnaire
MCMI
   Millon Clinical Multiaxial Inventory

McMurray
   M. circumduction maneuver
   M. meniscal tear test
   M. osteotomy
   M. sign
   M. twist maneuver
McMurtry
   M. kinematic index
   kinematic index of M.
MCP
   metacarpophalangeal
   MCP finger joint
      prosthesis
MCR
   midcarpal radial
   MCR portal
McRae line
McReynolds
   M. driver
   M. driver-extractor
   M. method
   M. open fracture reduction
      technique
   M. open tibia reduction
McShane-Leinberry-Fenlin open
   acromioplasty
MCU
   midcarpal ulnar
   MCU portal
McWhorter posterior shoulder
   approach
MD
   muscular dystrophy
   myotonic dystrophy
   MD brace
MDCN
   medial dorsal cutaneous nerve
MDI
   multidirectional instability
MDS MicroDebrider
M-DVPA
   Modified Dynamic Visual Processing
      Assessment
Mead
   M. bone rongeur
   M. mallet
   M. periosteal elevator
meal
   bone m.
MEAMS
   Middlesex Elderly Assessment of
      Mental state
mean
   m. flow velocity
   m. value
Mears sacroiliac plate
Meary
   M. line
   M. metatarsotalar angle

measure

    Canadian Occupational Performance M. (COPM)
    Child and Adolescent Social Perception M. (CASP)
    emergency closed manipulative m.
    functional assessment m. (FAM)
    functional independence m. (FIM)
    Gross Motor Function M. (GMFM)
    limited performance m.
    outcome m.
    parallel goniometric m.
    reconstructive m.
    standard goniometric m.

measured stress

measurement

    AccuSway balance m.
    Agliette m.
    alignment m.
    anthropometric m.
    appendicular bone mass m.
    arthrometer m.
    arthrometric knee laxity m.
    Blackburn-Peel m.
    bone density m.
    calcaneal compartment pressure m.
    clear space m.
    curve m.
    foot central compartment pressure m.
    functional capacity m.
    Insall-Salvati m.
    Kite m.
    limb accurate m. (LAM)
    Mehta rib angle m.
    motion m.
    nondynamometric trunk strength m.
    pain m.
    pedodynographic m.
    psychophysical m.
    range of motion m.
    roof arc m.
    Schober m.
    scoliometer m.
    skinfold m.
    spasticity m.
    spinal bone density m.
    tibiofibular overlap m.
    tissue pressure m.
    Zwipp subtalar joint instability m.

measurer

    Bunnell digital exertion m.

measuring

    m. gauge
    precise lesion m. (PLM)

mechanical

    m. agent
    m. allodynia
    m. axis

    combined m.
    m. dermatome
    m. dysfunction
    m. fixation
    m. instability
    m. instrument adjusting
    m. insufficiency
    m. low back pain syndrome
    m. modality
    m. pain threshold
    m. plate design

mechanics

    altered intervertebral m.
    altered regional m.
    body m.
    fracture m.
    walking m.

mechanism

    abductor m.
    adhesion/cohesion m.
    adjustable leg and ankle repositioning m. (ALARM)
    4-bar linkage prosthetic knee m.
    capsuloligamentous m.
    central extensor m. (CEM)
    clamping m.
    Cook-Gordon m.
    cranial-sacral respiratory m. (CSRM)
    digital extensor m.
    extensor hood m.
    fail-safe m.
    flexor m.
    fracture m.
    gliding m.
    Hosmer Dorrance voluntary control 4-bar knee m.
    humeral m.
    locomotor m.
    MicroStable liner locking m.
    neurotraumatic m.
    Noiles rotating hinge knee m.
    m. of correction
    m. of growth arrest
    m. of reflex immunologic competence
    physiological venous pump m.
    post-and-cam m.
    primary cranial sacral respiratory m.
    quadriceps m.
    screw-home m.
    slider crank m.
    tendo Achillis m.
    terminal extensor m. (TEM)
    UHR locking ring m.
    windlass m.

mechanoreceptor

    m. activity
    m. Golgi tendon organ
    joint capsule m.

M

mechanoreceptor (*continued*)
    pacinian m.
    Ruffini m.
Meckel cavity
meclofenamate sodium
Meclomen
Mecring acetabluar prosthesis
MED
    microendoscopic discectomy
Medak glove
Medarmor puncture-resistant glove
Mederma topical gel
Med-Fit
    M.-F. cranial-sacral table
    M.-F. Senior Circuit exercise
    machine
media (*pl. of* medium)
medial
    m. antebrachial cutaneous nerve
    m. articular nerve
    m. aspect
    m. aspiration
    m. bicipital sulcus
    m. bicortical screw
    m. border
    m. brachial cutaneous nerve injury
    m. brachial nerve
    m. calcaneal displacement osteotomy
    m. calcaneal tubercle
    m. capsular imbrication
    m. capsular ligament
    m. capsulorrhaphy
    m. clear space
    m. closing wedge phalangeal
    osteotomy
    m. collateral ligament (MCL)
    m. collateral sprain
    m. column calcaneal fracture
    m. column instability
    m. compartment
    m. compartment disruption
    m. compartment injury
    m. cortical overlap technique
    m. crossover toe
    m. deviation
    m. deviation of second toe
    m. disc protrusion
    m. displacement
    m. displacement osteotomy
    m. dorsal cutaneous nerve (MDCN)
    m. drainage
    m. elbow epicondyle test
    m. eminence
    m. eminence resection
    m. end
    m. epicondylar apophysis
    m. epicondyle
    m.-epicondylectomy
    m. epicondyle humeral fracture

m. epicondyle of humerus
m. epicondylitis
m. exostectomy
m. extensor expansion
m. femoral condyle (MFC)
m. gastrocnemius bursitis
m. genicular
m. geniculate artery
m. geniculate fascia
m. hamstring
m. head of gastrocnemius rupture
m. head-stem offset
m. heel-and-sole wedge
m. heel skive technique
m. heel wedge
m. heel wedge orthosis
m. hip rotation
m. humeral condyle
m. joint line (MJL)
m. longitudinal arch
m. malleolar fracture
m. malleolar/small bone fragment
    clamp
m. malleolus (MM)
m. malleolus cast
m. malleolus fixation
m. malleolus of tibia
m. malleolus resection
m. meniscectomy
m. meniscus
m. metacarpal bone
m. movement
m. nerve protector
m. neurovascular bundle
m. oblique
m. opening wedge osteotomy
m. outline
m. parapatellar arthrotomy
m. parapatellar capsular approach
m. parapatellar incision
m. patellar plica
m. patellofemoral ligament
    (MPFL)
m. plantar artery
m. plantar fasciocutaneous flap
m. plantar nerve
m. portal
m. proximal tibial angle
m. quadruple complex
m. ray adduction deformity
m. release
m. repair
m. rollover
m. rotation procedure
m. sesamoid
m. sesamoid ligament
m. shelf
m. shelf/medial plica
m. sole wedge

m. sole wedge orthosis
m. sole wedge shoe modification
m. stem pivot
m. sural cutaneous nerve
m. swivel dislocation
m. talocalcaneal bar
m. talocalcaneal ligament
m. talonavicular capsule
m. tennis elbow tendinosis
m. tibial epiphysiodesis
m. tibial flare
m. tibial stress syndrome
(MTSS)
m. tibial syndrome (MTS)
m. torsion
m. T-strap
m. ulnar collateral ligament
(MUCL)
m. unicortical screw
m. V-Y capsulotomy
m. wall
m. wall fracture
mediales (*pl. of* medialis)
medialis, *pl.* **mediales**
malleolus m.
m. pedis flap
vastus m. (VM)
medialization ratio
medial/lateral
m. femoral condyle
m. grind knee test
m. meniscus
medial/plantar hinge
median
m. nerve
m. nerve block
m. nerve compression
m. nerve entrapment
m. nerve injury
m. nerve palsy
m. neuropathy
m. raphe
m. sagittal plane
Medi-Band bandage
medical
m. adhesive
M. Design brace
M. Examination and Diagnostic
Coding System (MEDICS)
m. galvanism
m. manipulation
M. Research Council (MRC)
M. Research Council system
m. subcutaneous reflection
medication
antiinflammatory m.
beta blocker m.
nonsteroidal antiinflammatory m.
Occlusal-HP wart m.

medicinal leech
medicine
allopathic m.
alternative m.
American College of Sports M.
(ACSM)
American Medical Society for
Sports M. (AMSSM)
American Orthopaedic Society for
Sports M. (AOSSM)
m. ball
Chinese m.
complementary and alternative m.
(CAM)
dance m.
Doctor of Podiatric M. (DPM)
electrodiagnostic m.
evidence-based m. (EBM)
International Society of Arthroscopy,
Knee Surgery, and Orthopaedic
Sports M. (ISAKOS)
manual m.
Native American m.
occupational and environmental m.
(OEM)
osteopathic m.
physical m.
podiatric m.
sports m.
vertebral m.
MediCordz rehabilitation kit
MEDICS
Medical Examination and Diagnostic
Coding System
Medicus bed
Mediflow
M. waterbase pillow
M. Waterpillow
Mediloy
M. implant metal
M. implant metal prosthesis
mediolateral (ML)
m. position
m. radiocarpal angle
m. stress
m. tilt
mediotarsal amputation
Medipain 5
Medipedic Multicentric knee brace
Mediplast
Medi Plus compression stockings
Medipore H surgical tape
Medipren
Medi-Quick Topical Ointment
Medi-Rip dressing
MediRule II measuring device
Medisana Massager
Medi-Stim stimulator
meditation and mindfulness

M

medium, *pl.* **media**
    Amipaque contrast m.
    m. callus Podi-Burr
    m. carbide cone bur
    dermatophyte test m. (DTM)
    m. fine bur
    Microfil contrast m.
    m. nail Podi-Burr
    m. profile femoral prosthesis
Medium-Plus alpha liner
medium-viscosity cement
medius
    digitus m.
    lacertus m.
MEDLS
    Milwaukee Evaluation of Daily Living Skills
Medmetric
    M. knee ligament arthrometer
    M. KT-1000 knee laxity arthrometer
Medoff
    M. axial compression screw
    M. sliding plate
Medralone Injection
Medrol
    M. Dosepak
    M. Oral
medroxyprogesterone
Medtronic spinal cord stimulation system
medulla, *pl.* **medullae**
medullae (*pl. of* medulla)
medullary
    m. bone graft
    m. callus
    m. canal
    m. canal reamer
    m. cavity
    m. locking
    m. nail
    m. nail fixation
    m. nailing
    m. paraganglioma
    m. pin
    m. prosthesis
    m. saw
    m. venous malformation (MVM)
    m. vent tubing
medullectomy
medullization
medulloarthritis
medullostomy
    tarsal m.
MedX
    M. functional testing machine
    M. Mark II lumbar extension machine
    M. stretch machine

Meek
    M. clavicular strap
    M. pelvic traction belt
mefenamic acid
Mefoxin
Mega-Air bed
megahorn meniscus
megaprosthesis
Mega Tilt and Turn bed
Mehta rib angle measurement
Meige syndrome
melagra
melalgia
melamine resin
melanoma
    acral lentiginous m.
    Clark classification of m.
    lentigo maligna m.
    malignant m.
    metastatic m.
    nodular m.
    plantar malignant m.
melanosis circumscripta praeblastomatosa Dubreuilh
melanotic
    m. panaris
    m. whitlow of Hutchinson
Melaware flatware
Meleney
    M. infection
    M. synergistic gangrene
melioidosis
    musculoskeletal m.
melioidotic
Mellaril
mellitus
    diabetes m.
    insulin-dependent diabetes m.
    non-insulin-dependent diabetes m.
Melone distal radius fracture classification
melon-seed body
melorheostosis
melosalgia
meloxicam
melphalan
Melzack Pain Questionnaire
membrane
    anterior atlantooccipital m.
    atlantooccipital anterior m.
    basement m.
    cricothyroid m.
    m. instability
    interosseous m. (IOM)
    interposition m.
    intraosseous m.
    mucous m.
    obturator m.
    periprosthetic m.

Preclude spinal m.
spinal m.
suprasyndesmotic m.
synovial m. (SM)
m. tack
thickened synovial m.
trauma-induced m.
villous lipomatous proliferation of
    synovial m.
membranous
  m. bone
  m. ossification
  m. osteogenesis
memory
  m. board
  cine m.
  m. compression staple
  m. splint
Menadol
Mendel-Bekhterev
  M.-B. reflex
  M.-B. sign
Mendelsohn
  M. maneuver
  M. modification of matricectomy
    suture technique
Menelaus triceps transfer
Menest
Menghini Surecut bone biopsy needle
meningeal
  m. nerve
  m. syndrome
meningioma
meningism
meningismus
meningitides (*pl. of* meningitis)
meningitis, *pl.* **meningitides**
meningocele
meningococcal purpura
meningoencephalomyelitis
meningomyelitis
meningomyelocele
meniscal
  m. aponeurosis
  m. arrow
  m. autograft transplant
  m. clamp
  m. curette
  m. cutter
  m. cyst
  m. degeneration
  m. excision
  m. flounce
  m. injury
  m. lateral tear
  m. mirror
  m. radial tear
  m. repair
  m. repair needle

m. scissors
m. spoon
m. staple
m. transverse tear
meniscectomy
  arthroscopic m.
  m. knife
  lateral m.
  medial m.
  partial m.
  Patel medial m.
  m. scissors
  subtotal lateral m.
  total m.
menisci (*pl. of* meniscus)
meniscitis
meniscocapsular
  m. junction
  m. tear
meniscofemoral
  m. capsule
  m. ligament
meniscoid
  m. entrapment
  joint m.
  m. lesion
meniscopexy
meniscoplasty
meniscorrhaphy
meniscosynovial junction
meniscotibial
  m. capsule
  m. ligament
meniscotome
  Bircher m.
  curved m.
  Grover m.
  Storz m.
meniscotomy chisel
meniscus, *pl.* **menisci**
  M. Arrow fixation
  m. ArthroWand
  bridge of m.
  clefting of m.
  degenerative m.
  discoid lateral m.
  m. forceps
  frayed m.
  fraying of m.
  m. graft
  m. homolog
  m. hook
  m. knife
  lateral m.
  medial m.
  medial/lateral m.
  megahorn m.
  M. Mender II system
  peripheral m.

M

meniscus (*continued*)
resection of m.
m. retractor
m. scissors
m. suturing
torn m.
trapped m.
Mennell
M. sign
M. 2–stage lower back test
MENS
microamperage electrical nerve
stimulation
MENS unit
Mensor-Scheck
M.-S. hanging-hip operation
M.-S. technique
mentagrophytes
Trichophyton m.
mental
m. imagery
m. torticollis
Mentax
mentor
M. Self-Cath soft catheter
M. tissue expander
MEP
muscle energy procedure
mepacrine
Mepergan
meperidine and promethazine
Mephisto
M. Mobils professional shoe
M. speed lacing system
mepivacaine
MEPP
miniature end-plate potential
meprobamate
meptazinol
MERAC
musculoskeletal evaluation,
rehabilitation and conditioning
meralgia paresthetica
paresthetica
merbromin
merchant
M. and Dietz ankle score
M. congruence angle
M. patella view
M. radiograph
Mercurochrome
mercury (Hg)
millimeter of m. (mmHg)
meridian
M. Intersegmental table
M. ST femoral implant
component
m. therapy
Merit final flexion kit

Merkel cell
**Merland perimedullary arteriovenous
fistula classification**
Merle
M. d'Aubigné and Postel hip rating
scale
M. d'Aubigné and Postel
postoperative function score
M. d'Aubigné femoral reconstruction
M. d'Aubigné hip score
M. d'Aubigné hip status system
M. d'Aubigné resection
reconstruction
Merlin arthroscopy blade
Merocel pack
meropenem
Merrem I.V.
merry
M. Walker
M. Walker ambulation device
Mersilene
M. Kessler stitch
M. sling
M. suture
M. tape
Mersol
Meryon sign
Mesa spinal system
mesencephalic injury
mesenchyma (*var. of* mesenchyme)
mesenchymal
m. cell
m. chondrosarcoma
m. stem cell
m. tumor
mesenchyme, mesenchyma
mesenchymoma
pluripotential m.
mesenteric vasculitis
mesh
chromium-cobalt m.
m. graft
Marlex m.
metal m.
sintered titanium m.
stainless steel m.
tantalum m.
mesher
Zimmer skin graft m.
mesiodistal plane
mesocuneiform bone
mesotendineum (*var. of* mesotendon)
mesotendon, mesotendineum
mesothenar muscle
MESS
Mangled Extremity Severity Score
MESSIER
Matson Evaluation of Social Skills in
Individuals with Severe Retardation

Mestinon
mesylate
    benztropine m.
MET
    metabolic equivalent of task
metabolic
    m. bone disease
    m. equivalent of task
    (MET)
    m. syndrome
    m. variable
metabolism
    arachidonate m.
    energy m.
    purine m.
metacarpal (MC)
    m. amputation
    m. base
    m. beak
    m. block
    m. bone
    duplicated m.
    fifth m.
    first m.
    fourth m.
    fracture of fifth m.
    m. lengthening
    m. ligament
    m. neck
    m. neck fracture
    m. osteotomy
    second m.
    third m.
    thumb m.
metacarpectomy
metacarpi (*pl. of* metacarpus)
metacarpocapitate joint
metacarpocarpal joint
metacarpoglenoid ligament
metacarpohamate joint
metacarpophalangeal (MCP)
    m. arthroscopy
    m. articulation
    m. dislocation
    m. implant
    m. joint (MPJ)
    m. joint arthroplasty
    m. ligament
metacarpophysial
    m. joint
    m. joint extension contracture
metacarpotrapezoid joint
metacarpus, *pl.* **metacarpi**
metachromatic mucoid substance
metaepiphysis
metal
    m. acetabular liner
    Alivium implant m.
    biophase implant m.

Biotex implant m.
m. clamp
Coballoy implant m.
Co-Cr-Mo alloy implant m.
Co-Cr-W-Ni alloy implant m.
m. endurance limit
m. failure
m. fatigue
m. femoral head prosthesis
m. foot plate
Haynes-Stellite 21
    implant m.
m. hemi-toe implant
m. hybrid orthosis
implant m.
m. implant corrosion
m. locator
m. measuring triangle
Mediloy implant m.
m. mesh
Orthochrome implant m.
m. orthopaedic implant
m. pin
porous m.
Protasul implant m.
m. pusher
m. pylon
Sinterlock implant m.
m. splint
titanium alloy implant m.
vitallium implant m.
Zimaloy implant m.
metal-backed
    m.-b. acetabular component
    m.-b. acetabular component hip
    implant
    m.-b. acetabular cup
    m.-b. acetabular shell
    m.-b. patellar implant
    m.-b. plastic-on-metal
    prosthesis
    m.-b. socket
metallic
    m. bead
    m. debris
    m. implant
metalloproteinase
metalloproteinase-1
    tissue inhibitor of m.-1
metallosis
metal-on-metal
    m.-o.-m. articulating intervertebral
    disc prosthesis
    m.-o.-m. design
    m.-o.-m. device
metal-on-polymer device
Meta-Nail tibial nail system
metaphyseal (*var. of* metaphysial)
metaphyses (*pl. of* metaphysis)

M

metaphysial, metaphyseal
    m. abscess
    m. aclasis
    m. artery
    m. bone
    m. chondrodysplasia
    m. dysostosis
    m. fibrous cortical defect
    m. head resection
    m. head resection with prosthesis
    m. osteotomy
    m. shortening
    m. spike
    m. stapler
    m. tibial fracture
    m. tuberculosis
    m. wedge
metaphysial-articular nonunion
metaphysial-diaphysial
    m.-d. angle
    m.-d. junction
metaphysial-epiphysial angle
metaphysial-to-diaphysial width ratio
metaphysis, *pl.* **metaphyses**
    distal m.
    femoral m.
    fibular m.
    funnelization of m.
    tibial m.
metaphysitis
metaplasia
    cartilaginous m.
    fibrous m.
    osteocartilaginous m.
metaplastic ossification
metastases (*pl. of* metastasis)
metastasis, *pl.* **metastases**
    bone m.
    bony m.
    osteoblastic m.
    osteogenic m.
    Picker Magnascanner for bone m.
    spinal m.
metastatic
    m. bone lesion
    m. bone survey
    m. disease
    m. melanoma
    m. spinal tumor
Metasul
    M. hip implant
    M. hip joint component
    M. joint
    M. metal-on-metal hip
    M. metal-on-metal hip prosthesis
        system
metatarsal
    m. arch
    m. artery

    m. axis
    m. bar shoe modification
    m. base angle
    m. block
    m. bone
    m. callosity
    m. cookie
    m. cuneiform exostosis
    dorsiflexed m.
    m. flatfoot bar
    m. flat head
    m. fracture
    m. head extractor
    m. head osteotomy
    m. head resection
    m. joint
    m. length
    lesser m.
    m. ligament
    m. neck
    m. neck osteotomy
    m. oblique osteotomy
    m. ossification
    osteochondrosis of m.
    m. osteology
    m. overload syndrome
    m. pad
    m. parabola
    m. phalangeal angle
    m. proximal dome osteotomy
    m. ray
    m. Reverdin osteotomy
    m. shaft
    m. traction
    m. V-shaped osteotomy
metatarsalgia
    Morton m.
    secondary m.
    transfer m.
metatarsal-sesamoid arthrosis
metatarsal-tarsal joint
metatarsea
    syndesmitis m.
metatarsectomy
metatarsi (*pl. of* metatarsus)
metatarsocalcaneal angle
metatarsocuboid joint
metatarsocuneiform (MTC)
    m. angle
    m. arthrodesis
    m. articulation
    m. joint
    m. joint exostosis
    m. joint fusion
metatarsophalangeal (MTP)
    m. arthroplasty
    m. capsulotomy
    m. creaking
    m. crease

m. joint
m. joint arthrodesis
m. joint capsule
m. joint disarticulation
m. joint dislocation
m. joint fusion
m. joint ganglion
m. joint injury
m. joint synovitis
m. subluxation
metatarsophalangeal-interphalangeal scale
metatarsosesamoid
m. joint
m. ligament
metatarsotalar angle
metatarsus, *pl.* **metatarsi**
m. abductus
m. adductocavus
m. adductovarus
m. adductus (MTA)
m. adductus angle
m. adductus deformity
m. atavicus
m. internus
m. latus
pes cavus m.
m. primus adductus (MPA)
m. primus atavicus
m. primus declination angle
m. primus elevatus
m. primus osteotomy
m. primus rectus
m. primus varus (MPV)
m. primus varus deformity
m. quintus valgus
m. varus (MTV)
m. varus deformity
metatropic dwarfism
metaxalone
metazonal region
Met Bar shoe modification
Metcalf spring drop brace
meter, metre
Fischer pressure threshold m.
flow m.
pinch m.
pressure threshold m.
methacrylate
antibiotic-impregnated polymethyl m.
centrifuged methyl m.
methyl m.
polymethyl m. (PMMA)
m. resin
methadone
methaemoglobin (*var. of* methemoglobin)
methemoglobin, methaemoglobin
methicillin
methicillin-resistant *Staphylococcus aureus*
(MRSA)

methocarbamol and aspirin
method
Abbott m.
antegrade m.
anthropometric m.
ARM m.
Bardenheuer extension fracture
treatment m.
biofeedback-assisted m.
Bleck m.
Buck m.
Budin-Chandler femoral neck
anteversion measurement m.
bundle-nailing m.
Burkhalter-Reyes m.
cable cerclage m.
Callahan m.
Carrel m.
Caton m.
Chamberlain m.
Chaput m.
Cobb m.
contoured adduction trochanteric-
controlled alignment m.
(CAT-CAM)
cup and cone m.
depth caliper-meter stick m.
dynamic traction m.
Edinburgh m.
Elmslie-Trillat patellar realignment m.
Essex-Lopresti m.
extension block splinting m.
Fallat-Buckholz m.
Feldenkrais m.
Ferguson scoliosis measuring m.
Fick m.
Gohil-Cavolo m.
Grace m.
gravity m.
Greenspan scoliosis assessment m.
Hoffa tendon-shortening m.
Hoke triple-section m.
hold-relax m.
hole preparation m.
hydrogen washout blood flow m.
Ilizarov limb lengthening m.
immobilization m.
1-inclinometer m.
2-inclinometer m.
Insall patella alta m.
installation m.
Jahss 90-90 m.
keyhole m.
Lange tendon-lengthening m.
Lindsjö m.
Ling m.
McConnell taping technique m.
McKenzie m.
McReynolds m.

M

method (*continued*)
    Mose m.
    Mosley anterior shoulder repair m.
    nail length gauge m.
    Neufeld dynamic m.
    m. of perpendiculars
    OnTrack treatment m.
    Oxford m.
    Palmer m.
    pedicle m.
    Pilates exercise m.
    pin-and-plaster m.
    Ponseti clubfoot treatment m.
    Ranawat-Dorr-Inglis atlantoaxial
      impaction m.
    Ranawat-Dorr-Inglis total hip m.
    receptor-tonus m.
    retrograde m.
    Risser m.
    Russe-Gerhardt range of motion of
      living joints m.
    Schede femur fracture repair m.
    Schober lumbar flexion-extension
      measuring m.
    splinting m.
    Stamm m.
    Stimson gravity shoulder dislocation
      reduction m.
    Stulberg m.
    Tajima suture m.
    total mesenteric apron m.
    Trager m.
    Wagner limb lengthening m.
methohexital
methotrexate toxicity
methotrimeprazine
methyl
    m. methacrylate
    m. methacrylate adhesive
    m. methacrylate bead
    m. methacrylate bead implant
    m. methacrylate cement
    m. methacrylate implant material
    m. salicylate
methylcellulose
methylene
    m. bisphenyl diisocyanate
    m. blue
    m. blue dye
    m. diphosphonate (MPD)
methylmalonic acid
methylprednisolone
    m. acetate
    m. sodium succinate
methylsulfonylmethane
methyltestosterone
methylxanthine
Meticorten
metre (*var. of* meter)

Metrecom
    M. digitizer
    M. spinal analyzer
MetroGel Topical
metronidazole
metronome
METRx
    M. tubular retractor system
    M. X-Tube retractor
Mettler
    M. electrotherapy
    M. Trio neuromuscular electrical
      stimulator
metyrosine
Metzenbaum
    M. chisel
    M. gouge
    M. scissors
Meuli arthroplasty
Meurig Williams plate
Meyer
    M. cervical orthosis
    M. dysplasia
    M. line
Meyer-Betz
    M.-B. disease
    M.-B. syndrome
Meyerding
    M. bone skid
    M. chisel
    M. classification for
      spondylolisthesis (grade I-IV)
    M. curved osteotome
    M. gouge
    M. mallet
    M. retractor
    M. spondylolisthesis classification
      line
    M. spondylolisthesis (grade I-IV)
    M. straight osteotome
Meyers-McKeever tibial fracture
classification
Meyers quadratus muscle-pedicle bone
graft
Meyhoeffer bone curette
Meyn
    M. elbow reduction
    M. reduction of elbow dislocation
Meynet node
Meyn-Quigley maneuver
mezlocillin
MFA
    Musculoskeletal Function Assessment
    MFA questionnaire
MFC
    medial femoral condyle
MFH
    malignant fibrous histiocytoma
M-F heel protector

MG
  muscle group
  MG II knee prosthesis
  MG II total knee system
Mg
  magnesium
MGHL
  middle glenohumeral ligament
  MGHL cord
MGH osteotome
MgSO4
  magnesium sulfate
MH
  malignant hyperpyrexia
  malignant hyperthermia
MHOCE
  multiple hereditary osteochondral
  exostosis
Miacalcin
  M. injection
  M. nasal spray
Miami
  M. Acute Care (MAC)
  M. Acute cervical collar
  M. Acute collar cervical traction
  M. fracture brace
  M. J cervical collar
  M. J collar cervical traction
  M. TLSO scoliosis brace
Mibelli
  porokeratosis of M.
Micatin Topical
Mica 3x sleeve
mice (*pl. of* mouse)
Michaelis rhomboid
Michael Reese articulated prosthesis
Michel clip
Michele
  M. long-stem prosthesis
  M. test
  M. vertebral biopsy
  M. vertebral trephine
Michelson-Sequoia air drill
Michigan
  M. Bone Health Study
  M. Hand Outcomes
  M. Hand Outcomes Questionnaire
miconazole
MiCOR
  M. machine bone allograft
  M. precision bone allograft
micro
  M. QuickAnchor
  M. Series wire driver
  m. waveform
Micro-Aire
  M.-A. débridement of bone surface
  M.-A. drill
  M.-A. oscillating saw

M.-A. osteotome
  M.-A. reamer
microamperage
  m. electrical nerve stimulation
  (MENS)
  m. neural stimulation (MNS)
microanastomosis
microavulsion
MicroBite forceps
Microblator ArthroWand
microcirculation
microcoil
microcomputer upper limb exerciser
  (MULE)
microcrystalline collagen
microcurrent
  m. electrical neuromuscular
  stimulator unit
  m. electrode
  m. therapy
MicroDebrider
  MDS M.
  Topaz M.
microdecompression for spinal
stenosis
microdiscectomy, microdiskectomy
  arthroscopic m. (AMD)
microdiskectomy (*var. of* microdiscectomy)
  uniportal arthroscopic m.
microendoscope
microendoscopic
  m. discectomy (MED)
  m. surgical treatment
MicroFET2
  M. muscle tester
  M. muscle testing device
Micro-FET hand held dynamometer
Microfil contrast medium
Microfoam dressing
microfracture
microgeodic phalangeal syndrome
microinterlock
microirrigating cannula
microirrigator
MicroLite suture anchor
Microloc
  M. knee implant
  M. knee prosthesis
  M. knee system
microlumbar
  m. discectomy (MLD)
  m. disc excision
  m. discography
micromelic dwarfism
micrometric screw
Micro-Mill knee instrument system
MicroMite suture anchor
micromotion
  liner m.

M

Micronail intramedullary distal radius fixation system
microneedle holder
microneurography
microneurosurgical technique
micronutrient
Micro-One
    M.-O. dissecting forceps
    M.-O. hook
microoscillating saw
microparticulated protein product
MicroPhor iontophoretic drug delivery system
micropin
    Pischel m.
Microplasty minimally invasive hip program
microplate
    Luhr m.
micropodia
microprocessor
    Intertron therapy m.
microsagittal saw
microsaw
    Zimmer m.
microscissors
microscope
    double binocular operating m.
    operating m.
microscopic decompression
microscopy
    confocal m.
    hyperspectral near-infrared Raman imaging m.
    light m.
    transmission electron m.
Microsect
    M. curette
    M. shaver
MicroStable liner locking mechanism
microstaple
    Barouk m.
microsurgical
    m. anterior cervical foraminotomy
    m. discectomy (MSD)
    m. instrument
    m. thoracoscopic vertebrectomy
microtiter protein kinase assay
microtrauma
    cervical m.
    lumbar m.
    repetitive m.
    thoracic m.
Micro-Two forceps
microvalve
    hypobaric m.
microvascular
    m. clamp
    m. free muscle flap

    m. osseous transfer
    m. surgical anastomosis
microvasculature
Microvel prosthesis
microwave diathermy (MWD)
Micro-Z neuromuscular stimulator
Midas
    M. Rex acorn
    M. Rex bone cutter
    M. Rex bur
    M. Rex drill
    M. Rex instrumentation system
    M. Rex knife
    M. Rex pneumatic instrument
midaxillary
    m. line (MAL)
    m. line incision
midazolam
midbody of vertebra
midcalf
midcarpal
    m. arthrodesis
    m. arthroscopy
    m. injury
    m. instability (MCI)
    m. joint
    m. portal
    m. radial (MCR)
    m. radial portal
    m. ulnar (MCU)
    m. ulnar portal
Middeldorpf
    M. splint
    M. splint triangle
middiaphysial axis
middle
    m. atlantoepistrophic joint
    m. carpal joint
    m. column injury
    m. ear barotrauma
    m. finger
    m. finger amputation
    m. finger test
    m. glenohumeral ligament (MGHL)
    m. glenohumeral ligament cord
    m. raphe
    m. sacral artery
    m. sacral vein
    m. third (M/3)
    m. third of shaft
    m. thyroid vein
    m. tibial shaft fracture
Middlesex Elderly Assessment of Mental state (MEAMS)
midface fracture
midfacial fracture
midfemur

midfoot
    m. adductus
    m. arthritis
    m. arthrodesis
    m. arthropathy
    m. cavus
    m. deformity
    m. fracture
    m. joint
    m. scale
midheel line
Midland
    M. multifunctional mat platform
    M. tilt table
midlatency SEP
midlateral
    m. approach
    m. capsule
    m. portal
midline
    m. disc herniation
    M. Hi-Lo Mat Platform
    m. ligament
    m. medial approach
    m. raphe
midmalleolar line
midmedial capsule
midnight fracture
midpalmar
    m. abscess
    m. space
midpatellar
    m. portal
    m. tendon
Midrin
midsagittal
    m. plane
    m. splitting laminaplasty
midshaft
    m. fracture
    m. metatarsal osteotomy
midstance period of gait
midsternal line (MSL)
midsubstance tear
midtarsal
    m. dome osteotomy
    m. joint
    m. joint pain
    m. osteoarthritis
    m. V osteotomy
midtarsus
midthigh amputation
Midwest Regional Spinal Cord Injury Center
Mignon eosinophilic granuloma
migrating-type herniation
migration
    brace m.
    hallux m.

    instrument m.
    Luque rod m.
    m. of acetabular cup
    m. of prosthesis
    rod m.
    spinal cord m.
    staple m.
    trochanteric m.
migratory
    m. arthralgia
    m. arthritis
MII
    McDowell Impairment Index
Mikasa subacromial bursography
Mikhail bone block
Mikulicz
    M. knee angle
    M. operation
    M. pad
    M. procedure
    M. sponge
Mikulicz-Vladimiroff amputation
Milano Shoethotic footwear
Milch
    M. cuff resection of ulna
    M. cuff resection of ulna technique
    M. elbow fracture classification (I, II)
    M. elbow operation
    M. elbow technique
    M. fracture classification (I, II)
    M. medial condylar of elbow fracture classification (I, II)
    M. plate
    M. radioulnar joint repair
Miles
    M. bone chisel
    M. Nervine caplet
milestone
    motor m.
Milford mallet finger technique
miliare
    heloma m.
MiLIF
    minimally invasive lumbar interbody fusion
military
    M. Amputee Research Program (MARP)
    m. antishock trousers (MAST)
    m. brace maneuver
    m. brace position
    m. brace position shoulder test
    m. maneuver
    m. posture test
    m. tuck position
milk-alkali disease

M

milking
    m. maneuver
    m. of vessel
    m. sign
milkmaid's
    m. elbow
    m. elbow dislocation
Milkman
    M. osteomalacia syndrome
    M. pseudofracture
milk test
mill
    bone m.
    Lere bone m.
    Novio Magus bone m.
    OrthoBlend powered bone m.
mille
    m. pattes screw
    m. pattes technique
Millender arthroplasty
Millender-Nalebuff wrist arthrodesis
Miller
    M. Assessment for Preschoolers
    (MAP)
    M. flatfoot operation
    M. foot procedure
    M. rasp
Miller-Galante
    M.-G. hip prosthesis
    M.-G. I condylar total knee
    system
    M.-G. I hemiarthroplasty
    M.-G. II knee prosthesis
    M.-G. jig
    M.-G. knee
    M.-G. knee arthroplasty
    M.-G. revision knee system
Millesi
    M. modified nerve graft technique
    M. nerve graft
milliampere (mA)
millimeter (mm), millimetre
    m. of mercury (mmHg)
millimetre (*var. of* millimeter)
millimetric rule
milliner's needle
milling cutter
Millon
    M. Behavioral Health Inventory
    M. Clinical Multiaxial Inventory
    (MCMI)
Mills
    M. dressing
    M. elbow test
Miltex
    M. bone saw
    M. mallet
    M. nail nipper
    M. wire twister

Milwaukee
    M. cervicothoracolumbosacral
    orthosis
    M. Evaluation of Daily Living
    Skills (MEDLS)
    M. scoliosis brace
    M. scoliosis orthosis
    M. shoulder syndrome
mimicry
    somatic visceral disease m.
Mimix bone replacement system
mimocausalgia
Minaar
    M. classification of coalition
    M. classification system
mind-body therapy
mindfulness
    meditation and m.
mineralization
Miner osteotome
miner's elbow
Minerva
    M. cast
    M. cervical brace
    M. cervical jacket
    M. fixation
    M. orthosis
    M. vest
mini
    m. AO screw
    m. applier
    M. Bio-Phase suture anchor
    M. Fragment Set
    M. GLS anchor
    m. lag screw system (MLS)
    M. Mental State Examination
    (MMSE)
Mini-Acutrak small bone fixation
system
miniature
    m. end-plate potential (MEPP)
    m. multipurpose clamp
mini-C-arm
    XiScan m.-C-a.
mini-core disease
Minidyne
minifixator
    articulated m.
minifragment
    m. plate fixation
    m. screw
mini-Hoffmann external fixator
mini-Hohmann podiatric retractor
mini-Kessler external fixator
mini-Lambotte osteotome
mini-Lexer osteotome
minimal
    m. access spinal surgery (MASS)
    m. incision plantar fasciotomy

minimally
m. displaced fracture
m. invasive bone graft harvester
m. invasive dynamic condylar screw and plate
m. invasive lumbar interbody fusion (MiLIF)
m. invasive solution
m. invasive surgery (MIS)
m. invasive surgical technique
MiniMedBall hand exerciser
mini-meniscus blade
minimi
abductor digiti m. (ADM)
extensor digiti m. (EDM)
opponens digiti m. (ODM)
minimum incision surgery (MIS)
minimus
digitus pedis m.
mini-open rotator cuff repair
mini-Orthofix fixator
mini-pilon fracture
miniplate
Luhr m.
Mini-Revo Screws suture anchor
Mini-ROC anchor
Minislide sliding mat
ministaple
Bio-R-Sorb resorbable poly-L-lactic acid m.
ministem shaft
mini-Stryker power drill
mini-Ullrich bone clamp
Minneapolis hip prosthesis
Minnesota
Cognitive Assessment of M. (CAM)
M. Manual Dexterity Test
M. Rate of Manipulation test (MRMT)
M. Spatial Relations Test
minor
m. amputation
m. curve
m. lumbar curve pattern
M. sign
m. thoracic curve pattern
Minos air drill
6-minute walk functional capacity test
Mira
M. cautery
M. drill
M. reamer
mirabilis
Proteus m.
Mirage Spinal System
mirror
m. box
m. box pain management therapy
m. box therapy

dental m.
m. hand
meniscal m.
MIS
minimally invasive surgery
minimum incision surgery
MIS technique
misalignment
miserable misalignment syndrome
misoprostol
diclofenac sodium and m.
missed fracture
misshapen
missile injury
Mital
M. elbow release
M. elbow release operation
M. elbow release technique
Mitchell
M. bunionectomy
M. distal osteotomy
M. hallux valgus procedure
M. operation
M. osteotome
M. osteotomy/bunionectomy
M. posterior displacement osteotomy
M. step-down osteotomy
Mitek
M. absorbable anchor
M. anchor system
M. bone anchor
M. Fastin threaded anchor
M. GII easy anchor
M. GII Snap-Pak
M. GII suture anchor system
M. GL anchor
M. knotless anchor
M. ligament anchor
M. micro anchor
M. Micro QuickAnchor
M. Mini GLS anchor
M. Mini QuickAnchor
M. Panalok RC anchor
M. rotator cuff anchor
M. SuperAnchor instrument
M. Tacit QuickAnchor suture anchor
M. Tacit threaded anchor
M. VAPR tissue removal system
Mitella
Actimove M.
miter technique
Mithracin
mitochondria (*pl. of* mitochondrion)
mitochondrial myopathy
mitt
holding m.
impact m.

M

mitt (*continued*)
    motion control m.
    paraffin m.
    wash m.
mitten hand
Mittlemeier
    M. ceramic hip prosthesis
    M. noncemented femoral
      prosthesis
Mitutoyo digital caliper
MIV
    major injury vector
Mivacron
mivacurium
mixed
    m. amputation
    m. connective tissue disease
    m. connective tissue
      disorder
    m. cord syndrome
mixer
    MixEvac bone cement m.
MixEvac bone cement mixer
Mixter
    M. forceps
    M. ligature-carrier clamp
    M. right-angle clamp
Miya hook ligature carrier
Miyakawa knee procedure
Mize-Bucholz-Grogan posterolateral
  femur approach
Mizuno double-patch ventricular septal
  perforation repair technique
MJL
    medial joint line
MKG
    McDavid Knee Guard
    MKG support
MKS
    Mueller Knee Support
    MKS II brace
ML
    mediolateral
    ML lift
MLD
    microlumbar discectomy
MLS
    Maroteaux-Lamy syndrome
    mini lag screw system
MLSI
    multiple line-scan imaging
MM
    medial malleolus
mm
    millimeter
mmHg
    millimeter of mercury
MMSE
    Mini Mental State Examination

MMT
    manual muscle test
    manual muscle testing
MNCV
    motor nerve conduction velocity
MNS
    microamperage neural
    stimulation
Moberg
    M. advancement flap
    M. arthrodesis
    M. deltoid-to-triceps elbow
      reconstruction transfer
    M. dowel graft
    M. free muscle transfer
    M. key-grip tenodesis
    M. key-pinch procedure
    M. ninhydrin test
    M. osteotome
    M. Picking Up Test
    M. screw
    M. splint
Mobi-C
    M.-C artificial cervical disc
    M.-C cervical disc prosthesis
Mobic
Mobidin
Mobidisc artificial lumbar disc
mobile-bearing
    m.-b. knee
    m.-b. knee arthroplasty
    m.-b. knee implant
mobile wad
Mobilimb CPM device
mobility
    active m.
    m. aid
    coordinated m.
    fractured bone m.
    gait and m.
    hip m.
    intersegmental m.
    joint m.
    limited joint m. (LJM)
    lumbar sagittal m.
    muscle tissue m.
    passive m.
    passive joint m.
    rotation m.
    sacral m.
    sacroiliac joint m.
    sagittal m.
    segmental m.
    side-bending m.
    symphysial m.
    m. testing
    translation m.
    unisegmental m.
    vertical symphysial m.

mobilization
  augmented soft tissue m. (ASTM)
  Duran passive m.
  grade (1–5) of m.
  instrument-assisted soft tissue m.
    (IASTM)
  joint m.
  lateral band m.
  nonthrust m.
  soft tissue m.
  spinal joint m.
  m. with impulse
Mobils Professionals pedorthic footwear
modality
  deep heat m.
  electrical m.
  Fluidotherapy sterile dry heat m.
  mechanical m.
  nonthermal m.
  passive treatment m.
  superficial heat m.
  thermal m.
mode
  Gruen m.
  loading m.
model
  Bennett pain m.
  corpectomy m.
  Currey bone anisotropy m.
  Denis Browne 3-column m.
  family management m.
  foot m.
  joint m.
  lumbar spine m.
  M.'s of Media Representation of
    Disability
  Sandoz spinal degeneration 4-phase
    m.
  Tanner developmental m.
modeling, modelling
  Anderson m.
  cortical bone m.
  postoperative helmet m.
modelling (*var. of* modeling)
moderate-grade ulcer
Modic vertebral endplate lesion (1–2)
modification
  Aufranc m.
  Bloom-Raney m.
  Bonfiglio m.
  Bunnell m.
  Burwell-Scott m.
  C-D screw m.
  chevron m.
  Chrisman-Snook technique m.
  dietary m.
  Downey m.
  Fairbanks technique with Sever m.
  Frank and Johnson m.

  Gillette m.
  Green-Laird m.
  Helal m.
  Inclan m.
  Jacobs locking hook spinal rod
    instrumentation m.
  Kalish bunionectomy m.
  Kaplan m.
  Kleinert m.
  Kramer m.
  MacKinnon m.
  McGlamry and Feldman m.
  medial sole wedge shoe m.
  metatarsal bar shoe m.
  Met Bar shoe m.
  Neer m.
  plasty m.
  Seattle m.
  Seddon nerve injury grading m.
  Sequeira-Khanuja mini-incision total
    hip m.
  shoe m.
  Stauffer speech threshold level m.
  Strickland m.
  Thompson m.
modified
  M. American Shoulder and Elbow
    Surgeons Shoulder Patient
    Self-Evaluation Form patient
    questionnaire
  m. anterior approach to cervical
    thoracic junction
  m. Ashworth scale (MAS)
  m. Bauth thumb hypoplasia
    classification (I–V)
  m. Boyd amputation
  m. Boyd amputation of ankle and
    distal tibial physis
  m. Boyd ankle arthrodesis
  m. Boytchev procedure
  m. Brooks atlantoaxial subluxation
    tape repair technique
  m. Broström-Evans procedure
  m. Broström procedure
  m. Chrisman-Snook ankle
    reconstruction
  m. Cocklin toe operation
  m. Cotrel cast
  m. Crawford Campbell inlaid
    bone-grafting technique
  m. Darrach-type elevator
  M. Dynamic Visual Processing
    Assessment (M-DVPA)
  m. Fränkel classification
  m. Fukuda-type retractor
  M. Gait Abnormality Rating Scale
    (GARS-M)
  m. Grace plate
  m. Harris hip score

M

modified (*continued*)
    m. Hoffmann quadrilateral external fixator
    m. Hohmann bunionectomy
    m. Hohmann osteotomy
    m. Hoke-Miller flatfoot procedure
    m. Kalish osteotomy
    m. Keller resection arthroplasty
    m. Kessler 4-strand suture
    m. Kessler-Tajima suture
    m. Kienböck disease
    m. Lapidus arthrodesis
    m. Lapidus procedure
    m. Mau bunionectomy
    m. Mau osteotomy
    m. McBride bunionectomy
    m. mold and surface replacement arthroplasty
    m. Moore hip locking prosthesis
    m. Oppenheimer splint
    m. 2-portal endoscopic carpal tunnel release
    m. posterolateral approach
    m. Rankin scale
    m. Robert Jones dressing
    m. Rowe shoulder score
    m. Sillence classification
    m. Stahl classification of Kienböck disease (stage I-V)
    m. Stahl classification (stage I-V)
    m. tonsillar prong
    m. Wagner classification system
    m. Watson-Jones ankle tenodesis
    m. Wilson osteotomy
    m. Z bunionectomy
    m. Z osteotomy
Modny
    M. drill
    M. pin
modular
    M. Acetabular Revision System (MARS)
    m. acetabular revision system acetabular component
    m. Austin Moore hip prosthesis
    m. design
    m. hip implant component
    m. implant
    m. instrumentation
    m. Iowa Precoat total hip prosthesis
    m. large-head component
    m. Moniflex hip stem
    m. socket
    m. S-ROM total hip system
    m. unicompartmental knee prosthesis
modulation
    central m.
    peripheral m.

module
    Allen Diagnostic M. (ADM)
    Peak gait m.
    Skills Assessment M. (SAM)
    WeeFIM II 0-3 m.
Modulock posterior spinal fixation
modulus
    m. of elasticity
    Young m.
Moe
    M. alar hook
    M. bone curette
    M. bone impactor
    M. gouge
    M. intertrochanteric plate
    M. modified Cotrel cast
    M. modified Harrington rod
    M. osteotome
    M. scoliosis operation
    M. scoliosis technique
    M. square-end rod
    M. system
Moe-Kettleson distribution
Moeller-Barlow disease
Moeltgen flexometer
Mogensen procedure
mogul skier's palms
Mohammed internal fixation shoulder arthrodesis
Mohrenheim fossa
Mohr finger splint
Mohs chemosurery technique
Moire topographic scoliosis assessment
moist
    m. heat
    m. heat therapy
    Restore Clean 'N M.
moisturizer
    Betadine First Aid Antibiotics + M.
Molander-Olerud
    M.-O. ankle score
    M.-O. shoulder score
mold
    m. acetabular arthroplasty
    Aufranc concentric hip m.
    Biothotic orthotic m.
    caudad anterior m.
    cephalad anterior m.
molded
    AFO m.
    m. ankle-foot orthosis (MAFO)
    m. lumbosacral orthosis
    m. posterior plaster splint
    m. postpartum insole
    m. Thomas collar
molding
    compression m.
    elastomer skin m.

polyethylene compression m.
postoperative helmet m.
m. sock
Mold-In-Place back support
moleskin
m. padding
m. strip dressing
m. traction tape
Molestick padding
Molesworth osteotomy
molle
fibroma m.
heloma m. (HM)
Moloney line
Molt periosteal elevator
molybdenum
stainless steel and m. (SMO)
moment
anterior bending m.
m. arm
m. of force
3-point bending m.
posterior bending m.
momentum
angular m.
Momma-Too Maternity Support
Monarch knee brace
Monark
M. bicycle
M. Rehab Trainer
monarthric
monarthritis
viral m.
monarticular synovitis
Mönckeberg sclerosis
Mondini dysplasia
Moniflex hip stem
Monistat-Derm Topical
monitor
AccuGuide injection m.
blood pressure m. (BPM)
Brevio nerve conduction m.
M. Master monitor support
MyoTrac EMG biofeedback m.
NervePace nerve conduction m.
Polar wrist m.
Tabs Elite mobility m.
transcutaneous oxygen m. (TCOM)
Vantage Performance m.
monitored anesthesia control (MAC)
monitoring
blood pressure m.
fluorescein perfusion m.
intraoperative spinal cord m.
neurophysiologic m.
screw position perioperative m.
somatosensory evoked potential m.
spinal cord function
  intraoperative m.

MonitorMate monitor arm
monkey fist hand
monkey-paw
Monk hip prosthesis
monoamine oxidase-B inhibitor
monoarthritis
monoarticular septic arthritis
monoblock
m. femoral component
m. femoral stem prosthesis
monocane
Monocid
monoclonal gammopathy
monodactylism (*var. of* monodactyly)
monodactyly, monodactylism
Monodos orthosis
monofilament
calibrated m.
nylon m.
m. pressure test
Semmes-Weinstein m. (SWMF)
Softip m.
m. suture
m. wire
m. wire fixation
5.07 monofilament gauge
Monofixateur external fixator
Mono-Gesic
Monogram total knee instrument
monolithic
m. A1203 cup
m. A1203 cup prosthesis
monomalleolar ankle fracture
monomelic
mononeuritis multiplex
mononeuropathy
diabetic femoral m.
m. electrodiagnosis
embolic m.
m. multiplex
monophasic
m. action potential
m. endplate activity
m. waveform
monoplace hyperbaric chamber
monoplegia
monostotic m.
monopolar
m. cautery
m. electrothermal arthroscopy
m. needle recording electrode
m. sleeve
monosodium urate crystal (MSU)
monospherical total shoulder
  arthroplasty
monostotic
m. fibrous dysplasia
m. monoplegia
monosynaptic reflex arc

M

monotube
    M. external fixator system
    Howmedica m.
Monro bursa
Monteggia
    M. dislocation
    M. equivalent lesion
    M. forearm fracture
    M. fracture-dislocation
    M. fracture-dislocation of ulna
Montercaux fracture
Monticelli-Spinelli
    M.-S. circular external fixation
      system
    M.-S. distraction
    M.-S. distraction epiphysiolysis limb
      lengthening technique
    M.-S. distractor
    M.-S. fixator
    M.-S. frame
    M.-S. leg fixation
Montreal hip positioner
moon
    M. boot
    M. Boot brace
    M. Boot shoe
    M. Walker
Mooney
    M. brace
    M. cast
Moore
    M. bone drill
    M. bone elevator
    M. bone reamer
    M. driver
    M. femoral neck prosthesis
    M. fixation pin
    M. fracture
    M. hip endoprosthesis system
    M. hip prosthesis
    M. nail
    M. osteotomy
    M. osteotomy-osteoclasis
    M. posterior hip approach
    M. prosthesis extractor
    M. prosthesis-mortising chisel
    M. sliding nail plate
    M. stem
    M. technique
    M. template
    M. tibial plateau fracture
      classification
Moore-Southern approach
mooring
mop-end
    m.-e. Achilles tendon tear
    m.-e. appearance
    m.-e. mid-substance tear
Morand foot

morbidity
    surgical m.
morcel
morcellate
morcellation, morcellement
    Robinson m.
morcellement (*var. of* morcellation)
morcellize, morselize
morcellized, morselized
    m. bone
    m. bone graft
    m. cancellous graft
Moreira plate
Moreland
    M. femoral component extractor
    M. osteotome
    M. total hip revision instrumentation
Moreland-Marder-Anspach femoral stem removal
Morel-Lavallée
    M.-L. internal degloving lesion
    M.-L. lesion
Moretz prosthesis
Morfam Quality Jeanie Rub massager
Morgagni hyperostosis
Morgagni-Stewart-Morel syndrome
Morgan-Casscells meniscus suturing
morphealike lesion
morphine
    m. pump
    m. sulfate (MS)
Morpho Exerciser
morphogenesis
morphogenetic protein
morphologically
morphometry
    pedicle m.
Morquio
    M. disease
    M. sign
    M. syndrome
Morquio-Brailsford syndrome
Morquio-Ullrich
    M.-U. disease
    M.-U. syndrome
Morrey elbow arthroplasty rating system
Morris
    M. biphase screw
    M. retractor
Morrison
    M. neurovascular free flap
    M. technique
Morrissy
    M. percutaneous fixation of slipped
      epiphysis
    M. percutaneous slipped epiphysis
      fixation
Morscher cervical plate

Morse
- M. taper
- M. tapered prosthetic post
- M. taper lock
- M. taper lock of modular hip implant component

morsel

morselize (*var. of* morcellize)

morselized (*var. of* morcellized)

mortality
- surgical m.

mortise
- m. and tenon joint
- ankle m.
- bone m.
- cuneiform m.
- tibial m.
- m. view

mortising chisel

Morton
- M. disease
- M. foot
- M. interdigital neuroma
- M. interdigital neuroma test
- M. metatarsalgia
- M. neuralgia
- M. neurectomy
- M. neuroma
- M. neuroma neurolysis
- M. sign
- M. syndrome
- M. toe
- M. toe support

mosaic
- m. arthroplasty
- m. plantar verruca
- M. spinal implant system
- m. wart

mosaicplasty
- arthroscopic m.
- M. system
- m. technique

Moseley
- M. bone age graph
- M. fasciotome
- M. glenoid rim prosthesis
- M. straight line graph

Mose method

Mosley
- M. anterior shoulder repair
- M. anterior shoulder repair method

mosquito, *pl.* **mosquitos, mosquitoes**
- m. clamp
- m. forceps
- m. hemostat

mosquitoes (*pl. of* mosquito)

mosquitos (*pl. of* mosquito)

mosquito-tip grasping forceps

moss
- M. cage
- M. fixation system
- M. hook
- M. instrumentation
- M. rod
- M. screw
- M. technique

Moss-Miami
- M.-M. scoliosis instrumentation
- M.-M. transforaminal interbody fusion instrumentation

Mosso ergograph

mossy foot

Most Options system rotating hinge revision knee

Motech titanium spinal repair cage

moth-eaten destruction

Mother-Child Interaction checklist

Mother Jones dressing

Mother-To-Be back and abdominal support

motion
- accessory m.
- active and passive range of m.
- active ankle joint complex range of m.
- active-assisted range of m. (AAROM)
- active-assistive range of m. (AAROM)
- active integral range of m. (AIROM)
- active range of m. (AROM)
- m. activity
- AIM continuous passive m.
- alternating range of m. (ARM)
- m. analysis evaluation
- angular m.
- angulation m.
- ankle dorsiflexion range of m. (ADROM)
- ankle inversion-eversion range of m.
- AP translatory m.
- arc of m.
- axis of rib m.
- back range of m. (BROM)
- m. barrier
- bucket-handle rib m.
- cervical range of m. (CROM)
- constant massive m.
- continuous passive m. (CPM)
- m. control (MC)
- controlled ankle m. (CAM)
- controlled range of m. (CRM)
- m. control limiter
- m. control mitt
- m. control procedure
- coupled m.

M

motion (*continued*)
degrees of freedom joint m.
m. demand
distractive m.
double-flexion knee m.
end range of m.
Euler angle of wrist m.
frontal m.
full range of m. (FROM)
hindfoot m.
hip extension range of m.
incremental range of m. (IROM)
inherent m.
intersegmental m.
intervertebral m.
joint m.
m. limit
m. limitation
limitation of m. (LOM)
loss of m. (LOM)
lumbar range of m.
lumbopelvic m.
m. measurement
osteokinematic m.
m. palpation
m. palpation screen
passive intervertebral m. (PIVM)
passive range of m. (PROM)
pattern of m.
m. performance
physiologic range of joint m.
pistoning m.
plantarflexory m.
protective limitation of range of m.
pump-handle rib m.
m. quality
range of m. (ROM)
range of rotational m.
rectilinear m.
m. response
restricted range of m.
restriction of m.
rib m.
rotary m.
sacroiliac joint m.
sagittal m.
scapulothoracic m.
m. segment
shoulder range of m.
m. slack
sling suspension range of m.
stable to m.
subtalar m.
synergistic finger m.
synergistic wrist m.
m. testing
m. therapy
toe range of m.
total active m. (TAM)
total cervical range of m. (TCROM)
total eversion range of m.
total passive m. (TPM)
total range of m. (TROM)
translation m.
translatory m.
trial range of m.
triaxial m.
triplane m.
uninhibited ankle m.
valgus knee m.
m. velocity
winging m.
wrist m.
motion-preserving procedure
Motivator FTR2000 exerciser
motor
m. activity
m. activity log
m. and sensory neuropathy (I, II)
m. branch
m. conduction velocity
m. deficit
m. development
m. dysfunction
m. examination
m. fascicle
m. function
m. function assessment
m. function deficit
m. latency
m. loss
m. milestone
m. neglect testing
m. nerve conduction velocity (MNCV)
m. neurectomy
m. neurolysis
m. neuronal pool
m. neuron disease
m. neuropathy
m. point
m. point block
m. recovery
m. reflex
m. response
m. restlessness
sensory m.
m. speech disorder
m. strength
m. unit
m. unit action potential (MUAP)
m. unit fraction
m. unit potential (MUP)
m. vehicle accident (MVA)
m. weakness
motorcycle accident (MCA)
motorcyclist's knee

motorized
    m. bur
    m. meniscal cutter
    m. meniscal shaver
    m. reamer
    m. shaving system
    m. suction shaver
    m. trimmer
Moto-tool
Motricity Index
Motrin
    M. IB
    M. IB Sinus
    Junior Strength M.
mottled
mottling
Mouchet
    M. disease
    M. fracture
Mould arthroplasty
Moule screw pin
Mouradian
    M. humeral fixation system
    M. screw
mouse, *pl.* **mice**
    joint mice
mouse-ear appearance
MouseMitt Keyboarder padded wrist support
movable, moveable
    m. joint
move
    push-pull m.
moveable (*var. of* movable)
movement
    aberrant m.
    active hip m.
    adventitious m.
    adversive m.
    anterior-inferior m.
    anterior-posterior m.
    arcuate m.
    m. artifact
    AS m.
    ASEX m.
    ASIN m.
    M. Assessment Battery for Children
    M. Assessment of Infants (MAI)
    assistive m.
    associated m.'s
    atlas-axis m.
    caliper rib m.
    compensatory m.
    conjunct m.
    m. coordination test
    m. disorder
    dissociation m.
    dynamic m.

    external ilium m.
    freedom of m.
    Frenkel m.
    INEX m.
    inferior m.
    innominate m.
    intentional m.
    internal m.
    intersegmental m.
    isokinetic m.
    limitation of m. (LOM)
    medial m.
    passive m.
    PIEX m.
    PIIN m.
    posteroinferior external m.
    posteroinferior internal m.
    primary or intentional m.
    primary rotation m.
    quasi-independent Y-axis m.
    resistive m.
    sagittal m.
    m. science
    Swedish m.
    m. system
    total body m.
    trick m.
    unilateral posterior-anterior m.
    universal coronal m.
mover
    prime m.
moviegoer's knee
movie sign
moxa, moxibustion
    m. therapy
moxalactam
moxibustion (*var. of* moxa)
Moyer line
Moynihan towel clamp
MPA
    metatarsus primus adductus
M-Pact
    M-P. cast cutter
    M-P. cast spreader
    M-P. cast vacuum
    M-P. flexible orthotic
MPAI-3
    Mayo-Portland Adaptability Inventory 3
MPD
    methylene diphosphonate
MPFL
    medial patellofemoral ligament
MPGR
    multiplanar gradient recalled
MPJ
    metacarpophalangeal joint
MPM
    MPM antimicrobial wound cleanser
    MPM bandage

M

MPQ
McGill pain questionnaire
MP reconstruction prosthesis
M-Prednisol Injection
MPS
myofascial pain syndrome
MPV
metatarsus primus varus
MRA
magnetic resonance arteriography
MRAr
magnetic resonance arthrography
MRC
Medical Research Council
Musculoskeletal Research Centre
MRC muscle function classification
MRI
magnetic resonance imaging
dynamic MRI
flexion-extension MRI
FONAR Stand-Up MRI
gadolinium-enhanced MRI
Gyroscan superconducting MRI
positional MRI
MRI testing
MRI-compatible plate and screw system
MRI-directed surgery
MRMT
Minnesota Rate of Manipulation test
MRN
magnetic resonance neurography
MRS
magnetic resonance spectroscopy
MRSA
methicillin-resistant *Staphylococcus aureus*
MRSI
magnetic resonance spectroscopic imaging
MRT
manual resistance technique
MRV
magnetic resonance venography
MS
morphine sulfate
multiple sclerosis
MS Contin Oral
MSC cold pack
MSD
microsurgical discectomy
MSI
magnetic source imaging
MSI mapping
MSIR Oral
MSK
musculoskeletal
MSK radiology
MSL
midsternal line

MS322 muscle stimulator
MSTS
Musculoskeletal Tumor Society
MSU
monosodium urate crystal
MT
massage therapy
MT bar
MTA
metatarsus adductus
MTA brace
^{99m}Tc
technetium-99m
MTC
metatarsocuneiform
MTF
Musculoskeletal Transplant Foundation
mtMRI
magnetization transfer magnetic resonance imaging
MTP
metatarsophalangeal
MTP joint
MTS
medial tibial syndrome
MTS Mini Bionixtest system
MTSS
medial tibial stress syndrome
MTV
metatarsus varus
MUAP
motor unit action potential
Muay Thai boxing
mucate
isometheptene m.
MUCL
medial ulnar collateral ligament
mucoid degeneration
mucopolysaccharide
sulfated m.
mucopolysaccharidoses (*pl. of* mucopolysaccharidosis)
mucopolysaccharidosis, *pl.* **mucopolysaccharidoses**
mucous
m. cyst
m. membrane
mucus
Mudder sign
mud pack bath
Mueli wrist prosthesis
Mueller
M. anterolateral femorotibial ligament tenodesis
M. arthrodesis
M. ATF ankle brace
M. compression apparatus
M. compression blade-plate
M. cup

M. distractor
M. dual-lock hip prosthesis
M. femoral supracondylar fracture classification
M. fixation device
M. hinged knee brace
M. hip arthroplasty
M. humerus fracture classification
M. intertochanteric varus osteotomy
M. knee operation
M. knee procedure
M. Knee Support (MKS)
M. lateral compartment
M. Lite ankle brace
M. orthopaedic shoulder brace
M. patellar tendon graft
M. retractor
M. template
M. tibial fracture classification
M. total hip replacement prosthesis
M. transposition osteotomy
M. Ultralite brace
M. wrap-around knee brace
M. wrench
Mueller-Charnley hip prosthesis
Mueller-Weiss syndrome
Mulder
M. click
M. sign
MULE
microcomputer upper limb exerciser
Mulholland and Gunn criteria
Müller
M. intraarticular shoulder fusion
M. osteotomy
M. plate
M. prosthesis
M. saw
Mulligan silastic prosthesis
multangular
m. bone
greater m.
lesser m.
m. ridge fracture
Multi
M. Balance System (MBS)
M. Podus boot
M. Podus boot system
M. Podus foot system
multiaction pin cutter
multiarticular
multiaxial
M. Assessment of Pain (MAP)
m. joint
m. screw
multiaxis
m. ankle
m. foot
m. prosthesis

MultiBoot orthosis
Multicenter ACL Revision Study (MARS)
multicentric
m. osteogenic sarcoma
m. reticulohistiocytosis
multichannel pelvic phased-array coil
Multidex chronic wound treatment system
Multidimensional Pain inventory
multidirectional (*var. of* atraumatic multidirectional bilateral rehabilitation inferior)
m. instability (MDI)
multidisciplinary
m. approach
m. rehabilitation
multielectrode
multifidus
m. muscle
m. syndrome
Multiflex foot prosthesis
multifocal osteomyelitis
multifrequency
m. probe
m. transducer
multilead electrode
multileaf collimator
multilevel
m. fracture
m. fusion
m. laminectomy
Multi-Lig knee brace
Multi-Lock
M.-L. hand operating table
M.-L. hip prosthesis
M.-L. knee brace
multiloculated fluid collection
multipack
Ortho-ice m.
multipartite
m. fracture
m. patella
multipennate muscle
multiplace hyperbaric chamber
multiplanar
m. computed tomography scan
m. CT scan
m. deformity
m. gradient recalled (MPGR)
m. ligamentotaxis
m. virtual fluoroscopic imaging
multiplane echo probe
multiple
m. action cutter
m. cancellous chip graft
m. digits
m. discharge
m. enchondroma
m. enchondromatosis

M

multiple (*continued*)
  m. epiphysial dysplasia
  m. fingers
  m. flexible medullary nails
  m. fractures
  m. hereditary osteochondral exostosis (MHOCE)
  m. hook assembly
  m. hook assembly C-D instrumentation
  m. injuries
  m. line-scan imaging (MLSI)
  m. myeloma
  m. neurofibroma
  m. osteochondromatoses
  m. pinhole occluder
  m. pterygium syndrome
  m. rays
  m. ray amputation
  m. sclerosis (MS)
  m. synostoses syndrome
  m. tarsal coalitions
  m. traumas
multiple-axis knee joint
multiple-point sacral fixation
multiplex
  mononeuritis m.
  mononeuropathy m.
  myoclonus m.
  paramyoclonus m.
multipolar bipolar cup
Multipulse 1000 compression pump
multipurpose
  m. angled clamp
  m. curved clamp
multiradius unconstrained prosthesis
multiray fracture
multisegmental
  m. spinal distortion
  m. spinal stenosis
multisided blade handle
multisized reamer
multispan fracture hook
multistaged carrier flap
Multitak
  M. SS system
  M. suture snap system
multocida
  Pasteurella m.
Mumford
  M. distal clavicle open resection procedure
  M. distal clavicle resection
Mumford-Gurd arthroplasty
mummification necrosis
Munchmeyer disease
Munster cast
MUP
  motor unit potential

mupirocin
Murphy
  M. Achilles tendon advancement
  M. brace
  M. gouge
  M. heel cord advancement
  M. lateral approach
  M. nail
  M. osteotome
  M. skid
  M. sling
  M. splint
Murphy-Lane bone skid
Murray
  M. fixation
  M. knee prosthesis
Murray-Jones arm splint
Murray-Thomas arm splint
muscle
  abdominal m.
  abductor digiti minimi m.
  abductor digiti quinti m.
  abductor hallucis m.
  abductor pollicis brevis m.
  abductor pollicis longus m.
  accessory soleus m.
  adductor hallucis m.
  adductor pollicis m.
  Aeby m.
  agonist m.
  agonistic m.
  Albinus m.
  m. analysis
  anconeus m.
  m. and neurological stimulation electrotherapy device
  antagonistic m.
  anterior scalene m.
  anterior serratus m.
  anterior tibial m.
  appendicular skeletal m. (ASM)
  BBC m.'s
  m. belly
  biceps, brachialis, coracobrachialis m.'s
  biceps brachii m.
  biceps femoris m.
  bicipital m.
  m. biopsy clamp
  Bowman m.
  brachialis m.
  brachioradialis m.
  buccinator m.
  casserian m.
  Casser perforated m.
  Chassaignac axillary m.
  m. contractility
  m. contracture
  m. contusion

coracobrachial m.
corrugator m.
m. cramp
cricopharyngeal sphincter m.
de-epithelialized rectus abdominis m. (DRAM)
deltoid m.
digastric m.
m. disorder
dorsal interosseous m.
Dupré m.
ECRB m.
ECRL m.
ECU m.
EDB m.
EIP m.
elevator m.
emergency m.
m. energy
m. energy procedure (MEP)
m. energy technique
epimeric m.
epitrochleoanconeus m.
Eve vascularized seventh rib fascia cartilage and serratus m.
extensor carpi radialis brevis m.
extensor carpi radialis longus m.
extensor carpi ulnaris m.
extensor communis m.
extensor digiti minimi m.
extensor digiti quinti m.
extensor digitorum brevis m.
extensor digitorum communis m.
extensor digitorum longus m.
extensor hallucis brevis m.
extensor hallucis longus m.
extensor indicis m.
extensor pollicis brevis m.
extensor pollicis longus m.
extensor wad of 3 m.'s
external intercostal m.
external oblique m.
extrinsic m.
fascia of quadratus lumborum m.
m. fascicle
fast m.
femoral m.
m. fiber action potential
m. fiber conduction velocity
m. fibrillation
fibular m.
finger flexor m.
fixator m.
m. flap
flexor carpi radialis m.
flexor carpi ulnaris m.
flexor digiti quinti m.
flexor digitorum longus m.
flexor digitorum profundus m.

flexor digitorum sublimis m.
flexor digitorum superficialis m.
flexor hallucis brevis m.
flexor hallucis longus m.
flexor pollicis brevis m.
flexor pollicis longus m.
flexor wad of 5 m.'s
m. force
gastrocnemius m.
gastrocnemius-soleus m.
gluteus maximus m.
gluteus medius m.
gluteus minimus m.
gracilis m.
greater rhomboid m.
m. group (MG)
m. guarding
hamstring m.
handbag m.
m. hernia
hypothenar m.
iliacus m.
iliococcygeus m.
iliocostal m.
iliopsoas m.
m. imbalance
inferior gemelli m.
infraspinatus m.
m. innervation
m. insufficiency
internal oblique m.
interosseous m.
intervening m.
intraspinous m.
intrinsic m.
m. ischemia
Jung m.
Langer axillary arch m.
lateral malleolus m.
latissimus dorsi m.
lesser rhomboid m.
levator scapulae m.
long fibular m.
longissimus colli m.
longus capitis m.
longus cervicis colli m.
longus colli m.
lumbrical m.
Luschka m.
mesothenar m.
multifidus m.
multipennate m.
nonstriated m.
oblique m.
obturator externus m.
obturator internus m.
omohyoid m.
opponens digiti quinti m.
opponens pollicis m.

M

muscle (*continued*)

palmar interosseous m.
palmaris digitorum superficialis m.
palmaris longus m.
paraspinal m.
paravertebral m. (PVM)
m. patterning sequence
pectineal m.
pectoralis major m.
pectoralis minor m.
m. pedicle bone graft
peroneal m.
peroneus brevis m.
peroneus longus m.
peroneus quartus m.
peroneus tertius m.
Phillips m.
piriform m.
plantaris m.
platysma m.
m. play
pollicis longus m.
popliteal m.
postaxial m.
posterior deltoid m.
postural m.
preaxial m.
profundus m.
pronator quadratus m.
pronator teres m.
m. protein synthesis
psoas m.
quadrate m.
quadratus femoris m.
quadratus lumborum m.
quadratus plantae m.
quadriceps femoris m.
rectus abdominis m.
rectus femoris m.
red m.
m. reflex latency
m. reflex response
m. relaxant
released ulnar intrinsic m.
m. repositioning
rhomboid m.
rider's m.
Riolan m.
rotator m.
M. Rub
sacrococcygeal m.
sacrospinal m.
sartorius m.
scalene m.
scapulohumeral m.
scapulothoracic m.
SCM m.
semimembranosus m.
semispinal m.

semitendinosus m.
serratus anterior m.
m. sheath
short fibular m.
shunt m.
Sibson m.
skeletal m.
m. slide
m. sliding operation
slow m.
smooth m.
soleus m.
somatic m.
m. spasm
m. spasticity
sphincter m.
m. spindle
m. splitting approach
spurt m.
sternohyoid m.
sternomastoid m.
sternothyroid m.
m. strain
strap m.
m. stretch reflex
striated m.
striped m.
subclavius m.
subclavius m.
subcostal m.
suboccipital m.
subscapularis m.
subvertebral m.
supinator m.
supinator m.
supraspinatus m.
supraspinous m.
synergistic m.
teres major m.
teres minor m.
m. testing
thenar m.
third fibular m.
tibial m.
tibialis anterior m.
tibialis posterior m.
m. tissue mobility
toe extensor m.
toe flexor m.
m. tone
tonic m.
trachelomastoid m.
m. transfer
transversus abdominis m.
trapezius m.
triangular m.
triceps brachii m.
triceps surae m.
tricipital m.

twitch m.
unipennate m.
unstriated m.
vastus intermedius m.
vastus lateralis m.
vastus medialis m.
vestigial m.
voluntary m.
white m.
Wilson m.
yoked m.
muscle-balancing procedure
muscle-bound
muscle-plasty
Speed V-Y m.-p.
muscle-setting exercise
muscle-splitting incision
muscle-strengthening exercise
muscle-tendon
m.-t. attachment
m.-t. injury
m.-t. transplant
muscle-to-bone suture
muscular
m. atrophy
m. attachment
m. clamp
m. contraction
m. coordination
m. cramp
m. dystrophy (MD)
m. lesion
m. neurofibromatosis
m. reeducation
m. reflex
m. rehabilitation
m. tissue
m. torticollis
m. trophoneurosis
muscularity
musculature
axial m.
left erector spinae m.
paraspinal m.
paravertebral m.
peroneal m.
right erector spinae m.
musculoaponeurotic
musculocutaneous
m. amputation
m. free flap
m. nerve
m. nerve block
m. nerve injury
m. nerve paralysis
musculoelastic
musculofascial
musculointestinal
musculoligamentous

musculomembranous
musculophrenic
musculorum
dystonia m.
musculoskeletal (MSK)
m. analysis
m. evaluation, rehabilitation and conditioning (MERAC)
M. Function Assessment (MFA)
m. infection
m. loading
m. melioidosis
m. radiology
M. Research Centre (MRC)
M. Transplant Foundation (MTF)
m. trauma
M. Tumor Society (MSTS)
M. Tumor Society Rating Scale
musculospiral paralysis
musculotendinous
m. cuff
m. flap
m. junction
m. system
m. unit
musculotendinous-osseous link
Musgrave
M. footprint pedobarograph
M. Footprint System
mushroom
m. impactor
m. walker glide
mushy edema
musician's plight
muslin sling
Mustard iliopsoas muscle transfer
mute toe sign
mutilans
arthritis m.
m. rheumatoid arthritis
mutilation
MVA
motor vehicle accident
MVC
maximal voluntary contraction
MVE
maximum voluntary effort
MVM
medullary venous malformation
MVP
Biodex Multi-Joint System 3 MVP
MWD
microwave diathermy
M3-X extremity fixation system
myalgia
myasthenia
m. angiosclerotica
m. gravis
myatonia, myatony

M

myatony (*var. of* myatonia)
myatrophy
Mycelex
Mycelex-7
Mycelex-G
mycetoma
    Carter m.
    recurrent m.
Mycifradin Sulfate Topical
Mycitracin Topical
mycobacterial
    m. arthritis
    m. infection
Mycobacterium
    M. avium
    M. avium-intracellulare
      (MAI)
    M. chelonei
    M. fortuitum
    M. gordonae
    M. intracellulare
    M. kansasii
    M. marinum
    M. terrae
    M. tuberculosis
Mycocide
    M. NS
    M. NS antimicrobial solution
mycotic club nail
myectomy
myectopia (*var. of* myectopy)
myectopy, myectopia
myelalgia
myelapoplexy
myelasthenia
myelatelia
myelatrophy
myelauxe
myelencephalitis
myelinated
myelinopathy
myelinosis
myelitis
    acute transverse m.
myelo
    myelogram
    myelography
myeloblastoma
myelocele
myelocystocele
myelocystomeningocele
myelodiastasis
myelodysplasia
myelodysplastic kyphosis
myeloencephalitis
myelofibrosis
myelogenous callus
myelogram (myelo)
myelographic

myelography (myelo)
    air m.
    computer-assisted m. (CAM)
    iopamidol m.
    Isovue m.
    opaque m.
    oxygen m.
myelolipoma
myeloma
    multiple m.
    solitary m.
myelomalacia
myelomeningitis
myelomeningocele
myelomere
myeloneuritis
myeloparalysis
myelopathic symptom
myelopathy
    cervical m.
    cervical spondylotic m.
      (CSM)
    compressive m.
    m. incidence
    noncompressive m.
    nonstenotic cervical m.
    progressive subacute m.
    radiation-related m.
    spinal stenotic m.
    transverse m.
    vacuolar m.
myelophthisis
myeloplegia
myeloproliferative disorder
myeloradiculitis
myeloradiculopathy
myelorrhagia
myelorrhaphy
    commissural m.
myelosclerosis
myelosyphilis
myelotomy
    Bischof m.
Myers knee retractor
mylohyoid
myoasthenia
myoblast
myoblastoma
    granular cell m.
Myobock
    M. artificial hand
    M. system
myobradia
myocardiac (*var. of* myocardial)
myocardial, myocardiac
    m. bridging
    m. ischemia
myocele
myocelialgia

myocelitis
myocellulitis
myocerosis
myocervical collar
Myochrysine
myoclasis
myoclonia
myoclonic epilepsy
myoclonus
    action m.
    epileptic m.
    hereditary essential m.
    intention m.
    m. multiplex
    nocturnal m.
    palatal m.
    spinal m.
myocoele
myocrismus
myocutaneous
    m. flap
    transverse rectus abdominis m.
    (TRAM)
myocytoma
myodegeneration
myodemia
myodesis
myodiastasis
myodynamic
myodynamics
myodynia
myodysneuria
myodystonia
myodystrophia (*var. of* myodystrophy)
myodystrophy, myodystrophia
    myodystrophia fetalis
myoedema, myo-oedema
myoelastic
myoelectrical
myoelectrically silent
myoelectric control prosthesis
myoencephalopathy
myofascia
myofascial
    m. closure
    m. manipulation
    m. pain
    m. pain-dysfunction syndrome
    m. pain syndrome (MPS)
    m. release
    m. tenderness
    m. trigger point
    m. unit
    m. unwinding
myofasciitis
    interstitial m.
myofibril
myofibroblast
myofibroma

myofibrosis
myofibrositis
Myoflex
MyoForce test
myogelosis
myogenic
    m. paralysis
    m. tonus
    m. torticollis
myoglobinuria
    familial m.
myography
    acoustic m.
myohypertrophia
myoinositol level
myoischemia
myokerosis
myokinesis
myokymia
    exercise-induced m.
myokymic discharge
myolipoma
myologia
myology
myolysis
myoma
myomalacia
myomatosis
myomelanosis
myonecrosis
    clostridial m.
myoneuralgia
    postural m.
myoneural ischemia
myoneurasthenia
myoneurectomy
myoneuroma
myoneurosis
myonosus
myo-oedema (*var. of* myoedema)
myopachynsis
myopalmus
myoparalysis
myoparesis
myopathic
    m. arthrogryposis
    m. atrophy
    m. gait
    m. motor unit potential
    m. paralysis
    m. recruitment
    m. scoliosis
myopathophysiology
myopathy
    acquired m.
    benign congenital m.
    carcinomatous m.
    centronuclear m.
    congenital m.

M

myopathy (*continued*)
    exercise m.
    m. hand
    idiopathic polymyositis m.
    Kiloh-Nevin m.
    mitochondrial m.
    myotubular m.
    nemaline rod-body m.
    polymyositis m.
    postinfectious m.
    ragged red fiber m.
    rheumatoid arthritis m.
    sarcotubular m.
    steroid m.
    structural congenital m.
    Welander distal m.
    zebra body m.
    zidovudine-induced m.
myophagism
myoplastic muscle stabilization
myoplasty
myopsychopathy
myorrhaphy
myorrhexis
myosarcoma
Myoscan sensor
myoschwannoma
myosclerosis
myositis
    acute progressive m.
    cervical tension m.
    clostridial m.
    m. fibrosa
    focal nodular m.
    granulomatous m.
    inclusion body m.
    inflammatory m.
    ischemic m.
    nodular m.
    m. ossificans
    m. ossificans progressiva
    proliferative m.
    rheumatoid m.
    m. serosa
    streptococcal m.
    suppurative m.
    tension m.
    viral m.
myospasm, myospasmus
myospasmus (*var. of* myospasm)
Myossage lotion
myostasis
myosteoma
myosthenic
myosthenometer
myosuture

myosynizesis
myotasis
myotatic
    m. reflex
    m. unit
myotendinous junction
myotenontoplasty
myotenositis
myotenotomy
myotomal pain
myotome
myotomy
myotonia
    m. acquisita
    m. atrophica
    chondroplastic m.
    m. congenita
    m. congenita intermittens
    congenital m.
    drug-induced m.
    m. dystrophica
    m. hereditaria
    Schwartz-Jampel m.
myotonic
    m. discharge
    m. dystrophy (DM, MD)
    m. muscular dystrophy
    m. potential
myotonica
    dystrophia m. (DM)
myotonoid
myotonometer
myotonus
MyoTrac
    M. device
    M. EMG biofeedback monitor
    M. single-channel
myotrophic
myotrophy
myotube
myotubular myopathy
myovascular
Mysono 201 portable ultrasound
Mysotrol hand sanitizer
myxedema, myxoedema
myxoedema (*var. of* myxedema)
myxofibroma
myxoid
    m. chondrosarcoma
    m. cyst
    m. liposarcoma
myxoid-type liposarcoma
myxoma
    enchondromatous m.
    soft tissue m.
myxosarcoma

NA
  neuropathic arthropathy
Na
  sodium
NAAP
  National Arthritis Action Plan
nabumetone
Nada-Chair Back-Up portable back sling
NADPH
  nicotinamide-adenine dinucleotide
    phosphate
naevus (*var. of* nevus)
Nafcil Injection
nafcillin
Naffziger
  N. nerve root compression test
  N. sign
  N. syndrome
naftifine
Naftin
  N. cream
  N. gel
NAG
  natural apophysial glide
  reverse NAG
Nägele pelvis
nail
  adjustable n.
  Ainsworth modification of Massie n.
  Albizzia intramedullary n.
  Alta tibial n.
  annular elastic n.
  antegrade femoral n.
  antegrade/retrograde compression n.
  anteroposterior n.
  antibiotic cement-coated
    interlocking n.
  AO slotted medullary n.
  AP n.
  n. assembly
  Augustine boat n.
  n. avulsion
  Bailey-Dubow n.
  Barr bolt n.
  n. bed
  n. bed graft
  n. bed hematoma evacuation
  n. bed lesion
  bent n.
  Bickel intramedullary n.
  Biomet ankle arthrodesis n.
  blind medullary n.
  boat n.
  Böhler n.
  brittle n.

Brooker double-locking unreamed
  tibial n.
Brooker femoral n.
Brooker-Wills n.
n. bur
Calandruccio n.
cannulated n.
centromedullary n.
Chandler unreamed interlocking
  tibial n.
Chick n.
Christensen interlocking n.
closed Küntscher n.
closed unlocked n.
cloverleaf Küntscher n.
clubbed n.
C-nail flexible pediatric n.
condylocephalic n.
crutch and belt femoral closed n.
Curry hip n.
n. deformity
Delta femoral n.
Delta Recon n.
Delta tibial n.
Derby n.
Diamond n.
diamond-shaped medullary n.
digital n.
double-ended n.
double-hollow n.
n. drill
n. driver
n. dust
dynamic locking n.
dystrophic n.
Ender flexible medullary n.
Ender round elastic condylar n.
n. extender
extension n.
n. extension
extraction of broken femoral
  antegrade n.
extraction of unbroken antegrade
  femoral n.
femoral neck n.
fissured n.
Fixion intramedullary humeral n.
Fixion proximal femoral n.
4-flanged n.
flexible intramedullary n. (FIN)
flexible medullary n.
fluted Sampson n.
fluted titanium n.
n. fold
n. fold removal

N

nail (*continued*)
Gamma locking n.
Gamma trochanteric locking n.
golfer's n.'s
Green-Seligson-Henry n.
n. groove
n. groove callus
Grosse-Kempf interlocking
  medullary n.
Grosse-Kempf locking n.
GSH n.
Hackethal n.
Hagie pin n.
Hahn bone n.
Halder locking n.
half-and-half n.
hallux n.
Hansen-Street n.
Harrington n.
Harris condylocephalic n.
Harris hip n.
Harris medullary n.
Holt n.
hooked intramedullary n.
hooked medullary n.
Huckstep n.
IMSC multihole n.
ingrown n.
n. injury
Inro surgical n.
interlocking medullary n.
Intertan femoral fracture n.
intramedullary ANK n.
intramedullary elastic n.
intramedullary supracondylar
  multihole n.
Jewett n.
K n.
Ken sliding n.
Klemm n.
Knowles pin n.
Küntscher n. (K nail)
Laing H-beam n.
left-sided n.
n. length gauge method
Lewis n.
Lloyd adapter for Smith-Petersen n.
locking n.
long-edge medullary n.
Lottes triflanged medullary n.
Luck n.
Massie II n.
Massie sliding n.
n. matrix
n. matrix phenolization (NMP)
McKee tri-fin n.
McLaughlin n.
medullary n.
Moore n.

multiple flexible medullary n.'s
Murphy n.
mycotic club n.
nested n.
Neufeld n.
No-Lok self-locking n.
noncannulated n.
nonreamed n.
Nylok self-locking n.
onychocryptosis n.
Ony-Clear N.
open n.
open-section n.
Orthofix intramedullary n.
OrthoSorb pin n.
Palmer bone n.
Panta arthrodesis n.
parrot beak n.
pediatric fracture fixation with
  titanium elastic n.
PGP n.
Pidcock n.
pincer n.
Pitcock n.
n. plate
n. plate apparatus
n. plate device
n. plate fixation
n. plate removal
prebent n.
preoperative planning under
  intramedullary interlocking n.'s
Pugh sliding n.
reamed n.
Recon n.
retrograde intramedullary n.
ReVision n.
Richards reconstruction n.
right-sided n.
n. root
n. rotational guide
Rush flexible medullary n.
Rush pin n.
Russell-Taylor delta tibial n.
Russell-Taylor interlocking
  medullary n.
Rydell n.
Sage forearm n.
Sage radial n.
Sage triangular n.
Sampson medullary n.
Sarmiento n.
Schneider intramedullary n.
Seidel n.
Seidel humeral locking n.
self-broaching n.
self-locking n.
n. set
sliding n.

Slocum n.
slotted n.
Smillie n.
Smith-Petersen femoral neck n.
Smith-Petersen transarticular n.
specialized n.
spring-loaded n.
standard medullary n.
n. starter
static locking n.
Steinmann extension n.
Street forearm n.
striated n.
supracondylar medullary n.
n. suture
Sven-Johansson femoral neck n.
telescoping n.
Temple University n.
Terry n.
Thatcher n.
third-generation n.
Thompson n.
Thornton n.
titanium n.
titanium elastic n.
triangular medullary n.
triflanged Lottes n.
triflanged medullary n.
Trigen Intertan femoral fracture n.
TriGen TAN antegrade femoral n.
TriGen third generation knee n.
turtle neck n.
Uniflex humeral n.
Uniflex intramedullary n.
universal n.
Vector intertrochanteric n.
Venable-Stuck n.
vitallium Küntscher n.
V-medullary n.
watch crystal n.
Watson-Jones n.
Webb bolt n.
Williams n.
Winograd technique for ingrown n.
Z fixation n.
Zickel subcondylar n.
Zickel subtrochanteric n.
Zickel supracondylar medullary n.
Zimmer telescoping n.

nail-bending device
nail-driving guide
nail-extracting hook
nailing
    antegrade n.
    blind medullary n.
    bundle n.
    centromedullary n.
    closed Küntscher n.
    closed medullary n.

condylocephalic n.
crutch and belt femoral closed n.
diaphysial forearm fracture Nancy n.
elastic stable intramedullary n.
  (ESIN)
Ender n.
exchange n.
femoral n.
fixator-augmented n.
fracture repair with
  intramedullary n.
gradual elongation n. (GEN)
gradual elongation intramedullary n.
  (GEIN)
Grosse-Kempf interlocking
  medullary n.
Harris condylocephalic n.
interlocking n.
intramedullary n. (IMN)
Küntscher medullary n.
locked n.
Lottes n.
marrow n.
medullary n.
Nancy n.
open medullary n.
retrograde n.
static lock n.
tibiocalcaneal medullary n.
TriGen femoral antegrade n.
Verstreken computed-aided closed
  medullary n.
Zickel n.

nail-mounted
    n.-m. compression device
    n.-m. targeting
nail-patella syndrome
nail-pulling forceps
nail-screw sideplate assembly
Nakamura
    N. brace
    N. disease
naked trabecula
nalbuphine
Nalebuff arthrodesis
**Nalebuff-Millender swan-neck deformity
lateral band mobilization technique**
Nalfon
Nallpen Injection
naloxone hydrochloride
**Namaqualand spondyloepiphysial
dysplasia (NSED)**
nana
    pelvis n.
Nancy nailing
nandrolone
nanocolloid
NAP
    nerve action potential

N

napkin
>n. ring calcar allograft
>n. ring compression

Napoleon hat sign
naprapathy
Naprelan
Naprosyn
naproxen sodium
Nara arthroplasty
Naraghi-DeCoster reduction clamp
Narcan
NARHA
> North American Riding for Handicapped Association

Naropin
narrow
>n. AO dynamic compression plate
>n. Assistant Free retractor blade
>n. cobra retractor
>n. double-prong acetabular retractor
>n. inferior acetabular retractor
>n. proximal femoral elevator
>n. toebox shoe

narrow-base gait
narrow-blade retractor
narrowed joint space
narrowing
>arthritic ankle joint n.
>intervertebral disc n.
>n. of forefoot
>n. of spinal canal

narrow-neck mini-Hohmann retractor
nasal
>n. elevator
>n. spine

nascent motor unit potential
Nash-Moe vertebral rotation scoliosis assessment technique
nasoethmoid fracture
natatory
>n. cord
>n. ligament

national
>N. Academy on Aging Society
>N. Accessible Apartment Clearinghouse
>N. Aging Information Center
>N. Alliance for Research on Schizophrenia and Depression
>N. Arthritis Action Plan (NAAP)
>N. Arthritis Data Workgroup
>N. Association for Rights, Protection, and Advocacy
>N. Association of Medical Equipment Suppliers
>N. Center for Dissemination of Disability Research
>N. Center to Improve Practice through Technology, Media, and Materials
>N. Collegiate Athletic Association drug testing policy
>N. Collegiate Athletic Association prohibited drug
>N. Collegiate Athletic Association spine injury prevention rule
>N. Consumer Supporter Technical Assistance Center
>N. Council on Disability
>N. Down Syndrome Society
>N. Empowerment Center
>N. Football Head and Neck Injury Registry
>N. Foundation for Depressive Illness Inc.
>N. Headache Foundation
>N. Hospice Organization
>N. Information Center for Children and Youth with Disabilities
>N. Institute for Child Health and Human Development (NICHD)
>N. Institute of Arthritis and Musculoskeletal and Skin Diseases (NIAMS)
>N. Lymphedema Network
>N. Maternal and Child Health Clearinghouse
>N. Mental Health Consumers' Self-Help Clearinghouse
>N. Operating Committee on Standards for Athletic Equipment (NOCSAE)
>N. Organization for Rare Disorders (NORD)
>N. Osteoporosis Foundation
>N. Registry of Rehabilitation Technology supplier
>N. Rehabilitation Information Center
>N. Spinal Cord Injury Association (NSCIA)
>N. Stroke Association

Native American medicine
natural apophysial glide (NAG)
Natural-Hip
>N.-H. prosthesis
>N.-H. system
>N.-H. titanium hip stem

naturalism
Natural-Knee
>N.-K. II system
>N.-K. implant
>N.-K. unconstrained prosthesis

Natural-Lok acetabular cup prosthesis
naturopathy
Naughton-Dunn triple arthrodesis

Nauth
- N. traction apparatus
- N. traction device

navicular
- accessory n.
- n. arthritis
- bifurcate n.
- n. body
- n. bone
- cartilaginous n.
- n. cookie in shoe
- cornuate n.
- n. cuneiform ligament
- divided n.
- n. dorsal lip fracture
- n. drop test
- lip of n.
- n. osteonecrosis
- n. prominence
- protrusion of n.
- n. screw
- n. shoe cookie
- n. shoe pad
- tarsal n.
- n. to 1st metatarsal angle
- n. tuberosity
- n. tuberosity fracture
- n. wedging

naviculectomy
naviculocapitate
- n. fracture
- n. fracture syndrome

naviculocuneiform
- n. breach
- n. coalition
- n. fusion
- n. joint
- n. joint arthrodesis
- n. ligament

navigation
- StealthStation Treon plus electromagnetic surgical n.

Navigator power wheelchair
Navitrack computer-assisted surgery system
NCS
- nerve conduction study

NCT
- nerve compression test

NCV
- nerve conduction velocity

NDI
- neck disability index

2nd-look arthroscopy
NDT
- neurodevelopmental treatment

Neal-Robertson litter
near-anatomic position of joint
near-constant frequency train

near-far
- n.-f. fashion
- n.-f. suture

near-field potential
nearthrosis, neoarthrosis
NEB
- New England Baptist
    - NEB acetabular cup
    - NEB arthroplasty
    - NEB total hip prosthesis

Necelon surgical glove
necessity
- fracture of n.

neck
- basal n.
- n. brace
- n. component
- congenital wry n.
- crick in n.
- n. diameter
- n. disability index (NDI)
- femoral head and n.
- fibular n.
- n. fracture
- glenoid n.
- humeral n.
- n. hyperextension
- metacarpal n.
- metatarsal n.
- n. pain syndrome
- phalangeal n.
- n. pillow
- radial n.
- n. reflex
- n. roll
- n. shaft
- skeletal wry n.
- supple n.
- surgical n.
- swan-neck deformity of mid n.
- talar n.
- n. wrap
- wry n.

Neckcare pillow
Neck-Hugger cervical support pillow
neck-righting reflex
Neck-Roll aromatherapy hot/cold pack
neck-shaft angle (NSA)
neck-tongue syndrome
Necktrac
- N. traction
- N. traction device

necroses (*pl. of* necrosis)
necrosis, *pl.* **necroses**
- alcoholic avascular n.
- aseptic n.
- atraumatic n.
- avascular n. (AVN)
- bone n.

N

necrosis (*continued*)
    bony n.
    bulbar n.
    central n.
    coagulation n.
    coagulative n.
    corticosteroid-induced avascular n.
    dry n.
    epiphysial aseptic n.
    epiphysial ischemic n.
    gangrenous n.
    gummatous n.
    hyaline n.
    idiopathic avascular n.
    infectious bulbar n.
    ischemic n.
    mummification n.
    Paget quiet n.
    pressure n.
    radiographic avascular n.
    septic n.
    skin n.
    steroid-induced avascular n.
    superficial n.
    thermal n.
    total n.
    n. ustilaginea
    Zenker n.
necrotic
    n. bone
    n. skin
    n. tissue
necroticans
    osteochondritis n.
necrotizing fasciitis
necrotomy
    osteoplastic n.
needle
    acupuncture n.
    atraumatic n.
    Beath n.
    Bergstrom n.
    Bier lumbar puncture n.
    n. biopsy
    bone biopsy n.
    bore n.
    Bunnell tendon n.
    conventional cutting n.
    n. cord length
    cutting n.
    Deschamps n.
    diamond point n.
    discogram n.
    n. electrode
    Framer tendon-passing n.
    Gallie n.
    hand-honed reverse cutting n.
    Hawkeye suture n.
    n. holder

    hubbed n.
    Jamshidi n.
    K n.
    Keith n.
    Luer-Lok n.
    McGee prosthesis n.
    Menghini Surecut bone biopsy n.
    meniscal repair n.
    milliner's n.
    osteodysplasty of Melnick and N.'s
    n. placement
    Plum-Blossom acupuncture n.
    Quincke n.
    reverse cutting n.
    ribbed n.
    Seirin acupuncture n.
    Sklar ligature n.
    spinal n.
    Stimuplex block n.
    swaged n.
    taper cut n.
    tapered n.
    tendon n.
    The Painless One acupuncture n.
    Thomas n.
    Tuohy lumbar puncture n.
    Verbrugge n.
    Veress n.
needle-nose
    n.-n. rongeur
    n.-n. vise-grip pliers
needlescope
Neer
    N. acromioplasty
    N. acromioplasty for rotator cuff
    tear
    N. capsular shift procedure
    N. femur fracture classification
    N. hemiarthroplasty
    N. humeral replacement prosthesis
    N. humerus fracture classification
    N. II humeral component
    N. II shoulder system
    N. II total knee system
    N. II total shoulder system
    implant
    N. impingement sign
    N. lateral shoulder view
    N. modification
    N. open shoulder reduction
    N. posterior shoulder reconstruction
    N. ring
    N. shoulder fracture classification
    N. shoulder impingement test
    N. shoulder prosthesis (I, II)
    N. transscapular view
    N. umbrella prosthesis
    N. unconstrained shoulder
    arthroplasty

Neer-Horowitz
- N.-H. classification of humeral fracture
- N.-H. humerus fracture classification

Neff
- N. femorotibial nail system
- N. meniscus knife

Neftel disease

negative
- n. afterpotential
- n. casting
- n. congruence angle
- n. impression cast
- n. pressure wound therapy (NPWT)
- n. tropism
- n. ulnar variance (NUV)
- n. work

neglect
- hemispatial n.
- traumatic brain injury-related n.
- visual n.

neglected rupture

neiguan point acupressure

Neisseria
- N. gonorrhoeae
- N. sicca

Neivert osteotome

Nélaton
- N. ankle dislocation
- N. line
- N. operation
- N. rubber tube drain

Nelson
- N. finger exerciser
- N. rib retractor
- N. rib spreader
- N. scissors
- N. sign

nemaline rod-body myopathy

Nembutal

neoadjuvant chemotherapy

neoarthrosis (*var. of* nearthrosis)

neocartilage

Neo-Cortef

neocortex

NeoDecadron Topical

neoformans
- *Cryptococcus n.*

neoformation
- nodular n.

neolimbus

Neomixin Topical

neomycin
- n. and dexamethasone
- n. and hydrocortisone
- n. and polymyxin B
- n., polymyxin B, and hydrocortisone

neonatal
- n. flatfoot
- n. sandbag
- n. septic arthritis
- n. tracheostomy tube holder

Neopap

neoplasia
- bone n.
- interdigital n.

neoplasm

neoplastic
- n. fracture
- n. lesion
- n. osteoblast

Neoplush foam

neoprene
- n. ankle support
- n. back support
- n. dressing
- n. elbow sleeve
- n. fabric
- n. knee sleeve
- n. shoe
- n. wrist brace
- n. wrist orthosis
- n. wrist strap

Neoral Oral

Neosar injection

Neosporin
- N. Cream
- N. Topical Ointment

Ne-Osteo bone morphogenic protein

neotendon

neovascularization

Nephro-Calci

nerve
- abductor digiti minimi n.
- accessory n.
- n. action potential (NAP)
- antebrachial cutaneous n.
- anterior thoracic n.
- anterior tibial n.
- Arnold n.
- articular n.
- axillary n.
- n. block
- n. block infusion kit
- Bock n.
- calcaneal n.
- n. cap
- cervical spine n.'s 1-7 (C1-C7)
- cluneal n.
- common digital n.
- common peroneal n.
- n. compression test (NCT)
- n. conduction study (NCS)
- n. conduction velocity (NCV)
- n. conduction velocity test

N

nerve (*continued*)
  n. crossing
  cubital n.
  cutaneous n.
  deep peroneal n. (DPN)
  digital branch of plantar n.
  dorsal cutaneous n.
  dorsal scapular n.
  dorsomedial cutaneous n.
  n. ending
  n. entrapment site
  n. entrapment syndrome
  n. entubulation
  femoral cutaneous n.
  n. fiber action potential
  n. function test
  genitofemoral n.
  gluteal n.
  n. graft
  great sciatic n.
  n. growth factor
  n. hook
  hypoglossal n.
  iliohypogastric n.
  ilioinguinal n.
  inferior calcaneal n.
  inferior laryngeal n.
  n. injury
  intercostal n.
  intercostobrachial n.
  interdigital n.
  n. interference
  intermediate dorsal cutaneous n.
    (IDCN)
  intermetatarsal n.
  interosseous n.
  n. involvement testing
  laryngeal n.
  lateral antebrachial cutaneous n.
  lateral anterior thoracic n.
  lateral common digital n.
  lateral femoral cutaneous n.
  lateral plantar n.
  lateral superior genicular n.
  lumbar (spine) n.'s 1-5 (L1-L5)
  mandibular n.
  medial antebrachial cutaneous n.
  medial articular n.
  medial brachial n.
  medial dorsal cutaneous n. (MDCN)
  medial plantar n.
  medial sural cutaneous n.
  median n.
  meningeal n.
  musculocutaneous n.
  obturator n.
  n. palsy
  pectoral n.
  peroneal n.

  plantar n.
  popliteal n.
  posterior femoral cutaneous n.
  posterior interosseous n.
  posterior tibial n. (PTN)
  radial digital n.
  radial sensory n.
  recurrent laryngeal n.
  recurrent meningeal n.
  regeneration of n.
  n. root
  n. root block
  n. root compression
  n. root compromise
  n. root decompression
  n. root entrapment
  n. root injection
  n. root irritability
  n. root irritation
  n. root lesion
  n. rootlet ablation
  n. root sheath
  sacral n.
  saphenous n.
  scapular n.
  sciatic n.
  sensorimotor n.
  sensory n.
  n. separator
  n. sheath tumor
  sinuvertebral n.
  somatic n.
  spinal accessory n.
  n. stretching
  superficial peroneal n.
  superficial radial n. (SRN)
  superior gluteal n.
  superior laryngeal n.
  suprascapular n.
  sural n.
  sympathetic n.
  thoracic n.
  thoracodorsal n.
  tibial n.
  n. tracing
  n. transmission
  n. transposition
  n. transposition surgery
  n. trunk action potential
  tubulization of n.
  ulnar n. (UN)
  vertebral n.
  n. wrapping
NervePace nerve conduction monitor
nervi (*gen.* and *pl. of* nervus)
Nervocaine
Nervoscope device
nervus, *gen.* and *pl.* **nervi**
  nervi erigentes

Nesacaine
Nesacaine-MPF
nested
    n. nail
    n. step stool
netting
    splint pan n.
network
    National Lymphedema N.
Neubeiser adjustable forearm splint
Neufeld
    N. apparatus
    N. cast
    N. device
    N. dynamic method
    N. nail
    N. pin
    N. plate
    N. roller traction
    N. screw
NeuFlex metacarpophalangeal joint implant
Neuhauser variant
Neumann syndrome
Neurain drill
Neurairtome
    N. drill
    Hall N.
neural
    n. arch resection technique
    n. axis
    n. axis abnormality
    n. crest
    n. element
    n. foramen
    n. foraminal stenosis (NFS)
    n. foraminotomy
    n. injury
    n. nevus
    n. strength training
    n. tension
    n. tissue
    n. tube defect
    n. tube defect-related anomaly of vertebra
    n. tumor
neuralgia
    adhesive n.
    brachial n.
    geniculate n.
    glossopharyngeal n.
    intercostal n. (ICN)
    Morton n.
    obturator n.
    occipital n.
    prepatellar n.
    saphenous n.
    sciatic n.
    stump n.

    supraorbital n.
    tension n.
    traumatic prepatellar n.
    trigeminal n. (TGN)
    vagoglossopharyngeal n.
    vidian n.
neuralgic amyotrophy
neurapraxia
    cervical cord n. (CCN)
    Seddon n.
    traction n.
    transient n.
neurasthenia
neuraxial compression
neurectomy, neuroectomy
    adductor tenotomy and obturator n. (ATON)
    Eggers n.
    Morton n.
    motor n.
    obturator n.
    Phelps n.
    ulnar motor n.
neurilemmoma
neurinoma
neuritic
    n. amyotrophy
    n. atrophy
neuritides (*pl. of* neuritis)
neuritis, *pl.* **neuritides**
    axial n.
    brachial n.
    obturator nerve n.
    peripheral n.
    pudendal n.
    radicular n.
    sciatic n.
    suprascapular n.
    sural n.
    wallet n.
neuroablation
    cryogenic n.
neuroablative
Neuro-Aide testing device
neuroanastomosis
neuroarthropathic foot
neuroarthropathy
    atrophic n.
    Charcot n.
neuroarticular
    n. dysfunction
    n. subluxation
    n. syndrome
Neurobehavioral Functioning Inventory (NFI)
neurobiology
neuroblastoma
neurocentral synchondrosis
neurocirculation

N

NeuroCom
    N. Balance Master
    N. Equitest System
neurocompressive disorder
neurocutaneous hand flap
neurodermatitis
neurodevelopmental
    n. approach
    n. training
    n. treatment (NDT)
NeuroDrape surgical drape
neurodystrophic
neuroectodermal tumor
neuroectomy (*var. of* neurectomy)
neuroendocrine-immune connection
neurofibroma
    multiple n.
    nonplexiform cutaneous n.
    plexiform n.
neurofibromatosis
    forme of n.
    n. kyphoscoliosis
    kyphoscoliosis secondary to n.
    muscular n.
    n. (type 1, 2)
neurofibrosarcoma
neurofibrositis
neurofunctional subluxation
neurogenetic (*var. of* neurogenic)
neurogenic, neurogenetic, neurogenous
    n. arthrogryposis
    n. atrophy
    n. bladder (NGB)
    n. bowel
    n. claudication
    n. disease
    n. disorder
    n. fracture
    n. motor evoked potential (NMEP)
    n. scoliosis
    n. shock
    n. syndrome
    n. torticollis
neurogenous (*var. of* neurogenic)
neurography
    magnetic resonance n. (MRN)
neuroimmune hypothesis
neuroleptanalgesia
neuroleptic
neurologic
    n.
    n. assessment
    n. complication
    n. deficit
    n. deterioration
    n. disorder
    n. examination
    n. function
    n. pain

neurological (*var. of* neurologic)
    n. nerve conduction velocity examination
    n. physical therapy
    n. testing
neurologically intact
neurolysis
    alcohol n.
    chemical n.
    distal n.
    epidural n.
    external n.
    interfascicular n.
    internal n.
    intrathecal n.
    Morton neuroma n.
    motor n.
    phenol n.
neurolytic block
neuroma, *pl.* **neuromata, neuromas**
    amputation stump n.
    bulb n.
    cutaneous n.
    dorsal n.
    false n.
    incisional n.
    n. in continuity
    interdigital n. (IDN)
    Morton n.
    Morton interdigital n.
    posttraumatic n.
    refractory n.
    n. sign
    spindle n.
    stump n.
    sural n.
    traumatic n.
neuromas (*pl. of* neuroma)
neuromata (*pl. of* neuroma)
neuromatosis
neuromatous
neuromechanical
    n. correction
    n. lesion
    n. spinal chiropractic management
neuromeningeal pathway
neuromuscular
    n. block
    n. component
    n. disease
    n. electrical stimulation (NMES)
    n. electrical stimulation therapy
    n. facilitation
    n. gait pattern
    n. gait pattern change
    n. hamartoma
    n. III stimulator
    n. junction disorder
    n. proprioceptive process

n. reflex treatment
n. scoliosis
n. scoliosis orthotic treatment
n. transfer
neuromusculoskeletal
neuromyotonia
neuromyotonic discharge
neuron, neurone
fusimotor n.
serotonergic n.
neurone (*var. of* neuron)
neuronitis
Parsonage-Turner n.
neuropathic
n. ankle
n. arthritis
n. arthropathy (NA)
n. collapse
n. foot
n. foot deformity
n. forefoot ulceration
n. fracture
n. hyperkyphoscoliosis
n. joint
n. joint disease
n. joint dislocation
n. knee
n. motor unit potential
n. osteoarthropathy
n. recruitment
n. spinal arthropathy
n. ulcer
neuropathogenic
neuropathophysiology
normalization of n.
neuropathy
alcoholic n.
amyloid n.
brachial plexus n.
chemotherapy-related n.
compressive n.
diabetic n.
entrapment n.
epineurial n.
epineurial-perineurial n.
fascicular n.
femoral n.
hereditary motor sensory n.
  (HMSN)
hip pocket n.
hypertrophic interstitial n.
median n.
motor n.
motor and sensory n. (I, II)
periepineurial n.
peroneal n.
porphyritic n.
radiation-related n.
spontaneous median n.

sural n.
ulnar n.
neurophysiologic
n. effect
n. monitoring
neurophysiology
neuroplasty
neuroprosthesis
neuropsychological screening
neuroreflexive
neurorrhaphy
epineurial n.
perineurial n.
neuroses (*pl. of* neurosis)
neurosis, *pl.* **neuroses**
low back n.
torsion n.
neuroskeletal
neurostimulator
Biotens n.
Grass n.
responsive n.
Staodyne EMS + 2 n.
neurosuture
neurosyphilis
neurotendinous
neurotherapy
manual reflex n.
neurothlipsis
neuroticism
neurotization
neurotmesis
Seddon n.
neurotomy
neurotraumatic mechanism
neurotripsy
neurotrophic
n. atrophy
n. factor
n. food ulcer
n. fracture
n. joint
n. ulceration
Neurotube bioabsorbable nerve conduit
neurovascular
n. anatomy
n. bundle
n. complication
n. corn
n. dystrophy
n. free flap
n. hilum
n. impairment
n. injury
n. island graft
n. status (NVS)
n. structure
neurovasculare
heloma n.

N

neurovascularly intact
neutral
- n. angle
- n. anteversion
- n. drill guide
- n. hip position
- n. hook
- n. position splint
- n. rotation
- n. triangle
- n. wrist curl
- n. zone

neutralisation (*var. of* neutralization)
neutralization, neutralisation
- anterior n.
- n. parameter
- n. plate
- n. plate fixation

neutron radiography
nevi (*pl. of* nevus)
Neviaser
- N. acromioclavicular technique
- N. arthroplasty
- N. classification of frozen shoulder
- N. frozen shoulder classification
- N. old shoulder dislocation operation
- N. portal
- N. test

Nevin ankle brace
nevoid histiocytoma
nevus, naevus, *pl.* **nevi**
- balloon cell n.
- blue n.
- compound n.
- congenital n.
- despotic n.
- halo n.
- junctional n.
- neural n.

new
- n. bone
- n. bone formation
- N. England Baptist (NEB)
- N. England Baptist acetabular cup
- N. England Baptist hip arthroplasty
- N. England scoliosis brace
- n. happy bur
- N. Jersey ankle
- N. Jersey hemiarthroplasty prosthesis
- N. Jersey LCS shoulder prosthesis
- N. Jersey LCS total knee prosthesis
- N. Mind Set toe splint
- N. Schwinn 900 bicycle
- N. Schwinn elliptical bicycle
- N. York diagnostic criteria
- N. York diagnostic criteria classification

- N. York diagnostic criteria for rheumatoid arthritis
- N. York Orthopaedic front-opening orthosis
- N. York University (NYU)
- N. York University orthotic insert

NewBridge laminoplasty fixation system
newer-generation device
Newington
- N. brace
- N. orthosis

newly woven bone
Newman
- N. plate
- N. radial fracture
- N. radial neck and head fracture classification

Newman-Keuls procedure
new-onset limp
Newport
- N. hip system
- N. MC hip orthosis
- N. MC hip orthosis brace

Newton
- N. ankle prosthesis
- N. force

newtonian body
newton-meter
89-newton test
Nexerciser Plus
NexGen
- N. complete knee replacement system
- N. complete knee system
- N. component
- N. knee implant
- N. LPS Flex-Mobile bearing knee
- N. LPS-Mobile bearing knee
- N. offset stem extension

Nex-Link spinal fixation system
Nextep knee brace
Nexus
- N. hip prosthesis
- N. implant
- N. wheelchair seating system

NFI
- Neurobehavioral Functioning Inventory

NFS
- neural foraminal stenosis

NGB
- neurogenic bladder

NIAMS
- National Institute of Arthritis and Musculoskeletal and Skin Diseases

N'ice
- N. Stretch night splint
- N. Stretch night splint suspension system with Sealed Ice

NICHD
National Institute for Child Health and Human Development
Nicholas
N. corococlavicular congenital knee dislocation ligament technique
N. 5-in-1 knee reconstruction technique
N. 5-in-1 reconstruction
N. manual muscle tester
Nickelplast blank
nickel-titanium (NiTi)
Nicola
N. arthroplasty
N. forceps
N. incision
N. scissors
N. shoulder operation
N. shoulder tenodesis procedure
Nicoladoni suture
Nicolet Compass EMG instrument
Nicoll
N. bone
N. bone replacement material
N. cancellous bone graft
N. cancellous insert graft
N. extractor
N. fracture reconstruction
N. fracture repair procedure
N. plate
N. rasp
N. spinal fracture classification
N. tendon prosthesis
nicotinamide-adenine dinucleotide phosphate (NADPH)
nidi (*pl. of* nidus)
NIDJD
noninflammatory degenerative joint disease
nidus, *pl.* **nidi**
radiolucent n.
Niebauer
N. finger-joint replacement prosthesis
N. implant
N. metacarpophalangeal joint silastic prosthesis
N. trapeziometacarpal arthroplasty
N. trapezium replacement prosthesis
Niebauer-Cutter
N.-C. implant
N.-C. prosthesis
Niebauer-King congenital knee dislocation open reduction technique
Niemann-Pick disease
Nievergelt-Pearlman syndrome
nifedipine
niger
Aspergillus n.

night
n. brace
n. splint
n. splinting
N. Splint support
Nightimer carpal tunnel support
nightstick fracture
night-walker fracture
nigricans
acanthosis n.
Nikon SMZ 2T magnifying lens
Nilsson lateral ankle stabilization procedure
Nimmo receptor-tonus technique
ninhydrin print sweat test
nipper
English anvil nail n.
House-Dieter malleus n.
Miltex nail n.
n. nail drill
nipple
jogger's n.'s
Niro
N. bone-cutting forceps
N. wire-twisting forceps
Nirschl
N. lateral epicondylitis mini-open technique
N. tennis elbow release
Nirvana mattress
Nitalloy
2-nite
Sleepwell 2-n.
NiTi
nickel-titanium
NiTi alloy
nitidus
lichen n.
Nitinol flexible wire
nitrate
silver n. ($AgNO_3$)
nitrofurantoin
nitrofurazone
nitrogen
n. balance
urinary n.
nitroglycerin
nitroprusside
Nitro wheelchair
Nizoral
NMEP
neurogenic motor evoked potential
NMES
neuromuscular electrical stimulation
NMES therapy
NMP
nail matrix phenolization
NMR
nuclear magnetic resonance

N

no
n. man's land of hand
n. touch rule
Nobel knee test
nociception
nociceptive
n. receptor
n. response
n. transmission
nociceptor
n. agent
angry backfiring C n.
bombardment by n.
NOCSAE
National Operating Committee on Standards for Athletic Equipment
nocturnal myoclonus
node
Bouchard n.
gouty n.
Haygarth n.
Heberden n.
Meynet n.
n. of Ranvier
Osler n.
Parrot n.
Schmorl n.
nodosa
arthritis n.
panarteritis n.
polyarteritis n.
nodose rheumatism
nodosity
Heberden n.
nodular
n. fasciitis
n. melanoma
n. myositis
n. neoformation
n. tenosynovitis
nodularity
tendon n.
nodulation
nodule
Bouchard n.
Lisch n.
rheumatoid n.
Schmorl n.
synovial n.
tendon n.
NOF
nonossifying fibroma
NoHands Mouse-Foot-Operated Computer Mouse System
Noiles
N. fully constrained tricompartmental knee prosthesis
N. hinge
N. posterior stabilized knee
N. rotating hinge knee
N. rotating hinge knee mechanism
noir
tache n.
talon n.
noise
endplate n.
Nolan system collimator mounted contact shield
No-Lok
N.-L. bolt
N.-L. screw
N.-L. self-locking nail
nomenclature
dynamic listing n.
static listing n.
nomogram
nonabsorbable suture
nonadherent gauze dressing
nonambulation
no-name, no-fame bursa
nonarticular
n. arthritis
n. distal radial fracture
nonaugmented repair
nonbeaded guidepin
nonbeveled
nonbipedal
noncannulated nail
noncemented total hip arthroplasty
noncollared press-fit femoral stem implantation
noncompliance
noncompressive myelopathy
noncongruent metatarsophalangeal joint
noncontact manipulation
noncontained
n. disc
n. disc herniation
noncontiguous fracture
noncontractile
nondegenerative spondylolisthesis
nondepolarizing block
nondermatomal pattern
nondisplaced fracture
nondissociative
carpal instability n. (CIND)
nondynamometric
n. trunk performance test
n. trunk strength measurement
nonenzymatic connective tissue glycation
nonfenestrated stem
nonfluency
non-fused arthrodesis
nonfusion spine implant
nonglabrous skin
nonhinged
n. knee prosthesis
n. linked prosthesis

nonimpulsed base nerve transmission
noninflammatory degenerative joint
  disease (NIDJD)
noninstrumented anterior cervical
  discectomy
non-insulin-dependent diabetes
  mellitus
noninvasive
  n. halo
  lower extremity n.
  n. technique
nonisometric graft
nonlamellar bone
nonlamellated bone
nonlinear lesion
nonloadbearing
  n. bone fracture
  n. fractured bone
nonloop fixation
nonmanipulable subluxation
nonnarcotic analgesic
nonobscured anatomy
nonoperative
  n. orthopaedic management
  n. treatment
nonorganic physical sign
nonosseous
  n. tarsal coalition
  n. tissue trauma
nonossified tarsal navicular cartilage
nonossifying fibroma (NOF)
nonosteoconductive bonevoid filler
nonosteogenic fibroma
nonphysial fracture
nonpitting edema
nonplexiform cutaneous neurofibroma
nonporous-coated endoprosthesis
nonporous sheet
nonpreferred leg
nonradicular pattern
nonreactive nonunion
nonreamed nail
nonreconstructable
nonreplantable amputation
nonrigid connector
nonrotational burst fracture
nonself-tapping screw
nonspasmodic torticollis
nonspecific
  n. arthralgia
  n. cardiomyopathy
nonstanding lateral oblique view
nonstenotic cervical myelopathy
nonsteroidal
  n. antiinflammatory drug (NSAID)
  n. antiinflammatory medication
nonstriated muscle
nonstructural curve
nonsubluxated metatarsophalangeal joint

nonsubperiosteal cortical defect
nonsuppurative
  n. osteitis
  n. osteomyelitis
nonsurgical management
nonthermal modality
nonthreaded
  n. pin
  n. wire
nonthrust mobilization
nontotal-contact disorder
nontraumatic
  n. idiopathic osteonecrosis
  n. synovitis
nontubed
  n. closed distant flap graft
  n. open distant flap graft
nontuberculous mycobacterial
  infection
nonunion
  aseptic hypertrophic n.
  atrophic n.
  avascular n.
  bayonet n.
  bioelectrical repair of delayed union
    or n.
  defect n.
  draining infected n.
  dry infected n.
  elephant-foot fracture n.
  fracture fragment n.
  n. fracture trauma
  gap n.
  hamate hook n.
  horse-hoof fracture n.
  n. horse-hoof fracture
  hypertrophic vital n.
  hypervascular n.
  n. incidence
  infected nondraining n.
  n. long-bone fracture
  metaphysial-articular n.
  nonreactive n.
  n. of fracture site
  oligotrophic fracture n.
  n. osteomyelitis
  n. rate
  reactive n.
  scaphoid n.
  supracondylar n.
  symptomatic n.
  synovial n.
  talar body n.
  torsion wedge fracture n.
  n. torsion wedge fracture
  vascular n.
  wedge n.
nonunited fracture
nonwalking cast

N

nonweightbearing
- n. brace
- n. crutch walk
- n. crutch walking
- n. view
- n. x-ray

Nora lesion
19-norandrosterone
Norcet
Norco
NORD
- National Organization for Rare Disorders

NordiCare
- N. Back Therapy System
- N. Enabler exerciser
- N. Strider exerciser

NordicTrack
- N. Motion Analyzer
- N. ski exerciser

no-reflow phenomenon
Norflex
norfloxacin
Norgaard both hands view
Norgesic Forte
Norian SRS cement
Noritate Cream
Norland
- N. bone densitometer
- N. bone densitometry

normal
- n. anatomic position
- n. last shoe
- n. lordotic curve
- upper limits of n.

normalization of neuropathophysiology
Normalize press-fit hip prosthesis
Norman
- N. tibial bolt
- N. tibial pin

Normiflo
normoxia
Norm testing and rehabilitation system
Norpramin
north
- N. American blastomycosis
- N. American leech
- N. American Malignant Hyperthermia protocol
- N. American Riding for Handicapped Association (NARHA)

Northville brace
Northwick
- N. Park Index
- N. Park Index of Independence in ADL

Norton
- N. ball reamer
- N. scale

nortriptyline
Norwich press-fit prosthesis
Norwood iliotibial band tenodesis
nose
- anteater n.
- squashed n.

no-stretch RocketSoc brace
notariorum
- paralysis n.

notch
- acetabular n.
- A-frame n.
- clavicular n.
- coracoid n.
- costal n.
- cotyloid n.
- cuboid n.
- n. cut
- n. cutting guide
- incisural n.
- interclavicular n.
- intercondylar n.
- interpeduncular n.
- intervertebral n.
- radial sigmoid n.
- scapular n.
- sciatic n.
- semilunar n.
- sigmoid n.
- spinoglenoid n.
- suprasternal n.
- trochlear n.
- ulnar n.
- vertebral n.
- n. view
- n. width index (NWI)

notcher device
notching technique
notchplasty
- n. blade
- n. procedure

Nothnagel acroparesthesia
no-tie stretch lace
notochord
- persistent n.

no-touch technique
Nottingham Extended ADL index
nourished
NovaBone Bioglass bone grafting material
Novagel gel sheet
Novation ceramic articulation hip system
Novio Magus bone mill
Novocain Injection
Novus
- N. LC threaded interbody fusion cage
- N. LT titanium threaded interbody fusion cage

Noyes flexion rotation drawer knee test
nozzle
 suction n.
NPRS
 numerical pain rating system
NPWT
 negative pressure wound therapy
NRM
 nucleus raphe magnus
NRS
 numeric rating scale
NS
 Mycocide NS
 Stadol NS
NSA
 neck-shaft angle
NSAID
 nonsteroidal antiinflammatory
 drug
NSCIA
 National Spinal Cord Injury
 Association
NSED
 Namaqualand spondyloepiphysial
 dysplasia
N-telopeptide
N-Terface dressing
Nu
 N. Gauze bandage
 N. Gauze dressing
 N. Gauze packing
Nubain
nubbin
nuchal
 n. ligament
 n. region
 n. rigidity
nuclear
 n. arthrogram
 n. magnetic resonance
 (NMR)
 n. magnetic resonance scan
nucleatum
 Fusobacterium n.
nuclei (*pl. of* nucleus)
nucleoplasty wand
nucleotome
 N. probe
 N. system
nucleotomy
 laser n.
 percutaneous n.
nucleus, *pl.* **nuclei, nucleuses**
 n. dehydration
 force n.
 intermediolateral n.
 intermediomedial n.
 periaqueductal gray n.
 prosthetic disc n. (PDN)

 n. pulposus
 pulpy n.
 n. raphe magnus (NRM)
 sacral autonomic n. (SAN)
nucleuses (*pl. of* nucleus)
nudge
 n. control
 n. control on prosthesis
Nu-Knit absorbable hemostat
NuKO knee orthosis
numerical pain rating system
 (NPRS)
numeric rating scale (NRS)
Numorphan
Nuprin
NuPulse device
Nurick
 N. classification of spondylosis
 N. spondylosis classification
Nurolon suture
nursemaid's elbow
Nussbaum bracelet
NuStep
 N. exerciser
 N. total body recumbent stepper
nut
 n. alignment guide
 Close Encounter n.
 Kirschner traction bow n.
 locking n.
 nylon n.
 traction bow n.
 VDS hex n.
nutation
 counter n.
nutcracker
 n. fracture
 n. injury
 n. sign
NutraFill hydrophilic dressing
NutraStat wound dressing
nutrient
 n. artery
 n. flap
nutrition
 parenteral n.
 tissue n.
 total parenteral n. (TPN)
nutritional osteomalacia
NUV
 negative ulnar variance
Nuwave transcutaneous electrical nerve
 stimulator
NVS
 neurovascular status
NWI
 notch width index
NX
 Talwin NX

N

Nylatex
> N. strap
> N. wrap

Nylok self-locking nail

nylon
> n. monofilament
> n. nut
> n. suture
> n. teaspoon

Nytol
> Maximum Strength N.
> N. Oral

NYU
> New York University
> NYU orthosis insert

NYU-Hosmer
> NYU-H. electric elbow
> NYU-H. prehension actuator

OA
  opioid antagonist
  opsonic activity
  osteoarthritis
      OA knee brace
OAdjuster knee brace
OAR
  Ottawa ankle rule
oarsman's wrist
OAS
  Oral Analogue Scale
OASIS
  osteotomy analysis simulation software
  Outcome and Assessment Information
      Set
Oasis wound dressing
OAsys knee brace
oath hand
OATS
  osteochondral autograft transfer system
      OATS graft
      OATS procedure
      OATS technique
OAV
  oculoauriculovertebral
      OAV dysplasia
OAVD
  oculoauriculovertebral dysplasia
OAWO
  opening abductory wedge osteotomy
Ober
  O. anterior tendon transfer
  O. hip physical therapy release
  O. iliotibial band test
  O. incision
  O. operation
  O. posterior drainage
  O. tendon transfer for footdrop
      technique
obese
  o. bed
  o. knee osteoarthritis
  o. support
  o. walker
objective sign
OBLA
  onset of blood lactate accumulation
obligate translation
oblique
  o. amputation
  o. bandage
  o. closing wedge osteotomy
      (OCWO)
  o. displacement
  o. facet wiring

  o. fracture
  o. incision
  medial o.
  o. meniscal tear
  o. metacarpal line
  o. metatarsocuneiform joint
  o. midtarsal joint axis (OMJA)
  o. muscle
  o. osteotomy for tibial deformity
  o. osteotomy with derotation
  o. popliteal ligament
  o. proximal phalangeal osteotomy
  o. retinacular ligament
  o. retinacular ligament tightness test
  o. screw insertion
  o. slide osteotomy
  o. view
  o. wire
  o. wiring facet
obliquity
  o. fracture
  pelvic o.
  reverse o.
obliquus
  vastus medialis o. (VMO)
obliterans
  arteriosclerosis o.
  endarteritis o.
obliterating endarteritis
oblong polyethylene acetabular cup
O₂Boot
OBPI
  obstetric brachial plexus injury
O'Brien
  O. bone clamp
  O. capsular shift procedure
  O. goniometer
  O. pelvic halo operation
  O. radial fracture classification
  O. rib hook
  O. shoulder active compression test
  O. staple
observation hip
obstetric
  o. brachial plexus injury (OBPI)
  o. hand
obstetrician's hand
obtecta
  pelvis o.
obturator
  o. artery
  o. avulsion fracture
  blunt o.
  conical o.
  core biopsy o.

O

obturator (*continued*)
    o. externus muscle
    o. internus muscle
    o. internus tendon
    Keene o.
    o. membrane
    o. nerve
    o. nerve injury
    o. nerve neuritis
    o. neuralgia
    o. neurectomy
    o. oblique view
    o. sign
    o. sleeve
    o. sulcus
obturator/brim line
Obus back support
Obwegeser
    O. sagittal mandibular osteotomy
    O. sagittal mandibular osteotomy
      technique
Obwegeser-Dalpont internal screw
  fixation
OCAIRS
    Occupational Circumstances Assessment
    Interview Rating Scale
occipital
    o. bone
    o. condyle
    o. condyle fracture
    o. neuralgia
    o. region
occipital-atlantal joint
occipital-atlantoaxial complex
occipital-axis joint
occipital-fiber analysis
occipitoatlantal dislocation
occipitoatlantoaxial
    o. fusion
    o. joint
    o. joint complex
occipitocervical
    o. angle
    o. arthrodesis
    o. articulation
    o. fixation
    o. fusion
    o. junction
    o. lordosis
    o. plate
    o. stabilization
occluder
    multiple pinhole o.
Occlusal-HP wart medication
occlusal splint
occlusive dressing
occult
    o. fracture
    o. primary malignant tumor

    o. sacral fracture
    o. talar lesion
occulta
    spina bifida o. (SBO)
occupation
    sedentary o.
occupational
    o. and environmental medicine
      (OEM)
    o. behavior
    O. Circumstances Assessment
      Interview Rating Scale (OCAIRS)
    O. Performance History Interview
      (OPHI)
    O. Questionnaire (OQ)
    o. rating
    o. risk
    o. role
    o. science
    o. stress syndrome (OSS)
    o. therapy (OT)
    O. Therapy Activities of Daily
      Living (OTADL)
occupation-related disorder
OCD
    osteochondritis dissecans
ochronosis
ochronotic
    o. arthritis
    o. arthropathy
OCL
    Orthopaedic Casting Laboratory
    OCL volar splint
O'Connor
    O. finger dexterity test
    O. operating arthroscope
    O. tweezer dexterity test
OCT
    optimal cutting temperature
    OCT compound
OctaFix occipital fixation system
octagon roll
Octocaine Injection
octopus holder
OCTR
    open carpal tunnel release
ocular
    o. prosthesis
    o. scoliosis
    o. sign
oculoauriculovertebral (OAV)
    o. dysplasia (OAVD)
oculoplethysmography
Ocutricin Topical Ointment
OCWO
    oblique closing wedge osteotomy
Oden peroneal tendon subluxation
  classification
Odland ankle prosthesis

ODM
opponens digiti minimi
O'Donoghue
O. ACL reconstruction
O. cervical muscle strain test
O. cotton cast
O. dressing
O. facetectomy
O. knee splint
O. stirrup splint
O. triad knee repair procedure
triad of O.
unhappy triad of O.
odontoid
o. agenesis
o. condyle
o. condyle fracture
o. fracture internal fixation
o. fracture stabilization
o. hypoplasia
o. osteotomy
o. perpendicular line
o. process
o. process osteosynthesis
o. x-ray view
odontoid-axial area
odontoidectomy
ODQ
opponens digiti quinti
O'Driscoll posterolateral pivot test
OEC
Orthopedic Equipment Company
outdoor emergency car
OEC knee immobilizer
OEC lag screw component
OEC lag screw component with keyway
OEC Mini 6600 imaging system
OEC popliteal pad
OEC splint
OEC wrist/forearm support
Oehler symptom
OEM
occupational and environmental medicine
Oesch hook
off-axis bone damage
offloading knee brace
offset
o. cane
o. cap
o. drill hole
femoral o.
head-stem o.
o. hinge
o. link
medial head-stem o.
o. suspension feeder

offset-V
o.-V osteotomy
o.-V procedure
ofloxacin
Ogata technique
Ogden
O. Anchor soft tissue device
O. bone anchor
O. construct Ogden construct
O. epiphysial fracture classification
O. fracture classification system
O. knee dislocation classification
O. plate
O. plate system
O. tissue reattachment mini system
Ogee acetabular component
OGI
osteoarthritis global index
Ogival interbody cage (O.I.C.)
Ogston
O. line
O. operation
Oh
O. cemented hip prosthesis
O. press-fit hip prosthesis
Ohio
O. Medical Instruments (OMI)
O. Medical Instruments loop
Oh-Spectron prosthesis
OI
osteogenesis imperfecta
O.I.C.
Ogival interbody cage
O.I.C. PEEK cage implant
OIC
osteogenesis imperfecta congenita
OIF
Osteogenesis Imperfecta Foundation
oil
Decubitene oxygenated o.
massage o.
trypsin, balsam peru, and castor o.
ointment
Cortisporin topical o.
Dermagran o.
Elase-Chloromycetin o.
Eucalyptamint arthritis pain o.
Kerasal o.
Medi-Quick Topical O.
Neosporin Topical O.
Ocutricin Topical O.
Panafil o.
Panafil-White o.
papain, urea, chlorophyllin copper complex sodium o. (PUC)
PUC healing, debriding, and deodorizing o.

O

ointment (*continued*)
    Septa Topical O.
    Travase o.
    Whitfield's O.
OIT
    osteogenesis imperfecta tarda
Oklahoma
    O. ankle joint
    O. ankle joint orthosis
    O. ankle prosthesis
    O. cable system
OKQ
    Osteoporosis Knowledge
    Questionnaire
old
    o. fracture
    o. man's back
    o. smoothie bur
    o. unreduced dislocation
Olds pin
olecranal
olecranarthritis
olecranarthrocace
olecranarthropathy
olecranization
olecranoid
olecranon
    o. bursa
    o. bursitis
    o. fossa
    o. ligament
    o. osteochondritis
    o. process
    o. region
    o. tip fracture
oleic acid
oleoma
Olerud
    O. and Molander fracture
    classification
    O. ankle fracture clinical and
    radiologic score
    O. internal fixator
    O. pedicle fixation system
    O. PSF fixation system
    O. PSF rod
    O. PSF screw
    O. transpedicular fixation
oligoarthritis
    undifferentiated o.
oligoarticular
    o. arthritis
    o. disease
oligodendroglioma
oligotrophic fracture nonunion
olisthesis
    anterior o.
    degenerative o.
    lumbar o.

    progressive o.
    rotatory o.
olisthetic vertebra
olisthy
Olivecrona
    O. clip-applying and removing
    forceps
    O. rasp
olive-shaped bur
olive wire
Ollier
    O. approach
    O. arthrodesis approach
    O. disease
    O. dyschondroplasia
    O. incision
    O. lateral hip approach
    O. law
    O. layer
    O. operation
    O. osteochondromatosis
    O. rake retractor
    O. technique
    O. thick split free graft
Ollier-Thiersch skin graft
OLT
    osteochondral lesion of talus
O'Malley jaw fracture splint
Ombredanne mallet
Omed vented instrument guard
omega
    O. compression hip screw
    system
    O. Plus compression hip system
    O. splinting material
Omega-3 dietary supplement
omental flap
Omer-Capen carpectomy
OMI
    Ohio Medical Instruments
    OMI loop
OMJA
    oblique midtarsal joint axis
Ommaya
    O. reservoir device
    O. reservoir implant material
Omni
    O. knee brace
    O. Roller massager
Omniace RT3200N electromyographic amplifier
Omniderm dressing
Omnifit
    O. dual geometry microstructured
    prosthesis
    O. HA hip stem prosthesis
    O. HA hip stent
    O. knee prosthesis
    O. Plus hip system

O. PSL microstructured prosthesis
O. stem
O. total knee system

Omnifit-C stem

OmniFlex
O. hip prosthesis
O. knee orthosis

Omni-Flexor
O.-F. device
O.-F. wrist exerciser

Omnisense 7000S bone sonometer

Omnitron exercise testing

omoclavicular

omodynia

omohyoid
o. muscle
o. syndrome

omosternum

Omotrain active shoulder support

omovertebral bone

OMS Concentrate Oral

OMT
osteomanipulative therapy
osteopathic manipulative therapy

Oncovin injection

one
o. and one-half spica cast
o. wound-one scar concept

One-Alpha

one-half
o.-h. patellar tendon transplant
o.-h. spica cast

one-stage correction of spastic dislocated hip

Ongoing Ambulating AFO boot

onlay
o. bone graft
o. bone graft cast
o. cancellous iliac graft

On-Q
O.-Q PainBuster postoperative pain relief system
O.-Q Soaker catheter

onset
delayed o.
o. frequency
o. latency
o. of blood lactate accumulation (OBLA)

Ontario Cohort of Running-Related Injury

OnTrack
O. system
O. treatment method

onychauxis

onychectomy

onychoclavus

onychocryptosis nail

onychodystrophy

onychogryphosis, onychogryposis

onychogryposis (*var. of* onychogryphosis)

onycholysis

onychomadesis

onychomycosis
Candida o.
proximal subungual o. (PSO)
subungual o.
superficial white o. (SWO)

onychomycotic toenail

onychoosteodysplasia
hereditary o.

onychophosis

onychotomy

Ony-Clear
O.-C. Nail
O.-C. Spray

onyxis

OP-1
osteogenic protein 1
OP-1 implant/bone graft
OP-1 putty spinal fusion implant
OP-1 TM bone implant

opaque
o. arthrography
o. myelography
o. synovium

OPC Synergy

open
o. amputation
o. base wedge osteotomy
o. base wedge osteotomy/bunionectomy
o. biopsy
o. body
o. bone graft epiphysiodesis
o. carpal tunnel release (OCTR)
o. C-D hook
o. condylar plate fixation
o. disc surgery
o. dislocation
o. double-decked hook cervical system
o. drainage
o. exit foramen
o. fracture
o. fracture (I, II, III, IIIA, IIIB, IIIC)
o. fracture wound drain
o. kinematic chain
o. kinetic chain exercise
o. medullary nailing
o. midline posterior approach
o. nail
o. palm technique
o. pinning
o. reduction
o. reduction and internal fixation (ORIF)

O

open (*continued*)
    o. reduction of fracture
    o. stabilization
    o. stabilization of traumatic anterior
      shoulder instability
    o. tenotomy
    o. wedge
    o. wound
open-air splint
open-book
    o.-b. fracture
    o.-b. pelvic injury
open-bowl cement technique
open-break fracture
open-chain exercise
open-door expansive laminaplasty
open-end wrench
opening
    o. abductory wedge osteotomy
      (OAWO)
    Sierra 2-load voluntary o.
    voluntary o. (VO)
    o. wedge manipulation
    o. wedge manipulation and
      reapplication of plaster
    o. wedge osteotomy
open-packed position
open-section nail
open-staple capsulorrhaphy
open-toe shoe
opera-glass hand
Operand
operating
    o. microscope
    o. room
    o. time
operation
    Abbe o.
    Abbott o.
    Abbott-Lucas shoulder o.
    Adams hip o.
    Adelmann hand o.
    Akin o.
    Albee o.
    Albee-Delbert o.
    Albert knee o.
    Alouette o.
    Amstutz resurfacing o.
    Anderson o.
    Annandale o.
    anterior ankle shift o.
    Armistead ulnar lengthening o.
    ASIF screw fixation o.
    Aufranc-Turner o.
    Auto-Implant o.
    Avila o.
    Axer foot o.
    Badgley cervical spine o.
    Baker translocation o.

Bankart o.
Bankart-Putti-Platt dislocated
  shoulder o.
Barker hallux valgus o.
Barr tendon transfer o.
Barsky cleft hand closure o.
Barwell knee o.
Bateman shoulder o.
Bent o.
Berger interscapulothoracic
  amputation o.
Bier o.
Blundell-Jones hip o.
Bora o.
Bosworth hip shelf o.
Boyd o.
Brahms foot o.
bridle posterior tibial tendon
  transfer o.
Bristow o.
Brittain o.
Brockman foot o.
Brooks cervical fusion o.
Broström-Gould ankle instability o.
Brown knee approach o.
Buck o.
Bunnell posterior tibial tendon
  transfer o.
Butler fifth toe o.
Campbell ankle o.
Carmody-Batson o.
Carnesale hip approach o.
Cave o.
centralization of radius o.
Chopart o.
Cloward cervical spine fusion o.
Cocklin toe o.
Codivilla o.
Cole o.
Colonna shelf o.
Compere o.
Conn o.
Contour DF-80 total hip o.
Cotrel-Dubousset derotation o.
Credo o.
Crutchfield o.
Cubbins o.
Davies-Colley o.
Diamond-Gould syndactyly o.
Dickson o.
Dickson-Diveley clinic foot o.
Dieffenbach o.
Dunn hip o.
Dupuytren o.
Durham flatfoot o.
DuVries modified McBride hallux
  valgus o.
Dwyer clawfoot o.
Eden-Hybbinette o.

Eggers o.
Ellis Jones peroneal tendon o.
Elmslie-Cholmeley foot o.
Elmslie peroneal tendon o.
Elmslie-Trillat patellar o.
Evans ankle joint instability o.
Farmer in utero myelomeningocele
  repair o.
flap o.
Fontan o.
French supracondylar fracture o.
Frost foot o.
Galeazzi patellar o.
Gant o.
Gardner o.
Gelman foot o.
Girdlestone o.
Grice-Green o.
Gritti o.
Guyon o.
Haas o.
Hammon foot o.
hanging hip o.
hanging toe o.
Hark foot o.
Hauser patellar o.
Hey o.
Heyman o.
Heyman-Herndon clubfoot o.
Hibbs o.
Hoffa o.
Hoffa-Lorenz o.
Hoffmann metatarsal o.
Hohmann o.
Hoke Achilles tendon lengthening o.
Holmes o.
Houston o.
I-beam hip o.
Inclan modification of Campbell
  ankle o.
inside-out Bankart shoulder
  instability o.
intermetatarsal angle-reducing o.
Jewett o.
Jones cock-up toe o.
Joplin o.
Juvara foot o.
Kapel o.
Keller foot o.
Keller hallux valgus o.
Kellogg-Speed o.
Kessler posterior tibial tendon
  transfer o.
Kidner foot o.
Kirkaldy-Willis o.
Kirk distal thigh o.
Kondoleon o.
Kortzeborn hand o.
Kraske o.

Kreuscher o.
Krukenberg hand o.
Lambrinudi dropfoot o.
Lange o.
Langenbeck o.
Lapidus o.
Larrey o.
lateral acetabular shelf o.
limb-sparing o.
Lisfranc o.
Liston o.
Littler o.
Lorenz o.
Luck o.
Ludloff o.
Lund o.
MacAusland o.
MacNab patella o.
Magnuson o.
Mallory-Head revision o.
Mauck o.
Mayer trapezius transfer o.
Mayo hallux valgus modified o.
Mazur o.
McBride bunion hallux valgus o.
McKeever o.
Mensor-Scheck hanging-hip o.
Mikulicz o.
Milch elbow o.
Miller flatfoot o.
Mital elbow release o.
Mitchell o.
modified Cocklin toe o.
Moe scoliosis o.
Mueller knee o.
muscle sliding o.
Nélaton o.
Neviaser old shoulder dislocation o.
Nicola shoulder o.
Ober o.
O'Brien pelvic halo o.
Ogston o.
Ollier o.
Osgood o.
Overholt o.
over-the-top knee o.
Paci o.
Pauwels o.
Pheasant elbow o.
Phelps o.
Phemister o.
Putti-Platt o.
resurfacing o.
reverse Mauck knee o.
revision total hip o.
Ridlon o.
Rose foot o.
Roux-Goldthwait o.
Sayre hip o.

O

operation (*continued*)
    screw fixation o.
    Selig interinnomino-abdominal hindquarter amputation o.
    Skoog Dupuytren contracture o.
    Smith-Robinson spinal fusion o.
    Sofield femoral deficiency o.
    Souter hip o.
    Stener-Gunterberg high sacral amputation o.
    Stewart arm o.
    subcutaneous o.
    Suppan foot o.
    Sutherland hip o.
    Syme ankle o.
    tharies hip replacement o.
    T-plasty modification of Bankart shoulder o.
    Vulpius equinus deformity o.
    Weaver-Dunn acromioclavicular o.
    West and Soto-Hall patella o.
    Woodward o.
    Zadik foot o.
    Zickel subtrochanteric fracture o.

operative
    o. ankylosis
    o. arthroscopy
    o. arthrotomy
    o. leg holder
    o. legholder
    o. roentgenogram
    o. site

O'Phelan technique

OPHI
    Occupational Performance History Interview

ophthalmic
    Voltaren O.

Ophthetic

opiate receptor antagonist

Opiela brace

opioid
    o. antagonist (OA)
    o. receptor

opisthenar

opisthotonic position

opium
    o. alkaloid
    belladonna and o.
    o. tincture

OPLL
    ossification of posterior longitudinal ligament

Opmi microscopic drape

Oppenheim
    O. amyotonia
    O. brace
    O. disease
    O. gait
    O. reflex
    O. sign
    O. syndrome

Oppenheimer
    O. sign
    O. spring wire
    O. spring wire splint
    O. with reverse knuckle-bender splint

Oppociser
    O. exercise device
    O. hand exerciser

opponens
    o. bar
    o. digiti minimi (ODM)
    o. digiti quinti (ODQ)
    o. digiti quinti muscle
    o. orthosis
    o. pollicis
    o. pollicis muscle
    o. splint
    o. transfer

opponensplasty
    abductor digiti minimi o.
    abductor digiti quinti o.
    Bunnell o.
    Camitz o.
    Goldmar o.
    Groves o.
    Huber adductor digiti quinti o.
    Littler o.
    Phalen-Miller o.
    ring sublimis o.
    Riordan finger o.

opposite
    o. foot-strike phase
    o. foot-strike phase of gait
    o. toe-off phase
    o. toe-off phase of gait

opposition
    o. contracture
    finger o.
    o. test
    thumb o.

Opraflex
    O. drape
    O. dressing

OpSite wound dressing

opsonic activity (OA)

Opteform
    O. bone graft material
    O. 100HT bone graft

Optetrak
    O. comprehensive knee system
    O. total knee replacement system

optical
    o. stereophotogrammetry
    o. trapping

Opti-Curve therapeutic pillow

Opti-Fix
O.-F. femoral prosthesis
O.-F. hip stem
O.-F. II acetabular cup
O.-F. I, II prosthesis
O.-F. total hip system
OptiLock
O. distal radius plating system
O. periarticular plating system
optimal
o. alignment
o. cutting temperature (OCT)
OptiMax Supreme pressure reduction mattress
optimizing motion palpation
option
O. hip system
O. Orthotic Series
optoelectric
o. measuring apparatus
o. measuring system
o. signal detection apparatus
Optotrak motion measurement system
OPTP
Orthopaedic Physical Therapy Products
OPTP Slant
OQ
Occupational Questionnaire
O'Rahilly limb deficiency classification
oral
AllerMax O.
O. Analogue Scale (OAS)
Ansaid O.
Anxanil o.
Banophen O.
Belix O.
Benadryl O.
Calciferol O.
Cataflam O.
Ceftin O.
Cipro O.
Cytoxan O.
Delta-Cortef O.
Dormarex 2 O.
Dormin O.
Drisdol O.
Genahist O.
o. incontinence
Lamisil O.
Medrol O.
MS Contin O.
MSIR O.
Neoral O.
o. nutritional supplement
Nytol O.
OMS Concentrate O.
Oramorph SR O.
Pediapred O.
Phendry O.

Prelone O.
Roxanol SR O.
Sandimmune O.
Siladryl O.
Sleep-eze 3 O.
Sominex O.
terbinafine, o.
Toradol O.
Twilite O.
Unipen O.
Valium O.
VePesid O.
Voltaren O.
Voltaren-XR O.
Oralet
Fentanyl O.
Oramorph SR Oral
Orasone
Oratec chisel
Orateck device
orbicular
o. ligament
o. zone
orbit
angular process of o.
Orbital shoulder stabilizer brace
Orbiter treadmill
orbitosphenoid bone
order of activation
ordinal classification
Oregon Poly II ankle prosthesis
Oretorp retractable knife
Orfit splint
Orfizip
O. body jacket
O. knee cast
O. wrist cast
organ
Golgi tendon o.
mechanoreceptor Golgi tendon o.
organic dysfunction
organization
homuncular o.
National Hospice O.
World Health O. (WHO)
organizational
o. phase
o. phase of tendon healing
Orgaran
orientation
phalangeal articular o.
visual o.
o. WHO Handicap Scale
ORIF
open reduction and internal fixation
origin
adductor o.
deltoid o.
fever of undetermined o. (FUO)

O

origin (*continued*)
    flexor-pronator o.
    tripartite muscle o.
original
    O. Backnobber massage tool
    O. Backnobber muscle massager
    O. Index Knobber II
    O. Index Knobber II massager
    O. Index Knobber II massage tool
    O. Jacknobber II muscle-massage
    device
Orion anterior cervical plate
Orlando hip-knee-ankle-foot orthosis
ORLAU
    Orthotic Research and Locomotor
    Assessment Unit
    ORLAU swivel walker
Orlon with Lycra stump sock
Ormandy screw
Ormco pin
oropharyngeal approach
Orozco plate
orphenadrine
    orphenadrine, aspirin, and caffeine
    o. citrate
Orphengesic
Orthairtome
    O. II drill
    O. wire driver
Orthawear antiembolism stockings
orthesis
orthetics (*var. of* orthotics)
Orth-evac
    O.-e. autotransfusion system
    O.-e. postoperative transfusion
    system
Orthex
    O. cannulated bone screw
    O. reliever insole
    O. Relievers shoe insert
Orthion traction machine
ortho
    Ortho DX electromedical stimulator
    Ortho DX stimulator for knee
    rehabilitation
    ortho physical therapy
Ortho-Arch II orthotic
orthobiologic implant
Ortho-Biotic recliner
OrthoBlast
    O. osteoinductive bioimplant
    O. paste
OrthoBlend powered bone mill
OrthoBone pillow
Ortho-Cel pad
Orthochrome
    O. implant metal
    O. implant metal prosthesis
Orthocomp cement

Orthocord suture
orthodigita
Orthodoc presurgical planning system
orthodox procedure
orthodromic velocity
OrthoDyn bone substitute material
Orthodyne Enhancer unit
Orthofit (9000, 9001) orthotic
Orthofix
    O. apparatus
    O. Cervical-Stim bone growth
    stimulator
    O. external fixation device
    O. intramedullary nail
    O. ISKD device
    O. M-100 distractor
    O. monolateral femoral external
    fixator
    O. Ogden anchor
    O. pin
    O. prosthesis
    O. screw
Orthoflex
    O. dressing
    O. elastic plaster bandage
Ortho-Foam
    O.-F. elbow/heel pad
    O.-F. protector
Orthofuse implantable growth stimulator
OrthoGel liner
OrthoGen bone growth stimulator
Orthogenesis LPS limb preservation
    prosthesis system
Ortho-Glass
    O.-G. splint
    O.-G. synthetic material
orthognathia, orthognathism
orthognathic, orthognathous
orthognathism (*var. of* orthognathia)
orthognathous (*var. of* orthognathic)
orthogonally placed suture
Ortho-Grip silicone rubber handle
Ortho-ice multipack
Ortho-Jel impression material
orthokinetic exercise
orthokinetics
    orthopaedic o.
    O. travel chair
Ortho-last splint
Ortholav
    O. irrigation and suction device
    O. jet
Ortholen sheet
Ortholign spinal orthosis
Ortholoc
    O. Advantim revision knee system
    O. Advantim total knee system
    O. II unconstrained prosthesis
    O. implant metal prosthesis

OrthoLogic
    O. 1000 bone growth stimulation
    O. 1000 bone growth stimulator
orthomechanical
orthomechanotherapy
Orthomedics
    O. brace
    O. Stretch and Heel splint
    O. Ultra-Guard hip orthosis
orthomelic
Orthomerica
    O. TC AFO system
    O. UFO
Orthomet
    O. Axiom total knee system
    O. Perfecta total hip system
Orthomite II adhesive
Ortho-Mold
    O.-M. lumbar body
    O.-M. spinal brace
    O.-M. splint
orthomolecular medicine/megavitamin therapy
orthonormal diameter
orthopaedic, orthopedic
    o. bed
    o. bone file
    o. broach
    o. bur
    O. Casting Laboratory (OCL)
    o. cement
    o. chisel
    o. curette
    o. cutting instrument
    o. depth gauge
    o. dynamometer
    o. evaluation
    o. felt
    o. forceps
    o. goniometer
    o. gouge
    o. hammer
    o. hardware
    o. hemostat
    o. impactor
    o. knife
    o. mallet
    o. orthokinetics
    o. osteotome
    o. oxford shoe
    O. Physical Therapy Products (OPTP)
    O. Positioning Seat
    o. propeller
    o. prosthesis
    o. rasp
    o. reamer
    o. rehabilitation
    o. retractor

    o. rongeur
    o. scissors
    o. shoulder elevator
    o. stockinette
    o. strap clavicular splint
    o. surgical file
    o. surgical pliers
    o. surgical stripper
    O. Systems Inc. (OSI)
    o. table
    O. Trauma Association (OTA)
    O. Trauma Association classification
    O. Trauma Association fracture classification
orthopaedics, orthopedics
    Advanta O.
    damage-control o.
    Encore O.
    evidence-based o.
    pediatric o.
    Sulzer O.
OrthoPak
    O. bone growth stimulator system
    O. II bone growth stimulator
Ortho-Pal body support
orthopantogram imaging
OrthoPAT system
orthopedic (*var. of* orthopaedic)
    O. Equipment Company (OEC)
orthopedics (*var. of* orthopaedics)
orthopercussion
Orthoplast
    O. dressing
    O. fracture brace
    O. isoprene splint
    O. jacket
    O. plastic
    O. slipper cast
orthoPLUG soft bone plug
orthopod
orthopraxis
orthopraxy
orthoRAP
    o. ankleRAP
    o. backRAP
    o. backRAP postsurgical wound wrap
    o. hipRAP
    o. hipRAP postsurgical wound wrap
    o. kneeRAP wrap
    o. postsurgical wound wrap
    o. shoulderRAP postsurgical wound wrap
    o. wristRAP postsurgical wound wrap
orthoroentgenogram
orthoroentgenography
orthoses (*pl. of* orthosis)
Orthoset radiopaque bone cement

O

orthosis, *pl.* **orthoses**
 abduction hip o.
 accommodative o.
 Adjustable Advanced Reciprocating
  Gait O. (ARGO)
 A-frame o.
 airplane splint o.
 AliCork Foot O.
 AliMed o.
 Aliplast custom-molded
  foot o.
 ambulation training o.
 Amfit custom o.
 ankle o.
 ankle contracture o.
 ankle-foot o. (AFO)
 ankle-foot plastic o.
 ankle stabilizing o. (ASO)
 anteroposterior control o.
 Anti-Shox o.
 Atlanta brace o.
 Atlanta-Scottish Rite abduction o.
 bail-lock knee joint o.
 balanced forearm o. (BFO)
 balance padding o.
 bar-and-shoe o.
 Bauerfeind Malleolic Ankle O.
 Beaufort seating o.
 Bebax o.
 Bennett o.
 BioCast wrist/hand o.
 Biothotic foot o.
 Boston brace thoracolumbosacral o.
 Boston postoperative hip o.
 cable-twister o.
 calcaneal spur cookie o.
 Caligamed ankle o.
 caliper o.
 Canadian Knee O.
 CASH thoracolumbosacral o.
 C-bar o.
 cervical o.
 cervical thoracic o.
 cervicothoracic o. (CTO)
 cervicothoracolumbosacral o.
  (CTLSO)
 chairback lumbosacral o.
 clavicle o.
 cock-up splint o.
 Comfy Elbow O.
 Comfy knee o.
 Controller shoulder o.
 copolymer ankle-foot o.
 corrective o.
 Craig-Scott o.
 cranial remolding o.
 cruciform anterior spinal
  hyperextension o.
 Daytona cervical o.

 DDH o.
 Denis Browne bar foot o.
 developmental dislocated hip o.
 Diabetic D-Sole foot o.
 dial-lock o.
 dorsiflexion assist ankle joint
  ankle-foot o.
 o. drop-lock ring
 dual-photon electrospinal o.
 DuraBoot o.
 Dynamic elbow o.
 Dynamic foot o.
 Dynamic knee o.
 Dynamic wrist o.
 elastic knee cage o.
 elastic twister o.
 elbow o.
 elbow-wrist-hand o. (EWHO)
 Engen extension o.
 Engen palmar finger o.
 externally powered tenodesis o.
 E-Z arm abduction o.
 figure-of-8 thoracic o.
 Fillauer bar foot o.
 FirmFlex custom o.
 Flex Foam o.
 flexible o.
 flexion-extension control cervical o.
 flexor hinge o.
 floor-reaction ankle-foot o.
 foot o.
 Foot Levelers o.
 Frejka pillow o.
 front-opening o.
 Gator plastic o.
 Gillette joint o.
 Gillette modification of
  ankle-foot o.
 GunSlinger shoulder o.
 G/W Heel Lift, Inc. o.
 hallux valgus o.
 halo cervical o.
 halo extension o.
 halo traction o.
 halo-vest o.
 hand o.
 heat-molded petroplastic
  ankle-foot o.
 hindfoot o.
 hip o.
 hip guidance o. (HGO)
 hip-knee-ankle-foot o. (HKAFO)
 Hosmer VC 4-bar knee o.
 hyperextension o.
 Hyperex thoracic o.
 Ilfeld splint o.
 Ipomax o.
 Ipos forefoot relief o.
 Ipos heel relief o.

ischial weightbearing o.
J-24 cervical o.
J-45 contraflexion o.
Jewett-Benjamin cervical o.
Jewett contraflexion o.
Jewett hyperextension o.
Jewett postfusion o.
Jewett thoracolumbosacral o.
J-35 hyperextension o.
Jousto dropfoot splint, skid o.
J-55 postfusion o.
Kallassy o.
Kid-Dee-Lite o.
Klenzak o.
knee o.
knee-ankle-foot o. (KAFO)
knee extension o.
knee management o.
Knight-Taylor thoracolumbosacral o.
Kosair Scoliosis O. (KSO)
Kydex chairback o.
L.A. cervical o.
leather o.
Legg-Perthes disease o.
Lenox Hill knee o.
Lerman multiligamentous knee
   control o.
Levy & Rappel foot o.
L'Nard Multi Podus o.
L'Nard thoracolumbosacral o.
long leg o.
long opponens o.
long thoracic nerve injury o.
lower limb o. (LLO)
LSU reciprocation-gait o.
lumbosacral o. (LSO)
Lynco foot o.
Malibu cervical o.
Malleoloc ankle o.
Maple Leaf hip o.
Marlin cervical o.
medial heel wedge o.
medial sole wedge o.
metal hybrid o.
Meyer cervical o.
Milwaukee
   cervicothoracolumbosacral o.
Milwaukee scoliosis o.
Minerva o.
molded ankle-foot o.
   (MAFO)
molded lumbosacral o.
Monodos o.
MultiBoot o.
neoprene wrist o.
Newington o.
Newport MC hip o.
New York Orthopaedic
   front-opening o.

NuKO knee o.
Oklahoma ankle joint o.
OmniFlex knee o.
opponens o.
Orlando hip-knee-ankle-foot o.
Ortholign spinal o.
Orthomedics Ultra-Guard hip o.
o. overlapped uprights
overlapped uprights in o.
parapodium o.
passive prehension o. (PPO)
patellar tendon-bearing o.
   (PTBO)
patellar tendon weightbearing
   brace o.
patellar tracking o.
patellofemoral o.
pediatric pressure relief ankle
   foot o.
Phelps o.
pillow o.
plantar arch support o.
plantar fasciitis o. (PFO)
Plastazote cervical collar o.
plastic ankle-foot o.
plastic floor reaction ankle-foot o.
pneumatic o.
polypropylene ankle-foot o.
polypropylene glycol ankle-foot o.
   (PPG-AFO)
polypropylene
   glycol-thoracolumbosacral o.
   (PPG-TLSO)
poster o.
2-poster cervical o.
4-poster cervical o.
posterior leaf-spring ankle-foot o.
postoperative lumbosacral o.
prehension o.
pressure-relief ankle-foot o.
   (PRAFO)
pressure-relieving o.
Profile Sitting O.
Pro-glide o.
progressive ankle o.
prosthesis and o. (P&O)
PTB ankle-foot o.
PTB plastic o.
Pucci pediatrics hand o.
Pucci rehab knee o.
reciprocal finger prehension o.
reciprocating gait o. (RGO)
resting o.
rib belt o.
rigid o.
Rochester hip-knee-ankle-foot o.
SACH o.
sacroiliac o. (SIO)
safety pin o.

O

orthosis (*continued*)
- Sawa shoulder o.
- scapular winging o.
- scapulothoracic o.
- scapulothoracic fixation o.
- Scottish Rite hip o.
- Seattle o.
- Select joint o.
- semirigid polypropylene ankle-foot o.
- serial stretch orthoses
- serratus anterior palsy o.
- Shaeffer rigid o.
- short leg o.
- short opponens o.
- shoulder o. (SO)
- shoulder abduction o.
- shoulder-elbow-wrist-hand o. (SEWHO)
- single-photon electrospinal o.
- skull-occiput-mandibular immobilization o.
- Slim Option shoe o.
- soft collar cervical o.
- SOLEutions custom o.
- SOMI o.
- spinal o.
- Sport-Stirrup o.
- spring-loaded lock o.
- spring-wire ankle-foot o.
- standard shell ankle-foot o.
- standing frame o.
- static o.
- steel sole plate o.
- sternal-occipital-mandibular immobilizer o.
- sternooccipital mandibular immobilizer o.
- supramalleolar o. (SMO)
- Swede-O-Universal o.
- Swedish knee cage o.
- Tachdjian o.
- Taylor thoracolumbosacral o.
- tenodesis o.
- themoplastic ankle-foot o.
- therapeutic o.
- Thera-Pos elbow o.
- Therapy Carrot Finger O.
- Therapy Carrot finger contracture o.
- Thomas collar cervical o.
- Thomas heel o.
- thoracic o.
- thoracic spine o.
- thoracolumbar o.
- thoracolumbosacral o. (TLSO)
- Tib-Transformer o.
- TIRR foot-ankle o.
- ToeOFF o.
- tone-reducing ankle-foot o. (TRAFO)
- Toronto parapodium o.
- total contact o. (TCO)
- total contact bivalve ankle-foot o.
- total hip stabilization o.
- TPE ankle-foot o.
- TPE biomechanical foot o.
- Transpire wrist o.
- trilateral knee-ankle-foot o.
- trunk-hip-knee-ankle-foot o. (THKAFO)
- turnbuckle wrist o.
- UBC o.
- UCB foot o.
- UCBL o.
- UCOlite o.
- Ultrabrace knee o.
- underarm o.
- Universal plantar fasciitis o. (UFO)
- University of British Columbia O.
- University of California Berkeley O.
- University of California Berkeley Laboratory o.
- upper limb o. (ULO)
- VAPC dorsiflexion assist o.
- Vari-Duct hip and knee o.
- VertiLok spinal o.
- Viscoheel K, N o.
- Viscolas o.
- Viscolas heel o.
- von Rosen splint hip o.
- Walkabout o.
- weight-relieving o.
- Williams o.
- wrist-driven flexor hinge o.
- wrist-driven lateral prehension o.
- wrist-driven wrist-hand o.
- wrist-hand o. (WHO)
- XPE foot o.
- Zinco ankle o.

Orthosleep Pillow

OrthoSorb
- O. absorbable pin
- O. pin fixation
- O. pin nail
- O. rod

orthostatic

Orthotech Controller knee brace

Orthotec pressurized fluid irrigation system

orthotic
- Aerodyn o.
- Alden CDI o.
- Alznner o.
- Amfit o.
- Anti-Shox sports o.
- o. attachment implant
- BIOflex o.
- Biofoot o.
- BioSole-GEL o.

Biothotic o.
Blake inverted o.
Blanke inverted tibialis posterior tendon o.
Blue Line o.
o. coiled spring twister
custom-molded o.
DesignLine o.
o. device
Diab-A-Thotics o.
DressFlex o.
DSIS o.
D-Soles o.
Dual AFO Boot o.
Duraleve custom molded foot o.
Extreme foot o.
FirmFlex custom o.
FlexiSport o.
Foot Levelers custom o.
Footmaster o.
functional o.
Golden Comfort o.
Golden Fitness o.
Healthflex o.
inverted o.
Jamaica Sandalthotics o.
Kinetic Wedge o.
Lyte Fit o.
Magnathotic o.
Malibu Sandalthotics o.
mallet finger o.
Mayer o.
MBS snap-on o.
M-Pact flexible o.
Ortho-Arch II o.
Orthofit (9000, 9001) o.
ParFlex o.
o. plate
Powerstep o.
PRAFO adjustable o.
PreCustom O.
ProLite Plus runner's o.
prosthetic and o. (P&O)
Pro Support Systems o.
Pucci Air o.
QuikFormables o.
Rediform o.
O. Research and Locomotor Assessment Unit (ORLAU)
Rohadur o.
SACH o.
SAFE o.
Sandalthotics postural support o.
shoe o.
o. shoe insert
Slimthetics o.
Sof Sole motion control o.
Soft Super Sport o.
Soft Support Preforms o.

SOLEutions soft plus o.
SOLEutions sport shell o.
solid ankle cushioned heel o.
Sporthotics o.
Sport Preforms o.
Sport-Rite o.
stationary attachment flexible endoskeletal o.
Stratos o.
Superfeet Custom Pre-Fabricated O.
Superform Contours o.
Super Jock n' Jill store Superfeet o.
Supralen cradle o.
Supralen Schaefer o.
Swiss Balance o.
ThermoCork o.
Thermo HK/Rohadur o.
Thermo HK/Tepefom o.
Thinline uncovered o.
total contact shell ankle-foot o.
UCOheal o.
UltraStep o.
Universal Plantar Fasciitis O. (UFO)
Wire-Foam o.
orthotics, orthetics
orthotist
orthotome resector
Ortho-Trac
　　O.-T. adhesive skin traction bandage
　　O.-T. pneumatic vest
orthotripsy
　　OssaTron o.
Orthotron exerciser
OrthoTurn standing transfer aid
Ortho-Vent
　　O.-V. bandage
　　O.-V. traction
OrthoVise
　　O. orthopaedic instrument
　　O. with slap hammer
OrthoWedge healing shoe
Ortho-Yomy facebow
Ortolani
　　O. click
　　O. maneuver
　　O. pediatric hip dislocation test
　　O. sign
Orudis KT
Oruvail
os, *pl.* **ossa**
　　o. acromiale
　　o. acromiale pain syndrome
　　o. calcis pin fixation
　　o. coxa
　　O. ilium
　　o. peroneum
　　Oris pin
　　o. sacrum

O

os (*continued*)
   o. styloideum
   o. supratrochleare dorsale-related
     elbow pain
   ossa tarsi
   o. trigonum fracture
   o. trigonum pain syndrome
   o. vesalianum
Osada
   O. portable electric handpiece
     system
   O. portable handpiece system
   O. saw
Osborne
   O. fascia
   O. plate
   O. posterior hip approach
   O. punch
Osborne-Cotterill
   O.-C. elbow dislocation
   O.-C. elbow technique
Os-Cal 500
Oscar ultrasonic bone cement removal
  system
oscillating
   o. gouge
   o. saw
oscillation
   grade (I, II) o.
oscillator
   circadian o.
oscillococcinum
oscilloscope instrument
Osebold-Remondini syndrome
Osgood
   O. modified technique
   O. operation
   O. rotational osteotomy
Osgood-Schlatter
   O.-S. disease
   O.-S. knee brace
   O.-S. lesion
   O.-S. syndrome
Osher irrigating implant hook
OSI
   Orthopaedic Systems Inc.
   OSI arthroscopic leg holder
   OSI extremity elevator
   OSI laxity tester
   OSI modular table system
   OSI well leg Support
OSI-Schlein shoulder positioner
Osler node
OsmoCyte island wound-care
  dressing
osmolality
   plasma o.
Osmond-Clarke staged congenital vertical
  talus repair technique

osphyomyelitis
osphyotomy
OS-5/Plus 2 knee brace
OSS
   occupational stress syndrome
ossa (*pl. of* os)
OssaTron
   O. noninvasive extracorporeal shock
     wave therapy device
   O. orthotripsy
   O. Orthotripter device
   O. shock wave
   O. shock wave therapy system
OsSatura synthetic bone graft
  substitution material
osseoaponeurotic
osseocartilaginous thoracic
  cage
Osseodent surgical drill
osseofibrous
osseointegrated prosthesis
osseointegration
osseomucoid
osseous, osteal
   o. adjustment
   Association Research Circulation O.
   o. attachment
   o. bridge
   o. bridge prevention
   o. coalition
   o. defect
   o. drift
   o. dystrophy
   o. equinus
   o. foraminal encroachment
   o. homeostasis
   o. instability
   o. lacuna
   o. lamella
   o. lesion
   o. patella outgrowth
   o. pin
   o. prominence
   o. ring
   o. ring of Lacroix
   o. structure
   o. tissue
   o. trabecula
   o. tunnel
ossicle
   accessory o.
   talonavicular o.
ossiferous
ossific
ossificans
   myositis o.
   osteitis o.
   pelvospondylitis o.
   periostitis o.

ossification
- bilateral heterotopic o.
- bipartite o.
- Brooker classification of heterotopic o.
- cartilaginous o.
- ectopic o.
- enchondral o.
- endochondral o.
- endplate o.
- heterotopic o.
- hill-shaped o.
- iliac crest o.
- intramembranous o.
- mandible o.
- membranous o.
- metaplastic o.
- metatarsal o.
- o. of posterior longitudinal ligament (OPLL)
- periarticular heterotopic o.
- perichondral o.
- periosteal o.
- pisiform o.
- o. primary center
- o. secondary center
- trapezium o.
- trapezoid o.
- triquetrum o.

ossification-associated fracture
ossifluent abscess
ossiform
ossify
ossifying fibroma
ossimeter
- Küntscher o.

ossium
- fragilitas o.

Ostase
- Access O.

osteal (*var. of* osseous)
- o. resonance

ostealgia
ostealgic
osteanagenesis
ostectomy, osteoectomy
- fibular o.
- partial o.

osteitis, ostitis
- alveolar o.
- condensing o.
- o. deformans
- o. distal phalanx
- Garré o.
- o. necroticans pubis
- nonsuppurative o.
- o. ossificans
- pagetoid o.
- o. pubis

- o. pubis syndrome
- rarefying o.
- sclerosing nonsuppurative o.
- suppurative o.

ostemia
ostempyesis
osteoanagenesis, osteanagenesis
OsteoAnalyzer device
osteoanesthesia
osteoaneurysm
Osteoarc-Guide
osteoarthritic
- o. degeneration
- O. knee brace
- o. knee pain

osteoarthritis (OA)
- ankle o.
- atlantoaxial o.
- o. deformans
- o. deformans endemica
- degenerative o.
- endemic o.
- erosive o.
- o. global index (OGI)
- o. grading classification
- hyperplastic o.
- hypertrophic o.
- interphalangeal o.
- joint o.
- knee o.
- midtarsal o.
- obese knee o.
- o. padded night sleeve brace
- posttraumatic o.
- primary degenerative o.
- o. radiographic grading
- tarsometatarsal o.
- traumatic o.

osteoarthropathy
- hypertrophic o.
- hypertrophic pulmonary o.
- idiopathic hypertrophic o. (IHO)
- neuropathic o.
- pneumogenic o.
- pulmonary o.
- pustulotic o.
- tabetic o.

osteoarthroscopy
- hypertrophic o. (HOA)

osteoarthrosis
- posttraumatic o.

osteoarthrotomy
osteoarticular
- o. allograft
- o. allograft transplant
- o. defect
- o. graft
- o. pathology
- o. tuberculosis

O

Osteo Bi-Flex
osteoblast
    neoplastic o.
    o. proliferation fluorometric
       assay
osteoblastic
    o. bone regeneration
    o. lesion
    o. metastasis
    o. osteogenic sarcoma
osteoblastoma
    spinal o.
Osteobond copolymer bone cement
Osteo-B Plus
osteobunionectomy
osteocachexia
osteocalcin injection
osteocampsia
OsteoCap hip prosthesis
osteocartilaginous
    o. exostosis
    o. graft
    o. lesion
    o. loose body
    o. mass
    o. metaplasia
osteochondral
    o. allograft
    o. autograft
    o. autograft transfer system (OATS)
    o. autograft transfer system graft
    o. contusion
    o. defect
    o. fracture arthrography
    o. fracture of dome of talus
    o. fragment
    o. graft
    o. injury
    o. lesion
    o. lesion of talus (OLT)
    o. non-load-bearing bone fracture
    o. nonunion articular fracture
    o. prominence
    o. ridge
osteochondritis
    capitellar o.
    crushing o.
    o. deformans juvenilis
    o. deformans juvenilis dorsi
    o. dissecans (OCD)
    epiphysial o.
    o. juvenilis
    o. necroticans
    olecranon o.
    pulling o.
    puncture wound o.
    syphilitic o.
osteochondroarthropathy
osteochondrodesmodysplasia

osteochondrodysplasia
osteochondrodystrophia deformans
osteochondrodystrophy
osteochondrofibroma
osteochondrolysis
osteochondroma
    congenital o.
    epiphysial o.
    excision of o.
    intraarticular o.
    pedunculated o.
    sessile-type o.
osteochondromatoses
    multiple o.
osteochondromatosis
    Ollier o.
    synovial o.
    tumefactive synovial o.
osteochondromatous dysplasia
osteochondromyxoma
osteochondropathy
osteochondrophyte
osteochondrosarcoma
osteochondrosis
    o. deformans tibiae
    o. of metatarsal
osteochondrotic loose body
osteochrondral slice fracture
Osteo-clage cable system
osteoclasia (*var. of* osteoclasis)
osteoclasis, osteoclasia
    Blount technique for o.
    o. maneuver
osteoclast
    Collin o.
    Rizzoli o.
    o. tension staple
osteoclastic
    o. erosion
    o. giant cell
    o. resorption
osteoclast-mediated
    o.-m. bone
    o.-m. osteoporosis
osteoclastoma
osteoconduction
osteocutaneous free flap
osteocystoma
osteocyte
osteodesmosis
osteodiastasis
osteodistractor
    Ace/Normed o.
osteodynia
osteodysplasty of Melnick and Needles
osteodystrophia (*var. of* osteodystrophy)
osteodystrophy, osteodystrophia
    Albright hereditary o.
    azotemic o.

parathyroid o.
pulmonary o.
renal o.
osteoectasia
    familial o.
osteoectomy
osteoenchondroma
osteoepiphysis
osteofascial compartment
osteofibrochondrosarcoma
osteofibroma
osteofibromatosis
osteofibrosis
osteofibrous dysplasia
Osteofil
    O. allograft bone paste
    O. allograft paste
OsteoGen
    O. bone growth stimulation
    O. implantable bone growth
    stimulator
    O. resorbable osteogenic bone-filling
    implant
osteogenesis
    distraction o.
    endochondral o.
    o. imperfecta (OI)
    o. imperfecta congenita (OIC)
    O. Imperfecta Foundation (OIF)
    o. imperfecta tarda (OIT)
    membranous o.
    periosteal o.
osteogenetic (*var. of* osteogenic)
osteogenic, osteogenetic
    o. cell
    o. fibroma
    o. metastasis
    o. osteomalacia
    o. protein 1 (OP-1)
    o. protein-1 bone graft
    o. sarcoma
    o. scoliosis
osteogenicity
**Osteogenics BoneSource synthetic bone
replacement material**
OsteoGram
    O. bone density test
    O. 2000 densitometer
osteohalisteresis
osteohydatidosis
osteoid
    calcified o.
    o. osteoma
    o. seam
    unmineralized o.
osteoinduction
osteoinductive
    o. enhanced-graft gel
    o. therapy

osteokinematic motion
osteokinematics
osteolipochondroma
osteolipoma
Osteolock
    O. acetabular component
    O. HA femoral component
    O. hip prosthesis
    Precision O.
osteology
    metatarsal o.
osteolysis
    acetabular o.
    atraumatic o.
    debris-incited o.
    debris-induced o.
    familial expansile o.
    femoral o.
    Gorham massive o.
    malignant acetabular o.
    massive o.
    posttraumatic o.
    pubic o.
osteolytic sarcoma
osteoma
    cavalryman's o.
    compact o.
    o. durum
    o. eburneum
    giant osteoid o.
    intraarticular osteoid o.
    intracapsular osteoid o.
    ivory o.
    osteoid o.
    parosteal o.
    solitary o.
    o. spongiosum
    subperiosteal paraarticular-type
    osteoid o.
osteomalacia
    nutritional o.
    osteogenic o.
    renal tubular o.
    senile o.
osteomalacic pelvis
**osteomanipulative therapy
(OMT)**
**Osteomark bone-loss urine
test**
osteomatoid
osteomatosis
Osteomed screw
osteomesopyknosis
osteometry
**osteomusculocutaneous
flap**
osteomyelitic
    o. cloaca formation
    o. sinus

O

osteomyelitis
  Ackerman criteria for o.
  acute hematogenous o. (AHO)
  anaerobic o.
  ankle o.
  bacterial o.
  blastomycotic o.
  Brucella o.
  chloramphenicol o.
  cystic o.
  femoral o.
  Gaenslen o.
  Garré sclerosing o.
  hematogenous o.
  hemorrhagic o.
  iatrogenic o.
  long bone o.
  multifocal o.
  nonsuppurative o.
  nonunion o.
  pedal o.
  pin-tract o.
  postfracture o.
  posttraumatic chronic o.
  primary subacute o.
  probe test for o.
  pyogenic vertebral o.
  Salmonella o.
  sclerosing nonsuppurative o.
  secondary hematogenous o.
  spinal o.
  subacute hematogenous o.
  suppurative o.
  synovitis, acne pustulosis,
    hyperostosis, o. (SAPHO)
  tuberculous spinal o.
  tuberculous vertebral o.
  typhoid o.
  vertebral o.
osteomyelodysplasia
osteon, osteone
osteonal
  o. bone union
  o. lamellar bone
osteone (*var. of* osteon)
  O. air drill
osteonecrosis
  ARCO o.
  dysbaric o.
  femoral head o.
  Ficat and Arlet classification of
    major joint o.
  Ficat and Arlet radiographic
    classification of humeral head o.
    (stage I-IV)
  Ficat radiographic classification of
    femoral head o. (stage I-IV)
  idiopathic o.
  navicular o.

  nontraumatic idiopathic o.
  posttraumatic o.
  steroid-induced o.
osteoneuralgia
Osteonics
  O. acetabular cup
  O. acetabular dome hole plug
  O. HA femoral implant
  O. hip prosthesis
  O. jig
  O. Omnifit-C stem
  O. Omnifit-HA component
  O. Omnifit-HA hip stem
  O. Scorpio insert
  O. Scorpio posterior cruciate
    retaining total knee system
  Stryker Howmedica O.
osteoonychodysplasia
  hereditary o. (HOOD)
Osteopatch
  O. bone density test
  O. transdermal patch
osteopathia (*var. of* osteopathy)
  o. striata
osteopathic
  o. lesion
  o. manipulation
  o. manipulative therapy
    (OMT)
  o. manipulative treatment
  o. medicine
  o. scoliosis
osteopathology
osteopathy, osteopathia
  alimentary o.
osteopenia
  transient o.
osteopenic
  o. bone
  o. bone stock
osteoperiosteal
  o. bone graft
  o. flap
osteoperiostitis
osteopetrorickets
osteopetrosis
  malignant o.
osteophage
osteophlebitis
osteophore
osteophyma
osteophyte
  apophysial joint o.
  bony o.
  bridging o.
  coronoid o.
  o. elevator
  o. formation
  fringe of o.

jagged o.
marginal o.
posterior o.

osteophytic
o. bone lip
o. spur

osteophytosis
osteoplaque
osteoplastic
o. amputation
o. flap clamp
o. laminectomy
o. necrotomy
o. reconstruction

osteoplasty
osteoplysis
massive o.

osteopoikilosis
osteopoikilotic
osteoporosis
disuse o.
dual photon densitometry test for o.
femoral o.
idiopathic juvenile o.
idiopathic transient o.
juvenile o.
O. Knowledge Questionnaire (OKQ)
low-turnover o.
osteoclast-mediated o.
posttraumatic o.
o. pseudoglioma syndrome
regional migratory o.
secondary o.
senile o.
o. severity
Singh index of o.
transient o.

osteoporotic
o. ankle fracture
o. bone
o. fracture risk
o. spine

Osteopower modular handpiece system
osteoprogenitor
o. cell
o. stem cell

osteoprotegerin
osteoradiologist
osteoradionecrosis
osteorrhagia
osteorrhaphy
osteosarcoma
conventional o.
extraskeletal o.
intraosseous o.
low-grade central o.
parosteal o.
periosteal o.
postirradiation o.

recurrent parosteal o.
secondary o.
spinal o.
telangiectatic o.

OsteoSet
O. bone filler
O. bone graft substitute
O. resorbable bead kit

**OsteoSet-T medicated bone graft
substitute**
osteosis, ostosis
**OsteoSponge osteoinductive bone
allograft material**
osteospongioma
OsteoStat
O. disposable power tool
O. single-use power surgical
equipment

**OsteoStim implantable bone growth
stimulator**
osteosuture
osteosynovitis
Osteosynthesefragen
Arbeitsgemeinschaft für O. (AO)

osteosynthesis
anterior column o.
o. device
locked intramedullary o.
lumbar spine vertebral o.
odontoid process o.
o. pelvic ring injury repair
plate-screw o.
posterior column o.
thoracic spine vertebral o.
thoracolumbar spine vertebral o.
vertebral o.
Wagner multiple K-wire o.

osteotabes
osteotelangiectasia
osteothrombophlebitis
osteothrombosis
OsteoTite bone screw
osteotome
AcuDriver o.
Acufex o.
air compression o.
Albee o.
Alexander costal o.
Anderson-Neivert o.
Andrews o.
Army o.
arthroscopic o.
Aufranc o.
backcutting o.
bayonet o.
Blount o.
Bowen o.
box o.
Campbell o.

O

osteotome (*continued*)
  Cavin o.
  Cebotome o.
  Cherry o.
  Cinelli o.
  Clayton o.
  Cloward spinal fusion o.
  Cobb o.
  Compere o.
  Cottle o.
  Crane o.
  curved o.
  Dautrey o.
  Dingman o.
  disposable 1-piece o.
  Epker o.
  fine o.
  grooving o.
  guarded o.
  Hendel guided o.
  Hibbs curved o.
  Hibbs straight o.
  Hoke o.
  Joseph o.
  Lambotte o.
  Leinbach o.
  Lexer o.
  Meyerding curved o.
  Meyerding straight o.
  MGH o.
  Micro-Aire o.
  Miner o.
  mini-Lambotte o.
  mini-Lexer o.
  Mitchell o.
  Moberg o.
  Moe o.
  Moreland o.
  Murphy o.
  Neivert o.
  orthopaedic o.
  Padgett o.
  Parkes o.
  Peck o.
  Rhoton o.
  Rish o.
  rotary o.
  Sheehan o.
  Silver o.
  Simmons o.
  Smith-Petersen curved o.
  Smith-Petersen straight o.
  Stille o.
  straight o.
  Swanson o.
  Swiss pattern o.
  thin o.
  unguarded o.
  U.S. Army o.

  Weck o.
  West o.
osteotomize
osteotomized bone
osteotomy
  Abbott-Gill o.
  abduction o.
  abductory midfoot o.
  abductory wedge o.
  acetabular shelf o.
  adduction o.
  Agliette supracondylar o.
  Akin proximal phalangeal o.
  Akron midtarsal o.
  Amspacher-Messenbaugh closing
    wedge o.
  Amstutz-Wilson o.
  o. analysis simulation software
    (OASIS)
  o. and fusion
  angular o.
  angulation o.
  anterior calcaneal o.
  arcuate o.
  Austin o.
  Axer lateral opening wedge o.
  Axer varus derotational o.
  Baker-Hill o.
  Balacescu closing wedge hallux
    valgus o.
  ball-and-socket trochanteric o.
  Barouk microscrew with
    shortening o.
  barrel-stave skull o.
  basal chevron o.
  basal closing wedge o.
  base of neck o.
  base wedge o. (BWO)
  basilar closing wedge metatarsal o.
  basilar crescentic o.
  basilar plantarflexory metatarsal o.
  Bellemore-Barrett closing wedge o.
  Berens o.
  Berman-Gartland metatarsal o.
  Bernese periacetabular o.
  bicorrectional Austin o.
  bifurcation o.
  biplane Dwyer o.
  biplane trochanteric o.
  biplaning of o.
  block o.
  Blount displacement o.
  Blundell-Jones hip o.
  Blundell-Jones varus o.
  Bonney-Kessel dorsiflexionary
    tilt-up o.
  Booth wire fixation of sagittal split
    mandibular o.
  Brackett o.

Brett o.
o. bunionectomy
calcaneal L o.
calcaneal sliding corrective o.
Campbell tibial o.
Canale o.
canal innominate o.
capital crescentic shelf o.
Carstan reverse wedge o.
Cartam-Treander reverse wedge o.
cervical o.
cervical extension o.
Chambers o.
chevron o.
chevron-Akin double o.
chevron modification of Mitchell o.
Chiari innominate o.
closed base wedge o. (CBWO)
closed intramedullary o.
closed wedge dorsal o.
closing abductory-wedge o.
  (CAWO)
closing base-wedge o.
closing wedge greenstick dorsal
  proximal metatarsal o.
closing wedge high tibial o.
  (CWHTO)
Cole o.
compensatory basilar o.
compromise o.
controlled rotational o.
corrective lengthening o.
countersinking o.
Coventry distal femoral o.
Coventry proximal tibial o.
Coventry vagal o.
Crawford L-shaped o.
Crego femoral o.
crescentic base wedge o.
crescentic basilar first metatarsal o.
crescentic calcaneal o.
crescentic shelf o. (CSO)
crescent-shaped o.
cuboid-calcaneal o.
cuboid wedge o.
cuneiform o.
cup-and-ball o.
curved o.
cylindrical o.
decompressive o.
Dega pelvic o.
delayed femoral o.
derotational o.
dial pelvic o.
dial periacetabular o.
diaphysial o.
Dickson geometric o.
Dillwyn-Evans o.
Dimon o.

Dimon-Hughston intertrochanteric
  medial displacement o.
displacement anterior cavus V o.
distal Akin phalangeal o.
distal first metatarsal o.
distal L o.
distal oblique sliding o.
dome proximal tibial o.
dome-shaped o.
dorsal closing wedge o.
dorsal closing wedge proximal
  phalangeal o.
dorsal proximal metatarsal o.
dorsal V o.
dorsiflexion metatarsal o.
dorsiflexory wedge o.
double o.
Dunn o.
Dwyer o.
Dwyer calcaneal o.
elevating o.
Elizabethtown o.
Elmslie-Trillat o.
Emmon o.
epiphysial-metaphysial o.
Eppright dial o.
Estersohn o.
Evans anterior opening wedge
  calcaneal o.
eversion o.
extended slide trochanteric o.
extension o.
failed femoral o.
femoral derotation o.
Fernandez o.
fibular o.
Fish cuneiform o.
flexion o.
Fowler o.
free-floating o.
French lateral closing-wedge o.
Fulkerson oblique tibial tubercle o.
Gant o.
Ganz periacetabular o.
geometric supracondylar
  extension o.
Gerbert o.
Giannestras oblique metatarsal o.
Giannestras step-down modified o.
Gibson-Piggott o.
Gigli saw o.
Gleich o.
glenoid o.
Golden closing wedge o.
greater tuberosity o.
Greenfield o.
Green-Laird modification of
  Reverdin o.
Green-Reverdin o.

O

osteotomy (*continued*)

greenstick dorsal proximal metatarsal o.
Green-Watermann o.
Gudas scarf Z-plasty o.
Haas o.
Haddad metatarsal o.
Hass o.
Helal o.
high tibial o. (HTO)
Hirayma o.
Hohmann o.
Hohmann-Thomasen metatarsal o.
horizontal o.
iliac o.
Ingram o.
innominate o.
intertrochanteric varus o.
intraarticular o.
intracapsular o.
intraepiphysial o.
Irwin o.
Japas o.
Johnson chevron o.
Kalamchi o.
Kalish o.
Kaplan o.
Kawamura dome o.
Kawamura pelvic o.
Kelikian modified Z o.
Kelly-Keck o.
Kelly-Kelly o.
Kelly tendon lengthening o.
Kessel-Bonney extension o.
Koutsogiannis calcaneal displacement o.
Kramer modification of Hohmann o.
Lambrinudi o.
Langenskiöld o.
lateral closing wedge o.
lateral displacement o.
lateral opening wedge o.
Le Fort (I–III) o.
Lelièvre o.
Lichtblau o.
Lindgren oblique o.
Lindseth o.
linear o.
Lorenz o.
L-shaped o.
Ludloff o.
Macewen o.
malleolar o.
mandibular o.
Maquet dome o.
Marquardt angulation o.
Martin o.
Mau o.
Mayday distal first metatarsal o.

McKay o.
McMurray o.
medial calcaneal displacement o.
medial closing wedge phalangeal o.
medial displacement o.
medial opening wedge o.
metacarpal o.
metaphysial o.
metatarsal head o.
metatarsal neck o.
metatarsal oblique o.
metatarsal proximal dome o.
metatarsal Reverdin o.
metatarsal V-shaped o.
metatarsus primus o.
midshaft metatarsal o.
midtarsal dome o.
midtarsal V o.
Mitchell distal o.
Mitchell posterior displacement o.
Mitchell step-down o.
modified Hohmann o.
modified Kalish o.
modified Mau o.
modified Wilson o.
modified Z o.
Molesworth o.
Moore o.
Mueller intertochanteric varus o.
Mueller transposition o.
Müller o.
oblique closing wedge o. (OCWO)
oblique proximal phalangeal o.
oblique slide o.
Obwegeser sagittal mandibular o.
odontoid o.
offset-V o.
open base wedge o.
opening abductory wedge o. (OAWO)
opening wedge o.
Osgood rotational o.
Pauwels proximal o.
Pauwels valgus o.
Pauwels Y o.
pedicle subtraction o.
peg-in-hole o.
Peimer reduction o.
pelvic o.
Pemberton pericapsular o.
percutaneous o.
periacetabular o.
pericapsular o.
phalangeal o.
Phemister o.
o. pin
plantarflexor proximal metatarsal o.
plantarflexory o.
Platou o.

Ponte spinal scoliosis o.
posterior calcaneal displacement o.
posterior iliac o.
posterior spinal wedge o.
Potts eversion o.
Potts tibial o.
proximal chevron o.
proximal dome o.
proximal femoral o.
proximal first metatarsal o.
proximal metatarsal o.
proximal phalangeal o.
proximal phalanx o.
proximal tibial o.
radial recession o.
radial wedge o.
Rappaport fifth metatarsal
    proximal o.
rearfoot o.
reduction o.
Regnauld hallux o.
Reverdin o.
Reverdin-Green o.
Reverdin-Laird o.
reverse Austin o.
reverse closing base wedge o.
reverse Dillwyn-Evans calcaneal o.
rotational scarf o.
Roux o.
sagittal split o. (SSO)
sagittal Z o.
Sakoff fifth metatarsal
    metaphysial o.
Salter innominate o.
Salter pelvic o.
Samilson crescentic calcaneal o.
sandwich o.
Sarmiento intertrochanteric o.
scarf Z o.
Schanz femoral o.
Schanz irreducible hip dislocation
    angulation o.
Schanz-type proximal femoral
    valgization o.
Schede hip o.
Schwartz midfoot dorsiflexory o.
segmental alveolar o.
shortening o.
shortening metatarsal o.
Siffert tibia vara intraepiphysial o.
Simmonds-Menelaus metatarsal o.
Simmonds-Menelaus proximal
    phalangeal o.
Simmons o.
Smith-Petersen pedicle subtraction o.
Sofield o.
Southwick biplane trochanteric o.
Speed o.
spike o.

spinal o.
Sponsel oblique metatarsal o.
Stamm metatarsal o.
Steel triple innominate o.
Steel triradiate pelvic o.
step o.
step-cut o.
step-down o.
subcapital o.
subcondylar o.
subtraction o.
subtrochanteric o.
Sugioka transtrochanteric
    rotational o.
supracondylar femoral derotational o.
supracondylar varus o.
supramalleolar derotational o.
supramalleolar varus derotation o.
supratubercular wedge o.
Sutherland-Greenfield o.
Swanson o.
talar neck o.
talocalcaneal o.
tarsal wedge o.
tendon lengthening o.
Thompson telescoping V o.
through-and-through V-shaped
    horizontal o.
tibial tuberosity o.
total maxillary o.
translational o.
transpedal multiplanar wedge o.
transtrochanteric rotational o.
transtrochanteric valgus o. (TVO)
transverse chevron o.
transverse diaphysial o.
transverse metatarsal o.
transverse supracondylar o.
trapezoidal resection o.
Trillat o.
triplane o.
triple innominate o.
trochanteric o.
tubercle o.
U o.
unplanned valgus o.
V o.
valgization o.
valgus extension o.
valgus high tibial o.
valgus intertrochanteric-wedge o.
valgus subtrochanteric o.
valgus wedge o.
valgus Y-shaped o.
Vanore modification of
    Youngswick-Austin o.
varus derotational o. (VDO)
varus rotational o. (VRO)
varus rotation shortening o.

osteotomy (*continued*)
    varus supramalleolar o.
    vertical sagittal split o. (VSO)
    visor o.
    visor/sandwich o.
    volar o.
    V-shaped o.
    Wagdy double-V o.
    Waterman hallux limitus o.
    Weber humeral o.
    Weber subcapital rotation o.
    wedge o.
    Weil o.
    Weil MTP joint o.
    Whitman o.
    Wilson double oblique o.
    Wilson oblique displacement o.
    Wiltse ankle o.
    Wiltse varus supramalleolar o.
    Y o.
    Yancey o.
    Youngswick o.
    Yu o.
osteotomy/bunionectomy
    base wedge o./b.
    closed wedge o./b.
    crescentic base wedge o./b.
    Kelikian modified Z o./b.
    Mitchell o./b.
    open base wedge o./b.
    rotational scarf o./b.
    supertubercular wedge o./b.
osteotomy-osteoclasis
    Moore o.-o.
osteotribe
osteotripsy
osteotrite
Osteotron stimulator for bone union
osteotylus
OsteoView
    Digital O. 2000
    O. digital bone densitometer
    O. 2000 imaging system
    O. x-ray device
ostia (*pl. of* ostium)
ostitis (*var. of* osteitis)
ostium, *pl.* **ostia**
ostosis
ostraceous
ostracosis
Ostrum-Furst syndrome
Ostrup bone graft harvesting technique
Oswestry
    O. Disability Score
    O. index
    O. Low Back Pain Disability
Oswestry-O'Brien spinal stapler
OT
    occupational therapy

OTA
    Orthopaedic Trauma Association
    OTA fracture classification
OTADL
    Occupational Therapy Activities of
    Daily Living
Ottawa ankle rule (OAR)
Otto
    O. Bock 1A30 Greissinger Plus
    foot
    O. Bock 1D25 Dynamic Plus foot
    O. Bock dynamic prosthesis
    O. Bock MOBIS mobility system
    O. Bock 3R65 children's hydraulic
    knee joint
    O. Bock 3R60 EBS knee
    O. Bock 3R45 modular knee
    joint
    O. Bock 3R80 modular rotary
    hydraulic knee
    O. Bock Safety constant-friction
    knee
    O. Bock system electric hand
    O. disease
    O. pelvis
    O. pelvis dislocation
Otto-Chrobak hip disease
Oudard shoulder bone block procedure
out
    draped o.
    rule o. (R/O)
    step out, turn o. (SOTO)
    toeing o.
outcome
    O. and Assessment Information Set
    (OASIS)
    o. assessment
    functional o.
    o. measure
    Michigan Hand O.'s
outdoor
    o. emergency car (OEC)
    o. emergency care wrist/forearm
    support
Outerbridge
    O. chondral knee lesion
    classification
    O. degenerative arthritis staging
    O. ridge
    O. scale
Outerbridge-Kashiwagi procedure
outer malleolus
outflow cannula
outgrowth
    osseous patella o.
outlet
    cervical o.
    supraspinatus o.
    o. view

outline
    inferior o.
    medial o.
out-of-cast ankle brace
outpatient
    o. physical therapy
    o. rehabilitation
outpouching
    synovial o.
output
    cardiac o.
    urinary o.
outrigger
    o. arm
    o. cast
    dorsal wrist splint with o.
    Harrington distraction o.
    o. splint
    O. wire
outside-in technique
outside-the-boot brace
**outside-to-outside arthroscopy
  technique**
outsole
outstretched hand
out-toeing gait
outward rotation
**Ovadia-Beals tibial plafond fracture
  classification**
oval
    o. amputation
    o. curved-cup curette
    o. washer
Oval-8
    O.-8 kit
    O.-8 ring splint
    O.-8 sizing set
over-bed table
Overcast cast cover
overcorrection
overdistraction
Overdyke hip prosthesis
overextension
overflexion
overgrowth
    bony o.
    terminal o.
overhead
    o. exercise test
    o. olecranon traction
    o. pulley
overhinge
    variable flexion o.
Overholt
    O. clip-applying
      forceps
    O. operation
overhydration
    fluid o.

overlap
    tibiofibular o.
overlapped uprights in orthosis
overlapping fifth toe
overlay
    Bodyline sleeper mattress o.
    o. drafting
    o. mattress
    o. plate
    Stimulite honeycomb mattress o.
    x-ray o.
overload
    compression o.
    lateral forefoot o.
    progressive o.
    torsional o.
overmotivation
overpull
overreaching
overriding fifth toe
oversewn
oversize tennis shoe
over-straight toe
overstrain
overstretch weakness
over-the-door traction unit
over-the-top
    o.-t.-t. knee operation
    o.-t.-t. knee procedure
    o.-t.-t. position
Overton dowel graft
overtraining syndrome
over-tying wire
overuse
    o. injury
    o. injury assessment
    o. syndrome
Owen gauze dressing
Owens silk
oxacillin
oxaprozin
oxazepam
Oxford
    O. fixator
    O. meniscal unicompartmental knee
      system
    O. meniscal unicompartment
      prosthesis
    O. method
    O. method for scoring skeletal
      maturity
    O. uncompartmental device
    O. unicompartmental knee
oxiconazole
oxidation
    carbohydrate o.
    fat o.
oxide
    ethylene o.

O

oxidized
- o. zirconium
- o. zirconium alloy on implant

oximeter
- pulse o.

Oxiplex/SP
- O. bioresorbable product
- O. gel

Oxistat
- O. cream
- O. Topical

Oxycel oxidized cellulose
oxychlorosene
oxycodone
- o. and acetaminophen
- o. and aspirin
- o. hydrochloride

OxyContin

oxygen
- dysbaric o.
- epiphysial o.
- hyperbaric o. (HBO)
- o. myelography
- o. seizure
- o. tension
- o. therapy
- transcutaneous o.

OxyIR
oxymorphone hydrochloride
oxyphenbutazone
oxytoca
- *Klebsiella o.*

Oyst-Cal 500
Oystercal 500
oyster-shell brace
Ozer retractor

P/3
    proximal third
PA
    posteroanterior
Paas disease
Paced Auditory Serial Addition test
  (PASAT)
pachydactylia (*var. of* pachydactyly)
pachydactylous
pachydactyly, pachydactylia
pachyonychia congenita
pachyperiostitis
pachypodous
Pacifica thoracolumbar fusion interbody
  VBR
pacinian mechanoreceptor
Paci operation
pack
    Adaptic p.
    Arctic Blaze hot/cold p.
    Avitene p.
    Back-Ease aromatherapy hot/cold p.
    BodyIce cold p.
    Coldhot p.
    Colpacs p.
    cool p.
    CP2 inflatable cold p.
    DynaHeat hot p.
    gel p.
    Gelfoam p.
    Glacier P.
    hot moist p.
    hydrocollator steam p.
    ice p. (IP)
    I.C.E. Down cold p.
    instant cold p.
    Jack Frost hot/cold p.
    JoyBags therapeutic heat p.
    Kool Kit cold therapy p.
    Merocel p.
    MSC cold p.
    Neck-Roll aromatherapy hot/cold p.
    Polar P.
    Softouch Cold/Hot P.
    P. technique
    TheraBeads microwaveable moist
      heat p.
    Thera-Med cold p.
    Thermal P.
    ThermalSoft hot & cold p.'s
    Thermophore hot p.
    Ultimate Cold N' Hot P.
    vaginal p.
    Von-Loc personal ice p.
    Whitehall Glacier P.

Pack-Ehrlich deep iliac dissection
6-pack hand exercise
packing
    Adaptic p.
    gauze p.
    Nu Gauze p.
    wound p.
Pacs
    Boo-Boo P.
PACU
    postanesthesia care unit
pad
    abdominal lap p.
    ABD sterile abdominal p.
    Achilles heel p.
    Airex balance p.
    AirLITE support p.
    Aliplast p.
    alternating pressure p.
    antidecubitus p.
    aperture p.
    Aquaflex gel p.
    Aquatech cast p.
    Aquatherm bed p.
    Arthropor cup p.
    artificial fat p.
    balance p.
    Bauerfeind silicone heel p.
    buttocks p.
    buttress p.
    calcaneal fat p.
    Charnley foam suture p.
    cloverleaf met foot p.
    cold p.
    crest buttress p.
    dancer's p.
    digital p.
    dinner p.
    distal star p.
    elbow p.
    fat p.
    fibrocartilaginous p.
    finger p.
    fingertip p.
    foam p.
    Hapad heel p.
    Hapad longitudinal metatarsal
      arch p.
    Hapad medial arch p.
    Hapad prefabricated wool felt p.
    horseshoe heel p.
    horseshoe-shaped felt p.
    Hydrocollator p.
    infrapatellar fat p.
    internal gel p.

P

pad (*continued*)
J p.
Kager fat p.
knee-control orthosis p.
knuckle p.
lamb's wool p.
lateral p.
L-shaped p.
MagneCore magnetic
    therapy p.
metatarsal p.
Mikulicz p.
navicular shoe p.
OEC popliteal p.
Ortho-Cel p.
Ortho-Foam elbow/heel p.
painful heel p.
patellar orthosis p.
Pedi-Cushions p.
Pedifix crest p.
Pedifix hammertoe p.
Pen/Alps distal p.
plantar fat p.
prefabricated wool felt p.
retropatellar fat p.
pubic p.
Redigrip knee p.
reticulated polyurethane p.
retropatellar fat p.
Roho heel p.
scaphoid shoe p.
second skin p.
sensor p.
shock-absorbent heel p.
shoe heel p.
silicone p.
Silipos digital p.
Sof-Rol cast p.
Sof Sole Sof Gel heel p.
Sorbothane recoil p.
S'port Max stabilization p.
spur p.
Staph-Chek p.
supracondylar p.
Sure Sport p.
T-Foam bed p.
Thermapad p.
Thermophore moist heat p.
thickness of heel p.
Vac-Pac p.
valgus knee control p.
varus knee control p.
Zimfoam p.
padded
p. aluminum splint
p. board splint
p. bolster
p. button
p. clamp

p. plywood splint
p. tongue blade splint
padding
biplane p.
cast p.
contoured felt p.
cotton cast p.
Delta-Rol cast p.
felt p.
Kerlix cast p.
moleskin p.
Molestick p.
pressure relief p.
Protouch synthetic orthopaedic p.
QuickStick p.
Reston p.
Sifoam p.
splint p.
Therafoam p.
Thero-Skin gel p.
Webril cotton p.
Padgett
P. electric dermatome
P. osteotome
P. prosthesis
pad/protector
paediatric (*var. of* pediatric)
Pagddu procedure
Paget
P. disease
P. osteitis deformans
P. quiet necrosis
P. sarcoma
P. tumor test
Paget-associated osteogenic sarcoma
pagetoid
p. bone
p. osteitis
Paget-von Schrötter syndrome
Pagosid
pain
aches and p.'s
Achilles tendon p.
aching p.
acute p.
adolescent back p.
Agency for Healthcare Research and
    Quality guidelines for treatment of
    acute low back p.
AHRQ guidelines for treatment of
    acute low back p.
amputation-related bone p.
p., asymmetry, range, tone, special
    test (PARTS)
p. at rest
back p.
bandlike p.
Behavioral Assessment of P. (BAP)
boring p.

bunionette p.
burning p.
causalgic p.
cervical myofascial p.
chronic low back p. (CLBP)
chronic subtalar joint p.
contralateral p.
p. control infusion pump
cross leg p.
deafferentation p.
demi-pointe position ankle p.
dermatomal p.
discogenic neck p.
p. drawing
dull aching p.
p. dysfunction syndrome
endogenous p.
epicritic p.
exercise-induced breast p.
exercise-related leg p. (ERLP)
fibromyalgic p.
focal back p.
functional back p.
gate control theory of p.
glenohumeral p.
gouty p.
groin p.
growing p.
idiopathic anterior knee p.
idiopathic arm p.
impingement p.
p. induction
joint line p.
kinetic foot p.
lancinating p.
late operative site p. (LOSP)
low back p. (LBP)
machine-gunlike p.
manubriosternal joint p.
p. measurement
midtarsal joint p.
Multiaxial Assessment of P. (MAP)
myofascial p.
myotomal p.
neurologic p.
os supratrochleare dorsale-related
  elbow p.
osteoarthritic knee p.
patellofemoral p.
perimalleolar p.
periscapulitis shoulder p.
persistent p.
pes anserine bursitis p.
phantom breast p.
phantom limb p. (PLP)
pillar p.
plantar p.
postherpetic p.
postmastectomy p.

postoperative p.
posttraumatic p.
prickling p.
primary focus of p.
Pronex pneumatic device for
  cervical p.
p. provocation test
psoas bursitis p.
psychoprosthetic p.
radicular p.
recalcitrant p.
p. reduction
referred neuritic p.
referred trigger point p.
rest p.
Roland index of low back p.
scapulothoracic p.
sclerotomal p.
searing p.
shooting p.
somatic p.
splintlike p.
static foot p.
subtalar joint p.
sympathetically mediated p.
p. threshold gauge
ticlike p.
viselike p.
volley of p.
p. with weightbearing
pain-all-over syndrome
PainFree pump
pain-free walking time (PFWT)
painful
　　p. arc
　　p. arc sign
　　p. arc syndrome
　　p. femoral head prosthesis
　　p. gait
　　p. heel
　　p. heel pad
　　p. minor intervertebral dysfunction
　　　(PMID)
　　p. spur
　　p. stump
　　p. toe
pain-related sleep disturbance
pain-relieving body posture
paint
　　Betadine p.
　　Castellani p.
　　p. gun injury
　　p. thinner injury
paired
　　p. discharge
　　p. response
　　p. scintigraphy
　　p. stimulus
Pais fracture

P

Pak
    Apollo hot/cold P.
PAL
    posterior axillary line
Palacos
    P. bone cement
    P. cement adhesive
    P. radiopaque bone cement
    P. R bone cement
palatal myoclonus
palatine bone
Palex expansion screw
Paley fibular hemimelia classification
PAL-Guard postamputation limb guard
palindromic
    p. arthropathy
    p. rheumatism
palliation
palliative care
pallor
palm
    p. guard
    mogul skier's p.'s
    p. space
palmar
    p. advancement flap
    p. aponeurosis
    p. approach
    p. arch
    p. carpal ligament
    p. carpometacarpal ligament
    p. clip
    p. cock-up splint
    p. creaking
    p. crease
    p. cross-finger flap
    p. fascia
    p. fasciotomy
    p. fibromatosis
    p. flexion
    p. grasp reflex
    p. incision
    p. intercarpal deltoid ligament
    p. interosseous muscle
    p. luxation
    p. metacarpal ligament
    p. pinch
    p. plate
    p. radiocarpal ligament
    p. swab kit
    p. synovectomy
    p. tilt
    p. T-plate
    p. ulnocarpal ligament
    p. wrist
    p. wrist splint
palmaris
    p. digitorum superficialis muscle
    p. longus

    p. longus muscle
    p. longus tendon
palmature
Palmer
    P. all-inside TFCC repair technique
    P. bone nail
    P. method
    P. primary fracture
    P. screw
    P. transscaphoid perilunar dislocation
    P. triangular fibrocartilage complex
        lesion classification
Palmerian
    P. law
    P. philosophy
palm-to-axilla dressing
palm-up test
palpable band
palpation
    digital p.
    end-feel p.
    flat p.
    intersegmental range of motion p.
      (IRMP)
    motion p.
    p. of anterior superior iliac spine
    p. of iliac crest
    p. of posterior superior iliac spine
    optimizing motion p.
    pincer p.
    screening p.
    static p.
    p. testing
palpatory
    p. diagnosis
    p. examination
    p. skill
    p. technique
    p. technique for joint assessment
PALS
    pediatric advanced life support
palsy
    ataxic cerebral p.
    athetoid cerebral p.
    backpack p.
    Bell p.
    brachial plexus p.
    cerebral p.
    combined nerve p.
    creeping p.
    crutch p.
    cyclist's p.
    drummer-boy p.
    Duchenne-Erb p.
    dyskinetic cerebral p.
    Erb p.
    Erb-Duchenne p.
    flaccid cerebral p.
    handlebar p.

high median-high radial p.
high median-high ulnar p.
high ulnar-high radial p.
Hoke procedure for tibial p.
Klumpke p.
long thoracic nerve p.
low median-low ulnar p.
median nerve p.
nerve p.
peripheral nerve p.
peroneal nerve p.
posterior interosseous nerve p.
postnatal cerebral p.
prisoner's p.
progressive supranuclear p.
pseudobulbar p.
radial nerve p.
Saturday night p.
sciatic p.
spastic cerebral p.
tardy ulnar p.
thenar p.
thoracic nerve p.
tourniquet p.
ulnar nerve p.
wasting p.

Paltrinieri-Trentani
P.-T. prosthesis
P.-T. resurfacing

Palumbo
P. ankle stabilizer
P. dynamic patellar brace
P. knee brace
P. knee support
P. patella tracker
P. stabilizing brace

pamidronate
Panacryl suture
Panadol
Junior Strength P.

Panafil ointment
Panafil-White ointment
Panalok absorbable suture anchor
panaris
melanotic p.

panarteritis nodosa
panarthritis
panastragaloid arthrodesis
pancake
p. cast
p. hand

panclavicular
p. dislocation
p. fracture dislocation

pancreatic enzyme therapy
pandemic
panmetatarsal
p. head resection
p. tendon suspension

Panner disease
panni (*pl. of* pannus)
pannus, *pl.* **panni**
p. deformity
p. of synovium

Panogauze Hydrogel wound dressing
panosteitis
Panoview
P. arthroscope
P. arthroscopic system

panplexopathy
pan splint
pant
prophylactic abduction p.'s

Panta arthrodesis nail
pantalar
p. ankle fusion
p. arthrodesis

pantalocrural
p. arthritic destruction
p. arthritic involvement
p. osteoarthritic destruction

pantaloon
p. brace
p. spica cast
p. walking cast

Pantopaque
Pantopon
pantrapezial arthritis
pants-over-vest
p.-o.-v. capsulorrhaphy
p.-o.-v. technique

panty
Cadenza p.

PAOD
peripheral arterial occlusive disease

papain
p., urea, chlorophyllin copper
complex ointment sodium
p., urea, chlorophyllin copper
complex sodium ointment
(PUC)

Papavasiliou olecranon fracture classification
papaverine
papillary adenoma
Papineau
P. graft
P. open bone grafting technique

Paprosky acetabular defect classification system (type I, IIa, IIb, IIc, IIIa, IIIb)
papule
Gottron p.
piezogenic p.

papyrus
Edwin Smith p.

PAR
postanesthesia recovery

P

paraaminosalicylic acid
paraarticular
    p. arthrodesis
    p. calcification
Parabath
    P. paraffin heat treatment
    P. paraffin heat treatment
      system
parabola
    metatarsal p.
Para-Care paraffin therapy
 bath
paracervical
paracetamol-induced
    p.-i. renal injury
    p.-i. renal tubular injury
parachute
    Corkscrew P.
    p. jumper's dislocation
    p. reflex
    p. technique
    p. test
    p. therapy
parachutist ankle brace
Paradigm BioDevices
paradoxic (*var. of* paradoxical)
paradoxical, paradoxic
    p. ankle reflex
    p. breathing
    p. extensor reflex
    p. flexor reflex
    p. lumbrical-plus finger
    p. patellar reflex
    p. triceps reflex
paraesthesia (*var. of* paresthesia)
paraffin
    p. bath (PB)
    p. heat therapy
    p. implant material
    p. mitt
    p. treatment
    p. wax therapeutic
      application
Paraflex
Parafon
    P. Forte
    P. Forte DSC
paraganglioma
    medullary p.
paraglenoid sulcus
Paragon T2 ArthroWand
parainfluenzae
    Haemophilus p.
parajugular line
parallel
    p. goniometric measure
    p. pin kit
    p. pitch lines
    p. squat exercise

parallelism
parallelogram electrogoniometer
paralyses (*pl. of* paralysis)
paralysis, *pl.* **paralyses**
    adductor pollicis p.
    p. agitans
    atrophic muscular p.
    backpack p.
    brachial plexus p.
    Chaves-Rapp p.
    common peroneal nerve p.
    compression p.
    cruciate p.
    crutch p.
    Cruveilhier p.
    Dewar-Harris p.
    Dickson p.
    familial periodic p.
    femoral nerve p.
    flaccid p.
    gluteus medius p.
    Haas p.
    hand p.
    Henry p.
    intrinsic p.
    isolated p.
    musculocutaneous
      nerve p.
    musculospiral p.
    myogenic p.
    myopathic p.
    p. notariorum
    peripheral p.
    peripheral facial p.
    peroneal p.
    Pott p.
    pressure p.
    pseudohypertrophic
      muscular p.
    Remak p.
    rucksack p.
    segmental motor p.
    serratus anterior p.
    spastic p.
    spinal cord p.
    spinomuscular p.
    tourniquet p.
    ulnar nerve p.
    Volkmann ischemic p.
    wasting p.
    Whitman p.
    writer's p.
paralytic
    p. chest
    p. contracture
    p. foot
    p. kyphosis
    p. scoliosis
paramalleolar artery

ParaMax
    P. ACL guide system
    P. angled driver
paramedian
    p. approach
    p. sagittal plane
parameniscus
parameter
    angular p.
    anthropometric growth p.
    clinical p.
    neutralization p.
    radiographic p.
    rotational p.
    translational p.
paramethasone acetate
paramount
    P. total body plate-loaded machine
    P. 3-way press bench
paramyoclonus multiplex
paramyotonia
    ataxic p.
Paramyxoviridae
paranasal sinus fracture
paraneoplastic neuromuscular syndrome
paraosseous lesion
paraparesis
paraparetic gait
parapatellar
    p. approach
    p. arthrotomy
    p. incision
    p. plica
    p. synovitis
paraphysiological space
paraphysiologic zone
paraplegia
    ataxic p.
    incomplete p.
    postoperative p.
    Pott p.
    spastic p.
    traumatic p.
parapodium orthosis
pararectus approach
parasacral block
parasagittal
    p. groove
    p. scar
parascapular flap
paraspinal
    p. abscess
    p. approach
    p. calcification
    p. interface
    p. mapping
    p. muscle
    p. muscle spasm
    p. musculature

    p. point
    p. rod application
    p. skin temperature thermocouple
      instrument
paraspinous
    p. muscular spasm
    p. tumor
parasympathetic
    p. innervation
    p. nervous system (PNS)
parasympatholytic
paratenon
paratenonitis
parathenar incision
parathormone level
parathyroid
    p. gland
    p. osteodystrophy
paratonia
paratrooper's fracture
paravertebral
    p. abscess
    p. block (PVB)
    p. muscle (PVM)
    p. muscle spasm (PVMS)
    p. musculature
    p. sympathetic chain
paraxial hemimelia
Pare elbow dislocation reduction
parenteral nutrition
paresis
    limb-girdle-trunk p.
paresthesia, paraesthesia
    Berger p.
    intermittent p.
    saddle p.
paresthetica
    brachialgia statica p.
    cheiralgia p.
    meralgia p.
paretic leg
ParFlex orthotic
Parham
    P. band
    P. support
Parham-Martin
    P.-M. band
    P.-M. bone-holding clamp
    P.-M. fracture apparatus
    P.-M. fracture device
parietal
    p. bone
    p. pleura (PP)
    p. tendon sheath layer
    p. tuberosity
Paris
    elastic plaster of P.
    P. manual therapy table
    plaster of P. (POP)

P

park
P. aneurysm
transverse line of P.
Parkes osteotome
Parkinson disease
parkinsonian gait
Parona space
paronychia bur
parosteal
p. chondrosarcoma
p. lesion
p. osteogenic sarcoma
p. osteoma
p. osteosarcoma
parosteitis
parosteosis, parostosis
parostosis (*var. of* parosteosis)
paroxysmal burning
PAR-Q
Physical Activity Readiness
Questionnaire
parquetry set
**Parrish-Mann hammertoe
technique**
**Parrish microvascular decompression
procedure**
parrot
p. beak fingernail
p. beak nail
p. beak tear
p. foot
P. node
P. pseudoparalysis
parry fracture
pars, *pl.* **partes**
p. defect
p. interarticularis
p. interarticularis fracture
**Parsonage-Aldren-Turner
syndrome**
Parsonage-Turner
P.-T. neuronitis
P.-T. syndrome
2-part
2-p. Apley test
2-p. fracture
partes (*pl. of* pars)
1-, 2-, 3-, 4-part fracture
partial
p. adactyly
p. ankylosis
p. aphalangia
p. cervical vertebrectomy
p. discectomy
p. dislocation
p. fasciectomy
p. fibulectomy
p. hand amputation
p. hemimelia

p. matricectomy
p. meniscectomy
p. ossicular reconstruction/
replacement prosthesis
p. ossicular replacement prosthesis
(PORP)
p. ostectomy
p. patellectomy
p. sit-ups back exercise technique
p. thromboplastin time (PTT)
p. weightbearing (PWB)
partialis
rachischisis p.
partially
p. necrotic osseous trabecula
p. threaded pin
participation
sports p.
particle of bone
particulate
p. cancellous bone graft
p. synovitis
p. wear debris
partnership
P. implant
P. instrument
P. system
partridge
P. band
P. strap
PARTS
pain, asymmetry, range, tone, special
test
Partsch
P. chisel
P. gouge
4-part variant
Parvin
P. closed posterior elbow dislocation
reduction
P. gravity technique
P. maneuver
pas
marche à petits p.
PASA
proximal articular set angle
PASAT
Paced Auditory Serial Addition test
PASG
pneumatic antishock garment
passage
screw p.
wire p.
passer
Batzdorf cervical wire p.
Brand tendon p.
Bunnell tendon p.
Charnley wire p.
Concept 2-pin p.

curved p.
DeMayo suture p.
Framer tendon p.
Hewson suture p.
Incavo wire p.
ligature p.
Malis ligature p.
Shuttle Relay suture p.
suture p.
tendon p.
Wedeen wire p.
wire p.

passing suture
passivation metal instrument
passive
    p. accessory motion test
    p. assistance exercise
    p. dorsiflexion
    p. function
    p. gliding technique
    p. insufficiency
    p. intervertebral motion (PIVM)
    p. intervertebral motion testing
    p. joint manipulation
    p. joint mobility
    p. ligamentous system
    p. mobility
    p. mobility testing
    p. motion device
    p. motion machine
    p. movement
    p. night stretch splint
    p. patellar glide test
    p. patellar tilt test
    p. physiological test
    p. physiotherapy
    p. plantarflexion
    p. positioning device
    p. prehension orthosis (PPO)
    p. range of motion (PROM)
    p. range of motion exercise
    p. resistive exercise
    p. restraint
    p. spacer
    p. straight leg raising
    p. stretch
    p. stretch exercise
    p. tennis elbow test
    p. thermal device
    p. traction table
    p. treatment modality
Passow chisel
Passport instrumentation
paste
    absorbable collagen p.
    allograft p.
    bone p.
    Coe-pak p.
    electrode p.

Grafton Plus DBM p.
OrthoBlast p.
Osteofil allograft p.
Osteofil allograft bone p.
Regenafil allograft p.
Unna p.
Pasteurella multocida
PAT
    Physical Ability Test
Patau syndrome
patch
    Carrel p.
    p. dressing
    felt p.
    lidocaine p.
    Osteopatch transdermal p.
patella, *gen.* and *pl.* **patellae**
    absent p.
    p. alta
    apex patellae
    apex of head of p.
    p. baja
    ballottable p.
    p. ballottement
    p. bipartita
    bipartite p.
    p. bone saw
    chondromalacia patellae
    p. cubitus
    p. cup
    p. débridement
    dislocated p.
    p. displacement
    floating p.
    grasshopper p.
    head of p.
    high-riding p.
    jockey cap p.
    low-riding p.
    p. luxation
    maltracking p.
    multipartite p.
    plastic p.
    prosthetic p.
    P. Pusher
    skyline x-ray view of p.
    slipping p.
    squinting p.
    subluxing p.
    superior pole of p.
    p. tap test
    p. tendon and patella ligament
      length test
    p. tracker
    p. turndown approach
    undersurface of p.
patellae (*gen.* and *pl. of* patella)
patellalgia
Patellaligner knee brace

P

patellapexy
patellaplasty
patellar
    p. advancement
    p. affection
    p. aligner
    p. alignment
    p. apprehension sign
    p. apprehension test
    p. band
    P. Band knee protector
    p. bar
    p. bone-tendon-bone
      autograft
    p. bursa
    p. bursitis
    p. button
    p. cement clamp
    p. chondromalacia
    p. clonus
    p. clunk syndrome
    p. contour
    p. dislocation cast
    p. drill guide
    p. edge
    p. fat-pad
    p. fossa
    p. fracture
    p. glide
    p. glide test
    p. grind test
    p. groove
    p. hesitation sign
    p. inhibition test (PIT)
    p. instability
    p. intraarticular dislocation
    p. jerk
    p. ligament
    p. ligament-to-patella ratio
    p. malalignment syndrome
    p. orthosis pad
    p. pair syndrome
    p. plica
    p. plug
    p. portal
    p. realignment
    p. reamer guide
    p. reamer shaft
    p. reduction clamp
    p. reflex
    p. region
    p. resection guide
    p. resurfacing
    p. resurfacing implant
    p. retinacula release
    p. retinaculum
    p. retraction test
    p. rotation
    p. shelf

    p. skyline view
    p. sleeve fracture
    p. stabilizer
    p. stabilizing brace (PSB)
    p. subluxation
    p. taping
    p. tap knee swelling test
    p. tendinitis
    p. tendon
    p. tendon-bearing (PTB)
    p. tendon-bearing below-knee
      prosthesis
    p. tendon-bearing brace
    p. tendon bearing cast
    p. tendon-bearing orthosis (PTBO)
    p. tendon bearing socket
    p. tendon-bearing-supracondylar
    p. tendon-bearing-supracondylar-
      suprapatellar
      (PTB-SC-SP)
    p. tendon-bearing suspension
      (PTBS)
    p. tendon bone block
    p. tendon graft
    p. tendon repair
    p. tendon socket (PTS)
    p. tendon stabilization (PTS)
    p. tendon substitution
    p. tendon transfer (PTT)
    p. tendon weightbearing brace
      orthosis
    p. tendon weightbearing cast
    p. tracking
    p. tracking orthosis
    p. transplant
    p. tuberosity
patellectomy
    partial p.
    total p.
    West and Soto-Hall p.
patelloadductor reflex
patellofemoral
    p. alignment
    p. angle
    p. arthritis
    p. articulation
    p. brace
    p. compartment
    p. congruence
    p. crepitation
    p. disorder
    p. dysarthrosis
    p. dysfunction (PFD)
    p. dysplasia
    p. groove
    p. groove cartilage
    p. joint
    p. joint pain syndrome (PJPS)
    p. joint radiography

p. joint reaction force
p. ligament
p. orthosis
p. pain
p. pain syndrome (PPS)
p. realignment
p. stress syndrome
patellomeniscal ligament
patelloplasty
patelloquadriceps
p. tendon
p. tendon substitution
patellotibial ligament
Patel medial meniscectomy
Paterson
P. procedure
P. technique
PATH
Planning Alternative Tomorrows with Hope
pathfinder
P. pedicle screw
P. prosthetic foot
pathoanatomic cause
pathoanatomy
Pathocil
pathogenesis
pathognomonic sign
pathokinesiologic
pathologic, pathological
p. amputation
p. barrier
p. dislocation
p. fracture
pathological plica
p. reflex
p. spondylolisthesis
pathological (*var. of* pathologic)
pathology
bone p.
cervicothoracic p.
heel pad p.
osteoarticular p.
peripheral osteoarticular p.
pathomechanical state
pathomechanics
gait p.
juvenile flatfoot p.
kyphotic deformity p.
spinal fusion p.
pathomechanism
pathway
critical p.
neuromeningeal p.
patient
p. positioning
p. positioning and preparation
Test of Orientation for Rehabilitation P.'s (TORP)

patient-controlled
p.-c. analgesia (PCA)
p.-c. anesthesia (PCA)
patient-on-table friction
patient-resisted internal rotation
patient-table interface
Patrick
P. cross-leg maneuver
P. drill
P. hip joint disease test
P. sign
P. trigger area
Patrick/fabere test
Patten-Bottom-Perthes brace
pattern
AO fracture p.
calcaneal gait p.
cloverleaf p.
collimator plugging p.
compression p.
corduroy cloth p.
dermatomal p.
DISI collapse p.
dorsal intercalated segment instability collapse p.
double major curve p.
facilitation p.
filling p.
firing p.
fracture p.
full interference p.
gait p.
heel-toe p.
honeycomb p.
injury p.
interference p.
intermediate interference p.
kinematic gait p.
lamellar p.
left thoracolumbar major curve p.
locomotor p.
major lumbar curve p.
major thoracic curve p.
minor lumbar curve p.
minor thoracic curve p.
neuromuscular gait p.
nondermatomal p.
nonradicular p.
p. of motion
p. of thrust
plantar pressure p.
PNF p.
2-point step-to gait p.
polka-dot p.
posterior depression p.
primitive locomotor p.
proprioceptive neuromuscular facilitation p.
recruitment p.

P

pattern (*continued*)
    reduced interference p.
    right thoracic, left lumbar
      curve p.
    right thoracic, left thoracolumbar
      curve p.
    right thoracic minor curve p.
    single lumbar curve p.
    single ray p.
    single thoracic curve p.
    single-unit p.
    storiform p.
    stretch p.
    thoracolumbar curve p.
    whorled p.
patterning
    Aston p.
PattStrap knee support
patty
    cement p.
    cottonoid p.
pauciarticular arthritis
Paufique blade
Paulos ligament technique
Paulson knee retractor
Paulus plate
Pauly point
Pauwels
    P. femoral neck fracture
      classification
    P. fracture
    P. operation
    P. osteotomy technique
    P. proximal osteotomy
    P. valgus osteotomy
    P. vertical sheet vector
      angle
    P. Y osteotomy
Pauzat disease
Pavlik
    P. bandage
    P. harness
    P. harness splint
    P. sling
Pavlov ratio
Payr sign
PB
    paraffin bath
    peroneus brevis
Pb
    lead
P-BAP
    Behavioral Assessment of Pain
      Questionnaire
PBS
    peroneus brevis split
PC
    PC Performer knee
    PC Performer knee prosthesis

PCA
    patient-controlled analgesia
    patient-controlled anesthesia
    porous-coated anatomic
      PCA cutting guide
      PCA hip stem
      PCA medullary guide
      PCA Original prosthesis
      PCA primary total knee system
      PCA Standard prosthesis
      PCA total hip replacement
      PCA unconstrained tricompartmental
       prosthesis
      PCA unicompartmental knee
       prosthesis
      PCA Universal total knee instrument
       system
PCE
    physical capacity evaluation
    Smith PCE
PCL
    posterior cruciate ligament
      PCL Protension isometer
      PCL reconstruction
PCL-oriented
    PCL-o. placement
    PCL-o. placement marking
      hook
PDD
    progressive diaphysial dysplasia
pDEXA peripheral bone densitometer
PDGF
    platelet-derived growth factor
PDLS
    physical daily living skill
PDN
    prosthetic disc nucleus
      PDN device
PDS
    polydioxanone suture
      PDS band
      PDS II suture
      PDS knot
pDXA
    peripheral dual-energy x-ray
      absorptiometry
Peabody
    P. and Munro procedure
    P. splint
peacock
    P. neurovascular island pedicle flap
      technique
    P. transposing index ray
peak
    P. anterior compression plate
      system
    p. bone mass
    p. dorsiflexion torque
    P. Fixation System

P. gait module
p. height velocity (PHV)
p. latency
P. Motus Motion Measurement System
p. pressure
p. torque
p. torque test
peak-pressure analysis
Pean clamp
pear bur
pear-shaped
p.-s. body
p.-s. vertebra
Pearson
P. attachment to Thomas splint
P. intramedullary saw
P. splint attachment
Pease-Thomson traction
Pebax
P. counter unit
P. fastening strap
Pec-Dec machine
Peck osteotome
pectineal muscle
pectora (*pl. of* pectus)
pectoral
p. girdle
p. nerve
p. reflex
pectoralis
p. major flap
p. major muscle
p. major shoulder contraction test
p. major tear syndrome
p. minor muscle
p. muscle implant
pectoris (*gen. of* pectus)
pectus, *pl.* **pectora,** *gen.* **pectoris**
p. carinatum
p. excavatum
p. recurvatum
pedal
p. exerciser
p. hyperpigmented lesion
p. hypophalangism
p. macrodactylia
p. osteomyelitis
Pedar
P. in-shoe measurement system
P. pressure insole system
P. pressure measurement system
pedes (*pl. of* pes)
pedestal
Body P.
cast equipped with rubber p.
halo p.
IMP surgical leg p.
rubber p.

shelf p.
p. sign
surgical leg p.
pedestaled
pedestrian accident
PEDI
Pediatric Evaluation of Disability Inventory
Pediapred Oral
Pediaprofen
pediatric, paediatric
p. advanced life support (PALS)
p. blade-plate
p. C-D hook
Cleocin P.
p. Cotrel-Dubousset rod
P. Evaluation of Disability Inventory (PEDI)
p. flatfoot
p. fracture fixation with titanium elastic nail
p. gait, arms, legs, spine (pGALS)
p. gait, arms, legs, spine screening
p. nutritional formula
p. orthopaedics
p. physical therapy
PRAFO p.
p. PRAFO brace
p. pressure relief ankle foot orthosis
p. shoulder support
p. system
p. TSRH hook
P. Ultrasound Bone Analyzer
pedicle
adjoining p.
p. anatomy
p. axis angle
p. bone graft
p. C-D hook
p. clamp
p. connector
contralateral hypoplastic/agenetic p.
p. cortex disruption
p. diameter
p. entrance point
p. erosion
p. fat graft
p. finder
p. fracture
p. groin flap
p. implant
p. landmark
p. localization
p. location
lower thoracic p.
lumbar p.
p. marker
p. method
p. morphometry

P

pedicle (*continued*)
    p. of vertebral arch
    p. plate
    p. screw
    p. screw breakage
    p. screw-cable system
    p. screw construct
    p. screw cord length
    p. screw fixation
    p. screw hardware prominence
    p. screw insertion
    p. screw linkage design
    p. screw path length
    p. screw plating
    p. screw pull-out strength
    p. screw system
    p. sounder
    p. sounding probe
    p. subtraction osteotomy
    thoracic p.
    vertebral p.
pedicled
    p. fibular transfer
    p. transplant
Pedic sponge
pedicular
    p. fixation
    p. kinking
pediculosis
pedicure
Pedi-Cushions pad
Pedi-Dri topical powder
Pedifix
    P. crest pad
    P. forefoot compression sleeve
    P. hammertoe pad
Pedilen polyurethane foam
Pediplast
    P. cushion
    P. moldable footcare compound
Pedi-Pro Topical
pedis (*gen. of* pes)
Pedi-Wrap immobilizer
pedobarogram
pedobarograph
    Biokinetics p.
    Musgrave footprint p.
pedobarographic analysis
pedobarography
    dynamic p. (DPB)
pedodynamometer
pedodynograph
pedodynographic
    p. examination
    p. measurement
pedogram
pedograph
pedography
pedometer

Pedors orthopaedic shoe
pedorthic
pedorthics
    American Board for Certification in
    Orthotics and Prosthetics and P.
    (ABCOP)
pedorthist
pedoscope
Pedrialle template
pedunculated
    p. loose body
    p. osteochondroma
PEEK
    polyaryletheretherketone
PEER
    pronation eversion external rotation
Peet Z-plasty
pefloxacin
peg
    anchoring p.
    p. base plate
    Beath bone intramedullary p.
    bone p.
    p. bone graft
    p. device
    fiber-metal p.
    fibular p.
    fixation p.
    glenoid alignment p.
    Harrison-Nicolle polypropylene p.
    Kinemax removable fixation p.
    locking p.
    polyethylene p.
    Smith subtalar joint arthroereisis p.
    stringing p.
    subtalar arthroereisis p.
    (STA-peg)
peg-and-socket technique
pegboard
    p. lateral positioning device
    Purdue p.
pegged tibial prosthesis
pegging
    bone p.
peg-in-hole
    p.-i.-h. arthrorisis
    p.-i.-h. osteotomy
Peimer reduction osteotomy
Peiper–Isbert reaction
PEK
    polyetherketone
Pelite thermoplastic crepe material
Pelken sign
**Pellegrini-Stieda knee ligament
ossification disease**
pellet
    calcium hydroxyapatite p.
pelmatogram
pelves (*pl. of* pelvis)

pelvic

 p. abscess
 p. angle
 p. avulsion fracture
 p. band
 p. bench
 p. block
 p. brace
 p. brim
 p. C clamp
 p. circumference
 p. diaphragm
 p. discontinuity
 p. drainage
 p. effluent
 p. fixation
 p. floor exercise
 p. fracture frame
 p. frontal obliquity angle
 p. girdle
 p. hyperextension traction
 p. injury
 p. instability
 p. kinematic chain
 p. lateral shift
 p. lateral tilt
 p. obliquity
 p. osteotomy
 p. plane
 p. reconstruction kit
 p. region bursitis
 p. region contusion
 p. rim fracture
 p. ring
 p. ring disruption
 p. ring dysfunction
 p. ring fracture
 p. rock (PR)
 p. rock test
 p. rotation
 p. rotation motion gait determinant
 p. sheet
 p. shift motion gait determinant
 p. side-shift
 p. sling
 p. splint
 p. splinting
 p. straddle fracture
 p. tilt motion gait determinant
 p. traction belt
 p. unleveling

pelvic-femoral angle
pelvis, *pl.* **pelves**
 achondroplastic p.
 assimilation p.
 beaked p.
 bony p.
 caoutchouc p.
 cordate p.
 coxalgic p.
 dual drop p. (DDP)
 dwarf p.
 false p.
 frozen p.
 greater p.
 high-assimilation p.
 juvenile p.
 kyphorachitic p.
 kyphoscoliorachitic p.
 kyphoscoliotic p.
 kyphotic p.
 lesser p.
 lordotic p.
 low-assimilation p.
 Nägele p.
 p. nana
 p. obtecta
 osteomalacic p.
 Otto p.
 Prague p.
 pseudoosteomalacic p.
 rachitic p.
 Rokitansky p.
 rostrate p.
 rubber p.
 scoliotic p.
 split p.
 spondylolisthetic p.
 sprung p.
 p. spuria
 stove-in p.

pelvofemoral muscular dystrophy
pelvospondylitis ossificans
Pemberton
 P. acetabuloplasty
 P. pericapsular osteotomy
 P. spur-crushing clamp
PEMF
 pulsating electromagnetic field
 pulsed electromagnetic field
 PEMF bone growth stimulation
pen
 weighted p.
Pen/Alps distal pad
pencil
 p. and cup deformity
 electrosurgical p.
 p. grip
 skin p.
 sterile p.
 p. test
penciling of ribs on x-ray
pencil-tip drill
Penco Walker Sleds
pendulum exercise
penetrating
 p. drill
 p. fracture

P

penetration
anterior cortex p.
penetrator
Arthrex P.
Penfield
P. 4 dissector
P. periosteal elevator
penguin gait
penicillamine
penicillin
p. G
p. g benzathine and procaine combined
Penlac
P. Nail Lacquer
P. Nail Lacquer topical solution
Pennal pelvic fracture classification
pennation angle
Penn finger drill
Pennig dynamic wrist fixator
Pennsylvania bimanual work sample
Penrose drain
pentazocine
p. compound
p. hydrochloride
pentobarbital
Pentothal Sodium
pentoxifylline
PEOS
posterior element overuse syndrome
peptic ulcer
peptide
atrial natriuretic p. (ANP)
brain natriuretic p. (BNP)
chemotactic p.
peptido-leukotriene
Peptococcus
Peptostreptococcus
PER
pronation-external rotation
PER (I-IV) fracture
PER injury
PER primam healing
peracetic acid
percent
Kendall muscle grade p. (0–100)
perception
constant-touch p.
p. deficit
pressure p.
visual p.
Percocet
Percodan
Percodan-Demi
Percogesic
Percolone
PercScope percutaneous discectomy
percussion
p. elbow test

p. hammer
p. sign
p. tenderness
Percuss-O-Matic jackhammer device
percutaneous
p. Achilles tendon repair
p. autogenous dowel bone graft
p. bone biopsy
p. bone marrow infection
p. core bone biopsy
p. corticotomy
p. dorsal column stimulator implant
p. epiphysiodesis
p. fixation
p. heel cord lengthening
p. K wire
p. lumbar discectomy
p. muscle biopsy
p. needle placement
p. nucleotomy
p. osteotomy
p. pin
p. pin insertion
p. pinning
p. pinning of fracture
p. plantar fasciotomy (PPF)
p. reduction
p. stapling
p. tendo Achillis lengthening
p. tenotomy
p. transcaudal epidural endoscopy
p. transmalleolar drilling
p. transpedicular biopsy
p. vertebroplasty
Percy
P. amputating saw
P. amputation retractor
P. plate
Perdriolle spinal vertebral rotation scoliosis assessment
Perez postoperative pain scale
Perfecta
P. femoral stem
P. hip prosthesis
P. (I, II) hip prosthesis
P. total hip system
perfect circle
perfect-circle technique
PerFixation
P. screw
P. system
perforating
p. artery
p. bur
p. forceps
p. fracture
p. twist drill
perforation
attritional p.

cortical p.
femoral cortical p.
perforator
Boyd p.
Dodd p.
p. drill
performance
p. area
P. Assessment of Self-Care Skills
p. component
p. context
Fugl-Meyer Evaluation of Physical P.
functional p.
isokinetic p.
P. knee prosthesis
P. modular total knee system
motion p.
safety p.
Test of Infant Motor P. (TIMP)
P. unicompartmental knee system
P. Wrap knee support
performance-enhancing steroid
performer ultralight knee brace
perfringens
Clostridium p.
perfusion
digital blood p.
pulsatile hypothermic p.
pergolide
periacetabular osteotomy
Periactin
perianal
p. sensation
p. skin
periaqueductal
p. gray
p. gray nucleus
periarthritis
periarthrosis humeri
periarticular
p. abscess
p. calcification
p. fibrositis
p. fracture
p. heterotopic ossification
p. tissue
pericapsular osteotomy
pericapsulitis
pericellular halo
perichondral, perichondrial
p. circulation
p. ossification
p. ring
perichondrial (*var. of* perichondral)
perichondrium
pericyte
Zimmerman p.

peridiscal
p. bone destruction
p. rim enhancement
periepineurial neuropathy
perihamate injury
perilesional bone
Peri-Loc
P.-L. periarticular locked plating device
P.-L. prosthesis
perilunar
p. instability
p. transscaphoid dislocation
perilunate
p. carpal dislocation
p. fracture-dislocation (PLFD)
perilymphatic fistula (PLF)
perimalleolar pain
perimeniscal cyst
perimysia (*pl. of* perimysium)
perimysial
perimysiitis, perimysitis
perimysitis (*var. of* perimysiitis)
perimysium, *pl.* **perimysia**
p. externum
perineal
p. flexure
p. loop
p. post
p. sensation
perinealis
luxatio p.
perineometer
Peritron p.
perineum
perineural
p. block
p. fibroma (PNR)
p. fibrosis
p. tissue
perineuria (*pl. of* perineurium)
perineurial neurorrhaphy
perineurium, *pl.* **perineuria**
period
absolute refractory p.
functional refractory p.
incubation p.
latent p.
postinjury p.
refractory p.
relative refractory p.
silent p.
periodic arthralgia
periodization of training
PerioGlas bone graft material
perionychia (*pl. of* perionychium)
perionychium, *pl.* **perionychia**
perioperative
p. antibiotic therapy

P

545

perioperative (*continued*)
    p. autotransfusion system
    p. reduction
periostalgia
    chronic p.
periostea (*pl. of* periosteum)
periosteal
    p. arthritis
    p. band
    p. bone collar
    p. button
    p. cambium layer
    p. chondroma
    p. chondrosarcoma
    p. desmoid
    p. elevation
    p. elevator
    p. fibroma
    p. ganglion
    p. implantation
    p. lamella
    p. new bone
    p. new bone formation
    p. ossification
    p. osteogenesis
    p. osteosarcoma
    p. reaction
    round-tapped p.
    p. sarcoma
    p. sleeve
    p. tissue
    p. vessel
periosteitis (*var. of* periostitis)
periosteopathy
periosteoplastic amputation
periosteotome
    Alexander costal p.
    Alexander-Farabeuf p.
    Ballenger p.
    Brown p.
    costal p.
    elevator p.
    Fomon p.
    Joseph p.
periosteotomy
periosteum
    p.
periostitis, periosteitis
    florid reactive p.
    p. ossificans
    suppurative p.
periostotome
periostotomy
peripatellar
    p. retinacular support
    p. tendinitis
peripheral
    p. arterial occlusive disease (PAOD)
    p. arteriography

    p. artery
    p. capsule
    p. chemical sympathectomy
    p. dual-energy x-ray absorptiometry (pDXA)
    p. facial paralysis
    p. gangrene
    p. meniscus
    p. modulation
    p. nerve block
    p. nerve block anesthesia
    p. nerve cutaneous field
    p. nerve entrapment
    p. nerve glove
    p. nerve injury (PNI)
    p. nerve palsy
    p. nerve tumor classification
    p. nervous system (PNS)
    p. neuritis
    p. neurocompressive disorder
    p. osteoarticular pathology
    p. paralysis
    p. polyneuritis
    p. vascular disease (PVD)
    p. vascular insufficiency (PVI)
    p. vascular obstructive disease
    p. vascular surgery (PVS)
    p. vascular system (PVS)
peripisiform injury
peripolar zone
periprosthetic
    p. bone loss
    p. bone resorption
    p. fracture
    p. membrane
    p. radiolucency
periscapulitis shoulder pain
perispondylitis
    Gibney p.
peritendinitis, peritenonitis, peritenontitis
    Achilles p.
    p. crepitans
    p. serosa
peritendinous scar
peritendon (*var. of* peritenon)
peritenon, peritendon
peritenonitis (*var. of* peritendinitis)
peritenontitis (*var. of* peritendinitis)
peritoneum
peritrapezial
    p. arthritis
    p. injury
peritrapezoidal injury
peritrochanteric fracture
Peritron perineometer
periungual fibroma
Perkins
    P. traction
    P. vertical line

Perkins-Ombredanne line
Perlstein brace
Perma-Hand silk suture
Permalock
Perman cartilage forceps
permanent
    p. and total disability (PTD)
    p. callus
    p. disability
    p. implant
    p. partial disability (PPD)
    p. partial disability rating
permanganate
    potassium p. ($KMnO_4$)
peroneal
    p. artery
    p. bupivacaine injection
    p. compartment syndrome
    p. dislocation
    p. groove
    p. island flap
    p. muscle
    p. muscle spasm
    p. muscular atrophy (PMA)
    p. musculature
    p. nerve
    p. nerve entrapment
    p. nerve injury
    p. nerve palsy
    p. neuropathy
    p. paralysis
    p. retinaculum
    p. sign
    p. sinus
    p. spastic flatfoot
    p. strengthening exercise
    p. tendinitis
    p. tendon
    p. tendon displacement
    p. tendon impingement
    p. tendon procedure
    p. tendon sheath injection
    p. tendon subluxation
    p. tenolysis
    p. tenosynovitis
    p. tunnel
    p. tunnel compression test
    p. vein
peronealis
    trochlea p.
peroneum
    os p.
peroneus
    p. brevis (PB)
    p. brevis elongation
    p. brevis graft
    p. brevis muscle
    p. brevis split (PBS)
    p. brevis tendon

    p. brevis to longus anastomosis
    p. brevis transfer
    p. longus
    p. longus muscle
    p. longus tendinopathy (PLT)
    p. longus tendon
    p. quartus muscle
    p. tertius muscle
    p. tertius tendon
peroxide
    p. flush
    hydrogen p. (H_2O_2)
perpendicular
    method of p.'s
    p. strumming
perphenazine
Perrin-Ferraton disease
Perry
    P. extensile anterior distal humerus
      approach
    P. sensor
    P. technique
Perry-Nickel cranial halo
Persian slipper foot
persistent
    p. clonus
    p. notochord
    p. occiput/atlas disrelationship
    p. pain
    p. sciatic artery (PSA)
personal protective equipment (PPE)
perstans
    macularis eruptiva p.
Perthes
    P. disease
    P. epiphysis
    P. lesion
    P. procedure
    P. reamer
    P. tourniquet test
Perthes-Bankart lesion
pertrochanteric fracture
perturbation
perverted function
pes, *pl.* **pedes,** *gen.* **pedis**
    p. abductus
    p. adductus
    p. anserine bursitis
    p. anserine bursitis pain
    p. anserinus
    p. anserinus syndrome
    p. anserinus transplant
    p. arcuatus
    p. arcuatus clawfoot deformity
    p. calcaneus
    calcar pedis
    p. cavovalgus
    p. cavovarus
    p. cavus

P

pes (*continued*)
    p. cavus clawfoot deformity
    p. cavus metatarsus
    dorsalis pedis (DP)
    p. equinovalgus
    p. equinovarus
    p. equinovarus adductus
    p. equinus
    p. febricitans
    p. gigas
    p. planovalgus
    p. planovalgus deformity
    p. plantigrade planus
    p. planus deformity
    p. planus et valgus
    pollex pedis
    porta pedis
    p. pronatus
    tinea pedis
    p. varus

PET
  positron emission tomography
    PET electrotherapy
petaling the cast
petechia, *pl.* **petechiae**
  p.
petechiae (*pl. of* petechia, *pl. of*
 petechia)
Peterson traction
PET/Eurotech Generation 2000 table
petit
    P. inferior lumbar triangle
    p. pas gait
Petren gait
Petrie spica cast
pétrissage
petroclinoid ligament
petrolatum gauze
petroleum gauze dressing
petrosal bone
petrous temporal bone
Pettibon chiropractic procedure
PF
  plantar flexion
    PF Night Splint II splint
PFC
  press-fit condylar
    PFC curved unconstrained prosthesis
    PFC femoral prosthesis
    PFC hip stem
    PFC modular total knee system
    PFC offset tibial tray
    PFC Sigma knee system
    PFC TC3 modular knee system
    PFC total hip replacement system
PFD
  patellofemoral dysfunction
  polyurethane foam dressing
Pfeiffer syndrome

PFFD
  proximal femoral focal deficiency
  proximal focal femoral deficiency
Pfitzner theory of coalition formation
PFO
  plantar fasciitis orthosis
    PFO night splint
PFS
  post-facilitation stretch
  preservative-free solution
    Adriamycin PFS
    Folex PFS
PFT
  postoperative flexor tendon
    PFT traction brace
PFWT
  pain-free walking time
P/G
    Fulvicin P/G
PGA
  polyglycolic acid
    PGA rod
    PGA screw
pGALS
  pediatric gait, arms, legs, spine
    pGALS screening
PGA-PLA
  polyglycolic acid-polylactic acid
    PGA-PLA biomaterial
PGP
    PGP flexible nail system
    PGP nail
PGS-3000 pulsed galvanic stimulator
phagocytosis
phalangeal
    p. articular orientation
    p. articulation
    p. bone
    p. clamp
    p. condylectomy
    p. degloving
    p. diaphysial fracture
    p. dislocation
    p. fracture fixation
    p. head
    p. herniation
    p. hypoplasia
    p. implant
    p. malunion correction
    p. microgeodic syndrome
    p. neck
    p. osteotomy
    p. polydactyly
    p. synostosis
phalangectomy
    intermediate p.
phalanges (*pl. of* phalanx)
phalangis (*gen. of* phalanx)
phalangization

phalangophalangeal amputation
phalanx, *pl.* **phalanges,** *gen.* **phalangis**
    accessory p.
    delta p.
    distal p. (DP)
    osteitis distal p.
    proximal p. (PP)
    tufted p.
    waist of p.
Phalen
    P. carpal tunnel syndrome sign
    P. maneuver
    P. position
    P. wrist flexion test
Phalen-Miller opponensplasty
phantom
    p. breast pain
    p. frame
    Jaszczak p.
    p. limb
    p. limb pain (PLP)
    p. limb syndrome
    p. pain phenomenon
    Rollo p.
    p. sensation
phantosmia
pharmacodynamic
pharyngeal tissue
phase
    blood pool p.
    double-leg stance p.
    p. 2 elbow program
    fibroblastic p.
    flexor p.
    foot-strike p.
    granulation p.
    heel-contact p.
    heel-off p.
    heel-strike p.
    inflammatory p.
    initial contact p.
    inosculation p.
    maturation p.
    opposite foot-strike p.
    opposite toe-off p.
    organizational p.
    plasmatic p.
    propulsive p.
    push-off p.
    remodeling p.
    reparative p.
    stance p.
    swing p.
    toe-off p.
3-phase bone scan
pheasant
    P. discotome
    P. elbow operation
    P. elbow technique

Phelps
    P. brace
    P. neurectomy
    P. operation
    P. orthosis
    P. partial resection
    P. scapulectomy
    P. splint
Phemister
    P. acromioclavicular pin fixation
    P. biopsy trephine
    P. elevator
    P. medial approach to tibia
    P. medial epiphysiodesis approach
    P. onlay bone graft
    P. onlay bone graft technique
    P. operation
    P. osteotomy
    P. posteromedial approach
    P. rasp
Phemister-Bonfiglio femoral neck bone grafting technique
Phenaphen With Codeine
phencyclidine hydrochloride
Phendry Oral
Phenergan
phenobarbital
phenol
    camphor and p.
    p. cauterization
    p. chemosurgery
    P. EZ swab
    p. matricectomy
    p. neurolysis
phenol-alcohol matricectomy
phenolization
    nail matrix p. (NMP)
phenomena (*pl. of* phenomenon)
phenomenon, *pl.* **phenomena**
    bioelectric p.
    brake p.
    Burner p.
    catch-up p.
    combined flexion p.
    compression p.
    crankshaft p.
    gelling p.
    give-way p.
    glued-to-the-floor p.
    Gordon knee p.
    Gowers p.
    halisteresis p.
    Herendeen p.
    Holmes p.
    Holmes-Stewart p.
    Hunt paradoxical p.
    Kienböck p.
    lumbrical plus p.
    Lust p.

P

phenomenon (*continued*)
    magic angle p.
    no-reflow p.
    phantom pain p.
    pivot-shift p.
    pronation p.
    Queckenstedt p.
    radial p.
    Raynaud p.
    referred anatomic p.
    referred trigger point p.
    relaxation p.
    release p.
    Rust p.
    spontaneous vacuum p.
    staircase p.
    temporary cavity p.
    tibial p.
    toe p.
    vacuum p.
    Valleix p.
    vertebral steal p.
    Westphal p.
    windup p.
phentolamine
phenylbutazone
phenylephrine
    prilocaine and p.
phenylpropanolamine
phenyltoloxamine
    acetaminophen and p.
phenytoin
Philadelphia
    P. cervical collar
    P. collar cervical support
    P. collar cervical traction
    P. Plastizote cervical brace
    P. rigid collar
Philips
    P. Angiodiagnostics 96
      apparatus
    P. linear accelerator
    P. toe force gauge
Phillips
    P. head screw
    P. head screwdriver
    P. muscle
    P. recessed-head screw
    P. screw head
    P. splint
philosophy
    Palmerian p.
pHisoHex
phlebography
phlebolith
phlebothrombosis
phlogistic agent
phocomelia, phocomely
    complete p.

    distal p.
    proximal p.
phocomelic dwarfism
phocomely (*var. of* phocomelia)
Phoenix
    P. foot system
    P. Outrigger splint
    P. total hip prosthesis
phonological analysis
phonophoresis
    hydrocortisone p.
    p. plantarflexion
    ultrasound p.
Phoresor
    P. II iontophoretic drug delivery
      system
    P. PM900 iontophoresis system
phos
    alk p.
phosphatase
    alkaline p. (alk phos)
    bone-specific alkaline p. (BSAP)
    tartrate resistant acid p. (TRAP)
phosphate (PO$_4$)
    Aralen P.
    betamethasone sodium p.
    calcium p.
    chloroquine p.
    Cleocin P.
    Decadron P.
    Hexadrol P.
    Hydrocortone P.
    hydroxyapatite tetra-tri-calcium p.
    nicotinamide-adenine dinucleotide p.
      (NADPH)
    sodium p.
    technetium 99m p.
    tetracalcium p.
    tricalcium p.
phosphatidylcholine
    dipalmitoyl p.
phosphatidylserine
phosphokinase
    creatine p.
photoactive naphthalimide compound
photogrammetry
    x-ray p.
photon densitometry
photopenia
    hardware p.
photoplethysmography
    digital p.
phthinoid chest
PHV
    peak height velocity
phycomycosis
physeal (*var. of* physial)
physial, physeal
    p. angle

p. bar
p. bridge
p. cartilage
p. closure
p. damage
p. disruption
p. distraction
p. growth
p. injury
p. line
p. mamillary process
p. plate fracture
p. region
p. scar
p. stapling
physiatric
physiatrics
physiatrist
physiatry
physical
P. Ability Test (PAT)
p. activity
P. Activity Readiness Questionnaire (PAR-Q)
p. agent
p. capacity evaluation (PCE)
p. condition, upper limb function, lower limb function, sensory component, excretory function, support function (PULSES)
p. daily living skill (PDLS)
p. examination
p. impairment
p. inactivity
p. independence WHO Handicap Scale
p. medicine
p. medicine and rehabilitation (PM&R, PMR)
p. realignment
p. therapy (PT)
p. therapy table
p. training (PT)
p. work
p. work capacity (PWC)
physiognomy
PhysioGymnic exercise ball
physiologic, physiological
p. barrier
p. flatfoot
p. lock
p. lock of motion segment
p. range of joint motion
p. response
p. saline
p. valgus
physiological (*var. of* physiologic)
p. hyperactivity
p. venous pump mechanism

PhysioLogics Alpha Lipoic Acid
physiology
exercise p.
Fontan p.
physiolysis
central p.
Physio-Roll-R-Cise
Physio-Roll VisuaLiser exercise ball
Physio-Stim Lite bone growth stimulator
physiotherapeutic
physiotherapist
physiotherapy (PT)
active p.
aqua PT dry p.
individual p.
passive p.
physique
ectomesomorphic p.
ectomorphic p.
physis
distal tibial p.
p. fracture
modified Boyd amputation of ankle and distal tibial p.
Phytaid
phytoestrogen
Phytolyn
phytonadione
phytonutrient
PI
posteroinferior
piano key shoulder sign
piano-wire dorsiflexion brace
PIB
Pittsburgh Compound B
PICA
posterior inferior cerebellar artery
pick
P. chisel
dental p.
Picker Magnascanner for bone metastasis
picket
p. fence guide
P. Fence leg positioner
pick-up
p.-u. forceps
p.-u. test
Picot incision
picture
maximum pressure p.
picture-frame appearance
Pidcock
P. nail
P. pin
piecemeal
pie-crusting skin graft
Piedmont fracture

P

Pierrot
  P. and Murphy tendo Achillis
    insertion transplant
  P. and Murphy advancement insertion
PIEX
  posteroinferior external
    PIEX ilium
    PIEX movement
    PIEX subluxation
piezoelectric
  p. accelerometer
  p. potential
Piezoelectro-needleless stimulator
piezogenic papule
Piffard curette
pigeon
  p. breast
  p. chest
pigeon-toeing gait
pigmented
  p. nodular synovitis
  p. nodular synovitis of tendon sheath
  p. villonodular bursitis
  p. villonodular synovitis (PVNS, PVS)
  p. villonodular tenosynovitis
pigmenti
  incontinentia p.
pigtail tendon stripper
PIIN
  posteroinferior internal
    PIIN ilium
    PIIN movement
    PIIN subluxation
Pilates
  P. exercise method
  P. method exercise
pillar
  articular p.
  p. pain
  P. PEEK partial vertebral body
    replacement system
  P. PEEK VBR system
  p. tenderness
Pillet hand prosthesis
Pilliar
  P. prosthesis
  P. total hip replacement
Pillo
  Knee P.
Pillo-Pedic cervical traction pillow
pillow
  abduction p.
  antibacterial p.
  Bio-Gel decubitus p.
  Bodynapper Comfort P.
  Capello slim-line abduction p.
  Carter elevation p.
  Carter foam p.
  cervical sleep p.

cervical support p.
cervical traction p.
p. collar
Comfort Club tub p.
Comfort-U total body p.
Crescent Complete Sleeper p.
Crescent memory p.
Crescent-Pillo p.
D-Core support p.
Dream P.
elevation p.
Flip-Flop p.
foam p.
foot p.
p. fracture
Frejka p.
Mediflow waterbase p.
neck p.
Neckcare p.
Neck-Hugger cervical support p.
Opti-Curve therapeutic p.
OrthoBone p.
p. orthosis
p. orthosis for hip
Orthosleep P.
Pillo-Pedic cervical traction p.
Pillo-Wedge p.
Pron p.
shoulder abduction p.
Silicore foot p.
snooze p.
Softeze water p.
p. splint
Tempur-Pedic pressure relieving
  Swedish p.
T-Foam p.
Theracloud p.
Therapeutics Sleeping P.
Therasleep Cervical P.
Tricore cervical support p.
Wal-Pil-O neck p.
Pillo-Wedge pillow
pill rolling tremor
pilomotor
  p. dysfunction
  p. response
pilon
  p. fracture
  p. fracture classification
pilonidal dimple
Pil-O-Splint wrist splint
pilot
  p. bur
  p. drill
  P. point screw
pin

A p.
absorbable polymeric p.
absorbable polyparadioxanone p.

Ace p.
Acufex distractor p.
alignment p.
Allofix freeze-dried cortical bone p.
Apex p.
Arthrex Trim-It Spin P.
Arthrex zebra p.
arum fixation p.
ASIF screw p.
Asnis p.
Austin Moore p.
p. ball system
Barr p.
beaded hip p.
Beath p.
Belos compression p.
bevel-point Rush p.
Bilos p.
Biofix system p.
bioresorbable p.
Böhler p.
Böhler-Knowles hip p.
Böhler-Steinmann p.
Bohlman p.
breakaway p.
Breck p.
Bremer HIFix skull p.
buttress p.
calcaneal p.
calibrated p.
Canakis beaded hip p.
cancellous p.
Charnley p.
p. chuck
p. clamp
clavicle p.
cloverleaf p.
Co-Cr-Mo p.
collapsible p.
Compere threaded p.
Compton clavicle p.
Conley p.
cortical p.
Craig p.
p. crimper
Crowe pilot point on Steinmann p.
Crowe tip p.
Crutchfield p.
p. cutter
Davis p.
Day fixation p.
DCS p.
deluxe FIN p.
Denham p.
DePuy p.
derotational p.
distraction p.
drill p.
Ender p.

p. external fixator
Fahey p.
femoral guide p.
Fischer transfixing p.
Fisher half p.
p. fixation
fixation p.
Freebody p.
freeze-dried bone p.
friction lock p.
p. guard
p. guide
guide p.
Hagie hip p.
halo p.
Hansen p.
Hare p.
Hatcher p.
Haynes p.
p. headrest
Hegge p.
Hewson breakaway p.
hex head p.
HIFix skull p.
hip p.
Hoffmann apex fixation p.
Hoffmann transfixion p.
p. holder
hook p.
hook-end intramedullary p.
p. implant
Intraflex intramedullary p.
intramedullary p.
Jones compression p.
Jurgan p.
Kirschner wire p.
Knowles hip p.
Kronfeld p.
Küntscher p.
LIH hook p.
locating p.
locked intramedullary
  osteosynthesis p.
Lottes p.
marble bone p.
Markley retention p.
Matthews-Green p.
McBride p.
medullary p.
metal p.
Modny p.
Moore fixation p.
Moule screw p.
Neufeld p.
nonthreaded p.
Norman tibial p.
Olds p.
Oris p.
Ormco p.

P

pin (*continued*)
  Orthofix p.
  OrthoSorb absorbable p.
  osseous p.
  osteotomy p.
  partially threaded p.
  percutaneous p.
  Pidcock p.
  p. placement for treatment of pelvic
    fracture
  Pugh hip p.
  rasp p.
  resorbable polydioxanon p.
  resorbable polymer p.
  restorative p.
  p. retractor
  ReUnite orthopaedic p.
  Rhinelander p.
  Riordan p.
  Risser p.
  Rush intramedullary fixation p.
  Safir p.
  Sage p.
  Scand hip p.
  Schanz p.
  Schneider p.
  Schweitzer p.
  self-broaching p.
  self-tapering p.
  Serrato forearm p.
  Shriners p.
  p. site
  skeletal p.
  skull p.
  p. sleeve
  Smart P.
  SmartPin/PLLA p.
  Smillie p.
  Smith-Petersen fracture p.
  SMO Moore p.
  smooth Steinmann p.
  Snap fixation p.
  SOC p.
  socket p.
  spring p.
  Stader p.
  Steinmann fixation p.
  Street medullary p.
  strut-type p.
  p. suture
  Tachdjian p.
  tapered p.
  threaded Steinmann p.
  tibial p.
  titanium half p.
  p. track
  p. tract infection
  traction p.
  transarticular p.

  transcapitellar p.
  transfixing p.
  Trim-It drill p.
  Trim-It Spin P.
  trochanteric p.
  Turner p.
  Tutofix cortical p.
  union broach retention p.
  Varney p.
  p. vise
  von Saal medullary p.
  Watanabe costal p.
  Webb p.
  p. wheel
  wrench p.
  Z p.
  Zimfoam p.
  Zimmer p.
pin-and-plaster
  p.-a.-p. fixation
  p.-a.-p. method
pin-bone interface
pincement
pincer
  p. nail
  p. nail formation
  p. palpation
  p. testing
pincer-type impingement
pinch
  p. callus
  p. gauge
  P. Gauge and Jackson Strength
    Evaluation System
  p. grasp
  p. grip test
  key p.
  lateral squeeze p.
  p. meter
  palmar p.
  p. power
  p. restoration
  p. strength
  tip p.
  tip-to-tip p.
  p. tree
pinchometer
  Prestop p.
pinch-tuck stitch
ping-pong
  p.-p. bone
  p.-p. fracture
Pinkus
  fibroepithelioma of P.
Pinna-Cal ipriflavone
pinnacle
  P. acetabular cup system
  P. hip replacement
  P. Hip Solutions

Pinn-ACL guide system
Pinn anterior cruciate ligament guide
  system
pinning
    Asnis p.
    closed p.
    hip p.
    Knowles p.
    open p.
    percutaneous p.
    Sherk-Probst percutaneous p.
    Sofield p.
    Wagner closed p.
pinpoint ulceration
pinprick
    p. hyperalgesia test
    p. sensation
pin-seating forceps
pin-to-bar clamp
Pinto distractor
pin-tract osteomyelitis
pinwheel
    Cleanwheel disposable
     neurological p.
    Safe-T-Wheel p.
    P. System
    Wartenberg p.
Piotrowski sign
PIP
    proximal interphalangeal
    PIP flexion creaking
    PIP joint
PIP/DIP strap
piperacillin
piperacillin/tazobactam therapy
pipe tree
Pipkin
    P. fracture classification system
    P. posterior hip dislocation
     classification
    P. subclassification of
     Epstein-Thomas classification
Pipkin-type femoral head fracture
pi plate dorsal distal radius
  plate
PIR
    postisometric relaxation
Pirie
    P. bone
    talonavicular ossicle of P.
piriform, pyriform
    p. muscle
    p. sclerosis
    p. sclerosis of ilium
piriformis
    p. entry portal
    p. sign
    p. syndrome
    p. test

Pirogoff amputation
piroxicam
Pischel micropin
pisiform
    p. bone
    p. bursa
    p. metacarpal
     ligament
    p. ossification
pisohamate ligament
pisometacarpal ligament
pisotriquetral
    p. arthritis
    p. joint
pistol-grip hand drill
piston
    cannulated expulsion p.
    p. prosthesis
    p. sign
pistoning motion
PIT
    patellar inhibition test
pitch
    calcaneal p.
pitching injury
Pitcock nail
pitted
    p. cartilage
    p. keratolysis
pitting edema
Pittsburgh
    P. Compound B (PIB)
    P. pelvic frame
pituitary
    p. gigantism
    p. grasper
    p. rongeur
PIVM
    passive intervertebral motion
    PIVM testing
pivot
    Accu-Line dual p.
    calcar p.
    p. joint
    medial stem p.
    P. MIS system
    p. of calcar
    P. Plate rehabilitation
     plate
    P. Pole walking device
    p. shift sign
    p. sport activity
pivoting
    p. and cutting activity
    p. sports
pivot-shift
    p.-s. knee test
    p.-s. phenomenon
    p.-s. test

P

PJPS
    patellofemoral joint pain syndrome
    PJPS Severity Scale (PSS)
PKA
    posterior knee ankle
    PRAFO PKA
PLA
    polylactic acid
    PLA anchor
placement
    bone graft p.
    electrode p.
    glide hole for screw p.
    graft p.
    hand p.
    K wire p.
    needle p.
    PCL-oriented p.
    percutaneous needle p.
    plate p.
    portal p.
    posterolateral bone graft p.
    p. reflex
    rod p.
    sacral screw p.
    screw p.
    variable screw p. (VSP)
Placidyl
placing reflex
plafond
    p. fracture
    tibial p.
    varus p.
plagiocephaly
    deformational p.
plain
    Citanest P.
    p. gauze
    p. pattern plate
    p. rotary scissors
    p. screwdriver
    p. tissue forceps
Plak-Vac oral suction brush
plan
    Making Action P.'s (MAPs)
    McConnell patellofemoral treatment p.
    National Arthritis Action P. (NAAP)
    preoperative p.
plana
    coxa p.
    manus p.
    vertebra p.
1-plane
    1-p. bilateral external fixator
    1-p. bilateral frame
    1-p. deformity
    1-p. instability
    1-p. unilateral external fixator
    1-p. unilateral frame

2-plane
    2-p. bilateral external fixator
    2-p. bilateral frame
    2-p. deformity
    2-p. fluoroscopy
    2-p. roentgenogram
    2-p. unilateral external fixator
    2-p. unilateral frame
plane
    AC-PC p.
    anatomic p.
    axial p.
    coronal p.
    facet p.
    fascial p.
    flexion-extension p.
    Frankfort horizontal p.
    frontal p.
    Hensen p.
    Hodge p.
    horizontal p.
    internervous p.
    intertubercular p.
    p. joint
    Ludwig p.
    median sagittal p.
    mesiodistal p.
    midsagittal p.
    paramedian sagittal p.
    pelvic p.
    primary movement p.
    sagittal p.
    scapulothoracic guiding p.
    spinous p.
    sternoxiphoid p.
    subcostal p.
    suprasternal p.
    thigh-shank p.
    thoracic p.
    transverse p.
    varus-valgus p.
    vertical p.
3-plane deformity
planer
    calcar p.
    Rubin bone p.
    Rubin cartilage p.
plane-type acromioclavicular
    articulation
planigram (*var. of* tomogram)
planigraphy (*var. of* tomography)
planning
    P. Alternative Tomorrows with Hope
      (PATH)
    preoperative p.
    rehabilitation p.
planogram (*var. of* tomogram)
planography (*var. of* tomography)
Planostretch stockings

planovalgus
    collapsing pes p.
    p. deformity
    p. foot
    hypermobile pes p.
    pes p.
    talipes p.
plantalgia
plantar
    p. angulation
    p. aponeurosis
    p. approach
    p. arch support orthosis
    p. arterial arch
    p. artery
    p. artery flap
    p. axial view
    p. Babinski response
    p. bone
    p. bony prominence
    p. bromhidrosis
    p. buckling
    p. calcaneal spur
    p. calcaneocuboid ligament
    p. calcaneonavicular ligament
    p. calcaneonavicular ligament-tibialis
      posterior tendon advancement
    p. callosity
    p. capsular release
    p. capsule
    p. capsuloligamentous complex
    p. compartment
    p. condylectomy
    p. corn
    p. cuboideonavicular ligament
    p. cuneocuboid ligament
    p. cuneonavicular ligament
    p. dermatosis
    p. ecchymosis sign
    p. fascia
    p. fascial release
    p. fasciitis
    p. fasciitis night splint
    p. fasciitis orthosis (PFO)
    p. fasciitis orthosis splint
    p. fasciitis syndrome
    p. fasciitis taping
    p. fasciotomy
    p. fat pad
    p. fibromatosis
    p. flexion (PF)
    p. flexion-inversion test
    p. foot
    p. grasp reflex
    p. intercuneiform ligament
    p. keratosis
    p. lateral base
    p. ligament
    p. longitudinal incision

    p. malignant melanoma
    p. metatarsal angle
    p. metatarsal artery
    p. metatarsal ligament
    p. nerve
    p. pain
    p. plate
    p. plate injury
    p. plate release
    p. pressure
    p. pressure pattern
    p. reflex
    p. shift
    p. spring ligament
    p. stress ankle x-ray
    p. sweating
    p. tarsometatarsal ligament
    p. tendinopathy
    p. toe pulp
    p. transposition
    p. ulcer
    p. vault
    p. V infiltration block
    p. V-Y advancement flap
    p. wart
plantar-dorsiflexion
plantarflex
plantarflexed stress radiograph
plantarflexing
plantarflexion
    p. injury
    passive p.
    phonophoresis p.
    p. stress view
    p. torque
plantarflexion-inversion deformity
plantarflexor
    p. proximal metatarsal osteotomy
    p. reflex
plantarflexory
    p. motion
    p. osteotomy
plantar-hindfoot-midfoot bony mass
plantaris
    p. muscle
    talipes p.
    p. tendon
    p. tendon graft
plantar-lateral release
plantar-medial release
plantarward
plantigrade
    p. foot
    p. limb
    p. platform
planus
    flexible pes p.
    Gleich osteotomy for pes valgo p.
    lichen p.

P

planus (*continued*)
    pes plantigrade p.
    rigid pes p.
    talipes p.
Plaquenil
plasm (*var. of* plasma)
plasma, plasm
    p. beta-endorphin
    p. cell dyscrasia
    coagulated p.
    p. osmolality
    p. volume shift
plasmacytoma
    aggressive solitary p.
    extramedullary p. (EMP)
Plasmanate
plasma-sprayed
    low-pressure p.-s. (LPPS)
    p.-s. titanium
plasmatic
    p. phase
    p. phase of skin healing
plasmin
Plasmodium falciparum
Plastalume
    P. bulb-ended splint
    P. straight splint
Plastazote
    P. arch support
    P. blank
    P. cervical collar
    P. cervical collar orthosis
    P. foam
    P. foot bed
    P. insole
    P. orthotic device
    P. shoe liner
Plastazote-Kydex cervical immobilizer
plaster
    p. bandage
    Batchelor p.
    p. cast
    p. cast application burn
    p. cast jacket
    closing wedge manipulation and
      reapplication of p.
    Hapset hydroxyapatite bone graft p.
    p. of Paris (POP)
    p. of Paris bandage
    p. of Paris cast
    p. of Paris splint
    opening wedge manipulation and
      reapplication of p.
    p. saw
    p. slab splint
    p. sole
    p. sore
    p. toe cap
    Velpeau p.

    x-ray in p. (XIP)
    x-ray out of p. (XOP)
    Zoroc p.
plastic
    p. achillotenotomy
    p. ankle-foot orthosis
    p. ball implant
    p. body jacket
    p. bowing fracture
    p. cast
    p. collar
    p. deformation
    p. end cap
    p. femoral plug
    p. floor reaction ankle-foot orthosis
    p. heel cup
    p. leaf-spring (PLS)
    p. limited-motion joint
    low-temperature p.
    p. marrow canal restrictor
    Orthoplast p.
    p. patella
    p. repair
    p. strain
    thermolabile p.
    unitary p.
PlastiCast adjustable joint cast system
plasticity
    connective tissue p.
    cortical p.
Plasticor prosthesis
Plasti-Pore
    P.-P. ossicular replacement prosthesis
    P.-P. prosthetic material
Plastiport TORP prosthesis
Plast-O-Fit thermoplastic bandage
plasty
    Bosworth-type reverse p.
    Coleman p.
    Durham p.
    flap p.
    p. modification
    rotation p.
    side-swing p.
    skin p.
    transbone p.
    V-Y p.
    Y-V p.
plate
    acetabular reconstruction p.
    AcroMed VSP p.
    Acumed congruent clavicle p.
    alar p.
    Alta condylar buttress p.
    Alta distal fracture p.
    anchor p.
    angled compression p.
    Ant-Cer cervical p.
    Ant-Cer dynamic cervical p.

anterior cervical p. (ACP)
anterior sacroiliac joint p.
antiglide p.
AO-ASIF compression p.
AO contoured T p.
AO dynamic compression p.
AO hook p.
AO-Morscher p.
AO reconstruction p.
AO semitubular p.
AO small fragment p.
AO spoon p.
Armstrong p.
ASIF broad dynamic compression
  bone p.
ASIF reconstruction p.
athletic shoe carbon fiber p.
Atlantis anterior cervical p.
autocompression p.
avulsion of nail p.
axial p.
Badgley spinal p.
Bagby angled compression
  mandibular p.
barrel p.
Batchelor p.
Becton Colles fracture p.
p. bender
biodegradable p.
Blanchard traction device blade p.
Blount blade p.
bone flap fixation p.
Bosworth spine p.
Boyd side p.
bridge p.
broad AO dynamic compression p.
Burns p.
butterfly-shaped monoblock
  vertebral p.
buttress pie p.
buttress-type p.
Calandruccio side p.
Calcanea calcaneal fracture p.
calcaneal Y p.
cap-and-anchor p.
carbon fiber-reinforced p.
cartilaginous growth p.
Caspar cervical p.
cervical p.
cloverleaf p.
coaptation p.
cobra-head p.
Collison p.
compression p.
Concise side p.
condylar p.
connecting p.
Continuum total knee base p.
contoured anterior spinal p. (CASP)

contoured T-plate p.
cortical p.
craniocervical p.
crosslink p.
cruciform tibial base p.
C-shaped p.
p. cutter
3D p.
deck p.
Deltaloc Reveal anterior cervical p.
DePuy p.
Deyerle p.
dorsal p.
double cobra p.
double-H p.
Driessen hinged p.
p. driver
dual p.
DVR anatomic wrist fracture p.
Dwyer-Hall p.
dynamic compression p. (DCP)
eccentric dynamic compression p.
  (EDCP)
Eggers bone p.
Elliott femoral condyle blade p.
end p.
epiphysial growth p.
femoral p.
ferromagnetic metal p.
fibrocartilaginous p.
p. fixation
flat p.
flexor p.
foot p.
force p.
frontal p.
fusion p.
gait p.
Gallannaugh p.
Galveston p.
growth p.
Hagie sliding nail p.
Haid cervical p.
Haid Universal bone p.
half-circle p.
Harlow p.
Harms posterior cervical p.
Harris p.
heavy-duty femur p.
heavy side p.
Hicks lugged p.
Hoen skull p.
2-hole p.
3-hole p.
5-hole p.
6-hole p.
7-hole p.
11-hole p.
17-hole p.

P

plate (*continued*)

4-hole Alta straight p.
4-hole side p.
Holt nail p.
hook p.
hot p.
H-shaped p.
Hubbard side p.
Hungarian grip p.
Inner Lip P.
interfragmentary p.
intertrochanteric p.
Jergesen I-beam p.
Jergesen tapered p.
Jewett nail overlay p.
Jones compression p.
Kaneda p.
Kessel p.
L p.
Lane p.
Lawson-Thornton p.
Letournel p.
limited compression-dynamic
  compression p.
limited-contact dynamic
  compression p.
locking compression p.
LoCon-T distal radial p.
Louis p.
low-contact dynamic compression p.
low-profile dorsal p.
L-shaped p.
Luhr Microfixation cranial p.
Luhr pan p.
Lundholm p.
Luque II p.
Mancini p.
Massie p.
May anatomical bone p.
Mayo Clinic congruent elbow p.
McBride p.
McLaughlin p.
Mears sacroiliac p.
Medoff sliding p.
metal foot p.
Meurig Williams p.
Milch p.
minimally invasive dynamic condylar
  screw and p.
modified Grace p.
Moe intertrochanteric p.
Moore sliding nail p.
Moreira p.
Morscher cervical p.
Müller p.
nail p.
narrow AO dynamic compression p.
Neufeld p.
neutralization p.

Newman p.
Nicoll p.
occipitocervical p.
Ogden p.
Orion anterior cervical p.
Orozco p.
orthotic p.
Osborne p.
overlay p.
palmar p.
Paulus p.
pedicle p.
peg base p.
Percy p.
pi plate dorsal distal
  radius p.
Pivot Plate rehabilitation p.
p. placement
plain pattern p.
plantar p.
Polyax polyaxial locked p.
Polytechnic foot-pressure
  measuring p.
precurved p.
pressure p.
protection p.
proximal humerus p.
pterygoid p.
Pugh p.
pylon attachment p.
Pyramid anterior fixation p.
quadrangular positioning p.
reconstruction p.
resorbable p.
resorbable cervical mesh p.
Richards-Hirschhorn p.
Rohadur gait p.
roof p.
round-hole compression p.
Roy-Camille p.
SC-AcuFix ThinLine p.
Schneider cobra-head p.
Schweitzer spring p.
semitubular compression p.
Senn p.
serpentine p.
Sherman bone p.
side p.
Simmons p.
slide p.
slotted femur p.
Smith-Petersen intertrochanteric p.
SMO p.
Sorrells tibia protector plate Sorrells
  tibia protector p.
p. spacer washer
spinous process p.
spoon p.
spring p.

stabilization p.
stainless steel p.
static compression p.
Steffee pedicle p.
Steffee screw p.
stem base p.
subchondral p.
supracondylar p.
symmetrical thoracic vertebral p.
symmetric sacral p.
Synthes dorsal distal radius p.
Synthes pie p.
Tacoma sacral p.
tarsal p.
T buttress p.
tectal p.
Temple University p.
tendon p.
tension band p.
thoracolumbosacral p.
Thornton nail p.
tibial base p.
titanium hollow-screw
  osseointegrating reconstruction p.
  (THORP)
titanium mandibular p.
toe p.
Townley tibial plateau p.
Townsend-Gilfillan p.
transoral atlantoaxial reduction p.
  (TARP)
trial base p.
T-shaped AO p.
TSRH p.
tubular bone p.
Tupman femur fracture p.
twisted p.
UCBL foot p.
Unity 51 lumbosacral fixation p.
universal bone p. (UBP)
Uslenghi p.
variable screw p. (VSP)
variable screw placement p.
V blade p.
Venable p.
vertebral end p.
vitallium Luhr p.
V nail p.
volar T p.
VSP p.
Wainwright p.
Weber antiglide p.
Wenger p.
Whitman p.
Wilson p.
Window titanium and titanium alloy
  anterior cervical p.
wing p.
Wright p.

Wurzburg p.
X p.
X-10 Crosslink p.
X-shaped p.
Y bone p.
Y-shaped p.
Zimmer side p.
Zimmer Y p.
Z-shaped p.
Zuelzer hook p.
plateau
  bicondylar tibial p.
  p. fracture
  proximal tibial p.
  tibial p.
plateaued
plate-holding forceps
platelet
  p. concentrate
  p. count
platelet-derived growth factor (PDGF)
platelike atelectasis
plate-screw
  p.-s. fixation
  p.-s. osteosynthesis
  p.-s. system
plate-to-bone compression
platform
  p. crutch
  force p.
  Kistler force p.
  Midland multifunctional mat p.
  Midline Hi-Lo Mat P.
  plantigrade p.
  spinal imaging p. (SIP)
  Velcro-Lock mat p.
plating
  compression p.
  diaphysial p.
  Gotfried percutaneous compression
    p.
  pedicle screw p.
  posterior spinal p.
  stacked p.
  variable spinal p. (VSP)
Platinol
Platinol-AQ
Platinum stationary table
Platou osteotomy
platybasia
platysma muscle
platyspondylia, platyspondylisis
platyspondylisis (*var. of* platyspondylia)
play
  end p.
  excessive joint p.
  joint p.
  muscle p.
  return to p. (RTP)

P

playfulness
Test of P. (ToP)
Playmaker
P. functional knee brace
P. support
PlayTuf knee brace
PLB
primary lymphoma of bone
PLC
posterior ligamentous
complex
pledget
Betadine-soaked p.
p. dressing
Gelfoam p.
p. of gauze
pleomorphic
p. fibrous histiocytoma
p. lipoma
p. liposarcoma
p. rhabdomyosarcoma
pleonosteosis
Léri p.
plethysmograph
Electro-Diagnostic Instruments
Model 720 bilateral tetrapolar
impedance p.
plethysmography
digital p.
impedance p.
pleura, *pl.* **pleurae**
parietal p. (PP)
pleurae (*pl. of* pleura)
pleural injury
Plexidure insole
plexiform
p. fibrohistiocytic tumor
p. neurofibroma
Plexiglas
P. jig
P. spacer
PlexiPulse
P. DVT prophylaxis
system
P. intermittent pneumatic
compression device
plexitis
brachial p.
plexopathy
brachial p.
congenital p.
Klumpke p.
Plexur P bone void filler
plexus, *pl.* **plexus, plexuses**
p. block
brachial p.
cervical p.
fascial p.
lumbosacral p.

sacral p.
subdermal p.
PLF
perilymphatic fistula
posterolateral fusion
PLFD
perilunate fracture-dislocation
plica, *pl.* **plicae**
bucket-handle p.
infrapatellar p.
lateral p.
medial patellar p.
medial shelf/medial p.
parapatellar p.
patellar p.
pathological p.
suprapatellar p.
symptomatic synovial p.
p. syndrome
synovial p.
tendon p.
p. test
plicae (*pl. of* plica)
plicamycin
plication
capsular p.
disc p.
soft tissue p.
plicectomy
pliers
compaction p.
extraction p.
Howmedica Microfixation
System p.
locking p.
Luhr Microfixation System p.
needle-nose vise-grip p.
orthopaedic surgical p.
Power-Grip p.
slip-joint p.
Sontec p.
square-end p.
Storz Microsystems p.
Synthes Microsystems p.
wire bending p.
PLIF
posterior lumbar interbody fusion
plight
musician's p.
plinth
PLL
posterior longitudinal ligament
PLLA
polylevolactic acid
poly-L-lactic acid
poly-L-lactide acid
PLLA anchor
PLLA implant
PLLA Trim-It system

PLM
 precise lesion measuring
  PLM device
plombage
 bone p.
plot
 load-displacement p.
plotter
PLP
 phantom limb pain
PLS
 plastic leaf-spring
PLT
 peroneus longus tendinopathy
plug
 bone femoral p.
 bone-graft p.
 Buck p.
 calcaneal bone p.
 cement p.
 cortical cancellous allograft p.
 corticocancellous p.
 p. cutter
 Exeter P.
 femoral p.
 Grafton DBM Matrix p.
 orthoPLUG soft bone p.
 Osteonics acetabular dome hole p.
 patellar p.
 plastic femoral p.
 polyethylene femoral Buck p.
plumb
 p. line
 p. line analysis
plumbism
Plum-Blossom acupuncture needle
plunger
 dome p.
plunger-type femoral pressurizer
pluripotential
 p. mesenchymal tumor
 p. mesenchymoma
plus
 DHC P.
 Extra Strength Bayer P.
 Livotrit P.
 Lorcet P.
 lumbrical p.
 Nexerciser P.
 Osteo-B P.
 Quinsana P.
 Steri-Cuff P.
Plyoback Rebounder
plyometric
 p. exercise
 p. resistance
plyometrics
Plyo-Sled exerciser
Plystan prosthesis

P.M.
 Excedrin P.M.
PMA
 peroneal muscular atrophy
 progressive muscular atrophy
PMD
 progressive muscular dystrophy
PMID
 painful minor intervertebral dysfunction
PMMA
 polymethyl methacrylate
 PMMA bone cement
 PMMA centralizer
 PMMA implant
PM&R
 physical medicine and rehabilitation
PMR
 physical medicine and rehabilitation
 polymyalgia rheumatica
 posteromedial release
PMT
 PMT halo system
 PMT halo system brace
PneuGel
 P. ankle brace
 P. ankle wrap
 P. shoulder wrap
Pneu Knee brace
pneumarthrosis
pneumatic
 p. ankle tourniquet
 p. antishock garment (PASG)
 p. 4-bar linkage knee
 p. compression boot
 p. compression sleeve
 p. compression stockings
 p. compression therapy
 p. drill accessory
 p. external compression device
 p. garment
 p. massage
 p. orthosis
 p. pedal compression
 p. peripheral circulation improvement
  device (PPCID)
 p. resistance exercise
 p. splint
 p. tire injury
 p. tourniquet
 p. tourniquet cuff
pneumatocyst
 intraosseous p.
pneumoarthrogram sign
pneumoarthrography
pneumogenic osteoarthropathy
pneumoniae
 Diplococcus p.
 Klebsiella p.
 Streptococcus p.

P

pneumonitis
pneumothermomassage
pneumothorax
Pneu-trac
    P.-t. cervical collar
    P.-t. neck brace
PNF
    proprioceptive neuromuscular
    facilitation
      PNF exercise
      PNF pattern
      PNF technique
PNI
    peripheral nerve injury
PNR
    perineural fibroma
PNS
    parasympathetic nervous system
    peripheral nervous system
P&O
    prosthesis and orthosis
    prosthetic and orthotic
PO4
    phosphate
podalgia
podarthritis
podedema, podoedema
podiatric
    p. bur
    p. medicine
podiatrist
podiatry
    P. Institute
    P. Institute procedure
    P. Institute procedures for ankle
    arthrodesis
    P. Institute rasp
PodiAxis orthopaedic sole
Podi-Burr
    large callus P.-B.
    large nail P.-B.
    medium callus P.-B.
    medium nail P.-B.
    P.-B. nail bur
podismus (*var. of* podospasm)
poditis
pododynamometer
pododynia
podoedema (*var. of* podedema)
PodoFlex
    P. machine
    P. reflexology device
podogeriatrics
podogram
podograph
podologist
podology
podomechanotherapy
podometer

podopediatrics
podospasm, podospasmus, podismus
podospasmus (*var. of* podospasm)
Podospray
    Darco P.
    P. nail drill system
    P. podiatry drill
Pogon chair
Pogrund lateral meniscectomy
  approach
2-point
    2-p. discrimination
    2-p. discrimination test
    2-p. gait
    2-p. nerve block
    2-p. step-to gait pattern
3-point
    3-p. bending moment
    3-p. gait
    3-p. pressure cast
    3-p. pressure system
    3-p. pressure technique
    3-p. skeletal traction
4-point
    4-p. fixation
    4-p. gait
    4-p. IROM brace
    4-p. IROM splint
    4-p. SuperSport functional knee
    brace
    4-p. walker
point
    acupuncture p.
    anchoring p.
    p. and pressure systems
    associated myofascial trigger p.
    back shu paraspinal p.
    bleeding p.
    break p.
    cannulated drill p.
    carbon steel drill p.
    contact p.
    cookbook stimulation of acupuncture
    p.'s
    Crowe pilot p.
    Crutchfield drill p.
    dorsal p.
    drill p.
    electrodesiccated bleeding p.
    end p.
    entry p.
    Erb p.
    glenoid p.
    inflexion p.
    isometric p.
    Krackow p.
    material failure break p.
    Mathews drill p.
    motor p.

myofascial trigger p.
paraspinal p.
Pauly p.
pedicle entrance p.
pressure p.
primary myofascial trigger p.
referred p.
satellite myofascial trigger p.
secondary myofascial trigger p.
single reference p.
Steinmann pin with Crowe pilot p.
tender p. (TeP)
p. tenderness
trigger p. (TrP)
Trousseau spinous process p.
twist drill p.
universal drill p.
vector p.

pointed
p. awl
p. toe shoe

pointer
hip p.
shoulder p.

Pointer-Plus locator/stimulator
pointillage
6-point knee brace
point-of-reduction clamp
Poirier
space of P.

Poisson ratio
poker
p. back
p. spine

Poland
P. anomaly
P. classification of physial injury
P. epiphysial fracture classification
P. syndrome

polar
P. Care 500 cryotherapy device
P. Pack
P. Wrap cold therapy
P. wrist monitor
p. zone

Polaris
P. knee rehab brace
P. 5.5 spinal system
P. 6.35 spinal system

polarization
Polar-Mate coagulator
Polarus
P. humeral rod
P. Plus humeral fixation system
P. positional humeral fixation system

pole
Exerstrider walking p.
walking p.

policeman's heel

policy
P. and Review Committee for
Human Research
impaired competitor p.
National Collegiate Athletic
Association drug testing p.

poliodystrophy
Alpers progressive infantile p.

poliomyelitis treatment
polka-dot pattern
Polk finger goniometer
pollex, *pl.* **pollices**, *gen.* **pollicis**
p. abductus
adductor pollicis
pollicis longus muscle
opponens pollicis
p. pedis

pollices (*pl. of* pollex, *pl. of* pollicis)
pollicis (*gen. of* pollex)
pollicization
Buck-Gramcko p.
Gillies p.
Littler p.
Riordan p.

pollicized ray
Pollock sign
Polocaine
POLPSA
posterior labrocapsular periosteal sleeve
avulsion
POLPSA lesion

polyacetal resin
polyarteritis nodosa
polyarthric
polyarthritis
p. chronica villosa
juvenile p.
vertebral p.

polyarthropathy
polyarticular
p. juvenile rheumatoid arthritis
p. symmetric tophaceous joint
inflammation

polyaryletheretherketone (PEEK)
Polyax
P. locking plating system
P. polyaxial locked plate

polyaxial
p. cervical screw
p. joint
p. system

polybutester suture
polybutilate-coated polyester
Polycel bone composite
prosthesis
polycentric
P. and Wide-Track knee system
P. Hinged Ulnar Deviation Splint
p. knee prosthesis

P

polycentric (*continued*)
    p. rotation
    p. unconstrained prosthesis
polydactylia (*var. of* polydactyly)
polydactylism (*var. of* polydactyly)
polydactylous cleft foot
polydactyly, polydactylia,
  polydactylism
    central p.
    phalangeal p.
    postaxial p.
    preaxial p.
    short rib p.
    thumb p.
    Wassel classification of thumb p.
      (I-VI)
Polydek suture
Polyderm hydrophilic polyurethane foam
  dressing
Poly-Dial
    P.-D. insert
    P.-D. prosthesis
    P.-D. socket
Polydine
polydioxanone suture (PDS)
polydystrophy
    Hurler p.
polyester
    Dacron p.
    polybutilate-coated p.
    p. suture
polyether implant material
polyetherketone (PEK)
    p. polymer
polyethylene
    ArCom processed p.
    p. button
    carbon fiber-reinforced p.
    p. compression molding
    p. debris
    p. drain
    Durasul p.
    extruded bar p.
    p. femoral Buck plug
    p. femoral Buck plug procedure
    p. foam
    high molecular weight p.
      (HMWPE)
    p. implant material
    p. liner
    p. liner implant component
    p. patellar implant prosthesis
    p. peg
    porous p.
    p. proximal brim in quadrilateral
      contour
    p. sleeve
    p. socket
    p. suture

    p. talar prosthesis
    p. tibial insert
    ultrahigh molecular weight p.
      (UHMWPE)
polyethylene-faced
    p.-f. driver
    p.-f. mallet
Polyform splint
polygalactic acid suture
polyglactin suture
polyglycolic
    p. acid (PGA)
    p. acid-polylactic acid
      (PGA-PLA)
    p. acid suture
polyglycolide implant
polyglyconate suture
polylactic acid (PLA)
polylactide
    p. absorbable screw
    p. implant
polylevolactic acid (PLLA)
poly-L-lactic acid (PLLA)
poly-L-lactide acid (PLLA)
Poly-Lock bonding
PolyMem wound care dressing
polymer
    biodegradable synthetic p.
    carbon fiber-reinforced p.
      (CFRP)
    cold-curing p.
    Hylamer orthopaedic bearing p.
    polyetherketone p.
    self-curing p.
    viscoelastic p.
PolymerFriction total knee
polymeric
    p. debris
    p. dressing
polymerization of bone cement
polymetatarsalia, polymetatarsalism
polymetatarsalism (*var. of*
  polymetatarsalia)
polymethyl
    p. methacrylate (PMMA)
    p. methacrylate bone
      cement
polymethylmethacrylate
    p. biomaterial
    p. implant
polymorphic hamartoma
polymyalgia rheumatica (PMR)
polymyositis myopathy
polymyxin
    neomycin and p. B
polyneuritiformis
    heredopathia atactica p.
polyneuritis
    peripheral p.

polyneuropathy
    diabetic p.
    gait disorder, autoantibody, late-age onset, p. (GALOP)
    sensory p.
polyolefin elastomer
polyostotic
    p. bone lesion
    p. fibrous dysplasia
polyp
    fibroepithelial p.
polyphasic action potential
Polypin biodegradable pin implant
polypropylene
    p. ankle-foot orthosis
    p. glycol ankle-foot orthosis (PPG-AFO)
    p. glycol-thoracolumbosacral orthosis (PPG-TLSO)
    p. insert
    p. prosthesis
    p. suture
polyradiculoneuropathy
    acute inflammatory demyelinating p. (AIDP)
polyradiculopathy
    acute inflammatory p.
    diabetic p.
polyserositis
Polyskin dressing
Polysonic ultrasound lotion
Polysorb
    P. heel cup
    P. liner
    P. meniscal stapler XLS
    P. suture
Polysporin Topical
Polystim electrode
Polytechnic foot-pressure measuring plate
polytef
    polytetrafluoroethylene
polytetrafluoroethylene (polytef, PTFE)
    expanded p. (EPTFE)
    p. graft
polytomography
polytrauma algorithm
polyurethane
    p. bandage
    p. cast
    p. foam dressing (PFD)
    p. implant material
    p. liner
polyvinyl
    p. alcohol
    p. alcohol splint
    p. alcohol splinting material
    p. chloride (PVC)
    p. implant material

PolyWic dressing
pommel
    p. cushion
    p. horse gymnastics
Poncet
    P. disease
    P. rheumatism
poncho restraint
pond
    P. adjustable splint
    p. fracture
Ponseti
    P. clubfoot treatment method
    P. splint
    P. technique
Ponstel
Pontenza arthrodesis
Ponte spinal scoliosis osteotomy
Pontocaine With Dextrose Injection
pontoon spica cast
pool
    Aquaciser p.
    AquaMotion p.
    aquatic therapy p.
    Endless Pool physical therapy p.
    Ferno custom therapy p.
    motor neuronal p.
    SwimEx p.
    p. therapy
poor
    p. alignment
    p. bone stock
    p. cosmesis
POP
    plaster of Paris
    POP cast
    POP rivet
    POP Rivet fixation system
Popeye arm
popliteal
    p. angle
    p. artery
    p. block
    p. bursitis
    p. crease
    p. entrapment syndrome
    p. fascia
    p. flexion creaking
    p. fossa
    p. fossa block
    p. fossa entrapment
    p. fossa neural blockade
    p. hiatus
    p. ligament
    p. muscle
    p. nerve
    p. pressure sign
    p. pterygium syndrome

P

popliteal (*continued*)
    p. recess
    p. region
    p. sciatic nerve block
    p. space
    p. tendon
    p. vein
    p. vessel
popliteofibular ligament
popliteomeniscal fascicle
popliteus
    p. fossa muscle tendon
    p. tendinitis
popoff suture
Poppen
    P. forceps
    P. Gigli saw guide
    P. ridge sensitometer
popping
    joint p.
porcine
    p. graft material
    p. prosthesis
PORD
    posterior reduction device
porencephalic cyst
Porocoat
    P. AML noncemented prosthesis
    P. porous coating
    P. prosthetic material
    Tri-Lock total hip prosthesis
      with P.
Poro-in-between sole
porokeratoma
porokeratosis of Mibelli
poroma
    eccrine p.
Porometal noncemented femoral prosthesis
Poron
    P. cellular urethane
    P. 400 insole
poroplastic splint
porosity
    interfacial p.
porotic bone
porous
    p. cementless component
    p. coating
    p. ingrowth fixation
    p. metal
    p. polyethylene
    p. polyethylene graft
    p. prosthetic material
    p. sheet
    p. surfaced prosthesis
porous-coated
    p.-c. acetabular cup
    p.-c. anatomic (PCA)

    p.-c. anatomic guide
    p.-c. anatomic prosthesis
    p.-c. anatomic total hip
      replacement
    p.-c. anatomic total knee
    p.-c. component
    p.-c. femur prosthesis
    p.-c. hip prosthesis
    p.-c. implant
PORP
    partial ossicular replacement
      prosthesis
    Richards hydroxyapatite PORP
porphyria
porphyritic neuropathy
portable
    p. C-arm image intensifier
      fluoroscopy
    p. diagnostic kit
    P. Topical Hyperbaric Oxygen
      Extremity Chamber
portal
    1–2 p.
    3–4 p.
    4–5 p.
    p. accessory
    ankle p.
    anterior p.
    anterior superior p. (ASP)
    anterocentral arthroscopic p.
    anteroinferior p.
    anterolateral p.
    anteromedial p.
    arthroscopic entry p.
    Caspari arthroscopic p.
    central transpatellar tendon p.
    desktop therapy p.
    direct lateral p.
    inside-out technique for establishing
      ankle p.
    lateral transmalleolar p.
    MCR p.
    MCU p.
    medial p.
    midcarpal p.
    midcarpal radial p.
    midcarpal ulnar p.
    midlateral p.
    midpatellar p.
    Neviaser p.
    p. of Wilmington
    patellar p.
    piriformis entry p.
    p. placement
    posterior p.
    posteroinferior p.
    posterolateral p.
    posteromedial p.
    P. Pro 2 treatment chair

proximal midpatellar medial and lateral p.'s
radiocarpal p.
stab wound arthroscopic entry p.
straight posterior p.
subacromial p.
subtalar p.
superior p.
superolateral outflow p.
superomedial p.
suprapatellar p.
Swedish p.
transmalleolar p.
transpatellar tendon p.
transtendocalcaneus p.
6U p.
Wilmington arthroscopic p.

6-portal synovectomy
2-portal technique
3-portal technique
porta pedis
Porter-Richardson-Vainio
    P.-R.-V. arthroscopic synovectomy technique
    P.-R.-V. rheumatoid arthritis elbow synovectomy

portion
    accessory p.
    cord p.
    devitalized p.
    proximal p.

Portmann drill
portmanteau procedure
Portola Valley Scale
port-wine stain
Porzett splint
Posada fracture
Posey
    P. bar kit
    P. bed cradle
    P. belt
    P. drop seat
    P. grip
    P. Palm Cone
    P. sling

Positex knee wedge
position
    anatomic p.
    angular p.
    antiembolic p.
    arch and slouch p.
    barber chair p.
    bayonet fracture p.
    beach chair p.
    close-packed p.
    cotton-loader p.
    decubitus p.
    de Kleyn p.
    dorsal lithotomy p.

dorsal recumbent p.
dorsiflexion-plantar flexion p.
empty can p.
equinus p.
erect p.
figure-of-4 p.
fist p.
flexed p.
Fowler p.
frog-leg p.
full lateral p.
Gaynor-Hart p.
horizontal p.
p. in space
intrinsic minus p.
jackknife p.
James p.
jet-pilot p.
Jones p.
jumper's knee p.
90-90 kneeling p.
kneeling p.
Kraske p.
lateral decubitus p.
lateral park-bench p.
limb p.
lithotomy p.
loose-packed p.
lotus p.
mediolateral p.
military brace p.
military tuck p.
neutral hip p.
normal anatomic p.
p. of function
open-packed p.
opisthotonic p.
over-the-top p.
Phalen p.
prayer p.
prone p.
proximal bow p.
quasistatic stressed p.
rectus p.
recumbent p.
resting calcaneal stance p. (RCSP)
reverse Trendelenburg p.
scissors-leg p.
semi-Fowler p.
semisitting p.
p. sense
side-lying p.
side-posture p.
Sims p.
sitting p.
sniffer's p.
spinal fusion p.
subtalar joint neutral p. (STNP)
supine p.

P

position (*continued*)
    three-quarters prone p.
    tibial sesamoid p. (TSP)
    translational p.
    Trendelenburg p.
    x-ray p.
positional
    p. dyskinesia
    p. MRI
    p. release therapy
positioner
    acetabular cup p.
    Allen arthroscopic elbow p.
    Allen arthroscopic knee p.
    Allen arthroscopic wrist p.
    arm p.
    Bareskin knee p.
    Biomet Second Assistant
     knee p.
    cup p.
    De Mayo hip p.
    Grasshopper p.
    IMP universal knee p.
    IMP universal lateral p.
    Kirschenbaum foot p.
    knee p.
    leg p.
    Mark II Stulberg hip p.
    Mark II Stulberg leg p.
    Mark II Wixson hip p.
    McConnell shoulder p.
    McGuire pelvic p.
    Montreal hip p.
    OSI-Schlein shoulder p.
    Picket Fence leg p.
    Prep-Assist p.
    Profex arthroscopic leg p.
    Schlein shoulder p. (I-III)
    shoulder abduction p.
    Stulberg hip p.
    Stulberg Mark II leg p.
    SurgAssist leg p.
    Ther-A-Shapes p.
    universal knee p.
    universal lateral p.
    Vac-Pac p.
    Wixson hip p.
positioning
    patient p.
    proper neck p.
positive
    p. ability
    p. afterpotential
    p. impingement sign
    p. rim sign
    p. sharp wave
    p. supporting reflex
    p. tropism
    p. ulnar variance (PUV)

positron
    p. emission tomographic scan
    p. emission tomography (PET)
post
    p. dural puncture headache
    extrinsic rearfoot p.
    Galveston intrasacral p.
    iliac p.
    Isola spinal implant system
     iliac p.
    Luque-Galveston p.
    Morse tapered prosthetic p.
    perineal p.
    status p.
    thumb p.
    P. total shoulder arthroplasty
postactivation
    p. depression
    p. exhaustion
    p. facilitation
    p. potentiation
postacute sprain
Postalume finger splint
post-and-cam mechanism
postanesthesia
    p. care unit (PACU)
    p. recovery (PAR)
postaxial
    p. muscle
    p. polydactyly
postcalcaneal bursitis
postcast compression reflex
postcasting syndrome
postcompetition rehabilitation
postconcussive syndrome
postdiscectomy syndrome
Postel
    P. coxarthropathy
    P. hip status system
2-poster
    2-p. brace
    2-p. cervical orthosis
4-poster
    4-p. cervical brace
    4-p. cervical orthosis
    4-p. frame
posterior
    anterior and p. (AP)
    p. apprehension shoulder test
    p. apprehension test
    p. approach to sacrum and
     sacroiliac joint
    p. arch
    p. arch fracture
    p. atlantoaxial arthrodesis
    p. atlantoodontoid interval
    p. axillary line (PAL)
    p. bending moment
    p. bone block

p. bone graft
p. bow
p. calcaneal displacement osteotomy
p. capsule
p. capsulorrhaphy
p. capsulotomy
p. cervical fixation
p. cervical fusion
p. cervical line
p. cervical spinal instrumentation
p. colliculus
p. column fracture
p. column osteosynthesis
p. column sign
p. compartment
p. component
p. construct
p. cord syndrome
p. costotransversectomy approach
p. cruciate
p. cruciate condylar knee system
p. cruciate ligament (PCL)
p. cruciate ligament graft
p. cruciate ligament of knee
p. cruciate ligament reconstruction
p. cruciate ligament tear
p. cruciate sprain
p. curvature
p. deltoid muscle
p. deltoid-to-triceps transfer
p. depression pattern
p. distraction instrumentation
p. drainage
p. drawer knee test
p. drawer sign
p. element
p. element fracture
p. element overuse syndrome
  (PEOS)
p. endplate
p. facet
p. facet dislocation
p. facet displacement
p. femoral cutaneous nerve
p. fixation system biomechanics
p. flap
p. flap technique
p. fracture-dislocation
p. glenoid elevator
p. glenoid labrum
p. glenoplasty
p. glide
p. hiatal sign
p. hip dislocation
p. hook-rod spinal instrumentation
p. horn
p. horn meniscal tear
p. iliac osteotomy
p. iliofemoral technique

p. impingement
p. impingement syndrome
p. incision
p. inferior cerebellar artery (PICA)
p. inferior cerebellar artery index
p. innominate
p. innominate rotation
p. interosseous branch
p. interosseous nerve
p. interosseous nerve approach
p. interosseous nerve compression
  syndrome
p. interosseous nerve entrapment
p. interosseous nerve palsy
p. interspinous wiring
p. inverted-U approach
p. joint syndrome
p. knee ankle (PKA)
p. knee pull syndrome
p. labrocapsular periosteal sleeve
  avulsion (POLPSA)
p. labrocapsular periosteal sleeve
  avulsion lesion
p. leaf-spring ankle-foot orthosis
p. ligamentous complex (PLC)
p. ligamentous injury
p. lip
p. longitudinal fiber region
p. longitudinal ligament (PLL)
p. lower cervical spine stabilization
p. lower cervical spine surgery
p. lumbar interbody fusion (PLIF)
p. lumbar interbody fusion surgery
p. lumbar spine and sacrum surgery
p. malleolus
p. meniscofemoral ligament
p. midline approach
p. mold splint
p. nerve decompression
p. oblique fiber region
p. oblique meniscal tear
p. oblique sprain
p. occipitocervical approach
p. odontoid stabilization
p. osteophyte
p. pelvic tilt
p. pharyngeal abscess
p. plate osteosynthesis pelvic ring
  injury repair
p. portal
p. process fracture
p. radial collateral artery
p. reduction device (PORD)
p. release
p. rhizotomy
p. rod system
p. rotation on left side
p. rotation on right side
p. sacroiliac ligament

P

posterior (*continued*)
   p. sacroiliac spine
   p. sag knee test
   p. sag sign
   p. screw fixation
   p. segmental fixation
   p. shoulder approach
   p. shoulder dislocation
   p. shoulder impingement test
   p. shoulder instability
   p. spinal fusion (PSF)
   p. spinal plating
   p. spinal wedge osteotomy
   p. spur
   p. stability
   p. stress test
   p. subluxation test
   p. superior humeral head defect
   p. superior iliac spine (PSIS)
   superior labrum anterior and p.
     (SLAP)
   p. talar process fracture
   p. talofibular ligament (PTFL)
   p. tarsal tunnel syndrome
   p. thigh bar
   p. tibial (PT)
   p. tibial artery (PTA)
   p. tibialis tendinitis
   p. tibialis tendon lengthening
   p. tibial nerve (PTN)
   p. tibial nerve entrapment
   p. tibial pulse (PTP)
   p. tibial spine
   p. tibial tendinitis
   p. tibial tendinopathy
   p. tibial tendon (PTT)
   p. tibial tendon dysfunction
     (PTTD)
   p. tibial tendon insufficiency
   p. tibial tendon transfer
   p. tibiofibular ligament
   p. tibiotalar ligament
   p. translation
   p. transolecranon approach
   p. triangle
   p. tuberosity
   p. upper cervical spine
   surgery
   p. vertebral column resection
     (PVCR)
   p. wall fracture
posterior-anterior, posteroanterior
   p.-a. glide
   p.-a. pressure
   p.-a. screw
posterior-inferior, posteroinferior
   p.-i. capsular shift procedure
   p.-i. spine
posteriorly

posterior-superior, posterosuperior
   p.-s. humeral head lesion
   p.-s. oblique projection
posterior-to-anterior screw
posteroanterior (PA)
posterodistal
posteroinferior (PI)
   p. external (PIEX)
   p. external movement
   p. ilium major
   p. internal (PIIN)
   p. internal movement
   p. portal
   p. tibiofibular ligament
posteroinferior-external subluxation
posteroinferior-internal subluxation
posterolateral
   p. approach
   p. approach of Henry
   p. arthrodesis
   p. aspect
   p. bone graft
   p. bone graft placement
   p. bundle
   p. capsule
   p. compartment
   p. costotransversectomy incision
   p. costotransversectomy technique
   p. decompression
   p. decompression for spine tumor
   p. drainage
   p. drawer sign
   p. drawer test
   p. fusion (PLF)
   p. herniation
   p. interbody fusion
   p. lumbosacral fusion
   p. pivot test
   p. portal
   p. release
   p. rotary instability
   p. spine fusion
   p. structure
posteromedial
   p. approach
   p. bow
   p. bundle
   p. capsule
   p. compartment
   p. corner
   p. dislocation
   p. drainage
   p. drawer sign
   p. pivot-shift test
   p. portal
   p. region
   p. release (PMR)
   p. release of clubfoot
   p. rotary instability

posteroproximal
poster orthosis
posterosuperior
postexercise hypotension
post-facilitation stretch (PFS)
postfracture
    p. cyst
    p. lesion
    p. osteomyelitis
    p. swelling
    p. syndrome
postfusion brace
postganglionic technique
postherpetic pain
postinfectious
    p. arthritis
    p. myopathy
posting
    heel p.
    strip p.
    wedge p.
postinjection image
postinjury period
postirradiation
    p. fracture
    p. osteosarcoma
postisometric
    p. relaxation (PIR)
    p. relaxation traction technique
    p. stretch technique
postlaminectomy
    p. kyphosis
    p. 2-level spondylolisthesis
postmastectomy pain
postmenopausal
    p. arthritis
    p. bone loss
postmortem fracture
postnatal
    p. cerebral palsy
    p. gangrene
    p. skeletal growth deformity
postop
    postoperative
postoperative (postop)
    p. antibiotic
    p. bracing
    p. casting
    p. complication
    p. corticosteroid
    p. drainage-related hematoma
    p. dressing
    p. extubation
    p. flexor tendon (PFT)
    p. fracture
    p. helmet modeling
    p. helmet molding
    p. immobilization
    p. immobilizer

    p. infection
    p. lumbosacral orthosis
    p. pain
    p. paraplegia
    p. radiograph
    p. regimen
    p. shoe
    p. synovitis
    p. therapy
    p. wound care
postphlebitis syndrome
postpoliomyelitic contracture
postpolio syndrome (PPS)
postpyelomyelitis syndrome
postradiation kyphosis
postreduction x-ray
poststatic dyskinesia (PSDK)
postsurgical heel condition
posttetanic
    p. exhaustion
    p. facilitation
    p. potentiation
posttraumatic
    p. algodystrophic syndrome
    p. amnesia (PTA)
    p. angulation
    p. apoplexy
    p. arthritis
    p. arthrosis
    p. cavus
    p. chronic cord syndrome
    p. chronic osteomyelitis
    p. degenerative disease
    p. dystrophy
    p. edema
    p. epilepsy (PTE)
    p. flatfoot
    p. headache
    p. hemarthrosis
    p. kyphosis
    p. neuroma
    p. osteoarthritis
    p. osteoarthrosis
    p. osteolysis
    p. osteonecrosis
    p. osteoporosis
    p. pain
    p. sacroiliac dysfunction
    p. spinal deformity
    p. syringomyelia
postulnar bone
postural
    p. analysis
    p. balance
    p. complex
    p. component
    p. control
    p. development
    p. exteroceptor

P

postural (*continued*)
    p. fixation back maneuver
    p. instability
    p. interoceptor
    p. ischemia
    p. list
    p. muscle
    p. myoneuralgia
    p. receptor
    p. reflex
    p. strain
    p. sway
    p. syndrome
    p. tremor
    p. variation

Postura wheelchair cushion

posture
    batrachian p.
    benediction p.
    Brügger cogwheel analysis of p.
    cavus p.
    P. Curve lumbar cushion
    decorticate p.
    p. education
    forward flexion p.
    forward head p.
    p. of limb
    pain-relieving body p.
    P. Pump lordoticiser
    P. Pump Spine Trainer
    recumbent p.
    P. S'port
    P. Wedge seat cushion

Posture-Rite lap desk

posturing
    equinovarus p.

posturography
    computerized dynamic p. (CDP)

potassium (K)
    p. permanganate (KMnO₄)
    ticarcillin and clavulanate p.

potential
    action p. (AP)
    auditory evoked p. (AEP)
    bioelectric p.
    biphasic action p.
    bizarre repetitive p.
    brainstem auditory evoked p.
      (BAEP)
    brief, small, abundant p. (BSAP)
    brief, small, abundant, polyphasic p.
      (BSAPP)
    complex motor unit action p.
    compound mixed nerve action p.
    compound motor nerve action p.
    compound muscle action p. (CMAP)
    compound muscle-motor action p.
      (CMAP)
    compound sensory nerve action p.

    denervation p.
    dermatosensory evoked p.
    electrical p.
    electrokinetic p.
    endplate p. (EPP)
    evoked compound muscle action p.
    excitatory postsynaptic p.
    far-field p.
    fasciculation p.
    fibrillation p.
    giant motor unit action p.
    inhibitory postsynaptic p.
    irregular p.
    kilovoltage p.
    linked p.
    long-latency somatosensory evoked p.
    miniature end-plate p. (MEPP)
    monophasic action p.
    motor unit p. (MUP)
    motor unit action p. (MUAP)
    muscle fiber action p.
    myopathic motor unit p.
    myotonic p.
    nascent motor unit p.
    near-field p.
    nerve action p. (NAP)
    nerve fiber action p.
    nerve trunk action p.
    neurogenic motor evoked p.
      (NMEP)
    neuropathic motor unit p.
    piezoelectric p.
    polyphasic action p.
    pseudopolyphasic action p.
    regeneration motor unit p.
    resting membrane p.
    satellite p.
    sensory evoked p.
    sensory nerve action p. (SNAP)
    serrated action p.
    short-latency somatosensory
      evoked p.
    somatosensory evoked p. (SEP,
      SSEP)
    spinal evoked p.
    streaming p.
    tetraphasic action p.
    transcranial motor-evoked p.
      (TcMEP)
    triphasic action p.
    visual evoked p. (VEP)

potentiation
    postactivation p.
    posttetanic p.

potentiometer
    linear p.

Pott
    P. abscess
    P. ankle fracture

P. disease
P. dwarfism
P. gangrene
P. paralysis
P. paraplegia
P. puffy tumor
P. spinal curvature
Potter arthrodesis
Potts
P. eversion osteotomy
P. splint
P. tibial osteotomy
Potts-Smith dressing forceps
pouce
p. flottant
p. flottant thumb
pouch
antibiotic bead p.
bead p.
inflamed synovial p.
suprapatellar p.
pouch-type sling
Poulet disease
poundal
pound of traction
Poupart inguinal ligament
Pouteau wrist fracture
povidone-iodine solution
powder
Absorbine antifungal foot p.
Ammens foot p.
p. board
bromelain p.
Bromi-Talc Plus antiperspirant p.
Goody's Headache P.'s
Lotrimin AF spray p.
Pedi-Dri topical p.
thrombin p.
Zeasorb-AF p.
powdered bone graft
power
P. Anthro Shoe
p. bone saw
p. bur
p. drill
grasping p.
p. oscillating saw
P. Pillow cervical massager
pinch p.
P. Play knee brace
P. Pogo stationary exerciser
p. rasp
p. reamer
thumb pinch p.
P. Trainer cycle
P. Web hand exerciser
P. Web Jr. exerciser
p. wheelchair
Powerbelt exercise system

PowerCut drill blade
power-driven
p.-d. reamer
p.-d. saw
powered metaphysial stapler
Powerflex
P. CMP exerciser
P. tape
Power-Grip pliers
Powermatic table
POWERPoint orthotic shoe insert
PowerStar bipolar scissors
Powerstep
P. foot support
P. orthotic
PowerTrack II muscle testing instrument
PP
parietal pleura
proximal phalanx
PPCID
pneumatic peripheral circulation improvement device
PPCID slippers
PPD
permanent partial disability
PPD rating
PPE
personal protective equipment
PPF
percutaneous plantar fasciotomy
PPG-AFO
polypropylene glycol ankle-foot orthosis
PPG-AFO brace
PPG-TLSO
polypropylene glycol-thoracolumbosacral orthosis
PPG-TLSO brace
PPO
passive prehension orthosis
PPS
patellofemoral pain syndrome
postpolio syndrome
prospective payment system
PPT
professional protective technology
PPT flat insole
PPT gel stirrup ankle support
PPT insole system
PPT MXL soft molded insole
PPT orthotic device
PPT Plastizote insole
PPT RX firm molded insole
PPT sheet
PPT soft tissue orthotic system
PQ
pronator quadratus
PQ premium heel cup

P

PR
pelvic rock
practitioner
scientific p.
PRAFO
pressure-relief ankle-foot orthosis
PRAFO adjustable orthotic
PRAFO APU
PRAFO attachment
PRAFO EV
PRAFO KAFO
PRAFO pediatric
PRAFO PKA
Prague pelvis
pramipexole
Pratt
P. open radius reduction
P. symptom
P. T-clamp
P. technique
prayer
p. position
p. view
PRE
progressive-resistance exercise
progressive-resistive exercise
preacher curl
pre-Achilles
p.-A. bursa
p.-A. bursitis
p.-A. fat-pad
p.-A. mass
preassembled metal-backed socket
preaxial
p. muscle
p. polydactyly
prebent nail
precaution
cardiac p.'s
universal p.'s
precise lesion measuring (PLM)
precision
P. hip stem
P. Osteolock
P. Osteolock femoral component system
P. Osteolock femoral prosthesis
P. Osteolock fixation
P. Osteolock hip prosthesis
P. spinal cord stimulator
P. Strata hip system
P. total hip
Preclude spinal membrane
Precoat
P. hip prosthesis
P. Plus femoral prosthesis

precompression jig
precontoured unit rod
precurved
p. ball-tipped guidepin
p. plate
PreCustom Orthotic
Predcor-TBA Injection
prediction
Anderson-Green growth p.
growth p.
predictive salvage index (PSI)
predictor of injury
predislocation syndrome
predisposition
congenital p.
Prednicen-M
prednisolone
Prednisol TBA injection
prednisone
preemptive
p. analgesia
p. blockade technique
prefabricated wool felt pad
preganglionic
p. sympathectomy
p. technique
prehallux
external p.
p. osseous prominence
prehension
p. force
p. grasp
p. orthosis
preinterparietal bone
Preiser disease
preload
Prelone Oral
premalleolar
p. bursitis
p. fat pad
premanipulative testing
premature
p. closure
p. consolidation
Premier press fit prosthesis
Premphase
Prempro
prenatal dislocation
Prenyl jacket
preoperative
p. antibiotic
p. drawing
p. evaluation
p. management
p. plan
p. planning
p. planning under intramedullary interlocking nails
p. planning under pin fixators

p. roentgenography
p. tomography
preparation
bone-patellar tendon-bone p.
facet joint p.
graft p.
3M p.
patient positioning and p.
rod contour p.
skin p.
Spälteholz p.
wire contour p.
Prep-Assist
P.-A. legholder
P.-A. positioner
prepatellar
p. bursa
p. bursa inflammation
p. bursitis
p. neuralgia
Prep-IM
presacral block
Presbyterian Hospital T-clamp
preschooler
Miller Assessment for P.'s (MAP)
prescription (Rx)
ACSM Guidelines for Exercise
Testing and P.
P. Strength Desenex
preservation
lordosis p.
lumbar lordosis p.
preservative-free solution (PFS)
prespondylolisthesis
press
CamStar power leg p.
p. fit
leg p.
Shuttle MVP leg p.
supine chest p.
p. up
press-fit
p.-f. acetabular implant insertion
technique
p.-f. circumferential grommet
p.-f. condylar (PFC)
p.-f. condylar knee arthroplasty
p.-f. condylar total knee
p.-f. condylar total knee
prosthesis
p.-f. cup
p.-f. femoral component
p.-f. fixation
p.-f. stem
p.-f. total condylar knee system
pressure
p. algometer
ankle systolic p.
blood p. (BP)

bone marrow p. (BMP)
central posterior-anterior p.
compartmental p.
p. cushion
disc p.
Doppler ankle systolic p.
p. epiphysis
p. excursion index
forefoot peak p.
p. fracture
p. glove
hydrostatic p.
injection p.
intracompartmental p.
intradiscal p.
intramuscular p. (IMP)
lateral root p.
manual p.
p. necrosis
p. paralysis
peak p.
p. perception
plantar p.
p. plate
p. point
posterior-anterior p.
p. relief padding
p. relief shoe
P. Sentinel reamer
sequential p.
p. sore
systolic blood p.
p. therapy
p. threshold
p. threshold meter
tissue p.
toe p.
p. tolerance
tourniquet p.
p. transducer
p. transducer-monitor system
p. ulcer assessment
p. ulcer classification
p. ulcer cleansing
p. ulcer dressing
p. ulcer (grade I-IV)
p. ulcer management
p. ulcer prevention
p. ulcer-related maggot infestation
PressureGuard mattress
pressure-relief
p.-r. ankle-foot orthotic
(PRAFO)
p.-r. cushion
pressure-relieving orthosis
pressure-sensitive
p.-s. area
p.-s. tissue
Pressure-Specified Sensory Device

P

pressure-time integral
pressure-tolerant tissue
pressurized cement
pressurizer
>   acetabular p.
>   plunger-type femoral p.

Prestige cervical disc system
Preston
>   P. ligamentum flavum forceps
>   P. overhead pulley
>   P. pinch gauge
>   P. screw
>   P. Traveler CPM exerciser

Prestop pinchometer
pretarget filtration system
pretendinous
>   p. band
>   p. band of hand
>   p. cord

pretibial
>   p. bearing (PTB)
>   p. buttress (PTB)
>   p. edema (PTE)

Prevacare
>   P. moisturizing cream
>   P. spray

prevent
>   P. Recurrence of Osteoporotic
>   Fractures (PROOF)
>   P. Recurrence of Osteoporotic
>   Fractures Group

prevention
>   heat injury p.
>   heterotopic ossification p.
>   infection p.
>   Lower Extremity Amputation P.
>   (LEAP)
>   osseous bridge p.
>   pressure ulcer p.
>   rod rotation p.

prevertebral
>   p. abscess
>   p. space

PRICE
>   protection, restricted activity, ice,
>   compression, elevation

Price muscular biopsy clamp
prickling pain
Pridie
>   P. ankle arthrodesis
>   P. incision

prilocaine
>   p. and phenylephrine
>   lidocaine and p.

Primaderm dressing
Primapore wound dressing
primary
>   p. amputation
>   p. arthroplasty

p. bone union
p. center
p. closure
p. cranial sacral respiratory
  mechanism
p. curve
p. cystic arthrosis
p. degenerative arthritis
p. degenerative osteoarthritis
p. focus of pain
p. hip replacement
p. intention
p. lymphoma
p. lymphoma of bone (PLB)
p. movement plane
p. myofascial trigger point
p. or intentional movement
p. peroneus longus
  tendinopathy
p. progressive amyotrophy
p. repair
p. rotation movement
p. sequestrum
p. spongiosa
p. stem
p. subacute osteomyelitis
p. subtalar arthrodesis
p. tumor
p. x-ray beam

Primaxin
prime mover
Primer modified Unna boot
primitive
>   p. bone
>   p. dislocation
>   p. locomotor pattern
>   p. reflex

primus
>   digitus p.
>   P. flexible great toe implant
>   p. implant

princeps pollicis artery
principal stress
principle
>   anatomic fracture reduction p.
>   axial compression p.
>   biomechanical p.
>   Brügger cogwheel p.
>   Enneking p.
>   gliding p.
>   Lambotte p.
>   SAID p.
>   spherical gliding p.

prism
>   Fresnel p.

prisoner's palsy
Pritchard
>   P. II elbow prosthesis
>   P. total elbow prosthesis

Pritchard-Walker
P.-W. semiconstrained elbow
  prosthesis
P.-W. total elbow prosthesis
**Pritsch talar osteochondroma
  classification**
prizm
p. Electro-Mesh Sock electrode
p. Electro-Mesh Z-Stim-II stimulator
pro
P. Balance Master
P. Balance Master ADL evaluation
  device
P. Osteon 500 bone graft
  substitute
P. Support Systems orthotic
ProAdvantage knee
Pro-8 ankle brace
probability
bone cyst fracture p.
Pro-Banthine
probe
Acufex p.
angled p.
arthroscopic p.
bipolar circumactive p.
  (BICAP)
blunt-tip p.
Bunnell dissecting p.
Bunnell forwarding p.
calibrated p.
dissecting p.
free-spinning p.
gearshift p.
gold p.
intraosseous p.
LASE p.
laser Doppler p.
multifrequency p.
multiplane echo p.
Nucleotome p.
pedicle sounding p.
reverse-cutting meniscal p.
skin temperature monitoring p.
spinning p.
p. test
p. test for osteomyelitis
triple-frequency p.
ultrasonic p.
Woodson p.
probenecid
colchicine and p.
probe-to-bone test
problem area
procaine
procaine-phenol motor point injection
procallus formation
Procardia XL
Procase Ankle-Lock brace

procedure
Adams hallux valgus interphalangeus
  correction p.
Akin p.
Albee shelf p.
Albizzia leg-lengthening p.
anchovy tendon interposition p.
Anderson-Fowler paralytic clawhand
  correction p.
antenna p.
anterior floating p.
anterior stabilization p.
AO p.
arthroscopic transglenoid suture
  stabilization p.
articulatory p.
Auto-Implant p.
Axer-Clark muscle-tendon transfer
  for elbow paralysis p.
Badgley cervical discectomy and
  fusion combination p.
Baker Achilles tendon
  lengthening p.
BAK laparoscopic p.
Bankart p.
Barsky cleft hand repair p.
Bartlett p.
basic cranial adjusting p. (I, II)
Baxter-D'Astous proximal femoral
  resection-interposition
  arthroplasty p.
beefburger p.
Bell Tawse radial head p.
Berman-Gartland forefoot p.
BH Moore p.
Bilhaut-Cloquet polydactyly p.
Blair p.
Blatt capsulodesis p.
bone block p.
bony p.
Bose hip resurfacing p.
Bosworth hip shelf p.
Boyd-McLeod tennis elbow p.
Boytchev recurrent dislocated
  shoulder p.
Brahms p.
Braun gastric p.
bridle footdrop p.
bridle posterior tibial tendon p.
Bristow p.
Bristow-Helfet recurrent shoulder
  dislocation p.
Bristow-Latarjet anterior shoulder
  instability p.
Bristow-May dislocated shoulder p.
Brockman p.
Broström-Evans p.
Broström lateral ankle instability p.
Bryan p.

P

procedure (*continued*)
    buttressing p.
    Calandriello orthopedic p.
    callus distraction p.
    Campbell ankle p.
    capsular imbrication p.
    capsular shift p.
    Carticel implant p.
    Castle femoral resection p.
    cervical myelopathy anterior
      floating p.
    Chambers p.
    Chandler p.
    Charnley ankle fusion p.
    checkrein p.
    chevron p.
    Chiari shelf p.
    chiropractic adjustment p.
    Chrisman-Snook weave p.
    Clayton first metatarsophalangeal
      joint fusion p.
    Cobb tibialis posterior tendon
      dysfunction p.
    Cole p.
    Connolly p.
    Copeland-Howard shoulder p.
    core drilling p.
    Cotting ingrown nail p.
    Cotton p.
    Cracchiolo hallux limitus implant
      arthroplasty p.
    Cummins p.
    curative soft tissue p.
    Darrach extensor carpi ulnaris
      tendesis p.
    Das Gupta transbronchial needle
      aspiration p.
    debulking p.
    decompressive p.
    degloving p.
    denervation p.
    DePalma staple p.
    Dewar posterior cervical fixation p.
    Dickson-Diveley total joint
      replacement p.
    Dorrance push-back cleft palate p.
    Downey-McGlamery p.
    Downey-Rubin overlapping toe
      repair p.
    DREZ lesioning p.
    Durham p.
    DuVries p.
    Dwyer orthopaedic p.
    Eden-Hybbinette anterior glenoid
      bone block p.
    Eden-Lange trapezius p.
    Edwards transposing atrial
      septum p.
    eggshell p.

Elmslie-Cholmeley p.
Elmslie peroneal tendon p.
Elmslie-Trillat patellar p.
Elmslie weave p.
Engebretsen p.
Evans ankle instability p.
Eve reconstruction of gliding tissue
    defects p.
extraarticular Grice p.
failed p.
Fairbanks-Sever brachial plexus
    repair p.
femoral Buck plug p.
Fontan-type p.
forage core decompression
    biopsy p.
Fowler p.
Frank and Johnson modification of
    Heyman p.
Fried-Hendel p.
Froimson-Oh arm p.
Froimson tendon interposition
    thumb p.
Frost foot p.
Fulford subtalar arthrodesis p.
Gallie p.
Gartland forefoot reconstruction p.
Gelman foot p.
Gerard resurfacing p.
Gilbert p.
Gillquist p.
Gill shelf p.
Girdlestone orthopedic p.
Girdlestone-Taylor muscle transfer
    clawtoe repair p.
Gould ankle p.
gracilis p.
Grant, Surrall, and Lehman p.
Green p.
Green-Grice p.
Grice p.
Gritti-Stokes distal thigh p.
Gruca lower leg p.
Gurd distal clavicle open
    resection p.
Hall Kalamchi shelf p.
hallux valgus p.
Hammon foot p.
Hardinge vastus lateralis p.
Hark pes planus p.
Harmon p.
Hass p.
Hauser Achilles lengthening p.
Hauser heel cord p.
Hauser patellar tendon p.
Hawkins shoulder p.
Heifetz nail matrix excision p.
Hey Groves p.
Heyman p.

Heyman-Herndon p.
Hibbs lumbar fusion p.
His-Haas p.
Hitchcock arm p.
Hodor-Dobbs p.
Hoffer ankle p.
Hoffmann metatarsal p.
Hohmann hallux osteotomy p.
Hoke-Miller pes planus p.
Hoke tibial palsy p.
Howorth hip p.
Hughston lateral knee
  instability p.
IDET p.
iliac buttressing p.
Ilizarov p.
4-incision p.
5-incision p.
Inclan modification of Campbell
  ankle p.
Inclan-Ober p.
Ingram p.
Insall patellar instability repair p.
installation of orthosis p.
instillation p.
intercalary allograft p.
intermetatarsal angle-reducing p.
intraarticular p.
intradiscal electrothermal therapy p.
intradiscal electrothermal
  treatment p.
Jaffe p.
Jahss dorsal wedge osteotomy p.
James p.
Jansey toenail ablation p.
Johnson p.
Johnson-Spiegl p.
joint-destructive p.
joint salvage p.
Jones retinaculum reconstruction p.
J.R. Moore p.
Juvara closing abudetory wedge for
  feet p.
Kaplan modification of
  Ruiz-Mora p.
Karlsson ankle instability
  correction p.
Kehr p.
Kelikian lateral ankle suture
  anchor p.
Keller-Brandes p.
Keller bunionectomy p.
Kelly peroneal tendon dislocation p.
Kendrick below-knee amputation p.
Kessel-Bonney hallux osteotomy p.
Kidner excision of accessory
  navicular bone p.
King intraarticular hip fusion p.
Kortzeborn p.

Koutsogiannis sliding calcaneal
  osteotomy p.
Krukenberg reconstruction of
  BKA p.
kyphoplastic p.
Lance shelf p.
Lane p.
Lange p.
Langenskiöld central physeal bar
  excision p.
Lapidus p.
Larmon forefoot p.
Larsen lateral ankle stabilization p.
Latarjet p.
lateral sling p.
Lauenstein ulnar head resection p.
Lawton p.
Lee p.
Leeds spinal p.
Legg p.
lengthening over nails p.
Lepird metatarsus adductus p.
L'Episcopo obstetric brachial plexus
  injury repair p.
ligamentous weave p.
limb-salvage p.
Lindeman laryngeal diversion p.
Lindholm Achilles lengthening p.
Linton varicose vein p.
Lipscomb p.
Localio p.
loose p.
loose knee p.
Lorenz congenital clubfoot p.
Loughheed and White p.
lower cervical spine p.
Lowman shelf p.
Luck hand p.
Lynn Achilles lengthening p.
MacAusland p.
MacCarthy excision of sacrum p.
macrodactylia reduction p.
Magnuson-Stack shoulder p.
Mahan pediatric sedation p.
manipulative p.
Manktelow transfer p.
Mann hallux valgus repair p.
Maquet patellar realignment p.
Matson p.
Mau and Ludloff p.
Mauck knee p.
McBride p.
McCarthy hip p.
McCash hand p.
McCauley foot p.
McElvenny foot p.
McGlamry p.
McGlamry-Downey forefoot p.
McKay hip p.

P

procedure (*continued*)
McKeever p.
McLaughlin posterior shoulder dislocation repair p.
medial rotation p.
Mikulicz p.
Miller foot p.
Mitchell hallux valgus p.
Miyakawa knee p.
Moberg key-pinch p.
modified Boytchev p.
modified Broström p.
modified Broström-Evans p.
modified Hoke-Miller flatfoot p.
modified Lapidus p.
Mogensen p.
motion control p.
motion-preserving p.
Mueller knee p.
Mumford distal clavicle open resection p.
muscle-balancing p.
muscle energy p. (MEP)
Neer capsular shift p.
Newman-Keuls p.
Nicola shoulder tenodesis p.
Nicoll fracture repair p.
Nilsson lateral ankle stabilization p.
notchplasty p.
OATS p.
O'Brien capsular shift p.
O'Donoghue triad knee repair p.
offset-V p.
orthodox p.
Oudard shoulder bone block p.
Outerbridge-Kashiwagi p.
over-the-top knee p.
Pagddu p.
Parrish microvascular decompression p.
Paterson p.
Peabody and Munro p.
peroneal tendon p.
Perthes p.
Pettibon chiropractic p.
Podiatry Institute p.
polyethylene femoral Buck plug p.
portmanteau p.
posterior-inferior capsular shift p.
Proxiderm p.
Putti-Platt shoulder p.
realignment p.
reefing p.
Regnauld enclavement p.
Regnauld hallux p.
resurfacing p.
Reverdin-Green foot p.
Reverdin-Green-Laird p.
reverse Jones p.

reverse Mauck knee p.
reverse Putti-Platt p.
revision p.
Ridlon p.
Roaf, Kirkaldy-Willis, and Cattero p.
Rockwood acromioclavicular joint dislocation repair p.
Root p.
Rose foot p.
Roux-Goldthwait repair of recurrent patellar dislocation p.
Ruiz-Mora proximal phalangectomy for hammertoe p.
Ryerson triple arthrodesis of foot p.
sacroiliac buttressing p.
Saha recurrent anterior shoulder dislocation surgical p.
salvage p.
Samilson sliding osteotomy of calcaneus p.
sartorial slide p.
Sauvé-Kapandji p.
Scaglietti spondyloptosis reduction p.
Schrock pediatric scapula p.
Schrock scapula elevation repair p.
Selakovich sustenaculum tali p.
semitendinosus p.
sequential p.
Sgarlato hammertoe implant p.
sham p.
shelf p.
short lever specific contact p.
Silfverskiöld gastrocnemius soleus recession p.
Silver and Simon modification of Silfverskiöld p.
Silver bunionectomy p.
Skoog hyperhidrosis p.
sling p.
Slocum knee p.
Somerville hip p.
Souter hip p.
Southwick slide p.
spinal fusion p.
spinal locking p.
Spira scapulothoracic arthrodesis p.
Spittler ankle disarticulation p.
Spittler 2–stage syme ankle amputation p.
SPLATT p.
split anterior tibial tendon p.
stabilization of chevron p.
Stack shoulder p.
staged p.
staggered p.
Staheli acetabular shelf p.
Staheli hip osteotomy shelf p.
Stamm temporary gastrostomy p.

STA-peg p.
Steindler p.
Steytler-Van Der Walt metatarsus
  adductus osteotomy p.
Stone anoplasty p.
Strayer Achilles lengthening p.
Stromeyer Achilles tenotomy p.
Sutherland hip p.
Syme ankle p.
Tachdjian external fixation for cavus
  fixation p.
Taylor p.
tendon checkrein p.
terminal Syme p.
Thomas p.
Thomas-Thompson p.
Thompson-Terwilliger terminal Syme
  operation for ingrown toenail p.
Tikhoff-Linberg bone and soft tissue
  tumors p.
Tikhoff-Linberg radical arm p.
p. time
transpedicular wedge resection
  osteotomy p.
Trillat shoulder bone block p.
triple-wire p.
Tsai-Stillwell distal radioulnar joint
  repair p.
upper cervical spine p.
Valenti hallux limitus/rigidus p.
van Ness lower limb amputation
  with foot reversal p.
Verebelyi-Ogston decancellation p.
Vulpius lengthening of
  gastrocnemius muscle p.
Vulpius-Stoffel gastrocnemius
  intramuscular aponeurotic
  recession p.
wafer p.
Watson-Jones p.
Weaver-Dunn acromioclavicular joint
  stabilization p.
Webb p.
Weber anterior talofibular ligament
  reconstruction p.
Weston shelf p.
White slide lengthening of tendo
  Achillis p.
Whitman talectomy p.
Williams discectomy p.
Wilson angulation osteotomy for
  hallux valgus p.
Woodward release of high-riding
  scapula p.
Woodward scapula correction p.
yoke transposition p.
Youngswick-Austin metatarsal
  head p.
Youngswick metatarsal head p.

Yount gluteal-iliotibial fasciotomy p.
Yount knee flexion contracture
  release p.
Zadik foot p.
Zancolli biceps tendon transfer p.
Zancolli clawhand deformity p.
Zancolli lasso p.
Zarins-Rowe semitendinosus and
  iliotibial band knee repair p.
Zimmer minimally invasive solutions
  hip p.

process
abnormal posterior talar p.
absent spinous p.
acromion p.
articular p.
bifid spinous p.
BioCleanse tissue sterilization p.
bone destructive p.
bony p.
capitular p.
casting p.
Civinini p.
cleft spinous p.
clinoid p.
condyloid p.
conoid p.
coracoacromial p.
coracoid p.
coronoid p.
cubital p.
deficient spinous p.
dislocation of articular p.
Drummond segmental wire fixation
  through spinous p.
ensiform p.
inferior p.
intact spinous p.
intercondylar p.
internal p.
lateral p.
mammillary p.
mastoid p.
maxillary p.
neuromuscular proprioceptive p.
odontoid p.
olecranon p.
physial mamillary p.
proprioceptive p.
sacralized transverse p.
spinous p.
spurious articular p.
spurious spinous p.
styloid p.
superior p.
supracondylar p.
talar p.
talus lateral posterior p.
transverse p.

P

583

process (*continued*)
  Tutoplast p.
  unciform p.
  ungual p.
  Wisconsin segmental wire fixation
    through spinous processes
  xiphoid p.
  Zimmer PMMA precoat p.
processed carbon implant
procession
  fast imaging with steady p. (FISP)
ProCol bovine bioprosthesis tendon
procurvatum deformity
ProCyte transparent dressing
Proderm topical spray
Pro-Designed wrist guard
Prodisc
  P. I disc prosthesis
  P. II lumbar implant
  P. lumbar total disc replacement
  P. spinal disc prosthesis
Prodisc-C
  P.-C cervical artificial disc implant
  P.-C total disc replacement
product
  Body Glove orthopaedic p.
  cyclooxygenase p.
  Fortitude Ti titanium spinal fixation
    p.
  Fortitude Vue titanium spinal
    fixation p.
  Innovation Sports bracing p.
  Innovative Medical P.'s (IMP)
  Linvatec p.
  Linvatec arthroscopy p.
  microparticulated protein p.
  Orthopaedic Physical Therapy P.'s
    (OPTP)
  Oxiplex/SP bioresorbable p.
  resistive exercise p.'s (REP)
production
  bone p.
  torque p.
Profemur tapered stem total hip system
professional protective technology (PPT)
Profex
  P. arthroscopic leg positioner
  P. arthroscopic tourniquet
proficiency
  Bruininks-Oseretsky Test of
    Motor P.
profile
  acromial p.
  Functional Limitation P. (FLP)
  Hawaii Early Learning P. (HELP)
  P. hip prosthesis
  P. hip stem
  Maryland Foot Score P.
  PULSES p.

  reduced p.
  risk factor p.
  P. Sitting Orthosis
  Staheli pediatric lower extremity
    rotational p.
  surface p.
  P. total hip system
  wrist speed p.
profilometry
  stress p.
Profix
  P. confirming tibial insert
  P. metaphysial tibial stem
  P. mobile-bearing knee implant
  P. nonporous tibial base
  P. porous femoral component
  P. total knee replacement system
ProFlex wrist support
ProFlo vascular compression therapy
Profore
  P. Four-Layer bandage system
  P. wound dressing
ProForma prosthesis
profunda
  p. brachii artery
  p. femoris artery
profundus
  p. advancement
  p. artery fracture
  flexor digitorum p. (FDP)
  p. muscle
  p. tendon
Pro-glide
  P.-g. orthosis
  P.-g. splint
prognostic
  p. analysis
  p. factor
program, programme
  aquatic exercise p.
  aquatic stabilization p.
  Camp Diversity arthritis p.
  Carpal Care rehabilitative p.
  exercise p.
  flexibility conditioning p.
  home exercise p.
  home spinal stabilization p.
  independent exercise p.
  interdisciplinary vocational
    evaluation p.
  LEAP p.
  macrotrauma rehabilitation p.
  Microplasty minimally invasive hip
    p.
  Military Amputee Research P.
    (MARP)
  phase 2 elbow p.
  rehabilitation therapeutic p.
  Rothman Institute total hip p.

4-star exercise p.
stretching p.
TotalGym Exercise P.
trunk stabilization rehabilitation p.
Ultimate Hand Helper
strengthening p.
walking p.
weight-training p.
work hardening p.
programmable VariGrip II prosthetic control system
programme (*var. of* program)
progression
curve p.
kyphosis p.
p. of training
slow curve p.
p. to full weightbearing
p. walking component
progressiva
dysbasia lordotica p.
fibrodysplasia ossificans p.
fibrositis ossificans p.
fibrous dysplasia ossificans p.
myositis ossificans p.
progressive
P. Ambulation Scale
p. ankle orthosis
p. diaphysial dysplasia (PDD)
p. loading
p. lumbar extension rehabilitation
p. macrodactylia
p. muscle relaxation
p. muscular atrophy (PMA)
p. muscular dystrophy
(PMD)
p. myositis fibrosa
p. neurologic disorder
p. nuclear amyotrophy
p. olisthesis
p. osseous heteroplasia
p. overload
P. palm guard
p. perilunar instability
p. resistance brace
p. resistance training
p. spinal amyotrophy
p. subacute myelopathy
p. subluxation
p. supranuclear palsy
p. systemic sclerosis (PSS)
p. torsion spasm
p. weakness
p. weight
p. weightbearing
progressively larger reamer
progressive-resistance exercise (PRE)
progressive-resistive exercise (PRE)
Progress splint

proinflammatory state
projection
axial calcaneal p.
axial sesamoid p.
bursal p.
cephaloscapular p.
convergence p.
dorsoplantar p.
Harris-Beath p.
lateral p.
posterior-superior oblique p.
stress dorsiflexion p.
prolapse
disc p.
Prolene suture
proliferating zone
proliferation
angiofibroblastic p.
bizarre parosteal osteochondromatous
p. (BPOP)
fibroblastic p.
reactive periosteal p.
p. therapy
proliferative, proliferous
p. arthritis
p. fasciitis
p. myositis
p. synovitis
proliferous (*var. of* proliferative)
Proline Stomatex shoulder brace
ProLite Plus runner's orthotic
Prolixin
Prolo lumbar and cervical spine postoperative functional and economic status score
prolongation rod
prolonged insertional activity
prolotherapy
PROM
passive range of motion
promazine
promethazine
meperidine and p.
prominence
heel p.
navicular p.
osseous p.
osteochondral p.
pedicle screw hardware p.
plantar bony p.
prehallux osseous p.
rotational p.
tibial tubercle p.
prominent
p. heel
p. spur
Promogran matrix wound dressing
promontoria (*pl. of* promontorium)
promontorium, *pl.* **promontoria**

P

585

promontory
  sacral p. (SP)
Promos modular shoulder system
pronate
pronated
  p. foot
  p. pes cavus
  p. straight flatfoot
pronation
  p. and supination
  p. contracture
  p. control
  p. eversion external rotation (PEER)
  hindfoot p.
  p. injury
  p. of foot
  p. phenomenon
  rearfoot p.
  p. sign
  p. spring-control device
  subtalar p.
pronation-abduction
  p.-a. fracture
  p.-a. injury
pronation-eversion
  p.-e. fracture
  p.-e. injury
pronation-eversion-external
  p.-e.-e. rotation fracture
  p.-e.-e. rotation injury
  p.-e.-e. rotation injury of ankle
pronation-external
  p.-e. rotation (PER)
  p.-e. rotation (I-IV) fracture
  p.-e. rotation injury
pronation/spring control
pronation-supination
pronator
  p. drift
  p. drill
  p. quadratus (PQ)
  p. quadratus muscle
  p. reflex
  p. sign
  p. syndrome
  p. teres (PT)
  p. teres muscle
  p. teres release
  p. teres syndrome
  p. teres tendon
pronatory gait
pronatus
  pes p.
prone
  p. blocking technique
  p. extension test
  p. external rotation test
  p. knee-bend test
  p. knee flexion test

  p. position
  p. rectus test
  p. reduction
  p. sacral push
  p. scapular retraction exercise
Pronex
  P. home traction
  P. patient controlled pneumatic
    traction device
  P. pneumatic cervical traction
  P. pneumatic device for cervical
    pain
2-prong
  2-p. rake retractor
  2-p. stem finger prosthesis
3-prong
  3-p. headrest
  3-p. rake blade retractor
prong
  modified tonsillar p.
4-prong finger splint
5-prong rake blade retractor
pronometer
Pron pillow
Pronto cement
PROOF
  Prevent Recurrence of Osteoporotic
  Fractures
  PROOF group
ProOsteon
  P. bone graft material
  P. Implant 500
  P. implant 500 coralline
    hydroxyapatite bone void filler
  P. Implant 500 granules
Propac
  Champ Insulated P. II
Propacet
propagation velocity
proparacaine
Propel cannulated interference screw
propeller
  orthopaedic p.
proper
  p. digital nerve branch
  p. neck positioning
properitoneal space
properly seated
property
  elastic p.
  elongation p.
prophylactic
  p. abduction pants
  p. antibiotic
  p. antibiotic therapy
  p. anticoagulation
  p. bone graft
  p. fasciotomy
  p. operative stabilization

p. resection
p. skeletal fixation
p. taping
prophylaxes (*pl. of* prophylaxis)
prophylaxis, *pl.* **prophylaxes**
deep venous thrombosis p.
dextran p.
DVT p.
tetanus p.
propiomazine
Propionibacterium acnes
propionic acid
Proplast
P. HA
P. I, II porous implant material
P. prosthesis
P. prosthetic material
proportionate dwarfism
propoxyphene
p. and acetaminophen
p. and aspirin
p. hydrochloride
propranolol
proprioception
gravitational p.
p. of hand
proprioceptive
p. deficit
p. exercise
p. impairment
p. neuromuscular facilitation
(PNF)
p. neuromuscular facilitation
approach
p. neuromuscular facilitation
exercise
p. neuromuscular facilitation pattern
p. process
p. rehabilitation
p. training
proprioceptor
propriosensory training
proprius
extensor indicis p. (EIP)
p. tendon
Prop'R Toes hammertoe cushion
propulsion
p. biomechanics
p. gait
propulsive phase
prospective payment system (PPS)
prostaglandin
PROSTALAC
prosthesis of antibiotic-loaded acrylic
cement
PROSTALAC temporary hip
prosthesis
PROSTALAC total hip prosthesis
PROSTALAC total joint prosthesis

Prostaphlin
prosternation
prostheses (*pl. of* prosthesis)
prosthesis, *pl.* **prostheses**
above-knee p.
Accolade hip p.
acetabular p.
acrylic bar p.
ACS Gemini p.
ACS Profile p.
ACS Star p.
AcuMatch M Series modular
femoral hip p.
Advanced mobile-bearing p.
Advance PS total knee p.
Advantim total knee p.
Advantim unconstrained p.
Aequalis humeral p.
Aequalis reversed shoulder p.
Aequalis shoulder p.
Aesculap-PM noncemented
femoral p.
AGC femoral p.
AGC knee p.
AGC tibial p.
AHP digital p.
AHSC elbow p.
AHSC-Volz elbow p.
Airlite p.
Airprene hinged knee p.
AK p.
Alivium implant metal p.
Allen-Brown p.
all median-nerve hand p.
Allurion foot p.
alumina cemented total hip p.
alumina-on-alumina total hip p.
AMC total wrist p.
American Heyer-Schulte chin p.
American Heyer-Schulte Radovan
tissue expander p.
AMK unconstrained p.
AML Plus p.
AML tang femoral p.
AML total hip p.
Amstutz cemented hip p.
anametric total knee p.
Anatomic Precoat hip p.
anatomic surface p.
Anderson acetabular p.
p. and orthosis (P&O)
ankle p.
Apollo hip p.
APR acetabular p.
APR femoral p.
APR II p.
APRL hand p.
Arthropor cup p.
Arthropor II acetabular p.

P

prosthesis (*continued*)

Atlas modular humeral p.
Attenborough total knee p.
Aufranc cobra hip p.
Aufranc-Turner cemented hip p.
Austin Moore femoral head p.
Autophor ceramic total hip p.
Autophor femoral p.
Avanta MCP joint implant finger p.
Averett hip p.
Averill press fit p.
Balance hip p.
ball-and-socket ankle p.
Bankart shoulder p.
Bantam CDH p.
4-bar linkage on knee p.
4-bar polycentric knee p.
Bateman femoral neck p.
Bateman finger p.
Bateman Universal Proximal
  Femur p.
Bateman UPF II bipolar p.
BDH p.
Beachcomber waterproof p.
bead-blasted p.
Bechtol hip p.
Bechtol patellofemoral joint p.
Bechtol shoulder p.
Bechtol system p.
Bechtol total knee p.
Becker hand p.
Beck-Steffee total ankle p.
below-elbow p.
below-knee p.
Bi-Angular shoulder p.
Biaxial Weave composite p.
bicentric p.
bicompartmental knee implant p.
bicondylar ankle p.
bicondylar knee p.
Bi-Metric hip p.
Bi-Metric Interlok femoral p.
Bi-Metric porous primary femoral p.
Bio-Chromatic hand p.
Bioclad with pegs reinforced
  acetabular p.
BioFit Press-Fit acetabular p.
Bioglass p.
Bio-Groove acetabular p.
Bio-Groove Macrobond HA
  femoral p.
Biomet AGC knee p.
Biomet hip p.
Biometric p.
Biomet total toe p.
Bio-Modular shoulder p.
biophase implant metal p.
Biotex implant metal p.
bipolar femoral head p.

bipolar hip replacement p.
Björk p.
Blauth knee p.
Blazina p.
Bock knee p.
Bombelli-Mathys-Morscher hip p.
bone p.
bovine collagen material p.
Brigham p.
Bryan cervical disc p.
Bryan total knee implant p.
Buchholz p.
Buechel-Pappas total ankle p.
Byars mandibular p.
CAD/CAM p.
Caffinière trapeziometacarpal p.
Calandruccio cemented hip p.
calcar replacement femoral p.
Callender technique hip p.
Calnan-Nicolle finger p.
Calnan-Nicolle
  metatarsophalangeal p.
Calnan-Nicolle synthetic joint p.
camouflage p.
Canadian hip disarticulation p.
Capello press-fit p.
capitellocondylar unconstrained
  elbow p.
Carbon Copy high performance
  foot p.
Carbon Copy HP foot p.
Carbon Copy II foot p.
Carbon Copy II Light p.
Cardona keratoprosthesis p.
carpal lunate implant p.
carpal scaphoid implant p.
Cathcart Orthocentric hip p.
CDH Precoat Plus hip p.
cemented hip p.
cementless p.
Centralign precoat hip p.
ceramic femoral head p.
ceramic ossicular p.
Ceramion p.
CFLB p.
CFS hip p.
Charnley acetabular cup p.
Charnley cemented p.
Charnley-Hastings p.
Charnley low-friction hip p.
Charnley-Müller hip p.
Charnley total hip p.
Chatzidakis hinged Vitallium
  implant p.
CHD p.
Chopart partial foot p.
Choyce MK II keratoprosthesis p.
Christiansen hip p.
Cintor knee p.

Cirrus foot p.
clamshell p.
Clayton p.
C-Leg p.
C-Leg lower limb p.
Cloutier unconstrained knee p.
coated p.
Coballoy implant metal p.
cobalt-chromium alloy p.
Co-Cr-Mo alloy p.
Co-Cr-W-Ni alloy p.
Cofield shoulder p.
cold-mold p.
cold-weld femoral p.
collar-calcar support femoral p.
College Park TruStep foot p.
Compartmental II knee p.
p. component
p. component subsidence
compression-molded p.
computer-assisted
  design/computer-assisted
  manufacturing p.
Conaxial ankle p.
conoidal ankle p.
constrained hinged knee p.
constrained nonhinged knee p.
Continuum unconstrained p.
Contour internal p.
conventional single-axis knee p.
Coonrad-Morrey sloppy hinge
  elbow p.
Coonrad semiconstrained elbow p.
Corail press-fit p.
C-2 OsteoCap hip p.
CPT p.
crimped Dacron p.
cruciate condylar unconstrained p.
cruciate-retaining p.
cruciate-sacrificing p.
p. cup
custom p.
custom-threaded p.
Dacron p.
DANA shoulder p.
d'Aubigné femoral p.
Deane unconstrained knee p.
DeBakey p.
debonded femoral stem p.
Dee totally constrained elbow p.
p. dehiscence
de La Caffinière
  trapeziometacarpal p.
DeLaura knee p.
DeLaura-Verner knee p.
Delrin p.
DePalma hip p.
DePuy AML Porocoat stem p.
DePuy hip p.

Deune knee p.
digital p.
Dimension-C femoral stem p.
Dimension hip p.
direct-impact p.
distal radioulnar joint p.
doffing p.
donning p.
Dorrance hand p.
Dow Corning Wright finger joint p.
p. driver
DRUJ p.
dual-lock total hip p.
Duocentric p.
Duocondylar knee p.
Duo-Lock hip p.
duopatellar unconstrained p.
Dupaco knee p.
Duracon p.
Duraloc p.
Dycor Geriatric ADL single axis
  foot p.
Dynaplex knee p.
Eaton trapezium finger joint
  replacement p.
Edwards seamless p.
E-2 foot p.
Eftekhar-Charnley hip p.
Eftekhar long-stem p.
Eicher femoral p.
Eicher hip p.
Eilers-Armstrong unicompartmental
  knee p.
elbow p.
Endolite p.
Endo-Model hinged knee p.
Endo-Model rotating knee joint p.
Endo-Model sled p.
Endo rotating knee joint p.
energy storing foot p.
Engh porous metal hip p.
Englehardt femoral p.
English-McNab shoulder p.
Entegra p.
EPTFE graft p.
Eriksson knee p.
Evolution hip p.
Ewald unconstrained elbow p.
Exeter cemented hip p.
Exeter-Femora press fit p.
femoral neck p.
finger joint implant p.
Finney p.
Finney-Flexirod p.
Finn hinged knee p.
fixed femoral head p.
flanged revision p.
Flatt finger-joint p.
Flatt finger-thumb p.

prosthesis (*continued*)

Flex-Foot Modular III p.
Flex H/A total ossicular p.
Flex-Sprint p.
Flex-Walk p.
Flex-Walk II p.
fluid p.
foot p.
forearm lift assist p.
forged cobalt-chromium alloy p.
Free-Flow system p.
Freeman-high neck press fit p.
Freeman modular total hip p.
Freeman-Samuelson knee p.
Freeman-Swanson knee p.
F.R. Thompson femoral p.
fully constrained tricompartmental
  knee p.
Gaffney ankle p.
Galante hip p.
Gemini hip system p.
Genesis knee p.
GeoFlex knee p.
Geomedic total knee p.
geometric total knee p.
Gerard p.
Gianturco p.
Gilfillan humeral p.
Giliberty acetabular p.
Giliberty femoral neck p.
Giliberty hip p.
Gillette joint p.
Gillies p.
Girard keratoprosthesis p.
Gore-Tex knee p.
great toe implant p.
Greifer p.
Greissinger foot p.
Gripper acetabular cup p.
grit-blasted p.
Gritti-Stokes knee p.
GSB elbow p.
GSB expanded version for knee p.
Guepar hinged knee p.
Guilford-Wright p.
Gunston-Hult knee p.
Gunston polycentric knee p.
Gustilo hip p.
Gustilo knee p.
Gustilo unconstrained p.
Hamas upper limb p.
hand p.
hand-glove p.
Hanger ComfortFlex knee p.
Hanslik patellar p.
Harken p.
Harris cemented hip p.
Harris Design femoral p.
Harris-Galante porous hip p.

Harris Micromini p.
Hastings hip p.
Haynes-Stellite implant metal p.
HD-2 cemented total hip p.
heat-cured acrylic femoral head p.
Herbert knee p.
Hexcel knee p.
Hexcel total condylar p.
HG multilock hip p.
Hinderer malar p.
hinged constrained knee p.
hinged great toe replacement p.
hinged implant p.
hinged total knee p.
hip disarticulation p.
hip replacement p.
Hittenberger p.
homograft p.
Hosmer WALK p.
Howmedica Kinematic II knee p.
Howmedica PCA p.
Howorth p.
Howse p.
HPS II total hip p.
HSS total condylar knee p.
Hunter silastic p.
Hunter tendon p.
Hydra-Cadence knee p.
hydraulic knee unit p.
I-beam hemiarthroplasty hip p.
ICLH ankle p.
ICLH knee p.
Identifit hip p.
immediate postoperative p. (IPOP)
Impact modular porous p.
Impact total hip p.
Implant Technology LSF p.
Index p.
Indiana conservative p.
Indong Oh hip p.
Infinity modular hip p.
Insall-Burstein semiconstrained
  tricompartmental knee p.
p. inserter
Integral Interlok femoral p.
Integrity acetabular cup p.
Intelligent Prosthesis Plus p.
p. interface
Intermedics Natural-Knee knee p.
Inter-Op acetabular p.
Inter-Op hip p.
Interseal Variant (I–IV) p.
Iowa internal p.
Iowa total hip p.
ischial weightbearing p. (IWP)
Ishizuki unconstrained elbow p.
isoelastic pelvic p.
Ivalon p.
Jaffe press-fit p.

Jewett p.
Jobst p.
Johnson-Elloy Accord
  unconstrained p.
Johnston-Iowa hip p.
Jonas p.
Joplin toe p.
Judet press-fit hip p.
keeled p.
Keller bunionectomy with p.
Kessler p.
Kinematic fully constrained
  tricompartmental knee p.
Kinematic II rotating hinge total
  knee p.
Kinemax Plus knee p.
Kirschner Medical Dimension p.
Kirschner total shoulder p.
KMP femoral stem p.
knee p.
Koenig MPJ p.
K2 sensation p.
Kudo unconstrained elbow p.
Küntscher humeral p.
Lacey fully constrained
  tricompartmental knee p.
Lacey hinged knee p.
Laing hip cup p.
Lanceford p.
Landers-Foulks p.
LaPorta total toe p.
LCS meniscal bearing
  semiconstrained p.
LCS New Jersey knee p.
LCS rotating platform
  semiconstrained p.
LCS substituting semiconstrained p.
LCS universal APG
  semiconstrained p.
Leinbach femoral p.
Leinbach hip p.
Lewis expandable adjustable p.
  (LEAP)
Lewis Trapezio p.
Ling cemented hip p.
Link Endo-Model rotational knee p.
Link MP hip noncemented
  reconstruction p.
Lippman hip p.
Lisfranc below-knee p.
Liverpool elbow p.
Liverpool knee p.
Lo Bak spinal support p.
locking p.
London unconstrained elbow p.
Longevity V-Lign hip p.
Lo-Por vascular graft p.
Lord press-fit hip p.
Lord total hip p.

Lotus unicompartment p.
low-contact stress semiconstrained p.
lower extremity p.
lower limb p. (LLP)
low-neck femoral p.
low-profile femoral p.
Lubinus knee p.
lunate acrylic cement wrist p.
Lunceford-Pilliar-Engh hip p.
Lund prototype unicompartment p.
MacIntosh tibial plateau p.
MacNab-English shoulder p.
madreporic hip p.
Mallory p.
Mallory-Head I, II p.
Mallory-Head porous primary
  femoral p.
Mallory-Head total hip p.
manual locking knee p.
Marlex and methyl methacrylate p.
Marmor modular knee p.
Master step foot p.
Mathys p.
Matrol femoral head p.
Mayo semiconstrained elbow p.
Mayo total ankle p.
Mazas totally constrained elbow p.
McBride femoral p.
McKee-Farrar total hip p.
McKee femoral p.
McKee totally constrained elbow p.
McKeever patellar cap p.
McKeever vitallium knee p.
MCP finger joint p.
Mecring acetabluar p.
Mediloy implant metal p.
medium profile femoral p.
medullary p.
metal-backed plastic-on-metal p.
metal femoral head p.
metal-on-metal articulating
  intervertebral disc p.
metaphysial head resection with p.
MG II knee p.
Michael Reese articulated p.
Michele long-stem p.
Microloc knee p.
Microvel p.
migration of p.
Miller-Galante hip p.
Miller-Galante II knee p.
Minneapolis hip p.
Mittlemeier ceramic hip p.
Mittlemeier noncemented femoral p.
Mobi-C cervical disc p.
modified Moore hip locking p.
modular Austin Moore hip p.
modular Iowa Precoat total hip p.
modular unicompartmental knee p.

P

prosthesis (*continued*)

Monk hip p.
monoblock femoral stem p.
monolithic A1203 cup p.
Moore femoral neck p.
Moore hip p.
Moretz p.
Moseley glenoid rim p.
MP reconstruction p.
Mueli wrist p.
Mueller-Charnley hip p.
Mueller dual-lock hip p.
Mueller total hip replacement p.
Müller p.
Mulligan silastic p.
multiaxis p.
Multiflex foot p.
Multi-Lock hip p.
multiradius unconstrained p.
Murray knee p.
myoelectric control p.
Natural-Hip p.
Natural-Knee unconstrained p.
Natural-Lok acetabular cup p.
NEB total hip p.
Neer humeral replacement p.
Neer shoulder p. (I, II)
Neer umbrella p.
New Jersey hemiarthroplasty p.
New Jersey LCS shoulder p.
New Jersey LCS total knee p.
Newton ankle p.
Nexus hip p.
Nicoll tendon p.
Niebauer-Cutter p.
Niebauer finger-joint replacement p.
Niebauer metacarpophalangeal joint
  silastic p.
Niebauer trapezium replacement p.
Noiles fully constrained
  tricompartmental knee p.
nonhinged knee p.
nonhinged linked p.
Normalize press-fit hip p.
Norwich press-fit p.
nudge control on p.
ocular p.
Odland ankle p.
p. of antibiotic-loaded acrylic
  cement (PROSTALAC)
p. of antibiotic-loaded acrylic
  cement total joint prosthesis
Oh cemented hip p.
Oh press-fit hip p.
Oh-Spectron p.
Oklahoma ankle p.
Omnifit dual geometry
  microstructured p.
Omnifit HA hip stem p.

Omnifit knee p.
Omnifit PSL microstructured p.
OmniFlex hip p.
Opti-Fix femoral p.
Opti-Fix I, II p.
Oregon Poly II ankle p.
Orthochrome implant metal p.
Orthofix p.
Ortholoc II unconstrained p.
Ortholoc implant metal p.
orthopaedic p.
osseointegrated p.
OsteoCap hip p.
Osteolock hip p.
Osteonics hip p.
Otto Bock dynamic p.
Overdyke hip p.
Oxford meniscal unicompartment p.
Padgett p.
painful femoral head p.
Paltrinieri-Trentani p.
partial ossicular
  reconstruction/replacement p.
partial ossicular replacement p.
  (PORP)
patellar tendon-bearing
  below-knee p.
PCA Original p.
PCA Standard p.
PCA unconstrained
  tricompartmental p.
PCA unicompartmental knee p.
PC Performer knee p.
pegged tibial p.
Perfecta hip p.
Perfecta (I, II) hip p.
Performance knee p.
Peri-Loc p.
PFC curved unconstrained p.
PFC femoral p.
Phoenix total hip p.
Pillet hand p.
Pilliar p.
piston p.
Plasticor p.
Plasti-Pore ossicular replacement p.
Plastiport TORP p.
Plystan p.
Polycel bone composite p.
polycentric knee p.
polycentric unconstrained p.
Poly-Dial p.
polyethylene patellar implant p.
polyethylene talar p.
polypropylene p.
porcine p.
Porocoat AML noncemented p.
Porometal noncemented femoral p.
porous-coated anatomic p.

porous-coated femur p.
porous-coated hip p.
porous surfaced p.
Precision Osteolock femoral p.
Precision Osteolock hip p.
Precoat hip p.
Precoat Plus femoral p.
Premier press fit p.
press-fit condylar total knee p.
Pritchard II elbow p.
Pritchard total elbow p.
Pritchard-Walker semiconstrained
  elbow p.
Pritchard-Walker total elbow p.
Prodisc I disc p.
Prodisc spinal disc p.
Profile hip p.
ProForma p.
2-prong stem finger p.
Proplast p.
PROSTALAC temporary hip p.
PROSTALAC total hip p.
PROSTALAC total joint p.
Protasul femoral p.
Protasul-10 noncemented
  femoral p.
Protasul-64 WF Zweymuller
  femoral p.
Protek p.
provisional p.
proximal humeral p.
proximal third femoral p.
PTB-SC-SP p.
PTB supracondylar p.
PTB suprapatellar p.
PTS soft wedge p.
pyrocarbon p.
Quantum Foot p.
radial head implant p.
Radovan tissue expander p.
Ranawat-Burstein hip p.
Randelli shoulder p.
Rastelli p.
Reflection I p.
Reflection Interfit p.
Reflection V p.
Re-Flex VSP p.
Repiphysis p.
retaining knee p.
Reverdin p.
reversed shoulder p.
Richards hip p.
Richards maximum contact
  cruciate-sparing p.
Richard Smith p.
Richards Spectron metal-backed
  acetabular p.
Richards Zirconia femoral head p.
Ring knee p.

Ring total hip p.
Ring UPM press-fit p.
RMC p.
RM isoelastic hip p.
Robert Brigham semiconstrained p.
Robert Brigham total knee p.
Roper-Day p.
Rosenfeld hip p.
rotating femoral head p.
rotating hinge knee p.
rotating knee joint p.
Rothman Institute femoral p.
Roy-Camille p.
SACH foot p.
sacrificing knee p.
saddle p.
SAF p.
SAFE II p.
Saint Georg-Buchholz total ankle p.
Salzer ceramic p.
Sampson p.
Sarmiento STH-2 hip p.
Sauerbruch p.
Savastano hemiknee p.
Savastano unconstrained p.
Savastano unicompartment p.
Sbarbaro hip p.
Sbarbaro tibial plateau p.
Scarborough p.
Schlein semiconstrained elbow p.
Schlein total elbow p.
Schlein trisurface ankle p.
Schuknecht Gelfoam wire p.
Schuknecht Teflon wire piston p.
seating of p.
Seattle foot p.
Secur-Fit HA PSL X'tra p.
Select ankle p.
Select modular shoulder p.
self-bearing ceramic hip p.
self-centering Universal hip p.
semiconstrained tricompartmental
  knee p.
Sense-of-Feel p.
SensorHand p.
Sgarlato hammertoe implant p.
  (SHIP)
Sharrard-Trentani p.
Shaw-Sgarlato hammertoe implant p.
Sheehan knee p.
Sherfee p.
Shier knee p.
shoulder disarticulation p.
silastic ball spacer p.
silastic radial head p.
silastic thumb p.
Silflex intramedullary p.
silicone trapezium p.
single-axis ankle p.

P

prosthesis (*continued*)
  sintered implant p.
  Sinterlock implant metal p.
  Sivash hip p.
  SMA p.
  Smith ankle p.
  Smith-Petersen hip cup p.
  SMO p.
  solid ankle cushioned heel p.
  Solution p.
  Souter-Strathclyde elbow p.
  Souter unconstrained elbow p.
  Spectron hip p.
  Speed radius cap p.
  spherocentric fully constrained
   tricompartmental knee p.
  Spotorno hip p.
  Springlite lower limb p.
  S-ROM Arthropor (I-III) p.
  S-ROM Arthropor oblong p.
  S-ROM femoral stem p.
  S-ROM hip p.
  S-ROM super cup p.
  S-ROM ZZT (I, II) p.
  stainless steel implant metal p.
  Stanmore shoulder p.
  Stanmore totally constrained
   elbow p.
  STAR ankle joint p.
  stemmed tibial p.
  Stenzel rod p.
  Stevens-Street humeral replacement
   elbow p.
  St. Georg unicompartment p.
  STH-2 hip p.
  Street-Stevens humeral p.
  substituting knee p.
  suction suspension p.
  Sulzer p.
  SuperCup acetabular cup p.
  Sure-Flex p.
  surgical p.
  Surgitek p.
  Sutter double-stem silicone
   implant p.
  Sutter MCP finger joint p.
  Swanson finger joint p.
  Swanson flexible hallux valgus p.
  Swanson great toe p.
  Swanson metacarpal p.
  Swanson metatarsal p.
  Swanson silastic elbow p.
  Swanson T-shaped great toe
   silastic p.
  Swanson wrist p.
  Syme amputation p.
  Syme foot p.
  Synatomic total knee p.
  synthetic p.

Taperloc femoral p.
TARA total hip p.
Target p.
Tavernetti-Tennant knee p.
Teflon tri-leaflet p.
p. template
tendon p.
Thackray hip p.
tharies hip replacement p.
thermomechanical implant metal p.
T28 hip p.
Thompson femoral neck p.
Thompson hemiarthroplasty hip p.
Thompson-Parkridge-Richards p.
threaded titanium acetabular p.
  (TTAP)
threaded titanium alloy p.
  (TTAP)
thrust plate p. (TPP)
Ti-Bac II hip p.
tibial plateau p.
Ti/CoCr alloy hip p.
Ti-Con p.
Tillman p.
Titan cemented hip p.
titanium alloy hip p.
titanium alloy implant metal p.
titanium hip p.
titanium implant p.
titanium rod and buttress p.
Ti-Thread p.
TMA p.
toe p.
total articular replacement
  arthroplasty p.
Total Concept ankle/foot p.
total condylar p. (III)
total condylar III fully
  constrained p.
total condylar knee p.
total condylar semiconstrained
  tricompartmental p.
total hip replacement p.
total joint replacement p.
total knee replacement p.
Townley horizontal platform p.
Townley TARA p.
Townley total articular resurfacing
  arthroplasty p.
Townley total knee p.
TPR ankle p.
Trac II knee p.
transfemoral modular p.
transradial p.
transtibial immediate
  postoperative p.
trapezial p.
trapeziometacarpal joint
  replacement p.

trapezium implant p.
Trapezoidal-28 hip p.
Trapezoidal-28 internal p.
TR-28 hip p.
Triad p.
trial p.
TriAxial p.
triaxial semiconstrained elbow p.
tricompartmental knee p.
Tricon-M cruciate-sparing p.
Tricon-M patellar p.
trileaflet p.
Tri-Lock bone preservation stem
  hip p.
Tri-Lock press-fit p.
Trilogy p.
Trilogy AB acetabular p.
Tronzo total hip p.
trunnion-bearing hip p.
TruStep foot p.
TT Pylon p.
Turner p.
UCI ankle p.
UCI unconstrained p.
UHMWPE p.
ulnar head implant p.
Ultimate knee p.
unconstrained tricompartmental
  knee p.
unicompartmental knee p.
unicondylar p.
universal femoral head p.
universal hip p.
universal (I, II) p.
upper extremity myoelectric p.
upper limb p. (ULP)
Valls hip p.
Vanghetti limb p.
Varikopf hip p.
VerSys p.
vibrotactile sensory p.
Viladot p.
Vinertia implant metal p.
vitallium humeral replacement p.
vitallium-W implant metal p.
Volz wrist p.
Wadsworth unconstrained
  elbow p.
Wagner p.
Walldius vitallium mechanical
  knee p.
Waugh knee p.
Waugh total ankle replacement p.
Wayfarer modifiable foot p.
Weller total hip joint p.
well-seated p.
William Harris hip p.
Wright knee p.
Wright titanium p.

wrist joint implant p.
Xenophor femoral p.
Young hinged knee p.
Zimaloy femoral head p.
Zimaloy implant metal p.
Zimmer hip p.
Zimmer shoulder p.
Zimmer tibial p.
zirconia femoral head p.
zirconia orthopaedic p.
zirconium oxide ceramic p.
Z-stent p.
ZTT (I, II) acetabular cup p.
Zweymüller cementless hip p.
prosthesis-cement interface
prosthetic
  p. ambulation
  American Hand P.'s (AHP)
  p. and orthotic (P&O)
  p. arthroplasty
  Cirrus foot p.
  p. cone
  p. design
  p. disc nucleus (PDN)
  p. disc nucleus device
  p. evaluation questionnaire
  p. femorodistal graft
  p. finger
  p. fitting
  p. foam
  p. foot
  p. gait training
  p. hemiarthroplasty
  p. hook
  p. intervention
  p. joint replacement
  p. loosening
  p. patella
  P. Problem Inventory Scale
  P. Problem Inventory Scale
    classification
  p. replacement
  p. replacement for joint
  roll-over shape p.
  p. sock
  p. socket
  p. spacer
  p. speech aid
  p. stance phase shock
  p. stem lateral fin
  p. support
  Total Knee for Children p.
  p. training
prosthetist
prosthetist/orthotist
ProStretch exerciser
Protasul
  P. femoral prosthesis
  P. implant metal

P

595

Protasul-10 noncemented femoral prosthesis
Protasul-64 WF Zweymuller femoral prosthesis
Pro-Tec patellar tendon strap
protection
    digital artery p.
    Ionact antibacterial p.
    p. plate
    p., restricted activity, ice, compression, elevation (PRICE)
protective
    p. extension reaction
    p. limitation
    p. limitation of range of motion
    p. sensation
    p. shield
    p. weightbearing
protector
    Air-Limb amputation p.
    Alvarado collateral ligament p.
    ankle ligament p. (ALP)
    Cast Gard cast p.
    grooved p.
    Heelbo decubitus heel/elbow p.
    Jurgan Pin Ball pin p.
    medial nerve p.
    P. meniscus suturing system
    M-F heel p.
    Ortho-Foam p.
    Patellar Band knee p.
    Roho heel p.
    Seal-Tight cast p.
    ShowerSafe waterproof cast and bandage p.
    The Heeler inflatable heel p.
    tissue p.
Protecto splint
Protege manual flexion distraction table
protein
    bone morphogenetic p. (BMP)
    cartilage oligomeric matrix p. (COMP)
    C-reactive p. (CRP)
    dietary p.
    IGF binding p.
    p. malnutrition
    morphogenetic p.
    Ne-Osteo bone morphogenic p.
    osteogenic p. 1 (OP-1)
    soluble N-eythyl-maleimide sensitive factor attachment p. (SNAP)
protein-1
protein-based bone graft substitute
Protek prosthesis
proteoglycan
    p. matrix
    p. synthesis

Proteus
    P. mirabilis
    P. syndrome
prothelen set
ProThotics insole
prothrombin time (PT)
prothrombotic state
protocol
    Bruce p.
    Evans-Burkhalter p.
    Mann p.
    Marx osteoradionecrosis p.
    North American Malignant Hyperthermia p.
    p. of Walsh
proton density
Protonic brace
Protoplast cement
prototype design
Protouch synthetic orthopaedic padding
ProTrac
    P. alignment guide
    P. cruciate reconstruction system
    P. measurement device
    P. system for knee surgery
protraction
protractor
    arthrodial p.
    Demariniff p.
    triplanar p.
    Zimmer p.
protruded disc
protruding disc
protrusio
    p. acetabuli
    p. cage
    p. deformity
    p. ring
    p. shell
protrusion
    central disc p.
    disc p.
    p. distance
    lateral disc p.
    medial disc p.
    p. of navicular
protuberans
    dermatofibrosarcoma p. (DFSP)
    enchondroma p.
proud flesh
Providence Scoliosis System
provisional
    p. amputation
    p. calcification
    p. callus
    p. fixation
    P. Fixation TC-100 plating system
    p. prosthesis
    p. stabilization

Proxiderm
- P. procedure
- P. wound closure system

proximal
- p. and distal realignment
- p. and distal screw
- p. anular pulley
- p. anular pulley of thumb
- p. articular facet angle
- p. articular set angle (PASA)
- p. bow position
- p. carpal row
- p. cement spacer
- p. chevron osteotomy
- p. communicating branch
- p. compression test
- p. dome osteotomy
- p. drill-guide assembly
- p. end tibia fracture
- p. femoral elevator
- p. femoral epiphysiolysis
- p. femoral focal deficiency (PFFD)
- p. femoral fracture
- p. femoral metaphysial shortening
- p. femoral osteotomy
- p. femoral resection
- p. femur
- p. fibula
- p. fibular facet
- p. first metatarsal osteotomy
- p. focal femoral deficiency (PFFD)
- p. humeral fracture
- p. humeral prosthesis
- p. humerus
- p. humerus plate
- p. interlocking
- p. interphalangeal (PIP)
- p. interphalangeal articulation
- p. interphalangeal/distal interphalangeal
- p. interphalangeal joint
- p. interphalangeal joint approach
- p. intrinsic release
- p. latency
- p. level amputation
- p. locking
- p. medial brim
- p. metatarsal approach
- p. metatarsal osteotomy
- p. midpatellar medial and lateral portals
- p. nerve release
- p. phalangeal epiphysiodesis
- p. phalangeal osteotomy
- p. phalanx (PP)
- p. phalanx osteotomy
- p. phocomelia
- p. portion
- p. radioulnar articulation
- p. radioulnar joint
- p. radius
- p. reference axis
- p. row carpectomy
- p. set angle deviation
- p. stacked wire technique
- p. subungual onychomycosis (PSO)
- p. tendon rupture
- p. thigh band
- p. third (P/3)
- p. third femoral prosthesis
- p. third of radius and ulna
- p. third of shaft
- p. tibia
- p. tibial metaphysial fracture
- p. tibial osteotomy
- p. tibial plateau
- p. tibiofibular joint
- p. tibiofibular joint dislocation
- p. tibiofibular subluxation
- p. tibiofibular synostosis
- p. ulna
- p. Wagner metaphysial shortening

proximal-to-distal
- p.-t.-d. dissection technique
- p.-t.-d. ring

proximoataxia

proximolateral

prune-belly syndrome

PSA
- persistent sciatic artery

PSB
- patellar stabilizing brace

PSDK
- poststatic dyskinesia

pseudankylosis

pseudarthrosis, pseudoarthrosis
- ball-and-socket giant p.
- closed p.
- congenital tibial p.
- documented p.
- extraarticular p.
- failed back syndrome with documented p.
- fibular p.
- Girdlestone p.
- interspinous p.
- radial p.
- p. rate
- p. repair
- synovial p.
- tibial p.

pseudoacetabulum

pseudoachondroplasia

pseudoanaemia (*var. of* pseudoanemia)

pseudoanemia, pseudoanaemia
- athlete's p.
- dilutional p.

pseudoaneurysm

P

pseudoarthritis
  ball-and-socket giant p.
  congenital p.
pseudoarthrosis (*var. of* pseudarthrosis)
pseudoarticulation
pseudo-Babinski sign
pseudo-Bennett fracture
pseudoboutonnière deformity
pseudobulbar palsy
pseudocapsule chondrosarcoma
pseudo-Charcot joint
pseudoclaudication
pseudoclawing
pseudocortex
pseudocoxalgia
pseudocyst
  calcaneal p.
  p. of humerus
pseudodislocation of humerus
pseudoephedrine and ibuprofen
pseudoepiphysis
pseudoexostosis
pseudofacilitation
pseudofracture
  Milkman p.
pseudogamekeeper's injury
pseudogout
pseudohead
pseudo-Hurler deformity
pseudohypertrophic
  p. dystrophy
  p. muscular paralysis
pseudohypertrophy
pseudohypoparathyroidism
pseudo-Jones fracture
pseudomallei
  Pseudomonas p.
pseudometatarsal head
Pseudomonas
  P. aeruginosa
  P. pseudomallei
pseudomyotonic discharge
pseudoneoplastic lesion
pseudoneuroma
pseudoosteomalacic pelvis
pseudoosteomyelitis
pseudoparalysis
  congenital atonic p.
  Parrot p.
pseudoperiosteal reaction
pseudopodia (*pl. of* pseudopodium)
pseudopodium, *pl.* **pseudopodia**
pseudopolyphasic action potential
pseudo-Pott disease
pseudoradicular syndrome
pseudosarcomatous
  p. fasciitis (PSF)
  p. fibromatosis
  p. reaction

pseudostability test
pseudosubluxation
pseudotendon
pseudotumorous mucin deposition
pseudovarus
PSF
  posterior spinal fusion
  pseudosarcomatous fasciitis
PSI
  predictive salvage index
PSIS
  posterior superior iliac spine
PSO
  proximal subungual onychomycosis
psoas
  p. abscess
  p. bursitis
  p. bursitis pain
  p. muscle
  p. tendon syndrome
Psoralen-UVA therapy
psoriasis
  arthritis-associated p.
psoriatica
  arthropathia p.
psoriatic arthritis
PSS
  PJPS Severity Scale
  progressivesystemic sclerosis
psychogenic equinovarus
psychological adjustment
psychometrics
psychomotor
psychoneuroimmunology
psychophysical measurement
psychophysiologic
psychoprosthetic pain
psychosomatic
PT
  physical therapy
  physical training
  physiotherapy
  posterior tibial
  pronator teres
  prothrombin time
    PT pulse
    PT tilt table
PTA
  posterior tibial artery
  post traumatic amnesia
PTB
  patellar tendon-bearing
  pretibial bearing
  pretibial buttress
    PTB ankle-foot orthosis
    PTB brace
    PTB cast
    PTB plastic orthosis
    PTB socket

PTB supracondylar prosthesis
PTB suprapatellar prosthesis
PTBO
    patellar tendon-bearing
      orthosis
PTBS
    patellar tendon-bearing suspension
PTB-SC-SP
    patellar tendon-bearing-supracondylar-
      suprapatellar
    PTB-SC-SP prosthesis
PTD
    permanent and total disability
PTE
    posttraumatic epilepsy
    pretibial edema
pterotic bone
pterygium colli
pterygoid
    p. bone
    p. chest
    p. plate
PTFE
    polytetrafluoroethylene
    PTFE graft
PTFL
    posterior talofibular ligament
PTN
    posterior tibial nerve
PTP
    posterior tibial pulse
PTS
    patellar tendon socket
    patellar tendon stabilization
    PTS knee brace
    PTS soft wedge prosthesis
PTT
    partial thromboplastin time
    patellar tendon transfer
    posterior tibial tendon
    PTT insufficiency
PTTD
    posterior tibial tendon
      dysfunction
pubalgia
    athletic p.
pubic
    p. bone
    p. diastasis
    p. fascia
    p. osteolysis
    p. pad
    p. ramus
    p. symphysis
pubiotomy
pubis
    osteitis p.
    osteitis necroticans p.
    symphysis p. (SP)

puboanalis
pubocapsular ligament
pubococcygeus
pubofemoral ligament
puboischial area
puborectalis
PUC
    papain, urea, chlorophyllin copper
      complex ointment sodium
    PUC healing, debriding, and
      deodorizing ointment
Pucci
    P. Air orthotic
    P. pediatrics hand orthosis
    P. rehab knee orthosis
    P. splint
pucker sign
Puddu
    P. drill guide
    P. osteotomy system
    P. tendon technique
pudendal
    p. artery
    p. block
    p. nerve injury
    p. neuritis
puerperal synovitis
Pugh
    P. driver
    P. hip pin
    P. plate
    P. sliding nail
    P. traction
Pugil stick injury
Puka chisel
Pul-Ez
    P.-E. exerciser
    P.-E. shoulder pulley
pull
    p. screw
    spinous p.
pulled elbow
puller
    Ultra-Drive plug p.
pulley
    anular p. (A1–A4)
    cruciate p.
    p. exercise
    fibroosseous p.
    Flex Ranger stretch cable
      with p.
    Home Ranger shoulder p.
    overhead p.
    Preston overhead p.
    proximal anular p.
    Pul-Ez shoulder p.
    Range-Master p.
    p. reconstruction
    Saba p.

P

pulley (*continued*)
    shoulder p.
    weight and p.
pulling osteochondritis
pull-out (*var. of* pullout)
    p.-o. button
    p.-o. strength
    p.-o. suture
pullout, pull-out
    screw p.
pulmonary, pulmonic
    p. atelectasis
    p. barotrauma
    p. complication
    p. embolism
    p. osteoarthropathy
    p. osteodystrophy
pulmonic (*var. of* pulmonary)
pulp
    p. amputation
    p. approach
    finger p.
    p. flap
    plantar toe p.
    p. traction
pulposus
    herniated nucleus p. (HNP)
    nucleus p.
pulpy nucleus
pulsatile
    p. hypothermic perfusion
    p. jet lavage
    p. pneumatic plantar-compression device
    p. pressure lavage
pulsating
    p. electromagnetic field (PEMF)
    p. hematoma
Pulsavac
    P. III wound débridement system
    P. irrigation
    P. lavage
pulse
    blood volume p. (BVP)
    dorsalis pedis p.
    dorsal pedal p.
    DP p.
    intact peripheral p.'s
    p. irrigator
    p. oximeter
    posterior tibial p. (PTP)
    PT p.
    p. status-pull test
    p. volume recorder (PVR)
pulsed
    p. diathermy
    p. electric magnetic field bone growth stimulation

    p. electromagnetic field (PEMF)
    p. galvanic stimulator
    p. lavage
    p. short-wave therapy
    p. ultrasound
pulselessness
PULSES
    physical condition, upper limb function, lower limb function, sensory component, excretory function, support function
    PULSES profile
    PULSES Profile for Comprehensive Rehabilitation
Pulvertaft
    P. end-to-end suture
    P. fish-mouth stitch
    P. interweave suture
    P. weave tendon repair technique
pulvinar
    p. fibrofatty debris
    p. region
pulvule
    Darvon Compound-65 P.'s
pumice stone
pump
    Alzet continuous infusion osmotic p.
    ankle rehabilitation p.
    arthroscopic p.
    A-V Impulse foot p.
    p. bump
    p. bump area
    p. bump deformity
    p. bump exostosis
    cement p.
    compression p.
    continuous wave arthroscopy p.
    extremity p.
    EZ hand p.
    infusion p.
    intermittent extremity p.
    P. It Up pneumatic socket volume management system
    Jobst athrombotic p.
    knee p.
    Linvatec arthroscopic infusion p.
    morphine p.
    Multipulse 1000 compression p.
    pain control infusion p.
    PainFree p.
    sequential extremity p.
    Vacumix vacuum p.
    vacuum p.
    venous foot p.
pump-handle rib motion
PumpPals insole
punch
    Acufex rotary p.
    arthroscopic p.

p. biopsy
bone graft p.
bone hole p.
boxer's p.
Caspari suture p.
Casselberry suture p.
cervical laminectomy p.
Charnley femoral prosthesis
 neck p.
cruciate p.
Deyerle p.
p. drunk syndrome
p. forceps
Hirsch hypophysial p.
I-beam cement p.
keel bone p.
Kerrison p.
keyhole p.
Osborne p.
rotary p.
Rowe glenoid p.
Schlesinger p.
suction p.
suture p.
tibial p.
tubular p.

punctata
chondrodysplasia p. (CP)
keratosis p.

puncture
p. fracture
lumbar p. (LP)
spinal p.
p. wound
p. wound osteochondritis

Puno-Winter-Byrd (PWB)
P.-W.-B. system

purchase
p. and press the ground
bony p.
compression locking anchor with
 secondary p. (CLASP)
secondary p.
socket p.
toe-ground p.

Purdue pegboard

pure
p. limb apraxia limb
 asymmetry
p. syndactyly

PureFix hydroxyapatite
purine metabolism
Puros Accugraft
purposeful activity
purpura
p. fulminans
Henoch-Schönlein p.
meningococcal p.

pursestring suture

purulent
p. material
p. synovitis

push
p. cuff
knee-chest p.
P. medical brace
prone sacral p.
spinous p.

Push-Ease
P.-E. Quad Cuff
P.-E. wheelchair glove

pusher
Charnley femoral
 prosthesis p.
femoral component p.
hemispherical p.
hook p.
Jacobson suture p.
knot p.
metal p.
Patella P.
Revo loop handle knot p.
suture p.

push-off
p.-o. by great toe
great toe p.-o.
p.-o. phase
p.-o. phase of gait
p.-o. velocity

push-pull
p.-p. activity
p.-p. ankle stress view
p.-p. hip view
p.-p. instability
p.-p. move
p.-p. test

push-up
p.-u. block
p.-u. test

pustulotic osteoarthropathy
**putative segmental instantaneous axis of
rotation**
Puth abduction splint
Putti
P. Boneplast
P. bone rasp
P. knee arthrodesis
P. posterior bone block
P. posterior knee
 approach
scapular sign of P.
P. sign
P. splint

Putti-Platt
P.-P. arthroplasty
P.-P. instrumentation
P.-P. operation
P.-P. shoulder procedure

P

putty

> AliMed p.
> AlloMatrix bone graft p.
> AlloMatrix injectable p.
> BeOK hand exercise p.
> Blue Brand Therapy P.
> bone graft p.
> color-coded therapy p.
> exercise p.
> Flexi-Grip exercise p.
> Grafton DBM p.
> Grafton demineralized bone
>   matrix p.
> matrix Grafton p.
> Thera-Plast p.
> Therapy P.

PUV

> positive ulnar variance

PVB

> paravertebral block

PVC

> polyvinyl chloride
> PVC drain
> PVC tubing

PVCR

> posterior vertebral column resection

PVD

> peripheral vascular disease
> PVD dressing

PVI

> peripheral vascular insufficiency

PVM

> paravertebral muscle

PVMS

> paravertebral muscle spasm

PVNS

> pigmented villonodular
>   synovitis

PVR

> pulse volume recorder

PVS

> peripheral vascular surgery
> peripheral vascular system
> pigmented villonodular synovitis

PWB

> partial weightbearing
> Puno-Winter-Byrd
>   PWB transpedicular spine fixation
>   system

PWC

> physical work capacity

pyarthrosis

PYD

> pyridinium collagen crosslink
> pyridinoline

Pyle

> bone age according to Greulich and
>   P.
> P. disease

pylon

> AirStance p.
> p. attachment plate
> Icon p.
> impact-reducing p.
> P. intramedullary nail system
> metal p.
> Stratus impact-reducing p.
> vertical shock p.

pyocyanin

pyogenetic (*var. of* pyogenic)

pyogenic, pyogenetic, pyogenous

> p. arthritis
> p. bursitis
> p. discitis
> p. granuloma
> p. spinal infection
> p. spondylitis
> p. spondylodiscitis
> p. vertebral osteomyelitis

pyogenicum

> granuloma p.

pyogenous (*var. of* pyogenic)

pyomyositis

> staphylococcal p.

Pyramesh cage

pyramid

> P. anterior fixation plate
> P. anterior plate
> P. anterior plate fixation system
> p. attachment
> suction p.

pyramidal fracture

pyrazinamide

Pyrenochaeta romeroi

pyridinium collagen crosslink (PYD)

pyridinoline (PYD)

pyridoxine

pyriform (*var. of* piriform)

Pyrilinks-D urine assay

pyrocarbon

> p. implant
> p. prosthesis

pyrolytic

> p. carbon
> p. carbon device

pyrophosphate

> p. arthropathy
> technetium 99m p.
> technetium stannous p.

Pyrost bone graft material

Q
  Q angle
  Q disc
  Q Star Voyager pressure reduction
    mattress
Q-angle
  quadriceps angle
QCT
  quantitative computed tomography
QDR-2000 bone densitometer
QDR-1500, -2000 densitometer
QF
  quadratus femoris
qi
  q. gong therapy
  q. stagnation
QIF
  Quadriplegia Index of Function
qigong
Qingyangshen
QLV
  quasilinear viscoelastic
  QLV theory
QNA
  quadriceps neutral angle
QNST
  Quick Neurological Screening Test
Q-Ray bracelet
QRS
  Quantronic Resonance System
  QRS pulsating magnetic field
QSAC
  quadrant sparing acetabular component
QSART
  Quantitative Sudomotor Axon Reflex
  Test
QSGT
  quadruple semitendinosus and gracilis
  tendons
  QSGT graft
QST
  quantitative sensory testing
quad
  q. bar
  q. board
  q. cane
quadrangular
  q. cartilage
  q. positioning plate
quadrant
  Q. advanced shoulder brace
  q. hip scouring test
  q. of death
  q. sparing acetabular component
  (QSAC)

quadrate
  q. ligament
  q. ligament of Denucé
  q. muscle
quadratus
  q. femoris (QF)
  q. femoris fascia
  q. femoris muscle
  q. lumborum muscle
  q. lumborum syndrome
  q. plantae muscle
  pronator q. (PQ)
quadriceps (*pl.* quadriceps, quadricepses)
  q. active test
  q. angle (Q-angle)
  q. aponeurosis
  q. apron
  q. atrophy
  q. contraction test
  q. contracture
  q. contusion
  q. De Lorme boot
  q. expansion syndrome
  q. femoris muscle
  q. femoris muscle cast
  q. inhibition test
  q. jerk
  q. mechanism
  q. muscle group
  q. neutral angle
  (QNA)
  q. reflex
  q. strengthening exercise
  q. tendon
  q. tendon graft
  q. wasting
quadricepses (*pl. of* quadriceps)
quadricepsplasty
  Coonse-Adams q.
  Judet q.
  Thompson q.
  V-Y q.
quadriceps-setting exercise
quadriceps-sparing, minimally invasive
  total knee instrument
Quadriflex
quadrilateral
  q. brim
  q. frame
  q. ischial weightbearing
    socket
  q. space syndrome
quadriparesis
  spastic q.
quadripartite bone

quadriplegia
    Q. Index of Function (QIF)
    spastic q.
    transient q.
quadriplegic
quadruped
    q. back exercise technique
    q. fracture
quadruple
    q. amputation
    q. complex
    q. semitendinosus and gracilis tendons (QSGT)
    q. semitendinosus and gracilis tendons graft
Quadtro
    Q. cushion
    Q. cushion with Isoflap valve
QualCare knee brace
QualCraft
    Q. ankle support
    Q. short elastic wrist support
    Q. splint
    Q. strap
quality
    Agency for Healthcare Research and Q. (AHRQ)
    motion q.
    q. of life
    Q. of Well-Being Scale
quantitative
    q. computed tomography (QCT)
    q. mechanical pain testing
    q. sensory testing (QST)
    Q. Sudomotor Axon Reflex Test (QSART)
    q. ultrasound (QUS)
quantity
    scalar q.
    vector q.
Quantronic Resonance System (QRS)
quantum
    Q. foot
    Q. Foot prosthesis
    Q. 400 traction
Quartzo device
quasi-independent Y-axis movement
quasilinear
    q. viscoelastic (QLV)
    q. viscoelastic theory
quasistatic stressed position
quazepam
Quebec Back Pain Disability Scale
Queckenstedt
    Q. maneuver
    Q. phenomenon
    Q. sign
    Q. spinal stenosis test

Queckenstedt-Stookey subarachnoid channel block test
Quengel
    Q. apparatus
    Q. cast
    Q. device
    Q. hinge
Quénu-Küss tarsometatarsal injury classification
Quénu nail plate removal technique
Quervain disease
question
    Enneking q.
questionnaire
    American Academy of Orthopaedic Surgeons/Hip Society Q.
    American Shoulder and Elbow Surgeons q.
    Behavioral Assessment of Pain Q. (P-BAP)
    Children's Comprehensive Pain Q. (CCPQ)
    Cincinnati knee scoring q.
    Clinical Analysis Q. (CAQ)
    Community Integration Q. (CIQ)
    Coping Strategies Q. (CSQ)
    DASH q.
    Diabetic Quality of Life Q.
    Disabilities of Arm, Shoulder, and Hand q.
    disability screening q.
    Foot Function Index q.
    Foot Health Status Q.
    Functional Index Q. (FIQ)
    Functional Status Q. (FSQ)
    Headache Assessment Q. (HAQ)
    International Knee Ligament Standard Evaluation q.
    Jan van Breemen function q.
    Kenny Self-Care Q.
    Lambeth disability screening q.
    Levine Orthopaedic Outcomes Q.
    Lysholm knee scoring q.
    McGill pain q. (MPQ)
    McMaster-Toronto Arthritis Patient Preference Disability Q.
    Melzack Pain Q.
    MFA q.
    Michigan Hand Outcomes Q.
    Modified American Shoulder and Elbow Surgeons Shoulder Patient Self-Evaluation Form patient q.
    Occupational Q. (OQ)
    Osteoporosis Knowledge Q. (OKQ)
    Physical Activity Readiness Q. (PAR-Q)
    prosthetic evaluation q.
    Roland-Morris Q. (RMQ)

Short Musculoskeletal Function Assessment q.
Shoulder Pain and Disability Index patient q.
Shoulder Severity Index patient q.
Simple Shoulder Test patient q.
Subjective Shoulder Rating Scale patient q.
Varni-Thompson Pediatric Pain Q.

Questus leading edge grasper-cutter

Quetelet index

quick

Q. Neurological Screening Test (QNST)
q. stretch

QuickAnchor

Micro Q.
Mitek Micro Q.
Mitek Mini Q.

Quickbox container

QuickCast

Q. splint
Q. wrist immobilizer

QuickDraw bone harvester

Quickie

Q. Carbon wheelchair
Q. EX wheelchair
Q. GPS wheelchair
Q. GP Swing-Away wheelchair
Q. GPV wheelchair
Q. Kidz wheelchair
Q. Recliner wheelchair
Q. Shark pediatric wheelchair
Q. Ti wheelchair

Quick-Sil silicone system

QuickStick padding

QuickTack periosteal fixation system

quiescence

quiet hip disease

Quigley traction

QuikFormables orthotic

Quik splint

Quinby pelvic fracture classification

Quincke needle

quinine

Hyland's Leg Cramps with Q.

Quinsana Plus

quinti

abductor digiti q. (ADQ)
extensor digiti q. (EDQ)
Huber transfer of abductor digiti q.
opponens digiti q. (ODQ)

quotient

acetabular head q.

QUS

quantitative ultrasound

QUS-2 calcaneal ultrasonometer

Q

RA
    rheumatoid arthritis
        RA factor
        RA test
rabbeting
Rabideau Kitchen Evaluation-Revised (RKE-R)
race-pace exercise
rachicentesis, rachiocentesis
rachigraph
rachilysis
rachiocentesis (*var. of* rachicentesis)
rachiochysis
rachiodynia
rachiokyphosis
rachiometer
rachiomyelitis
rachioparalysis
rachiopathy
rachioplegia
rachioscoliosis
rachiotome, rachitome
rachiotomy
rachisagra
rachischisis
    r. partialis
    r. totalis
rachitic
    r. cat-back
    r. pelvis
    r. rosary sign
    r. scoliosis
rachitome (*var. of* rachiotome)
rack
    Hausmann weight r.
racket amputation
racquetball
racquet-shaped incision
radial
    r. agenesis
    r. antebrachial region
    r. artery
    r. artery injury
    r. bearing
    r. bone
    r. bursa
    r. carpal collateral ligament
    r. clubhand
    r. collateral ligament (RCL)
    r. collateral ligament complex (RCLC)
    r. column
    r. deficiency
    r. deviation

r. digital nerve
r. drift
r. epicondylalgia
r. forearm flap
r. fracture reduction
r. head
r. head anlage
r. head-capitellum view
r. head dislocation (RHD)
r. head fracture
r. head implant prosthesis
r. head subluxation (RHS)
r. hemimelia
R. Hinged Ulnar Deviation Splint
r. laminectomy
r. malalignment
r. malleolus
r. meniscal tear
r. metacarpal ligament
midcarpal r. (MCR)
r. neck
r. neck fracture
r. neck fracture fixation
r. nerve glove
r. nerve injury
r. nerve palsy
r. phenomenon
r. pseudarthrosis
r. ray defect
r. recession osteotomy
r. reflex
r. sensory nerve
r. sensory nerve entrapment syndrome
r. shaft
r. sigmoid notch
r. slab splint
r. styloid fracture
r. sulcus
r. trial
r. tuberosity
r. tunnel
r. tunnel supinator syndrome
r. tunnel syndrome
r. wedge osteotomy
r. wrist extensor
r. wrist extensor tendinitis
radial-based flap
radialis
    flexor carpi r. (FCR)
    malleolus r.
    r. sign
radialized

R

radiate
r. carpal ligament
r. ligament of head of rib
r. sternocostal ligament
radiation
r. therapy
thorny r.
radiation-related
r.-r. myelopathy
r.-r. neuropathy
radiatum
ligamentum r.
radical
r. approach
r. compartmental excision
r. flexor release
r. nail bed ablation
r. palmar fasciectomy
r. resection
radices (*pl. of* radix)
radicis (*gen. of* radix)
radicotomy
radicular
r. artery
r. neuritis
r. pain
r. symptom
radiculectomy
radiculitis
acute brachial r.
cervical r.
radiculomyelopathy
radiculoneuritis
radiculopathy
cervical r.
4-level r.
lumbosacral r.
radicurogram
radii (*gen.* and *pl. of* radius)
radioactive
r. iodine-labeled fibrinogen
r. xenon clearance
radiocapitate ligament
radiocapitellar
r. articulation
r. joint
r. joint ganglion
r. line
r. subluxation
radiocarpal
r. angle
r. arthritis
r. arthrodesis
r. arthroscopy
r. articulation
r. dislocation
r. instability

r. joint
r. ligament
r. portal
radiodense mass
radiodiagnostic study
radiogram
radiograph, skiagraph, skiagram, roentgenogram, roentgenograph
anterior drawer stress r.
cross-table lateral r.
dorsoplantar r.
frog-leg lateral r.
Judet r.
lateral weightbearing r.
lumbopelvic r.
Merchant r.
plantarflexed stress r.
postoperative r.
skyline r.
spot r.
stress r.
tangential standing r.
Velpeau axillary r.
weightbearing dorsoplantar r.
weightbearing tangential r.
West Point axillary lateral r.
radiographic, roentgenographic
r. avascular necrosis
r. examination
r. grid
r. parameter
radiography, skiagraphy, roentgenography
biplanar r.
Broden subtalar stress r.
carpometacarpal joint r.
elbow r.
flat plate r.
flexion-extension r.
neutron r.
patellofemoral joint r.
scanogram r.
serendipity view in shoulder r.
shoulder r.
stress r.
upright skeletal r.
radiohumeral
r. articulation
r. bursa
r. bursitis
r. epicondylitis
r. joint
radioisotope
r. clearance assay
r. gallium scan
r. indium-labeled white blood cell scan
r. technetium scan
r. thallium

radiology
American Chiropractic College of R. (ACCR)
MSK r.
musculoskeletal r.
radiolucency
periprosthetic r.
radiolucent
r. awl
r. lesion
r. line
r. nidus
r. roll
r. sound
r. splint
r. wrist fixation system
radiolunate
r. arthrodesis
r. fusion
r. joint
long r. (LRL)
short r. (SRL)
radiolunotriquetral ligament
radionucleotide imaging
radionuclide bone scan
radiopaque bone cement
radioscaphocapitate (RSC)
r. ligament
r. ligament laxity
radioscaphoid
r. articulation
r. fusion
r. joint
r. ligament
radioscapholunate
r. joint
r. ligament
radiosurgery
stereotactic r.
radiotherapy, roentgenotherapy
radiotranslucent rod
radiotriquetral ligament
radioulnar
r. articulation
r. dislocation
r. dissociation
distal r. (DRU)
r. joint
r. joint injury
r. subluxation
r. surface
r. synostosis (type I, II)
radius, *gen.* and *pl.* **radii**
absent r.
anular ligament of r.
distal r.
Kapandji fracture of r.
r. of angulation
r. of curvature

proximal r.
thrombocytopenia-absent r. (TAR)
thrombocytopenia-absent r.
Trimed system for fracture of distal r.
radix, *pl.* **radices,** *gen.* **radicis**
Radley-Liebig-Brown
R.-L.-B. ischium gluteal approach
R.-L.-B. resection of body of pubic bone approach
Radovan tissue expander prosthesis
RAF
rheumatoid arthritis factor
ragged
r. red fiber
r. red fiber myopathy
Ragnell retractor
rail
Bed-Bar support r.
Lumex Tub-Guard safety r.
Raimiste organic hemiplegia sign
Raimondi hemostatic forceps
Rainbow cast sandal
raise
crossed straight leg r.
resisted straight leg r.
single-leg toe r.
raising
contralateral straight leg r.
crossed straight leg r. (CSLR)
diurnal variation in straight leg r.
passive straight leg r.
straight leg r. (SLR)
well-leg r.
rake-handle effect
rake retractor
rales and rhonchi
Ralks
R. bone drill
R. fingernail drill
raloxifene
Raman spectroscopic imaging
rami (*pl. of* ramus)
ramp
Graftech structural allograft anterior r.
Graftech structural allograft posterior r.
r. load
ramus, *pl.* **rami**
dorsal r.
inferior r.
ischiopubic r.
pubic r.
Ranawat
R. neurologic deficit (I, II, IIIA, IIIB) classification
R. pneumatoid spondylitis classification

R

Ranawat-Burstein
 R.-B. hip prosthesis
 R.-B. porous stem
Ranawat-Dorr-Inglis
 R.-D.-I. atlantoaxial impaction method
 R.-D.-I. total hip method
Rancho
 R. Los Amigos
 R. Los Amigos ankle foot control device
 R. Los Amigos anklet foot control apparatus
 R. Los Amigos Cube System
 R. Los Amigos external fixation instrument
 R. Los Amigos National Rehabilitation Center
 R. Los Amigos Scale
 R. Los Amigos swivel hinge
Rand
 R. Functional Limitations Battery
 R. Physical Capacities Battery
Randelli shoulder prosthesis
random pattern flap
Raney
 R. bone drill
 R. flexion jacket brace
 R. perforator drill
 R. saw guide
Raney-Crutchfield
 R.-C. cervical traction tongs
 R.-C. tong traction
range
 interquantile r.
 r. of excursion
 r. of extension
 r. of motion (ROM)
 r. of motion brace
 r. of motion exercise
 r. of motion measurement
 r. of motion rehabilitation
 r. of motion restriction
 r. of motion testing
 r. of motion therapeutic stretching
 r. of motion therapy
 r. of rotational motion
Range-Master pulley
Ransford
 R. loop
 R. Pain Drawing
Ranvier
 R. disc
 groove of R.
 node of R.
 zone of R.
Rapamune
raphe, rhaphe
 anterolateral r.

 median r.
 middle r.
 midline r.
Rapid Assessment of Disease Activity in Rheumatology
RAP-n-roll
Rappaport fifth metatarsal proximal osteotomy
rarefaction
rarefying osteitis
RAS
 rhythmic auditory stimulation
Rascal scooter
rasp (*var. of* raspatory)
 Acufex convex r.
 Alexander r.
 Alexander-Farabeuf r.
 angled r.
 Arthrofile orthopaedic r.
 Aufricht glabellar r.
 Austin Moore r.
 Bacon r.
 bell r.
 Bristow r.
 Brown r.
 carbon-tungsten r.
 Charnley r.
 convex r.
 Coryllos r.
 Cottle r.
 custom r.
 DePuy r.
 diamond r.
 Doyen costal r.
 Doyen rib r.
 Endotrac r.
 Epstein bone r.
 Farabeuf bone r.
 Farabeuf-Lambotte r.
 femoral r.
 first rib r.
 Fisher r.
 Fomon r.
 Gallagher r.
 glabellar r.
 Good r.
 Hylin r.
 interbody r.
 Israel r.
 Jansen r.
 Joseph nasal r.
 Key r.
 Kleinert-Kutz r.
 Koenig r.
 Langenbeck r.
 Lewis periosteal r.
 Mallory-Head r.
 Maltz r.
 Mathieu r.

Miller r.
Nicoll r.
Olivecrona r.
orthopaedic r.
Phemister r.
r. pin
Podiatry Institute r.
power r.
Putti bone r.
rib r.
Rubin r.
Thompson r.
triangular r.
ulnar r.
Yasargil micro r.
Zollner r.
raspatory, rasp
Rastelli prosthesis
rasterstereographic analysis
rasterstereography
ratchet
r. clamp
r. flexor tenodesis splint
R. Lock variable flexion knee lock
ratcheting T-handle
ratchet-type brace
ratchety weakness
rate
basal metabolic r. (BRM)
erythrocyte sedimentation r. (ESR)
firing r.
fusion nonunion r.
heart r.
implant survival r.
nonunion r.
pseudarthrosis r.
resting heart r. (RHR)
sedimentation r.
steady state heart r. (SSHR)
vertebral osteosynthesis fusion r.
volumetric wear r.
Westergren sedimentation r. (WSR)
rated perceived exertion (RPE)
Rath treatment table
rating
Fitzgerald r.
HSS knee ligament r.
Mazur ankle r.
McGuire r.
occupational r.
r. of perceived exertion (RPE)
permanent partial disability r.
PPD r.
ratio
abduction-to-adduction r. (AB:AD)
abductor-to-adductor r. (AB:AD)
acetabular depth to femoral head
diameter r. (AD:FHD)
ankle-brachial pressure r.

arch-height r.
Blackburne r.
Blackburn-Peel r.
bone age r.
bone and limb growth velocity r.'s
Brattström condylar height r.
canal-to-calcar-isthmus r.
carpal height r.
Dorr r.
external rotation-to-internal rotation
r. (ER:IR)
femoral head-to-neck r.
femur length-to-abdominal
circumference r. (FL:AC)
Grace method of metatarsal length
r.
Insall r.
Insall-Salvati r.
medialization r.
metaphysial-to-diaphysial width r.
patellar ligament-to-patella r.
Pavlov r.
Poisson r.
respiratory exchange r.
r. scale in rehabilitation testing
Ratliff avascular necrosis classification
rat-tooth forceps
Rauchfuss sling
rave
fracture en r.
raw bone
ray
r. amputation
r. axis
border r.
R. cage implant
central r.
finger r.
long-axis r.
metatarsal r.
multiple r.'s
Peacock transposing index r.
pollicized r.
r. resection
R. screw
stiff r.
transposing index r.
**Rayhack ulnar shortening osteotomy
technique**
Raymond shoulder immobilizer
Raynaud
R. disease
R. gangrene
R. phenomenon
R. syndrome
Rayport muscular biopsy clamp
Ray-Tec sponge
razor
RazorVac ArthroWand

RBANS
 Repeatable Battery for the Assessment
 of Neuropsychological status
RBMT
 Rivermead Behavioral Memory Test
RBMT-E
 Rivermead Behavioral Memory
 Test-Extended Version
RC
 rehabilitation counseling
 role checklist
RCB
 rotator cuff buttress
RCL
 radial collateral ligament
RCLC
 radial collateral ligament complex
RCSP
 resting calcaneal stance position
reabsorption
reach
 R. Easy massager
 McGill standing overhead arm r.
reacher
 Double Duty cane r.
 E-Z R.
reaction
 Collis horizontal r.
 compensation r.
 epidermophytid r.
 equilibrium r.
 exaggeration r.
 r. force
 foreign body r.
 giant cell r.
 ground r.
 host immune r.
 hunting r.
 implant r.
 Peiper–Isbert r.
 periosteal r.
 protective extension r.
 pseudoperiosteal r.
 pseudosarcomatous r.
 r. time
 vagal r.
 Vojta r.
reactive
 r. arthritis
 r. bone formation
 low-surface r.
 r. nonunion
 r. periosteal proliferation
 r. synovitis
Read gouge
Real-EaSE neck and shoulder relaxer
realignment
 distal r.
 Elmslie-Trillat knee extensor r.

Galeazzi patella r.
Genutrain PE patellar r.
Hauser lateral retinacular
 release r.
Hughston hypoplastic dislocation of
 patella r.
Insall proximal r.
patellar r.
patellofemoral r.
physical r.
r. procedure
proximal and distal r.
Roux-Goldthwait patella r.
sagittal r.
Reality Orientation Chart
reamed
 r. nail
 sequentially r.
reamer
 acetabular r.
 acorn r.
 Aequalis r.
 Anspach r.
 Arthrex coring r.
 Aufranc r.
 Austin Moore r.
 ball r.
 blunt tapered T-handled r.
 bone r.
 r. brace
 brace-type r.
 calcar r.
 Campbell r.
 cannulated Henderson r.
 chamfer r.
 Charnley deepening r.
 Charnley expanding r.
 Charnley taper r.
 Charnley trochanter r.
 cheese-grater hemispherical r.
 Christmas tree r.
 r. clamp
 concave-surface r.
 congruous cup-shaped r.
 conical r.
 Con-Nex r.
 corrugated r.
 cup r.
 debris-retaining r.
 deepening r.
 DePuy r.
 end-cutting r.
 expanding r.
 female r.
 femoral head bone removal r.
 fenestrated r.
 flexible medullary r.
 fluted r.
 grater r.

Gray r.
grooving r.
r. guide
Hall Versipower r.
handle-type r.
Harris brace-type r.
Harris center-cutting acetabular r.
hemispherical r.
hollow mill r.
humeral r.
Indiana r.
Intracone intramedullary r.
intramedullary r.
Küntscher r.
male r.
medullary canal r.
Micro-Aire r.
Mira r.
Moore bone r.
motorized r.
multisized r.
Norton ball r.
orthopaedic r.
Perthes r.
power r.
power-driven r.
Pressure Sentinel r.
progressively larger r.
Richards r.
rigid r.
Rush rod awl r.
Smith-Petersen r.
spherical r.
spiral cortical r.
spiral trochanteric r.
spot-face r.
step-cut r.
straight power r.
Swanson r.
tapered r.
tapered hand r.
T-handled r.
triangular bone r.
triple r.
trochanteric r.
Wagner acetabular r.
reaming
r. awl
immediate tibial nailing without r.
reamputation
reanastomosis of blood supply
rear-entry ACL drill guide
rearfoot
r. deformity
r. ligament
r. osteotomy
r. pronation
r. stability system (RSS)
r. supination

r. valgus
r. varus
re-arthroscoped
reassessment
reattachment
Amstutz r.
Doll trochanteric r.
Harris 4-wire trochanter r.
4-wire trochanter r.
Rebel knee brace
rebound
r. hyperextension
r. phenomenon of Holmes
r. tenderness
rebounder
Plyoback R.
recalcitrant
r. neuropathic ulcer
r. pain
r. plantar fasciitis
recalled
multiplanar gradient r. (MPGR)
ReCap femoral resurfacing system
receiver operating characteristic (ROC)
recent dislocation
receptor
delta r.
epicritic r.
epsilon r.
kappa r.
nociceptive r.
opioid r.
postural r.
sensory nerve action potential r.
(SNARE)
sigma r.
SNAP r.
stretch r.
receptor-tonus method
recess
acetabular r.
anular periradial r.
Flatt r.
lateral r.
popliteal r.
ulnar synovial r.
recession
Bleck iliopsoas r.
endoscopic gastrocnemius r.
gastrocnemius r.
gastrocnemius-soleus r.
iliopsoas r.
Strayer gastrocnemius r.
Strayer gastrocnemius-soleus r.
tongue-in-groove r.
ulnar r.
recip
recipient
reciprocal

recipient (recip)
  r. site
  r. team
reciprocal (recip)
  r. arm raise back exercise technique
  r. finger prehension orthosis
  r. innervation
  r. isokinetic testing
  r. planing instrument
  r. relaxation
  r. stimulation
reciprocating
  r. gait orthosis (RGO)
  r. motor saw
  r. power handpiece
reciprocator
  LSU r.
Recklinghausen disease of bone
recliner
  HydroSoothe r.
  Ortho-Biotic r.
reclining frame wheelchair
recoil
  elastic r.
recombinant human erythropoietin
  (rHuEPO)
Recon
  R. nail
  R. proximal drill guide bolt
reconstituted depolymerized heparin
reconstruction
  ACL r.
  Allman modification of Evans
    ankle r.
  allograft r.
  Andrews iliotibial band r.
  ankle r.
  anterior capsulolabral r. (ACLR)
  anterior cruciate ligament r.
  arthroscopically assisted anterior
    cruciate ligament r.
  arthroscopic transhumeral r.
  augmented r.
  autogenous patellar tendon r.
  backfilling r.
  Bankart anterior capsolabral r.
  bifurcate vein graft for
    vascular r.
  bilobed flap r.
  Bristow shoulder r.
  Broström ligament r.
  Brown knee joint r.
  Bunnell technique of pulley r.
  capsular r.
  capsular-shift r.
  Cho anterior cruciate ligament r.
  Chrisman-Snook ankle ligament r.
  Clancy-Andrews r.
  Clancy cruciate ligament r.

complex acetabular r.
cruciate ligament r.
double-tunnel PCL r.
Eaton-Littler ligament r.
Ellison lateral knee r.
Elmslie r.
endoscopic anterior cruciate
  ligament r.
Eriksson cruciate ligament r.
Evans calcaneal r.
Evans lateral ankle r.
exogenous r.
extraarticular r.
Galveston r.
Goldner thumb r.
hand r.
Harmon hip r.
hindfoot r.
House upper limb r.
Hughston lateral compartment r.
index metacarpophalangeal
  joint r.
5-in-1 knee r.
Insall anterior cruciate ligament r.
intraarticular r.
joint r.
Jones-Ellison ACL r.
juxtacubital r.
Kleinert technique of pulley r.
Krukenberg hand r.
Kugelberg r.
Lange Achilles tendon r.
Larson ligament r.
lateral compartment r.
Lee r.
L'Episcopo hip r.
ligament r.
Lister technique of pulley r.
MacIntosh over-the-top ACL r.
Merle d'Aubigné femoral r.
Merle d'Aubigné resection r.
modified Chrisman-Snook ankle r.
Neer posterior shoulder r.
Nicholas 5-in-1 r.
Nicoll fracture r.
O'Donoghue ACL r.
r. of posterolateral structures using
  semitendinosus tendon
osteoplastic r.
PCL r.
r. plate
posterior cruciate ligament r.
pulley r.
Rosenberg endoscopic anterior
  cruciate ligament r.
Sauvé-Kapandji distal radioulnar
  joint r.
Silfverskiöld Achilles tendon r.
S-K distal radioulnar joint r.

2-stage tendon graft r.
sternoclavicular joint r.
sural island flap for foot and ankle r.
surgical r.
Swanson midfacial defect r.
tenoplastic r.
thumb r.
Torg knee r.
Verdan osteoplastic thumb r.
Vulpius Achilles tendon r.
Watson-Jones r.
Whitman femoral neck r.
Zancolli upper limb r.
reconstructive measure
recorder
pulse volume r. (PVR)
recording
r. electrode
intramuscular r.
recovery
fluid attenuation inversion r. (FLAIR)
functional r.
motor r.
r. phase rehabilitation
postanesthesia r. (PAR)
r. room
recreational
r. terminal device
r. therapy (RT)
recrudescence
recruitment
r. frequency
r. interval
myopathic r.
neuropathic r.
r. pattern
rectangle
Hartshill r.
Luque r.
rectangular
r. amputation
r. awl
r. frame
rectified socket
rectilinear
r. bone scan
r. motion
rectus
r. abdominis flap
r. abdominis muscle
r. adductor syndrome
r. femoris
r. femoris contracture
r. femoris flap
r. femoris graft
r. femoris muscle
r. femoris tendon

r. foot type
r. hallux
metatarsus primus r.
r. position
r. sheath
recumbency
recumbent
r. bicycle
r. cycle
r. position
r. posture
recurrent
r. disorder
r. hyperextension
r. laryngeal nerve
r. laryngeal nerve injury
r. median nerve block
r. meningeal nerve
r. mycetoma
r. parosteal osteosarcoma
r. patellar dislocation
r. synovitis
recurvatum
r. angulation deformity
cubitus r.
genu r.
pectus r.
r. test
red
R. Cross freeze-dried allograft
r. light neon laser
r. marrow
r. muscle
r. response
r., white, blue sign
r., yellow, blue (RYB)
r., yellow, blue wound color classification
Reddihough scale
redesign
job r.
Redi-Around finger splint
Rediform orthotic
Redigrip
R. knee pad
R. pressure bandage
Redi-Trac
R.-T. traction apparatus
R.-T. traction device
Redi-Vac cast cutter
Redler small bone caliper Redler small bone caliper
Redondo thoracolumbar fusion interbody VBR
red-red meniscal zone
redressement forcé
redresser
dual pin r.
redressment

reduced
> r. interference pattern
> r. profile

reducible

reduction
> Ace bandage r.
> Agee force-couple splint r.
> Allen lung volume r.
> anatomic r.
> Aston cartilage r.
> balloon-assisted endplate r. (BAER)
> Barsky macrodactyly r.
> Becton metacarpophalangeal open r.
> Bell Tawse pediatric Monteggia fracture open r.
> calcaneal fracture r.
> closed r.
> concentric r.
> congruent r.
> cotton elbow r.
> Crego hip r.
> Crosby calcaneal fracture r.
> Cubbins open shoulder r.
> r. deformity
> delayed open r.
> Eaton closed carpometacarpal joint r.
> Essex-Lopresti open radial head fracture r.
> external fixation r. (EX-FI-RE)
> fall r.
> femoral neck fracture r.
> Ferguson hip r.
> r. fixation
> Flynn femoral neck fracture r.
> force-couple splint r.
> r. forceps
> Fowles open elbow r.
> fracture r.
> fracture-dislocation r.
> frame of r.
> Hankin lung volume r.
> Hankin posterior elbow r.
> Hastings open radius r.
> hip r.
> incomplete r.
> indirect r.
> internal fixation, closed r.
> Kaplan open metacarpophalangeal joint r.
> Kinast indirect multifragmenting femur fracture r.
> King open radial head r.
> Kocher shoulder r.
> Lange hip r.
> Lorenz hip r.
> Lowell hip r.
> macrodactylia r.
> manual fracture r.

> McBride hallux abductovalgus r.
> McBride hallux valgus r.
> McKeever open r.
> McReynolds open tibia r.
> Meyn elbow r.
> Neer open shoulder r.
> r. of fracture
> open r.
> r. osteotomy
> pain r.
> Pare elbow dislocation r.
> Parvin closed posterior elbow dislocation r.
> percutaneous r.
> perioperative r.
> Pratt open radius r.
> prone r.
> radial fracture r.
> Ridlon hip r.
> r. ring
> Scaglietti congenital dislocation of hip open r.
> shoulder r.
> side posture r.
> spondylolisthesis r.
> stable r.
> sternoclavicular joint r.
> Stimson r.
> surgical r.
> swan-neck finger deformity r.
> r. syndactylia
> r. technique
> tibiofibular joint r.
> trial r.
> Wayne County General Hospital r.
> Wayne County intertrochanteric fracture r.

Redutemp

red-white meniscal zone

Reebok
> R. shoe
> R. Slide System
> R. Step System

Reece
> R. orthopaedic shoe
> R. osteotomy guide

Reed cast belt

reeducation
> muscular r.

reefing
> capsular r.
> r. procedure

reel foot

reeling gait

Reese
> R. dermatome
> R. osteotomy guide system

reevaluate

reexploration

reference
    biomechanical frame of r.
    r. electrode
    frame of r.
referencing
    sway r.
referred
    r. anatomic phenomenon
    r. neuritic pain
    r. point
    r. trigger point pain
    r. trigger point phenomenon
refill
    capillary r.
reflection
    Campbell triceps r.
    R. ceramic acetabular system
    R. Interfit prosthesis
    R. Interfit shell
    R. I prosthesis
    R. I, V, FSO acetabular cup
    R. liner
    medical subcutaneous r.
    vertebral neural r.
    R. V prosthesis
Re-Flex
    R.-F. VSP artificial foot
    R.-F. VSP prosthesis
reflex
    absent r.
    r. action
    adductor r.
    anal r.
    ankle jerk r.
    antagonistic r.
    R. anterior cervical plate system
    aponeurotic r.
    r. arc
    arthrokinetic r.
    asymmetric incurvatum r.
    asymmetric tonic neck r. (ATNR)
    attitudinal reflexes
    automatic neonatal walking r.
    axon r.
    Babinski r.
    Bekhterev deep r.
    Bekhterev-Mendel r.
    Benedek r.
    biceps r.
    blink r.
    body righting r.
    brachioradialis r.
    Brain r.
    Brudzinski r.
    bulbocavernosus r.
    Chaddock r.
    R. Comfort insole
    cremasteric r.
    crossed adductor r.

crossed extensor r.
crossed flexor r.
cry r.
cutaneous axon r.
deep tendon r. (DTR)
delayed r.
deltoid r.
depressed r.
derotational r.
r. development
digital r.
dorsal r.
elbow r.
equilibrium r.
r. examination
R. exercise and rehabilitation
  equipment
extensor thrust r.
external hamstring r.
external oblique r.
femoral r.
finger-thumb r.
flexor withdrawal r.
r. function
gluteal r.
Gordon r.
grasp r.
great toe r.
R. Gun
H r.
r. hammer
hamstring r.
heel-tap r.
Hirschberg r.
Hoffmann r.
hyperactive r.
hypoactive deep tendon r.
hypothenar r.
r. immunologic competence
incurvatum r.
interscapular r.
inverted radial r.
jaw opening r. (JOR)
knee flexion r.
knee jerk r.
lengthening r.
lumbar r.
Mayer r.
Mendel-Bekhterev r.
motor r.
muscle stretch r.
muscular r.
r. muscular contraction
myotatic r.
neck r.
neck-righting r.
r. neurovascular dystrophy
Oppenheim r.
palmar grasp r.

reflex (*continued*)
    parachute r.
    paradoxical ankle r.
    paradoxical extensor r.
    paradoxical flexor r.
    paradoxical patellar r.
    paradoxical triceps r.
    patellar r.
    patelloadductor r.
    pathologic r.
    pectoral r.
    placement r.
    placing r.
    plantar r.
    plantarflexor r.
    plantar grasp r.
    positive supporting r.
    postcast compression r.
    postural r.
    primitive r.
    pronator r.
    quadriceps r.
    radial r.
    r. rebound component of whiplash
    Remak r.
    righting r.
    Romberg r.
    scapular r.
    scapulohumeral r.
    slow stretch r.
    sole r.
    sole-tap r.
    somatoautonomic r.
    somatosomatic r.
    Stookey r.
    stretch r.
    sudomotor startle r.
    supinator jerk r.
    suprapatellar r.
    r. sympathetic dystrophy (RSD)
    r. sympathetic dystrophy syndrome
      (RSDS)
    tarsophalangeal r.
    tendon r.
    r. therapy
    r. threshold
    tibioadductor r.
    tilting r.
    toe r.
    tonic neck r.
    r. tracheostomy management
    triceps surae r.
    ulnar r.
    vertebra prominens r.
    vertical suspension r.
    vestibulospinal r.
    viscerosomatic r.
    von Bekhterev r.
    wrist flexion r.

ReFlexion first MPJ implant system
reflexogenic, reflexogenous
reflexogenous (*var. of* reflexogenic)
reflexology
refractory
    r. neuroma
    r. period
refracture
Refsum
    R. disease
    R. syndrome
refusion
Regal Acrylic/Stretch prosthetic
  sock
Regenafil allograft paste
regenerated fibroblast
regeneration
    r. flexion exercise
    r. motor unit potential
    r. of nerve
    osteoblastic bone r.
    tibial bone defect r.
    r. torus
regimen
    postoperative r.
region
    axillary r.
    basilar r.
    calcaneal r.
    cervical r.
    deltoid r.
    diaphysial r.
    elbow r.
    femoral r.
    gluteal r.
    H r.
    hookian r.
    hypochondriac r.
    iliac r.
    infraclavicular r.
    infrascapular r.
    infraspinous r.
    ischiorectal r.
    lumbar r.
    metazonal r.
    nuchal r.
    occipital r.
    olecranon r.
    patellar r.
    physial r.
    popliteal r.
    posterior longitudinal
      fiber r.
    posterior oblique fiber r.
    posteromedial r.
    pulvinar r.
    radial antebrachial r.
    sinus tarsi r.
    superomedial r.

true acetabular r.
ulnar antebrachial r.
volar antebrachial r.

regional
r. anesthesia
r. block
r. migratory osteoporosis

registration
sensory r.

registry
Joint Theater Trauma R. (JTTR)
National Football Head and Neck Injury R.

Regitine

Regnaud rigidus classification (I-III)

Regnauld
R. enclavement procedure
R. free phalangeal base autograft for hallux limitus
R. free phalangeal bone autograft
R. great toe degeneration
R. hallux osteotomy
R. hallux procedure
R. hallux rigidus classification
R. modification of Keller arthroplasty

0.01% Regranex Gel

regular
r. stem
R. Strength Bayer Enteric 500 Aspirin

rehab
rehabilitation
2 + 2 Rehab Collar
Rehab TROM brace

rehabilitation (rehab)
acute phase r.
aquatic r.
r. assessment
r. care
community r.
r. counseling (RC)
cryotherapy r.
day treatment r.
electrical stimulation r.
R. Engineering and Assistive Technology Society of North America (RESNA)
r. flexibility exercise
free weight r.
functional phase r.
r. goal
home r.
R. Impairment Category (RIC)
r. intervention
multidisciplinary r.
r. muscle strengthening
muscular r.
Ortho DX stimulator for knee r.

orthopaedic r.
outpatient r.
physical medicine and r. (PM&R, PMR)
r. planning
postcompetition r.
progressive lumbar extension r.
proprioceptive r.
PULSES Profile for Comprehensive R.
range of motion r.
recovery phase r.
remote locomotor r.
Safety Assessment of Function and the Environment for R. (SAFER)
Stage model of industrial r.
subacute r.
Synergy joint r.
r. therapeutic program
r. treatment
vocational r.

rehabilitator
Ankle Isolator ankle r.

Reichenheim elbow surgical stabilization technique

Reichert-Mundinger stereotactic device

Reimers
R. hip instability index
R. hip position migration index

reimplantation

Reiner
R. bone rongeur
R. plaster knife

Reinert acetabular extensile approach

reinforcement
acetabular r.
Bragard r.
r. ring

reinnervation

Reintegration to Normal Living index

reinterpretation
hypnotic r.

Reiter
R. disease
R. syndrome

ReJuveness scar treatment

rekindling test

Relafen

relapsing ankle sprain

relation to subadjacent segment

relative
r. refractory period
r. response attributable to maneuver (RRAM)
r. risk

Relax-A-Bac posture support

relaxant
muscle r.
skeletal muscle r.

R

relaxation
    ferromagnetic r.
    r. phenomenon
    postisometric r. (PIR)
    progressive muscle r.
    reciprocal r.
    r. response
    r. training
relaxed skin tension line
relaxer
    Real-EaSE neck and shoulder r.
relaxing incision
Re-Lax-O chiropractic table
release
    adductor tendon and lateral
      capsular r.
    Agee carpal tunnel r.
    Agee endoscopic carpal tunnel r.
    anterior hip r.
    anterior shoulder r.
    anterior transoral atlantoaxial r.
    anterolateral r.
    Baxter nerve r.
    Beaty recurrent patellar dislocation
      lateral r.
    bipolar r.
    brevis r.
    Brown 2-portal carpal tunnel r.
    capsular r.
    carpal tunnel r. (CTR)
    Chow endoscopic carpal tunnel r.
    circumferential r.
    clubfoot r.
    complete subtalar r. (CSR)
    direct-vision carpal tunnel r.
    distal intrinsic r.
    distal soft tissue r. (DSTR)
    Dupuytren contracture r.
    Eberle contracture r.
    endoscopic carpal tunnel r.
      (ECTR)
    Endotrac endoscopic carpal
      tunnel r.
    extensor hood r.
    fascial r.
    Ferkel bipolar muscular
      torticollis r.
    flexor hallucis longus tendon r.
    flexor plate r.
    flexor-pronator origin r.
    Guyon tunnel r.
    hamstring r.
    Heyman-Herndon r.
    Heyman-Herndon-Strong capsular r.
    immediate r.
    Inglis-Cooper r.
    interleukin-1 beta r.
    John Barnes myofascial r.
    joint r.
    key r.
    Kinetix instrument for carpal
      tunnel r.
    lateral capsular r.
    lateral extensor r.
    lateral retinaculum r.
    leg compartment r.
    ligamentous r.
    Little r.
    McKay-Simons complete
      subtalar r.
    medial r.
    Mital elbow r.
    modified 2-portal endoscopic carpal
      tunnel r.
    myofascial r.
    Nirschl tennis elbow r.
    Ober hip physical therapy r.
    r. of fibroosseous tunnel
    r. of trigger finger
    open carpal tunnel r. (OCTR)
    patellar retinacula r.
    r. phenomenon
    plantar capsular r.
    plantar fascial r.
    plantar-lateral r.
    plantar-medial r.
    plantar plate r.
    posterior r.
    posterolateral r.
    posteromedial r. (PMR)
    pronator teres r.
    proximal intrinsic r.
    proximal nerve r.
    radical flexor r.
    retinacular r.
    retrogeniculate hamstring r.
    Sengupta proximal quadriceps
      femoris r.
    Siegel hip r.
    Snow-Littler cleft hand r.
    soft tissue r.
    spinal fascial r.
    sustained r. (SR)
    tarsal tunnel r. (TTR)
    tendon r.
    tennis elbow r.
    triceps surae r.
    trigger finger r.
    trigger thumb r.
    Turco clubfoot r.
    Turco clubfoot posteromedial r.
    Ueba r.
    ulnar nerve r.
    unipolar r.
    Z-plasty r.
released ulnar intrinsic muscle
Reliance CM femoral implant
    component

relief
    Deep R.
    Extra Strength Deep R.
    Solarcaine Aloe Extra Burn R.
    Tylenol Extended R.
reliever
    Arthritis Foundation Pain R.
    Cama Arthritis Pain R.
relieving incision
relocation test
Relton-Hall frame
Remak
    R. paralysis
    R. reflex
remedial exercise
remediation
    biokinetic r.
Remeron
remifentanil
remobilization
remodeling
    bone r.
    cortical bone r.
    cranial vault r.
    haversian bone r.
    r. phase
    simultaneous r.
remolding
    cranial r.
remote
    r. locomotor rehabilitation
    r. pedicle flap
removable cast
removal
    Cameron femoral component r.
    cast r.
    cement r.
    Collis-Dubrul femoral stem r.
    femoral component r.
    femoral stem r.
    Harris femoral component r.
    implant r.
    Moreland-Marder-Anspach femoral
      stem r.
    nail fold r.
    nail plate r.
    r. of excess cement
    stem r.
    Winograd nail plate r.
remover
    Biomet Ultra-Drive cement r.
    Craig pin r.
    Wart stick plantar wart r.
Remular-S
renal
    r. osteodystrophy
    r. tubular osteomalacia
Renaut body
Renee knee creak sign

Renolux convertible car seat
reoperation
REP
    resistive exercise products
    REP Bands exercise band
repair
    Achilles tendon r. (ATR)
    ACL r.
    acromioclavicular joint r.
    all-inside r.
    arthroscopic Bankart r.
    Atasoy-type flap for nail injury r.
    augmented r.
    Bankart dislocated shoulder
      capsular r.
    Becker tendon r.
    biceps tendon rupture r.
    bioabsorbable tack r.
    bioelectrical r.
    bone graft r.
    Bosworth tendo calcaneus r.
    Boyd-Anderson biceps tendon r.
    brachial plexus r.
    Broström lateral ankle ligament r.
    Bunnell tendon r.
    capsule r.
    capsulolabral r.
    Caspari transglenoid r.
    delayed primary r.
    dog-ear r.
    Drummond scoliosis r.
    dural r.
    DuVries hammertoe r.
    dynamic r.
    end-to-end tendon r.
    end-to-side r.
    epineural r.
    extensor tendon r.
    fascicular r.
    femoral fracture Ogden construct r.
    first toe Jones r.
    fixed hammertoe deformity r.
    flexor tendon r.
    fracture r.
    Froimson-Oh upper limb tendon
      interposition r.
    Genzyme Tissue R.
    glenohumeral dislocation r.
    group fascicular r.
    hammertoe r.
    inferior tibiofibular r.
    5-in-1 knee ligament r.
    inside-out meniscal r.
    Jones first toe r.
    Kessler modified Achilles tendon r.
    Kleinert flexor tendon r.
    Kocher-Langenbeck posterior
      approach for acetabular fracture r.
    Krackow Achilles tendon r.

R

repair (*continued*)

Lange tendon lengthening and r.
ligamentous and capsular r.
(LCR)
Lindholm open surgical tendon r.
Lindholm tendo calcaneus r.
Lynn tendo calcaneus r.
MacIntosh over-the-top anterior
cruciate ligament r.
MacNab shoulder r.
Ma-Griffith percutaneous Achilles
tendon r.
Ma-Griffith ruptured Achilles
tendon r.
Marshall anterior cruciate
ligament r.
mattress double anchor footprint
rotator cuff tear r.
McLaughlin posterior dislocated
shoulder r.
medial r.
meniscal r.
Milch radioulnar joint r.
mini-open rotator cuff r.
Mosley anterior shoulder r.
nonaugmented r.
r. of forearm malunions with distal
radioulnar joint instability
r. of spring ligament
osteosynthesis pelvic ring injury r.
patellar tendon r.
percutaneous Achilles tendon r.
plastic r.
posterior plate osteosynthesis pelvic
ring injury r.
primary r.
pseudarthrosis r.
Revo rotator cuff r.
rod fracture r.
rotator cuff r.
Scuderi ruptured quadriceps
tendon r.
semitendinosus augmentation of
patellar tendon r.
sesamoid fracture r.
Sever-L'Episcopo shoulder r.
shoulder r.
1-sided dog-ear r.
Smith-Petersen cervical-thoracic
kyphosis r.
Speed sternoclavicular r.
Staples elbow r.
Staples ligament r.
suture anchor shoulder r.
sutureless avascular meniscal r.
tendon r.
Teuffer tendo calcaneus r.
tissue r.
total extraperitoneal r.

transacromial coracoacromial
ligament r.
transglenoid suture r.
triad knee r.
triple ligamentous r.
Tsuge tendon r.
vertical loop suture technique for
meniscus r.
volar plate r.
Watson-Jones fracture r.
Wisconsin wiring scoliosis r.

reparative

r. granuloma
r. phase

**Repeatable Battery for the Assessment
of Neuropsychological status (RBANS)**

repeated

r. quick stretch (RQS)
r. quick stretch from elongation
(RQS-E)
r. quick stretch superimposed upon
an existing contraction
(RQS-SEC)

reperfusion injury

repetition

r. maximum (RM)
r. strain injury (RSI)
r. time (TR)

1-repetition maximum (1-RM)

repetitive

r. discharge
r. exercise
r. loading
r. microtrauma
r. nerve stimulation
r. nerve stimulator (RNS)
r. osseous impingement
r. strain disorder
r. stress disorder
r. stress injury
r. stress syndrome (RSS)
r. trauma
r. trauma disorder (RTD)

Repicci II knee replacement

Repiphysis prosthesis

replacement

allograft ligament r.
alumina bioceramic joint r.
Amstutz total hip r.
anatomic porous r. (APR)
Ascension MCP total joint r.
Ascension PIP total joint r.
Averill total hip r.
bicompartmental r.
Bigliani/Flatow complete shoulder r.
r. bone
calcar r.
Capello total hip r.
cementless total hip r.

Charnley total hip r.
dynamic double tendon r.
elbow r.
electrolyte r.
Engh total hip r.
ESKA Implant artificial joint r.
Ewald total elbow r.
facet r.
failed joint r.
hip r.
Howse total hip r.
hybrid total hip r.
hypnotic r.
intercalary segmental r.
Kirschner Medical Dimension hip r.
Leeds-Keio Dacron mesh r.
ligament r.
Marmor r.
PCA total hip r.
Pilliar total hip r.
Pinnacle hip r.
porous-coated anatomic total hip r.
primary hip r.
Prodisc-C total disc r.
Prodisc lumbar total disc r.
prosthetic r.
prosthetic joint r.
Repicci II knee r.
revision hip r.
Ring UPM total hip r.
Ring UPM total knee r.
SAF hip r.
Scandinavian total ankle r. (STAR)
Scarborough total hip r.
self-articulating femoral hip r.
self-bearing ceramic total hip r.
Stanmore knee r.
Stanmore total hip r.
surface r.
tharies hip r.
tile plate facet r.
r. tissue
total ankle r. (TAR)
total cervical disc r. (TCDR)
total hip r. (THR)
total joint r. (TJR)
total knee r. (TKR)
tricompartmental r.
TR-28 total hip r.
unicompartmental knee r.
universal head r. (UHR)
Vanguard Uni unicompartmental
   knee r.
vertebral body r. (VBR)
replantable amputation
replantation
autogenous meniscal cartilage r.
r. bandage
limb r.

r. of amputated digit
r. of finger
RepliCare wound dressing
Replica total hip replacement system
repolarization
report
Juvenile Arthritis Functional
   Assessment R. (JAFAR)
repositioner
Wilson Cook prosthesis r.
repositioning
muscle r.
reproducibility
reproducible
Repro head halter
requirement
therapeutic r.
rerouted tendon
rerouting
Blair-Omer flexor pollicis longus r.
r. insertion
Zancolli biceps tendon r.
Rescudose
Roxanol R.
research
Alvarado Orthopaedic R.
Foundation for Chiropractic
   Education and R. (FCER)
National Center for Dissemination
   of Disability R.
Policy and Review Committee for
   Human R.
The Institute for Rehabilitation R.
   (TIRR)
resect
resectable
resecting fracture
resection
anterior tarsal r.
r. area
r. arthrodesis
r. arthroplasty
Badgley iliac wing r.
bar r.
bone r.
bony bridge r.
calcaneal r.
calcaneonavicular bar r.
Carrell distal fibula r.
caudal lamina r.
Clayton procedure with
   panmetatarsal head r.
cuff r.
Darrach distal ulna r.
r. dermodesis
Dillwyn-Evans relapsed club foot r.
distal femoral r.
DuVries metatarsal head r.
en bloc r.

resection (*continued*)
    epiphysial bar r.
    extraarticular r.
    femoral r.
    fibular head r.
    first rib r.
    Girdlestone hip r.
    Guller sigmoid r.
    Gurd distal clavicle r.
    Henry femoral neck r.
    Hoffmann panmetatarsal head r.
    iliac wing r.
    Ingram bony bridge r.
    innominate bone r.
    intercalary r.
    intralesional r.
    Kashiwagi ulnohumeral r.
    Kotz modular femur and tibia r.
      (KMFTR)
    kyphos r.
    Langenskiöld bony bridge r.
    Lewis intercalary r.
    local radical r.
    Malawer fibula tumor r. (type I, II)
    Mankin knee r.
    marginal r.
    Mayo metatarsal head r.
    medial eminence r.
    medial malleolus r.
    metaphysial head r.
    metatarsal head r.
    Mumford distal clavicle r.
    r. of distal femur
    r. of meniscus
    panmetatarsal head r.
    Phelps partial r.
    posterior vertebral column r.
      (PVCR)
    prophylactic r.
    proximal femoral r.
    radical r.
    ray r.
    Rockwood sternoclavicular joint r.
    Thompson r.
    Tikhoff-Linberg shoulder girdle r.
    transoral odontoid r.
    tumor r.
    vertebral body stapling wedge r.
    vertebral column r.
    wafer distal ulna r.
    Weaver-Dunn distal clavicle r.
    wedge r.
    wedge matrix r. (WMR)
resection-arthrodesis
resection-realignment
resector
    Accu-Line femoral r.
    Accu-Line tibial r.
    r. blade

femoral r.
full-radius r.
orthotome r.
synovial r.
tibial r.
residence ridge
residua (*pl. of* residuum)
residual
    r. cement
    r. disc tissue
    r. heel equinus
    r. hindfoot equinus
    r. latency
    r. limb
    r. tension
residuum, *pl.* **residua**
resilience
resin
    Delrin acetal r.
    melamine r.
    methacrylate r.
    polyacetal r.
Resist-A-Band exercise band
resistance
    growth hormone r.
    intralesional vascular r.
    isometric r.
    isotonic r.
    manual r.
    plyometric r.
    strength against r.
    R. Support Formula
    Thera-Band system of progressive r.
    r. training
resistant clubfoot
Resist-A-Tube exercise band
resisted
    r. active flexion
    r. dorsiflexion
    r. external rotation
    r. straight leg raise
    r. straight leg raise test
resistive
    r. chair exercise kit
    r. exercise
    r. exercise products (REP)
    r. exerciser
    r. exercise table
    r. movement
    r. tennis elbow test
    r. weighed column
RESNA
    Rehabilitation Engineering and
    Assistive Technology Society of
    North America
resonance
    field focusing nuclear magnetic r.
      (FONAR)
    hydatid r.

nuclear magnetic r. (NMR)
osteal r.
resonator
Jacobson r.
resorbable
r. ceramic
r. cervical mesh plate
r. graft containment system
r. plate
r. polydioxanon pin
r. polymer pin
r. polymer screw
r. scaffold
resorption
bone r.
bony r.
osteoclastic r.
periprosthetic bone r.
tuftal r.
resource
Assessment of Living Skills and
R.'s (ALSAR)
respiratory exchange ratio
Respond II muscle stimulator
response
acute inflammatory r.
average evoked r.
axon r.
biochemical r.
blink r.
brainstem auditory evoked r.
(BAER)
cellular level r.
decremental r.
delayed r.
evoked r.
foreign body r.
F-wave r.
galvanic skin r.
horizontal suspension r.
hunting r.
hyperactive r.
incremental r.
r. interval
late r.
motion r.
motor r.
muscle reflex r.
nociceptive r.
paired r.
physiologic r.
pilomotor r.
plantar Babinski r.
red r.
R. rehabilitation and fitness
equipment
relaxation r.
sensory r.
spinal neuropeptide r.

tissue-level r.
traction r.
vertical suspension r.
visual evoked r.
responsive neurostimulator
rest
bed r.
Chiroflow back r.
Core Hibak R.
Core Lobak R.
Core Sitback R.
foot r.
hand r.
rest, ice, compression, elevation
(RICE)
kidney r.
Mayfield head r.
r. pain
pain at r.
Restcue bed
resting
r. calcaneal stance position (RCSP)
r. foot sling
r. forefoot supination angle
r. heart rate (RHR)
r. length
r. membrane potential
r. orthosis
r. pan splint
r. shear stiffness
r. tremor
r. zone
restless leg
restlessness
motor r.
Reston
R. dressing
R. padding
restoration
R. acetabular system
functional r.
R. GAP acetabular cup
intrinsic r.
R. modular revision hip system
pinch r.
R. Secur-Fit X'tra acetabular shell
Restoration-HA hip system
restorative pin
restore
R. ACL guide system
R. AF
R. AF antifungal lotion
R. AF antimicrobial skin cleanser
R. AF antimicrobial solution
R. CalciCare dressing
R. Clean 'N Moist
R. cuff tear implant
R. orthobiologic soft-tissue implant
Restoril

restraint
    active r.
    passive r.
    poncho r.
    universal canvas body r.
restricted
    r. inversion
    r. range of motion
restriction
    extension r.
    flexion r.
    intercostal r.
    lateral flexion r.
    r. of motion
    range of motion r.
    rotational r.
    skin r.
    soft tissue r.
    talocrural r.
restrictive bandage
restrictor
    BioStop G bone cement r.
    cement r.
    femoral canal r.
    plastic marrow canal r.
result
    false-negative r.
resurfacing
    Achilles tendon r.
    Amstutz r.
    bone r.
    r. operation
    Paltrinieri-Trentani r.
    patellar r.
    r. procedure
    Salzer joint r.
resurrection bone
retainer
    Thermoskin heat r.
retaining knee prosthesis
retardation
    deafness, onychoosteodystrophy,
      mental r. (DOOR)
    growth r.
    healing r.
    Matson Evaluation of Social Skills
      in Individuals with Severe R.
      (MESSIER)
retention
    r. drill
    r. suture
reticula (*pl. of* reticulum)
reticular, reticulated
    r. bone bruise
    r. cell sarcoma
reticularis
    livedo r.
reticulated (*var. of* reticular)
    r. polyurethane pad

reticulin stain
reticulocytosis
    cerebroside r.
reticuloendothelial system
reticuloendotheliosis
reticulohistiocytosis
    multicentric r.
reticulum, *pl.* **reticula,** *gen.* **retinaculi**
    endoplasmic r. (ER)
    sarcoplasmic r. (SR)
retinacula (*pl. of* retinaculum)
retinacular
    r. artery
    r. hood
    r. ligament
    r. release
retinaculi (*gen. of* retinaculum)
retinaculum, *pl.* **retinacula**
    caudal r.
    extensor r.
    flexor r.
    hypertrophic flexor r.
    inferior extensor r.
    inferior peroneal r.
    patellar r.
    peroneal r.
    superior extensor r.
    superior peroneal r. (SPR)
    r. tendinum
    Weitbrecht r.
retraction
retractor
    Adson cerebellar r.
    Adson hemilaminectomy r.
    Allport r.
    Alm wound r.
    amputation r.
    APC hip r.
    appendiceal r.
    Army-Navy r.
    Aufranc cobra r.
    Badgley laminectomy r.
    Balfour self-retaining r.
    Ballantine hemilaminectomy r.
    Bankart r.
    Beckman r.
    Bennett bone r.
    Bennett tibial r.
    Bertin hip r.
    beveled tubular r.
    blade-point r.
    blade-spike r.
    Blount anvil r.
    Blount knee r.
    Bodnar r.
    Boyle-Davis r.
    Busenkell posterior hip r.
    Campbell nerve root r.
    Carroll-Bennett r.

Carroll hand r.
Caspar r.
cerebellar r.
Chandler knee r.
Charnley horizontal r.
Charnley initial incision r.
Charnley knee r.
Charnley pin r.
Charnley self-retaining r.
Cherry laminectomy r.
Cloward blade r.
cobra r.
Collis r.
Collis-Taylor r.
Cooley rib r.
crank frame r.
Crego r.
curved r.
Cushing r.
Darrach r.
Deaver r.
deep r.
D'Errico r.
digital self-retaining r.
Doane knee r.
double bent Hohmann acetabular r.
double-ended right-angle r.
double-hook Lovejoy r.
Downey hemilaminectomy r.
Dozier radiolucent Bennett r.
dual nerve root suction r.
East-West r.
Elite Farley r.
extra-depth posterior acetabular r.
extra-large hip r.
Fahey r.
fat pad r.
Finochietto rib r.
flat r.
FlexPosure endoscopic r.
Fukuda humeral head r.
Gelpi r.
Gifford mastoid r.
handheld r.
Hays hand r.
heavy-duty 2-tooth r.
Heiss soft tissue r.
Hendren self-retaining r.
Henning meniscal r.
Hibbs r.
Hoen r.
Hohmann bone r.
Holscher knee r.
Holscher root r.
Holzheimer r.
humeral head r.
inferoposterior acetabular capsule r.
Inge r.
Israel r.

R

Kasdan r.
Kirschenbaum r.
Kleinert-Ragnell r.
knee r.
Kocher r.
Lange bone r.
Lange-Hohmann bone r.
Langenbeck r.
large Cobra r.
Love nerve root r.
lower hand r.
Lowman hand r.
Luongo hand r.
Markham-Meyerding r.
Mark II Chandler total knee r.
Mark II concave total knee r.
Mark II lateral collateral ligament r.
Mark II modular weight r.
Mark II S total knee r.
Mark II Stubbs short prong
  collateral ligament r.
Mark II wide PCL knee r.
Mark II Z knee r.
Mayo-Collins r.
McCullough r.
McIvor ENT r.
meniscus r.
METRx X-Tube r.
Meyerding r.
mini-Hohmann podiatric r.
modified Fukuda-type r.
Morris r.
Mueller r.
Myers knee r.
narrow-blade r.
narrow cobra r.
narrow double-prong acetabular r.
narrow inferior acetabular r.
narrow-neck mini-Hohmann r.
Nelson rib r.
Ollier rake r.
orthopaedic r.
Ozer r.
Paulson knee r.
Percy amputation r.
pin r.
2-prong rake r.
3-prong rake blade r.
5-prong rake blade r.
Ragnell r.
rake r.
rib r.
ribbon r.
Richardson r.
ring r.
Rosenberg r.
Rowe humeral head r.
Sauerbruch r.
Scholten sternal r.

retractor (*continued*)
Scoville r.
Seeburger r.
self-retaining r.
Senn r.
sharp r.
Sherwin knee r.
Sims r.
single-prong broad
  acetabular r.
skid humeral head r.
Smillie knee r.
Smillie meniscus
  hook r.
Sofamor tubular r.
Sofield r.
soft tissue blade r.
Southwick 2-tined r.
standard 2-inch blade r.
standard 4-inch blade r.
stiff ribbon r.
tang r.
Taylor r.
thin glenoid r.
tibial r.
tubular r.
Tupper hand-holder and r.
upper hand r.
U-shaped r.
Verbrugge-Hohmann bone r.
Volkmann rake r.
Wagner r.
Watanabe r.
Weitlaner r.
Weitlaner self-retaining r.
Wichman r.
Williams self-retaining r.
Wilson gonad r.
Wink r.
Yasargil Leyla r.
Z r.
retractor-narrow
bent Hohman r.-n.
retractor-wide
bent Hohman r.-w.
retraining
vastus medialis obliquus r.
VMO r.
retrieved insert
retriever
Carroll tendon r.
Hewson suture r.
Kleinert-Kutz tendon r.
magnetic r.
retroacetabular lesion
retro-Achilles bursa
retrocalcaneal
r. bursa
r. bursitis

r. disorder
r. exostosis
r. spur
retrocalcaneobursitis
retrodisplaced fracture
retroflection (*var. of* retroflexion)
retroflexion, retroflection
tibial r.
retrogeniculate hamstring release
retrograde
r. AXT
r. Beaver blade
r. degeneration
r. drilling
r. intramedullary nail
r. meniscal blade
r. method
r. nailing
retrograde-cutting hook-shaped knife
retrolisthesed fragment
retrolisthesis positional dyskinesia
**retromedullary arteriovenous
  malformation**
retropatellar
r. fat pad
r. fat pad contracture
retroperitoneal
r. approach
r. decompression
r. fibrosis
r. hemorrhage
r. space
retropharyngeal
r. abscess
r. approach
r. fascial cleft
r. space
retropulsed
r. bone excision
r. bony fragment
retropulsion of gait
retroreflective marker
retrosacral fascia
RetroScrew
Arthrex R.
retrospondylolisthesis
retrosternal
r. abscess
r. dislocation
retrotorsion
femoral r.
tibial r.
retrovascular cord
retroversion
angle of r.
femoral r.
r. of acetabular cup
sacrum r.
tibial r.

Rett syndrome
return
    r. of sensation
    r. to play (RTP)
    r. to play consideration
return-to-play
    r.-t.-p. injury assessment
    r.-t.-p. musculoskeletal assessment
    r.-t.-p. sidelines decision making
reulceration
ReUnion fracture system
ReUnite
    R. hand fixation
    R. orthopaedic pin
    R. orthopaedic screw
    R. resorbable orthopaedic fixation
      system
revascularization
    endosteal r.
    r. of graft
revascularized tissue
Revelation hip system
Reverdin
    R. bunionectomy
    R. epidermal free graft
    R. osteotomy
    R. prosthesis
Reverdin-Green
    R.-G. bunionectomy
    R.-G. foot procedure
    R.-G. osteotomy
Reverdin-Green-Laird procedure
Reverdin-Laird
    R.-L. bunionectomy
    R.-L. osteotomy
Reverdin-McBride bunionectomy
Revere pedicle screw
reversal
    isotonic r. (IR)
    r. of antagonist (ROA)
    r. of cervical lordosis
    r. of fore-aft shear phase of
      gait
    stabilizing r.
reverse
    r. Austin osteotomy
    r. Bankart lesion
    r. Barton fracture
    r. Bigelow maneuver
    r. buckling
    r. closing base wedge osteotomy
    r. Colles fracture
    r. cross-finger flap
    r. cutting needle
    r. Dillwyn-Evans calcaneal
      osteotomy
    r. forearm island flap
    r. Hill-Sachs defect
    r. Hill-Sachs lesion

    r. Hill-Sachs sign
    r. Jones procedure
    r. knuckle-bender splint
    r. Lachman test
    r. Lasègue test
    r. last shoe
    r. lunge back exercise technique
    r. Mauck knee operation
    r. Mauck knee procedure
    r. Monteggia fracture
    r. NAG
    r. obliquity
    r. obliquity fracture
    r. Phalen test
    r. pivot shift
    r. pivot-shift knee test
    r. Putti-Platt procedure
    r. tennis elbow
    r. Thomas heel
    r. Trendelenburg position
    r. undercutting lengthening
    r. wedge technique
    r. windlass
    r. wrist curl
reverse-cutting meniscal probe
reversed shoulder prosthesis
reverse-flow flap
reverse-threaded screw
reversible ischemic neurologic disability
  (RIND)
revised
    Symptoms Checklist 90 R.
      (SCL-90R)
    Vineland Adaptive Behavior Scales,
      R. (VABS)
revision
    r. arthroplasty
    exploration and r.
    hip r.
    r. hip arthroplasty
    r. hip replacement
    R. hip stem
    jumbo uncemented cup acetabular
      component r.
    Mallory-Head total hip r.
    R. nail
    r. of shoulder arthroplasty
    r. of total hip
    r. procedure
    stump r.
    total hip r.
    r. total hip operation
Revo
    R. knot
    R. loop handle knot pusher
    R. retrievable cancellous screw
    R. rotator cuff repair
    R. rotator cuff repair system
    R. suture anchor

Rezaian
R. external fixation apparatus
R. external fixation device
R. interbody device
R. spinal fixation
R. spinal fixator
RGO
reciprocating gait orthosis
rhabdomyolysis
exertional r.
rhabdomyoma
rhabdomyosarcoma, rhabdosarcoma
alveolar r.
embryonal r.
pleomorphic r.
rhabdosarcoma (*var. of*
rhabdomyosarcoma)
R-Hab lighter weight ankle
rhachotomy
Capener lateral r.
decompression r.
lateral r.
rhaphe (*var. of* raphe)
RHD
radial head dislocation
rHead
r. implant system
r. Recon implant
rheobase
rheostosis
rheumatic
r. fever
r. granuloma
r. scoliosis
rheumatica
polymyalgia r. (PMR)
rheumatism
articular r.
Besnier r.
chronic r.
Heberden r.
lumbar r.
Macleod r.
Macleod capsular r.
nodose r.
palindromic r.
Poncet r.
tuberculous r.
World Health
Organization/International League
Against R. (WHO/ILAR)
rheumatismal edema
rheumatoid
r. arthritis (RA)
r. arthritis factor (RAF)
r. arthritis myopathy
r. arthritis synovitis
r. cyst
r. deformity

r. disease
r. disorder
r. foot
r. myositis
r. nodule
r. spondylitis
r. vasculitis
rheumatologic disorder
rheumatologist
rheumatology
American College of R. (ACR)
Rapid Assessment of Disease
Activity in R.
Rheumatrex
Rhinelander pin
Rhino Triangle polypropylene hip
abduction brace
rhizomelia
rhizomelic spondylosis
rhizomelic-type chondrodysplasia
rhizomesomelic bone dysplasia
rhizotomy
intradural dorsal spinal root r.
posterior r.
selective posterior r. (SPR)
RHOCS
right-handed orthogonal coordinate
system
rhomboid, rhomboidal
r. flap
r. ligament
Michaelis r.
r. muscle
rhomboidal (*var. of* rhomboid)
rhonchi (*pl. of* rhonchus)
rhonchus, *pl.* **rhonchi**
rales and rhonchi
sibilant r.
sonorous rhonchi
Rhoton
R. elevator
R. enucleator
R. needle holder
R. osteotome
RHR
resting heart rate
RHS
radial head subluxation
rHuEPO
recombinant human erythropoietin
Rhus toxicodendron
rhythm
scapulohumeral r.
rhythmic, rhythmical
r. auditory stimulation (RAS)
r. handgrip work
r. initiation
r. initiation technique
r. stabilization

rhythmical (*var. of* rhythmic)
rib
    r. approximator
    bed of r.
    r. belt
    r. belt orthosis
    bicipital r.
    bucket-handle r.
    r. cage
    cervical r.
    r. contractor
    r. contusion
    costochondral junction
      of r.'s
    r. cutter
    r. drill
    r. dysplasia
    r. elevator
    false r.
    r. fixation
    floating r.
    r. forceps
    r. fracture
    r. graft
    r. hump
    hypoplastic first r.
    interarticular ligament of head of r.
    r. motion
    radiate ligament of head of r.
    r. rasp
    r. retractor
    r. ribbon
    rudimentary r.
    slipping r.
    spurious r.
    sternal r.
    Stiller r.
    r. tethering
    true r.
    vertebral r.
    vertebrocostal r.
    vertebrosternal r.
    vertical expandable prosthetic
      titanium r. (VEPTR)
ribbed
    r. hook
    r. needle
ribbed-sole shoe
Ribbing disease
Ribble bandage
ribbon
    r. retractor
    rib r.
    r. sign
rib-hump scoliosis index
rib-vertebral angle
RIC
    Rehabilitation Impairment
    Category

Rica
    R. bone drill
    R. wire guidepin
Ricard amputation
RICE
    rest, ice, compression,
      elevation
rice
    r. body
    joint r.
    R. Krispies crepitation
rich
    Rolaids Calcium R.
Richards
    R. angle guide
    R. arthrodesis
    R. bone clamp
    R. classic compression hip screw
    R. Colles external fixator
    R. drill guide
    R. fixation staple
    R. fixator system
    R. hip endoprosthesis system
    R. hip prosthesis
    R. hydroxyapatite PORP
    R. lag screw
    R. lag screw device
    R. locking rod
    R. Lovejoy bone drill
    R. mallet
    R. maximum contact (RMC)
    R. maximum contact cruciate-sparing
      prosthesis
    R. modular hip system
    R. modular stem
    R. pistol-grip drill
    R. reamer
    R. reconstruction nail
    R. sideplate
    R. Solcotrans orthopaedic
      drainage-reinfusion system
    R. Spectron metal-backed acetabular
      prosthesis
    R. Zirconia femoral head
      prosthesis
Richards-Hirschhorn plate
Richard Smith prosthesis
Richardson
    R. retractor
    R. rod
    R. subtalar arthrodesis
Riche-Cannieu
    R.-C. anastomosis
    R.-C. connection
Riches artery forceps
Richet
    R. bandage
    R. tibial-astragalocalcaneal canal
Richie brace

R

Richmond
    R. bolt
    R. subarachnoid screw
    R. subarachnoid screw sensor
    R. subarachnoid twist drill
Richter
    R. bone drill
    R. bone screwdriver
rickets
    adult r.
    florid r.
    vitamin D-dependent r. (VDDR)
    vitamin D-resistant r. (VDRR)
rickshaw rehabilitation exerciser
Ridaura
Rideau hip contracture release technique
Ridenol
rider's
    r. bone
    r. bursa
    r. leg
    r. muscle
    r. sprain
    r. tendon
ridge
    dorsal r.
    epicondylar r.
    greater multangular r.
    longitudinal r.
    osteochondral r.
    Outerbridge r.
    residence r.
    talar r.
    trapezial r.
    vastus lateralis r.
Ridlon
    R. hip reduction
    R. operation
    R. plaster knife
    R. procedure
Riecken PQ premium heel cup
rifampicin (*var. of* rifampin)
rifampin, rifampicin
rig
    Leg Extension Power R.
right
    r. and left ankle indices
    r. ankle bur
    r. erector spinae musculature
    r. lateral flexion
    r. lower extremity (RLE)
    r. lower limb (RLL)
    r. posterior innominate
    r. rotation
    r. thoracic curve
    r. thoracic curve with hypokyphosis
    r. thoracic, left lumbar curve pattern
    r. thoracic, left thoracolumbar curve pattern

    r. thoracic minor curve pattern
    r. upper extremity (RUE)
    r. upper limb (RUL)
    r. ventricular cardiomyopathy
right-angle
    r.-a. dental drill
    r.-a. hook
right-hand
    r.-h. dominance
    r.-h. dominant
right-handed orthogonal coordinate system (RHOCS)
righting
    r. reflex
    trunk r.
right/left
    r./l. discrimination
    r./l. timing
right-sided
    r.-s. nail
    r.-s. submandibular transverse incision
    r.-s. thoracotomy
rigid
    r. bar
    r. below-knee cast
    r. body
    r. collar
    r. curve
    r. curve scoliosis
    r. dressing
    r. equinovarus deformity
    r. flatfoot
    r. flatfoot deformity
    r. foot
    r. foot cavus
    r. frame wheelchair
    r. gait
    r. internal fixation
    r. metal pelvic band
    r. neck hyperextension
    r. orthosis
    r. pedicle screw
    r. pes planus
    r. postoperative brace
    r. reamer
    r. rockerbottom (RRB)
    r. round back
    r. sound
rigidity
    C-D instrumentation r.
    cogwheel r.
    Cotrel pedicle screw r.
    nuchal r.
    spinal fixation r.
    torsional r.
rigidus
    hallux r.

R

Rik
R. fluid mattress
R. FootHugger fluid heel boot
Riley-Day syndrome
rim
acetabular r.
alar r.
r. enhancement thickness
glenoid r.
r. lesion
sclerotic marginal r.
r. sign
tibial r.
Rimadyl
Rincoe human action bionic ankle
RIND
reversible ischemic neurologic disability
ring
Ace-Colles half r.
arterial r.
r. block anesthesia
carbon fiber half r.
cartilaginous r.
Charnley centering r.
congenital r.
constriction r.
cricoid r.
r. curette
r. cushion
doughnut r.
drop-lock r.
epiphysial r.
r. external fixator
extracapsular arterial r.
fibroosseous r.
r. finger
r. finger–small finger syndactyly
Fischer r.
foam r.
r. forceps
r. fracture
half r.
halo r.
Ilizarov r.
invalid r.
ischial weightbearing r.
R. knee prosthesis
Lacroix osseous r.
Luque r.
Neer r.
orthosis drop-lock r.
osseous r.
pelvic r.
perichondral r.
protrusio r.
proximal-to-distal r.
reduction r.
reinforcement r.
r. retractor

r. sign
r. structure
r. sublimis opponensplasty
r. syndrome
R. total hip prosthesis
unstable pelvic r.
R. UPM press-fit prosthesis
R. UPM total hip replacement
R. UPM total knee replacement
V1 halo r.
ringer
R. arthroscopy
R. lactate
RingLoc
R. acetabular series
R. hip liner
R. instrument
ringman's shoulder
Riolan
R. bone
R. muscle
Riordan
R. clubhand classification
R. finger flexion
R. finger opponensplasty
R. pin
R. pollicization
R. sign
R. tendon transfer technique
Ripped Fuel
rise
single heel r.
r. time
Riseborough-Radin
R.-R. fracture classification system
R.-R. intercondylar fracture
classification
risedronate
riser
stress r.
Rish osteotome
risk
ergonomic r.
r. factor profile
fracture r.
heat injury r.
occupational r.
osteoporotic fracture r.
relative r.
Risser
R. bone maturation index of
scoliosis
R. category
R. classification
R. frame
R. grade
R. localizer scoliosis cast
R. method
R. pin

Risser (*continued*)
    R. sign (grade 1-4)
    R. stage
    R. technique
    R. turnbuckle cast
Risser-Ferguson technique
Ritchie
    R. brace
    R. rheumatoid arthritis index
Rivermead
    R. ADL index
    R. Behavioral Memory Test
      (RBMT)
    R. Behavioral Memory
      Test-Extended Version (RBMT-E)
    R. Mobility Index (RMI)
    R. Motor Assessment
Riverside
    University of California R. (UCR)
rivet
    r. gun
    POP r.
Rizzoli osteoclast
RKE-R
    Rabideau Kitchen Evaluation-Revised
RLE
    right lower extremity
RLL
    right lower limb
1-RM
    1-repetition maximum
RM
    repetition maximum
    RM isoelastic hip prosthesis
RMC
    Richards maximum contact
    RMC knee replacement device
    RMC prosthesis
RMI
    Rivermead Mobility Index
3R80 modular hydraulic knee joint
RMQ
    Roland-Morris Questionnaire
RNS
    repetitive nerve stimulator
R/O
    rule out
ROA
    reversal of antagonist
road burn injury
Roaf, Kirkaldy-Willis, and Cattero
  procedure
Robaxin
Robaxisal
Robert
    R. Brigham semiconstrained
      prosthesis
    R. Brigham total knee prosthesis
    R. Jones bandage

R. Jones dressing
R. Jones splint
R. ligament
R. true AP thumb view
Roberts
    R. approach
    R. fat grafting technique
Robinow syndrome
Robinson
    R. anterior cervical discectomy
    R. anterior cervical fusion
    R. arthrometer
    R. arthroplasty
    R. cervical spine fusion
    R. morcellation
    R. spinal arthrodesis
Robinson-Smith
    R.-S. anterior cervical approach
    R.-S. anterior cervical technique
    R.-S. spinal arthrodesis
Robinson-Southwick
    R.-S. cervical spine fusion technique
    R.-S. fusion
Robins-Riley spinal fusion
Robodoc robot
robot
    Robodoc r.
robotic surgery
robust rheumatoid arthritis
ROC
    receiver operating characteristic
    ROC anchor
Rocabado posture gauge
Rocaltrol
Rocephin
Rochester
    R. bone trephine device
    R. compression system
    R. harvest bone cutter
    R. hip-knee-ankle-foot orthosis
    R. lamina elevator
    R. recipient bone cutter
    R. spinal elevator
Rochester-Carmalt forceps
Rochester-Ochsner forceps
Rochester-Pean forceps
rock
    R. ankle exercise board
    pelvic r. (PR)
    R. & Roller exercise board
rocker
    r. balance square
    r. bar
    r. board
    r. boot
    Carolina r.
    r. knife
    Uniplane r.
rocker-bottom (*var. of* rockerbottom)

rockerbottom, rocker-bottom
    r. deformity
    r. flatfoot
    r. foot
    rigid r. (RRB)
    r. shoe
    r. sole
RocketSoc ankle brace
rocking
    knee-chest r.
Rockwood
    R. acromioclavicular injury
      classification (I-VI)
    R. acromioclavicular joint dislocation
      repair procedure
    R. anterior acromioplasty
    R. classification
    R. posterior capsulorrhaphy
    R. shoulder screw
    R. sternoclavicular joint resection
Rockwood-Green orthopaedic casting
  technique
rocky boat exerciser
rod
    alignment guide r.
    Alta advance tibial/humeral r.
    Alta CFX reconstruction r.
    Alta tibial-humeral r.
    aluminum master r.
    Amset R-F r.
    autoreinforced polyglycolide r.
    Bailey-Dubow r.
    r. bender
    r. bending
    Bickel intramedullary r.
    r. breakage
    centralizing r.
    r. clamp
    cold rolled r.
    compression r.
    concave r.
    r. contour preparation
    convex r.
    Cotrel-Dubousset r.
    Dacron-impregnated silicone r.
    degradable polyglycolide r.
    delta r.
    distraction r.
    r. distraction device
    double-L spinal r.
    dual square-ended Harrington r.
    Edwards D-L modular screw r.
    Edwards-Levine r.
    Edwards modular system
      Universal r.
    Ender r.
    Enneking r.
    fixateur interne r.
    flared spinal r.

    fluted medullary r.
    r. fracture repair
    guide r.
    Harrington compression r.
    Harrington distraction r.
    Harris condylocephalic r.
    hinge r.
    r. holder
    Hunter silastic r.
    impactor r.
    impingement r.
    intramedullary alignment r.
    Isola spinal implant system eye r.
    Jacobs distraction r.
    Jacobs locking hook spinal r.
    K r.
    Kaneda r.
    Knodt distraction r.
    Küntscher r. (K rod)
    L r.
    r. linkage
    locking-hook spinal r.
    long alignment r.
    L-shaped r.
    Luque r.
    Luque-Galveston r.
    r. migration
    Moe modified Harrington r.
    Moe square-end r.
    Moss r.
    Olerud PSF r.
    OrthoSorb r.
    pediatric Cotrel-Dubousset r.
    PGA r.
    r. placement
    Polarus humeral r.
    precontoured unit r.
    prolongation r.
    radiotranslucent r.
    Richards locking r.
    Richardson r.
    r. rotation prevention
    round-ended distraction r.
    Rush r.
    Russell-Taylor delta r.
    Sage r.
    Sampson r.
    Schneider r.
    screw alignment r.
    Selby I, II r.
    Serrato forearm r.
    Shaw-SHIP r.
    Sheffield r.
    silicone-dacron tendon r.
    r. sleeve
    r. sleeve fixation
    spinal fixation r.
    square-ended distraction r.
    stainless steel r. (SST)

R

rod (*continued*)
    Stenzel r.
    straight threaded r.
    surgical r.
    R. TAG suture anchor system
    telescoping medullary r.
    r. template
    tendon r.
    threaded r.
    U Luque vertebral r.
    unit spinal r.
    V-A alignment r.
    VDS compression r.
    VSF r.
    Williams r.
    Wiltse screw r.
    Wiltse system aluminum master r.
    Wiltse system spinal r.
    Wissinger r.
    Zickel r.
    Zielke r.
rod-hook construct
rod-mounted
    r.-m. targeting apparatus
    r.-m. targeting device
rod-sleeve instrumentation
Roeder manipulative aptitude test device
roentgen
    r. stereophotogrammetric analysis (RSA)
    r. stereophotogrammetry
roentgenogram
    biplane r.
    lateral r.
    operative r.
    2-plane r.
    templating r.
roentgenograph (*var. of* radiograph)
roentgenographic (*var. of* radiographic)
roentgenography
    intraoperative r.
    preoperative r.
    stress r.
roentgenometrics
roentgenotherapy (*var. of* radiotherapy)
roentgen-stereophotogrammatic study
rofecoxib
Roger
    R. Anderson compression device
    R. Anderson external fixation apparatus
    R. Anderson external fixation device
    R. Anderson external fixator
    R. Anderson fixation
    R. Anderson pin fixation appliance
    R. Anderson splint
    R. Anderson stabilization device

    R. Anderson system
    R. Anderson table
    R. Anderson traction
Rogers cervical fusion technique
Rogozinski
    R. hook
    R. screw system
    R. spinal fixation
    R. spinal fixation system
    R. spinal rod system
Rohadur
    R. gait plate
    R. orthotic
Roho
    R. bed
    R. heel pad
    R. heel protector
    R. Pack-It cushion
    R. pediatric seating system
    R. solid seat insert
ROI intersomatic implant
Rokitansky pelvis
Rolaids Calcium Rich
Roland
    R. index of low back pain
    R. low back pain index
Roland-Morris Questionnaire (RMQ)
Rolando fracture
role
    r. checklist (RC)
    intrinsic transverse connector r.
    occupational r.
Rolfing
    R. therapy
    R. treatment
Rolimeter
    Aircast R.
roll
    cervical r.
    chest r.
    r. control bolster
    cotton r.
    Dutchman's r.
    Feldenkrais foam r.
    Fluftex gauze r.
    hip r.
    lumbar r.
    McKenzie cervical r.
    McKenzie lumbar r.
    McKenzie night r.
    neck r.
    octagon r.
    radiolucent r.
    Skillbuilder half r.
    r. stitch
    towel r.
    Tumble Forms r.
Roll-A-Bout 4-wheel walker
Rollator Nova walker

R

rollback
    femoral r.
rolled felt
roller
    r. bandage
    r. injury
    Sorbothane rice sheller r.
RollerBack self-massage device
rolling
    skin r.
Rollocane
Roll-On
    Biofreeze R.-O.
Rollo phantom
roll-over
    r.-o. shape
    r.-o. shape prosthetic
rollover
    medial r.
Rolyan
    R. AquaForm wrist and thumb
      spica splint
    R. arm elevator
    R. foot support
    R. Gel Shell spica splint
    R. Reach N Range Pulley System
    R. TakeOff Sprint brace
    R. tibial fracture brace
Rolz device
ROM
    range of motion
    ROM knee brace
    ROM therapy
    ROM walker brace
Roman arch
Romano
    R. curved drilling system
    R. curved surgical drill
Romberg
    R. dorsal column of spinal cord
      test
    R. reflex
    R. sign
    R. symptom
Romberg-Howship symptom
Rome criteria
romeroi
    Pyrenochaeta r.
ROM therapy
rongeur
    Adson r.
    angled jaw r.
    angled pituitary r.
    angular bone r.
    Bacon bone r.
    Baer bone r.
    Bane bone r.
    Bane-Hartmann bone r.
    basket r.

bayonet r.
Beyer r.
Blumenthal bone r.
bone-nibbling r.
bone punch r.
Bruening-Citelli r.
Campbell r.
cervical r.
Cicherelli bone r.
Cintor bone r.
Cleveland bone r.
Cloward intervertebral disc r.
Codman-Kerrison laminectomy r.
Cohen r.
Colclough laminectomy r.
Corbett bone r.
curved bone r.
Cushing disc r.
Dale first rib r.
Dean bone r.
Decker r.
Defourmentel bone r.
disc r.
double-action r.
downbiting r.
duckbill r.
Echlin bone r.
Echlin duckbill r.
Echlin-Luer r.
Ferris-Smith r.
Ferris-Smith-Kerrison laminectomy r.
Ferris-Smith-Spurling disc r.
Fisch bone r.
flat-bottomed Kerrison r.
r. forceps
Friedman bone r.
Guleke bone r.
Hartmann bone r.
Hein r.
Hoen r.
Horsley bone r.
Husk bone r.
Jackson intervertebral disc r.
Kerrison downbiting r.
Kleinert-Kutz bone r.
Kleinert-Kutz synovectomy r.
Lebsche r.
Leksell laminectomy r.
Leksell-Stille thoracic r.
Lempert bone r.
Liston bone r.
Liston-Littauer r.
Luer bone r.
Markwalder bone r.
Marquardt bone r.
mastoid r.
McIndoe bone r.
Mead bone r.
needle-nose r.

rongeur (*continued*)
  orthopaedic r.
  pituitary r.
  Reiner bone r.
  Ruskin r.
  Ruskin-Liston bone r.
  Ruskin-Rowland bone r.
  Schell bone r.
  Schlesinger cervical r.
  Schlesinger intervertebral
    disc r.
  Semb bone r.
  Semb-Stille bone r.
  Shearer r.
  single-action r.
  Smith-Petersen r.
  Spurling r.
  Spurling-Kerrison upbiting and
    downbiting r.
  Stille r.
  Stille-Horsley bone r.
  Stille-Luer bone r.
  Stille-Luer duckbill r.
  Stille-Luer-Echlin r.
  Stille-Ruskin bone r.
  straight bone r.
  straight pituitary r.
  Super Cut laminectomy r.
  synovial r.
  upbiting r.
  upcut r.
  Watson-Williams intervertebral
    disc r.
  Weil-Blakesley intervertebral
    disc r.
  Wilde intervertebral disc r.
rongeured
Rood technique
roof
  acetabular r.
  r. arc measurement
  center of femoral head and external
    acetabular r. (CE)
  r. impingement
  intercondylar r.
  r. plate
  r. wedge
roofplasty
roofplate (*var. of* roof plate)
roof-reinforcement ring hip arthroplasty
  component
room
  Allender vertical laminar
    flow r.
  Charnley laminar flow r.
  operating r.
  recovery r.
  surgical dressing r. (SDR)
  training r.

Roos
  R. overhead exercise shoulder test
  R. rib cutter
  R. transaxillary first rib resection
    approach
root
  r. anomaly
  r. canal broach
  cervical r.
  r. infiltration
  nail r.
  nerve r.
  R. procedure
  r. tension sign
rootlet
Roper-Day prosthesis
rope stretching device
ropey
ropiness
ropinirole
ropivacaine
rose
  R. foot operation
  R. foot procedure
Rosen
  R. bur
  R. elevator
  R. splint
Rosenberg
  R. endoscopic anterior cruciate
    ligament reconstruction
  R. knee view
  R. retractor
Rosenfeld hip prosthesis
Rosenthal
  R. classification
  R. classification of nail injury
Roser line
Roser-Nélaton line
rosette
  r. Beaver blade
  R. strain gauge
rostrate pelvis
rostrocaudal spacing
Rotablator rotating bur
Rotaflex exerciser
Rotaglide
  R. knee implant
  R. lubricating solution
  R. total knee system
rotary
  r. ankle instability
  r. basket
  r. basket forceps
  r. bur
  r. control
  r. deviation
  r. displacement
  r. drawer test

R

r. instability test
r. joint
r. motion
r. osteotome
r. punch
r. stability

rotated
externally r.
internally r.

rotating
r. basket shaver
r. bur
r. drill
r. femoral head prosthesis
r. hinge
r. hinge knee prosthesis
r. knee joint prosthesis
r. patellar implant
r. turner

rotation
abduction and external r. (ABER)
abduction-external r. (AER)
abnormal instantaneous axis of r.
adduction-internal r.
anatomical hip center of r.
anterior innominate r.
axial r.
r. axis
axis of r.
Borggreve limb r.
center of axial r.
cervical general r.
cervical specific r.
r. device
r. drawer test
eccentric axis of ankle r.
r. exercise
external r.
flexion, abduction, external r. (faber)
flexion, adduction, internal r. (fadir)
foot r.
forced passive internal r.
functional axial r.
Hermodsson internal r.
hip r.
horizontal external r.
instantaneous axis of r. (IAR)
intentional r.
internal-external r.
internal femoral r.
intersegmental r.
inversion-eversion r.
inward r.
ipsilateral r.
knee r.
lateral hip r.
left r.
lumbar r.
medial hip r.

r. mobility
neutral r.
outward r.
patellar r.
patient-resisted internal r.
pelvic r.
r. plasty
polycentric r.
posterior innominate r.
pronation eversion external r.
  (PEER)
pronation-external r. (PER)
putative segmental instantaneous axis
  of r.
r. recurvatum test
resisted external r.
right r.
sagittal r.
spine r.
supination-external r. (SER)
synchronous scapuloclavicular r.
r. testing
tibiofibular r.
vertebral r.

rotational
r. alignment
r. burst fracture
r. contracture
r. correction
r. deformity
r. flap
r. instability
r. kyphosis
r. malalignment
r. malposition
r. manipulation
r. parameter
r. prominence
r. restriction
r. scarf osteotomy
r. scarf osteotomy/bunionectomy
r. scoliosis

rotation-compression maneuver
rotationplasty
Borggreve r.
tibial hindfoot osteomusculocutaneous
  r.
van Ness r.
Winkelmann femoral bone sarcoma
  r.

rotator
r. cuff
r. cuff buttress (RCB)
r. cuff calcific tendinitis
r. cuff calcified deposit
r. cuff contusion
r. cuff degeneration
r. cuff function
r. cuff imbalance

rotator (*continued*)
   r. cuff impingement
   r. cuff impingement syndrome
   r. cuff injury
   r. cuff lesion
   r. cuff repair
   r. cuff tear
   r. cuff tear arthroplasty
   r. cuff tendinopathy
   r. cuff tendon
   external r.
   Hosmer above-knee r.
   Howmedica monotube
     external r.
   internal r.
   r. interval capsule closure
   Jarit r.
   long external r.
   r. muscle
   short external r.
   r. unit
rotatores syndrome
rotatory
   r. atlantoaxial subluxation
   r. load
   r. olisthesis
   r. torque
rotatory-variable-differential transducer
Rotes joint mobility scale
Rothman
   R. Institute femoral prosthesis
   R. Institute total hip program
Roto-Rest bed
RotorloC absorbable rotator cuff suture anchor
rotoscoliosis
rototome
Rotter-Erb syndrome
roughened cartilage
roughening
roughen the surface
rouleaux formation
round
   r. bur
   r. cell liposarcoma
   r. cell-type liposarcoma
   r. ligament
   r. shoulder
   r. shoulder deformity
roundback stem
round-ended distraction rod
round-hole compression plate
round-tapped
   r.-t. elevator
   r.-t. periosteal
Rousek
   R. extender
   R. extraction set
   R. extractor

Rousso everting skin closure stitch
Roussy-Lévy
   R.-L. disease
   R.-L. syndrome
Rouviere ligament
Roux
   R. osteotomy
   R. sign
Roux-duToit staple capsulorrhaphy
Roux-Goldthwait
   R.-G. operation
   R.-G. patella realignment
   R.-G. repair of recurrent patellar dislocation procedure
row
   carpal r.
   proximal carpal r.
Rowe
   R. blanket
   R. calcaneal fracture classification (type 1a, 1b, 1c, 2a, 2b, 3-5)
   R. disimpaction forceps
   R. fusion
   R. glenoid punch
   R. glenoid-reaming forceps
   R. humeral head retractor
   R. modified-Harrison forceps
   R. posterior shoulder approach
   R. shoulder instability score
   R. shoulder view
Rowe-Harrison bone-holding forceps
rower's rump
Rowe-Zarins shoulder immobilization
rowing and sculling
Roxanol
   R. Rescudose
   R. SR Oral
Roxicodone
Roxilox
Roxiprin
Royalite body jacket
Roy-Camille
   R.-C. plate
   R.-C. posterior screw plate fixation
   R.-C. prosthesis
Roylan ergonomic hand exerciser
Royle-Thompson tendon transfer technique
RPE
   rated perceived exertion
   rating of perceived exertion
RQS
   repeated quick stretch
RQS-E
   repeated quick stretch from elongation
RQS-SEC
   repeated quick stretch superimposed upon an existing contraction

RRAM
    relative response attributable to
    maneuver
RRB
    rigid rockerbottom
RSA
    roentgen stereophotogrammetric
    analysis
RSC
    radioscaphocapitate
RSD
    reflex sympathetic dystrophy
RSDS
    reflex sympathetic dystrophy syndrome
RSI
    repetition strain injury
RSS
    rearfoot stability system
    repetitive stress syndrome
RT
    recreational therapy
RTD
    repetitive trauma disorder
RTP
    return to play
rub
    friction r.
    Jeanie R.
    Muscle R.
rubber
    r. band traction
    r. bolster
    r. drain
    r. held cup
    r. pedestal
    r. pelvis
    r. shod
    r. shod clamp
    r. sling
    r. sole cast walker
    r. spacer
    r. walking heel
    r. wedge walker
**Rubbermaid adjustable bath/shower
    seat**
Rubex
Rubin
    R. bone planer
    R. cartilage planer
    R. gouge
    R. rasp
Rubinstein-Taybi syndrome
rubor
rubrum
    Trichophyton r.
rucksack paralysis
rudimentary
    r. bone
    r. rib

RUE
    right upper extremity
Ruedi-Allgower
    R.-A. pilon fracture classification
    R.-A. tibial plafond fracture
Ruedi fracture
Ruffini mechanoreceptor
rugby jersey finger
rugger
    r. jersey sign
    r. jersey spine
Ruiz-Mora
    R.-M. correction
    R.-M. proximal phalangectomy for
    hammertoe procedure
RUL
    right upper limb
rule
    millimetric r.
    National Collegiate Athletic
    Association spine injury prevention
    r.
    no touch r.
    Ottawa ankle r. (OAR)
    r. out (R/O)
ruler
    Berndt hip r.
    ulnar r.
Rumel
    R. aluminum bridge splint
    R. myocardial clamp
    R. rubber clamp
    R. thoracic clamp
rump
    rower's r.
    runner's r.
runner
    heel-toe r.
    Sprint R.
runner's
    r. bump
    r. knee
    r. rump
    r. toe
running
    marathon r.
    r. suture
    treadmill r.
running-related injury
rupture
    Achilles tendon r. (ATR)
    adductor longus muscle r.
    anterior talofibular ligament r.
    buttonhole r.
    closed r.
    collateral ligament r.
    crescentic r.
    cruciate ligament r.
    distal biceps brachii tendon r.

rupture (*continued*)
    extracapsular r.
    flexor tendon r.
    gastrocnemius r.
    infrapatellar tendon r.
    intracapsular r.
    longitudinal ligament r.
    medial head of gastrocnemius r.
    neglected r.
    proximal tendon r.
    snap of the whip r.
    spontaneous r.
    stress r.
    subscapularis r.
    syndesmosis r.
    tendon r.
    transverse ligament r.
    ulnar collateral ligament r.

ruptured
    r. disc
    r. disc excision

rush
    R. bender
    R. bone clamp
    R. driver
    R. driver-bender-extractor
    R. extender
    R. flexible medullary nail
    R. intramedullary fixation pin
    R. mallet
    R. pin nail
    R. pin reamer awl
    R. rod
    R. rod awl reamer

Ruskin
    R. bone-cutting forceps
    R. bone-splitting forceps
    R. rongeur
    R. rongeur forceps

Ruskin-Liston
    R.-L. bone-cutting forceps
    R.-L. bone rongeur

Ruskin-Rowland
    R.-R. bone-cutting forceps
    R.-R. bone rongeur

Russe
    R. bone graft
    R. classification
    R. scaphoid fracture technique

Russe-Gerhardt range of motion of living joints method

Russell
    R. fibular head autograft
    R. skeletal traction
    R. splint

Russell-Silver dwarfism

Russell-Taylor
    R.-T. classification
    R.-T. delta rod
    R.-T. delta tibial nail
    R.-T. femoral interlocking nail system
    R.-T. interlocking medullary nail
    R.-T. screw

Russian
    R. forceps
    R. waveform

rust
    R. amputation saw
    R. disease
    R. phenomenon
    R. sign
    R. syndrome

Rüter classification

Rutkow inguinal hernia repair technique

R-Value exercise ball

Rx
    prescription
    Rx Comfort sock

RYB
    red, yellow, blue
    RYB wound color classification

Rydell nail

Ryder needle holder

Ryerson
    R. bone graft
    R. technique
    R. triple arthrodesis
    R. triple arthrodesis of foot procedure

SAARD
  slow-acting antirheumatic drug
Saba pulley
saber
  S. Bisector ArthroWand
  s. shin
  s. shin deformity
  s. tibia
saber-cut
  s.-c. approach
  s.-c. incision
Sabolich above-knee socket
SAC
  short arm cast
  Standardized Assessment of Concussion
sac
  bursal s.
  common dural s.
  thecal s.
SACH
  solid ankle cushioned heel
  SACH foot
  SACH foot adapter
  SACH foot prosthesis
  SACH orthosis
  SACH orthotic
Sachs nerve separator
saclike cavity
sacra (*pl. of* sacrum)
sacral
  s. agenesis
  s. ala
  s. alar screw
  s. approach
  s. arcuate line
  s. artery
  s. autonomic nucleus (SAN)
  s. bar
  s. bar technique
  s. base angle
  s. base distortion
  s. block
  s. bone
  s. bone tip
  s. bursa
  s. canal
  s. cyst
  s. dermatome
  s. fracture
  s. fusion screw fixation
  s. horizontal plane line (SHPL)
  s. inclination
  s. mobility
  s. nerve
  s. nerve root sparing

  s. pedicle screw
  s. pedicle screw fixation
  s. plexus
  s. plexus injury
  s. promontory (SP)
  s. screw placement
  s. segment
  s. slope
  s. spine
  s. spine decompression
  s. spine fixation
  s. spine fusion
  s. spine modular instrumentation
  s. spine stabilization
  s. support
  s. tilt
  s. triangle
  s. tuberosity
  s. vertebra
sacralgia
sacralis
  hiatus totalis s.
sacralization
sacralized transverse process
sacrectomy
  total s.
sacrificing knee prosthesis
sacrococcygeal
  s. abscess
  s. articulation
  s. chordoma
  s. joint
  s. ligament
  s. muscle
  s. teratoma
sacrodynia
sacrofemoral angle
sacrohorizontal angle
sacroiliac (SI)
  s. approach
  s. articulation
  s. belt
  s. binder
  s. block
  s. buttressing procedure
  s. disarticulation
  s. dislocation
  s. dysfunction
  s. extension fixation
  s. flexion fixation
  s. fracture
  s. hypermobility syndrome
  s. joint
  s. joint arthropathy
  s. joint disease

S

sacroiliac (*continued*)
s. joint fixation test
s. joint fusion
s. joint inflammatory
spondyloarthropathy
s. joint injury
s. joint locking
s. joint mobility
s. joint motion
s. joint stress test
s. joint syndrome
s. ligament
s. line
s. orthosis (SIO)
s. subluxation
sacroiliac-iliosacral dysfunction
sacroiliac-symphysis line
sacroiliitis
sacrolisthesis
sacrooccipital technique
(SOT)
sacropelvic fixation
sacrospinal
s. ligament
s. muscle
sacrospinale
ligamentum s.
sacrospinous ligament
sacrotomy
sacrotuberale
s. ligament
ligamentum s.
sacrotuberous ligament
sacrovertebral angle
sacrum, *pl.* **sacra**
dome-shaped s.
os s.
s. retroversion
teeter-totter s.
transverse process of s.
saddle
s. back
basal block cervical s.
s. block anesthesia
cervical s.
s. clamp
Cloward surgical s.
s. cushion
s. paresthesia
s. prosthesis
s. sore
saddlebag
Seidel s.
saddle-shaped joint
***S*-adenosylmethionine (SAMe)**
SAF
self-articulating femoral
SAF hip replacement
SAF prosthesis

SAFE
solid ankle flexible endoskeletal
stationary attachment flexible
endoskeletal
SAFE foot
SAFE II prosthesis
SAFE orthotic
SAFER
Safety Assessment of Function and
the Environment for Rehabilitation
Safe-T mate anti-rollback device
Safe-T-Wheel pinwheel
safety
S. Assessment of Function and the
Environment for Rehabilitation
(SAFER)
ergonomic s.
s. performance
s. pin orthosis
s. pin splint
safety-bolt suture
Safe-Wrap gauze
SAFHS
sonic accelerated fracture healing
system
SAFHS ultrasound device
Safir pin
SAFK
single-axis friction knee
sag
sling seat s.
s. test
tibial s.
sage
S. arthroscopic foot joint
cheilectomy
S. driver-extractor
S. forearm nail
S. pin
S. radial nail
S. rod
S. triangular nail
Sage-Clark foot joint cheilectomy
Sager traction splint
Sage-Salvatore classification I-III of
acromioclavicular joint injury
sagittal
s. alignment
s. anatomic alignment
s. balance
s. band
s. conventional spin-echo
proton-density sequence
s. deformity
s. imbalance
s. kyphosis
s. mobility
s. motion
s. movement

s. pedicle angle
s. pedicle diameter
s. plane
s. plane displacement
s. plane imaging
s. plane imbalance
s. plane instability
s. realignment
s. roll spondylolisthesis
s. rotation
s. spinal canal diameter
s. split osteotomy (SSO)
s. stress test
s. stress x-ray
s. surgical saw
s. translation
s. Z osteotomy
Saha
S. latissimus dorsi transfer technique
S. recurrent anterior shoulder
dislocation surgical procedure
S. trapezius muscle transfer
technique
Sahara
S. clinical bone sonometer
S. portable bone densitometer
SAID
specific adaptation to imposed demand
SAID principle
sailboarder injury
Saint Georg-Buchholz total ankle
prosthesis
Sakellarides calcaneal fracture treatment
Sakoff fifth metatarsal metaphysial
osteotomy
SAL
single axis locking
SAL knee
Salenius meniscus knife
Saleto-200, 400, 600, 800
Salflex
Salgesic
salicylate
choline s.
magnesium s.
methyl s.
sodium s.
triethanolamine s.
salicylic
s. acid
s. acid and lactic acid
s. acid and propylene glycol
salicylsalicylic acid
salient angle
saline
s. acceptance test
s. load test
physiologic s.
s. solution

saline-enhanced
s.-e. arthrography
s.-e. MR arthrogram
s.-e. MR arthrography of shoulder
SALK
single-axis locking knee
Salmonella
Salmonella arthritis
Salmonella osteomyelitis
Salmonine Injection
salsalate
Salsitab
salt
gold s.
Salter
S. epiphysis fracture
S. hip dysplasia surgical technique
S. innominate osteotomy
S. pediatric avascular necrosis of
hip criteria
S. pelvic osteotomy
Salter-Harris
S.-H. classification of epiphysial
plate injury
S.-H. distal tibial-fibular physis
fracture
S.-H. epiphysial fracture (I-VI)
S.-H. tibial-fibular physis injury
Salter-Harris-Rang epiphysial fracture
classification (1a, b, c, 2a, b, c, 3a, b,
4a, b, 5-9)
Salter-Thomson Perthes disease (A, B)
classification
Saltiel brace
salvage
s. ankle arthrodesis
diabetic limb s.
s. fusion
limb s.
s. procedure
Salzer
S. ceramic prosthesis
S. joint resurfacing
SAM
Skills Assessment Module
spinal analysis machine
structural aluminum malleable
SAM spinal analysis machine
SAM splint
SAMe
S-adenosylmethionine
same-day microsurgical arthroscopic
lateral approach laser-assisted (SMALL)
Samilson
S. crescentic calcaneal osteotomy
S. sliding osteotomy of calcaneus
procedure
sliding plane osteotomy of S.
Sam Jr. posture analyzer

S

Sammons biplane goniometer
sample
> Pennsylvania bimanual work s.
> Valpar Component Work S.'s

Sampson
> S. medullary nail
> S. prosthesis
> S. rod

Samuels forceps
SAN
> sacral autonomic nucleus

SANC
> short arm navicular cast

sand
> s. toe
> s. toe injury

sandal
> Benefoot & Birkenstock orthotic s.
> Exercise S.
> Rainbow cast s.

sandalthotics
> Foot Levelers s.
> S. postural support orthotic

sandbag
> neonatal s.

sandbagging long bone fracture
Sanders
> S. calcaneal fracture
> S. calcaneal fracture (I-IV)
>   classification
> S. calcaneal fracture (type I-IV)
> S. CT Classification
> S. highly comminuted calcaneal
>   fracture
> S. nondisplaced calcaneal fracture
> S. 3-part calcaneal fracture
> S. 4-part calcaneal fracture
> S. split calcaneal fracture

San Diego spastic hip acetabuloplasty
Sandimmune
> S. injection
> S. Oral

Sandoz
> S. 4-phase model of spinal
>   degeneration
> S. spinal degeneration 4-phase
>   model

sandwiched iliac bone graft
sandwich osteotomy
Sanfilippo syndrome
Sangeorzan
> S. foot and ankle internal
>   fixation
> S. navicular fracture classification
>   (1–4)

sanguineous
Sani-Grinder
sanitizer
> Mysotrol hand s.

Sani Vac
Santa Casa distractor
Santyl
SaO2
> arterial oxygen saturation

SAOF
> Self-Assessment of Occupational
>   Functioning

saphenous
> s. artery
> s. flap
> s. nerve
> s. neuralgia
> s. vein

SAPHO
> synovitis, acne pustulosis, hyperostosis,
>   osteomyelitis
> SAPHO syndrome

sapphire
> S. table
> S. View arthroscope

Saratoga exercise cycle
sarcoid
> s. arthritis
> Boeck s.

sarcoidosis
sarcoma
> alveolar soft part s. (ASPS)
> bicompartmental soft tissue s.
> botryoid s.
> chondroblastic s.
> clear cell s.
> deep intracompartmental soft tissue
>   s.
> epithelioid s.
> Ewing s.
> extracompartmental soft tissue s.
> fascial s.
> femoral s.
> fibroblastic s.
> giant cell s.
> high-grade surface osteogenic s.
> human osteogenic s.
> intracortical osteogenic s.
> Kaposi s.
> malignant myeloid s.
> multicentric osteogenic s.
> osteoblastic osteogenic s.
> osteogenic s.
> osteolytic s.
> Paget s.
> Paget-associated osteogenic s.
> parosteal osteogenic s.
> periosteal s.
> reticular cell s.
> small cell osteogenic s.
> soft tissue s.
> subcutaneous intracompartmental soft
>   tissue s.

synovial s. (SS, SYS)
synovial cell s.
sarcomatous change
sarcopenia
sarcoplasmic reticulum (SR)
sarcotubular myopathy
sargramostim
Sarmiento
S. fracture brace
S. intertrochanteric fracture technique
S. intertrochanteric osteotomy
S. nail
S. short leg patellar tendon-bearing cast
S. STH-2 hip prosthesis
Sarot needle holder
sartorial slide procedure
sartorius
s. muscle
s. tendon
SAS
short arm splint
shoulder arm system
SAS II brace
SAS shoe
Saso Variable Speed Massager
Sat-A-Lite contoured wedge seat cushion
sateen knee immobilizer
satellite
s. myofascial trigger point
s. potential
Saticon tube camera
Satinsky clamp
Satterlee
S. amputation saw
S. bone saw
saturation
arterial oxygen s. (SaO$_2$)
fat s.
Saturday night palsy
Saturn carpal tunnel splint
saturnina
arthralgia s.
saucerization
discoid meniscus s.
Saucony shoe
Sauerbruch
S. prosthesis
S. retractor
S. rib elevator
S. rib forceps
S. rib shears
Saunders
S. cervical HomeTrac
S. mobilization wedge
S. traction
sausage
s. digit
s. digit sign

s. finger
s. toe
Sauvé-Kapandji (S-K)
S.-K. distal radioulnar joint reconstruction
S.-K. procedure
S.-K. wrist arthroplasty
Savastano
S. hemiknee prosthesis
S. unconstrained prosthesis
S. unicompartment prosthesis
saver
intraoperative Cell S.
knee s.
saw
Adams s.
Adson wire s.
Aesculap s.
air-driven oscillating s.
amputation s.
Bailey wire s.
bayonet s.
Beaver s.
Bier amputation s.
Bishop s.
bone s.
Charriere amputation s.
Charriere bone s.
circular s.
Cottle s.
counter rotating s.
crescentic s.
crosscut s.
Delrin-handle bone s.
DeMartel wire s.
electric cast s.
end-cutting reciprocating s.
Engel plaster s.
fine-tooth electric s.
Gigli s.
s. guide
Hall air-driven oscillating s.
Hall sagittal s.
Hall Versipower oscillating s.
Hall Versipower reciprocating s.
hand s.
Herbert s.
Horsley bone s.
humeral s.
intramedullary s.
Langenbeck bone s.
Langenbeck metacarpal s.
Lebsche wire s.
Leica model 1600 water-cooled diamond s.
Luck-Bishop bone s.
medullary s.
Micro-Aire oscillating s.
microoscillating s.

S

saw (*continued*)
    microsagittal s.
    Miltex bone s.
    Müller s.
    Osada s.
    oscillating s.
    patella bone s.
    Pearson intramedullary s.
    Percy amputating s.
    plaster s.
    power bone s.
    power-driven s.
    power oscillating s.
    reciprocating motor s.
    Rust amputation s.
    sagittal surgical s.
    Satterlee amputation s.
    Satterlee bone s.
    single-blade s.
    single-sided bone s.
    Skil S.
    Sklar bone s.
    Stryker s.
    Tuke s.
    twin-blade oscillating s.
    Weiss amputation s.
    Zimmer oscillating s.

Sawa
    S. shoulder brace
    S. shoulder orthosis

sawblade
    Stablecut s.

sawcut

Sayre
    S. bandage
    S. elevator
    S. hip operation
    S. jacket
    S. splint
    S. suspension apparatus
    S. suspension traction

Sbarbaro
    S. hip prosthesis
    S. spica cast
    S. tibial plateau prosthesis

SBO
    spina bifida occulta

SC
    sternoclavicular
    SC joint
    SC suspension

SC-AcuFix
    SC-A. anterior cervical plate
      system
    SC-A. ThinLine plate

scaffold
    bioabsorbable mesh s.
    collagen s.
    Integra Mozaik osteoconductive s.
    s. matrix
    resorbable s.

Scaglietti
    S. closed reduction of
      spondiglolisthesis technique
    S. congenital dislocation of hip
      open reduction
    S. spondyloptosis reduction procedure

scalar
    s. classification
    s. quantity

scale
    abbreviated injury s. (AIS)
    Abnormal Involuntary Movement S.
      (AIMS)
    Activity Index and Meaningfulness
      of Activity S.
    Adelaar-Williams-Gould 10-point s.
    Adolescent and Pediatric Pain Tool
      S.
    Adult Nowicki Strickland Internal
      External Control S. (ANSIE)
    Adult Playfulness S.
    Alberta Infant Motor S.'s (AIMS)
    Allen Semantic Differential S.
    American Orthopaedic Foot and
      Ankle Society Ankle-Hindfoot S.
    American Spinal Injury Association
      impairment s.
    Angus-Cowell s.
    ankle-hindfoot s.
    AOFAS Lesser Metatarsophalangeal-
      Interphalangeal S.
    Arthritis Impact Measurement S.
      (AIMS)
    Arthritis Quality of Life S.
    Ashworth s. (1–5)
    ASIA impairment s.
    balance beam s.
    BASC s.
    Behavior Assessment Rating S.
      (BARS)
    Berg Balance S. (BBS)
    Borg Numerical Pain S.
    Boyd modification of Tardieu
      spastic measurement s.
    Braden risk assessment s.
    Broberg-Morrey elbow function s.
    Charnley-Merle d'Aubigné disability
      grading s.
    Charnley pain and function
      grading s.
    Children's Handwriting Evaluation S.
      (CHES)
    Clyde Mood s.
    Crowe hip s.
    DASH s.
    Disabilities of Arm, Shoulder, and
      Hand s.

disability s.
economic self-sufficiency WHO
  Handicap S.
Edinburgh Rehabilitation Status S.
  (ERSS)
Exercise Self-Efficacy S.
Expanded Disability Status S.
  (EDSS)
foot and ankle severity s. (FASS)
French s. (F)
Gait Abnormality Rating S. (GARS)
Geissling rating s.
Glasgow coma s. (GCS)
Graphic Rating S. (GRS)
hallux metatarsophalangeal
  interphalangeal s. (HMIS)
Harris hip s.
Health O Meter S.
hierarchial ADL s.
Hospital for Special Surgery s.
International Knee Documentation
  Committee knee s.
Japanese Orthopaedic Association S.
JOA S.
Johnson-Boseker s.
Karlsson and Peterson scoring s.
Kellgren knee s.
Kenna Knee S.
Kitaoka clinical rating s.
Klein-Bell Activities of Daily
  Living S.
Knox Preschool Play S.
Köhler hip protrusion grading s.
Kurtzke Expanded Disability s.
Leisure Boredom S. (LBS)
Lesser
  Metatarsophalangeal-Interphalangeal
  S. (LMIS)
Likert and Borg s.
Lincoln-Oseretsky Motor
  Development S.
linear analog pain s.
Lower Extremity Functional S.
  (LEFS)
Lysholm-Gillquist knee subjective
  function s.
Lysholm knee function scoring s.
Mathew s.
McGill pain s.
Merle d'Aubigné and Postel hip
  rating s.
metatarsophalangeal-interphalangeal s.
midfoot s.
modified Ashworth s. (MAS)
Modified Gait Abnormality Rating
  S. (GARS-M)
modified Rankin s.
Musculoskeletal Tumor Society
  Rating S.

Norton s.
numeric rating s. (NRS)
Occupational Circumstances
  Assessment Interview Rating S.
  (OCAIRS)
S.'s of Cognitive Ability for
  Traumatic Brain Injury (SCATBI)
Oral Analogue S. (OAS)
orientation WHO Handicap S.
Outerbridge s.
Perez postoperative pain s.
physical independence WHO
  Handicap S.
PJPS Severity S. (PSS)
Portola Valley S.
Progressive Ambulation S.
Prosthetic Problem Inventory S.
Quality of Well-Being S.
Quebec Back Pain Disability S.
Rancho Los Amigos S.
Reddihough s.
Rotes joint mobility s.
Severin hip dysplasia s.
Social Integration World Health
  Organization Handicap S.
Social Interaction S. (SIS)
Sports Activity S.
Stanford Hypnotic Clinical S.
Steinberg depression rating s.
subjective shoulder rating s. (SSRS)
Symptoms and Sports Participation
  Rating S.
Tardieu spasticity measurement s.
Tegner Activity S. (0-10)
Tegner activity rating s.
The Experience of Leisure S.
  (TELS)
The Knee Society clinical-rating s.
UCLA Shoulder Rating s.
visual analog s. (VAS)
Volpicelli functional ambulation s.
Wechsler Adult Intelligence S.
  (WAIS)
Wechsler Memory S.
Work Environment Impact S.
  (WEIS)

scalene
  s. block
  s. fat-pad
  s. maneuver
  s. muscle
scalenotomy
scalenus anterior syndrome
scalloping
  endosteal s.
  s. of vertebra
  vertebral s.
scalpel
  Bard-Parker s.

scalprum
scan
  adenosine thallium s.
  bone s.
  CT s.
  DEXA s.
  DXA s.
  gallium-67 s.
  gallium citrate s.
  intrathecally enhanced CT s.
  isotope bone s.
  lead-line s.
  leukocyte s.
  multiplanar computed tomography s.
  multiplanar CT s.
  nuclear magnetic resonance s.
  3-phase bone s.
  positron emission tomographic s.
  radioisotope gallium s.
  radioisotope indium-labeled white
    blood cell s.
  radioisotope technetium s.
  radionuclide bone s.
  rectilinear bone s.
  technetium-99m diphosphonate s.
  technetium-99m methylene
    diphosphate bone s.
  technetium-99m pyrophosphate s.
  technetium-99m sulfur colloid s.
  thallium s.
  triple-phase isotope bone s.
  white blood cell s.
Scand hip pin
**Scandinavian total ankle replacement
  (STAR)**
scanner
  Acoma s.
  All-Tronics s.
  s. gantry
  iStep FIT digital s.
  thermographic s.
scanning
  s. densitometry
  s. EMG
scanogram
  s. of lower extremity
  s. radiography
scanography
scaphocapitate
  s. fusion
  s. interval
  s. joint
  s. syndrome
scaphocapitolunate (SCL)
  s. arthrodesis
scaphoid
  s. arch
  avascular necrosis of s.
  bipartite s.

  s. bone
  carpal s.
  s. cookie in shoe
  s. fracture
  s. humpback deformity
  s. lift test
  s. nonunion
  s. scapula
  s. screw guide
  s. shift test
  s. shoe cookie
  s. shoe pad
  s. tuberosity injury
  waist of s.
scaphoiditis
scaphoid-lunate (*var. of* scapholunate)
scapholunate (SL), scaphoid-lunate
  s. advanced collapse (SLAC)
  s. angle
  s. arthritis collapse (SLAC)
  s. dissociation
  s. gap
  s. instability
  s. interosseous ligament
  s. joint
  s. ligament tear syndrome
scaphotrapeziotrapezoid arthrodesis
scaphotrapezoid interosseous ligament
scaphotrapezoid-trapezial (STT)
  s.-t. joint
scapula, *pl.* **scapulae**
  alar s.
  s. alata
  body of s.
  s. elevata
  elevated s.
  glenoid fossa of s.
  Graves s.
  locked s.
  scaphoid s.
  snapping s.
  winged s.
  winging of s.
scapulae (*pl. of* scapula)
scapulalgia
scapular
  s. approximation test
  s. border
  s. dysfunction
  s. elevation
  s. elevation test
  s. flap
  s. fracture
  s. graft
  s. ligament
  s. nerve
  s. notch
  s. peroneal atrophy
  s. reflex

s. sign of Putti
s. winging
s. winging orthosis
scapulary
scapulectomy
Das Gupta s.
Phelps s.
scapuloclavicular
s. articulation
s. injury
s. joint
scapulocostal syndrome
scapulodynia
scapulohumeral
s. atrophy
s. bursa
s. ligament
s. muscle
s. reflex
s. rhythm
scapulolateral view
scapuloperoneal
s. syndrome (SPS)
s. syndrome type Kaesar
scapulopexy
scapulothoracic (ST)
s. arthrodesis
s. bursitis
s. dissociation
s. fixation orthosis
s. fusion
s. guiding plane
s. joint (STJ)
s. motion
s. muscle
s. orthosis
s. pain
scapulovertebral border
scar
area s.
s. band
s. formation
hypertrophic s.
keloid s.
linear s.
parasagittal s.
peritendinous s.
physial s.
s. tissue
Scarborough
S. prosthesis
S. total hip replacement
scarf
s. bandage
s. osteotomy bunionectomy
s. Z osteotomy
s. Z osteotomy bunionectomy
s. Z-plasty
scarlatinal synovitis

Scarpa fascia
scarring
s. and furrowing
s. cosmesis
s. effect
epineural s.
SCATBI
Scales of Cognitive Ability for Traumatic Brain Injury
SCATBI Assessment
SCC
short calcaneocuboid
SCC ligament
SCD
sequential compression device
SCD stockings
SCDD
symptomatic cervical disc disease
SCFE
slipped capital femoral epiphysis
Schaffer squeeze
Schamroth sign
Schanz
S. collar
S. collar brace
S. disease
S. dressing
S. femoral osteotomy
S. irreducible hip dislocation angulation osteotomy
S. pin
S. screw
S. syndrome (1, 2)
Schanz-type proximal femoral valgization osteotomy
Schatzker
S. tibial plateau fracture
S. tibial plateau fracture classification (I-VI)
S. tibial plateau fracture classification system (I-VI)
Schauwecker
S. patellar tension band wire
S. patellar wiring
S. patellar wiring technique
Schede
S. bone curette
S. femur fracture repair method
S. hip osteotomy
Scheie syndrome
Schell bone rongeur
schenckii
Sporothrix s.
Scher nail biopsy
Scheuermann
S. disease of thoracic and lumbar spine
S. dystrophic spondylosis
S. juvenile kyphosis (SJK)

S

Scheuermann (*continued*)
  S. kyphoscoliosis
  S. kyphosis syndrome
Schiek belt
Schink metatarsal spreader
Schlatter disease
Schlatter-Osgood disease
Schlein
  S. clamp
  S. elbow arthroplasty
  S. semiconstrained elbow
    prosthesis
  S. shoulder positioner (I-III)
  S. total elbow prosthesis
  S. trisurface ankle prosthesis
Schlesinger
  S. cervical punch forceps
  S. cervical rongeur
  S. intervertebral disc rongeur
  S. punch
  S. rongeur forceps
  S. sign
Schmeisser
  S. spica
  S. spica cast
Schmid
  S. disease
  S. metaphysial dysostosis
Schmidt rod holder
Schmitt fan
Schmorl
  S. hernia
  S. node
  S. nodule
  S. nucleus pulposus disease
Schneider
  S. apparatus
  S. cobra-head plate
  S. cobra head plate arthrodesis
  S. driver-extractor
  S. fixation
  S. hip arthrodesis
  S. intramedullary nail
  S. nail driver
  S. pin
  S. rod
**Schnute osteitis pubis wedge resection
  technique**
Schober
  S. lumbar flexion-extension
    measuring method
  S. lumbar spine mobility measuring
    technique
  S. lumbar spine range of motion
    test
  S. measurement
  S. test of lumbar flexion
  S. true flexion measurement
    technique

**Schoemaker congenital hip dislocation
  line**
Scholten sternal retractor
School Setting Interview (SSI)
Schreiber patellar reflex test maneuver
Schrock
  S. hip arthroplasty
  S. pediatric scapula procedure
  S. scapula elevation repair
    procedure
Schrudde rotational flap
Schuind external fixation
Schuknecht
  S. Gelfoam wire prosthesis
  S. Teflon wire piston prosthesis
Schüller syndrome
Schultze acroparesthesia
Schwann
  S. cell
  S. tumor
schwannoma
  cellular s.
  collagenous s.
  malignant s.
Schwartz
  S. clip-applying forceps
  S. midfoot dorsiflexory osteotomy
  S. temporary clamp-applying forceps
Schwartze chisel
Schwartz-Jampel
  S.-J. myotonia
  S.-J. syndrome
Schwartz-Jampel-Aberfeld syndrome
Schwarz finger extension bow
Schweitzer
  S. pin
  S. spring plate
Schwinn
  S. Air-Dyne bicycle
  S. bi-directional Windjammer upper
    body cycle
  S. elliptical full body exercise
    machine
  S. Fitness Advisor
  S. Spinner bicycle
  S. 900 stationary bicycle
SCI
  spinal cord injury
sciage
sciatic
  s. foramen
  s. function index (SFI)
  s. leg block
  s. nerve
  s. nerve block
  s. nerve injury
  s. nerve irritation
  s. nerve palsy hematoma
  s. neuralgia

s. neuritis
s. notch
s. palsy
s. scoliosis
s. tension sign

sciatica
discogenic s.

science
exercise s.
movement s.
occupational s.

scientific practitioner
scientist-practitioner
scintigram
bone s.

scintigraphy
bone s.
combined s.
indium-111 s.
paired s.
triphase technetium s.

scintiscan
scissors
Acufex s.
adventitial s.
arthroscopic s.
Aslan endoscopic s.
Babcock wire-cutting s.
Bantam wire-cutting s.
Beebe wire-cutting s.
Bellucci alligator s.
blunt-tip iris s.
cartilage s.
collar and crown s.
Crafoord thoracic s.
crown and collar s.
curved Mayo s.
Dean s.
dissecting s.
Fiskars s.
s. gait
Giertz-Stille s.
Halsey nail s.
Harvey wire-cutting s.
hook rotary s.
iris s.
Jones s.
Kay s.
Koenig nail-splitting s.
Laschal suture s.
s. leg
loop s.
Martin cartilage s.
Mayo s.
McIndoe s.
meniscal s.
meniscectomy s.
meniscus s.
Metzenbaum s.

s. nail drill
Nelson s.
Nicola s.
orthopaedic s.
plain rotary s.
PowerStar bipolar s.
serrated s.
Sistrunk s.
Slip-N-Snip s.
Smillie meniscal s.
Smith s.
Stephen s.
straight s.
suture s.
tissue s.
Walton s.
Webster meniscectomy s.
Weck microsuture cutting s.
Weller cartilage s.
wire-cutting s.

scissors-leg
s.-l. gait
s.-l. position

SCIWORA
spinal cord injury without radiographic abnormality

SCL
scaphocapitolunate
SCL arthrodesis

scleroderma
focal s.

scleroses (*pl. of* sclerosis)
sclerosing
s. nonsuppurative osteitis
s. nonsuppurative osteomyelitis

sclerosis, *pl.* **scleroses**
amyotrophic lateral s. (ALS)
Baló concentric s.
bone s.
diaphysial s.
discogenic vertebral s.
endplate s.
Mönckeberg s.
multiple s. (MS)
piriform s.
progressive systemic s. (PSS)
subchondral s.
systemic s.
tuberous s.
zonal s.

sclerotic
s. bone
s. line
s. marginal rim
s. segment

sclerotomal pain
sclerotome pain chart
SCL-90R
Symptoms Checklist 90 Revised

S

SCM
    sternocleidomastoid
    synovial chondromatosis
        SCM muscle
SCOI
    Southern California Orthopaedic
     Institute
        SCOI arthroscopic biceps tenodesis
        SCOI shoulder brace
scoliokyphosis
scoliometer measurement
scoliosis
    adolescent s.
    adolescent idiopathic s. (AIS)
    adult s.
    s. angle
    Brissaud s.
    s. cast
    cicatricial s.
    Cobb-Webb angle of s.
    Cobb-Webb method for measuring
     degree of curve in s.
    compensatory s.
    congenital s.
    s. correction
    s. correction with Dwyer cable
    coxitic s.
    curve pattern of s.
    curve progression in s.
    degenerative lumbar s.
    de novo s.
    dextrorotary s.
    double major curve s.
    double thoracic curve s.
    Dwyer anterior endoscopic correction
     of s.
    electrical surface stimulation
     treatment for s.
    empyemic s.
    endoscopic correction of s.
    familial idiopathic s. (FIS)
    Ferguson method for measuring
     spinal curvature s.
    s. fixation
    fracture with s.
    functional s.
    Galen s.
    genetic s.
    habit s.
    hysterical s.
    idiopathic s.
    infantile idiopathic s.
    inflammatory s.
    ischiatic s.
    juvenile idiopathic s.
    King 2-curve classification of s.
     (type I-V)
    King-Moe classification of s.
    kyphosing s.

    Lenke 3–component classification
     (I-V) of adolescent idiopathic s.
    levoscoliosis s.
    Lippman-Cobb classification (I-VII)
     of curvature in s.
    lumbar s.
    myopathic s.
    neurogenic s.
    neuromuscular s.
    ocular s.
    s. operating frame
    osteogenic s.
    osteopathic s.
    s. overlap brace
    paralytic s.
    rachitic s.
    S. Research Society
    rheumatic s.
    rigid curve s.
    Risser bone maturation index of s.
    rotational s.
    sciatic s.
    s. spinal fusion
    static s.
    structural s.
    s. surgery
    thoracic curve s.
    thoracogenic s.
    thoracolumbar idiopathic s.
    thoracolumbar spine s.
    uncompensated rotary s.
    Winter-King-Moe s.
scoliotic
    s. curve
    s. curve fixation
    s. pelvis
ScoliTron instrument
scooter
    Go-Ped motorized s.
    K9 S.
    Lark s.
    Rascal s.
Scoot-Gard mat
scope
    Doppler s.
    Endoflex endoscopic lumbar
     discectomy s.
    Harris s.
    Hughston knee s.
    Liviscope s.
    Lysholm knee joint instability s.
SCORE
    Simple Calculated Osteoporosis Risk
    Estimation
score
    AAOS Knee Society Clinical
     Rating S.
    AOFAS s.
    ASES shoulder s.

Ashworth scale of muscle spasticity s. (0-4, 1-5)
Bandi patellofemoral pain s. (1–5)
Carter Rowe shoulder s.
Catterall hip s.
Champion trauma s. (CTS)
Charnley hip s.
composite knee s.
Constant-Murley shoulder assessment s.
Dupont Bunion Rating S.
Fries rheumatoid arthritis s.
Fulkerson functional knee s.
functional rating s.
Green and OBrien wrist function s.
Harris hip s. (HHS)
Hospital for Special Surgery knee s.
HSS knee s.
Hughston knee s.
IKDC s.
Injury Severity S. (ISS)
Iowa hip s.
Kapandji thumb opposition s.
Knee Society s.
Kofoed ankle s. (KAS)
Kurtzke Expanded Disability Status scale s.
Larson hip s.
Lysholm-Gillquist knee subjective function s.
Lysholm knee s. (1–5)
Mangled Extremity Severity S. (MESS)
Marshall knee s.
Maryland foot s.
Mayo Clinic forefoot s.
Mayo elbow performance s.
Mayo hip s.
McGuire ankle s.
Merchant and Dietz ankle s.
Merle d'Aubigné and Postel postoperative function s.
Merle d'Aubigné hip s.
modified Harris hip s.
modified Rowe shoulder s.
Molander-Olerud ankle s.
Molander-Olerud shoulder s.
Olerud ankle fracture clinical and radiologic s.
Oswestry Disability S.
Prolo lumbar and cervical spine postoperative functional and economic status s.
Rowe shoulder instability s.
Sherman foot s.
skeletal injury s.
Tachdjian flatfoot s.

Tegner knee reconstruction activity s.
Tegner meniscal knee injury s.
thoracolumbar injury severity s. (TLISS)
trauma s.
scored cartilage
scoring
Scorpio total knee system
Scotchcast
S. 2 cast tape
S. length splinting system
scotoma, *pl.* **scotomata**
absolute s.
scotomata (*pl. of* scotoma)
Scott
S. ankle splint
S. double-strap ankle support
S. elastic ankle strap
S. glenoplasty technique
S. hinged knee support
S. humeral splint
S. lumbar spondylolysis direct repair wiring
S. lumbar spondylosis wiring technique
S. posterior glenoplasty
S. RCE osteotomy guide
S. total knee revision arthroplasty
S. uniform tennis elbow splint
S. wrist wrap
Scottish
S. Rite brace
S. Rite hip orthosis
S. Rite splint
scotty
s. dog sign
S. stainless ankle joint
scout film
Scoville
S. curette
S. retractor
Scranton transmalleolar arthrodesis
scraper
Bradley femoral canal preparation s.
scraping toe gait
scratch test
screen
ACL S.
Allen Cognitive Level S. (ACLS)
dynamic mobility s.
Lanex s.
motion palpation s.
split s.
screening
gait, arms, legs, spine s.
GALS s.
Integrated Shape Imaging System scoliosis s.

S

screening (*continued*)
    ISIS scoliosis s.
    neuropsychological s.
    s. palpation
    pediatric gait, arms, legs, spine s.
    pGALS s.

screw
    Absolute absorbable s.
    Ace s.
    AcroMed s.
    alar s.
    s. alignment bar
    s. alignment rod
    Alta cancellous s.
    Alta cortical s.
    Alta cross-locking s.
    Alta lag s.
    Alta supracondylar s.
    Alta transverse s.
    Ambi hip s.
    Amset R-F s.
    anchor s.
    s. angle guide
    s. angulation
    AO-ASIF s.
    AO cancellous s.
    AO cortex s.
    AO lag s.
    AO spongiosa s.
    Arthrex sheathed interference s.
    arthrodesis s.
    ASIF cancellous s.
    ASIF cortical s.
    ASIF malleolar s.
    Aten olecranon s.
    Autogenesis automator for
      Ilizarov s.
    axial compression s.
    s. backout
    Barouk cannulated bone s.
    Basile hip s.
    Bechtol s.
    bicortical s.
    Bio-Absorbable interference s.
    BioCuff C bioresorbable
      cannulated s.
    Bio-Interference tibial s.
    Biologically Quiet interference s.
    Bionx absorbable cannulated s.
    Bionx self-reinforced PLLA smart s.
    BioRCI bioabsorbable s.
    bioresorbable s.
    BioScrew absorbable interference s.
    BioSorbFX SR self-reinforced plate
      and s.
    blocking s.
    Bold compression s.
    Bone Mulch s.
    Bosworth coracoclavicular s.

    breakable s.
    s. breakage
    buttress thread s.
    Campbell cannulated s.
    cancellous bone s.
    cannulated bone s.
    cannulated cancellous lag s.
    cannulated hip s.
    captured interlocking s.
    carpal scaphoid s.
    Carrell-Girard s.
    Caspar cervical s.
    CD Horizon M8 multiaxial s.
    chrome-cobalt s.
    Clearfix s.
    Cohort bone s.
    Collison s.
    compression hip s.
    compression lag s.
    s. compressor
    Concise compression hip s.
    coracoclavicular s.
    cortex s.
    cortical ASIF s.
    cortical bone s.
    cortical cancellous s.
    Cotrel pedicle s.
    Coventry s.
    crossing s.'s
    cross-locking s.
    crown drill s.
    cruciate head bone s.
    cruciform head bone s.
    Cubbins s.
    s. depth calibrator
    s. depth gauge
    DePuy interference s.
    s. design
    Deyerle interlocking s.
    distal locking s.
    distraction s.
    double-threaded Herbert s.
    dual-threaded s.
    Duo-Drive s.
    Dwyer spinal s.
    Dynamic condylar s. (DCS)
    dynamic hip s. (DHS)
    ECT bone s.
    Edwards modular system
      spinal/sacral s.
    Eggers s.
    encased s.
    Endo-Fix bioabsorbable
      interference s.
    Endo-Fix L s.
    s. epiphysiodesis
    s. epiphysiodesis for
      hemiepiphysiodesis of distal tibial
      epiphysis

expansion s.
Fabian s.
femoral head cork s.
fixateur interne s.
s. fixation
fixation s.
s. fixation operation
flute of cannulated s.
foreign body s.
FRS s.
s. fusion
Garden s.
Gentle Threads interference s.
Glasgow s.
glenoid fixation s.
Guardsman femoral interference s.
Hahn s.
Hall spinal s.
Hamilton s.
s. head
headless bone s. (HBS)
Heck s.
Hedrocel titanium s.
Henderson lag s.
Herbert bone s.
Herbert scaphoid s.
Herbert-Whipple bone s.
hex s.
hexagonal slot-cap s.
hip compression s.
hollow mill Asnis cannulated s.
hook trial set s.
Howmedica ICS s.
Howmedica universal compression s.
iliac s.
iliosacral s.
Ilizarov s.
s. implantation
InCompass polyaxial s.
InCompass thoracolumbar spine
  fixation s.
s. insertion
s. insertion technique
Instrument Makar biodegradable
  interference s.
Integrity acetabular cup s.
interference s.
interfragmentary lag s.
interlocking s.
Intrafix s.
Isola spinal implant system iliac s.
Isola vertebral s.
Jeter lag/position s.
Jewett pick-up s.
Johannson lag s.
Jones s.
Kostuik s.
Kurosaka interference-fit s.
LactoSorb s.

lag s.
Lane bone s.
lateral to medial s.
Leinbach olecranon s.
Leone expansion s.
Linvatec absorbable s.
Lippman s.
locking s.
locking-head s.
Long Beach pedicle s.
s. loosening
Lorenzo s.
Luhr s.
lumbar pedicle s.
Lundholm s.
Luque II s.
Luque pedicle s.
machine s.
malleolar s.
s. malposition
Marion s.
Martin s.
maxillofacial bone s.
McLaughlin carpal scaphoid s.
medial bicortical s.
medial unicortical s.
Medoff axial compression s.
micrometric s.
mille pattes s.
mini AO s.
minifragment s.
Moberg s.
Morris biphase s.
Moss s.
Mouradian s.
multiaxial s.
navicular s.
Neufeld s.
No-Lok s.
nonself-tapping s.
Olerud PSF s.
Ormandy s.
Orthex cannulated bone s.
Orthofix s.
Osteomed s.
OsteoTite bone s.
Palex expansion s.
Palmer s.
s. passage
PathFinder pedicle s.
pedicle s.
PerFixation s.
PGA s.
Phillips head s.
Phillips recessed-head s.
Pilot point s.
s. placement
s. placement C-guide
polyaxial cervical s.

S

screw (*continued*)
polylactide absorbable s.
s. position perioperative monitoring
posterior-anterior s.
posterior-to-anterior s.
Preston s.
Propel cannulated interference s.
proximal and distal s.
pull s.
s. pullout
Ray s.
resorbable polymer s.
ReUnite orthopaedic s.
Revere pedicle s.
reverse-threaded s.
Revo retrievable cancellous s.
Richards classic compression hip s.
Richards lag s.
Richmond subarachnoid s.
rigid pedicle s.
Rockwood shoulder s.
Russell-Taylor s.
sacral alar s.
sacral pedicle s.
Schanz s.
Selby I, II s.
self-tapping bone s.
SemiFix s.
set s.
Sharpey s.
sheathed interference s.
Shelton bone s.
Sherman bone s.
Simmons double-hole spinal s.
Simmons-Martin s.
sliding compression hip s.
small fragment s.
small-headed s.
spherical-headed s.
spongiosa s.
s. stabilization
stainless steel s.
Steffee plate and s.
step s.
Storz s.
s. stripout
Stryker lag s.
subarticular s.
superior thoracic pedicle s.
supracondylar s.
Swiss cancellous s.
syndesmotic s.
Synthes compression hip s.
Talon compression hip s.
tangoRS smart s.
4-tap s.
s. tap
Thatcher s.
thoracolumbar pedicle s.

Thornton s.
threaded cancellous s.
thumb s.
tibial head s.
tibia-pro-fibula s.
s. tip
titanium s.
titanium alloy cancellous bone s.
s. toggle
s. torque
Townley bone graft s.
Townsend-Gilfillan s.
traction tongs s.
transarticular s.
transfixion s.
translaminar facet s.
transpedicular s.
transverse s.
triangulated pedicle s.
Trinion meniscus s.
TSRH pedicle s.
tulip pedicle s.
TunneLoc bone mulch s.
Twist-Off S.
UCR thoracolumbar fusion posterior
  fixation pedicle s.
unicortical s.
universal fixation s.
Uppsala s.
Vari-Angle s.
varus derotational osteotomy with
  adolescent pediatric hip s.
varus-valgus adjustment s.
VDS s.
Venable s.
Vilex F-Series dual-thread s.
Virgin hip s.
vitallium s.
VSF s.
Wagner-Schanz s.
Weiss jack s.
Wiltse pedicle s.
wood s.
Woodruff s.
Wurzburg s.
Yuan s.
Zimmer compression hip s.
Zuelzer s.
screw-and-keel fixation
screw-and-plate fixation
screw-and-wire fixation
screwdriver
Allen head s.
automatic s.
Becker s.
Bio-Interference s.
Bosworth s.
cannulated s.
Children's Hospital s.

Collison s.
cross-slot s.
cruciform s.
Cubbins bone s.
DePuy s.
Dorsey screw-holding s.
double-slot s.
European-style s.
Flatt self-retaining s.
Hall s.
heavy cross-slot s.
hex head s.
Johnson s.
Ken s.
Lane s.
light cross-slot s.
Lok-it s.
Massie s.
Master s.
Phillips head s.
plain s.
Richter bone s.
self-retaining s.
Sherman s.
single cross-slot s.
single-slot s.
skull plate s.
straight hex s.
Stryker s.
torque s.
Trinkle s.
universal hex s.
White s.
Williams s.
Woodruff s.
Zimmer s.
screw-holding forceps
screw-home mechanism
screw-in ceramic acetabular cup
Screw-Lok tap
screw-plate
s.-p. approach
Calandruccio impaction s.-p.
s.-p. fixation
s.-p. technique
Zimmer impaction s.-p.
screw-rod device
screw-to-screw compression construct
Scrip Muscle Master massager
scroll bone
scrub
Betadine s.
Exidine S.
Hibiclens s.
Techni-Care surgical s.
SCS
spinal canal stenosis
spinal cord stimulator

SCSP
supracondylar-suprapatellar
Scuderi
S. quadriceps tendon repair technique
S. ruptured quadriceps repair technique
S. ruptured quadriceps tendon repair
sculling
rowing and s.
Scully
S. Hip S'port
S. Hip S'port hip device
sculp
Concise cementing s.
s. knife
Scultet (*var. of* Scultetus)
Scultetus, Scultet
S. bandage
S. binder
S-curve
Hadley S-c.
scurvy line
S-cutting block
Scytalidium
S. dimidiatum
S. hyalinum
SDB
subdeltoid bursitis
SDD
sterile dry dressing
SDR
surgical dressing room
S.D. Sorb Stapler
Seaber forceps
seal-fin deformity
seal limb
Seal-Tight cast protector
seam
osteoid s.
searing pain
seat
antithrust s.
Backjoy s.
s. belt injury
Carrie car s.
Comfy toilet lift s.
s. cushion
Dream Ride car s.
ischial-bearing s.
Maddacare child bath s.
Orthopaedic Positioning S.
Posey drop s.
Renolux convertible car s.
Rubbermaid adjustable bath/ shower s.
Snug s.
Special S.
Spelcast car s.

seat (*continued*)
    Tall-ette toilet s.
    Tubsider Kneeling S.

seated
    S. Cable Row exerciser
    s. flexion test
    s. hamstring curl
    properly s.
    s. root test
    s. scapular retraction exercise

seating
    s. aid
    s. chisel
    s. cushion
    s. of prosthesis
    trial s.
    s. wedge

Seattle
    S. foot prosthesis
    S. modification
    S. modification of Kocher incision
    S. orthosis
    S. safety knee
    S. splint

Sebileau periosteal elevator
SEBT
    Star Excursion Balance Test

secobarbital
    amobarbital and s.

Seconal Injection
second
    s. cervical vertebra
    cycle per s.
    s. impact syndrome
    s. intention
    s. metacarpal
    s. metatarsal artery
    s. metatarsophalangeal joint
      arthrodesis
    s. skin pad

secondary
    s. amputation
    s. bone union
    s. center
    s. closure
    s. curve
    s. disability
    s. erythromelalgia
    s. fracture
    s. hematogenous osteomyelitis
    s. hip-spine syndrome
    s. intention
    s. metatarsalgia
    s. myofascial trigger point
    s. osteoporosis
    s. osteosarcoma
    s. posttraumatic syringomyelia
    s. purchase
    s. stabilizer

second-generation cementing technique
Secretan syndrome
section
    bar s.
    calcaneonavicular bar s.

sectioning
    sequential s.

Secure Yet Gentle surgical dressing system
Secur-Fit HA PSL X'tra prosthesis
SED
    spondyloepiphysial dysplasia
    SED congenita
    SED tarda

sedation therapy
Seddon
    S. coin tactile test
    S. dorsal spine costotransversectomy
    S. nerve injury classification
    S. nerve injury grading modification
    S. neurapraxia
    S. neurotmesis
    S. technique

sedentary
    s. lifestyle
    s. occupation
    s. work

Sedillot periosteal elevator
sedimentation rate
Seeburger
    S. first metatarsophalangeal joint
      implant
    S. retractor

segment
    apical s.
    central s.
    motion s.
    physiologic lock of motion s.
    relation to subadjacent s.
    sacral s.
    sclerotic s.
    spinal s.
    subadjacent s.
    vertebral motion s.

segmental
    s. alveolar osteotomy
    s. bone defect
    s. bone loss
    s. compression construct
    s. curve
    s. deficiency
    s. dysfunction
    s. fixation
    s. fracture
    s. hyperextension
    s. kyphosis
    s. level
    s. mobility
    s. mobility testing

s. motion testing
s. motor paralysis
s. spinal cord disorder
s. spinal correction system (SSCS)
s. spinal instrumentation (SSI)
s. tendon graft
segmentally demineralized bone technology
segmentation
s. defect
supernumerary lumbar s.
Segond tibial avulsion fracture
Séguin fracture
Seidel
S. bone-holding clamp
S. humeral locking nail
S. intramedullary fixation
S. nail
S. saddlebag
Seinsheimer subtrochanteric fracture classification (I-VI)
Seirin acupuncture needle
seismotherapy
seizing forceps
seizure
acute repetitive s. (ARS)
oxygen s.
Selakovich sustenaculum tali procedure
Selby
S. I, II fixation system
S. I, II hook
S. I, II rod
S. I, II screw
select
S. ankle prosthesis
S. joint
S. joint orthosis
S. modular shoulder prosthesis
S. shoulder system
selection
bone plate s.
Edwards modular system construct s.
selective
s. nerve root injection
s. posterior rhizotomy (SPR)
Theraform S.'s
s. thoracic spine fusion
Selectively Lockable knee brace
selegiline
selenium sulfide
self-adhering varus/valgus wedge
self-aligning
s.-a. knee
s.-a. mobile-bearing knee implant
self-articulating
s.-a. femoral (SAF)
s.-a. femoral hip replacement

Self-Assessment of Occupational Functioning (SAOF)
self-bearing
s.-b. ceramic hip prosthesis
s.-b. ceramic total hip replacement
self-broaching
s.-b. nail
s.-b. pin
self-care
self-centering
s.-c. bone-holding forceps
s.-c. implant
s.-c. Universal hip prosthesis
self-curing polymer
self-efficacy
exercise s.-e.
self-help ability
self-locking nail
self-mutilation
self-propelling wheelchair
self-reinforcing polylevolactic acid (SR-PLLA)
self-retaining
s.-r. bone-holding forceps
s.-r. clamp
s.-r. retractor
s.-r. screwdriver
self-sealing
s.-s. cannula
s.-s. implant
self-sustained natural apophysial glides
self-tapering pin
self-tapping bone screw
Selig interinnomino-abdominal hindquarter amputation operation
Sellors rib contractor
Selsun
S. Blue
S. Gold for Women
Selverstone rongeur forceps
Semb
S. bone forceps
S. bone-holding clamp
S. bone rongeur
S. rib forceps
Semb-Stille bone rongeur
SEMG, sEMG
surface electromyography
semicanal of humerus sulcus
semicircular flap amputation
semiconstrained
s. total elbow arthroplasty
s. tricompartmental knee prosthesis
SemiFix screw
semiflexion
semi-Fowler position

S

semilunar
  s. bone
  s. cartilage
  s. cartilage knife
  s. notch
  s. sulcus
semilunaris
  linea s.
semiluxation
semimembranosus
  s. bursitis
  s. insertion syndrome
  s. muscle
  s. tendinitis
  s. tendon
semimembranous complex
semiopen sliding tenotomy
semirigid
  s. ankle brace
  s. fiberglass cast (SRF)
  s. polypropylene ankle-foot orthosis
  s. postoperative dressing
  s. shell
semisitting position
semispinal muscle
semisupinated oblique view
semi-suture-loop technique
semitendinosus
  s. augmentation of patellar tendon
    repair
  s. muscle
  s. procedure
  s. technique
  s. tendon
  s. tendon transfer
  s. tenodesis
semitendinosus-gracilis graft
semitendinous graft
semitubular
  s. blade-plate
  s. compression plate
Semmes-Weinstein
  S.-W. monofilament (SWMF)
  S.-W. monofilament pressure
    esthesiometry
  S.-W. monofilament pressure test
Senegas
  S. hip approach
  S. transtrochanteric lateral approach
    to hip
senescence
Sengupta proximal quadriceps femoris
  release
senile
  s. hallux valgus
  s. hip disease
  s. osteomalacia
  s. osteoporosis
  s. subcapital fracture

senilis
  coxa s.
  malum coxae s.
Senn
  S. plate
  S. retractor
senna
sensation
  altered s.
  catching s.
  diminished s.
  epicritic s.
  exteroceptive s.
  light touch s.
  loss of protective s.
    (LOPS)
  perianal s.
  perineal s.
  phantom s.
  pinprick s.
  protective s.
  return of s.
  sharp s.
  shocklike s.
  touch s.
  vibration s.
sense
  joint position s. (JPS)
  knee joint position s.
  position s.
  vibration s.
Sense-of-Feel prosthesis
sensibility
  articular s.
  s. recovery sequence
sensitivity
  vibration s.
sensitometer
  Poppen ridge s.
sensomotor (*var. of* sensorimotor)
sensor
  capacitive s.
  DermaTemp infrared
    thermographic s.
  magnetic s.
  Myoscan s.
  s. pad
  Perry s.
  Richmond subarachnoid
    screw s.
  Servo Pro force s.
Sensorcaine
Sensorcaine-MPF
SensorHand prosthesis
sensorimotor, sensomotor
  s. deficit
  s. nerve
  s. stimulation approach
sensorineural abnormality

sensory
- s. awareness
- s. component
- s. deficit
- s. delay
- s. evoked potential
- s. examination
- s. fascicle
- s. function
- s. impairment
- s. integration
- S. Integration and Praxis test (SIPT)
- s. loss
- s. motor
- s. motor stimulation (SMS)
- s. nerve
- s. nerve action potential (SNAP)
- s. nerve action potential receptor (SNARE)
- s. nerve action potential receptor complex
- s. nerve conduction velocity (SNCV)
- S. Organization Test (SOT)
- s. organization testing (SOT)
- s. peak latency
- s. polyneuropathy
- s. registration
- s. response
- s. stimulation kit

sensory-motor training
sentinel fracture
Senuva lotion
Seoffert triple arthrodesis
SEP
- somatosensory evoked potential
- midlatency SEP

separation
- AC joint s.
- acromioclavicular s.
- articular mass s.
- atlantoaxial s.
- degree of s.
- fracture fragment s.
- gravitational platelet s. (GPS)
- lamellar s.
- shoulder s.
- sternoclavicular joint s.
- surgical s.
- transepiphysial s.

separator
- abduction knee s.
- finger s.
- Horsley s.
- nerve s.
- Sachs nerve s.
- toe s.

sepses (*pl. of* sepsis)
sepsis, *pl.* **sepses**
septa (*pl. of* septum)

Septacin implant
septal forceps
septi (*gen. of* septum)
septic
- s. arthritis
- s. bursitis
- s. discitis
- s. finger joint
- s. knee
- s. necrosis

SeptiCare antimicrobial wound cleanser
Septisol solution
Septobal bead
septum, *pl.* **septa,** *gen.* **septi**
- Bigelow s.
- fascial s.
- intermuscular s.
- J s.
- Septa Topical Ointment
- vertical s.

Sequeira-Khanuja mini-incision total hip modification
sequela, *pl.* **sequelae**
sequelae (*pl. of* sequela)
sequence
- axial fat-suppressed turbo spin-echo T2-weighted s.
- Carr-Purcell s.
- Carr-Purcell-Meiboom-Gill s.
- coronal T1-weighted s.
- fat-suppressed turbo spin-echo T2-weighted s.
- muscle patterning s.
- sagittal conventional spin-echo proton-density s.
- sensibility recovery s.
- standard imaging s.
- T2-weighted dual-echo s.

sequencing bead patterns set
sequential
- s. compression
- s. compression device (SCD)
- s. compression device stockings
- s. extremity pump
- s. foot compression device (SFCD)
- s. pneumatic compression boot
- s. pneumatic pump traction
- s. pressure
- s. procedure
- s. sectioning

sequentially reamed
sequester
sequestered disc
sequestra (*pl. of* sequestrum)
sequestral
sequestrated disc
sequestration
sequestrectomy
sequestrotomy

S

sequestrum, *pl.* **sequestra**
    avascular s.
    bone s.
    bony s.
    button s.
    s. forceps
    kissing sequestra
    primary s.
    tuberculous s.
SER
    supination-external rotation
    SER (I-IV) fracture
sera (*pl. of* serum)
Seradge hand exercises
Serafin technique
Serax
serendipity
    s. view
    s. view in shoulder radiography
serial
    s. casting
    s. stretch orthoses
    s. wedge cast
series (*pl. of* series)
    Davis s.
    lumbosacral s.
    Option Orthotic S.
    RingLoc acetabular s.
    Valpar Component Work Sample s.
    x-ray s.
Serola sacroiliac belt
seroma
seronegative
    s. arthropathy
    s. enthesopathy and arthropathy
      syndrome
    s. rheumatoid arthritis
seropositive rheumatoid arthritis
serosa
    myositis s.
    peritendinitis s.
serosanguineous
serotonergic neuron
serotonin (ST)
    s. syndrome
serous
    s. abscess
    s. synovitis
serpentine
    s. foam collar
    s. foot
    s. incision
    s. plate
serrated
    s. action potential
    s. fine-cutting knife
    s. scissors
Serratia marcescens
serration

Serrato
    S. forearm pin
    S. forearm rod
serratus
    s. anterior flap
    s. anterior muscle
    s. anterior muscle syndrome
    s. anterior palsy orthosis
    s. anterior paralysis
sertraline
serum, *pl.* **serums, sera**
    s. calcium
serums (*pl. of* serum)
service
    Carticel cartilage-cell culturing s.
Servo Pro force sensor
Servox device
sesamoid
    accessory s.
    bipartite tibial s.
    s. bone
    s. clamp
    s. disruption
    fibular s.
    s. fracture
    s. fracture repair
    hallucal s.
    hallux s.
    s. hyperostosis
    s. injury
    lateral s.
    s. ligament
    medial s.
    tibial s.
    tibial hallux s.
sesamoidectomy
    s. dissector
    fibular s.
    lateral s.
sesamoiditis
sesamoidometatarsal joint
sesamophalangeal ligament
sessile
sessile-type osteochondroma
set
    acetabular trial s.
    Ackerman bone biopsy s.
    ACL guide s.
    aluminum contouring template s.
    s. angle
    s. angle of toe
    AO minifragment s.
    Bankart shoulder repair s.
    bone drill s.
    Brown-Mueller T-fastener s.
    Catalyst anterior instrument s.
    Craig vertebral biopsy s.
    Entrex small joint arthroscopy
      instrument s.

grid maze s.
hand evaluation s.
Harmony PLIF instrument s.
Henning instrument s.
Hollywood bed extension hook s.
Lido lift and work s.
Mini Fragment S.
nail s.
Outcome and Assessment
  Information S. (OASIS)
Oval-8 sizing s.
parquetry s.
prothelen s.
Rousek extraction s.
s. screw
sequencing bead patterns s.
SmartPin instrument s.
Stille bone drill s.
Stille-pattern trephine and bone
  drill s.
vari-balance board s.
volumeter s.

set-hold adjustment
Seton hip brace
Setopress dressing
setter
bone plug s.
setting
bone s.
Mache electromyogram s.
Seutin plaster shears
severance
severe s.
severe
s. kyphoscoliosis
s. rigid thoracic curve
s. severance
Sever heel pain disease
Severin
anatomical classification
  system of S.
S. hip criteria
S. hip dysplasia scale
S. radiographic residual hip
  dysplasia classification
severity
osteoporosis s.
Sever-L'Episcopo
S.-L. repair of shoulder
S.-L. shoulder repair
S.-L. tendon transfer
SEWHO
shoulder-elbow-wrist-hand orthosis
sex-linked muscular dystrophy
sextant rod insertion system
SFA
superficial femoral artery
SFCD
sequential foot compression device

SFEMG
single-fiber electromyography
SFI
sciatic function index
S-flap incision
Sgarlato
S. device
S. hammertoe implant procedure
S. hammertoe implant prosthesis
  (SHIP)
S. toe implant
shadow
elliptical overlap s.
s. shield
shadowing
acoustical s.
Shadow-Line ACF spine retractor system
Shaeffer rigid orthosis
Shaffner orthopaedic inserter
shaft
bone s.
Cloward drill s.
distal third of s.
femoral s.
flexible nailing of the femoral s.
s. fracture
metatarsal s.
middle third of s.
ministem s.
neck s.
patellar reamer s.
proximal third of s.
radial s.
shaken impact injury
sham procedure
shank
s. bone
extended steel s.
steel s.
Zimmer-Hudson s.
shape
Erlenmeyer flask s.
familial s.
s. memory alloy (SMA)
roll-over s.
shaped
knuckle s.
Shapiro classification
sharing
Edwards modular system load s.
sharp
S. acetabular angle
acetabular angle of S.
s. dissection
s. retractor
s. sensation
s. trocar
s. worm hook
sharp/dull discrimination

S

Sharpey
> S. fiber
> S. screw

sharp-pointed wire

Sharp-Purser cervical cord compression test

SharpShooter
> S. tissue repair system
> S. tissue repair technique

Sharrard
> S. iliopsoas transfer technique
> S. posterior transfer of iliopsoas
> S. psoas tendon transfer
> S. tendon transfer technique

Sharrard-Trentani prosthesis

Sharrard-type kyphectomy

Shar-Tek foot positioning grid

shaver
> arthroscopic s.
> automated s.
> Cuda s.
> cutting s.
> Dyonics s.
> Grierson meniscal s.
> Microsect s.
> motorized meniscal s.
> motorized suction s.
> rotating basket s.
> sucker s.
> synovial s.

shaving
> arthroscopic s.
> femoral condylar s.
> s. system

Shaw-Sgarlato hammertoe implant prosthesis

Shaw-SHIP
> S.-SHIP rod
> S.-SHIP rod hammertoe implant

Shea
> S. drill
> S. prosthesis placement instrument

shear
> anterior s.
> s. fracture
> lateral s.
> s. maneuver
> s. stiffness
> s. strain
> s. stress
> s. test
> s. testing
> vertical s.

ShearBan low-friction interface

Shearer rongeur

shearing
> s. callosity
> s. callus

> s. force
> s. injury
> S. posterior chamber implant material

shearling surface

shear-off device

shears
> airplane s.
> Baer rib s.
> Bethune-Coryllos rib s.
> Bethune rib s.
> biarticular bone s.
> Brunner rib s.
> Brunn plaster s.
> Collins rib s.
> Cooley rib s.
> Esmarch plaster s.
> Felt s.
> Giertz rib s.
> Giertz-Shoemaker rib s.
> Gluck rib s.
> Hercules plaster s.
> Lefferts rib s.
> Liston s.
> Liston-Key-Horsley rib s.
> Sauerbruch rib s.
> Seutin plaster s.
> Stille plaster s.

sheath
> arthroscopic s.
> carotid s.
> digital flexor tendon s.
> Endius bipolar s.
> fascia s.
> femoral s.
> fibroosseous s.
> flexor tendon s.
> giant cell tumor of tendon s.
> muscle s.
> nerve root s.
> pigmented nodular synovitis of tendon s.
> rectus s.
> synovial s.
> tendinous s.
> tendon s.
> tenosynovial s.
> visceral tendon s.

sheathed
> s. interference screw
> s. knife

sheath/liner
> Silipos Distal Dip prosthetic s./l.

Sheehan
> S. chisel
> S. gouge
> S. knee prosthesis
> S. osteotome

sheepskin

sheet
    Alpha flat s.
    Antishear gel s.
    Barrier lower extremity s.
    s. cork
    iodoform-impregnated plastic s.
    Korex cork s.
    laparotomy s.
    nonporous s.
    Novagel gel s.
    Ortholen s.
    pelvic s.
    porous s.
    PPT s.
    sterile s.
sheeting
    Carboplast II s.
    circumferential pelvic antishock s.
    silastic s.
    sterile s.
Sheffield
    S. hand elevator
    S. Ring Fixator
    S. rod
    S. support
shelf
    s. acetabuloplasty
    s. flexion
    lateral s.
    medial s.
    patellar s.
    s. pedestal
    s. procedure
shell
    acetabular s.
    AFO standard s.
    s. allograft
    calf s.
    s. impactor
    s. implant material
    Inter-Op acetabular s.
    IROM splint with s.'s
    metal-backed acetabular s.
    protrusio s.
    Reflection Interfit s.
    Restoration Secur-Fit X'tra
      acetabular s.
    semirigid s.
    S-ROM contained s.
    thigh s.
    total hip arthroplasty with internal
      eccentric s.'s (tharies)
    total hip articular replacement by
      internal eccentric s.'s (tharies)
    Unna paste s.
shelling off of cartilage
Shelton
    S. bone screw
    S. femoral fracture classification

shelving
Shenton line
Shenton-Ménard line
Shepherd
    S. internal screw fixation
    S. posterior process of talus
      fracture
shepherd's crook deformity
Sher diabetic shoe inlay
Sherfee prosthesis
Sherform silicone insole
Sherk-Probst percutaneous pinning
Sherlock threaded suture anchor
Sherman
    S. block test
    S. bone plate
    S. bone screw
    S. foot score
    S. remote podiatric vacuum
      system
    S. screwdriver
Sherman-Stille drill
Sherrington reciprocal innervation law
Sherwin knee retractor
ShiatsuBACK back support
Shiatsu therapeutic massage
shield
    AME pin site s.
    arthroscopic s.
    bunion s.
    contact s.
    Nolan system collimator mounted
      contact s.
    protective s.
    shadow s.
    Sof-Gel palm s.
    Sportelli system collimator mounted
      contact s.
shielding
    stress s.
Shier knee prosthesis
Shifrin wire twister
shift
    anterior talus s.
    capsular s.
    glenohumeral s.
    inferior capsular s.
    laser-assisted capsular s.
    lateral lumbar s.
    lateral pivot s.
    lateral trunk s.
    pelvic lateral s.
    plantar s.
    plasma volume s.
    reverse pivot s.
    s. sign
    spinal cord s.
    talar s.
    s. test

S

shift (*continued*)
    trochanteric s.
    trunk s.
shifter
    AliMed Conductive Patient S.
shifting
    vessel s.
Shikata grafting technique
shin
    barked s.
    s. bone
    saber s.
    s. splint
shingling
SHIP
    Sgarlato hammertoe implant prosthesis
Shirley drain
shirt
    EZ T orthopaedic s.
shirt-stud abscess
shish kebab technique
shock
    s. absorption
    s. artifact
    neurogenic s.
    prosthetic stance phase s.
    spinal s.
    s. treatment
    vasogenic s.
shock-absorbent
    s.-a. heel pad
    s.-a. sole
shock-absorbing shoe
shocklike sensation
Shockmaster heel cushion
shockwave therapy (SWT)
shod
    rubber s.
shoe
    accommodative s.
    AccuTread s.
    Acor Quikform I, II s.
    Ambulator H1200 healing s.
    ambulatory s.
    Anywear s.
    Apex Ambulator s.
    Ariat s.
    arthritic s.
    Asics Gel-MC s.
    Balmoral laced s.
    Bebax s.
    Bevin s.
    Birkenstock s.
    Blucher laced s.
    broad-toed s.
    Brooks sports and running s.
    calcaneal spur pad in s.
    Canfield s.
    cast s.

Comed postoperative s.
s. cookie
corrective s.
custom-made s.
custom-molded s.
cutout s.
Dansko s.
Darco Medical-Surgical s.
Darco OrthoWedge healing s.
Darco Softie s.
Darco surgical s.
Darco Wedge s.
depth inlay s.
depth orthopaedic s.
s. dermatitis
diabetic pressure relief s.
Dynaslipper night s.
extended-counter s.
extended steel-shank s.
s. extension
extra-depth s.
s. filler
GaitKeeper cast s.
s. gear
GentleStep s.
Goldenberg footplate s.
healing s.
s. heel pad
HeelWedge healing s.
H1209 healing s.
H1215 healing s.
high heel s.
Hi-Top s.
ill-fitting s.
infant clown cast s.
s. insert
Ipos heel relief s.
Ipos postoperative s.
J&J postoperative s.
laced blucher of s.
s. lift
s. lining
low-heeled s.
low quarter Blucher s.
Markell Mobility S.'s
Markell open-toe s.
Markell tarso medius straight s.
Markell tarso pronator outflare s.
Mephisto Mobils professional s.
s. modification
Moon Boot s.
narrow toebox s.
navicular cookie in s.
neoprene s.
normal last s.
open-toe s.
orthopaedic oxford s.
s. orthotic
OrthoWedge healing s.

oversize tennis s.
Pedors orthopaedic s.
pointed toe s.
postoperative s.
Power Anthro S.
pressure relief s.
Reebok s.
Reece orthopaedic s.
reverse last s.
ribbed-sole s.
rockerbottom s.
SAS s.
Saucony s.
scaphoid cookie in s.
shock-absorbing s.
Softie s.
soft-vamp s.
s. sole
space s.
stiff-soled s.
straight last s.
s. stretcher
tarsal pronator s.
Terrmocork diabetic s.
Thera-Medic s.
therapeutic s.
torque heel s.
Tru-Fit custom-molded s.
Tru-Mold s.
Urban Walkers s.
vamp of s.
Vibram rockerbottom s.
Viking postoperative s.
WACH orthopaedic s.
s. wear
Weaver rockerbottom s.
s. wedge
wedge adjustable cushioned heel s.
wedged s.
wide toe box s.
wooden s.
wooden-soled s.
Xsensibles s.
X-Static silver fiber diabetic s.
Zimmer postoperative s.
Zohar s.

shoe-foot interface
Shoemaker lateral transfibular approach
shooting pain
short

s. arm brace
s. arm cast (SAC)
s. arm fiberglass cast
s. arm gauntlet cast
s. arm navicular cast (SANC)
s. arm splint (SAS)
s. arm sugar-tong splint
s. bone
s. calcaneocuboid (SCC)

s. calcaneocuboid ligament
s. coarse bur
s. curette
s. external rotator
s. fibula
s. fibular muscle
s. fine bur
s. head of biceps
s. leg
s. leg caliper brace
s. leg cast (SLC)
s. leg double-upright brace
s. leg gait
s. leg orthosis
s. leg plaster cast
s. leg splint (SLS)
s. leg syndrome
s. leg walker
s. leg walking brace
s. leg walking cast (SLWC)
s. lever accessory movement
  technique
s. lever specific contact procedure
S. Musculoskeletal Function
  Assessment (SMFA)
S. Musculoskeletal Function
  Assessment questionnaire
s. oblique fracture
s. opponens orthosis
s. plantar ligament (SPL)
s. radiolunate (SRL)
s. radiolunate ligament
s. rib polydactyly
s. segment spinal fusion
s. stature
s. thumb
s. walking cast
s. Z bunionectomy

short-acting block anesthesia
shortened foot
shortening

Achilles tendon s.
closed femoral diaphysial s.
s. collectomy
s. contraction
digital s.
distal Wagner femoral
  metaphysial s.
femoral metaphysial s.
fibula s.
fibular s.
Hoffa tendon s.
leg s.
metaphysial s.
s. metatarsal osteotomy
s. osteotomy
proximal femoral metaphysial s.
proximal Wagner metaphysial s.
skeleton s.

S

shortening (*continued*)
    tibial diaphysial s.
    Wagner femoral metaphysial s.
short-latency somatosensory evoked potential
short-limb dwarfism
short-radius kyphosis
short-range elastic component
short-segment
    s.-s. pedicle screw instrumentation (SSPI)
    s.-s. posterior fixation
    s.-s. transpedicular fixation (SSTF)
shortwave diathermy (SWD)
shot
    fast low-angle s. (FLASH)
    s. wadding
shotgun injury
Shotokan karate
shoulder
    s. abduction immobilizer
    s. abduction orthosis
    s. abduction pillow
    s. abduction positioner
    s. abduction test
    s. amputation
    s. ankylosis
    apprehension s.
    s. apprehension sign
    archer's s.
    s. arm system (SAS)
    s. arthrodesis
    s. arthroplasty
    baseball s.
    s. blade
    s. bone
    bull's eye s.
    s. clock
    s. complex
    s. contracture
    s. controller
    s. cuff
    s. deformity
    s. depression test
    s. disarticulation
    s. disarticulation prosthesis
    s. dislocation
    s. dome
    double contrast arthrotomography of s.
    drop s.
    s. dystopia
    S. Ease abduction support
    flail s.
    floating s.
    football player's s.'s
    frozen s.
    s. girdle

    hatchet-head s.
    s. holder
    s. horn
    s. impingement sign
    s. instability
    s. joint
    s. joint effusion
    knocked-down s.
    s. ladder
    s. lesion
    loose s.
    Neviaser classification of frozen s.
    s. orthosis (SO)
    S. Pain and Disability Index patient questionnaire
    s. pointer
    s. pulley
    s. radiography
    s. range of motion
    s. reduction
    s. repair
    ringman's s.
    s. ROM arc
    round s.
    s. saddle sling
    saline-enhanced MR arthrography of s.
    s. separation
    S. Severity Index patient questionnaire
    Sever-L'Episcopo repair of s.
    s. spica cast
    s. spica splint
    s. strap contusion
    stubbed s.
    s. subluxation
    s. subluxation inhibitor (SSI)
    s. subluxation inhibitor brace
    swimmer's s.
    tennis s.
    terrible triad of s.
    S. Therapy Kit
    weightlifter's s.
    s. wheel
shoulder-elbow-wrist-hand orthosis (SEWHO)
shoulder-girdle syndrome
shoulder-hand-finger syndrome
shoulder-hand syndrome
shoulder-pad sign
shoulder-to-head check
ShowerSafe
    S. waterproof cast and bandage cover
    S. waterproof cast and bandage protector
SHPL
    sacral horizontal plane line

Shriners pin
shrinker
    stump s.
shuck carpal ligament test
shucking
shuffling gait
shunt muscle
Shur-Band self-closure elastic
  bandage
shuttle
    S. Balance trainer
    S. cardiomuscular conditioner
    Caspari s.
    S. MiniClinic resistance system
    S. MVP leg press
    S. Relay suture passer
    s. walking test (SWT)
Shutt Mantis retrograde forceps
Shwachman-Diamond syndrome
Shy-Drager syndrome
SI
    sacroiliac
    SI belt
    SI joint
sialoprotein
    bone s.
sibilant rhonchus
Sibson
    S. fascia
    S. muscle
sicca
    caries s.
    Neisseria s.
    synovitis s.
sickle-cell anemia
sickle-shape Beaver blade
sick scapula syndrome
side
    s. bending
    crest sign s.
    s. cutter
    s. lunge back exercise technique
    s. plate
    posterior rotation on left s.
    posterior rotation on right s.
    s. posture reduction
side-bending
    s.-b. barrier
    s.-b. mobility
side-cut pin cutter
side-cutting
    s.-c. basket forceps
    s.-c. blade
    s.-c. bur
    s.-c. Swanson bar
1-sided dog-ear repair
side-glide test
side-jump test
Sidekick foot support

sideline
    s. assessment
    s. assessment of concussion
    s.'s triage
side-lying
    s.-l. back exercise technique
    s.-l. hip abductor
    s.-l. iliac compression test
    s.-l. position
side-opening laminar hook
sideplate
    s. barrel
    barreled s.
    compression s.
    Richards s.
    sliding compression screw with s.
side-posture position
side-shift
    pelvic s.-s.
side-specific chiropractic adjustment
side-swing plasty
sideswipe
    s. elbow fracture
    s. injury
Siegel hip release
Sielke instrumentation
Siemens
    S. linear accelerator
    S. Sonocur Basic extracorporeal
    shockwave therapy system
Sierra
    S. 2-load voluntary opening
    S. posterior occipitocervicothoracic
    stabilization system
Siffert tibia vara intraepiphysial
  osteotomy
Sifoam padding
sighting device
sigma receptor
sigmoid notch
sign
    abduction s.
    Achilles bulge s.
    adduction s.
    Adson radial pulse loss s.
    alien hand s.
    Allen s.
    Allis s.
    Amoss s.
    André-Thomas ulnar nerve
    paralysis s.
    Anghelescu vertebral tuberculosis s.
    anteater nose s.
    antecedent s.
    anterior drawer s.
    anterior foot draw s.
    anterior hiatal s.
    anterior tibial s.
    anvil s.

S

sign (*continued*)
 Apley s.
 apprehension s.
 arterial occlusion s.
 arthroscopic drivethrough s.
 augmented Tinel s.
 Baastrup s.
 Babinski s.
 bamboo spine s.
 Barlow hip dysplasia s.
 Bassett s.
 Battle skull fracture s.
 bayonet s.
 Beevor s.
 Beevor umbilical movement s.
 benediction attitude s.
 bite s.
 blister of bone s.
 Bloomberg s.
 bone bruise s.
 bone-in-bone s.
 bottle s.
 Bouchard s.
 boutonnière deformity s.
 bowstring s.
 bow-tie s.
 Bragard meniscal injury s.
 Brudzinski s.
 Bryant s.
 Burton s.
 C s.
 camelback s.
 Carman meniscus s.
 cement-wedge s.
 chaddock s.
 Chinese red line s.
 Clark s.
 Clarke knee grind s.
 clawhand s.
 Cleeman s.
 click s.
 cockade image s.
 Codman s.
 cogwheel s.
 Collier s.
 comma s.
 commemorative s.
 Comolli s.
 contralateral s.
 Coopernail s.
 cortical ring s.
 cotton-wool s.
 Cram bowstring s.
 crescent s.
 crest s.
 crowded carpal s.
 Cupid's bow s.
 Cupid's bow contour s.
 Dawbarn s.

 deep lateral femoral notch s.
 Dejerine s.
 Demianoff s.
 Desault s.
 Destot pelvic fracture s.
 dimple s.
 divot s.
 doll's eye s.
 double-arc s.
 double camelback s.
 double PCL s.
 double posterior collateral
  ligament s.
 drawer s.
 drivethrough s.
 drooping shoulder s.
 drop-arm s.
 Dupuytren s.
 Earle s.
 Egawa s.
 elbow fat-pad s.
 Erichsen s.
 eye s.
 fabere s.
 fadir s.
 Fairbanks s.
 Fajersztajn crossed sciatic s.
 fallen fragment s.
 fallen-leaf s.
 fan s.
 fat-blood interface s.
 fat-pad s.
 FBI s.
 finger in balloon s.
 Finkelstein s.
 fishtail s.
 fish vertebra s.
 flag s.
 fleck s.
 flipped meniscus s.
 fluid s.
 fluid-fluid level s.
 Forestier bowstring s.
 fragment-in-notch s.
 Fränkel s.
 Froment nerve palsy s.
 Froment paper s.
 Gaenslen s.
 Gage s.
 Galant s.
 Galeazzi hip dislocation s.
 gear-stick s.
 glenolabral ovoid mass s.
 GLOM s.
 Goldthwait s.
 Gordon reflex s.
 Gottron s.
 Gowers s.
 grab s.

Guilland s.
gun barrel s.
hair-on-end s.
half-moon s.
halo s.
hanging heel s.
Harris-Beath footprinting mat s.
Hawkins impingement s.
head-at-risk s.
heel pad s.
heel varus s.
Helbing s.
hiatal s.
Hill-Sachs s.
Hirschberg s.
Hoffa s.
Hoffmann s.
Homans s.
Hoover s.
hot-cross-bun skull s.
Hueter s.
Huntington s.
H vertebra s.
iliac apophysis s.
impingement s.
incomplete ring s.
intravertebral vacuum cleft s.
inverted Napoleon hat s.
ivory phalanx s.
J s.
jerk s.
jump s.
Kanavel s.
Kaplan s.
Keen s.
Kehr s.
Kellgren s.
Kernig s.
Kerr s.
Klippel-Feil s.
Lachman s.
lamp cord s.
Langoria s.
Lasègue s.
lateral capsular s.
lateral femoral notch s.
lateral gap s.
Laugier s.
Leichtenstern s.
Léri s.
Lhermitte s.
Light V s.
Linder s.
long tract s.
Lorenz s.
Ludington s.
Ludloff s.
Maisonneuve s.
Marie-Foix s.

Martel s.
masses s.
Matev s.
McMurray s.
Mendel-Bekhterev s.
Mennell s.
Meryon s.
milking s.
Minor s.
Morquio s.
Morton s.
movie s.
Mudder s.
Mulder s.
mute toe s.
Naffziger s.
Napoleon hat s.
Neer impingement s.
Nelson s.
neuroma s.
nonorganic physical s.
nutcracker s.
objective s.
obturator s.
ocular s.
Oppenheim s.
Oppenheimer s.
Ortolani s.
painful arc s.
patellar apprehension s.
patellar hesitation s.
pathognomonic s.
Patrick s.
Payr s.
pedestal s.
Pelken s.
percussion s.
peroneal s.
Phalen carpal tunnel syndrome s.
piano key shoulder s.
Piotrowski s.
piriformis s.
piston s.
pivot shift s.
plantar ecchymosis s.
pneumoarthrogram s.
Pollock s.
popliteal pressure s.
positive impingement s.
positive rim s.
posterior column s.
posterior drawer s.
posterior hiatal s.
posterior sag s.
posterolateral drawer s.
posteromedial drawer s.
pronation s.
pronator s.
pseudo-Babinski s.

S

sign (*continued*)
   pucker s.
   Putti s.
   Queckenstedt s.
   rachitic rosary s.
   radialis s.
   Raimiste organic hemiplegia s.
   red, white, blue s.
   Renee knee creak s.
   reverse Hill-Sachs s.
   ribbon s.
   rim s.
   ring s.
   Riordan s.
   Risser s. (grade 1-4)
   Romberg s.
   root tension s.
   Roux s.
   rugger jersey s.
   Rust s.
   sausage digit s.
   Schamroth s.
   Schlesinger s.
   sciatic tension s.
   scotty dog s.
   shift s.
   shoulder apprehension s.
   shoulder impingement s.
   shoulder-pad s.
   somatic s.
   Soto-Hall s.
   Speed s.
   spilled cup s.
   spilled teacup s.
   spine s.
   spur s.
   stair s.
   Stemmer lymphedema s.
   stepladder s.
   step-off vertebral body s.
   stork s.
   straight leg tension s.
   Strümpell s.
   Strunsky anterior arch of foot s.
   suction s.
   sulcus shoulder s.
   supinator fat pad s.
   swallow-tail s.
   swan-neck deformity s.
   teardrop s.
   terminal J s.
   Terry Thomas s.
   theater s.
   thermoregulatory s.
   thick patella s.
   Thomas scaphoid-lunate gap s.
   Thompson Achilles tendon test s.
   Thurston-Holland s.
   tibialis s.

   Tinel s.
   Tinel-Hoffmann s.
   toe spread s.
   toggle s.
   too many toes s.
   tooth s.
   Trendelenburg pelvis s.
   tripod s.
   trolley track s.
   trough line s.
   tuck s.
   tumbling bullet s.
   Turyn back pain s.
   Uhthoff multiple sclerosis s.
   V s.
   vacant glenoid s.
   vacuum phenomenon s.
   Valleix entrapment neuropathy s.
   Vanzetti sciatica s.
   Waddell nonorganic back pain s.
   Waldenström pediatric femoral head
      fracture s.
   Walker-Murdoch Marfan syndrome s.
   Wartenberg little finger abduction s.
   Wartenberg ulnar paralysis s.
   Werenskiold physial separation s.
   wet leather s.
   Wilson osteochondritis dissecans s.
   Wimberger bilateral metaphysial s.
   windshield wiper s.
   wink s.
   winking owl s.
   wrist s.
   Yergason biceps tendon injury s.
SignaDRESS hydrocolloid dressing
signal
   hyperintense s.
   hypointense s.
   intervertebral disc nucleus s.
   s. void
Sigvaris stockings
Siladryl Oral
Silapap
   Children's S.
   Infants' S.
silastic
   s. ball
   s. ball spacer prosthesis
   s. ball therapy
   s. button
   s. drain
   s. finger implant
   s. finger joint
   s. gel dressing
   S. HP-100
   S. HP-100 prosthetic finger
   S. HP-100 prosthetic finger joint
   s. lunate arthroplasty
   s. radial head prosthesis

s. sheeting
s. thumb prosthesis
s. toe implant

silence
electrical s.

silent
s. fascicle
s. hip stage
myoelectrically s.
s. period
s. thrombosis

Silesian
S. bandage
S. bandage prosthetic support
S. belt

Silflex intramedullary prosthesis
Silfverskiöld
S. Achilles tendon lengthening
S. Achilles tendon reconstruction
S. gastrocnemius soleus recession procedure
S. heads of origin of gastrocnemius transplant
S. Morquito variant syndrome
S. osteochondrodystrophy disease
S. syndrome
S. technique
S. tight calf test

silhouette
s. capsulectomy
S. pedicle screw system
S. spinal system
S. therapeutic massage

silicone
s. arthritis
s. breast implant
s. elastomer rubber ball implant
s. gel
s. gel socket insert
s. implant arthroplasty
s. insole
s. material
s. MP implant
s. pad
s. rubber arthroplasty
s. rubber sphere
s. spacer
s. synovitis
s. thermoplastic splinting (STS)
s. trapezium prosthesis
Wonderflex s.
s. wrist arthroplasty

silicone-dacron tendon rod
silicone-only suspension (SOS)
Silicore foot pillow
Silipos
S. digital pad
S. Distal Dip prosthetic sheath/liner
S. gel

S. mesh cap
S. mesh tubing
S. Silicone Wonder Cup
S. suspension sleeve

silk
s. mesh gauze dressing
Owens s.
s. suture

SilkTouch CO$_2$ laser
Sillence osteogenesis imperfecta classification
SiloLiner gel liner
Silon silicone thermoplastic splinting material
Silopad
S. body sleeve
S. toe sleeve

Silosheath
S. gel
S. sock

silver (Ag)
S. and Simon modification of Silfverskiöld procedure
S. bunionectomy
S. bunionectomy procedure
s. dollar
s. dollar technique
s. nitrate (AgNO$_3$)
S. osteotome
s. sulfadiazine

silver-fork
s.-f. deformity
s.-f. fracture

Silver-Thera
S.-T. stocking electrode
S.-T. stockings

Simmonds Achilles tendon rupture test
Simmonds-Menelaus
S.-M. metatarsal osteotomy
S.-M. proximal phalangeal osteotomy

Simmonds-Thompson Achilles tendon rupture test
Simmons
S. and Segil classification system
S. cervical spine fusion
S. chisel
S. crimper
S. double-hole spinal screw
S. Multi-Matic orthopaedic bed
S. osteotome
S. osteotomy
S. plate
S. plating system
S. spinal arthrodesis
S. Vari-Hite orthopaedic bed

Simmons-Martin screw
Simonart band

S

simple
- s. bone cyst
- s. button patellar implant
- S. Calculated Osteoporosis Risk Estimation (SCORE)
- s. dislocation
- s. fifth metatarsal fracture classification
- s. fracture
- s. joint
- s. knee test (SKT)
- s. metatarsus adductus
- s. reaction time (SRT)
- S. Shoulder Test patient questionnaire
- s. shoulder test thermal alteration Thomas traction
- s. suture
- s. syndactyly
- s. synovitis

simplex
- S. cement adhesive
- herpes s.
- hidroacanthoma s.
- S. P bone cement

Simpson
- S. arthrectomy catheter
- S. sugar-tong splint

Simpulse
- S. pulsing lavage
- S. S/I lavage

Sims
- S. position
- S. retractor

simulator
- Baltimore Therapeutic Equipment work s.
- Ergos work s.
- Lido WorkSET work s.
- Spinal Physiotherapy S.
- Work Seat driving s.

simultaneous
- S. Interview Technique (SIT)
- s. remodeling

S incision

Sinding-Larsen-Johansson
- S.-L.-J. knee growth plate lesion
- S.-L.-J. patella inflammation syndrome
- S.-L.-J. patellar tendinitis disease

Sine-Aid IB

Sinequan

Singh
- S. index of osteoporosis
- S. osteoporosis classification
- S. osteoporosis index
- trabecular index of S.

single
- s. axis
- s. axis locking (SAL)
- s. clamp
- s. cross-slot screwdriver
- s. heel rise
- s. limb support
- s. lumbar curve pattern
- s. overhand thoracic curve
- s. pearl-face hip joint
- s. photon emission computed tomography (SPECT)
- s. plantar verruca
- s. proximal portal technique
- s. ray pattern
- s. reference point
- s. reference point instrument
- s. smooth-face hip joint
- s. thoracic curve pattern

single-action rongeur

single-axis
- s.-a. ankle joint
- s.-a. ankle prosthesis
- s.-a. friction knee (SAFK)
- s.-a. knee unit
- s.-a. locking knee (SALK)
- s.-a. Syme Dycor foot

single-blade saw

single-cannula system

single-channel
- MyoTrac s.-c.
- s.-c. surface EMG

single-column fracture

single-condylar graft

single-contrast arthrogram

single-fiber
- s.-f. electromyography (SFEMG)
- s.-f. EMG
- s.-f. needle electrode

single-heel rise test

single-incision fasciotomy

single-leg
- s.-l. spica cast
- s.-l. toe raise

single-level spinal fusion

single-limb stance

single-lobed skin flap

single-onlay cortical bone graft

single-organ athlete

single-panel knee immobilizer

single-photon electrospinal orthosis

single-point cane

single-prong broad acetabular retractor

single-rod construct

single-row exercise

single-sided bone saw

single-slot screwdriver

single-stage
   s.-s. osteomyelitis repair technique
   s.-s. tendon graft
   s.-s. tissue transfer
single-stemmed
   s.-s. silicone hemiprosthesis
   s.-s. toe implant
single-unit pattern
single-use device
sinogram
sinography
sintered
   s. implant prosthesis
   s. titanium mesh
sintering
   cobalt-chrome power s.
   s. of cobalt-chrome powder coating
Sinterlock
   S. implant
   S. implant metal
   S. implant metal prosthesis
sinus, *pl.* **sinus, sinuses**
   air s.
   cervical ligament of tarsal s.
   coccygeal s.
   dermal s.
   s. fracture
   s. histiocytosis
   lunate s.
   Motrin IB S.
   osteomyelitic s.
   peroneal s.
   talar s.
   tarsal s.
   s. tarsi
   s. tarsi region
   s. tarsi syndrome
   tentorial s.
   s. tract
   traumatic s.
sinuses (*pl. of* sinus)
sinusoidal
sinuvertebral nerve
SIO
   sacroiliac orthosis
SIP
   spinal imaging platform
SIPE
   swimming-induced pulmonary edema
SIPT
   Sensory Integration and Praxis test
Siremobil Iso-C3D fluoroscope
Sir Henry Platt shoulder transverse approach
sirolimus
SIS
   Social Interaction Scale
sismotherapy
sisomicin

Sisson fracture reducing elevator
Sistrunk scissors
SIT
   Simultaneous Interview Technique
sit-and-reach
   s.-a.-r. box
   s.-a.-r. test
site, situs
   donor s.
   Evans calcaneal lengthening
     osteotomy s.
   fracture s.
   harvest s.
   hook s.
   nerve entrapment s.
   nonunion of fracture s.
   operative s.
   pin s.
   recipient s.
   tibial insertion s.
sit/stand chair
Sit-Straight wheelchair cushion
sitter
   floor s.
sitting
   s. duct stretch test
   s. flexion
   s. flexion test
   s. knee extension
   s. position
   s. root lumbar spine test
   s. side bend
sit-to-stand
   s.-t.-s. test
   s.-t.-s. training parallel bar unit
sit-up test
situs (*var. of* site)
Sivash hip prosthesis
size
   crosslink plate s.
sized orthotics for children (SOCS)
sizer
   Brannock Device shoe s.
SJA
   subtalar joint axis
SJF
   subtalar joint function
SJK
   Scheuermann juvenile kyphosis
Sjögren syndrome
S-K
   Sauvé-Kapandji
     S-K distal radioulnar joint
     reconstruction
     S-K reconstruction of distal
     radioulnar joint
skate
   arm s.

S

skateboard
skater's gait
Skelaxin
skeletal
    s. age
    s. amyloidosis
    s. bed
    s. defect
    s. deformity
    s. disruption
    s. dysplasia
    s. extension
    s. growth factor
    s. hyperostosis syndrome
    s. hypoplasia
    s. hypoplasia disease
    idiopathic s.
    s. infection
    s. injury score
    s. limb deficiency
    s. maturation
    s. maturity
    s. muscle
    s. muscle fiber
    s. muscle relaxant
    s. pin
    s. repair system (SRS)
    s. stabilization
    s. tissue
    s. traction
    s. tuberculosis
    s. wry neck
skeletal-extraskeletal angiomatosis
skeletally
    s. immature
    s. immature achondroplast
skeleton
    appendicular s.
    articulated s.
    axial s.
    bony s.
    s. hand
    s. shortening
skeletonize
Skelid
skew
    s. flap
    s. foot
skewer
skewering
skewfoot
    complex s.
    s. deformity
ski
    impact-release binding on s.
    walker s.'s
skiagram (*var. of* radiograph)
skiagraph (*var. of* radiograph)
skiagraphy (*var. of* radiography)

skid
    bone s.
    hip s.
    s. humeral head retractor
    Meyerding bone s.
    Murphy s.
    Murphy-Lane bone s.
skier's
    s. fracture
    s. injury
    s. thumb
skijump view
Skil-Care
    S.-C. cushion
    S.-C. cushion grip
    S.-C. reclining wheelchair
skill
    ambulation s.'s
    articulatory s.
    S.'s Assessment Module (SAM)
    Assessment of Communication and
      Interaction S.'s (ACIS)
    Assessment of Motor and Process
      S.'s (AMPS)
    bed mobility s.
    donning-doffing s.
    gross motor s.'s
    Kohlman Evaluation of Living S.'s
      (KELS)
    Milwaukee Evaluation of Daily
      Living S.'s (MEDLS)
    palpatory s.
    Performance Assessment of
      Self-Care S.'s
    physical daily living s. (PDLS)
    Test of Visual-Motor S.'s (TVMS)
    Test of Visual-Perception S.'s
      (TVPS)
Skillbuilder half roll
skilled nursing facility (SNF)
Skillern radius fracture
Skil Saw
skin
    s. adherence
    s. blood flow determination
    s. breakdown
    s. bridge
    S. Care kit
    s. closure
    s. coverage
    s. creaking
    s. crease
    dorsal s.
    s. expander
    s. flap
    s. glue
    s. graft
    s. hook
    hypertrophic s.

s. incision
s. marker
s. necrosis
necrotic s.
nonglabrous s.
s. pencil
perianal s.
s. plasty
s. preparation
s. resistance test
s. restriction
s. rolling
s. slapping
s. slough
s. staple
s. stroker
s. tag
s. tape
s. temperature monitoring probe
s. tension line
s. traction
s. trauma
undermined s.
s. wrinkling test
skin-contact instrumentation
skinfold
s. caliper
s. measurement
skin-gliding test
Skinner pelvic menstruation line
skin-slough
incisional s.-s.
SkinTemp collagen skin dressing
skin-tight cast
skive
skived incision
skiving knife
Sklar
S. bone drill
S. bone saw
S. ligature needle
S. pin cutter
S. wire tightener
Skoog
S. Dupuytren contracture operation
S. female genitalia construction technique
S. hyperhidrosis procedure
S. nasal dorsum technique
S. procedure for release of Dupuytren contracture
SKT
simple knee test
skull
base of s. (BOS)
hot-cross-bun s.
s. pin
s. plate screwdriver

s. tongs
s. traction
skull-occiput-mandibular
s.-o.-m. immobilization (SOMI)
s.-o.-m. immobilization orthosis
skyline
s. radiograph
s. view
s. x-ray view of patella
Skytron
S. bed
S. operating room table
SL
scapholunate
SL cage
SLAC
scapholunate advanced collapse
scapholunate arthritis collapse
slack
motion s.
tissue s.
s. wrist
Slam'r wheelchair
slant
foam s.
OPTP S.
SLAP
superior labrum anterior and posterior
SLAP lesion
slap
foot s.
s. foot gait
s. hammer
slapped
back s.
slapping
s. gait
skin s.
Slatis
S. pelvic fixation
S. pelvic fracture frame
slatted plinth table
SLC
short leg cast
SLE
systemic lupus erythematosus
SLE arthropathy
sled
Penco Walker S.'s
walker s.'s
Sleeper Gripper prosthetic device
Sleep-eze 3 Oral
Sleepinal
Sleepwell 2-nite
sleeve
arthroscope s.
arthroscopy s.
BioCompression Pneumatic S.
circumferential ligamentous s.

S

sleeve (*continued*)
    compression s.
    cylindrical s.
    drill s.
    Edwards-Levine s.
    Edwards modular system spinal s.
    Edwards polyethylene s.
    elbow s.
    Electro-Mesh s.
    epX suspension s.
    excursion amplifier s.
    forefoot s.
    forefoot compression s.
    s. fracture
    gel suspension s.
    heel s.
    Iceflex Endurance suction
      suspension s.
    knee s.
    Knit-Rite suspension s.
    malleolar gel s.
    Mica 3x s.
    monopolar s.
    neoprene elbow s.
    neoprene knee s.
    obturator s.
    Pedifix forefoot compression s.
    periosteal s.
    pin s.
    pneumatic compression s.
    polyethylene s.
    rod s.
    Silipos suspension s.
    Silopad body s.
    Silopad toe s.
    stabilization s.
    Super Grip s.
    thermal s.
    s. type
2-sleeve technique
slide
    flexor pronator s.
    Glassman-Engh-Bobyn trochanteric s.
    head-first s.
    muscle s.
    s. plate
    trochanteric s.
slideboard
    Activ s.
slider crank mechanism
sliding
    s. AFO
    s. arthrodesis
    s. barrel hook
    s. bone graft
    s. compression hip screw
    s. compression screw with sideplate
    s. fixation device
    s. flap

    s. hammer
    s. knot
    s. mat
    s. nail
    s. nail device
    s. plane osteotomy of Samilson
    s. tenotomy
    s. Z-plasty
slightly movable articulation
SlimLine cast boot
Slim Option shoe orthosis
Slimrest
    Core S.
Slimthetics orthotic
sling
    AliMed hemi arm s.
    Ampoxen s.
    s. and reef technique
    arm elevator s.
    Barton s.
    Böhler-Braun leg s.
    collar-and-cuff s.
    cradle arm s.
    CVA S.
    s. dressing
    envelope arm s.
    finger s.
    Fits-All s.
    FoamWrap finger s.
    foot s.
    s. frame
    Glisson s.
    hanging cast s.
    Harris Hemi Arm S.
    Harris splint s.
    s. immobilization
    s. immobilizer
    Jacksonville s.
    Kenny-Howard shoulder s.
    knee s.
    Kodel knee s.
    leg s.
    Legg-Perthes s.
    lymphedema s.
    Mersilene s.
    Murphy s.
    muslin s.
    Nada-Chair Back-Up portable
      back s.
    Pavlik s.
    pelvic s.
    Posey s.
    pouch-type s.
    s. procedure
    Rauchfuss s.
    resting foot s.
    rubber s.
    s. seat sag
    s. seat wheelchair

shoulder saddle s.
sling-and-swathe s.
Slingers arm s.
slinger-style envelope s.
soft tissue coaptation s.
stockinette s.
strap s.
subcutaneous fat s.
s. suspension range of motion
s. suture
swath and s.
Teare surgical s.
Thomas buckle s.
Thomas Kodel s.
thumb s.
triangular arm s.
universal s.
Uni-Versatil s.
Velpeau shoulder s.
Vogue arm s.
volar ulnar s.
Weil pelvic s.
Westfield-style envelope s.

sling-and-swathe
s.-a.-s. bandage
s.-a.-s. sling

sling-dressing
Velpeau s.-d.

Slingers arm sling
slinger-style envelope sling
Slingshot shoulder immobilizer
slip
s. angle
s. angle spondylolisthesis
central s.
conjoined gastrocnemius soleus
fascial s.
flexor digitorum s.
s. joint
lateral s.
s. of tendon

slip-joint pliers
Slip-N-Snip scissors
slip-on finger splint
slipped
s. capital femoral epiphysis (SCFE)
s. disc
s. elbow
s. under femoral epiphysis (SUFE)
s. vertebral apophysis

slipper
Acu-Pressure s.
s. cast
Kite s.
PPCID s.'s
WalkCare s.'s

slipping
s. patella
s. rib

s. rib cartilage
s. rib syndrome

slit catheter technique
sliver of bone
SLL
spinolaminar line

Slocum
S. ALRI test
S. anterior rotary drawer knee test
S. knee maneuver
S. knee procedure
S. knee rotatory instability
maneuver
S. lateral pivot-shift knee test
S. meniscal clamp
S. nail
S. pes anserinus transplant
S. rotary instability of knee test
S. spinal fusion technique
S. splint

Slo-Mo ball
slope
dorsal radial s.
sacral s.
tibial s.

slot
acetabular s.
S. distraction device
glenoid s.
s. table

slot-graft
slotted
s. acetabular augmentation
s. bolt
s. femur plate
s. mallet
s. nail
s. obturator-cannula system
s. tendon stripper

slough
skin s.

slow
s. axoplasmic transport
s. cautery
s. curve progression
s. distraction
s. muscle
s. stretch
s. stretch reflex
s. union

**slow-acting antirheumatic drug
(SAARD)**
SL-Plus stem
SLR
straight leg raising
SLR test
SLR with Bragard test
SLR with external rotation test
SLR with Kernig test

S

SLS
  short leg splint
slumping
  excessive thoracic s.
slump lumbar spine test
slurry
  autogenous bone s.
  bone s.
  matrix-bone marrow s.
SLWC
  short leg walking cast
Sly syndrome
SM
  synovial membrane
SMA
  shape memory alloy
  SMA prosthesis
SMALL
  same-day microsurgical arthroscopic
  lateral approach laser-assisted
  SMALL fluoroscopic discectomy
small
  s. cell osteogenic sarcoma
  s. egress cannula
  s. fracture
  s. fragment screw
  s. lamina spreader
  s. nail spicule bur
  s. patella syndrome
  s. plate forceps
  s. step distraction
small-base quad cane
small-diameter wire
small-headed screw
small-joint stiffness
smart
  S. Balance Master
  S. Balance Master system
  S. Pin
  S. Screw bioabsorbable
    implant
SmartBrace
  S. brace
  S. wrist splint
SmartKnit seamless diabetic sock
SmartPin instrument set
SmartPin/PLLA pin
SmartPReP PRP system
SmartTack fixation
SmartWrap elbow brace
Smedberg
  S. brace
  S. hand drill
  S. twist drill
Smedley dynamometer
SMFA
  Short Musculoskeletal Function
  Assessment
SMI 3000, 5000 bed

smile
  inverted s.
Smillie
  S. cartilage chisel
  S. cartilage knife
  S. knee retractor
  S. meniscal knife
  S. meniscal scissors
  S. meniscectomy chisel
  S. meniscus hook retractor
  S. nail
  S. pin
Smillie-Beaver
  S.-B. blade
  S.-B. knife
Smith
  S. and Ross central slip tenodesis
    test
  S. and Ross early boutonnière
    deformity test
  S. ankle fracture
  S. ankle prosthesis
  S. automatic perforated drill
  S. bone clamp
  S. cartilage knife
  S. dislocation
  S. flexor pollicis longus
    abductorplasty
  S. & Nephew bracing and support
    system
  S. & Nephew medium barbed
    staple
  S. & Nephew reflection acetabular
    cup implant component
  S. & Nephew small barbed staple
  S. PCE
  S. physical capacities evaluation
  S. scissors
  S. STA-peg
  S. subtalar joint arthroereisis
    peg
  S. technique
Smith-Davis Converta-Hite orthopaedic bed
Smith-Lemli-Opitz syndrome
Smith-Petersen
  S.-P. anterior hip approach
  S.-P. cervical-thoracic kyphosis
    repair
  S.-P. chisel
  S.-P. cup
  S.-P. cup arthroplasty
  S.-P. curved gouge
  S.-P. curved osteotome
  S.-P. femoral neck nail
  S.-P. fracture pin
  S.-P. gooseneck gouge
  S.-P. hemiarthroplasty
  S.-P. hip cup prosthesis

S.-P. impactor
S.-P. intertrochanteric plate
S.-P. nail with Lloyd adapter
S.-P. pedicle subtraction osteotomy
S.-P. reamer
S.-P. rongeur
S.-P. sacroiliac joint fusion
S.-P. SI joint technique
S.-P. spine technique
S.-P. straight gouge
S.-P. straight osteotome
S.-P. synovectomy
S.-P. transarticular nail

Smith-Petersen anterior hip surgical exposure
Smith-Richards instrumentation
Smith-Robinson
S.-R. anterior cervical discectomy
S.-R. anterior discectomy with horseshoe-shaped graft technique
S.-R. anterior fusion
S.-R. cervical disc approach
S.-R. cervical interbody fusion
S.-R. interbody arthrodesis
S.-R. spinal fusion operation

Smithwick clip-applying forceps
SMO
stainless steel and molybdenum supramalleolar orthosis
SMO Moore pin
SMO plate
SMO prosthesis

smooth
s. broach
s. cobalt-chromium
s. endoprosthesis
s. muscle
s. muscle hypertrophy
s. Steinmann pin
s. transfixion wire

smoother
Gore s.

smoothie junior bur
smooth-tipped jeweler's forceps
SMPS
sympathetically maintained pain syndrome

SMS
sensory motor stimulation

SMT
spinal manipulative therapy

SNAGS
sustained natural apophysial glides

SNAP
sensory nerve action potential
soluble N-eythyl-maleimide sensitive factor attachment protein
SNAP receptor

snap
s. finger
s. fit
S. fixation pin
S. Lock wire/pin extractor
s. of the whip rupture

snap-fit
s.-f. apparatus
s.-f. device

snap-lock brace
snap-off compression (SOC)
Snap-Pak
Mitek GII S.-P.

snapping
s. hip
s. hip syndrome
s. knee syndrome
s. scapula
s. scapula syndrome
tendon s.
s. tendon
s. thumb flexor

SNARE
sensory nerve action potential receptor
SNARE complex

snare
Zimmer s.

SNCV
sensory nerve conduction velocity

Sneppen talar fracture
SNF
skilled nursing facility

sniffer's position
snooze pillow
snowboarder's
s. ankle
s. fracture

snowboarding injury
Snow-Littler cleft hand release
snowstorm knee
SNS
sympathetic nervous system

snuffbox
anatomic s.

snug
S. seat
s. traction
s. wrap

SO
shoulder orthosis

soak
Betadine s.
Epsom salts s.

soap
Betadine s.

SOC
snap-off compression
SOC pin

S

social
> S. Integration World Health Organization Handicap Scale
> S. Interaction Scale (SIS)

society
> American Orthopaedic Foot and Ankle S. (AOFAS)
> Hip S.
> International Cartilage Repair S. (ICRS)
> International Spine Intervention S. (ISIS)
> Musculoskeletal Tumor S. (MSTS)
> National Academy on Aging S.
> National Down Syndrome S.
> Scoliosis Research S.

sock
> Active s.
> AFO brace s.
> s. aid
> ankle-foot orthosis brace s.
> arthritis s.
> Bio-Wick s.
> Carolon AFO s.
> cast s.
> Comfort Ag prosthetic s.
> Comfort n' Care Seamfree s.'s
> Creative diabetic s.'s
> Dero hole-in-1 prosthetic s.
> diabetic s.
> edema s.
> electrode s.
> gel stump s.
> molding s.
> Orlon with Lycra stump s.
> prosthetic s.
> Regal Acrylic/Stretch prosthetic s.
> Rx Comfort s.
> Silosheath s.
> SmartKnit seamless diabetic s.
> Soft Walk gel s.
> Spandex Lycra 3-ply stump s.
> Strassburg s.
> STS molding s.
> stump s.
> Thorlo s.'s
> Venosan support s.

Sock-Assist device
socket
> adjustable postoperative protective prosthetic s. (APOPPS)
> all-alumina s.
> all-polyethylene s.
> AML s.
> anatomic medullary locking s.
> Arthropor II porous s.
> check s.
> Cinch suction sleeve for BK prosthetic s.

> Clearpro suction s.
> concave loading s.
> endoskeletal s.
> flexible s.
> Flo-Tech prosthetic s.
> s. gauge
> hard s.
> Icex s.
> intermediate s.
> ischial containment s.
> ischial-gluteal weightbearing s.
> metal-backed s.
> modular s.
> patellar tendon s. (PTS)
> patellar tendon bearing s.
> s. pin
> Poly-Dial s.
> polyethylene s.
> preassembled metal-backed s.
> prosthetic s.
> PTB s.
> s. purchase
> quadrilateral ischial weightbearing s.
> rectified s.
> Sabolich above-knee s.
> standard s.
> supracondylar s.
> suspension-type s.
> temporary s.
> total contact s.
> universal frame outer s. (UFOS)
> University of California cuff suspension PTB s.
> unrectified s.
> variable circumference suprapatellar s. (VCSPS)
> s. wrench

Socon spinal system
SOCS
> sized orthotics for children
> SOCS AFO system
> SOCS pad system

sodium (Na)
> ardeparin s.
> bromfenac s.
> butabarbital s.
> Butisol S.
> cefazolin s.
> s. etidronate
> fondaparinux s.
> s. hyaluronate
> s. hyaluronate wound gel
> s. hypochlorite solution
> meclofenamate s.
> naproxen s.
> papain, urea, chlorophyllin copper complex ointment s. (PUC)
> Pentothal S.
> s. phosphate

s. salicylate
thiopental s.
s. thiosulfate
warfarin s.

Sof

S. Airr insole
S. Matt pressure relieving mattress
S. Sole motion control orthotic
S. Sole Sof Gel heel pad

Sofamor

S. spinal device
S. tubular retractor

Sofflex

S. mattress
S. mattress system

Sof-Gel palm shield

Sofield

S. femoral deficiency leg-lengthening
technique
S. femoral deficiency operation
S. osteotomy
S. pinning
S. retractor

SofPulse device

Sof-Rol

S.-R. cast pad
S.-R. dressing

SofSole Airr insole

soft

s. bone
s. bulky dressing
s. callus stage
s. collar
s. collar cervical orthosis
s. copolymer foam
s. corn
s. corset
s. cosmetic cover
s. dressing
s. fibroma
s. socket insert
S. Super Sport orthotic
S. Support Preforms orthotic
s. tissue
s. tissue abnormality
s. tissue abscess
s. tissue biomechanics
s. tissue blade retractor
s. tissue calcification
s. tissue coaptation sling
s. tissue compromise
s. tissue contracture
s. tissue coverage
s. tissue envelope
s. tissue flap
s. tissue graft
s. tissue healing
s. tissue hinge
s. tissue injury

s. tissue integrity
s. tissue interface
s. tissue interposition
s. tissue irritability
s. tissue lesion
s. tissue maladaptation
s. tissue manipulation
s. tissue mass
s. tissue massage
s. tissue mobilization
s. tissue myxoma
s. tissue plication
s. tissue release
s. tissue restriction
s. tissue sarcoma
s. tissue stretching
s. tissue tumor
s. touch hand exerciser
S. Touch stockings
S. Walk gel sock

softball sliding injury
SofTec rigid brace
Softeze water pillow
SoftFlex

S. computer glove
S. Wrist Wear

Softie shoe
Softip monofilament
Softouch Cold/Hot Pack
Softsplint foot splint
soft-vamp shoe
software

Achieve s.
Image-I analysis s.
osteotomy analysis simulation s.
(OASIS)
Yochum chiropractic s.

Sof-Wick dressing
Sofwire cable system
Solanas posterior cervicothoracic fixation
system
solani

Fusarium s.

Solarcaine Aloe Extra Burn Relief
Solcotrans

S. autotransfusion system
S. orthopaedic drainage-refusion
system

sole

Ambulator Bio-Rocker s.
s. insert
s. of foot
plaster s.
PodiAxis orthopaedic s.
Poro-in-between s.
s. reflex
rockerbottom s.
shock-absorbent s.
shoe s.

S

sole (*continued*)
    Texon s.
    Vibram s.
sole-tap reflex
soleus
    accessory s.
    s. complex
    gastrocnemius s.
    s. muscle
    s. syndrome
SOLEutions
    S. custom orthosis
    S. custom orthotic device
    S. prefab orthotic device
    S. soft plus orthotic
    S. sport shell orthotic
Solganal
solid
    s. ankle cushioned heel (SACH)
    s. ankle cushioned heel foot
    s. ankle cushioned heel orthotic
    s. ankle cushioned heel prosthesis
    s. ankle flexible endoskeletal
    (SAFE)
    s. ankle joint
    s. buckling implant material
    s. freeform fabrication
    s. hex bolt
    s. silicone exoplant implant
    material
solitary
    s. bone cyst
    s. enchondroma
    s. fibromatosis
    s. myeloma
    s. osteoma
Solitens transcutaneous electrical nerve stimulation unit
soluble *N*-eythyl-maleimide sensitive factor attachment protein (SNAP)
Solu-Cortef
Solu-Medrol injection
Solurex L.A.
Soluspan
    Celestone S.
solution
    acid-citrate-dextrose s.
    antibiotic and saline s.
    antiseptic s.
    bacitracin s.
    Betadine scrub s.
    Boropak astringent s.
    Bunnell s.
    Burroughs s.
    carbol-fuchsin s.
    colloid s.
    crystalloid s.
    Dakin s.
    dextrose s.

    Duofilm S.
    Esterom s.
    extravasation irrigation s.
    ferumoxide injectable s.
    Fungi-Nail antifungal s.
    Fungoid AF Topical S.
    heparinized Ringer lactate s.
    Hibiclens s.
    iodophor s.
    irrigating s.
    irrigation s.
    LazerSporin-C s.
    Lotrimin AF S.
    minimally invasive s.
    Mycocide NS antimicrobial s.
    Penlac Nail Lacquer topical s.
    Pinnacle Hip S.'s
    povidone-iodine s.
    preservative-free s. (PFS)
    S. prosthesis
    Restore AF antimicrobial s.
    Rotaglide lubricating s.
    saline s.
    Septisol s.
    sodium hypochlorite s.
    sterile saline s.
SOM
    sternal-occipital-mandibular
Soma
    S. compound
    S. Gonio system
    S. pulley system
    S. sacroiliac stabilization
    belt
somatectomy
    subtotal s.
somatic
    s. dysfunction
    s. innervation
    s. muscle
    s. nerve
    s. pain
    s. sign
    s. therapy
    s. visceral disease mimicry
somatization
somatoautonomic
    s. reflex
    s. reflex hypothesis
somatoprosthetics
somatosensory
    s. deficit
    s. evoked potential (SEP, SSEP)
    s. evoked potential monitoring
    s. postural control
    s. test
somatosomatic reflex
somatovisceral correction
Sombra

Somerville
  S. anterior hip approach
  S. bikini incision hip joint
    technique
  S. hip procedure
SOMI
  skull-occiput-mandibular immobilization
  sternal-occipital-mandibular
    immobilization
    SOMI brace
    SOMI orthosis
Sominex Oral
Sommaserene
Songer cable
sonic accelerated fracture healing system
  (SAFHS)
SonoAce PICO portable digital color
  ultrasound system
Sonocut ultrasonic aspirator
sonographic abnormality
sonography
Sonoma anterior cervical plate system
sonometer
  clinical bone s.
  Omnisense 7000S bone s.
  Sahara clinical bone s.
  SoundScan 2000 bone s.
  SoundScan Compact bone s.
  UBIS 5000 quantitative ultrasound
    bone s.
  UBIS 5000 ultrasound bone s.
sonorous rhonchi
Sontec pliers
Sony CCD/RGB DXC-151 color video
  camera
Sorbie calcaneal fracture
  classification
Sorbie-Questor
  S.-Q. elbow
  S.-Q. total elbow prosthesis
    system
sorbitol level
Sorbothane
  S. antivibration glove
  S. heel cushion
  S. II heel cup
  S. insole
  S. orthotic device
  S. recoil pad
  S. rice sheller roller
  S. wrap
Sorbsan
sore
  plaster s.
  pressure s.
  saddle s.
Soren
  S. ankle fusion
  S. foot arthrodesis

soreness
  delayed-onset muscle s. (DOMS)
Sorrells
  S. hip arthroplasty
  S. hip arthroplasty retractor system
  S. posterior condylar chisel
  S. tibia protector plate Sorrells tibia
    protector plate
Sorrel-type snowboard boot
SOS
  silicone-only suspension
    SOS Safe Salon Pedicure Kit
    SOS total hip system
    SOS total knee system
SOT
  sacrooccipital technique
  Sensory Organization Test
  sensory organization testing
SOTO
  step out, turn out
    SOTO technique
Soto-Hall
  S.-H. bone graft
  S.-H. maneuver
  S.-H. sign
  S.-H. spine pain test
sound
  flexible s.
  radiolucent s.
  rigid s.
  tearing s.
sounder
  ball-tipped pedicle s.
  pedicle s.
SoundScan
  S. 2000 bone sonometer
  S. Compact bone sonometer
source
  fiberoptic light s.
  light s.
  Wolf light s.
sourcil fracture
Souter
  S. hip operation
  S. hip procedure
  S. unconstrained elbow prosthesis
Souter-Strathclyde
  S.-S. elbow prosthesis
  S.-S. total elbow system
southern
  s. access
  S. California Orthopaedic Institute
    (SCOI)
Southwick
  S. biplane trochanteric osteotomy
  S. clamp
  S. lateral slip angle
  S. pin-holding apparatus
  S. pin-holding device

S

Southwick (*continued*)
    S. screw extractor
    S. slide procedure
    S. 2-tined retractor
Southwick-Robinson anterior cervical approach
Sox
    Champion Power S.
SP
    sacral promontory
    symphysis pubis
    SP Walker cast
Spa Bed
space
    s. available for cord
    Barouk button s.
    cartilage s.
    costoclavicular s.
    dead s.
    disc s.
    epidural s.
    fascial s.
    first web s.
    haversian s.
    hypoplastic disc s.
    increased lateral
      joint s.
    intercondylar s.
    intercostal s.
    intermetatarsal s.
    interpeduncular s.
    interphalangeal joint s.
    intervertebral s.
    joint s.
    lateral joint s.
    medial clear s.
    midpalmar s.
    narrowed joint s.
    s. of Poirier
    palm s.
    paraphysiological s.
    Parona s.
    popliteal s.
    position in s.
    prevertebral s.
    properitoneal s.
    retroperitoneal s.
    retropharyngeal s.
    s. shoe
    subacromial s.
    subcoracoid s.
    suprasternal s.
    thenar s.
    tibiocalcaneal s.
    tibiofibular
      clear s.
    tibiotalar clear s.
    web s.
spaced apart tangs

spacer
    acetabular s.
    AlloCraft PL allograft s.
    s. bar
    Barouk s.
    bayonet s.
    s. between toes
    bone s.
    Button S.
    ceramic vertebral s.
    Graftech structural allograft
      cervical s.
    Hourglass vertebral body s.
    s. inserter
    InterSpace hip s.
    InterSpace knee s.
    joint s.
    Kinemax s.
    passive s.
    Plexiglas s.
    prosthetic s.
    proximal cement s.
    rubber s.
    silicone s.
    Telescopic Plate Spacer implantable
      titanium s.
    temporary articulating
      methylmethacrylate antibiotic s.
      (TAMMAS)
    tibial s.
    titanium s.
    toe s.
    TraXis Ti alloy s.
    TraXis Vue alloy s.
    trial s.
    true s.
    XPand R radiolucent corpectomy s.
spacer-tensor jig
spacing
    rostrocaudal s.
spade
    s. finger
    s. hand
Spahr metaphysial dysostosis
Spälteholz
    S. bone-clearing technique
    S. preparation
Spandex Lycra 3-ply stump sock
spanner gauge
spanning external fixator
Sparine
sparing
    glycogen s.
    sacral nerve root s.
Spark handheld dynamometer
Spartan jaw wire cutter
spasm
    arterial s.
    carpal pedal s.

muscle s.
paraspinal muscle s.
paraspinous muscular s.
paravertebral muscle s. (PVMS)
peroneal muscle s.
progressive torsion s.
spasmodic torticollis
spastic
s. abasia
s. cerebral palsy
s. diparesis
s. diplegia
s. disorder
s. equinovalgus
s. equinus
s. equinus gait
s. flatfoot
s. gait
s. hand
s. hemiplegia
s. hindfoot valgus deformity
s. intrinsic contracture
s. paralysis
s. paraplegia
s. quadriparesis
s. quadriplegia
s. thumb-in-palm deformity
s. varus hindfoot
spasticity
Ashworth score of muscle s. (0-4, 1-5)
s. measurement
muscle s.
s. treatment
wrist s.
spatial contiguity
spatula
cement s.
s. foot
s. forceps
spatulate thumb
SPD
synpolydactyly
spear
s. tackle
s. tackler's spine
spearing
injurious energy input s.
special
s. Colles splint
Heel Spur S.
S. Seat
specialist
American Board of Physical Therapy S. (ABPTS)
specialized nail
specific
s. adaptation to imposed demand (SAID)

s. adjustment
s. curve
s. thrust manipulation
specimen
cadaveric s.
SPECT
single photon emission computed tomography
Spectazole
spectinomycin
Spectrobid
Spectron
S. EF total hip system
S. hip prosthesis
spectroscopy
fluorescence correlation s. (FCS)
Fourier transform infrared s.
magnetic resonance s. (MRS)
x-ray fluorescence correlation s. (XFCS)
Spectrum tissue repair system
speech aid
speed
S. arthroplasty
S. brace
S. hand splint
S. osteotomy
s. play training
S. radial head fracture classification
S. radius cap prosthesis
S. shoulder test
S. sign
S. sternoclavicular repair
S. V-Y muscle-plasty
speed-lock clamp
Spelcast car seat
Spencer Achilles tendon lengthening
Spence rongeur forceps
Spenco
S. arch support
S. boot
S. insole
S. liner
S. orthotic device
S. Second Skin dressing
S. shoe insert
Spetzler cervical spine anterior transoral approach
SpF spinal fusion stimulator
SPH contact acetabular component
sphenoid, sphenoidal
s. fossa
s. hamulus
wing of s.
sphenoidal (*var. of* sphenoid)
sphenoiditis
sphenoidostomy
sphenoidotomy

S

sphenopalatine ganglion block
sphere
    silicone rubber s.
spherical
    s. bur
    s. gliding principle
    s. reamer
spherical-headed screw
Spherisorb dressing
spherocentric
    s. fully constrained tricompartmental knee prosthesis
    s. knee system
spheroidal joint
sphincter
    s. muscle
    s. tone
sphygmomanometer, sphygmometer
sphygmometer (*var. of* sphygmomanometer)
spica, *pl.* **spicae**
    s. bandage
    s. cast
    freedom thumb s.
    hip s.
    Schmeisser s.
    s. splint
    thumb s.
spicae (*pl. of* spica)
spicule
    bone s.
spider finger
Spiegleman acromioclavicular splint
Spiessel internal screw fixation of mandible
spike
    ball-tip s.
    endplate s.
    Gissane s.
    heel s.
    metaphysial s.
    s. of bone
    s. osteotomy
    supracollicular s.
    s. washer implant
spiked
    s. Darrach-type elevator
    s. ligament washer
spilled
    s. cup sign
    s. teacup sign
spina, *gen.* and *pl.* **spinae**
    s. bifida
    s. bifida aperta
    s. bifida occulta (SBO)
    erector spinae
    thoracolumbar erector spinae

spinae (*gen.* and *pl. of* spina)
spinal
    s. abscess
    s. accessory nerve
    s. accessory nerve injury
    s. analysis
    s. analysis machine (SAM)
    s. anesthesia
    s. angulation
    s. arteriography
    s. artery
    s. arthritis
    s. arthrodesis
    s. axial load
    s. axis
    s. bone density measurement
    s. brucellosis
    s. canal
    s. canal stenosis (SCS)
    s. clearance
    s. column
    s. contour
    s. contusion
    s. cord
    s. cord angiography
    s. cord atrophy
    s. cord block
    s. cord canal
    s. cord compression
    s. cord function intraoperative monitoring
    s. cord injury (SCI)
    s. cord injury without radiographic abnormality (SCIWORA)
    s. cord irritation
    s. cord-meningeal complex
    s. cord migration
    S. Cord Motor Index and Sensory Indices
    s. cord paralysis
    s. cord shift
    s. cord stimulator (SCS)
    s. cord syndrome
    s. cord tethering
    s. cord tract
    s. coronal plane deformity
    s. curvature
    s. decompression
    s. deformity instability
    s. degeneration
    s. distraction
    s. dysarthria
    s. dysraphism
    s. evoked potential
    s. extension test
    s. fascial release
    s. fixation
    s. fixation rigidity
    s. fixation rod

s. fluoroscopy
s. fracture
s. fusion
s. fusion cage tang
s. fusion device
s. fusion pathomechanics
s. fusion position
s. fusion procedure
s. fusion stimulator
s. fusion system
s. fusion technique
s. hitch
s. hydatidosis
s. imaging platform (SIP)
s. implant
s. implant design
s. implant load to failure
s. infection
s. infection biopsy
s. injection therapy
s. injury operative stabilization
s. instability
s. instrumentation
s. joint mobilization
s. learning
s. level
s. lipoma
s. load bearing
s. locking procedure
s. malignancy
s. manipulation
s. manipulative therapy
  (SMT)
s. manual therapy
s. membrane
s. metastasis
s. mobilization technique
s. muscular atrophy (I–III)
s. myoclonus
s. needle
s. neuropeptide response
s. orthosis
s. osteoblastoma
s. osteomyelitis
s. osteosarcoma
s. osteotomy
s. osteotomy stabilization
S. Physiotherapy Simulator
s. posterior ligament
s. process apophysis
s. puncture
s. rod cross-bracing
s. segment
s. shock
s. stenotic myelopathy
s. stereotaxy
S. Technology bivalve TLSO
  brace
s. transverse ligament

s. tuberculosis
s. tumor
s. turning frame
SpinalPak
S. bone growth stimulator
S. II spine fusion stimulator
S. spine fusion stimulator
Spinal-Stim
S.-S. bone growth stimulation
S.-S. bone growth stimulator
spindle
anulospiral ending of muscle s.
s. cell lipoma
s. effect
muscle s.
s. neuroma
spine
achondroplastic s.
adjustment of s.
alar s.
angular s.
anterior column of s.
anterior inferior iliac s. (AIIS)
anterior maxillary s.
anterior occipitocervical s.
anterior superior iliac s. (ASIS)
anterior tibial s.
anterior upper s.
s. apparatus
axial loading of s.
bamboo s.
s. board
cervical s. (C-spine)
Chance fracture thoracolumbar s.
Charcot s.
chiropractic manual manipulation
  of s.
Civinini s.
cleft s.
coccygeal s.
3-column s.
convexity of s.
costotransversectomy for tumor of s.
s. deformity
degenerative lumbar s.
fixation dysfunction of lumbar s.
s. flexion
s. frame
full cervical s. (FCS)
gait, arms, legs, and s. (GALS)
gibbous deformity of s.
iliac s.
ischial s.
s. kinematics
kinetic cervical s.
kissing s.'s
laminectomized s.
lower cervical s.
lower lumbar s.

S

spine (*continued*)
    lower thoracic s.
    lumbar s. (L-spine)
    lumbosacral s.
    lytic s.
    mandibular s.
    maxillary s.
    nasal s.
    osteoporotic s.
    palpation of anterior superior
      iliac s.
    palpation of posterior superior
      iliac s.
    pediatric gait, arms, legs, s.
      (pGALS)
    poker s.
    posterior-inferior s.
    posterior sacroiliac s.
    posterior superior iliac s. (PSIS)
    posterior tibial s.
    S. Power pelvic stabilizer belt
    s. rotation
    rugger jersey s.
    sacral s.
    Scheuermann disease of thoracic
      and lumbar s.
    s. sign
    spear tackler's s.
    thoracic s. (T-spine)
    thoracolumbar s.
    thoracolumbosacral s.
    trochanteric s.
    upper thoracic s.
    variable screw placement
      system-instrumented lumbar s.
SpineCor
    S. nonrigid brace
    S. system
SpineScope
    Clarus S.
spin-lock MRI technique
spinning probe
spinocerebellar
    s. ataxia
    s. degeneration
    s. tract
spinoglenoid
    s. ligament
    s. notch
spinographic angle
spinography
spinolaminar
    s. angle
    s. line (SLL)
spinomuscular paralysis
spinopelvic
    s. transiliac fixation (STIF)
    s. transiliac fixation system
    s. transiliac fixation technique

Spinoscope noninvasive imaging system
spinothalamic tract
spinous
    s. plane
    s. process
    s. process fracture
    s. process osteotomy for spinal
      stenosis
    s. process plate
    s. process wire
    s. process wiring
    s. pull
    s. push
spiral
    s. bandage
    s. cortical reamer
    s. CT
    s. drill
    s. fracture
    s. groove syndrome
    s. humeral groove
    s. joint
    s. line of femur
    s. oblique fracture
    s. oblique retinacular ligament
    s. oblique retinacular ligament
      reconstruction splint
    s. stay
    s. sulcus
    s. technique
    s. trochanteric reamer
Spira scapulothoracic arthrodesis
  procedure
Spirec drill
spiritual healing
spirometer
    Buhl s.
Spittler
    S. ankle disarticulation procedure
    S. 2–stage syme ankle amputation
      procedure
SPL
    short plantar ligament
SPLATT
    split anterior tibialis tendon transfer
    split anterior tibial tendon
    SPLATT procedure
    SPLATT transfer
splayfoot deformity
splaying
    forefoot s.
    s. of toe
splint
    Abbott s.
    abduction finger s.
    abduction humeral s.
    abduction pillow cover s.
    abduction thumb s.
    Abouna mallet finger s.

abutment s.
acrylic cap s.
acrylic template s.
active s.
Adam and Eve rib belt s.
Adams s.
adjustable s.
Adjusta-Wrist s.
A-Force dorsal night s.
Agnew s.
Ainslie acrylic s.
air s.
AirFlex carpal tunnel s.
Airfoam s.
airplane s.
air pressure s.
Air-Soft S.
Alemdaroglu s.
AliMed diabetic night s.
AliMed turnbuckle elbow s.
Alumafoam s.
aluminum bridge s.
aluminum fence s.
aluminum finger cot s.
aluminum foam s.
aluminum hand s.
aluminum wire s.
anchor s.
Anderson s.
angle s.
ankle-foot orthotic s.
anterior acute flexion elbow s.
anterior shin s.
any-angle s.
Aquaplast s.
armchair s.
Asch s.
s. attachment
backboard s.
balanced s.
Balkan femoral s.
ball-peen s.
banana finger extension s.
Banana Split S.
banjo s.
Barlow cruciform infant s.
baseball finger s.
basic hand s.
Basswood s.
Bavarian s.
Baylor adjustable cross s.
Baylor metatarsal s.
Bend-A-Boot foot s.
birdcage s.
Bloom s.
Blount s.
Blue Line ThumbStay s.
Blue Line UNO s.
Blue Line Wrist Control s.

board s.
Böhler-Braun s.
Böhler wire s.
Bond arm s.
s. bone
Boston thoracic s.
Bosworth s.
boutonnière s.
Bowlby arm s.
bracketed s.
Brady balanced-suspension s.
Brady leg s.
Brant aluminum s.
Brooke Army Hospital s.
Browne s.
Buck extension s.
Buck traction s.
buddy s.
Budin hammertoe s.
Budin toe s.
Bunnell active hand and finger s.
Bunnell finger extension s.
Bunnell gutter s.
Bunnell outrigger s.
Bunnell reverse knuckle-bender s.
Bunnell safety-pin s.
Bunny boot foot s.
Burnham finger s.
Burnham thumb s.
Cabot leg s.
Cabot posterior s.
calibrated clubfoot s.
Campbell traction s.
cap s.
Capener coil s.
Capener finger s.
Carl P. Jones traction s.
Carpal Lock cock-up s.
Carpal Lock wrist s.
carpometcarpal s.
Carter s.
cartilage elastic pullover kneecap s.
Chandler felt collar s.
clavicular cross s.
Clayton greenstick s.
clubfoot s.
CMC s.
coaptation s.
cock-up arm s.
cock-up hand s.
cock-up wrist s.
Colles s.
Comforfoam s.
Comforter S.
Comfy elbow s.
composite spring elastic s.
compression sleeve shin s.
Comprifix ankle s.
Cone s.

S

splint (*continued*)
constant tension s.
contact s.
Converse s.
cool IROM s.
Cordon-Colles fracture s.
Cosmolon closure for s.
counterrotational s.
countertraction s.
Craig abduction s.
Cramer wire s.
CTS Gripfit s.
cubital tunnel s.
Culley ulnar s.
Curry walking s.
Darco foot s.
Darco Medical-Surgical shoe and
  toe alignment s.
Davis metacarpal s.
Delbet s.
Denis Browne s. (DBS)
Denis Browne clubfoot s.
Denis Browne hip s.
Denis Browne talipes hobble s.
DePuy aeroplane s.
DePuy any-angle s.
DePuy coaptation s.
DePuy open-spindle s.
DePuy open-thimble s.
DePuy-Pott s.
DePuy rocking leg s.
DePuy rolled Colles s.
dermal interposition s.
derotator s.
DeRoyal LMB finger s.
digit s.
Digit-Aide fifth toe s.
DonJoy knee s.
DonJoy wrist s.
dorsal extension block s.
dorsal wrist s.
dorsiflexion foot s.
Dorsiwedge night s.
double-occlusal s.
double sugar-tong s.
dropfoot s.
drop wrist s.
Dupuytren s.
Duran-Houser wrist s.
Dyna knee s.
dynamic s.
Early Fit night s.
Easton cock-up s.
Easy Access foot s.
Eaton s.
Eggers contact s.
Elastomull s.
elbow extension s.
elbow flexion s.

elephant-ear clavicular s.
Engelmann thigh s.
Engen palmar wrist s.
Erich s.
Extend-It finger s.
extension block s.
Ezeform s.
felt collar s.
fence s.
Ferciot tiptoe s.
fiberglass s.
Fillauer night s.
finger cot s.
finger extension clockspring s.
finger flexion s.
Finger-Hugger s.
finger sled s.
finger s. (type 501, 502, 504, 602)
Firm D-Ring wrist support s.
flat s.
flexor hinge s.
fold-over finger s.
footdrop night s.
forearm s.
Formatray mandibular s.
Forrester s.
Foster s.
Fox clavicular s.
Fractomed s.
fracture s.
Framer s.
Freedom neutral position s.
Freedom Omni Progressive s.
Freedom Progressive Resting s.
Freedom SportsFit s.
Freedom ultimate grip s.
Frejka pillow s.
Friedman s.
frog-leg s.
Froimson s.
full-hand s.
full-occlusal s.
functional s.
Funsten supination s.
Futuro s.
gait lock s. (GLS)
Gallows s.
Galveston s.
Ganley s.
Gibson s.
Gilchrist s.
Gilmer s.
Gordon s.
Gunning s.
gutter s.
hairpin s.
half ring leg s.
half-shell s.
hallux valgus night s.

Hammond s.
hand cock-up s.
Hanna night s.
Hare compact traction s.
Harrington outrigger s.
Harris s.
Hart extension finger s.
Heal Well night s.
Heel Free s.
hinged cylinder s.
hinged Thomas s.
HIPciser abduction s.
Hirschtick utility shoulder s.
Hodgen hip s.
Hodgen leg s.
humeral fracture abduction s.
HV NightSplint s.
HV SoftSplint s.
Ilfeld s.
Ilfeld-Gustafson s.
incremental range of motion s.
infant abduction s.
inflatable elbow s.
Innoboot s.
IROM bilateral s.
IROM Regal s.
Isoprene plastic s.
Jacoby bunion s.
Jacoby heel s.
James s.
Jet-Air s.
Joint-Jack finger s.
Jonell countertraction finger s.
Jonell thumb s.
Jones arm s.
Jones metacarpal s.
Jones traction s.
Joseph s.
Kanavel cock-up s.
Karfoil s.
Kazanjian s.
Keller-Blake half-ring s.
Keller-Blake leg s.
Kenny-Howard s.
Kerr abduction s.
Keystone s.
kinetic s.
Kleinert s.
Klenzak double-upright s.
knee brace s.
knee immobilizer s.
knuckle-bender s.
lace-lock ankle s.
ladder s.
Lambrinudi s.
leaf s.
Levis arm s.
Lewin finger s.
Lewin-Stern finger s.

Lewin-Stern thumb s.
Liberty One s.
s. liner
Link Stack Split S.
Link toe s.
Liston s.
live s.
LMB finger s.
LMB wire-foam economical
  resting s.
Lockhart toe s.
long arm s. (LAS)
long leg s.
loop-lock cock-up s.
Love s.
Lynx wrist, hand, finger orthosis
  arm positioner s.
Lytle metacarpal s.
magnet s.
Magnuson abduction humeral s.
malleable metal finger s.
Malmö hip s.
Mason s.
Mason-Allen Universal hand s.
Mayer s.
McGee s.
McIntire s.
McLeod padded clavicular s.
memory s.
metal s.
Middeldorpf s.
Moberg s.
modified Oppenheimer s.
Mohr finger s.
molded posterior plaster s.
Murphy s.
Murray-Jones arm s.
Murray-Thomas arm s.
Neubeiser adjustable forearm s.
neutral position s.
New Mind Set toe s.
N'ice Stretch night s.
night s.
occlusal s.
OCL volar s.
O'Donoghue knee s.
O'Donoghue stirrup s.
OEC s.
O'Malley jaw fracture s.
open-air s.
Oppenheimer spring wire s.
Oppenheimer with reverse
  knuckle-bender s.
opponens s.
Orfit s.
Ortho-Glass s.
Ortho-last s.
Orthomedics Stretch and Heel s.
Ortho-Mold s.

S

splint (*continued*)
orthopaedic strap clavicular s.
Orthoplast isoprene s.
outrigger s.
Oval-8 ring s.
padded aluminum s.
padded board s.
padded plywood s.
padded tongue blade s.
s. padding
palmar cock-up s.
palmar wrist s.
pan s.
s. pan netting
passive night stretch s.
Pavlik harness s.
Peabody s.
Pearson attachment to Thomas s.
pelvic s.
PF Night Splint II s.
PFO night s.
Phelps s.
Phillips s.
Phoenix Outrigger s.
pillow s.
Pil-O-Splint wrist s.
plantar fasciitis night s.
plantar fasciitis orthosis s.
Plastalume bulb-ended s.
Plastalume straight s.
plaster of Paris s.
plaster slab s.
pneumatic s.
4-point IROM s.
Polycentric Hinged Ulnar
  Deviation S.
Polyform s.
polyvinyl alcohol s.
Pond adjustable s.
Ponseti s.
poroplastic s.
Porzett s.
Postalume finger s.
posterior mold s.
Potts s.
Pro-glide s.
Progress s.
4-prong finger s.
Protecto s.
Pucci s.
Puth abduction s.
Putti s.
QualCraft s.
QuickCast s.
Quik s.
Radial Hinged Ulnar Deviation S.
radial slab s.
radiolucent s.
ratchet flexor tenodesis s.

Redi-Around finger s.
resting pan s.
reverse knuckle-bender s.
Robert Jones s.
Roger Anderson s.
Rolyan AquaForm wrist and thumb
  spica s.
Rolyan Gel Shell spica s.
Rosen s.
Rumel aluminum bridge s.
Russell s.
safety pin s.
Sager traction s.
SAM s.
Saturn carpal tunnel s.
Sayre s.
Scott ankle s.
Scott humeral s.
Scottish Rite s.
Scott uniform tennis elbow s.
Seattle s.
shin s.
short arm s. (SAS)
short arm sugar-tong s.
short leg s. (SLS)
shoulder spica s.
Simpson sugar-tong s.
slip-on finger s.
Slocum s.
SmartBrace wrist s.
Softsplint foot s.
special Colles s.
Speed hand s.
spica s.
Spiegleman acromioclavicular s.
spiral oblique retinacular ligament
  reconstruction s.
spreading hand s.
spring cock-up s.
spring-wire safety pin s.
Stack s.
Stader s.
static s.
Stax fingertip s.
stirrup plaster s.
Stock finger s.
strap clavicular s.
Stretch and Heel night s.
Stromeyer s.
structural aluminum malleable s.
Stuart Gordon hand s.
Stubbs acromioclavicular s.
sugar-tong plaster s.
surgical s.
suspension s.
swan-neck s.
Swanson dynamic toe s.
Swanson hand s.
synergistic wrist motion s.

Synergy s.
Taylor s.
tennis elbow s.
tension night s. (TNS)
T-finger s.
therapeutic s.
thermoplastic s.
Thomas full-ring s.
Thomas hinged s.
Thomas knee s.
Thomas leg s.
Thomas posterior s.
Thomas suspension s.
Thompson modification of Denis
  Browne s.
Thumbkeeper s.
thumb spica s.
thumb web s.
ThumSaver CMC Long s.
ThumSaver CMC Short s.
ThumSaver MP s.
ThumZ'Up thumb s.
Toad finger s.
Tobruk s.
toe alignment s.
Toronto s.
torsion bar s.
traction s.
triangular pillow s.
turnbuckle elbow s.
ulnar gutter s.
universal acromioclavicular s.
universal gutter s.
universal support s.
Urias air s.
Urias pressure s.
U-splint s.
U-stirrup s.
Valentine s.
Van Arsdale triangular s.
Velcro extenders s.
VersaWrist wrist s.
Vesely s.
volar plaster s.
Volkmann s.
von Rosen abduction s.
von Rosen cruciform s.
Wanchik neutral
  position s.
Weil s.
well-leg s.
well-padded s.
Wertheim s.
Wheaton bunion s.
Wilson s.
Winter s.
wire grip finger s.
wire grip toe s.
wraparound s.

WristJack wrist s.
wrist motion s.
wrist rest s.
yucca wood s.
Zimfoam s.
Zimmer airplane s.
Zimmer clavicular cross s.
Zim-Trac traction s.
Zollinger s.
Zucker s.
splintage
splinted in position of function
splintered fracture
splinting
  dynamic s.
  s. material
  s. method
  night s.
  pelvic s.
  silicone thermoplastic s. (STS)
  Strong dorsal extension block PIP
    joint s.
  s. therapy
splintlike pain
split
  s. anterior tibialis tendon transfer
    (SPLATT)
  s. anterior tibial tendon
    (SPLATT)
  s. anterior tibial tendon procedure
  s. calvarial bone graft
  s. foot
  s. fracture
  s. hand
  s. heel approach
  s. heel fracture
  s. heel incision
  s. incision
  longitudinal tendon s.
  s. patellar approach
  s. pelvis
  peroneus brevis s. (PBS)
  s. Russell skeletal traction
  s. screen
  s. stirrup
  s. table
split-depression fracture
split-finger hook
split-hand deformity
split-nail deformity
split-thickness
  s.-t. skin excision (STSE)
  s.-t. skin graft (STSG)
spoke-wheel configuration
sponastrime dysplasia
spondylalgia
spondylarthritis
spondylectomy
  margin-free s.

S

spondylexarthrosis
spondylitis
>ankylosing s.
>Bekhterev rheumatoid s.
>Bekhterev-Strümpell s.
>s. deformans
>hypertrophic s.
>juvenile-onset ankylosing s.
>Kümmell s.
>Marie-Strümpell s.
>pyogenic s.
>rheumatoid s.
>tuberculous s.

spondylizema
spondyloarthropathy
>destructive s.
>inflammatory s.
>sacroiliac joint inflammatory s.

spondyloarthrosis
spondylodesis
>ventral derotation s. (VDS)

spondylodiscitis
>pyogenic s.

spondylodynia
spondyloepimetaphysial
>s. dysplasia
>s. dysplasia, (sponastrime type)

spondyloepiphyseal (*var. of* spondyloepiphysial)
spondyloepiphysial, spondyloepiphyseal
>s. dysplasia (SED)
>s. dysplasia congenita
>s. dysplasia of Maroteaux
>s. dysplasia tarda

spondylogenic
spondylolisthesis
>anteroinferior s.
>5 classifications of s.
>congenital s.
>degenerative s.
>doweling s.
>dysplastic s.
>Gill-Manning-White surgical treatment of s.
>high-grade s.
>isthmic s.
>lumbosacral s.
>Meyerding classification for s. (grade I-IV)
>Meyerding s. (grade I-IV)
>nondegenerative s.
>pathologic s.
>postlaminectomy 2-level s.
>s. reduction
>s. reduction fixation
>sagittal roll s.
>slip angle s.
>symptomatic s.

>traumatic s.
>Wiltse and Winter surgical treatment of s.

spondylolisthetic
>s. change
>s. pelvis

spondylolysis
>cervical s.
>contralateral s.

spondylomalacia
spondylometer
spondylopathy
spondylophyte
spondyloptosis
spondylopyosis
spondyloschisis
spondylosis
>central spine s.
>cervical s.
>s. deformans
>degenerative s.
>dystrophic s.
>hyperostotic s.
>lumbar s.
>Nurick classification of s.
>rhizomelic s.
>Scheuermann dystrophic s.
>thoracolumbar s.

spondylosyndesis
spondylotherapy
spondylotic
>s. bar
>s. spur

spondylotomy
sponge
>absorbable gelatin s.
>Adaptic s.
>bone wax and gelatin s.
>buffing s.
>s. clamp
>EZ Bend s.
>gauze s.
>Helistat absorbable collagen hemostatic s.
>Instat collagen s.
>laparotomy s.
>Mikulicz s.
>Pedic s.
>Ray-Tec s.
>Spongostan absorbable gelatin s.
>s. stick
>Telfa s.
>s. test
>Vistec x-ray-detectable s.

sponge-holding forceps
spongialization
spongiosa
>primary s.
>s. screw

spongiosum
osteoma s.
Spongostan absorbable gelatin sponge
spongy
s. appearance
s. bone
Sponsel oblique metatarsal osteotomy
spontaneous
s. activity
s. amputation
s. fracture
s. hyperemic dislocation
s. median neuropathy
s. postfracture epiphysiodesis
s. rupture
s. vacuum phenomenon
s. wrist clunk
spoon
maroon s.
meniscal s.
s. plate
Sporanox
Sporothrix schenckii
sporotrichosis
sport
S.'s Activity Scale
s.'s anemia
s.'s anemia exercise
s.'s chiropractic
s.'s injury
lateral motion racket s.
s.'s medicine
s.'s medicine law
s.'s participation
pivoting s.'s
S.'s Plus II back belt
S. Preforms orthotic
stop-and-go s.'s
s.'s tape
s.'s terminal device
S'port
S. Max back support
S. Max sacroiliac belt
S. Max stabilization pad
Posture S.
Scully Hip S.
SportCord exercise and rehabilitation system
Sportelli system collimator mounted contact shield
Sporthotics orthotic
Sport-Rite
S.-R. Olympian device
S.-R. orthotic
S.-R. Runner device
Sports-Caster I, II knee brace
Sportscreme
Sports-Grip bar

sportsman's
s. groin
s. hernia
s. toe
SportsRAC arm care system
Sportstim
S. muscle stimulation electrode
S. stimulator
Sport-Stirrup orthosis
SporTX
S. pulsed direct current stimulator
S. stimulation device
spot
café au lait s.
de Morgan s.
s. film
s. radiograph
s. view
s. weld
spot-face reamer
Spotorno
cementless S. (CLS)
S. cementless hip arthroplasty stem
S. hip prosthesis
S. index
spotted bone disease
SPR
selective posterior rhizotomy
superior peroneal retinaculum
Sprague orthopaedic arthroscopic technique
sprain
acromioclavicular s.
ankle s.
anterior cruciate s.
anterior talofibular s.
calcaneofibular s.
chronic ankle s.
chronic foot s.
deltoid s.
deltoid ligament s.
fibular collateral s.
foot s.
s. fracture
hyperanteflexion s.
inversion ankle s.
joint s.
lateral ankle s.
lateral collateral s.
ligament rupture s.
medial collateral s.
postacute s.
posterior cruciate s.
posterior oblique s.
relapsing ankle s.
rider's s.
syndesmotic s.

S

sprain (*continued*)
   talocrural s.
   talonavicular s.
   tibiofibular s.
sprained ankle syndrome
Spratt
   S. bone curette
   S. mastoid curette
spray
   air plasma s. (APS)
   AliCool splint s.
   s. and stretch
   s. and stretch technique
   Aqua S.
   Dermagran s.
   Fluori-Methane topical s.
   HandClens ultra antiseptic s.
   L'Aprina topical s.
   low-pressure plasma s. (LLPS)
   Miacalcin nasal s.
   Ony-Clear S.
   Prevacare s.
   Proderm topical s.
   Stopain Spray topical
      analgesic s.
   vasocoolant s.
spread
   s. foot
   Fowler s.
   s. hand
spreader
   Bailey rib s.
   s. bar
   Beeson cast s.
   Beeson plaster s.
   Blount bone s.
   Blount laminar s.
   Bobechko s.
   bone s.
   Burford-Finochietto rib s.
   Burford rib s.
   calcaneal s.
   Cloward s.
   Haglund-Stille plaster s.
   Harrington s.
   Henning cast s.
   Henning plaster s.
   Inge s.
   laminar s.
   Lilienthal rib s.
   M-Pact cast s.
   Nelson rib s.
   Schink metatarsal s.
   small lamina s.
   TSRH eyebolt s.
   Weinraub joint and calcaneal s.
spreading
   s. forceps
   s. hand splint

Sprengel high-grade dislocation of scapula deformity
spring
   s. angled adjustable barbell
   s. cock-up splint
   compression s.
   s. finger
   s. fixation
   Gruca-Weiss s.
   internal fixation s.
   s. ligament
   s. ligament complex
   s. lumbar spine test
   s. pin
   s. plate
   s. swivel thumb
   Weiss s.
Springlite
   S. Advantage DP
   S. G foot component
   S. II foot component
   S. lower limb prosthesis
   S. low profile Symes II
   S. polyolefin BK cover
   S. polyurethane AK, BK conical
      cover
   S. super low profile Symes II
   S. toe filler
spring-loaded
   s.-l. knee lock
   s.-l. lock orthosis
   s.-l. nail
spring-mounted electromagnet
spring-wire
   s.-w. ankle-foot orthosis
   s.-w. safety pin splint
sprint
   S. Climber
   S. cross trainer
   S. Runner
sprinter's fracture
Spri Xercise board
sprung pelvis
SPS
   scapuloperoneal syndrome
   stiff person syndrome
S.P. 100 transcutaneous electrical neural stimulator
spur
   acromial s.
   anterior impingement s.
   bone s.
   calcaneal s.
   calcific s.
   cartilaginous s.
   chondroosseous s.
   degenerative s.
   fibrous s.
   s. formation

heel s.
impingement s.
inferior s.
osteophytic s.
s. pad
painful s.
plantar calcaneal s.
posterior s.
prominent s.
retrocalcaneal s.
s. sign
spondylotic s.
subacromial s.
traction s.
uncovertebral s.
spur-crushing clamp
spuria
pelvis s.
spurious
s. ankylosis
s. articular process
s. rib
s. spinous process
s. torticollis
Spurling
S. cervical foraminal compression
maneuver
S. cervical nerve root impingement
maneuver
S. cervical nerve root impingement
test
S. cervical spine test
S. rongeur
Spurling-Kerrison
S.-K. rongeur forceps
S.-K. upbiting and downbiting
rongeur
spurring
anterior s.
bony s.
degenerative s.
inferior s.
spurt
adolescent growth s.
s. muscle
Spurway brittle bones syndrome
Spurway-Eddowes brittle bones
syndrome
squamooccipital bone
squamous cell
squamous-type bone
square
S. Module Seating System
rocker balance s.
square-ended
s.-e. distraction rod
s.-e. hook
square-end pliers
square-hole broach

square-hollow chisel
square-shaped
s.-s. awl
s.-s. wrist test
squashed nose
squat
s. jump
s. lift
s. test
squatting
s. ability
s. test
squeeze
s. ball
s. dynamometer
s. exerciser
Schaffer s.
s. test
squinting patella
SR
sarcoplasmic reticulum
sustained release
Indocin SR
SRF
semirigid fiberglass cast
SRL
short radiolunate
SRL ligament
SRN
superficial radial nerve
S-ROM
S-ROM acetabular cup
S-ROM Arthropor (I-III) prosthesis
S-ROM Arthropor oblong prosthesis
S-ROM contained shell
S-ROM femoral stem prosthesis
S-ROM hip prosthesis
S-ROM hip replacement system
S-ROM modular femoral component
S-ROM modular stem
S-ROM modular total knee system
S-ROM Poly-Dial insert
S-ROM proximally modular total
hip system
S-ROM Super Cup
S-ROM super cup prosthesis
S-ROM ZZT (I, II) prosthesis
SR-PLLA
self-reinforcing polylevolactic acid
SRS
skeletal repair system
SRS injectable cement
SRT
simple reaction time
SS
suture system
synovial sarcoma
SSCS
segmental spinal correction system

S

SSEP
somatosensory evoked potential

S-shaped
S-s. deformity
S-s. foot
S-s. incision

SSHR
steady state heart rate

SSI
School Setting Interview
segmental spinal instrumentation
shoulder subluxation inhibitor
anterior-posterior fusion with SSI
SSI brace

SSO
sagittal split osteotomy

S-Soles insole

SSPI
short-segment pedicle screw
instrumentation

SSRS
subjective shoulder rating scale

SST
stainless steel rod

SSTF
short-segment transpedicular fixation

ST
scapulothoracic
serotonin

stab
s. incision
s. wound
s. wound arthroscopic entry portal

stabilimetry

stability
angular screw s.
ankle s.
elbow s.
glenohumeral joint s.
immediate postoperative s. (IPS)
knee s.
lateral s.
ligamentous s.
limits of s. (LOS)
lumbar spine rotational s.
posterior s.
rotary s.
tibiotalar s.
S. total hip system

stabilization
anterior short-segment s.
s. approach
atlantoaxial s.
cervical spine s.
cervicothoracic junction s.
definitive s.
distal radioulnar joint s.
dynamic lumbar s.
flexion compression spine injury s.

foot s.
fracture s.
iliac crest bone graft s.
interbody s.
lower cervical spine posterior s.
myoplastic muscle s.
occipitocervical s.
odontoid fracture s.
s. of chevron procedure
open s.
patellar tendon s. (PTS)
s. plate
posterior lower cervical spine s.
posterior odontoid s.
prophylactic operative s.
provisional s.
rhythmic s.
sacral spine s.
screw s.
skeletal s.
s. sleeve
spinal injury operative s.
spinal osteotomy s.
subluxation s.
thoracolumbar spine s.
time to s.
s. training
TSRH crosslink s.
wire s.

stabilizer
Ace Pelvic S.
ankle s.
Dynamic foot s.
foot s.
forearm s.
Freedom thumb s.
Heel Hugger therapeutic heel s.
kneecap s.
KT-1000 foot s.
Palumbo ankle s.
patellar s.
secondary s.
Verteflex arthrotonic s.

stabilizing
s. bar
s. hinge
s. reversal

stable
s. burst fracture
s. cervical spine injury
s. gait
s. hinge joint
s. reduction
s. to motion
s. vertebra

Stablecut sawblade

Stableloc
S. Colles fracture external fixator
S. external wrist fixation system

S. II external fixation
S. II external fixation system
stack
S. shoulder procedure
S. splint
stacked plating
stacking cone
Stader
S. pin
S. pin guide
S. splint
Stadol NS
2-stage
2-s. hip fusion
2-s. Syme amputation
2-s. tendon grafting technique
2-s. tendon graft reconstruction
stage
distractive-flexion s. (DFS)
Enneking disease s.
Greulich-Pyle skeletal maturation s.
hard callus s.
implant s.
late s.
S. model of industrial rehabilitation
Risser s.
silent hip s.
soft callus s.
1-stage amputation
staged procedure
Stagesic
staggered procedure
staggering gait
staging
Cierny-Mader osteomyelitis s. (type I-V)
Enneking malignant bone tumor s.
Functional Assessment S. (FAST)
HAVS s. (0–4)
Lichtman lunatomalacia s.
Outerbridge degenerative arthritis s.
Stockholm hand-arm vibration syndrome (1–4) s.
Waldenström s.
Stagnara
S. gouge
S. intraoperative wake-up test
stagnation
foot s.
qi s.
Staheli
S. acetabular shelf procedure
S. congenital hip dislocation containment technique
S. hip osteotomy shelf procedure
S. pediatric hip extension test
S. pediatric lower extremity rotational profile

S. pediatric lower extremity test
S. pediatric technique
Stahl
S. Kienbock disease classification
S. lunate disease index
S. lunatomalacia classification (I-V)
S. lunatomalacia staging system
stain
Gram s.
port-wine s.
reticulin s.
Verhoeff s.
stainless
s. steel
s. steel alloy
s. steel and molybdenum (SMO)
s. steel clamp
s. steel equipment
s. steel implant metal prosthesis
s. steel mesh
s. steel plate
s. steel rod (SST)
s. steel screw
s. steel staple
s. steel wire
stair
s. running test
s. sign
staircase phenomenon
StairClimber assist device
stairclimber's foot
stair-climbing exercise
StairMaster exercise system
stairstep
cervical s.
s. fracture
STALIF
stand alone lumbar intervertebral fusion
STALIF interbody construct
STALIF single incision (360°)
STALIF TT VBR
stall bar
Stamm
S. metatarsal osteotomy
S. method
S. procedure for intraarticular hip fusion
S. temporary gastrostomy procedure
stamp
Gelfoam s.
stamping gait
stance
s. angle
calcaneal s.
double-leg s.
frontside snowboard s.
initial s.
late s.

S

stance (*continued*)
  s. phase
  s. phase of gait
  s. phase walking
  single-limb s.
  terminal s.
  through s.
stand
  s. alone lumbar intervertebral fusion (STALIF)
  Atlas adjustable s.
  Cherf cast s.
  Grand Stand support s.
  heel s.
  IMP turnstile casting s.
  stork s.
  turnstile casting s. (TCS)
  Versa-Helper floor s.
standard
  s. deviation
  S. E-Z-On Vest
  s. goniometric measure
  s. imaging sequence
  s. 2-inch blade retractor
  s. 4-inch blade retractor
  s. medullary nail
  s. shell ankle-foot orthosis
  s. socket
  s. thoracotomy
  s. U patellar support
standardized
  S. Assessment of Concussion (SAC)
  s. growth curve
standing
  s. apprehension test
  s. arm elevation test
  s. dorsoplantar view
  s. flexion
  s. flexion test
  s. frame orthosis
  s. Gillet sacroiliac joint motion test
  s. knee bend PSIS-sacrum contact
  s. lateral view
  s. side bend
  s. stability walking component
  s. weightbearing view
Stanford Hypnotic Clinical Scale
Stanisavljevic knee reconstruction technique
Stanmore
  S. knee replacement
  S. shoulder arthroplasty
  S. shoulder prosthesis
  S. total hip replacement
  S. totally constrained elbow prosthesis
Staodyne EMS + 2 neurostimulator
stapedial tenotomy

STA-peg
  subtalar arthroereisis peg
  STA-peg implant
  STA-peg procedure
  Smith STA-peg
Sta-Pen
  Steady Write S.-P.
Staph-Chek
  S.-C. pad
  S.-C. Synergy fabric
staphylococcal
  s. arthritis
  s. pyomyositis
staphylococci (*pl. of* staphylococcus)
staphylococcus, *pl.* **staphylococci**
  S. aureus
  S. epidermidis
staphylorrhaphy elevator
staple
  s. arthrorisis
  Arthrotek meniscus s.
  automatic s.
  barbed s.
  bioabsorbable s.
  Biomet s.
  Blount fracture s.
  Bostick s.
  capsulorrhaphy s.
  s. capsulorrhaphy
  C-Jaws cervical compressive s.
  Coventry s.
  Day fixation s.
  DePalma s.
  Downing s.
  s. driver
  duToit shoulder s.
  Ellison fixation s.
  epiphysial s.
  s. extractor
  Fastlok implantable s.
  s. fixation
  GIA s.
  s. gun
  Hernandez-Ros bone s.
  s. holder
  Howmedica Vitallium s.
  s. inserter
  s. introducer
  Johannesberg s.
  Krackow HTO blade s.
  3M s.
  memory compression s.
  meniscal s.
  s. migration
  O'Brien s.
  osteoclast tension s.
  Richards fixation s.
  skin s.
  Smith & Nephew medium barbed s.

Smith & Nephew small barbed s.
stainless steel s.
Stone 4-point s.
Stryker soft tissue s.
s. suture
TA metallic s.
TA Premium (30, 55, 90) s.
Uni-Clip s.
vitallium s.
Wiberg fracture s.
Zimaloy s.

stapler

Auto Suture s.
Biologically quiet s.
Closer s.
Dwyer spinal mechanical s.
GIA s.
Hall double-hole spinal s.
metaphysial s.
Oswestry-O'Brien spinal s.
powered metaphysial s.
S.D. Sorb S.
tabletop Stone s.

Staples

S. elbow arthrodesis
S. elbow repair
S. ligament repair

stapling

anterior vertebral s.
Blount s.
epiphysial s.
intervertebral body s.
percutaneous s.
physial s.

STAR

Scandinavian total ankle replacement
STAR ankle joint prosthesis
STAR technique

star

S. Excursion Balance Test (SEBT)
s. gait

starch

s. bandage
s. test

Stardox wrist brace

4-star exercise program

Stark

S. bone graft
S. first metatarsophalangeal joint arthrodesis
S. iliac bone to mandibular body graft

Starrett pin vise

starter

nail s.

stasimorphia

stasis ulcer

Statak

S. anchor system
S. curette
S. soft tissue attachment device

state

gradient-recalled acquisition in steady s. (GRASS)
Middlesex Elderly Assessment of Mental s. (MEAMS)
pathomechanical s.
proinflammatory s.
prothrombotic s.
United S.'s (U.S.)

static

s. alignment
s. arthropathy
s. back
s. compression
s. compression plate
s. evaluation
s. fatigue
s. fixation
s. foot deformity
s. foot pain
s. footprint
s. lifting
s. listing
s. listing nomenclature
s. locking nail
s. lock nailing
s. orthosis
s. palpation
s. scoliosis
s. splint
s. stretch
s. stretching
s. tendon transfer
s. traction

statically

Staticin Topical

station

s. and gait
Aquatrend water workout s.
gait and s.
s. test
unsteadiness of gait and s.

stationary

s. angle guide
s. ankle flexible endoskeleton foot
s. arthropathy
s. attachment flexible endoskeletal (SAFE)
s. attachment flexible endoskeletal orthotic

stature

short s.

status

ambulatory s.
hydration s.

S

status (*continued*)
    intact neurovascular s.
    s. loading
    neurovascular s. (NVS)
    s. post
    Repeatable Battery for the
    Assessment of Neuropsychological
    s. (RBANS)
Stauffer speech threshold level
  modification
Stax fingertip splint
stay
    length of s. (LOS)
    spiral s.
    s. wire
StayFuse implant
stay-retractor
    Freebody s.-r.
S-T Cort
STC 900-series travel chair
steady
    s. state heart rate (SSHR)
    S. Write Sta-Pen
steal
    s. effect
    s. syndrome
stealth
    S. anchor
    S. frame
    S. image-guided system
    S. knee brace
StealthStation
    S. Treon plus electromagnetic
    surgical navigation
    S. Treon plus neurosurgical
    instrument
    S. with FluoroNav
    S. with Iso-C 3D
steam sterilization
Stedman awl
steel
    S. approach
    austenitic stainless s.
    martensitic stainless s.
    S. pelvic correction
    S. rule of thirds
    s. shank
    s. sole plate orthosis
    stainless s.
    S. triple innominate osteotomy
    S. triple osteotomy of innominate
    bone
    S. triradiate pelvic osteotomy
steering wheel injury
Steffee
    S. instrument
    S. pedicle plate
    S. pedicle screw-plate system
    S. plate and screw

    S. screw plate
    S. spinal fusion instrumentation
    technique
    S. spinal instrumentation
    S. thumb arthroplasty
    S. variable spine plating system
Steichen digital neurovascular free flap
Steinbach mallet
Steinberg
    S. depression rating scale
    S. infiltration block
Steinbrocker rheumatoid arthritis
  classification
Steindler
    S. elbow arthrodesis
    S. elbow flexion effect
    S. elbow flexorplasty
    S. plantar release stripping
    S. procedure
    S. ungual matricectomy
Steinert
    S. disease
    S. epiphysial fracture classification
Steinhauser bone clamp
Steinmann
    S. extension nail
    S. fixation pin
    S. meniscal injury test
    S. pin fixation
    S. pin with ball bearing
    S. pin with Crowe pilot point
    S. pin with pin chuck
    S. tendon forceps
    S. traction
Steinman tenderness displacement test
Stelazine
Stelkast Surpass ceramic-on-ceramic
  acetabular system
stellate
    s. fracture
    s. nail bed laceration
    s. sympathetic ganglion block
Stellbrink fixation device
stem
    Aequalis s.
    APR hip s.
    APR I femoral s.
    Aufranc-Turner s.
    s. base plate
    Biomet revision hip s.
    calcar replacement s.
    collarless s.
    s. component
    Continuum hip s.
    contoured femoral s.
    Corail HA-coated s.
    CRM s.
    s. deformation
    Engh-Glassman femoral s.

Epoch femoral s.
Exeter s.
Extend s.
s. extractor
s. failure
fenestrated s.
F2L Multineck femoral s.
GHE Eska femoral s.
Harris-Galante s.
HG multilock hip s.
hydroxyapatite-coated s.
implant s.
intramedullary s.
Iowa s.
Kirschner s.
KMP femoral s.
Linear hip s.
Link MP microporous hip s.
Link MP reconstruction hip s.
long s.
Mallory-Head femoral s.
modular Moniflex hip s.
Moniflex hip s.
Moore s.
Natural-Hip titanium hip s.
nonfenestrated s.
Omnifit s.
Omnifit-C s.
Opti-Fix hip s.
Osteonics Omnifit-C s.
Osteonics Omnifit-HA hip s.
PCA hip s.
Perfecta femoral s.
PFC hip s.
Precision hip s.
press-fit s.
primary s.
Profile hip s.
Profix metaphysial tibial s.
Ranawat-Burstein porous s.
regular s.
s. removal
Revision hip s.
Richards modular s.
roundback s.
SL-Plus s.
Spotorno cementless hip
 arthroplasty s.
S-ROM modular s.
straight femoral s.
Taperloc femoral s.
trial s.
Ultima calcar s.'s
Ultima Fx s.'s
Zimmer bone s.
Stemex
stemmed tibial prosthesis
Stemmer lymphedema sign
Stener gamekeeper's thumb lesion

**Stener-Gunterberg high sacral
 amputation operation**
stenosed
stenoses (*pl. of* stenosis)
stenosing tenosynovitis
stenosis, *pl.* **stenoses**
achondroplastic s.
ankylosing spinal s.
central canal s.
cervical s.
combined s.
congenital s.
constitutional s.
degenerative s.
foraminal s.
lateral recess s. (LRS)
microdecompression for spinal s.
multisegmental spinal s.
neural foraminal s. (NFS)
spinal canal s. (SCS)
spinous process osteotomy for
 spinal s.
vertebral canal s.
stent
Dacron s.
s. dressing
Omnifit HA hip s.
synthetic s.
stenting
Stenver
S. petrous temporal view
S. temporal bone view
Stenzel
S. rod
S. rod prosthesis
step
CUBEx multifunctional s.
s. defect
s. drill
equinus s.
s. exercise
s. length
s. osteotomy
s. out, turn out (SOTO)
s. screw
s. time
s. width
step-cut
s.-c. lengthening
s.-c. osteotomy
s.-c. reamer
s.-c. transection
step-down
s.-d. drill
s.-d. osteotomy
Stephen
S. scissors
S. spreader bar
stepladder sign

S

step-off
>s.-o. between bone fracture fragments
>s.-o. of fracture
>s.-o. vertebral body sign

steppage gait

stepper
>Diamondback 1100 recumbent s.
>Diamondback 1100 self-generated s.
>Diamondback 100 upright s.
>NuStep total body recumbent s.

step-up
>lateral s.-u.

stereoarthrolysis

stereognosis

stereolithography spinal cage

stereophotogrammetry
>optical s.
>roentgen s.

stereotactic
>s. arc
>s. radiosurgery

stereotaxic anterior capsulotomy

stereotaxy
>spinal s.

Steri-Clamp
>S.-C. clamp
>IMP S.-C.
>Innovative Medical Products S.-C.

Steri-Cuff
>S.-C. disposable tourniquet cuff
>S.-C. Plus

sterile
>s. condition
>s. dry dressing (SDD)
>s. loosening
>s. matrix
>s. pencil
>s. saline solution
>s. sheet
>s. sheeting
>s. towel

sterilization
>ethylene oxide s.
>gas s.
>steam s.
>tissue s.

Steri-Strip skin closure

Sterivap cement gun

sterna (*pl. of* sternum)

sternal
>s. approximator
>s. attachment component
>s. rib

sternalis syndrome

sternal-occipital-mandibular (SOM)
>s.-o.-m. immobilization (SOMI)
>s.-o.-m. immobilizer orthosis

sternal-occipital-manubrial immobilizer

Sternberg memory test

sternochondral articulation

sternoclavicular (SC)
>s. angle
>s. articulation
>s. disc
>s. joint
>s. joint dislocation
>s. joint injury
>s. joint reconstruction
>s. joint reduction
>s. joint separation
>s. joint stress test
>s. ligament
>s. syndrome

sternocleidomastoid (SCM)
>s. muscle fibromatosis

sternocostal
>s. joint
>s. ligament

sternohyoid muscle

sternomastoid muscle

sternooccipital mandibular immobilizer orthosis

sternothyroid muscle

sternotomy

sternoxiphoid plane

sternum, *pl.* **sterna**
>duplicate s.
>s. fracture
>xiphoid process of s.

sternum-splitting approach

steroid
>anabolic s.
>epidural s.
>s. injection
>s. myopathy
>performance-enhancing s.
>tapering dose s.
>s. therapy

steroid-induced
>s.-i. avascular necrosis
>s.-i. bone disease
>s.-i. osteonecrosis

Stevens-Street
>S.-S. elbow prosthesis template
>S.-S. humeral replacement elbow prosthesis

Stewart
>S. arm operation
>S. distal clavicular excision
>S. fifth metatarsal fracture classification (I-V)
>S. styloidectomy

Stewart-Milford traumatic pediatric hip dislocation classification (I-IV)

Stewart-Morel syndrome

Steytler-Van Der Walt metatarsus adductus osteotomy procedure

St. Georg unicompartment prosthesis
sthenometry
STH-2 hip prosthesis
stick
>
> Back Revolution S.
> dressing s.
> FMS Intracell s.
> Intracell massage s.
> Intracell Sprinter s.
> sponge s.
> switching s.
> s. tie ligature
> weighted walking s.

Stickler syndrome
Stieda
>
> S. medial femoral condyle avulsion
>   fracture
> S. posterior process of talus

STIF
>
> spinopelvic transiliac fixation
> STIF system

stiff
>
> s. gait
> s. man syndrome
> s. person syndrome (SPS)
> s. ray
> s. ribbon retractor
> s. toe

stiff-knee gait
stiff-legged gait
stiffness
>
> axial s.
> fusion s.
> joint s.
> resting shear s.
> shear s.
> small-joint s.
> tensile s.
> torsional s.

stiff-soled shoe
stifle joint
stigmatic electrode
Stiles-Bunnell flexor digitorum
  superficialis transfer technique
Still disease
Stille
>
> S. bone biter
> S. bone chisel
> S. bone drill
> S. bone drill set
> S. bone gouge
> S. brace
> S. bur
> S. hand drill
> S. osteotome
> S. plaster shears
> S. rongeur

Stille-Horsley
>
> S.-H. bone forceps

S.-H. bone rongeur
S.-H. rib forceps
Stille-Liston bone-cutting forceps
Stille-Luer
>
> S.-L. bone rongeur
> S.-L. duckbill rongeur
> S.-L. rongeur forceps

Stille-Luer-Echlin rongeur
Stille-pattern trephine and bone drill
  set
Stiller rib
Stille-Ruskin bone rongeur
Stille-Sherman bone drill
Stilphostrol
stilus (*var. of* stylus)
stim
>
> StIM neuromuscular stimulator
>   system

Stimoceiver implant material
Stimprene
>
> S. electrotherapy brace
> S. wrap

Stimson
>
> S. anterior shoulder reduction
>   technique
> S. figure-of-8 dressing
> gravity method of S.
> S. gravity shoulder dislocation
>   reduction method
> S. posterior hip dislocation
>   reduction maneuver
> S. reduction

stimulating
>
> s. electrode
> s. massage

stimulation (stim)
>
> antidromic s.
> continuous s.
> controlled disc s. (CDS)
> cranial electrical s. (CES)
> cycled s.
> direct electrical nerve s. (DENS)
> double simultaneous sensory s.
> electrical bone-growth s. (EBGS)
> electronic muscle s. (EMS)
> electrical nerve s.
> electrical surface s.
> electronic bone s. (EBI)
> electrotherapeutic point s. (ETPS)
> external-coil electrical s.
> functional electrical s. (FES)
> functional neuromuscular s. (FNS)
> galvanic s.
> high-voltage pulsed s. (HVPS)
> high-voltage pulsed galvanic s.
>   (HVPGS)
> IFC s.
> inferential current s.
> interferential electrical s.

S

709

stimulation (*continued*)
 lateral electrical surface s. (LESS)
 magnetic s.
 marrow s.
 microamperage electrical nerve s. (MENS)
 microamperage neural s. (MNS)
 neuromuscular electrical s. (NMES)
 OrthoLogic 1000 bone growth s.
 OsteoGen bone growth s.
 PEMF bone growth s.
 pulsed electric magnetic field bone growth s.
 reciprocal s.
 repetitive nerve s.
 rhythmic auditory s. (RAS)
 sensory motor s. (SMS)
 Spinal-Stim bone growth s.
 transcutaneous electrical nerve s. (TENS)
stimulation-ultrasound
 Amrex SynchroSonic muscle s.-u.
stimulator (stim)
 Acupoint s.
 AcuTENS transcutaneous nerve s.
 AME bone growth s.
 Amrex muscle s.
 Back Hammer muscle s.
 Biolectron bone growth s.
 BioStim Digital NMS muscle s.
 bone growth s.
 Cervical-Stim noninvasive cervical spine bone growth s.
 constant direct current s.
 dorsal column s. (DCS)
 EBI Medical SpinalPak II spine fusion s.
 electrical bone-growth s. (EBGS)
 Electro-Acuscope 85 s.
 electronic muscle s. (EMS)
 EMS 2000 neuromuscular s.
 Endo Multi-Mode s.
 Freedom Micro Pro s.
 galvanic electrode s.
 G5 Porta-Plus muscle s.
 IFC s.
 implanted bone growth s.
 inferential current s.
 Intelect electric s.
 Intelect Legend s.
 Intelect 600MP microcurrent s.
 interferential s.
 Magnum 100 s.
 Magnum 101 Plus s.
 Master-Stim interferential s.
 Maxima II transcutaneous electrical nerve s.
 Medi-Stim s.

Mettler Trio neuromuscular electrical s.
 Micro-Z neuromuscular s.
 MS322 muscle s.
 neuromuscular III s.
 Nuwave transcutaneous electrical nerve s.
 Ortho DX electromedical s.
 Orthofix Cervical-Stim bone growth s.
 Orthofuse implantable growth s.
 OrthoGen bone growth s.
 OrthoLogic 1000 bone growth s.
 OrthoPak II bone growth s.
 OsteoGen implantable bone growth s.
 OsteoStim implantable bone growth s.
 PGS-3000 pulsed galvanic s.
 Physio-Stim Lite bone growth s.
 Piezoelectro-needleless s.
 Precision spinal cord s.
 prizm Electro-Mesh Z-Stim-II s.
 pulsed galvanic s.
 repetitive nerve s. (RNS)
 Respond II muscle s.
 SpF spinal fusion s.
 spinal cord s. (SCS)
 spinal fusion s.
 SpinalPak bone growth s.
 SpinalPak II spine fusion s.
 SpinalPak spine fusion s.
 Spinal-Stim bone growth s.
 Sportstim s.
 SporTX pulsed direct current s.
 S.P. 100 transcutaneous electrical neural s.
 Stimuplex-S nerve s.
 Super Stimm MF s.
 Surgi-Stim s.
 SynchroSonic s.
 SysStim 226 muscle s.
 Theramini 1, 2 electrotherapy s.
 Theratouch 4.7 s.
 ThermaStim muscle s.
 Trio-Stim neuromuscular s.
stimulator/ultrasound
 Intelect Combo s./u.
stimuli (*pl. of* stimulus)
Stimulite honeycomb mattress overlay
stimulus (stim), *pl.* **stimuli**
 s. artifact
 maximal s.
 paired s.
 submaximal s.
 subthreshold s.
 supramaximal s.
 test s.

threshold s.
unconditional s.
Stimuplex block needle
Stimuplex-S nerve stimulator
Stinchfield resisted hip flexion test
stinger injury
sting mat
stippled epiphysis
stippling
stirrup
    Allen s.
    Böhler s.
    s. brace
    Comfort Cast s.
    s. plaster splint
    split s.
    Swivel-Strap ankle s.
    traction s.
    walking s.
stitch
    Allgöwer s.
    apical s.
    baseball s.
    Bunnell tendon repair s.
    half s.
    intracuticular s.
    Kessler tendon repair s.
    Mersilene Kessler s.
    pinch-tuck s.
    Pulvertaft fish-mouth s.
    roll s.
    Rousso everting skin closure s.
stitcher
    Acufex meniscal s.
Stiwer
    S. bone-holding forceps
    S. hand drill
STJ
    scapulothoracic joint
    subtalar joint
St Joseph Adult Chewable Aspirin
1st metatarsal head (FMH)
STNP
    subtalar joint neutral position
stock
    bone s.
    S. finger splint
    osteopenic bone s.
    poor bone s.
Stockholm
    S. hand-arm vibration syndrome
    (1–4) staging
    S. HAVS sensorineural component
    (0SN, 1SN, 2SN, 3SN)
    S. HAVS severity staging system
stockinette
    s. bandage
    basket s.
    bias-cut s.

Buck traction s.
orthopaedic s.
s. sling
s. tube
tubular s.
Velpeau s.
stocking-glove distribution
stockings
    antiembolic s.
    CircAid elastic s.
    compression s.
    dropfoot redression s.
    elastic s.
    Jobst s.
    long leg s.
    Medi Plus compression s.
    Orthawear antiembolism s.
    Planostretch s.
    pneumatic compression s.
    SCD s.
    sequential compression device s.
    Sigvaris s.
    Silver-Thera s.
    Soft Touch s.
    TED s.
    thromboembolic s.
    Zimmer antiembolism s.
Stokes amputation
stone
    S. anoplasty procedure
    s. arthrodesis
    s. basket screw mounted handle
    S. bunionectomy
    S. clamp-locking device
    S. 4-point staple
    pumice s.
Stookey reflex
stool
    foot s.
    nested step s.
    Swedish support s.
stop
    s. action brace
    Elite posterior adjustable s.
Stopain Spray topical analgesic spray
stop-and-go sports
stopwatch
storage
    energy s.
storiform pattern
stork
    s. leg
    s. sign
    s. stand
    s. standing lumbar spine test
    s. test
Storz
    S. meniscotome
    S. Microsystems drill bit

S

Storz (*continued*)
    S. Microsystems plate cutter
    S. Microsystems pliers
    S. oblique arthroscope
    S. screw
stout-neck curette
stove-in pelvis
stovepipe leg
straddle
    s. fracture
    s. injury
StraddleSitter seating aid
straight
    s. basket forceps
    s. bone rongeur
    s. chisel
    s. curette
    s. femoral stem
    s. gouge
    s. hex screwdriver
    s. incision
    s. last shoe
    s. lateral instability
    s. leg raising (SLR)
    s. leg raising exercise
    s. leg raising test
    s. leg tension sign
    s. osteotome
    s. periosteal elevator
    s. pituitary rongeur
    s. posterior portal
    s. power reamer
    s. scissors
    s. spine syndrome
    s. stem femoral component
    s. threaded rod
    s. walker brace
strain
    acute foot s.
    articular s.
    back s.
    compression s.
    coronary ligament s.
    elastic s.
    s. energy
    fibulocalcaneal ligament s.
    foot s.
    s. fracture
    s. gauge
    muscle s.
    plastic s.
    postural s.
    shear s.
    tensile s.
    thoracolumbosacral s.
    TLS s.
strain/counterstrain technique
strain-gauge extensometer
strain-sprain injury

strain-stress curve
strap
    Band-It tennis elbow s.
    Beta Pile II, III splint s.
    buddy s.
    Butterfly cushion with s.
    capsular s.
    Cho-Pat Achilles tendon s.
    Cho-Pat Dual Action Knee S.
    Cho-Pat elbow s.
    Cho-Pat ITB S.
    s. clavicular splint
    counterforce s.
    crotch s.
    D-ring s.
    Eclipse Gel elbow s.
    elastic s.
    external elastic s.
    extremity mobilization s.
    FoamWrap ThumDuction s.
    foot drop s.
    fork s.
    Gel-Bank patellar s.
    iliotibial band s.
    infrapatellar s.
    ITB s.
    Lema s.
    Levine patellar tendon s.
    S. Lok ankle brace
    Meek clavicular s.
    s. muscle
    neoprene wrist s.
    Nylatex s.
    Partridge s.
    Pebax fastening s.
    PIP/DIP s.
    Pro-Tec patellar tendon s.
    QualCraft s.
    Scott elastic ankle s.
    s. sling
    stretch-out s.
    suprapatellar s.
    suspension s.
    Synergistic suspension s.
    valgus corrective ankle s.
    varus corrective ankle s.
    Velcro s.
strapping
    adhesive s.
    AliStrap Velcro-type s.
    garter s.
    loop & hook s.
    Low-Dye s.
Strassburg sock
Strata hip system
strategy
    cuing s.
    diagnostic s.
Stratis ST ACL reconstruction system

Stratos orthotic
stratum corneum
Stratus impact-reducing pylon
Straub phlebography technique
Strayer
    S. Achilles lengthening
     procedure
    S. flexor slide tendon
     technique
    S. gastrocnemius recession
    S. gastrocnemius-soleus recession
    S. lengthening
streaming potential
streblodactyly
street
    S. forearm nail
    S. medullary pin
Streeter dysplasia
Street-Stevens humeral prosthesis
strength
    2/5 s.
    3/5 s.
    4/5 s.
    5/5 s.
    s. against resistance
    Aspirin Free Anacin Maximum S.
    axial gripping s.
    Bayer Low Adult S.
    bending s.
    bone s.
    bone-screw interface s.
    BUE s.
    C-D instrumentation fixation s.
    cervical extension s.
    Cotrel pedicle screw fixation s.
    s. curve
    Ecotrin Low Adult S.
    extensor hallucis longus s.
    extra s. (ES)
    extrinsic muscle s.
    fatigue s.
    fixation s.
    graft s.
    grip s.
    hand grasp s.
    hand grip s.
    intrinsic muscle s.
    isometric cervical extension s.
    Lovett clinical scale of
     zero-normal s.
    motor s.
    pedicle screw pull-out s.
    pinch s.
    pull-out s.
    tensile s.
    s. test eccentric bilateral
    s. testing
    torsional gripping s.
    s. training

    ultimate s.
    yield s.
strength-duration curve
strengthened
    gas atomized dispersion s.
    (GADS)
strengthening
    s. exerciser
    rehabilitation muscle s.
    wrist extensor s.
    wrist flexor s.
streptococcal myositis
Streptococcus
    S. faecalis
    S. pneumoniae
streptokinase
streptomycin
stress
    arch s.
    bending s.
    biomechanical s.
    contact s.
    cyclic mechanical s.
    s. distribution
    s. dorsiflexion projection
    s. examination
    fatigue s.
    s. film
    s. fracture
    heat s.
    hyperextension s.
    s. injury
    laxity to varus s.
    longitudinal arch s.
    low-contact s. (LCS)
    measured s.
    mediolateral s.
    principal s.
    s. profilometry
    s. radiograph
    s. radiography
    s. riser
    s. roentgenography
    s. rupture
    shear s.
    s. shielding
    supraphysiologic s.
    tensile s.
    s. test
    s. testing
    torsional s.
    s. transfer
    transverse arch s.
    valgus s.
    varus-valgus s.
    s. view
    von Mises s.
    s. x-ray
stress-corrosion cracking

S

stressor
Stress-Ray varus-valgus device
stress-relaxation
    intraoperative s.-r.
stress-strain curve
stress-testing arthrometer
stretch
    S. and Heel night splint
    s. cable
    carpal tunnel s.
    crossed-leg pike down s.
    diagonal s.
    elastic s.
    general capsular s.
    heel cord s.
    s. injury
    low-load prolonged s. (LLPS)
    passive s.
    s. pattern
    post-facilitation s. (PFS)
    quick s.
    s. receptor
    s. reflex
    repeated quick s. (RQS)
    slow s.
    spray and s.
    static s.
    s. test
    triplane s.
    vapocoolant spray and s.
    wrist and finger flexor s.
    wrist extensor s.
stretcher
    hamstring s.
    shoe s.
stretching
    bullet tissue s.
    s. contraindication
    gastrocnemius-soleus s.
    nerve s.
    s. program
    range of motion therapeutic s.
    soft tissue s.
    static s.
    s. velocity
stretch-out strap
Stretch-Rite exerciser system
striata
    osteopathia s.
striatal
    s. lesion
    s. toe
striated
    s. muscle
    s. nail
Strickland
    S. flexor tendon repair
      technique
    S. modification

stride
    S. Analyzer
    s. length
    s. length of gait
    s. time
strike
    heel s.
    knee s.
    s. phase of gait
striker
    forefoot s.
    forefoot-to-rearfoot s.
string drawing board
stringiness
stringing peg
strip
    corticocancellous bone s.
    Fas-Trac s.
    gastrocnemius-soleus fascial s.
    s. posting
    Thera-Band s.
stripe
    vertebral s.
striped muscle
stripout
    screw s.
stripper
    Acufex microsurgical tendon s.
    Brand tendon s.
    Bunnell tendon s.
    cartilage s.
    Fischer tendon s.
    orthopaedic surgical s.
    pigtail tendon s.
    slotted tendon s.
    tendon s.
stripping
    Steindler plantar release s.
stroke
    heat s.
    s. knee test
    s. test
    s. volume
stroker
    skin s.
stroke-related deconditioning
stroking
    deep s.
stroller
    adapted s.
stroma, *pl.* **stromata**
    fibrovascular connective tissue s.
stromata (*pl. of* stroma)
Stromeyer
    S. Achilles tenotomy procedure
    S. splint
Stromgren
    S. ankle brace
    S. support

Strong dorsal extension block PIP joint splinting
Stronghands hand exerciser
Stroop word color identification test
structural
- s. aluminum malleable (SAM)
- s. aluminum malleable splint
- s. bone graft
- s. component
- s. congenital myopathy
- s. curve
- s. derangement
- s. intersegmental distortion
- s. scoliosis

structure
- articular s.
- contiguous vertebral s.
- cordlike s.
- extraarticular s.
- graft s.
- Hedrocel tantalum metal s.
- intraarticular s.
- keystone s.
- ligamentous s.
- neurovascular s.
- osseous s.
- posterolateral s.
- ring s.
- uniaxial s.
- waist of anatomical s.
- Wolff law of bone s.

structured bone
strumming
- perpendicular s.

Strümpell
- S. disease
- S. sign

Strümpell-Marie disease
Strunsky anterior arch of foot sign
strut
- s. bone graft
- fibrotic s.
- Littig s.
- s. plate fixation
- s. spinal fusion technique

Struthers
- arcade of S.
- ligament of S.

2-strut tibial graft technique
strut-type pin
Stryker
- S. bed
- S. camera
- S. cartilage knife
- S. CPM exerciser
- S. dermatome
- S. drill
- S. fracture frame
- S. Howmedica Osteonics

- S. Intracompartmental Pressure Monitor System
- S. knee joint laxity device
- S. knee laxity arthrometer
- S. lag screw
- S. leg exerciser
- S. notch humeral head view
- S. power instrumentation
- S. saw
- S. screwdriver
- S. SE3 drive system
- S. soft tissue staple
- S. surgical hand table
- S. turning frame
- S. viewing arthroscope

STS
- silicone thermoplastic splinting
- STS molding sock

STSE
- split-thickness skin excision

STSG
- split-thickness skin graft

STT
- scaphotrapezoid-trapezial
- superficial tibiotalar
- STT joint
- STT ligament

Stuart Gordon hand splint
stubbed shoulder
Stubbs
- S. acromioclavicular splint
- S. elastic wrist support
- S. 4-way clavicle brace

stucco keratosis
stuck finger
student's elbow
studio cycling
study
- air-contrast s.
- anatomopathological s.
- bone density s.
- cinematographic gait s.
- cohort s.
- Cornwall hip fracture s.
- Doppler s.
- double-contrast s.
- electrophysiologic s.
- evoked potential s.
- fluorescein s.
- injection s.
- in vivo s.
- Johns Hopkins National Low Back Pain S.
- kinematic s.
- Michigan Bone Health S.
- Multicenter ACL Revision S. (MARS)
- nerve conduction s. (NCS)
- radiodiagnostic s.

study (*continued*)
    roentgen-stereophotogrammatic s.
    sudomotor s.
Stulberg
    S. hip classification
    S. hip positioner
    S. Mark II leg positioner
    S. method
stump
    amputation s.
    s. edema
    foot s.
    s. hallucination
    s. neuralgia
    s. neuroma
    s. of bone
    painful s.
    s. revision
    s. shrinker
    s. sock
    s. wrapping
stuttering of gait
STx
    STx lumbar traction device
    STx Saunders lumbar disc
      device
stylet, stylette
    blunt s.
stylette (*var. of* stylet)
stylohyoid
styloid
    s. fracture
    s. process
styloidectomy
    Stewart s.
styloideum
    os s.
stylus, stilus
    tibial s.
Styrofoam filler block
subacromial
    s. bursa
    s. bursa adhesion
    s. bursa injection
    s. bursitis
    s. bursography
    s. decompression
    s. impingement syndrome
    s. portal
    s. space
    s. spur
subacromiodeltoid bursa
subacute
    s. hematogenous osteomyelitis
    s. rehabilitation
    s. subperiosteal hemorrhage
subadjacent segment
subaponeurotic abscess
subarachnoid block

subarticular
    s. cyst
    s. screw
subastragalar
    s. amputation
    s. dislocation
    s. fusion
subaxial
    s. injury
    s. posterior cervical spinal fusion
    s. subluxation
subcalcaneal bursitis
subcapital
    s. fracture
    s. osteotomy
subchondral
    s. bone
    s. bone cyst
    s. lesion
    s. lucency
    s. plate
    s. sclerosis
subclavian
    s. artery
    s. artery injury
    s. steal syndrome
    s. vein
    s. vein injury
subclavicular approach
subclavius
    s. muscle
    s. muscle
    s. tendon graft
subcondylar
    s. deformity
    s. osteotomy
subcoracoid
    s. bone
    s. bursitis
    s. shoulder dislocation
    s. space
subcortical defect
subcostal
    s. muscle
    s. plane
subcrural joint
subcutaneous
    s. abscess
    s. anterior transposition
    s. calcaneal bursa
    s. drain
    s. fat sling
    s. fracture
    s. granuloma anulare
    s. infrapatellar bursa
    s. intracompartmental soft tissue
      sarcoma
    s. operation
    s. palmar fasciotomy

s. patellar bursa
s. pseudosarcomatous fibromatosis
s. synovial bursa
s. tenotomy
s. tissue
s. trochanteric bursa
subcuticular suture
subdeltoid
s. bursa
s. bursa adhesion
s. bursitis (SDB)
subdermal plexus
subdural button
subfascial
s. abscess
s. incision
s. transposition
subgaleal abscess
subglenoid shoulder dislocation
subgluteal
s. bursitis
s. hematoma
subjacent
subjective
S. Shoulder Rating Scale (SSRS)
S. Shoulder Rating Scale patient
questionnaire
sublaminar
s. fixation
s. wire
s. wiring
sublesional ulceration
subligamentous dissection
Sublimaze injection
sublimis
s. bridge syndrome
flexor digitorum s. (FDS)
s. tendon
s. tenodesis
subluxated metatarsophalangeal
joint
subluxation
anterosuperior s.
anterosuperior-external s.
anterosuperior-internal s.
arytenoid s.
AS s.
ASEX s.
ASIN s.
atlantoaxial s. (AAS)
atlantoaxial rotatory s.
atlantooccipital s.
calcaneocuboid s.
compensatory structural s.
congenital hip s.
Crowe s.
facet s.
facilitated s.
fixation s.

foraminal encroachment s.
functional s.
glenohumeral joint s.
hip s.
joint s.
Madelung s.
manipulable s.
metatarsophalangeal s.
neuroarticular s.
neurofunctional s.
nonmanipulable s.
patellar s.
peroneal tendon s.
PIEX s.
PIIN s.
posteroinferior-external s.
posteroinferior-internal s.
progressive s.
proximal tibiofibular s.
radial head s. (RHS)
radiocapitellar s.
radioulnar s.
rotatory atlantoaxial s.
sacroiliac s.
shoulder s.
s. stabilization
subaxial s.
talar s.
tibiofibular s.
unilateral facet s.
unilateral interfacetal s.
vertebral s.
Volkmann s.
wrist s.
subluxed vertebra
subluxing patella
submandibular
submaximal stimulus
subneural apparatus
suboccipital muscle
subperiosteal
s. abscess
s. amputation
s. cortical defect
s. dissection
s. exposure
s. fracture
s. giant cell reparative granuloma
s. new bone
s. new bone formation
s. paraarticular-type osteoid osteoma
subphrenic abscess
subplatysmal abscess
subsartorial tunnel
subscapular
s. angle
s. artery injury
s. nerve injury
s. tendinitis

S

subscapularis
- s. bursitis
- s. capsular lengthening
- s. muscle
- s. rupture
- s. tendon
- s. tendon transfer

subsidence
- benign s.
- component s.
- prosthesis component s.
- vertical s.

subspinous dislocation

substance
- androgenic-enhancing s.
- bone s.
- metachromatic mucoid s.

substitute
- AlloCraft bone spacer s.
- AlloMatrix injectable putty bone graft s.
- BCP synthetic bone s.
- BiCalPhos synthetic bone s.
- Biobrane synthetic skin s.
- Biocoral bone graft s.
- bone s.
- bone graft s. (BGS)
- Boplant Surgibone bovine bone s.
- dermal s.
- Healos bone graft s.
- OsteoSet bone graft s.
- OsteoSet-T medicated bone graft s.
- Pro Osteon 500 bone graft s.
- protein-based bone graft s.

substituting knee prosthesis

substitution
- arthroscopy-assisted patellar tendon s.
- Carrell fibular s.
- creeping s.
- extensor s.
- Marshall patelloquadriceps tendon s.
- patellar tendon s.
- patelloquadriceps tendon s.
- tendon s.

subsulfate
- ferric s.

subsurface white band

subtalar
- s. arthralgia
- s. arthrodesis
- s. arthroereisis peg (STA-peg)
- s. arthrosis
- s. arthrotomy
- s. articulation
- s. capsulotomy
- s. coalition
- s. distraction bone block fusion
- s. interosseous ligament
- s. inversion test
- s. joint (STJ)
- s. joint arthritis
- s. joint axis (SJA)
- s. joint dislocation
- s. joint function (SJF)
- s. joint incongruency
- s. joint instability
- s. joint neutral position (STNP)
- s. joint pain
- s. laxity
- s. MBA implant
- s. motion
- s. portal
- s. pronation
- s. supination
- s. tilt
- s. varus

subtendinous
- s. iliac bursa
- s. prepatellar bursa

subthreshold
- s. force
- s. stimulus

subtotal
- s. lateral meniscectomy
- s. maxillectomy
- s. plantar fasciectomy
- s. somatectomy

subtraction osteotomy

subtrochanteric
- s. femoral fracture
- s. osteotomy

subungual, subunguial
- s. abscess
- s. exostosis
- s. fibroma
- s. granuloma
- s. hematoma
- s. onychomycosis

subunguial (*var. of* subungual)

subvertebral muscle

succinate
- methylprednisolone sodium s.

sucker shaver

suction
- s. ArthroWand
- autotransfusion s.
- s. biter
- s. cannula
- s. drainage
- irrigation s.
- s. nozzle
- s. punch
- s. pyramid
- s. sign
- s. socket suspension

s. suspension prosthesis
s. tip
s. tube
Yankauer s.
suction-bubble technique
suction-irrigation
s.-i. system
s.-i. technique
Sudeck
S. atrophy
S. disease
S. syndrome
sudomotor
s. activity
s. activity test
s. function
s. startle reflex
s. study
SUFE
slipped under femoral
epiphysis
Sufenta injection
sufentanil citrate
sugar-tong
s.-t. cast
s.-t. plaster splint
s.-t. traction
Sugioka transtrochanteric rotational osteotomy
suit
body exhaust s.
G s.
Sukhtian-Hughes
S.-H. fixation
S.-H. fixation device
sulbactam
ampicillin and s.
sulci (*gen.* and *pl. of* sulcus)
sulconazole
sulcus, *gen.* and *pl.* **sulci**
s. angle
bicipital s.
calcaneal s.
s. calcanei
carpal s.
cuboid s.
gluteal s.
humerus s.
inferior costal s.
interarticular s.
intertubercular s.
lateral bicipital s.
malleolar s.
medial bicipital s.
obturator s.
s. of talus
s. of wrist
paraglenoid s.
radial s.

semicanal of humerus s.
semilunar s.
s. shoulder sign
spiral s.
supraacetabular s.
talar s.
s. test
sulfadiazine
silver s.
sulfamethoxazole
trimethoprim s.
Sulfamylon
sulfate, sulphate
ferrous s.
glucosamine s.
magnesium s. (MgSO$_4$)
morphine s. (MS)
sulfated mucopolysaccharide
sulfide, sulphide
selenium s.
sulfinpyrazone
sulfoxide, sulphoxide
dimethyl s. (DMSO)
sulindac
Sully shoulder stabilizer brace
sulphate (*var. of* sulfate)
sulphide (*var. of* sulfide)
sulphoxide (*var. of* sulfoxide)
Sulzer
S. Orthopaedics
S. Orthopaedics instrument
S. prosthesis
Summit minipolyaxial screw system
Sunday staphylorrhaphy elevator
Sunderland
S. classification of nerve injury
(1st-5th degree)
S. first-degree – fifth-degree nerve
injury
S. nerve injury first- through
fifth-degree classification
sunrise knee x-ray view
sunset knee x-ray view
Supartz joint fluid therapy
super
S. Cut laminectomy rongeur
S. Grip sleeve
S. Jock n' Jill store Superfeet
orthotic
S. Stimm MF stimulator
Valorin S.
s. wedge
s. wrap
superabduction
Superblade blade
SuperCup acetabular cup prosthesis
superextension
Superfeet Custom Pre-Fabricated Orthotic

superficial
- s. circumflex iliac artery
- s. femoral artery (SFA)
- s. heat modality
- s. infection
- s. medial ligament
- s. necrosis
- s. palmar arch
- s. peroneal nerve
- s. posterior compartment
- s. posterior sacrococcygeal ligament
- s. radial nerve (SRN)
- s. temporal artery
- s. temporal vein
- s. tibiotalar (STT)
- s. tibiotalar ligament
- s. transverse ligament
- s. transverse metacarpal ligament
- s. transverse metatarsal ligament
- s. TV metacarpal ligament
- s. TV metatarsal ligament
- s. varicosity
- s. white onychomycosis (SWO)

superficialis
- s. arcade
- flexor digitorum s. (FDS)
- s. tendon

superflexion

Superform Contours orthotic

Superglue adhesive

superincumbent

superior
- anterior and s. (AS)
- s. border
- s. costotransverse ligament
- s. dislocation
- s. endplate
- s. extensor retinaculum
- s. extensor retinaculum of foot
- s. glide
- s. gluteal nerve
- s. gluteal neurovascular bundle
- s. labrum anterior and posterior (SLAP)
- s. labrum anterior and posterior lesion
- s. laryngeal artery
- s. laryngeal nerve
- s. laryngeal nerve external branch
- s. leaf
- s. nuchal line
- s. peroneal retinaculum (SPR)
- s. pole of patella
- s. portal
- s. process
- s. radioulnar joint
- S. Sleeprite Hi-Lo orthopaedic bed
- s. sulcus tumor
- s. thoracic pedicle screw

- s. thyroid artery
- s. thyroid vein
- s. tibial articulation
- s. tibiofibular joint
- s. vena cava

Superman back exercise

supermarket elbow

supernumerary
- s. bone
- s. digit
- s. lumbar segmentation
- s. thumb
- s. toe

superoinferior tilt

superolateral outflow portal

superomedial
- s. calcaneonavicular ligament
- s. fragment
- s. portal
- s. region

SuperQuad assistive device

supersensitivity
- Cannon Law of Denervation S.
- denervation s.

Super-Seven exercise

SuperSkin thin film dressing

Superstabilizer
- S. cemented stem extender
- S. press-fit stem extender

supertubercular wedge osteotomy/bunionectomy

supinate

supination
- s. contracture
- s. deformity
- hindfoot s.
- s. injury
- s. of foot
- pronation and s.
- rearfoot s.
- subtalar s.
- s. torque

supination-adduction
- s.-a. fracture
- s.-a. injury

supination-eversion
- s.-e. fracture
- s.-e. injury

supination-external
- s.-e. rotation (SER)
- s.-e. rotation (I-IV) fracture
- s.-e. rotation injury

supination-inversion rotation injury

supination-outward rotation injury

supination-plantarflexion injury

supinator
- s. fat pad sign
- s. fossa
- s. jerk

s. jerk reflex
s. muscle
s. muscle
s. syndrome

supine
s. chest press
s. C-Trax traction
s. C-Trax traction system
s. iliac gapping test
s. long sitting test
s. position
s. position driver
s. position for hip arthroplasty
s. straight leg raising test

Suppan foot operation
supplement
Coromega dietary s.
Omega-3 dietary s.
oral nutritional s.

supplementation
zinc s.

supple neck
supplier
National Association of Medical
Equipment S.'s
National Registry of Rehabilitation
Technology s.

supply
blood s.
longitudinal blood s.
reanastomosis of blood s.

support
Accommodator arch s.
Accu-Back back s.
Achillotrain active Achilles tendon
s.
Active Ankle s.
Act joint s.
Act knee s.
AliMed-Freedom arthritis s.
AliMed wrist/thumb s.
ankle stabilizing orthosis s.
Anna-Dote Positioning S.
arch s.
Arizona universal leg s.
ASO s.
back s.
Back-Huggar lumbar s.
BackThing lumbar s.
Band-It magnetic elbow s.
base of s. (BOS)
Bauerfeind s.
BIOflex Magnet Back S.
BioSkin DP wrist s.
BioWrap lumbosacral/sacral s.
Birkenstock Blue Footbed arch s.
Birkenstock high-flange arch s.
Body Gard neoprene s.
boomerang wrist s.

Carabelt lower back s.
Carpal-Lock wrist s.
Castech extremity s.
cavus foot s.
cervical s.
ChinUpps cervicofacial s.
Chiroflow adjustable back s.
Cho-Pat knitted compression s.
cock-up wrist s.
ComfAlign spinal s.
Comfort Cool neoprene s.
Comprifix active ankle s.
Compro Plus Knee s.
Core Reflex wrist s.
Core Universal elastic knee s.
Core Universal elbow s.
Core Universal rib s.
Corfit System 7000 Series
Lumbosacral S.
Cryo/Cuff compression s.
cutout knee s.
Cybertech 1000 back s.
DayTimer carpal tunnel s.
Deltoid-Aid arm s.
DePuy s.
Desk-rest arm s.
double limb s.
Epi-Lock elbow s.
Epipoint elbow s.
Epitrain active elbow s.
Epitrain knitted elbow s.
Epitrain Viscoped s.
Ergo Cush back s.
Ergoflex Premiere back s.
external s.
Ezy Wrap lumbosacral s.
Fits-All s.
FlexLite hinged knee s.
Foot Hugger foot s.
fork strap prosthetic s.
Freedom accommodator arch s.
Freedom arthritis s.
Freedom back s.
Freedom elastic long wrist s.
Friedman s.
Futuro wrist s.
s. garment
Genutrain P3 knee s.
geriatric chair trunk s.
horizontal platform s. (HPS)
Houston halo cervical s.
Innovation Sports bracing s.
Juzo s.
Kallassy ankle s.
Kerr-Lagen abdominal s.
Knee Sleeve knee s.
lateral buttress s.
Lo Bak spinal s.
Loving Comfort maternity s.

S

support (*continued*)
    Loving Comfort postpartum s.
    Lumbotrain lumbosacral s.
    Malleoloc ankle s.
    Malleo-Med soft ankle s.
    Malleotrain ankle s.
    ManuTrain active wrist s.
    Markwort ankle s.
    McDavid knee guard s.
    MKG s.
    Mold-In-Place back s.
    Momma-Too Maternity S.
    Monitor Master monitor s.
    Morton toe s.
    Mother-To-Be back and
      abdominal s.
    MouseMitt Keyboarder padded
      wrist s.
    Mueller Knee S. (MKS)
    neoprene ankle s.
    neoprene back s.
    Nightimer carpal tunnel s.
    Night Splint S.
    obese s.
    Obus back s.
    OEC wrist/forearm s.
    Omotrain active shoulder s.
    Ortho-Pal body s.
    OSI well leg S.
    outdoor emergency care
      wrist/forearm s.
    Palumbo knee s.
    Parham s.
    PattStrap knee s.
    pediatric advanced life s. (PALS)
    pediatric shoulder s.
    Performance Wrap knee s.
    peripatellar retinacular s.
    Philadelphia collar cervical s.
    Plastazote arch s.
    Playmaker s.
    Powerstep foot s.
    PPT gel stirrup ankle s.
    ProFlex wrist s.
    prosthetic s.
    QualCraft ankle s.
    QualCraft short elastic wrist s.
    Relax-A-Bac posture s.
    Rolyan foot s.
    sacral s.
    Scott double-strap ankle s.
    Scott hinged knee s.
    Sheffield s.
    ShiatsuBACK back s.
    Shoulder Ease abduction s.
    Sidekick foot s.
    Silesian bandage prosthetic s.
    single limb s.
    Spenco arch s.

    S'port Max back s.
    standard U patellar s.
    Stromgren s.
    Stubbs elastic wrist s.
    SureStep ankle s.
    TakeOff elbow s.
    Taylor clavicle s.
    Thera-Back back s.
    therapeutic spinal s.
    Thermoskin 4-way elastic knee s.
    tibial fracture brace proximal s.
      (TFB-PS)
    Valeo back s.
    ViscoPed S s.
    ViscoSpot s.
    walking with s.
    walking without s.
    well-leg s.
    Whitman arch s.
    WorkAbout Carpal Mate wrist s.
    WorkMod back s.
    wrist hand extension compression s.
      (WHECS)
    WrisTimer carpal tunnel
      syndrome s.
    WrisTimer CTS s.
    WrisTimer PM CTS s.
supported extension exercise
supporter
supporting bone
suppression
    chemical shift selective s.
      (CHESS)
Supprettes
    Aquachloral S.
    B&O S.
suppurative
    s. arthritis
    s. flexor tenosynovitis
    s. joint infection
    s. myositis
    s. osteitis
    s. osteomyelitis
    s. periostitis
    s. synovitis
supraacetabular
    s. compression external fixation
    s. sulcus
supraclavicular
    s. approach
    s. brachial block anesthesia
    s. fossa
    s. fossa artery
supracollicular spike
supracondylar
    s. amputation
    s. cuff
    s. femoral derotational osteotomy
    s. humeral fracture

intramedullary s. (IMSC)
s. medullary nail
s. nonunion
s. pad
s. plate
s. process
s. process syndrome
s. screw
s. socket
s. varus osteotomy
s. Y-shaped fracture
supracondylar-suprapatellar (SCSP)
supraganglionic injury
supraglenoid tuberosity
suprahyoid
Supralen
S. cradle orthotic
S. Schaefer orthotic
supralevator abscess
supramalleolar
s. derotational osteotomy
s. flap
s. open amputation
s. orthosis (SMO)
s. varus derotation osteotomy
s. venous ulcer
supramaximal stimulus
supranaviculare
supraoccipital bone
supraorbital neuralgia
suprapatellar
s. bursitis
s. cannula
s. cuff
s. plica
s. plica snap test
s. portal
s. pouch
s. reflex
s. strap
s. tendinitis
supraphysiologic stress
suprapubic
suprascapular
s. nerve
s. nerve entrapment
s. nerve entrapment test
s. nerve injury
s. nerve syndrome
s. neuritis
supraspinal ligament
supraspinatus
s. calcification
s. implant
s. isolation test
s. muscle
s. outlet
s. rotator cuff tear test

s. syndrome
s. tendinitis
s. tendon
supraspinous
s. ligament
s. muscle
suprasternal
s. bone
s. notch
s. plane
s. space
suprasyndesmotic
s. fracture
s. membrane
s. screw fixation
supratectal transverse fracture
supratubercular
s. wedge osteotomy
s. wedge osteotomy bunionectomy
suprofen
sural
s. island flap
s. island flap for foot and ankle reconstruction
s. nerve
s. neuritis
s. neuroma
s. neuropathy
Surbaugh legholder
sure
S. Sport pad
S. Step ankle brace
SureClosure
S. closure
S. device
S. skin stretching system
Sure-Flex
S.-F. III prosthetic foot
S.-F. prosthesis
SureStep
S. ankle support
S. ankle support system
Suretac
S. bioabsorbable shoulder fixation device
S. drill
S. guidewire
S. shoulder fixation
surface
apposing articular s.'s
articular s.
Bazooka support s.
cancellous bone s.
s. cement
ceramic-on-ceramic bearing s.
concave articular s.
contiguous articular s.'s
distal concave articular s.
eburnated bone s.

surface (*continued*)
s. electrode
s. electromyography (SEMG, sEMG)
endosteal s.
erosion of articular s.
facet s.
freshen the s.
irregular articular s.
Micro-Aire débridement of bone s.
s. profile
radioulnar s.
s. replacement
s. replacement hip arthroplasty
roughen the s.
shearling s.
s. shoe interaction
volar s.
wear-resistant s.
weightbearing s.
surfer's
s. knee
s. knot
Surfit adhesive
Surgairtome air drill
SurgAssist
S. leg positioner
S. surgical legholder
surgeon
American Academy of Orthopaedic
S.'s (AAOS)
American Association of Hip and
Knee S.'s (AAHKS)
American Shoulder and Elbow S.'s
(ASES)
surgeon's thumb
surgery
ablative s.
adult scoliosis s.
American Association for Hand S.
(AAHS)
anterior cervicothoracic junction s.
anterior lower cervical spine s.
anterior minimally invasive s.
(AMIS)
arthroscopic laser s.
cervical disc s.
cervicothoracic junction s.
closed s.
computer-assisted orthopaedic s.
(CAOS)
curative s.
CyberKnife image-guided s.
failed flatfoot s.
first ray s.
fusionless s.
fusionless scoliosis s.
H-block nail s.
heel spur s.
Hospital for Special S. (HSS)

hypotensive s.
intradural tumor s.
joint-preservation s.
joint replacement s.
kyphosis correction s.
lateral column lengthening s.
limb-salvage s.
lower extremity bypass s.
lower posterior lumbar spine and
sacrum s.
McCash hand s.
minimal access spinal s. (MASS)
minimally invasive s. (MIS)
minimum incision s. (MIS)
MRI-directed s.
nerve transposition s.
open disc s.
peripheral vascular s. (PVS)
posterior lower cervical spine s.
posterior lumbar interbody fusion s.
posterior lumbar spine and
sacrum s.
posterior upper cervical spine s.
ProTrac system for knee s.
robotic s.
scoliosis s.
traumatic unidirectional Bankart
lesion s.
ulnar nerve transposition s.
Unilink system for hand s.
vascular s.
video-assisted lumbar s.
video-assisted thoracic spine s.
Surgibone
Bioplant S.
S. implant
Unilab S.
surgical
s. ablation
s. anastomosis
s. approach
s. autoimmunization
s. corset
s. dressing room (SDR)
s. exposure
s. extirpation
s. fixation
s. galvanism
s. glove
s. hand tray
s. knife handle
s. leg pedestal
s. loupe
s. morbidity
s. mortality
s. neck
s. neck fracture
s. orthopaedic drill
s. pin driver

s. prosthesis
s. reconstruction
s. reduction
s. rod
s. separation
S. Simplex P adhesive
S. Simplex P radiopaque bone cement
S. Simplex P radiopaque cement
s. splint
s. staple applier
s. technique
s. treatment
Surgicel
S. fibrillar hemostat
S. implant
S. Nu-Knit absorbable hemostat
Surgiflo hemostatic matrix
Surgilase CO₂ laser
Surgilast tubular elastic dressing
SurgiLav machine
Surgi-Stim
S.-S. postsurgical therapy system
S.-S. stimulator
Surgitek prosthesis
Surgitube tubular gauze
Surgivac drain
Surmontil
surprise shoulder test
survey
bone s.
metastatic bone s.
susceptibility testing
suspension
balanced s.
below-knee s.
Children's Advil oral s.
Children's Motrin oral s.
Collis horizontal s.
Collis vertical s.
corset s.
cuff s.
s. feeder
finger trap s.
flexible hinge s.
hip disarticulation s.
hip hemipelvectomy s.
horizontal s.
knee disarticulation s.
panmetatarsal tendon s.
patellar tendon-bearing s. (PTBS)
SC s.
silicone-only s. (SOS)
s. splint
s. strap
suction socket s.
total elastic s. (TES)
s. traction
transfemoral s.

suspension-type socket
suspensory
sustained
s. ankle clonus
s. loading
s. natural apophysial glides (SNAGS)
s. pressure technique
s. release (SR)
sustentacula (*pl. of* sustentaculum)
sustentacular fragment
sustentaculum, *pl.* **sustentacula**
s. tali
s. tali fracture
Sutherland
S. hip operation
S. hip procedure
S. lateral transfer
Sutherland-Greenfield osteotomy
Sutherland-Rowe incision
Sutter
S. device
S. double-stem silicone implant prosthesis
S. implant
S. MCP finger joint prosthesis
S. silicone metacarpophalangeal joint
S. silicone metacarpophalangeal joint arthroplasty
Sutter-CPM
S.-CPM knee apparatus
S.-CPM knee device
sutural bone
suture
s. abscess
Acufex bioabsorbable Suretac s.
Allgöwer-Donati s.
s. anchor
s. anchor shoulder repair
s. anchor technique
baseball s.
Becker core s.
Bell s.
Bio-FASTak s.
BioSorb s.
Biosyn synthetic monofilament s.
Bondek s.
braided s.
bregmatomastoid s.
bulb s.
bundle s.
Bunnell crisscross s.
Bunnell figure-of-8 s.
Bunnell pullout nonabsorbable s.
Bunnell wire pullout s.
button s.
caprolactam s.
Caprosyn s.
Carrel s.

S

725

suture (*continued*)
  Chinese fingertrap s.
  core s.
  cotton s.
  Dacron s.
  Dafilon s.
  Dagrofil s.
  Dexon s.
  Donati vertical mattress s.
  double right-angle s.
  Dupuytren s.
  end-to-end s.
  epitenon s.
  Ethibond s.
  Ethicon s.
  Ethiflex s.
  Ethilon s.
  far-near s.
  fascial s.
  figure-of-8 s.
  finger trap s.
  fishmouth end-to-end s.
  s. fixation
  Gillies s.
  Gore-Tex nonabsorbable s.
  grasping s.
  guy s.
  s. hole drill
  horizontal mattress s.
  interrupted s.
  intradermal s.
  jugal s.
  Kessler grasping s.
  Kessler 4-strand s.
  Kessler-Tajima s.
  Krackow s.
  lambdoid s.
  lashing s.
  lateral trap s.
  Le Dentu s.
  linen s.
  locking horizontal mattress s.
  lockout s.
  Mason-Allen s.
  mattress s.
  Maxon s.
  McLaughlin modification of Bunnell
    pullout s.
  Mersilene s.
  modified Kessler 4-strand s.
  modified Kessler-Tajima s.
  monofilament s.
  muscle-to-bone s.
  nail s.
  near-far s.
  Nicoladoni s.
  nonabsorbable s.
  Nurolon s.
  nylon s.

  s. of Krause
  Orthocord s.
  orthogonally placed s.
  Panacryl s.
  s. passer
  passing s.
  PDS II s.
  Perma-Hand silk s.
  pin s.
  polybutester s.
  Polydek s.
  polydioxanone s. (PDS)
  polyester s.
  polyethylene s.
  polygalactic acid s.
  polyglactin s.
  polyglycolic acid s.
  polyglyconate s.
  polypropylene s.
  Polysorb s.
  popoff s.
  Prolene s.
  pull-out s.
  Pulvertaft end-to-end s.
  Pulvertaft interweave s.
  s. punch
  pursestring s.
  s. pusher
  retention s.
  running s.
  safety-bolt s.
  S. Saver device
  s. scissors
  silk s.
  simple s.
  sling s.
  staple s.
  subcuticular s.
  s. system (SS)
  Tajima modified Kessler s.
  Teflon-coated s.
  tendon s.
  Tevdek s.
  transosseous s.
  Tycron s.
  UltraFix MicroMite anchor s.
  undyed s.
  USP #1, #2, #3 s.
  USP 2-0 (3) size s.
  USP 3-0 (2) size s.
  USP 4-0 (1.5) size s.
  USP 5-0 (1) size s.
  vertical mattress s.
  Vicryl s.
  violet monofilament s.
  wire s.
SutureLasso
  Arthrex S.
sutureless avascular meniscal repair

suture-loop technique
Suture-Self dressing
suturing
> Johnson medial meniscal s.
> meniscus s.
> Morgan-Casscells meniscus s.

Sven-Johansson
> S.-J. extractor
> S.-J. femoral neck nail

swab
> Phenol EZ s.

Swafford-Lichtman median nerve division
swaged needle
swallow-tail sign
swan-neck
> s.-n. chisel
> s.-n. deformity of mid neck
> s.-n. deformity sign
> s.-n. finger deformity
> s.-n. finger deformity reduction
> s.-n. gouge
> s.-n. splint

Swann-Morton surgical blade
Swanson
> S. carpal lunate implant
> S. carpal scaphoid implant
> S. congenital limb anomalies classification
> S. convex condylar arthroplasty
> S. dynamic toe splint
> S. elevator
> S. finger joint
> S. finger joint implant
> S. finger joint prosthesis
> S. flexible hallux valgus prosthesis
> S. great toe implant
> S. great toe prosthesis
> S. Grip-X hand exerciser
> S. hand splint
> S. interpositional wrist arthroplasty
> S. lunate awl
> S. mallet
> S. metacarpal prosthesis
> S. metacarpophalangeal implant
> S. metatarsal broach
> S. metatarsal prosthesis
> S. metatarsophalangeal joint arthroplasty
> S. midfacial defect reconstruction
> S. osteotome
> S. osteotomy
> S. PIP joint arthroplasty
> S. radial head implant
> S. radial head implant arthroplasty
> S. radiocarpal implant
> S. reamer
> S. scaphoid awl
> S. silastic elbow prosthesis
> S. silicone wrist arthroplasty

> S. small joint implant
> S. technique
> S. trapezium implant
> S. T-shaped great toe silastic prosthesis
> S. ulnar head implant
> S. wrist joint implant
> S. wrist prosthesis

swashbuckler approach to distal femur
swath, swathe
> s. and sling
> arm s.

swathe (*var. of* swath)
sway
> anteroposterior lateral s.
> s. back
> body s.
> lateral s.
> postural s.
> s. referencing

swaying gait
SWD
> shortwave diathermy

sweating
> excessive s.
> plantar s.

sweat test
Swede-O
> S.-O Ankle Loc brace
> S.-O Arch-Lok

Swede-O-Universal
> S.-O-U. brace
> S.-O-U. orthosis

Swediauer disease
Swedish
> S. approach
> S. gymnastics
> S. Helparm
> S. knee cage
> S. knee cage orthosis
> S. massage
> S. movement
> S. portal
> S. support stool

sweep knee test
swelling
> boggy s.
> fusiform soft tissue s.
> joint s.
> postfracture s.

SwimEx
> S. aquatic therapy
> S. aquatic therapy bodyCushion
> S. hydrotherapy system
> S. pool

swimmer's
> s. shoulder
> s. view

S

swimming-induced pulmonary edema (SIPE)
swimming pool granuloma
swing
    s. ankle/foot test
    s. phase
    s. phase of gait
    s. time
SwingAlong walker caddy
Swinger car bed
swing-phase
    s.-p. acceleration
    s.-p. control
swing-through gait
swing-to gait
Swiss
    S. Balance orthotic
    S. ball
    S. ball therapy
    S. cancellous screw
    S. MP joint implant
    S. pattern osteotome
switching stick
swivel
    s. clamp
    s. dislocation
    s. utensil
    s. walker
Swivel-Strap
    Aircast S.-S.
    S.-S. ankle brace
    S.-S. ankle stirrup
SWMF
    Semmes-Weinstein monofilament
SWO
    superficial white onychomycosis
swollen disc
SWT
    shockwave therapy
    shuttle walking test
Sydney line
symbrachydactyly
Syme
    S. amputation prosthesis
    S. ankle disarticulation amputation
    S. ankle operation
    S. ankle procedure
    S. Dycor prosthetic foot
    S. foot prosthesis
Symes
    Springlite low profile S. II
    Springlite super low profile S. II
symmetric, symmetrical
    s. sacral plate
    s. thumb duplication
    s. tonicity
    s. vertebral fusion
etrical (*var. of* symmetric)
    s. thoracic vertebral plate

symmetry
    weightbearing s.
sympathectomy, sympathetectomy, sympathicectomy
    cervical s.
    chemical s. (CS)
    lumbar s.
    peripheral chemical s.
    preganglionic s.
sympathetectomy (*var. of* sympathectomy)
sympathetic
    s. block
    s. blockade
    s. chain
    s. component
    s. dysfunction
    s. innervation
    s. nerve
    s. nervous system (SNS)
    s. reflex dystrophy
    s. trunk
sympathetically
    s. maintained pain syndrome (SMPS)
    s. mediated pain
sympathicectomy (*var. of* sympathectomy)
sympathicotonia
symphalangism, symphalangy
symphalangy (*var. of* symphalangism)
symphyses (*pl. of* symphysis)
symphysial mobility
symphysis, *pl.* **symphyses**
    amphiarthrodial s.
    pubic s.
    s. pubis (SP)
    s. pubis diastasis
symptom
    S.'s and Sports Participation Rating Scale
    S.'s Checklist 90 Revised (SCL-90R)
    functionally debilitating s.
    irritable s.
    s. magnification syndrome
    myelopathic s.
    Oehler s.
    Pratt s.
    radicular s.
    Romberg s.
    Romberg-Howship s.
    s. validation
symptomatic
    s. cervical disc disease (SCDD)
    s. implant
    s. nonunion
    s. spondylolisthesis
    s. synovial plica
    s. torticollis

symptomatology
Syms
    S. traction
    S. tractor
Synalgos-DC
Synaptic 2000 pain management system
synarthrodial joint
synarthrophysis
synarthroses (*pl. of* synarthrosis)
synarthrosis, *pl.* **synarthroses**
Synatomic total knee prosthesis
synchondritic fracture
synchondroses (*pl. of* synchondrosis)
synchondrosis, *pl.* **synchondroses**
    neurocentral s.
    tibiofibular s.
synchondrotomy
synchronized fibrillation
synchronous scapuloclavicular rotation
synchrony
    arm heel-strike s.
SynchroSonic
    S. stimulator
    S. U/HVG50 ultrasound/stimulator
syncope
    heat s.
syndactylia (*var. of* syndactyly)
    reduction s.
syndactylism (*var. of* syndactyly)
syndactylization
syndactylized finger
syndactyly, syndactylia, syndactylism
    burn s.
    complete s.
    complex s.
    complicated complex s.
    incomplete s.
    pure s.
    ring finger–small finger s.
    simple s.
syndesmectomy
syndesmectopia
syndesmitis metatarsea
syndesmopexy
syndesmophyte
syndesmoplasty
syndesmorrhaphy
syndesmoses (*pl. of* syndesmosis)
syndesmosis, *pl.* **syndesmoses**
    s. rupture
    s. screw lucency
    s. sprain of ankle
    tibiofibular s.
syndesmotic
    s. avulsion
    s. diastasis
    s. ligament
    s. screw
    s. sprain

syndesmotomy
syndrome
    Aarskog-Scott s.
    accessory navicular pain s.
    acetabular rim s.
    acute exertional compartment s.
      (AECS)
    acute locked-back s.
    acute low back s.
    Adair-Dighton s.
    Adamantiades-Behçet s.
    adult tethered cord s.
    Albright s.
    Albright-McCune-Sternberg s.
    alcohol fat embolism s.
    Alpers s.
    altitude s.
    anterior cervical cord s.
    anterior compartment s. (ACS)
    anterior impingement s.
    anterior interosseous s.
    anterior interosseous nerve s.
    anterior tarsal tunnel s.
    anterior tibial s.
    anterior tibial compartment s.
    anterolateral impingement s.
    anteversion s.
    anular constricting band s.
    Apert s.
    Arnold-Chiari s.
    arthroonychodysplasia s.
    ataxia telangiectasia s.
    athletic heart s.
    Baastrup s.
    Babinski-Fröhlich s.
    Babinski-Nageotte s.
    Bamberger-Marie s.
    Barré-Lieou s.
    Basser migraine-vertigo s.
    Beals s.
    Behavioral Assessment of the
      Dysexecutive S. (BADS)
    Behçet s.
    Behr s.
    benign hypermobile joint s.
    benign joint hypermobility s.
      (BJHS)
    Bertolotti s.
    bicipital shoulder s.
    bilateral acute radicular s.
    bilateral chronic radicular s.
    bioenergy imbalance s. (BIS)
    black heel s.
    blue foot s.
    blue toe s.
    body cast s.
    Breschet-Gorham s.
    Brissaud s.
    broad thumb–big toe s.

S

syndrome *(continued)*

Brown-Séquard s.
Brügger sternosymphysial s.
Bruns s.
bunionette pain s.
bunion pain s.
burner s.
burning-feet s.
Caffey s.
Caffey-Silverman s.
calcaneal spur s.
Calvé-Legg-Perthes s.
Caplan s.
carpal tunnel s. (CTS)
Carpenter s.
Carter-Wilkinson criteria for
  hypermobility s.
cast s.
cauda equina s.
central cord s.
central heel pad s.
central herniation s.
cervical acceleration/deceleration s.
cervical dorsal outlet s.
cervical rib s.
cervicoencephalic s.
cervicogenic s.
Cestan-Chenais s.
Charcot s.
Charlin s.
choke s.
Christian s.
chronic anterior exertional
  compartment s. (CAECS)
chronic compartment s. (CCS)
chronic exertional compartment s.
  (CECS)
chronic heel pain s. (CHPS)
chronic intractable benign pain s.
  (CIBPS)
chronic musculoskeletal pain s.
  (CMPS)
Claude s.
clenched fist s.
clumsy hand s.
Cobb s.
Coffin-Lowry s.
common peroneal nerve s.
compartment s.
complex regional pain s. (CRPS)
complex regional pain s. 2
  (CRPS 2)
complex regional pain s. (type I)
compression s.
computer-assisted carpal tunnel s.
congenital band s.
Conradi-Hünermann s.
constriction band s.
conus medullaris s.

copper deficiency s.
coracoid impingement s.
cord-traction s.
Cornelia de Lange s. (CdLS)
Costen s.
costoclavicular s. (CCS)
costosternal s.
Cowden s.
CREST s.
crossover s.
Crouzon s.
crush s.
cubital fossa s.
cubital tunnel s.
cuboid s.
Cushing s.
cyclops s.
dancing bear s.
Davidenkow scapuloperoneal s.
dead arm s.
de Barsy s.
deconditioning s.
de Lange s.
derangement s.
deSanctis-Cacchione s.
diffuse idiopathic skeletal
  hyperostosis s.
DiGeorge s.
disc s.
DISH s.
DOOR s.
double crush s.
Down s.
droopy shoulder s.
drug-related fetal hydantoin s.
Duplay periarthritis s.
Dyggve-Melchior-Clausen s.
Dyke-Davidoff-Masson s.
dysfunction s.
dysplastic nevus s.
Eagle s.
Eagle-Barrett s.
Eaton-Lambert s.
Eddowes brittle bones s.
Edwards s.
Ehlers-Danlos s. (EDS)
Ekbom restless leg s.
Ekman brittle bones s.
Ellis-van Creveld s.
empty can s.
entrapment s.
eosinophilia-myalgia s. (EMS)
Erb-Goldflam s.
Erdheim s.
exercise-induced compartment s.
exertional anterior compartment s.
  (EACS)
exertional deep posterior
  compartment s. (EDPCS)

extraarticular pain s.
fabella s.
facet joint s.
facioauriculovertebral s.
failed back s. (FBS)
failed back surgery s. (FBSS)
failed surgery s.
Fanconi s.
Fanconi-Albertini-Zellweger s.
far-out L5 nerve root
  compression s.
fat embolism s. (FES)
fat pad s.
FAV s.
Fazio-Londe s.
fetal alcohol s.
fibromyalgia s. (FMS)
fibulocalcaneal pain s.
filum terminale s.
flatback s.
flexor carpi ulnaris s.
flexor origin s.
floppy infant s.
forearm compartment s.
fragile X s.
Freeman-Sheldon s.
frozen shoulder s.
Funk tibialis posterior tendon
  dysfunction s.
GALOP s.
Gardner s.
Gardner-Diamond s.
general adaption s. (GAS)
gluteus maximus pain s.
gluteus medius pain s.
Goldenhar s.
Gorham s.
Gorham-Stout s.
Gowers-Welander musclar
  dystrophy s.
gracilis s.
Grisel s.
Grix-Blankenship-Peterson s.
Guillain-Barré s.
Guyon canal s.
Guyon tunnel s.
Haglund s.
Hajdu-Cheney s.
hammer digit s.
hammer toe s. (HTS)
hammer toe pain s.
hamstring s.
hand-arm vibration s. (HAVS)
hand-foot s.
hand-foot-uterus s.
heart-and-hand s.
heel compression s.
heel pain s.
heel spur s.

heel spur/plantar fasciitis s.
Heerfordt s.
hip joint s.
HLA B27 related
  spondyloarthropathy s.
Hoffa s.
Hoffmann s.
hungry bone s.
Hurler s.
Hurler-Scheie s.
hyoid s.
hyperflexed toe compartment s.
hypermobile joint s.
hypermobility s. (HMS)
hyperostosis s.
hypersensitivity s.
hypothenar hammertoe s.
idiopathic skeletal hyperostosis s.
iliacus s.
iliocostalis lumborum s.
ilioinguinal s.
iliotibial band s. (ITBS)
iliotibial band friction s. (ITBFS)
impingement s.
infrapatellar contracture s. (IPCS)
inguinal ligament s.
internal snapping hip s.
interosseous nerve s.
intersection s.
Isaac s.
Jaccoud s.
Jackson cerebellar s.
Jackson-Gorham s.
Jackson-Weiss s.
Jadassohn-Lewandowsky s.
Jaffe-Campanacci s.
Jarcho-Levin s.
Johanson-Blizzard s.
Karsch-Neugebauer s.
Kast s.
Kearns-Sayre s.
Kenny-Caffey s.
Kinsbourne s.
kissing spines s.
Klippel-Trenaunay s. (KTS)
Klippel-Trenaunay-Weber s.
Kniest s.
Kocher-Debré-Semelaigne s.
Kugelberg-Welander s.
Kuskokwim congenital hip
  contracture s.
kyphotic decompression s.
lacertus s.
Lambert-Eaton s. (LES)
Lambert-Eaton myasthenic s.
  (LEMS)
Larsen s.
lateral column s.
lateral gutter s.

S

syndrome (*continued*)

lateral hyperpressure s.
lateral patellar compression s.
Laurence-Biedl s.
Laurence-Moon s.
Laurence-Moon-Biedl s.
Lawrence-Seip s.
leg-foot-toe s.
Legg-Calvé-Perthes s.
Legg-Calvé-Waldenström s.
LEOPARD s.
Leriche s.
Léri-Weill s.
levator scapulae s.
Linberg restrictive thumb-index
  tenosynovitis s.
Lobstein brittle bones s.
local adaptation s. (LAS)
Looser-Milkman s.
lumbago-mechanical instability s.
lumbar flat back s.
lumbar myofascial pain s.
lumbar thecoperitoneal shunt s.
lumbosacral mechanical s.
Maffucci-Kast s.
manubriosternal joint pain s.
Marfan s.
Marie-Léri s.
Maroteaux-Lamy s. (MLS)
Mazabraud s.
McArdle s.
McCune-Albright s.
McFarland s.
mechanical low back pain s.
medial tibial s. (MTS)
medial tibial stress s. (MTSS)
Meige s.
meningeal s.
metabolic s.
metatarsal overload s.
Meyer-Betz s.
microgeodic phalangeal s.
Milkman osteomalacia s.
Milwaukee shoulder s.
miserable misalignment s.
mixed cord s.
Morgagni-Stewart-Morel s.
Morquio s.
Morquio-Brailsford s.
Morquio-Ullrich s.
Morton s.
Mueller-Weiss s.
multifidus s.
multiple pterygium s.
multiple synostoses s.
myofascial pain s. (MPS)
myofascial pain-dysfunction s.
Naffziger s.
nail-patella s.

naviculocapitate fracture s.
neck pain s.
neck-tongue s.
nerve entrapment s.
Neumann s.
neuroarticular s.
neurogenic s.
Nievergelt-Pearlman s.
occupational stress s. (OSS)
omohyoid s.
Oppenheim s.
os acromiale pain s.
Osebold-Remondini s.
Osgood-Schlatter s.
osteitis pubis s.
osteoporosis pseudoglioma s.
os trigonum pain s.
Ostrum-Furst s.
overtraining s.
overuse s.
Paget-von Schrötter s.
pain-all-over s.
pain dysfunction s.
painful arc s.
paraneoplastic neuromuscular s.
Parsonage-Aldren-Turner s.
Parsonage-Turner s.
Patau s.
patellar clunk s.
patellar malalignment s.
patellar pair s.
patellofemoral joint pain s. (PJPS)
patellofemoral pain s. (PPS)
patellofemoral stress s.
pectoralis major tear s.
peroneal compartment s.
pes anserinus s.
Pfeiffer s.
phalangeal microgeodic s.
phantom limb s.
piriformis s.
plantar fasciitis s.
plica s.
Poland s.
popliteal entrapment s.
popliteal pterygium s.
postcasting s.
postconcussive s.
postdiscectomy s.
posterior cord s.
posterior element overuse s. (PEOS)
posterior impingement s.
posterior interosseous nerve
  compression s.
posterior joint s.
posterior knee pull s.
posterior tarsal tunnel s.
postfracture s.
postphlebitis s.

postpolio s. (PPS)
postpyelomyelitis s.
posttraumatic algodystrophic s.
posttraumatic chronic cord s.
postural s.
predislocation s.
pronator s.
pronator teres s.
Proteus s.
prune-belly s.
pseudoradicular s.
psoas tendon s.
punch drunk s.
quadratus lumborum s.
quadriceps expansion s.
quadrilateral space s.
radial sensory nerve entrapment s.
radial tunnel s.
radial tunnel supinator s.
Raynaud s.
rectus adductor s.
reflex sympathetic dystrophy s.
 (RSDS)
Refsum s.
Reiter s.
repetitive stress s. (RSS)
Rett s.
Riley-Day s.
ring s.
Robinow s.
rotator cuff impingement s.
rotatores s.
Rotter-Erb s.
Roussy-Lévy s.
Rubinstein-Taybi s.
Rust s.
sacroiliac hypermobility s.
sacroiliac joint s.
Sanfilippo s.
SAPHO s.
scalenus anterior s.
scaphocapitate s.
scapholunate ligament tear s.
scapulocostal s.
scapuloperoneal s. (SPS)
Schanz s. (1, 2)
Scheie s.
Scheuermann kyphosis s.
Schüller s.
Schwartz-Jampel s.
Schwartz-Jampel-Aberfeld s.
secondary hip-spine s.
second impact s.
Secretan s.
semimembranosus insertion s.
seronegative enthesopathy and
 arthropathy s.
serotonin s.
serratus anterior muscle s.

short leg s.
shoulder-girdle s.
shoulder-hand s.
shoulder-hand-finger s.
Shwachman-Diamond s.
Shy-Drager s.
sick scapula s.
Silfverskiöld s.
Silfverskiöld Morquito variant s.
Sinding-Larsen-Johansson patella
 inflammation s.
sinus tarsi s.
Sjögren s.
skeletal hyperostosis s.
slipping rib s.
Sly s.
small patella s.
Smith-Lemli-Opitz s.
snapping hip s.
snapping knee s.
snapping scapula s.
soleus s.
spinal cord s.
spiral groove s.
sprained ankle s.
Spurway brittle bones s.
Spurway-Eddowes brittle bones s.
steal s.
sternalis s.
sternoclavicular s.
Stewart-Morel s.
Stickler s.
stiff man s.
stiff person s. (SPS)
straight spine s.
subacromial impingement s.
subclavian steal s.
sublimis bridge s.
Sudeck s.
supinator s.
supracondylar process s.
suprascapular nerve s.
supraspinatus s.
sympathetically maintained pain s.
 (SMPS)
symptom magnification s.
synovial plica s.
talofibular pain s.
tarsal tunnel s. (TTS)
temporomandibular joint s.
temporomandibular joint
 pain-dysfunction s.
tension neck s.
tensor fasciae latae s.
Terracol s.
tethered cord s. (TCS)
tethered patellar tendon s.
thoracic inlet s.
thoracic insufficiency s.

S

syndrome (*continued*)
  thoracic outlet s. (TOS)
  tibiofibular pain s.
  Tietze s.
  TMJ s.
  transient bone marrow edema s.
  transversospinalis s.
  trapezius myofascial pain s.
  traumatic compartment s.
  triangular fibrocartilage tear s.
  trigger finger s.
  trochanteric s.
  tunnel of Guyon s.
  Turner s.
  twelfth rib s.
  Uhthoff s.
  ulnar cubital tunnel s.
  ulnar impaction s.
  ulnar styloid impaction s.
  ulnar tunnel s.
  ulnocarpal abutment s.
  ulnocarpal impaction s.
  ulnolunate abutment s.
  unbalanced wrist s.
  unilateral acute radicular s.
  unilateral chronic radicular s.
  valgus extension overload s.
  van der Hoeve brittle bones s.
  van der Hoeve-de Klyn brittle
    bones s.
  VATER s.
  vertebral steal s.
  vertebral subluxation s.
  vibration white finger s.
  vibrator hand s.
  viscerospinal s.
  volar compartment s.
  von Hippel-Lindau s.
  Vrolik brittle bones recessive s.
  Waldenström s.
  Wallenberg s.
  washboard s.
  Weber s.
  Werdnig-Hoffmann s.
  whiplash s.
  whiplash-shaken infant s.
  whistling face s.
  windblown hand and whistling face
    s.
  winged scapula s.
  Wright s.
  wrist pain s.
  xiphodynia s.
  yellow nail s.
  Ziehen-Oppenheim s.
Synercid
    ia
    detrusor-sphincter s.
    st

synergistic
  s. finger motion
  s. gangrene
  s. muscle
  S. suspension strap
  s. wrist motion
  s. wrist motion splint
synergy
  S. flexible splinting material
  S. hinge system
  S. joint rehabilitation
  limb s.
  OPC S.
  S. spine rehab system
  S. splint
  S. Therapeutic System
**SynFix-LR stand alone anterior
  interbody fusion device**
syngraft
synosteosis (*var. of* synostosis)
synostosis, synosteosis
  s. between radius and ulna
  cervical s.
  congenital radioulnar s.
  fibula protibial s.
  phalangeal s.
  proximal tibiofibular s.
  radioulnar s. (type I, II)
  tibiofibular s.
synostotic
Synovator arthroscopic blade
synovectomy
  Albright s.
  arthroscopic s.
  arthroscopically assisted s.
  s. blade
  carpal s.
  dorsal s.
  s. of peroneal tendons
  palmar s.
  6-portal s.
  Porter-Richardson-Vainio rheumatoid
    arthritis elbow s.
  Smith-Petersen s.
  volar s.
  Wilkinson knee s.
synovial
  s. articulation
  s. biopsy
  s. bursa
  s. cavity
  s. cell sarcoma
  s. chondroma
  s. chondromatosis (SCM)
  s. cyst
  s. disease
  s. fistula
  s. fluid
  s. fold

s. fringe
s. frond
s. hernia
s. herniation
s. histopathology
s. injury
s. joint
s. membrane (SM)
s. nodule
s. nonunion
s. osteochondromatosis
s. outpouching
s. plica
s. plica syndrome
s. pseudarthrosis
s. resector
s. rongeur
s. sarcoma (SS, SYS)
s. shaver
s. sheath
s. stromal cell
s. tag
s. tap
s. tumor

synoviocyte
synoviogram
synovioma
malignant s.
synoviorthesis
synovitis
synovitis, acne pustulosis,
hyperostosis, osteomyelitis
(SAPHO)
benign transient s.
boggy s.
bursal s.
chronic hemorrhagic villous s.
chronic purulent s.
crystal-induced s.
dendritic s.
de Quervain s.
diffuse pigmented villonodular s.
(DPVNS)
disseminated pigmented
villonodular s.
dry s.
extraarticular pigmented
villonodular s.
filarial s.
Finkelstein test for s.
florid s.
focal pigmented villonodular s.
foreign body of s.
fungous s.
hemorrhagic villous s.
s. hyperplastica
hypertrophic s.
inflammatory s.
lead s.

localized nodular s. (LNS)
metatarsophalangeal joint s.
monarticular s.
nontraumatic s.
parapatellar s.
particulate s.
pigmented nodular s.
pigmented villonodular s. (PVNS,
PVS)
postoperative s.
proliferative s.
puerperal s.
purulent s.
reactive s.
recurrent s.
rheumatoid arthritis s.
scarlatinal s.
serous s.
s. sicca
silicone s.
simple s.
suppurative s.
tendinous s.
transient s.
traumatic s.
tuberculous s.
vaginal s.
vibration s.
villonodular s. (VNS)
villous s.

synovium
cartilage s.
exuberant s.
opaque s.
pannus of s.
synpolydactyly (SPD)
Synthaderm dressing
Synthes
S. CerviFix system
S. compression hip screw
S. dorsal distal radius plate
S. drill
S. fixation system
S. guidepin
S. ligament washer
S. LISS
S. Microsystems drill bit
S. Microsystems plate cutter
S. Microsystems plate-holding
forceps
S. Microsystems pliers
S. mini L-plate
S. pie plate
S. Schuhli implant system
S. Universal Spine System
S. USS Fracture System
S. USS II fracture system
S. wire guide
syntheses (*pl. of* synthesis)

S

synthesis, *pl.* **syntheses**
    activity s.
    muscle protein s.
    s. of continuity
    proteoglycan s.
synthetic
    s. augmentation
    s. bone implant
    s. cancellous bone void filler
    s. cortical bone
    s. cortical bone void filler
    s. graft bypass to ankle
    s. material
    s. prosthesis
    s. stent
    s. testosterone
Synvisc injection therapy
syphilitic
    s. abscess
    s. amyotrophy
    s. osteochondritis
Syracuse
    S. anterior spinal fixation
    S. I-plate
syringe
    cement s.
    s. grip
    Terumo s.
syringes (*pl. of* syrinx)
syringohydromyelia
syringoma
    chondroid s.
syringometaplasia
syringomyelia
    posttraumatic s.
    secondary posttraumatic s.
syrinx, *pl.* **syringes**
    s. cavity
SYS
    synovial sarcoma
SysStim 226 muscle stimulator
Systec irrigation
system
    ABG cement-free hip s.
    above-knee suction enhancement s.
    Accu-Cut osteotomy guide s.
    Accu-Flo ultrafiltration s.
    Acculength arthroplasty
      measuring s.
    Accu-SPINA cervical
      decompression s.
    AccuSway balance measurement s.
    Ace intramedullary femoral nail s.
    ACET s.
    acetabular cup s.
    acetabular prosthesis s.
    AcroContin drug delivery s.
    AcroMed VSP fixation s.
    Acryl-X-II bone cement removal s.

Acryl-X orthopaedic cement
    removal s.
Action traction s.
Acufex microsurgical rear-entry or
    front-entry femoral guide s.
AcuFix anterior cervical plate s.
AcuMatch integrated hip s.
Acumed great toe s.
Acuson imaging s.
Acustar surgical navigation s.
Acutrak fusion s.
Acutrak headless compression
    screw s.
Acutrak screw s.
Acutrak small bone fixation s.
Adjustaback wheelchair backrest s.
Advance PS total knee s.
Advantim revision knee s.
Advantim total knee s.
Aequalis s.
Aesculap ABC cervical plating s.
Affinity Anterior Cervical Cage S.
AGC Biomet total knee s.
AGC knee replacement s.
Agee-WristJack fracture reduction s.
Agility total ankle s.
AIM femoral nail s.
Air-Back spinal s.
Aircast Knee S.
air inflation s.
Airtrac ambulatory cervical/lumbar
    traction s.
Alcon Closure S.
AlgoMed infusion s.
Allen shoulder/wrist arthroscopy
    traction s.
Allen spinal s.
Alliance rehabilitation s.
S. Alloclassic hip system
Allofit acetabular cup s.
Allo-Pro hip s.
All-Pro ScanX-12 digital imaging s.
Alphatec mini lag-screw s.
Alphatec small fragment s.
Alta modular trauma s.
Altius M-INI occipitocervicothoracic
    spinal fixation s.
Altius M-INI spinal fixation s.
Ambi compression hip screw s.
AMK fixed bearing knee s.
AMK total knee s.
AML total hip s.
Amplatz anchor s.
Amset anterior locking plate s.
Amset R-F fixation s.
anatomically based exercise s.
anatomic medullary locking hip s.
Anderson s.
AnkleTough rehabilitation s.

Anspach 65K Universal
   instrument s.
anterior cervical plate fixation s.
   (ACFS)
anterior Kostuik-Harrington
   distraction s.
anterior locking plate s. (ALPS)
anterior plate s. (APS)
antimigration s. (AMS)
AOFAS hallux rating s.
Apex Universal Drive and
   Irrigation S.
Apollo DXA bone densitometry s.
Apollo hip s.
Apollo knee prosthesis s.
Apollo total knee s.
APR II hip s.
APR total hip s.
Aqua-Cel heating pad s.
Aquaciser hydrodynamic
   measurement s.
Aquaciser 100R underwater
   treadmill s.
Aquanex hydrodynamic
   measurement s.
AquaSens fluid monitoring s.
Aqua Spray wet nail débridement s.
ARCO classification s.
Ariel computerized exercise s.
Array spinal s.
Arthrex bioabsorbable PLLA
   Trim-It s.
Arthrex bioabsorbable Trim-It s.
Arthrex instruments and s.'s
Arthrex Trim-It screw fixation s.
ArthroCare arthroscopic s.
Arthro-Flo arthroscopic irrigation s.
Arthro-Lock s.
ArthroProbe laser s.
articular-ligamentous s.
Artisan cement s.
Ascent total knee s.
ASIF s.
Asnis 3 cannulated screw s.
Asnis 2 guided-screw s.
Association Research Circulation
   Osseous classification s.
Atavi atraumatic spine fusion s.
Atavi atraumatic spine surgery s.
Atavi TiTLE rod fixation s.
Atlantis cervical plate s.
Atlantis Vision anterior cervical
   plate s.
Atlas cable s.
AuRA cemented total hip s.
autonomic nervous s. (ANS)
Autovac TC orthopaedic
   autotransfusion s.
A-V Impulse s.

AVS spinal s.
axial spinal s.
Axiom modular knee s.
Axiom total knee s.
Axis fixation s.
AxyaWeld bone anchor s.
AxyaWeld J-tip suture welding s.
BacFix s.
Back Bull lumbar support s.
Back Revolution S.
Back Trainer spinal exercise s.
Bad Wildungen Metz spine s.
BAK/C Cervical Interbody
   Fusion S.
BAK interbody fusion s.
BAK/T thoracic interbody fusion s.
Balance Error Scoring S. (BESS)
Balance Master training and
   assessment s.
Balboa thoracolumbar fusion
   posterior fixation anterior buttress
   plate s.
Bassett electrical stimulation s.
Bateman UPF II bipolar knee s.
Batson vertebral brain s.
Bechtol patella s.
Bechtol total hip prosthesis s.
Becker orthopaedic spinal s. (BOSS)
Becker orthopaedic thermoformable
   ankle s.
Bigliani/Flatow shoulder s.
bilateral variable screw placement s.
Biodex Balance S.
Biodex Unweighing Support S.
Biodynamic Molding S.
Biofix absorbable fixation s.
Bio Flote air flotation s.
Bio-1000 knee brace s.
Biomechanical Ankle Platform S.
   (BAPS)
Biomet M2A metal-on-metal
   articulation for hip replacement s.
Biomet Maxim knee s.
Biomet revision knee s.
Biomet Ultra-Drive ultrasonic
   revision s.
Biomet Vision FootRing s.
Bio-Modular total shoulder s.
Bionicare 1000 stimulator s.
bioresorbable drug delivery s.
Biosensor biomechanical testing s.
BioZone nutrition s.
BMP cabling and plating s.
body logic rehabilitation s.
Body Masters MD 510 hi-lo
   pulley s.
Body Response s.
Bolin wedge filter s.
bone density and arthritis testing s.

system (*continued*)
Bone Foam surgical patient positioning s.
bone staple s.
Boston Classification S.
Boston elbow s.
Bottoms-Up posture s.
Bowden cable suspension s.
Brasseler orthopaedic power s.
Bremer halo s.
Bridge Hip s.
Bridwell-Lenke allograft incorporation grading s.
Brighton electrical stimulation s.
Browlift Bone Bridge s.
Buechel-Pappas total ankle replacement s.
Cable-Ready cable grip s.
cable suspension s.
Calandruccio external fixation s.
California soft spinal s.
cannula s.
cannulated guided hip screw s.
Cannulated Plus screw s.
capsuloligamentous s.
CarboJet CO_2 lavage s.
carbon Monotube long bone fracture external fixation s.
Cascade Up and About s.
CD Horizon Sextant S.
CD Horizon Sextant rod insertion s.
CDS s.
Cemex s.
central nervous s. (CNS)
Cervifix s.
Charnley-Howorth Exflow s.
Charnley-Merle d'Aubigné disability grading s.
Charnley total hip s.
Chattanooga balance s.
Chiba spinal s.
C-2 hip s.
Chirotech x-ray s.
Chonstruct chondral repair s.
Cincinnati Knee Rating S.
CircPlus bandage/wrap s.
Circul'Air shoe process s.
Circulator boot s.
CKS knee s.
Clanton turf toe grading s.
closed drainage s.
CLS hip s.
Coblation spinal surgery s.
Codman ACP s.
Codman anterior cervical plating s.
Codman Ti-frame posterior fixation s.
Cofield total shoulder s.
Cohort anterior plate s.

Colorado internal fixation s.
Combi Multi-Traction S.
combined magnetic field s.
ComfortWalk foot s.
Command hip instrumentation s.
Command joint replacement instrument s.
Compass stereotactic s.
compliant prestress s. (CPS)
Concept arthroscopy power s.
Concept beach chair shoulder positioning s.
Concept Precise ACL guide s.
Concept rotator cuff repair s.
Concept self-compressing cannulated screw s.
Concept Sterling arthroscopy blade s.
Concise compression hip screw s.
concurrent force s.
Conserve hip s.
Constant and Murley shoulder scoring s.
ConstaVac autoreinfusion s.
contact laser delivery s.
Contact SPH cups s.
Continuum knee s. (CKS)
Contour Meniscus Arrow bioresorbable repair s.
Coombs bone biopsy s.
Coordinate complete revision knee s.
CO_2 powered gun s.
Corail hip s.
Corin hip arthroplasty s.
Corkscrew rotator cuff repair s.
Cormet hip resurfacing s.
Counter Rotation S. (CRS)
CPT hip s.
CRM s.
Crowe congenital hip dysplasia classification s.
CRS Tibial Torsion S.
cruciate condylar knee s.
Cryo/Cuff Knee Compression Dressing S.
C-Tek anterior cervical plate s.
curved Küntscher nail s.
Cybex I, II, II+ isokinetic exercise s.
Cybex 340 isokinetic rehabilitation and testing s.
Cybex training s.
Dallas grading s.
Dall-Miles cable/crimp cerclage s.
Dall-Miles cable grip s.
DataHand s.
d'Aubigné hip status s.
deep bonding s. (DBS)

Deknatel orthopaedic autotransfusion s.
Deltaloc Reveal anterior cervical plating s.
DEPA diabetic foot ulcer scoring s.
device for transverse traction s.
Diab-A-Foot protection s.
Digital Biofeedback S.
Dimension hip s.
Discovery elbow s.
double-cannula s.
double inflow cannula s.
DTT s.
dual-lock total hip replacement s.
Dual Range Limiter S.
Dupont distal humeral plate s.
Duraloc acetabular cup s.
Durasul head s.
Dwyer-Wickham electrical stimulation s.
DynaFix external fixation s.
DynaFlex multilayer compression s.
Dynalok classic minimal access surgery s.
Dyna-Lok pedicle screw s.
Dyna-Lok plating s.
dynamic stabilizing innersole s. (DSIS)
Dynamic wound closure s.
Dynasplint shoulder s.
Dynesys dynamic stabilization of spinal segments s.
Eagle rigid anterior cervical plate s.
Easyspine pedicle screw and rod s.
Easyspine posterior fixation s.
EBI Medical Array spinal s.
ECT internal fracture fixation s.
EDG s.
Edintrak II s.
Edwards modular s.
ElastaTrac home lumbar traction s.
Electri-Cool cold therapy s.
electrotherapy s.
Elite hip s.
EMG biofeedback s.
Endius endoscopic access s.
Endius TriFix thoracolumbar pedicle screw s.
Endolite transtibial s.
endoscopic carpal tunnel release s.
endoskeletal alignment s. (EAS)
Endotrac blade s.
Endotrac carpal tunnel release s.
Envision anterior cervical plate s.
EPIC functional evaluation s.
EquiTest CDP testing s.
E-Series hip s.
Eska modular hip s.
Evans fracture classification s.

Ewald elbow arthroplasty rating s.
Exact-Fit ATH hip replacement s.
Exeter total hip s.
EX-FI-RE s.
Exogen bone healing s.
Exogen 2000 sonic accelerated fracture healing s.
Expedium anterior spine s.
Extend total hip s.
facet screw s.
facial grading s.
facilitated spinal s.
FASTak suture anchor s.
FAST1 intraosseous infusion s.
felt apron Bowden cable suspension s.
Fenlin total shoulder s.
Fernandez point-score wrist assessment s.
Fernandez scale posttraumatic wrist assessment s.
Ferno AquaCiser underwater treadmill s.
F3 hand, foot, wrist fracture fragment plating s.
Fillauer endoskeletal alignment s.
Fillauer modular shuttle lock s.
filtration s.
FIN s.
Finn knee s.
Fitnet joint testing s.
fixateur interne fixation s.
FlexiTherm Thermographic S.
Flowtron pneumatic compression system BioCryo s.
FluoroNav virtual fluoroscopy s.
FluoroScan imaging s.
FMP acetabular s.
Foamart foot impression s.
Foot screw s.
Foot-Station 3-D foot imaging s.
Foundation total knee and hip s.
Fowler knee s.
FP5000 pump s.
Freehand prosthesis s.
Freeman-Swanson knee s.
F-Scan foot force and gait analysis s.
F-Scan in-shoe s.
F-Scan pressure measurement s.
fusimotor s.
fusion and reconstruction s. (FRS)
Gateway Expedium anterior spine s.
Gateway thoracolumbar s.
GDLH posterior spinal s.
GD Regainer S.
Gem total knee s.
Genesis II foot s.
Genesis II foot/ankle s.

S

system (*continued*)

Genesis II total knee s.
genital s.
Genucom ACL laxity analysis s.
Genucom knee flexion analysis s.
Geomedic s.
Gillette double-flexure ankle joint s.
Glider II patient transfer s.
Global Fx shoulder fracture s.
Global total shoulder arthroplasty s.
Golden mean testing s.
Golf Exercise S.
Gonstead pelvic marking s.
Graf stabilization s.
graft containment s.
Granberg cervical traction s.
gravitational platelet separation s.
gravity extension locking s.
  (GELS)
Gray revision instrument s.
Green-O'Brien evaluation s.
Guardian limb salvage s.
Guldmann Overhead Trac S.
Haid UBP s.
Hajdu staging s.
Hall mandibular implant s.
Hall modular acetabular reamer s.
halo cervical traction s.
Hannover scoring s.
Harrington rod and hook s.
Harris hip status s.
Hausmann Work-Well work
  hardening s.
haversian s.
HBS s.
HCMI Chiropractic S.
headless bone screw s.
Herbert bone screw s.
Heritage hip s.
Hermes Evolution tricompartmental
  knee s.
Hermes total knee s.
Hexcel total condylar knee s.
Hipokrat bimodular shoulder s.
Histofreezer cryosurgical s.
HJD total hip s.
Hoffmann external fixation s.
hook probe s.
Hot/Ice S. III
Howmedica knee s.
Howmedica total ankle s.
Howmedica VSF fixation s.
HybridFit total hip s.
HybridFit total knee s.
hydraulic test s.
HydroFlex arthroscopy irrigating s.
HydroTrack underwater treadmill s.
hypobaric transfemoral s.
hypobaric transtibial s.

ICRS arthroscopic knee, shoulder,
  and ankle joint staging s.
Ilizarov limb-lengthening s.
immune s.
Impact modular total hip s.
Impact total hip s.
Impingement-Free Tibial Guide S.
implantable internal s.
InCompass spinal fixation s.
Indiana tome carpal tunnel
  syndrome release s.
In-Fast bone screw s.
Infinity hip s.
InFix interbody fusion s.
Inglis-Pellicci elbow arthroplasty
  rating s.
Innomed arthroplasty measuring s.
Innovative COR/T implant s.
4-in-1 positioning block s.
Insall-Burstein II modular total
  knee s.
Insight knee positioning and
  alignment s.
Instratek titanium cannulated small
  bone screw s.
instrumentation s.
In-Tac bone-anchoring s.
Integral hip s.
integrated shape and imaging s.
InteliJET fluid management s.
Inteq small joint suturing s.
Interax total knee s.
interbody fusion cage s.
Intermedics natural hip s.
internal fixation plate-screw s.
International 10-20 EEG scalp
  electrode placement s.
International Listing S.
Iowa hip status rating s.
Ipos arch support s.
IPS total hip s.
irrigation s.
ISKD s.
Isobar LP low profile pedicle
  screw s.
Isola fixation s.
Isola spinal instrumentation s.
Issys inverted polyaxial pedicle
  screw s.
Itrel II, III spinal cord
  stimulation s.
Jacobson s.
Joint Active S.'s (JAS)
joint coordinate s. (JCS)
Judet hip status s.
Julstro Self-Treatment s.
Jurgan Pin Ball s.
J-Vac closed drainage s.
Kaltenborn joint mobilization s.

Kaneda anterior spinal/scoliosis s.
(KASS)
Kellgren-Lawrence grading s.
Kendall A-V impulse s.
Keramos ceramic/ceramic total
hip s.
K-Fix fixator s.
K2 hemi toe implant s.
Kinamed Exact-Fit ATH s.
Kin-Con isokinetic exercise s.
Kinematic II condylar and stabilizer
total knee s.
Kinematic II rotating hinge knee s.
Kinemax modular condylar and
stabilizer total knee s.
Kinemax Plus total knee s.
Kinemetric guide s.
KineTec ECT s.
Kinetik great toe implant s.
King-Moe idiopathic scoliosis
classification s.
Kirschner II-C shoulder s.
Kirschner integrated shoulder s.
knee extensor s.
knee signature s.
Knee Society Total Knee
Arthroplasty Roentgenographic
Evaluation and Scoring S.
KobyGard s.
Koby Isogard surgical treatment s.
Kofoed scoring s.
Kostuik-Harrington distraction s.
Kurtzke functional s.
Kyle fracture classification s.
Langenskiöld grading s.
Larson hip status s.
LCR s.
LCS mobile bearing knee s.
LCS total knee s.
Leibinger Profyle hand s.
less invasive stabilization s. (LISS)
Liberty spinal s.
Lido Active Multijoint S.
Lidoback isokinetic dynamometry s.
Lido Passive Multijoint S.
Lifeline Wall Gym 2000 fitness s.
Linear total hip s.
Link custom partial pelvis
replacement s.
Link Endo-Model rotational knee s.
Link Lubinus SP II hip
replacement s.
Link Saddle Prosthesis Endo-Model
hip replacement s.
LiteNest portable seating s.
locomotor s.
LoCon-T distal radial plating s.
Lone Star retractor s.
Lordex lumbar spine s.

Lorenz osteosynthesis s.
Lubinus AP hip s.
Lubinus SP II anatomically adapted
hip s.
Luhr fixation s.
Lumbo 90 home care traction s.
lumbosacral cartilaginous s.
Luque II fixation s.
Lynco biomechanical orthotic s.
Mackinnon-Dellon staging s.
MacReflex infrared motion
analysis s.
MacroPore OS spinal s.
Madajet XL jet-injection
anesthesia s.
Magerl hook-plate s.
Magerl plate-screw s.
Magna-FX cannulated screw s.
Malcolm-Lynn radiolucent spinal
retraction s.
Malcolm-Rand radiolucent headrest
and retraction s.
Malibu thoracolumbar fusion
posterior fixation pedicle screw s.
Mallory-Head modular calcar s.
manual gun s.
Maramed Miami fracture brace s.
Mark III halo s.
Mark II Sorrells hip arthroplasty
retractor s.
Mason fracture classification s.
matrix seating s.
Mattrix spinal cord stimulation s.
Maxim Modular Knee S.
Mayo Clinic congruent elbow
plate s.
Mayo Clinic Forefoot Scoring S.
Mayo hip scoring s.
McCain TMJ arthroscopic s.
Medical Examination and Diagnostic
Coding S. (MEDICS)
Medical Research Council s.
Medtronic spinal cord stimulation s.
Meniscus Mender II s.
Mephisto speed lacing s.
Merle d'Aubigné hip status s.
Mesa spinal s.
Meta-Nail tibial nail s.
Metasul metal-on-metal hip
prosthesis s.
METRx tubular retractor s.
MG II total knee s.
Microloc knee s.
Micro-Mill knee instrument s.
Micronail intramedullary distal
radius fixation s.
MicroPhor iontophoretic drug
delivery s.
Midas Rex instrumentation s.

S

system (*continued*)

Miller-Galante I condylar total knee s.
Miller-Galante revision knee s.
Mimix bone replacement s.
Minaar classification s.
Mini-Acutrak small bone fixation s.
mini lag screw s. (MLS)
Mirage Spinal S.
Mitek anchor s.
Mitek GII suture anchor s.
Mitek VAPR tissue removal s.
modified Wagner classification s.
Modular Acetabular Revision S. (MARS)
modular S-ROM total hip s.
Moe s.
Monotube external fixator s.
Monticelli-Spinelli circular external fixation s.
Moore hip endoprosthesis s.
Morrey elbow arthroplasty rating s.
MosaicPlasty s.
Mosaic spinal implant s.
Moss fixation s.
motorized shaving s.
Mouradian humeral fixation s.
movement s.
MRI-compatible plate and screw s.
MTS Mini Bionix test s.
Multi Balance S. (MBS)
Multidex chronic wound treatment s.
Multi Podus boot s.
Multi Podus foot s.
Multitak SS s.
Multitak suture snap s.
musculotendinous s.
Musgrave Footprint S.
M3-X extremity fixation s.
Myobock s.
Natural-Hip s.
Natural-Knee II s.
Navitrack computer-assisted surgery s.
Neer II shoulder s.
Neer II total knee s.
Neff femorotibial nail s.
NeuroCom Equitest S.
NewBridge laminoplasty fixation s.
Newport hip s.
NexGen complete knee s.
NexGen complete knee replacement s.
Nex-Link spinal fixation s.
Nexus wheelchair seating s.
NoHands Mouse-Foot-Operated Computer Mouse S.
NordiCare Back Therapy S.
form testing and rehabilitation s.

Novation ceramic articulation hip s.
Nucleotome s.
numerical pain rating s. (NPRS)
OctaFix occipital fixation s.
OEC Mini 6600 imaging s.
Ogden fracture classification s.
Ogden plate s.
Ogden tissue reattachment mini s.
Oklahoma cable s.
Olerud pedicle fixation s.
Olerud PSF fixation s.
Omega compression hip screw s.
Omega Plus compression hip s.
Omnifit Plus hip s.
Omnifit total knee s.
On-Q PainBuster postoperative pain relief s.
OnTrack s.
open double-decked hook cervical s.
Optetrak comprehensive knee s.
Optetrak total knee replacement s.
Opti-Fix total hip s.
OptiLock distal radius plating s.
OptiLock periarticular plating s.
Option hip s.
optoelectric measuring s.
Optotrak motion measurement s.
Orth-evac autotransfusion s.
Orth-evac postoperative transfusion s.
Orthodoc presurgical planning s.
Orthogenesis LPS limb preservation prosthesis s.
Ortholoc Advantim revision knee s.
Ortholoc Advantim total knee s.
Orthomerica TC AFO s.
Orthomet Axiom total knee s.
Orthomet Perfecta total hip s.
OrthoPak bone growth stimulator s.
OrthoPAT s.
Orthotec pressurized fluid irrigation s.
Osada portable electric handpiece s.
Osada portable handpiece s.
Oscar ultrasonic bone cement removal s.
OSI modular table s.
OssaTron shock wave therapy s.
osteochondral autograft transfer s. (OATS)
Osteo-clage cable s.
Osteonics Scorpio posterior cruciate retaining total knee s.
Osteopower modular handpiece s.
OsteoView 2000 imaging s.
Otto Bock MOBIS mobility s.
Oxford meniscal unicompartmental knee s.
Panoview arthroscopic s.

Paprosky acetabular defect classification s. (type I, IIa, IIb, IIc, IIIa, IIIb)
Parabath paraffin heat treatment s.
ParaMax ACL guide s.
parasympathetic nervous s. (PNS)
Partnership s.
passive ligamentous s.
PCA primary total knee s.
PCA Universal total knee instrument s.
Peak anterior compression plate s.
Peak Fixation S.
Peak Motus Motion Measurement S.
Pedar in-shoe measurement s.
Pedar pressure insole s.
Pedar pressure measurement s.
pediatric s.
pedicle screw s.
pedicle screw-cable s.
Perfecta total hip s.
PerFixation s.
Performance modular total knee s.
Performance unicompartmental knee s.
perioperative autotransfusion s.
peripheral nervous s. (PNS)
peripheral vascular s. (PVS)
PFC modular total knee s.
PFC Sigma knee s.
PFC TC3 modular knee s.
PFC total hip replacement s.
PGP flexible nail s.
Phoenix foot s.
Phoresor II iontophoretic drug delivery s.
Phoresor PM900 iontophoresis s.
Pillar PEEK partial vertebral body replacement s.
Pillar PEEK VBR s.
pin ball s.
Pinch Gauge and Jackson Strength Evaluation S.
Pinnacle acetabular cup s.
Pinn-ACL guide s.
Pinn anterior cruciate ligament guide s.
Pinwheel S.
Pipkin fracture classification s.
Pivot MIS s.
PlastiCast adjustable joint cast s.
plate-screw s.
PlexiPulse DVT prophylaxis s.
PLLA Trim-It s.
PMT halo s.
Podospray nail drill s.
point and pressure s.'s
3-point pressure s.
Polaris 5.5 spinal s.

Polaris 6.35 spinal s.
Polarus Plus humeral fixation s.
Polarus positional humeral fixation s.
polyaxial s.
Polyax locking plating s.
Polycentric and Wide-Track knee s.
POP Rivet fixation s.
Postel hip status s.
posterior cruciate condylar knee s.
posterior rod s.
Powerbelt exercise s.
PPT insole s.
PPT soft tissue orthotic s.
Precision Osteolock femoral component s.
Precision Strata hip s.
press-fit total condylar knee s.
pressure transducer-monitor s.
Prestige cervical disc s.
pretarget filtration s.
Profemur tapered stem total hip s.
Profile total hip s.
Profix total knee replacement s.
Profore Four-Layer bandage s.
programmable VariGrip II prosthetic control s.
Promos modular shoulder s.
prospective payment s. (PPS)
Protector meniscus suturing s.
ProTrac cruciate reconstruction s.
Providence Scoliosis S.
Provisional Fixation TC-100 plating s.
Proxiderm wound closure s.
Puddu osteotomy s.
Pulsavac III wound débridement s.
Pump It Up pneumatic socket volume management s.
Puno-Winter-Byrd s.
PWB transpedicular spine fixation s.
Pylon intramedullary nail s.
Pyramid anterior plate fixation s.
Quantronic Resonance S. (QRS)
Quick-Sil silicone s.
QuickTack periosteal fixation s.
radiolucent wrist fixation s.
Rancho Los Amigos Cube S.
rearfoot stability s. (RSS)
ReCap femoral resurfacing s.
Reebok Slide S.
Reebok Step S.
Reese osteotomy guide s.
Reflection ceramic acetabular s.
Reflex anterior cervical plate s.
ReFlexion first MPJ implant s.
Replica total hip replacement s.
resorbable graft containment s.
Restoration acetabular s.

system (*continued*)

Restoration-HA hip s.
Restoration modular revision hip s.
Restore ACL guide s.
reticuloendothelial s.
ReUnion fracture s.
ReUnite resorbable orthopaedic
   fixation s.
Revelation hip s.
Revo rotator cuff repair s.
rHead implant s.
Richards fixator s.
Richards hip endoprosthesis s.
Richards modular hip s.
Richards Solcotrans orthopaedic
   drainage-reinfusion s.
right-handed orthogonal coordinate s.
   (RHOCS)
Riseborough-Radin fracture
   classification s.
Rochester compression s.
Rod TAG suture anchor s.
Roger Anderson s.
Rogozinski screw s.
Rogozinski spinal fixation s.
Rogozinski spinal rod s.
Roho pediatric seating s.
Rolyan Reach N Range Pulley S.
Romano curved drilling s.
Rotaglide total knee s.
Russell-Taylor femoral interlocking
   nail s.
SC-AcuFix anterior cervical plate s.
Schatzker tibial plateau fracture
   classification s. (I-VI)
Scorpio total knee s.
Scotchcast length splinting s.
Secure Yet Gentle surgical
   dressing s.
segmental spinal correction s.
   (SSCS)
Selby I, II fixation s.
Select shoulder s.
sextant rod insertion s.
Shadow-Line ACF spine retractor s.
SharpShooter tissue repair s.
shaving s.
Sherman remote podiatric vacuum s.
shoulder arm s. (SAS)
Shuttle MiniClinic resistance s.
Siemens Sonocur Basic
   extracorporeal shockwave
   therapy s.
Sierra posterior
   occipitocervicothoracic
   stabilization s.
Silhouette pedicle screw s.
Silhouette spinal s.
Simmons and Segil classification s.

Simmons plating s.
single-cannula s.
skeletal repair s. (SRS)
slotted obturator-cannula s.
Smart Balance Master s.
SmartPReP PRP s.
Smith & Nephew bracing and
   support s.
Socon spinal s.
SOCS AFO s.
SOCS pad s.
Sofflex mattress s.
Sofwire cable s.
Solanas posterior cervicothoracic
   fixation s.
Solcotrans autotransfusion s.
Solcotrans orthopaedic
   drainage-refusion s.
Soma Gonio s.
Soma pulley s.
sonic accelerated fracture healing s.
   (SAFHS)
SonoAce PICO portable digital
   color ultrasound s.
Sonoma anterior cervical plate s.
Sorbie-Questor total elbow
   prosthesis s.
Sorrells hip arthroplasty retractor s.
SOS total hip s.
SOS total knee s.
Souter-Strathclyde total elbow s.
Spectrum EF total hip s.
Spectrum tissue repair s.
spherocentric knee s.
spinal fusion s.
SpineCor s.
spinopelvic transiliac fixation s.
Spinoscope noninvasive imaging s.
SportCord exercise and
   rehabilitation s.
SportsRAC arm care s.
Square Module Seating S.
S-ROM hip replacement s.
S-ROM modular total knee s.
S-ROM proximally modular total
   hip s.
Stability total hip s.
Stableloc external wrist fixation s.
Stableloc II external fixation s.
Stahl lunatomalacia staging s.
StairMaster exercise s.
Statak anchor s.
Stealth image-guided s.
Steffee pedicle screw-plate s.
Steffee variable spine plating s.
Stelkast Surpass ceramic-on-ceramic
   acetabular s.
STIF s.
StIM neuromuscular stimulator s.

Stockholm HAVS severity staging s.
Strata hip s.
Stratis ST ACL reconstruction s.
Stretch-Rite exerciser s.
Stryker Intracompartmental Pressure Monitor S.
Stryker SE3 drive s.
suction-irrigation s.
Summit minipolyaxial screw s.
supine C-Trax traction s.
SureClosure skin stretching s.
SureStep ankle support s.
Surgi-Stim postsurgical therapy s.
suture s. (SS)
SwimEx hydrotherapy s.
sympathetic nervous s. (SNS)
Synaptic 2000 pain management s.
Synergy hinge s.
Synergy spine rehab s.
Synergy Therapeutic S.
Synthes CerviFix s.
Synthes fixation s.
Synthes Schuhli implant s.
Synthes Universal Spine S.
Synthes USS Fracture S.
Synthes USS II fracture s.
Tae Bo aerobic workout s.
TAG anchor s.
Talar-Fit implant s.
Tamarack anterior thoracolumbar plating s.
Tamarack flexure joint s.
Taperloc hip s.
Targon PH proximal humerus intramedullary nail s.
TEC interface s.
TempFix external fixation s.
The Healthy Back S.
Thera-Band resistive therapy s.
Therabath paraffin heat therapy s.
Thera-Ciser light exercise s.
Thera-Ciser therapeutic exercise s.
Thera-Wedge s.
Thompson hip endoprosthesis s.
Thompson leg check s.
THORP s.
tibia coordinate s.
tibial torsion s.
Ti-Fit total hip s.
titanium hollow-screw plate s.
Tokuhashi metastatic spine tumor preoperative scoring s.
Tokuhashi metastatic spine tumor prognostic evaluation s.
top-loading screw and rod s.
Torus external fixation s.
Total Condylar Knee s.
Total Gym rehabilitation s.
total posterior element s. (TOPS)

Townley anatomic knee s.
TransFix ACL s.
TransFix femoral fixation s.
TraumaJet wound debridement s.
trephine autologous bone harvesting s.
triangle blade s.
Triathlon knee s.
Triax monotube external fixation s.
Trigen Meta-Nail tibial nail s.
Trilogy acetabular cup s.
Trim-It screw s.
Tri-Motion Knee S.
Trio medialized rod s.
triple envelope s.
Tri-Wedge total hip s.
True/Fit femoral intramedullary rod s.
True/LOK external fixation s.
TSRH crosslink s.
TSRH fixation s.
TSRH spinal implant s.
TSRH universal spinal instrumentation s.
TurnAide therapeutic s.
Turning Board Exercise S.
Tylok high-tension cable s.
UBP s.
Ulson fixator s.
Ultima hip replacement s.
Ultima total hip s.
Ultimax distal femoral intramedullary rod s.
Ultra-Drive bone cement removal s.
Ultra-Drive ultrasonic revision s.
UltraFix RC suture anchor s.
Ultra-Guard FS hip bracing s.
Ultra-Guard hip orthosis s.
UltraPower drill s.
ultrasound bone imaging s. (UBIS)
Ultra-X external fixation s.
unicompartmental knee s.
Unicondylar Geomedic hemi-knee s.
Uniflex nailing s.
unilateral variable screw placement s.
Uniportal fascial release s.
UniSyn modular hip s.
Unity lumbosacral fixation s.
universal bone plate s.
Universal Spine S.
Up and About s.
V.A.C. Freedom wound-healing s.
Vanguard complete knee s.
Vapr s.
variable axis knee s.
variable screw placement s.
Vector low back analysis s.
Vermont pedicle fixation s.

S

system (*continued*)
    Verruca-Freeze freezing s.
    Versaback back s.
    Versa-Fx femoral hip fixation s.
    Versalok low back fixation s.
    VerSys hip s.
    VertAlign spinal support s.
    Vertetrac ambulatory traction s.
    Vicon 3-dimensional gait
        analysis s.
    Vilex cannulated screw s.
    Vilex screw s.
    Vivatek treatment s.
    VSF fixation s.
    VSP s.
    Wagner revision hip s.
    WalkAide s.
    WarmTouch patient warming s.
    Warm-Up active wound therapy s.
    wedge TAG suture anchor s.
    West Point Ankle Grading S.
    Whiteside Ortholoc modular knee s.
    Wiltse pedicle screw fixation s.
    Window anterior cervical plate s.
    Wisconsin spinal fracture s.
    Woodpecker total hip broaching s.
    wound closure s.
    Wrightington Frusto-Conical hip cup
        and stem s.

    Xact ACL graft-fixation s.
    Xia hook s.
    Y-knot tying s.
    Zenith Electrotherapy ultrasound s.
    Zephir anterior cervical plate s.
    Zickel fracture classification s.
    Zimmer anatomic hip s.
    Zimmer collarless polished taper
        hip s.
    Zimmer CPT 12/14 hip s.
    Zimmer crossover instrumentation s.
    Zimmer-Hall drive s.
    Zimmer hip implant s.
    Zimmer Pulsavac wound
        débridement s.
    Zimmer tharies surface
        arthroplasty s.
    Zimmer unicompartmental high-flex
        knee s.
    ZMR hip s.
    ZMS intramedullary fixation s.
    Zone Specific II meniscal repair s.
    Zuni exercise s.
    Zweymüller hip s.
systemic
    s. lupus erythematosus (SLE)
    s. sclerosis
systolic blood pressure
systremma

T

thoracic

T buttress plate
T condylar fracture
T fracture

TA

TA metallic staple
TA Premium (30, 55, 90) staple

TAA

total ankle arthroplasty

tabes dorsalis

tabetic

t. arthropathy
t. foot
t. gait
t. osteoarthropathy

Tab Grabber

table

Adapta physical therapy t.
adjusting t.
Advocate electric flexion distraction t.
Air-Drop chiropractic t.
Air-Flex chiropractic t.
Albee orthopaedic t.
Allen hand/arm surgery t.
AlphaStar t.
Amsco fracture t.
AMIS extension t.
AM-MI orthopaedic t.
Anatomotor traction/massage t.
Andrews spinal surgery t.
Andrews SST-3000 spinal surgery t.
anteroposterior t.
Apollo TM electric flexion t.
APS Hi-Lo electric lift t.
ATT-300 LAT traction t.
Back Specialist chiropractic t.
Back Specialist electric t.
Back Specialist manual t.
bariatric mat t.
Bell t.
Berstein cast t.
cast t.
Chick CLT operating t.
Chick fracture t.
Chick-Langren orthopaedic t.
Chiro-Manis chiropractic t.
circumductor t.
Cobb attachment for Albee-Compere
 fracture t.
craniosacral t.
crank t.
Crystal adjusting t.
cutout t.
DDP t.

DePuy graft preparation t.
Diamond biomechanical t.
Ergo style flexion t.
Eurotech Diamond t.
Eurotech Emerald t.
Eurotech Platinum t.
Eurotech Sapphire t.
EZ-Up inversion t.
flexion-distraction chiropractic t.
fluoroscopic t.
fracture t.
friction-reduced examination t.
friction-reduced segmented t.
Galaxy 900HS adjusting t.
Galaxy McManis hylo t.
Gemini chiropractic t.
Green-Anderson growth t.
Hercules TM drop-adjusting t.
Hessco 300, 500 series
 hydrotherapy t.
Hill Air-Drop HA90C t.
hi-lo t.
HLT-405 instrument adjusting t.
horseshoe therapy t.
hydromassage t.
inner t.
intersegmental traction chiropractic t.
Jackson spinal surgery and
 imaging t.
Knavel t.
knee-chest t.
Leander chiropractic t.
Leander motorized flexion t.
Legend Hy-Lo adjusting t.
Legend stationary adjusting t.
Lloyd chiropractic t.
long axis traction chiropractic t.
Magnum 101 Plus t.
Marquet fracture t.
Massage Time Pro hydromassage t.
mat t.
McKenzie Repex t.
Med-Fit cranial-sacral t.
Meridian Intersegmental t.
Midland tilt t.
Multi-Lock hand operating t.
orthopaedic t.
over-bed t.
Paris manual therapy t.
passive traction t.
PET/Eurotech Generation 2000 t.
physical therapy t.
Platinum stationary t.
Powermatic t.
Protege manual flexion distraction t.

table (*continued*)
    PT tilt t.
    Rath treatment t.
    Re-Lax-O chiropractic t.
    resistive exercise t.
    Roger Anderson t.
    Sapphire t.
    t. short leg
    Skytron operating room t.
    slatted plinth t.
    slot t.
    split t.
    Stryker surgical hand t.
    t. tie
    tilt t.
    Titan Apollo electric flexion t.
    Titan Meridian intersegmental
      traction t.
    Titan Nova manual flexion-extension
      multiflex t.
    Topaz manual flexion t.
    Tri W-G t.
    TX-1–TX-15 traction t.
    VAX-D therapy t.
    Verteflex Intersegmental
      Traction T.
    Winco folding treatment t.
    Zenith chiropractic t.
    Zenith-Cox flexion/distraction t.
    Zenith Hylo t.
    Zenith stationary t.
    Zenith Thompson t.
    Zenith VertiLift t.
table-skeletal
    t.-s. fixation
    t.-s. fixation frame
tablet
    bonemeal t.
    Tums E-X Extra
      Strength T.
tabletop Stone stapler
taboparesis
Tabs Elite mobility monitor
Tab-Strap knee immobilizer
Tac-3
Tac-40
Tachdjian
    T. external fixation for cavus
      fixation procedure
    T. flatfoot grade
    T. flatfoot score
    T. fractional lengthening
    T. hamstring lengthening
    T. orthosis
    T. pediatric ankle fracture
      classification
    T. pin
    ...oir
...readed anchor

tack
    biodegradable surgical t.
    t. breakage
    membrane t.
    T. test
    T. Test
tack-and-pin forceps
tackle
    spear t.
tackler's
    t. arm
    t. exostosis
Tacoma sacral plate
tacrine HCl
Tacticon
    T. peripheral neuropathy kit
    T. peripheral neuropathy screening
      device
    T. quantitative sensory testing
tactile
    t. anesthesia
    t. discrimination
Tae Bo aerobic workout system
TAG
    tissue anchor guide
    TAG anchor system
tag
    skin t.
    synovial t.
tai
    t. chi
    t. chi chuan exercise
tailbone
tailor's
    t. ankle
    t. bunion
    t. bunionectomy
    t. bunionette
Tait vascular graft
Tajima
    T. modified Kessler suture
    T. suture method
    T. suture technique
Takakura tarsal index
Take-apart forceps
TakeOff elbow support
Take-Out Extractor
taking off shoe test (TOST)
TAL
    tendo Achillis lengthening
Talacen
talalgia
talar
    t. avulsion fracture
    t. axis-first metatarsal base angle
      (TAMBA)
    t. beak
    t. beaking
    t. body

t. body fusion
t. body nonunion
t. canal
t. declination angle
t. dislocation
t. dome
t. head
t. malunion
t. neck
t. neck exostosis
t. neck fracture
t. neck injury classification (I–III)
t. neck osteotomy
t. neck tunnel
t. osteochondral fracture
t. process
t. ridge
t. shift
t. sinus
t. subluxation
t. sulcus
t. tilt
t. tilt angle
t. tilt eversion test
t. tilt inversion test
t. triple arthrodesis

Talar-Fit implant system
talectomy
Trumble t.
tali (*gen.* and *pl. of* talus)
talipedic
talipes
t.
t. calcaneocavus
t. calcaneovalgus
t. calcaneovarus
t. calcaneus
t. cavovalgus
t. cavovarus
t. cavus
t. cavus deformity
t. equinovalgus
t. equinovarus (TEV)
t. equinus
flexible t.
t. planovalgus
t. plantaris
t. planus
t. tendinoplasty
t. transversoplanus
t. valgus
t. varus

Tall-ette toilet seat
Talma disease
talocalcaneal, talocalcanean
t. angle (TCA)
anteroposterior t. (APTC)
t. coalition
t. fusion

t. index
t. index classification
t. joint
t. ligament
t. ligament disruption
t. osteotomy

talocalcanean (*var. of* talocalcaneal)
talocalcaneonavicular
t. complex
t. joint
t. ligament articulation

talocrural
t. alignment
t. angle
t. fusion
t. joint
t. restriction
t. sprain

talocruralis
talofibular
t. articulation
t. joint
t. ligament
t. pain syndrome

talometatarsal angle
talon
T. compression hip screw
t. noir

talonavicular (TN)
t. angle
t. arthrodesis
t. articulation
t. bone
t. capsule
t. capsulotomy
t. dislocation
t. fusion
t. joint
t. ligament
t. ossicle
t. ossicle of Pirie
t. sprain

talotibial exostosis
talus, *gen.* and *pl.* **tali**
t. alignment
beaking of head of t.
t. body fracture
congenital vertical t. (CVT)
flattop t.
t. foot deformity
t. lateral posterior process
t. lateral tubercle
osteochondral fracture of dome of t.
osteochondral lesion of t. (OLT)
Stieda posterior process of t.
sulcus of t.
sustentaculum tali
valgus tilt of t.
vertical t.

T

Talwin
  T. compound
  T. NX
TAM
  total active motion
Tamarack
  T. anterior thoracolumbar plating
  system
  T. flexure joint
  T. flexure joint system
TAMBA
  talar axis-first metatarsal base
  angle
TAMMAS
  temporary articulating
  methylmethacrylate antibiotic
  spacer
tamp
  bone t.
  inflatable bone t. (IBT)
  KyphX Elevate inflatable bone t.
  KyphX Exact inflatable bone t.
  KyphX inflatable bone t.
  KyphX Xpander inflatable bone t.
  tension band wire t.
Tandearil
tandem
  t. connector
  t. gait
  t. gait test
tang
  t. distractor
  t. distractor tool
  t. retractor
  spaced apart t.'s
  spinal fusion cage t.
  vertebral space t.
tangential
  t. hand
  t. incision
  t. layer
  t. standing radiograph
  t. x-ray view
tangoRS smart screw
**Tanita Professional Body Composition
  Analyzer**
tank
  Hubbard physical therapy t.
  therapy t.
Tanner developmental model
**Tanner-Whitehouse bone-age reference
  value**
tantalum
  t. ball marker
  t. mesh
tap
  AO t.
  t. drill
  dynamic condylar screw t.

t. elbow test
screw t.
Screw-Lok t.
synovial t.
tape
  anthropometric measuring t.
  benzoin adherent t.
  bias-cut t.
  cast t.
  Delta-Lite casting t.
  DynaSport athletic t.
  Elastikon elastic t.
  EnduraFIX t.
  Expandover athletic t.
  fiberglass-free cast t.
  foam t.
  graded Gore-Tex t.
  Gulick II t.
  Leukotape sports t.
  Lightplast athletic t.
  Medipore H surgical t.
  Mersilene t.
  moleskin traction t.
  Powerflex t.
  Scotchcast 2 cast t.
  skin t.
  sports t.
  t. traction
  TufStuf II cast t.
  Ultra-Light athletic t.
  umbilical t.
  Zonas porous t.
taper
  t. cut needle
  Eurotaper 12/14 t.
  fiber metal t.
  Morse t.
  VerSys fiber metal t.
tapered
  collarless, polished, t. (CPT)
  t. hand reamer
  t. needle
  t. pin
  t. reamer
tapering dose steroid
taper-jaw forceps
Taperloc
  T. femoral component
  T. femoral prosthesis
  T. femoral stem
  T. hip system
taping
  basket-weave ankle t.
  buddy t.
  figure-of-8 t.
  Gibney t.
  Kinesio elastic therapeutic t.
  Low-Dye t.
  patellar t.

plantar fasciitis t.
prophylactic t.
t. technique

tapir

bouche de t.

tapotement
tapping test of arm disability
4-tap screw
TAR

thrombocytopenia-absent radius
total ankle replacement

TARA

total articular replacement arthroplasty
total articular resurfacing arthroplasty
TARA total hip prosthesis

Taractan
Taratynov disease
tarda

osteogenesis imperfecta t. (OIT)
SED t.
spondyloepiphysial dysplasia t.

Tardieu spasticity measurement scale
tardive muscular dystrophy
tardy ulnar palsy
target

t. of manipulation
T. prosthesis
t. ulcer

targeter

bone screw t.
IMP bone screw t.

targeting

t. bead
distal t.
t. drill guide
nail-mounted t.

Targon PH proximal humerus
intramedullary nail system
Tarlov cyst
TARP

transoral atlantoaxial reduction plate

tarsal

t. amputation
t. arthrodesis
t. bar
t. bone
t. bone fracture
t. bridge
t. canal
t. canal artery
t. coalition
t. dislocation
t. joint
t. joint infection
t. medullostomy
t. navicular
t. navicular bursitis
t. plate
t. pronator shoe

t. sinus
t. sinus artery
t. tunnel
t. tunnel release (TTR)
t. tunnel syndrome (TTS)
t. twist test
t. wedge osteotomy

tarsalgia
tarsectomy
tarsectopia, tarsectopy
tarsectopy (*var. of* tarsectopia)
tarsi (*gen.* and *pl. of* tarsus)
tarsitis
tarsoclasia, tarsoclasis
tarsoclasis (*var. of* tarsoclasia)
tarsoepiphysial aclasis
tarsometatarsal (TMT)

t. amputation (TMA)
t. angle
t. articulation
t. dislocation
t. fracture-dislocation
t. joint
t. joint injury
t. junction
t. ligament
t. osteoarthritis
t. truncated-wedge arthrodesis

tarsophalangeal reflex
tarsotibial amputation
tarsotomy
tarsus, *gen.* and *pl.* **tarsi**

ligament of t.
ossa tarsi
sinus tarsi

tartrate

levorphanol t.
t. resistant acid phosphatase (TRAP)

task

T. Force on Standards of Physical
Therapy
metabolic equivalent of t. (MET)
walking t.

taut

t. band
t. foot

Tavernetti-Tennant knee prosthesis
Tawse

Bell T.

Taylor

T. apparatus
T. back brace
T. clavicle support
T. percussion hammer
T. procedure
T. retractor
T. spinal frame
T. spinal retractor blade
T. spine brace

T

Taylor (*continued*)
    T. splint
    T. technique
    T. thoracolumbosacral orthosis
Taylor-Knight brace
Tazicef
Tazidime
tazobactam
TB
    tuberculosis
T-Bar
    T-B. guide
    T-B. trigger point massager
TBI
    traumatic brain injury
TBM
    total bone matrix
    Accell TBM
TBW
    total body water
Tc
    technetium
TCA
    talocalcaneal angle
    transcondylar axis
    tricyclic antidepressant
TCAD
    tricyclic antidepressant
TCAT
    Toglia Category Assessment
    Test
TCC
    total contact cast
    total contact casting
TCDR
    total cervical disc replacement
T-cell
    T-c. depletion
    T-c. receptor antibody
TCL
    tibial collateral ligament
    transverse carpal ligament
T-clamp
    Pratt T-c.
    Presbyterian Hospital T-c.
TcMEP
    transcranial motor-evoked
    potential
TCO
    total contact orthosis
TCOM
    transcutaneous oxygen monitor
TCROM
    total cervical range of motion
TCS
    tethered cord syndrome
    turnstile casting stand
TDWB
    touchdown weightbearing

TEA
    Test of Everyday Attention
    total elbow arthroplasty
tea
    Chiro-Klenz t.
tea-and-toast diet
TEA-Ch
    Test of Everyday Attention for
    Children
teacup fracture
Teale amputation
team
    donor t.
    t. handball
    recipient t.
tear
    acute meniscal t.
    anterior horn meniscal t.
    anterior oblique meniscal t.
    bowstring t.
    bucket-handle t.
    cleavage t.
    complex meniscal t.
    concentric t.
    degenerative meniscal t.
    deltoid ligament t.
    dural t.
    flap meniscal t.
    full-thickness cuff t.
    horizontal meniscal t.
    horse-tail Achilles tendon t.
    iatrogenic dural t.
    incomplete t.
    interstitial meniscal t.
    intraoperative dural t.
    Johnson-Jahss classification of
      posterior tibial tendon t.
    labral t.
    lateral t.
    longitudinal displaced complete t.
    longitudinal incomplete
      intrameniscal t.
    longitudinal meniscal t.
    longitudinal split t.
    L-shaped rotator cuff t.
    meniscal lateral t.
    meniscal radial t.
    meniscal transverse t.
    meniscocapsular t.
    midsubstance t.
    mop-end Achilles tendon t.
    mop-end mid-substance t.
    Neer acromioplasty for rotator
      cuff t.
    oblique meniscal t.
    parrot beak t.
    posterior cruciate ligament t.
    posterior horn meniscal t.
    posterior oblique meniscal t.

radial meniscal t.
rotator cuff t.
TFC t.
through-and-through t.
transverse t.
triangular fibrocartilage t.
vertical longitudinal t.
V-shaped rotator cuff t.

teardrop
    t. fracture
    t. line
    t. sign

**teardrop-shaped flexion-compression
fracture**

Teare surgical sling

tearing sound

teaspoon
    nylon t.

TEC
    Total Environment Control
    TEC interface system
    TEC liner

Techmedica implant

technetium (Tc)
    t. labeled methylene diphosphonate
    t. 99m phosphate
    t. 99m pyrophosphate
    t. stannous pyrophosphate

technetium-99m (^{99m}Tc)
    t.-99m diphosphonate scan
    t.-99m methylene diphosphate bone
    scan
    t.-99m pyrophosphate scan
    t.-99m sulfur colloid scan

Techni-Care surgical scrub

technique
    abduction traction t.
    abductor slide t.
    Abumi screw insertion t.
    accessory movement t.
    Ace-Colles frame for radial
    dysplasia repair t.
    Achilles tendon taping t.
    Achilles tendon V-Y turndown t.
    active-release t. (ART)
    adduction traction t.
    Agee carpal tunnel release t.
    Albizzia minimally invasive
    intramedullary nail femoral
    lengthening t.
    Alexander musculoskeletal
    relaxation t.
    Allgöwer suture t.
    Amstutz hip resurfacing
    arthroplasty t.
    Anderson screw placement t.
    Andrews t.
    anterior decompression t.
    anterior iliofemoral t.

anterior quadriceps musculocutaneous
    flap t.
AO-ASIF compression t.
AO surgical t.
Armistead distraction osteogenesis t.
arthrographic capsular distension and
    rupture t.
Asher physical build assessment t.
ASIF screw fixation t.
Asnis cannulated screw fixation t.
Atasoy V-Y t.
Avila t.
avulsion t.
axial pin t.
back-slapping t.
Badgley anterior cervical discectomy
    and fusion t.
bag-of-bones t.
Bailey-Badgley cervical spine
    interbody fusion t.
Bailey-Dubow rod insertion t.
Baker t.
Barbour t.
barrier t.
Barsky bilateral cleft lips repair t.
basic t.
Basmajian iliopsoas
    electromyography t.
Batch-Spittler-McFaddin through-knee
    amputation t.
Baumgaertel and Gotzen calcaneal
    fracture reduction t.
Baumgard-Schwartz tennis elbow t.
Beckenbaugh biaxial wrist implant t.
Becker otoplasty t.
Becton fracture fixation t.
Bell Tawse open reduction t.
bilateral arm raise back exercise t.
Blair ankle fusion in
    osteonecrosis t.
Bleck midcalf lengthening by
    recession t.
Blount tracing t.
Bobath t.
Böhler calcaneal fracture
    reduction t.
Bohlman cervical fusion t.
Bohlman triple-wire cervical
    fusion t.
bone marrow stimulating t.
Bonfiglio modification of Phemister
    bone graft of femoral neck t.
Bonola cross-arm double-flap thumb
    repair t.
Bora t.
Borggreve-Hall tibial rotation
    plasty t.
Bosworth t.
Bowers genital reassignment t.

T

technique (*continued*)

Boyd-Anderson distal biceps tendon repair t.
Boyd-McLeod tennis elbow t.
Boyes brachioradialis transfer t.
Brady-Jewett proximal radial resection t.
Brand tendon transfer t.
bridge back exercise t.
Brooks atlantoaxial t.
Brooks-Jenkins atlantoaxial fusion t.
Broström injection t.
Brown endoscopic carpal tunnel release t.
Brügger rocking t.
Brumm t.
Bruser lateral knee t.
Bryan-Morrey triceps-sparing humerus fracture repair t.
Buck-Gramcko dorsal rotational advancement flap t.
Bugg-Boyd Achilles tendon repair t.
Buncke microsurgical t.
Bunnell atraumatic t.
Bunnell tendon suturing t.
Bunnell tendon transfer t.
bur-down t.
Burgess transtibial amputation t.
Burkhalter modification of Stiles-Bunnell t.
Burkhalter transfer t.
Burow skin flap t.
Burrows distal ulna shortening osteotomy t.
Calandruccio t.
Callahan posterior spinal fusion t.
Camino catheter t.
Camitz palmaris longus tendon reconstruction t.
Campbell opening-wedge thoracostomy t.
Canale distal humerus fracture pinning t.
cannulated reaming t.
Capello acetabular reconstruction t.
Carnesale extremity amputation t.
Carrell fibular substitution t.
Caspar anterior cervical plating t.
CBP t.
cementless t.
central semi suture-loop meniscal repair t.
central slip-sparing t.
central splitting t.
cerclage t.
cervical screw insertion t.
cervical spondylotic myelopathy fusion t.

cervical spondylotic myelopathy laminar door t.
CHESS MRI t.
chevron t.
Chiari pelvis osteotomy t.
Childress ankle fixation t.
chiropractic manipulative reflex t. (CMRT)
Cho tendon t.
Chow transbursal carpal tunnel release t.
Chrisman-Snook ankle t.
Cincinnati pelvic osteotomy t.
Clancy ligament t.
Clark transfer t.
Cloward anterior cervical discectomy and fusion t.
Cobb scoliosis measuring t.
Codivilla tendon lengthening t.
Cofield rotator cuff reconstruction t.
Coleman flatfoot t.
Cole orthopaedic surgical t.
Collis broken femoral stem t.
Coltart fracture t.
combination of isotonics therapeutic exercise t.
compression t.
Connolly bone regeneration t.
contoured anterior spinal plate t.
contract-relax t.
conventional t.
Conyers t.
Coonse-Adams V-Y quadriceps turndown knee t.
coracoclavicular t.
costotransversectomy t.
cotyloplasty t.
counterstrain t.
Cox flexion-distraction t.
Craig Handicap Assessment and Reporting T. (CHART)
craniosacral therapy t.
Crego tendon transfer t.
Cubbins shoulder dislocation t.
Cuniard and Campell t.
Curtis flexion contracture release t.
Cyriax diagnosis of soft tissue lesions t.
Davis drainage t.
DeBastiani t.
decompression t.
decortication t.
DePalma modified patellar t.
Dewar-Barrington clavicular dislocation t.
Dewar-Harris shoulder t.
Dewar posterior cervical fusion t.
Deyerle femoral fracture t.
Dickinson calcaneal bursitis t.

Dickson transplant t.
Dimon-Hughston medial displacement
  osteotomy hip fracture t.
distraction t.
distraction osteogenesis t.
Doll trochanteric reattachment t.
Doppler t.
double-looped semitendinous and
  gracilis hamstring graft knee
  reconstruction t.
double portal t.
double-rod t.
dowel graft t.
doweling spondylolisthesis t.
Drez modification of Eriksson ankle
  joint arthroscopy t.
drilling t.
Drummond interspinous wiring t.
Dunn acromioclavicular joint t.
DuVries deltoid ligament
  reconstruction t.
Eastwood anesthesia t.
Eaton-Littler carpometacarpal thumb
  repair t.
Eberle contracture release t.
Eftekhar broken femoral stem t.
Eggers tendon transfer t.
Ellis Jones peroneal tendon t.
Ellison iliotibial band transfer for
  ACL repair t.
Ellis skin traction t.
Ender femoral fracture t.
epidural cortisone injection t.
Eriksson brachial block t.
Eriksson ligament t.
Essex-Lopresti axial fixation t.
Essex-Lopresti calcaneal fracture t.
European compression t. (ECT)
Evans ankle reconstruction t.
excision-curettage t.
extraarticular t.
extramedullary nail extraction by
  proximal stacked wire t.
extremity mobilization t.
facet excision t.
facilitatory t.
Fahey t.
Fairbanks
  uvulopalatopharyngoplasty t.
far-near near-far suture t.
Farmer t.
Ferkel torticollis t.
FHL release t.
Fielding modification of Gallie
  atlantoaxial instability spine
  fusion t.
finger t.
Fish cuneiform osteotomy t.
fixation t.

flat-cut t.
Flatt hand surgery t.
flexor hallucis longus release t.
Flynn t.
Forbes modification of Phemister
  graft t.
Ford triangulation t.
Fowler t.
Fowles dislocation t.
freehand suturing t.
French fracture t.
Froimson bicipital groove keyhole t.
Frost posterior tibialis t.
functional squats back exercise t.
funnel t.
fusion t.
Gaenslen split-heel t.
Gallie atlantoaxial fusion t.
Gallie wire fixation t.
Gallie wiring t.
Galveston spinopelvic
  reconstruction t.
Ganley forefoot osseous
  reconstruction t.
Garceau tendon t.
Ger t.
Giannestras modification of Lapidus
  hallux valgus t.
Gill sliding graft t.
gliding hole first t.
gluteal/hamstring raise back
  exercise t.
Goldberg clavicle fracture repair t.
Goldner-Clippinger multangular bone
  excision t.
Goldstein spinal fusion t.
Gonstead t.
Gordon joint injection t.
Graston soft tissue t.
great toe arthroplasty implant t.
  (GAIT)
Green-Banks t.
Greulich-Pyle skeletal age
  estimation t.
Grice-Green subtalar extraarticular
  arthrodesis t.
Grosse-Kempf tibial locked
  nailing t.
Guhl ankle arthroscopy t.
Guttmann t.
Hackethal stacked nailing humeral
  shaft t.
Hall preformed metal crown t.
Hamas endoscopic facial
  rejuvenation t.
hamstring fixation t.
Hardinge hip prosthesis
  measurement t.
Harmon transfer t.

T

technique (*continued*)

Harms anterior scoliosis t.
Harms thoracic spine fracture repair t.
Harriluque t.
Harrington-Luque t.
Hauser patellar realignment t.
Hendler unitunnel ACL repair t.
Henning inside-to-outside meniscal repair t.
Henry acromioclavicular t.
Hermodsson internal rotation t.
Hey Groves fascia lata t.
Hey Groves-Kirk t.
Hey Groves ligament reconstruction t.
Heyman t.
high-velocity low-amplitude thrust t.
HIO t.
hip hinge back exercise t.
Hirschhorn compression t.
Hitchcock biceps tendon t.
Hodgson hypospadias repair t.
Hohl-Moore tibial plateau fracture repair t.
Hoke-Kite arthrodesis t.
hold-relax t.
hole-in-1 t. (HIO)
Hollywood roll t.
Hori umbilicus reconstruction t.
hot dog t.
Howard differential ureteral catheterization t.
Hungerford t.
Huntington tibial t.
Ilizarov t.
Ilizarov ankle fusion t.
Ilizarov limb-lengthening t.
inferior capsular split t.
injection t.
Insall-Hood reconstruction t.
Insall ligament reconstruction t.
inside-out tissue repair t.
inside-to-outside t.
interference screw t.
intrafocal reduction t.
inverting knot t.
ischemic tourniquet t.
Isobaric epidural/spinal anesthesia t.
isometric t.
Jacobs locking hook spinal rod t.
Jansey shoulder arthrodesis t.
Jeffery t.
Johnson pelvic fracture t.
Johnson staple t.
Kapandji pinning t.
Kapandji-Sauvé t.
Kapel elbow dislocation t.
Kaplan t.
Kashiwagi elbow arthroplasty t.

Kaufer tendon t.
Kaufmann subpial transection t.
Kennedy ligament t.
Kessler suture t.
keyhole tenodesis t.
King contrast venography t.
King-Richards dislocation t.
Kite and Lovell t.
Klein t.
Kloehn craniofacial remodeling t.
kneeling reciprocal back exercise t.
Krackow locking loop t.
Krackow locking suture t.
Krackow-Thomas-Jones t.
Kumar spica cast t.
Küntscher intramedullary nailing t.
Lambrinudi t.
Lapidus hammertoe t.
Larson posterolateral instability of knee repair t.
Leadbetter t.
Lee laryngotracheal stenosis management t.
Lehman endoscopic pancreatic sphincterotomy t.
Leibolt pantalar arthrodesis t.
Lewit stretch t.
Lichtman modification of stahl t.
Lichtman staging of Kienböck disease t.
Liebolt radioulnar t.
Lindholm Achilles tendon rupture repair t.
line-to-line reaming t.
Lippman-Cobb t.
Lipscomb t.
Lister flexor tendon pulley reconstruction t.
Little t.
Littler-Cooley opponensplasty t.
Littler swanneck deformity repair t.
Lloyd-Roberts fracture t.
local standby anesthesia t.
locking-suture t.
Locksley occipitocervical fusion t.
Losee modification of MacIntosh ACL repair t.
Losee sling and reef ACL repair t.
Louisiana ankle wrap t.
Low-Dye taping t.
Ludloff congenital hip dislocation repair t.
lumbar accessory movement t.
Luque instrumentation concave t.
Luque instrumentation convex t.
Luque sublaminar wiring t.
Lyden real-time cerebral angiography t.
Lynn Achilles tendon repair t.

MacIntosh laryngoscopy t.
Magerl screw placement t.
Magerl translaminar facet screw
   fixation t.
Magilligan femoral anteversion
   measuring t.
Magnuson anterior dislocation of
   shoulder repair t.
Ma-Griffith Achilles tendon rupture
   repair t.
Maitland manual spinal therapy t.
Majestro-Ruda-Frost tendon t.
Malawer excision t.
Mallory t.
manipulative t.
Mankin t.
Mann t.
Manske radioulnar osteoclasis t.
manual push-pull t.
manual resistance t. (MRT)
Marks-Bayne t.
Marshall ligament repair t.
Marshall-McIntosh ACL repair t.
Martin patellar wiring t.
Matti-Russe scaphoid nonunion bone
   graft t.
Mazet knee disarticulation t.
McConnell patellar taping t.
McElvenny orthopaedic t.
McFarland-Osborne hip joint lateral
   incision t.
McReynolds open fracture
   reduction t.
medial cortical overlap t.
medial heel skive t.
Mendelsohn modification of
   matricectomy suture t.
Mensor-Scheck t.
microneurosurgical t.
Milch cuff resection of ulna t.
Milch elbow t.
Milford mallet finger t.
mille pattes t.
Millesi modified nerve graft t.
minimally invasive surgical t.
MIS t.
Mital elbow release t.
miter t.
Mizuno double-patch ventricular
   septal perforation repair t.
modified Brooks atlantoaxial
   subluxation tape repair t.
modified Crawford Campbell inlaid
   bone-grafting t.
Moe scoliosis t.
Mohs chemosurery t.
Monticelli-Spinelli distraction
   epiphysiolysis limb lengthening t.
Moore t.

Morrison t.
mosaicplasty t.
Moss t.
muscle energy t.
Nalebuff-Millender swan-neck
   deformity lateral band
   mobilization t.
Nash-Moe vertebral rotation scoliosis
   assessment t.
neural arch resection t.
Neviaser acromioclavicular t.
Nicholas corococlavicular congenital
   knee dislocation ligament t.
Nicholas 5-in-1 knee
   reconstruction t.
Niebauer-King congenital knee
   dislocation open reduction t.
Nimmo receptor-tonus t.
Nirschl lateral epicondylitis
   mini-open t.
noninvasive t.
notching t.
no-touch t.
OATS t.
Ober tendon transfer for footdrop t.
Obwegeser sagittal mandibular
   osteotomy t.
t. of Cobb
Ogata t.
Ollier t.
open-bowl cement t.
open palm t.
O'Phelan t.
Osborne-Cotterill elbow t.
Osgood modified t.
Osmond-Clarke staged congenital
   vertical talus repair t.
Ostrup bone graft harvesting t.
outside-in t.
outside-to-outside arthroscopy t.
Pack t.
Palmer all-inside TFCC repair t.
palpatory t.
pants-over-vest t.
Papineau open bone grafting t.
parachute t.
Parrish-Mann hammertoe t.
partial sit-ups back exercise t.
Parvin gravity t.
passive gliding t.
Paterson t.
Paulos ligament t.
Pauwels osteotomy t.
Peacock neurovascular island pedicle
   flap t.
peg-and-socket t.
perfect-circle t.
Perry t.
Pheasant elbow t.

T

technique (*continued*)

Phemister-Bonfiglio femoral neck bone grafting t.
Phemister onlay bone graft t.
PNF t.
3-point pressure t.
Ponseti t.
2-portal t.
3-portal t.
Porter-Richardson-Vainio arthroscopic synovectomy t.
posterior flap t.
posterior iliofemoral t.
posterolateral costotransversectomy t.
postganglionic t.
postisometric relaxation traction t.
postisometric stretch t.
Pratt t.
preemptive blockade t.
preganglionic t.
press-fit acetabular implant insertion t.
prone blocking t.
proximal stacked wire t.
proximal-to-distal dissection t.
Puddu tendon t.
Pulvertaft weave tendon repair t.
quadruped back exercise t.
Quénu nail plate removal t.
Rayhack ulnar shortening osteotomy t.
reciprocal arm raise back exercise t.
reduction t.
Reichenheim elbow surgical stabilization t.
reverse lunge back exercise t.
reverse wedge t.
rhythmic initiation t.
Rideau hip contracture release t.
Riordan tendon transfer t.
Risser t.
Risser-Ferguson t.
Roberts fat grafting t.
Robinson-Smith anterior cervical t.
Robinson-Southwick cervical spine fusion t.
Rockwood-Green orthopaedic casting t.
Rogers cervical fusion t.
Rood t.
Royle-Thompson tendon transfer t.
Russe scaphoid fracture t.
Rutkow inguinal hernia repair t.
Ryerson t.
sacral bar t.
sacrooccipital t. (SOT)
Saha latissimus dorsi transfer t.
Saha trapezius muscle transfer t.
Salter hip dysplasia surgical t.

Sarmiento intertrochanteric fracture t.
Scaglietti closed reduction of spondiglolisthesis t.
Schauwecker patellar wiring t.
Schnute osteitis pubis wedge resection t.
Schober lumbar spine mobility measuring t.
Schober true flexion measurement t.
Scott glenoplasty t.
Scott lumbar spondylosis wiring t.
screw insertion t.
screw-plate t.
Scuderi quadriceps tendon repair t.
Scuderi ruptured quadriceps repair t.
second-generation cementing t.
Seddon t.
semi-suture-loop t.
semitendinosus t.
Serafin t.
SharpShooter tissue repair t.
Sharrard iliopsoas transfer t.
Sharrard tendon transfer t.
Shikata grafting t.
shish kebab t.
short lever accessory movement t.
side lunge back exercise t.
side-lying back exercise t.
Silfverskiöld t.
silver dollar t.
Simultaneous Interview T. (SIT)
single proximal portal t.
single-stage osteomyelitis repair t.
Skoog female genitalia construction t.
Skoog nasal dorsum t.
2-sleeve t.
sling and reef t.
slit catheter t.
Slocum spinal fusion t.
Smith t.
Smith-Petersen SI joint t.
Smith-Petersen spine t.
Smith-Robinson anterior discectomy with horseshoe-shaped graft t.
Sofield femoral deficiency leg-lengthening t.
Somerville bikini incision hip joint t.
SOTO t.
Spälteholz bone-clearing t.
spinal fusion t.
spinal mobilization t.
spin-lock MRI t.
spinopelvic transiliac fixation t.
spiral t.
Sprague orthopaedic arthroscopic t.
spray and stretch t.
2-stage tendon grafting t.

Staheli congenital hip dislocation containment t.
Staheli pediatric t.
Stanisavljevic knee reconstruction t.
STAR t.
Steffee spinal fusion instrumentation t.
Stiles-Bunnell flexor digitorum superficialis transfer t.
Stimson anterior shoulder reduction t.
strain/counterstrain t.
Straub phlebography t.
Strayer flexor slide tendon t.
Strickland flexor tendon repair t.
strut spinal fusion t.
2-strut tibial graft t.
suction-bubble t.
suction-irrigation t.
surgical t.
sustained pressure t.
suture anchor t.
suture-loop t.
Swanson t.
Tajima suture t.
taping t.
Taylor t.
tension band wiring t.
Teuffer Achilles tendon repair t.
third-generation cementing t.
Thomas-Thompson-Straub rotational transfer of vastus lateralis t.
thoracic lymphatic pump t.
thoracolumbar spondylosis surgical t.
threaded-hole-first t.
Tohen tendon t.
Torg Jones fracture repair t.
Torg tarsal navicular stress fracture repair t.
transiliac bar t.
triangulation t.
triple bundle t.
triple-wire t.
Tullos t.
Turco clubfoot release t.
unassisted locking-suture t.
unitunnel t.
unlocking spiral t.
vacuum cement mix t.
vasomotor t.
Vastamäki pectoralis major tendon transfer t.
Vastamäki wrist arthroscopy t.
Veleanu-Rosianu-Ionescu obturator neurectomy t.
Verdan intrasynovial flexor tendon t.
vertical loop suture t.
Vidal-Adrey femoral fracture t.
Viladot subtalar arthrocrisis t.

Wadsworth triceps tendon release t.
Wagner open reduction t.
Wagoner cervical spine t.
Warner-Farber ankle fixation t.
Watkins intertransverse process lumbar spine fusion t.
Watson-Cheyne wedge excision of toenail t.
Watson wrist salvage t.
Weaver-Dunn acromioclavicular t.
Weber-Vasey olecranon tension band wiring t.
Weber-Vasey traction-absorption wiring of olecranon fracture t.
Wellmerling femoral neck fracture t.
Wertheim-Bohlman occipitocervical fusion t.
Wertheim-Bohlman posterior cervical t.
Whiteside intraarticular infusion t.
Whitesides intracompartmental tissue pressure t.
Whitesides-Kelly lateral retropharyngeal cervical spine t.
wick t.
wick catheter t.
Williams flexion back exercise t.
Williams-Haddad femoral nerve block for hip fracture t.
Wilson t.
Wilson-Jacobs tibial fracture fixation t.
Windsor-Insall-Vince tissue grafting t.
Winograd ingrown nail t.
Winter spondylolisthesis reduction t.
wire removal t.
Wisconsin wire t.
Woodward scapula correction t.
Zancolli biceps tendon rerouting t.
Zarins-Rowe ACL reconstruction t.
Zeier transfer t.
Zielke t.

TechnoGel insole
technology
Footwear Integration T. (FIT)
professional protective t. (PPT)
segmentally demineralized bone t.
TruePoint PET-CT t.
work evaluation systems t.
tectal plate
Tectonic magnet
tectoral ligament
TED
thromboembolic disease
TED hose
TED stockings
teeter-totter sacrum
teeth (*pl. of* tooth)

759

Teflon
- T. cannula
- T. implant
- T. tri-leaflet prosthesis

Teflon-coated
- T.-c. driver
- T.-c. suture

Tegaderm dressing

Tegner
- T. activity rating scale
- T. Activity Scale (0-10)
- T. knee reconstruction activity score
- T. meniscal knee injury score

Tei-Shin

Tekscan in-shoe monitoring device

Telamon carbon implant

telangiectasia
- ataxia t.
- calcinosis, Raynaud, esophageal motility disorders, sclerodactyly, t. (CREST)

telangiectatic osteosarcoma

Telectronics
- T. electrical stimulation apparatus
- T. electrical stimulation device

teleroentgenography

telescopic
- T. Plate Spacer implantable titanium spacer
- t. view guide

telescoping
- t. brace
- t. medullary rod
- t. nail
- t. tubular device

telethermometer

Telfa
- T. bolster
- T. gauze
- T. gauze dressing
- T. sponge

Telos fracture table extension

TELS
- The Experience of Leisure Scale

TEM
- terminal extensor mechanism

temafloxacin

temazepam

temper
- T. Foam
- T. Foam cube
- T. Foam cushion
- t. tantrum elbow

temperature
- capillary refill, sensation, motor function, t. (CSMT)
- t. differential
- optimal cutting t. (OCT)
- wet globe t.

Temperlite saw blade

TempFix external fixation system

template
- acetabular cup t.
- Charnley t.
- femoral condylar t.
- malleable t.
- Moore t.
- Mueller t.
- Pedrialle t.
- prosthesis t.
- rod t.
- Stevens-Street elbow prosthesis t.
- thermoplastic t.
- tibial track t.
- transparent t.

templating roentgenogram

temple
- T. University nail
- T. University plate

temporal
- t. bone
- t. bone fracture
- t. dispersion
- t. fascia graft

temporalis fascia flap

temporary
- t. articulating methylmethacrylate antibiotic spacer (TAMMAS)
- t. callus
- t. cavity phenomenon
- t. cerclage wire
- t. external fixator
- t. external transpedicular fixation
- t. prosthetic fitting
- t. socket

temporomandibular
- t. disorder
- t. joint (TMJ)
- t. joint arthralgia
- t. joint dislocation
- t. joint pain-dysfunction syndrome
- t. joint syndrome

Tempra

Tempur-Pedic
- T.-P. mattress
- T.-P. pressure relieving Swedish mattress
- T.-P. pressure relieving Swedish pillow

tenacula tendinum

tenaculum-reducing forceps

tenalgia crepitans

tender
- t. point (TeP)
- t. point examination

Tenderlett device
tenderness
    bony t.
    costovertebral angle t. (CVAT)
    CVA t.
    joint line t.
    myofascial t.
    percussion t.
    pillar t.
    point t.
    rebound t.
tendines (*pl. of* tendo)
tendinis (*gen. of* tendo)
tendinitis, tendonitis, tenonitis
    abductor t.
    Achilles t.
    acute calcific t.
    adductor t.
    anterior tarsal t.
    biceps t.
    bicipital t.
    birefringent lipid crystals in t.
    calcific t.
    chronic Achilles t.
    chronic noninsertional tendo
      calcaneus t.
    de Quervain t.
    digital flexor t.
    extensor carpi ulnaris t.
    flexor carpi ulnaris t.
    hamstring t.
    infrapatellar t.
    infraspinatus t.
    insertional tendo calcaneus t.
    patellar t.
    peripatellar t.
    peroneal t.
    popliteus t.
    posterior tibial t.
    posterior tibialis t.
    radial wrist extensor t.
    rotator cuff calcific t.
    semimembranosus t.
    subscapular t.
    suprapatellar t.
    supraspinatus t.
    triceps t.
    ulnar wrist extensor t.
    wrist extensor t.
    wrist flexor t.
tendinopathy, tendopathy
    Achilles t.
    Blazina patellar t.
    insertion t.
    peroneus longus t. (PLT)
    plantar t.
    posterior tibial t.
    primary peroneus longus t.
    rotator cuff t.

tendinoplasty, tenontoplasty, tenoplasty,
  tendoplasty
    talipes t.
tendinosis, tendonosis
    angiofibroblastic hyperplasia t.
    calcific t.
    insertional Achilles t.
    lateral elbow t.
    medial tennis elbow t.
tendinosuture
tendinotrochanteric ligament
tendinous
    t. attachment
    t. fiber
    t. sheath
    t. synovitis
tendinum
    chiasma t.
    retinaculum t.
    tenacula t.
tendo, *pl.* **tendines,** *gen.* **tendinis**
    t. Achillis
    t. Achillis lengthening (TAL)
    t. Achillis mechanism
    t. calcaneus
    t. calcaneus lengthening
    theca tendinis
tendolysis (*var. of* tenolysis)
tendon
    abductor digiti quinti t.
    abductor hallucis t.
    abductor pollicis brevis t.
    abductor pollicis longus t.
    accessory communicating t.
    Achilles t.
    adductor hallucis t.
    adductor pollicis brevis t.
    adherent profundus t.
    t. advancement
    anchoring t.
    anterior tibial t.
    aponeurosis of t.
    attenuation of t.
    attrition of t.
    attrition rupture of t.
    avulsion of biceps t.
    biceps brachialis t.
    biceps brachii t.
    biceps femoris t.
    bicipital t.
    t. bowing
    t. bowing in arthritis
    brachialis t.
    brachial plexus t.
    brachioradialis t.
    calcaneal t.
    t. cartilage
    t. centralization
    t. checkrein procedure

T

tendon (*continued*)
    common extensor t.
    conjoined t.'s
    digital extensor t.
    digital flexor t.
    digiti quinti proprius t.
    digitorum communis t.
    t. disorder
    t. displacement
    distal rupture of biceps t.
    ECRB t.
    ECRL t.
    ECU t.
    EDB t.
    EHL t.
    EIP t.
    elbow extensor t.
    evertor t.
    t. excursion
    extensor carpi radialis brevis t.
    extensor carpi radialis longus t.
    extensor carpi ulnaris t.
    extensor digiti minimi t.
    extensor digiti quinti t.
    extensor digitorum brevis t.
    extensor digitorum communis t.
    extensor digitorum longus t.
    extensor hallucis longus t.
    extensor indicis proprius t.
    extensor pollicis brevis t.
    extensor pollicis longus t.
    extensor quinti t.
    t. fixation
    flexor carpi radialis t.
    flexor carpi ulnaris t.
    flexor digitorum communis t.
    flexor digitorum longus t.
    flexor digitorum profundus t.
    flexor digitorum sublimis t.
    flexor digitorum superficialis t.
    flexor hallucis brevis t.
    flexor hallucis longus t.
    flexor pollicis brevis t.
    flexor pollicis longus t.
    flexor profundus t.
    flexor sublimis t.
    t. forceps
    gastrocnemius t.
    gastrocnemius-soleus t.
    G-lengthening of semitendinosus t.
    Golgi t.
    t. gouge
    t. grabber
    gracilis t.
    t. graft
    hamstring t.
    t. harvester
    t. healing
    Hector t.

    hilum of t.
    iliopsoas t.
    t. inflammation
    infrapatellar t.
    infraspinatus t.
    interosseous t.
    t. interposition
    t. interposition arthroplasty
    t. irregularity
    t. jerk
    t. leader
    t. lengthening
    t. lengthening osteotomy
    long head biceps t.
    lumbrical t.
    midpatellar t.
    t. needle
    t. nodularity
    t. nodule
    obturator internus t.
    palmaris longus t.
    t. passer
    patellar t.
    patelloquadriceps t.
    peroneal t.
    peroneus brevis t.
    peroneus longus t.
    peroneus tertius t.
    plantaris t.
    t. plate
    t. plica
    popliteal t.
    popliteus fossa muscle t.
    posterior tibial t. (PTT)
    postoperative flexor t. (PFT)
    ProCol bovine bioprosthesis t.
    profundus t.
    pronator teres t.
    proprius t.
    t. prosthesis
    quadriceps t.
    quadruple semitendinosus and
      gracilis t.'s (QSGT)
    reconstruction of posterolateral
      structures using semitendinosus t.
    rectus femoris t.
    t. reflex
    t. release
    t. release in camptodactyly
    t. repair
    rerouted t.
    rider's t.
    t. rod
    rotator cuff t.
    t. rupture
    sartorius t.
    semimembranosus t.
    semitendinosus t.
    t. sheath

t. sheath endoscopy
slip of t.
t. snapping
snapping t.
split anterior tibial t. (SPLATT)
t. stripper
sublimis t.
subscapularis t.
t. substitution
superficialis t.
supraspinatus t.
t. suture
synovectomy of peroneal t.'s
t. thickening
thumb extensor t.
thumb flexor t.
tibial t.
tibialis anterior t.
tibialis posterior t.
toe extensor t.
t. transfer
t. transplant
t. transposition
t. trapping
triceps brachii t.
t. tucker
t. tunneler
V-Y lengthening of Achilles t.
wrist extensor t.
t. Z-lengthening around knee and
  ankle
Z-lengthening of biceps t.
tendon-bearing
patellar t.-b. (PTB)
tendon-bearing-supracondylar
patellar t.-b.-s.
tendon-bearing-supracondylar-suprapatellar
patellar t.-b.-s.-s. (PTB-SC-SP)
tendon-bone
t.-b. allograft
t.-b. attachment
bone-patellar t.-b. (BPB, BPTB)
t.-b. bridge
tendon-braiding forceps
tendon-holding forceps
tendonitis (*var. of* tendinitis)
tendonosis (*var. of* tendinosis)
tendon-passing forceps
tendon-pulling forceps
tendon-retrieving forceps
tendon-seizing forceps
tendon-to-bone attachment
tendon-tunneling forceps
tendopathy (*var. of* tendinopathy)
tendoplasty (*var. of* tendinoplasty)
tendoscopy
tendosuspension
Hibbs t.
Jones t.

tendosynovial (*var. of* tenosynovial)
tendosynovitis (*var. of* tenosynovitis)
tendotomy (*var. of* tenotomy)
tendovaginitis (*var. of* tenosynovitis)
tenectomy, tenonectomy
tennis
t. elbow
t. elbow arm band
t. elbow release
t. elbow splint
t. elbow test
t. fracture
t. heel
t. leg
t. shoulder
t. thumb
t. toe
tenocyte
tenodesis
Andrews iliotibial band t.
Andrews lateral t.
anterolateral femorotibial ligament t.
band t.
biceps t.
calcaneal t.
Chrisman-Snook ankle t.
Darrach ulnar t.
t. effect
Eggers spastic quadriplegia crouch
  gait repair t.
Ellison iliotibial band t.
Evans ankle t.
extensor hallucis longus t.
femorotibial ligament t.
Fowler dynamic hand t.
hallucis brevis t.
iliotibial band t.
interphalangeal t.
key-grip t.
keyhole t.
MacIntosh extraarticular ruptured
  anterior cruciate ligament t.
MacIntosh iliotibial band t.
Moberg key-grip t.
modified Watson-Jones ankle t.
Mueller anterolateral femorotibial
  ligament t.
Norwood iliotibial band t.
t. of heel cord
t. orthosis
SCOI arthroscopic biceps t.
semitendinosus t.
sublimis t.
t. test
triple t.
Watson-Jones ankle t.
Westin tendo Achillis t.
tenodynia
Teno Fix tendon repair device

T

tenography
tenolysis, tendolysis
    flexor t.
    peroneal t.
tenomyoplasty, tenontomyoplasty
tenomyotomy
tenonectomy (*var. of* tenectomy)
tenonitis
tenontodynia
tenontomyoplasty, tenomyoplasty
tenontomyotomy
tenontophyma
tenontoplastic
tenontoplasty (*var. of* tendinoplasty)
tenontothecitis
tenoperiostitis
tenophyte
tenoplastic reconstruction
tenoplasty
tenorrhaphy
tenositis
tenostosis
tenosuspension
tenosuture
tenosynography
tenosynovectomy
    dorsal t.
    flexor t.
tenosynovial, tendosynovial
    t. giant cell tumor
    t. injection
    t. sheath
tenosynovitis, tendosynovitis,
tendovaginitis, tenovaginitis
    adhesive t.
    bicipital t.
    t. crepitans
    de Quervain stenosing t.
    flexor hallucis longus t.
    gonococcic t.
    gonorrheal t.
    granulomatous t.
    t. hypertrophica
    infectious t.
    localized nodular t.
    nodular t.
    peroneal t.
    pigmented villonodular t.
    stenosing t.
    suppurative flexor t.
    tuberculous peroneal t.
    villonodular t.
    villonodular pigmented t.
    villous t.
tenotomized
tenotomy, tendotomy
    Achilles t.
    adductor t.
    Braun shoulder t.

    curb t.
    extensor t.
    fenestrated t.
    flexor t.
    Fowler central slip t.
    graduated t.
    inverted-Y Achilles t.
    t. knife
    Lichtblau t.
    open t.
    percutaneous t.
    semiopen sliding t.
    sliding t.
    stapedial t.
    subcutaneous t.
    transverse t.
    Z-plasty t.
tenovaginitis (*var. of* tenosynovitis)
    inflammatory t.
tenoxicam
TENS
    transcutaneous electrical nerve
    stimulation
    TENS therapy
    TENS unit
tensegrity
tensile
    t. force
    t. stiffness
    t. strain
    t. strength
    t. stress
Tensilon
    T. test
    T. test for myasthenia gravis
tensing test
tensiometer
    Acufex t.
tensiometry
tension
    adverse neurodynamic t. (ANDT)
    t. band
    t. band fixation
    t. band of knee
    t. band plate
    t. band wire
    t. band wire tamp
    t. band wiring technique
    capsular-ligamentous t.
    t. curve
    t. force
    t. fracture
    graft t.
    heel t.
    t. isometer
    t. loading
    t. myositis
    t. neck syndrome
    neural t.

t. neuralgia
t. night splint (TNS)
oxygen t.
residual t.
tension-band wiring
tensioner
cable t.
Dwyer t.
Kirschner wire t.
tension-free Millesi nerve graft
tensor, *pl.* **tensores**
t. fasciae latae (TFL)
t. fasciae latae anchovy
t. fasciae latae muscle flap
t. fasciae latae syndrome
tensores (*pl. of* tensor)
tent frame
tentorial sinus
tenuous vascularity
Tenzel elevator
TeP
tender point
Teq-Trode electrode
teratologic dislocation
teratoma
sacrococcygeal t.
terbinafine
t. HCl
t. hydrochloride cream
terbinafine, oral
terbinafine, topical
teres
anterior pronator t.
t. major muscle
t. minor muscle
pronator t. (PT)
terminal
t. device
t. extensor mechanism (TEM)
t. head
t. J sign
t. knee extension
t. latency
t. overgrowth
t. stance
t. Syme procedure
Terracol syndrome
terrae
Mycobacterium t.
Terra-Round
Trowbridge T5 T.-R.
terrible triad of shoulder
Terrmocork diabetic shoe
Terry
T. nail
T. Thomas sign
TERT
total end-range time
tertiary amputation

Terumo syringe
TES
total elastic suspension
TES belt
test
abduction external rotation t.
abduction load and shift t.
abduction stress t.
accordion t.
Achilles squeeze t.
Achilles tendon t.
acromioclavicular joint
compression t.
acromioclavicular joint distraction
t.
active bending t.
active knee extension t.
active release shoulder t.
actual leg length t.
Adams forward-bending t.
Adams position t.
Adams scoliosis t.
adduction load and shift t.
adduction stress t.
Adson thoracic outlet t.
AKE t.
Alcohol Use Disorders
Identification t.
Allen blood supply to hand t.
Allis leg length t.
ALRI t.
Anderson medial-lateral grind t.
Andrews anterior instability t.
ankle clonus t.
ankle dorsiflexion t.
anterior apprehension shoulder t.
anterior drawer t. (ADT)
anterior rotary drawer t.
anteroposterior stress t.
antinuclear antibody t.
anvil t.
AO pseudoisochromatic color plate
t.
Apley compression t.
Apley distraction t.
Apley grinding t.
Apley knee t.
Apley scratch shoulder t.
apparent leg-length discrepancy t.
apprehension of shoulder t.
ARA t.
arch-up t.
arm fossa t.
arthrometer t.
axial compression t.
axial load t.
axial manual traction t.
axon reflex t.
Babinski t.

T

test (*continued*)
    ballottable patella t.
    ballottement t.
    Barlow pediatric hip instability t.
    Barlow provocative t.
    Beals periarticular laceration saline
        load t.
    Beery Visual Motor Integration T.
    Behavioral Inattention T. (BIT)
    Bekhterev sciatica t.
    Bekhterev sitting t.
    belly-press t.
    bench t.
    Bennett Hand Tool Dexterity T.
    Benton Constructional Praxis T.
    Berg balance t.
    biceps jerk reflex t.
    Bielschowsky 3–step head tilt t.
    big toe t.
    Biodex Balance System t.
    block t.
    blot t.
    Booth transverse humeral
        ligament t.
    bounce home knee t.
    bowstring low back t.
    Boyes boutonniére deformity t.
    bracelet t.
    brachial plexus tension t.
    Bragard meniscal injury t.
    Bragard sciatica t.
    break t.
    brush knee swelling t.
    bulge knee t.
    Bunnell-Littler wrist contracture t.
    Burke t.
    Burn bench malingering t.
    calcidiol t.
    calf squeeze t.
    Callaway shoulder dislocation t.
    Caplan Indented Paragraph
        Reading T.
    carpal compression t.
    Carroll t.
    catch and clunk t.
    Centinela supraspinatus shoulder t.
    cerebellar function t.
    cervical compaction t.
    cervical sidegliding t.
    Chaddock t.
    Charpy impact t.
    chest expansion chest and spine
        arthritis t.
    Chiene line bilateral greater
        trochanter t.
    Children's Paced Auditory Serial
        Addition T. (CHIPASAT)
    Childress duck waddle knee t.
    chin-to-chest t.

circle draw t.
Clarke patellar compression t.
clock balance t.
clunk shoulder t.
Cognitive Performance T. (CPT)
cold pressor t.
Coleman lateral block t.
Combat Task T.
compression t.
concealed straight leg raising t.
conduction velocity t.
confrontational t.
Conner Continuous Performance T.
Contextual Memory T. (CMT)
continuous performance t. (CPT)
contralateral straight leg raising t.
costoclavicular syndrome t.
Cotton ankle instability t.
Cotton fibular bone hook t.
cough t.
Cozen elbow dislocation t.
Craig hip t.
cram sciatic nerve root pressure t.
crank shoulder t.
creep t.
crossed straight leg raise t.
crossover impingement of
    shoulder t.
Cybex isokinetic t.
d'Ambrosia t.
de Kleyn t.
Derefield leg length t.
Derefield-Thompson leg length t.
Deyerle sciatic tension t.
dial t.
digital Allen t.
digital response t.
dipyridamole handgrip t.
disc space saline acceptance t.
distal compression t.
distracted straight-leg raising t.
distraction t.
dorsal drawer t.
dorsiflexion-eversion t.
double leg raise t.
Downey fingertip texture
    discrimination t.
drawer t.
drop arm rotator cuff t.
dual photon densitometry t.
Duchenne lower extremity t.
duck waddle t.
Dugas dislocated shoulder t.
Duncan prone rectus femoris
    dysfunction t.
Dunn multiple comparison t.
Durkan carpal compression t.
Dvorak flexion-rotation t.
Dynatron 2000 muscle t.

Eden thoracic outlet t.
elbow flexion t.
elbow jerk reflex t.
elevated arm stress t. (EAST)
Elithorn perceptual maze t.
Elson middle slip finger t.
Ely heel-to-buttock t.
empty beer can shoulder t.
endpoint of orthopaedic t.
eversion stress t.
excessive laxity t.
external recurvatum knee t.
external rotation-abduction stress t.
  (EAST)
external rotation recurvatum knee t.
external rotation stress t.
extrinsic entrapment t.
extrinsic tightness t.
faber t.
fabere t.
fadir t.
fadire t.
Fastex proprioceptive and agility t.
Feagin shoulder dislocation t.
femoral nerve stretch t. (FNST)
femoral nerve traction hip t.
fibular bone hook t.
fibular compression t.
figure-of-4 t.
figure-of-8 t.
finger extension t.
fingertips-to-floor t.
finger-to-finger t.
finger-to-nose t. (FNT)
Finkelstein tendonitis of wrist t.
first metatarsus rise t.
FirstSTEP Developmental
  Screening T.
fist-edge-palm t.
fist-palm-side t.
fist-ring t.
flathand t.
flexion, abduction, external rotation,
  extension t.
flexion, abduction, internal
  rotation t.
flexion, adduction, internal
  rotation t.
flexion-rotation-drawer t.
flexion-rotation-drawer knee
  instability t.
flexion spinal radiography t.
flexor pronator syndrome t.
flip t.
fluctuation t.
foot placement t.
foraminal compression t.
forced adduction t.
forearm supination t.

forefoot adduction correction t.
forefoot block t.
Fortin finger low back pain t.
Fowler foot arch prosthesis t.
FRD t.
Froment ulnar nerve function t.
fulcrum t.
Gaenslen sacroiliac joint and lumbar
  vertebrae inflammation t.
Galeazzi pediatric hip dysplasia t.
Galveston Orientation and Amnesia
  T. (GOAT)
Garrick popliteus tendon t.
George vertebrobasilar
  insufficiency t.
Gerber subscapularis t.
Gilchrist t.
Gillet marching sacroiliac joint
  motion t.
gluteus maximus tensing t.
Goldman-Fristoe articulation t.
golfer's elbow t.
Gordon calf squeeze t.
gracilis t.
gravity drawer knee t.
gravity stress t.
grimace t.
grind shoulder t.
grip strength t.
Grooved Pegboard T.
Hamilton ruler t.
hand function t.
Harris Infant Neuromotor T. (HINT)
Hautant t.
Hawkins-Kennedy shoulder
  impingement t.
heel-palm t.
heel-rise t.
heel-tap t.
heel-tip t.
heel-to-knee t.
heel-to-shin t.
Helfet t.
hip abduction stress t.
hip quadrant t.
hip scouring t.
Hoffa t.
9-hole peg t.
Homans venous thrombosis of
  leg t.
Hoover paralyzed leg t.
hop t.
Hughston external rotation
  recurvatum t.
Hughston knee jerk t.
Hughston-Losee jerk t.
Hughston plica knee t.
Hughston posterolateral drawer
  knee t.

T

test (*continued*)

Hughston posteromedial drawer knee t.
hyperabduction thoracic outlet t.
hyperextension elbow t.
iliac compression t.
iliacus t.
iliopsoas t.
impingement of shoulder t.
impingement reduction t.
inhibition t.
inspiration and expiration breathing thoracic spine t.
interdigital neuroma t.
intrinsic tightness t.
inversion stress t.
ischemic forearm exercise t.
Jack t.
jackknife t.
Jackson compression t.
Jacob shift t.
Jakob knee t.
Jakob shoulder t.
Jamar grip strength t.
Jansen t.
Jebsen hand function t.
Jebsen-Taylor hand function t.
jerk knee t.
Jobe relocation shoulder t.
jogging in place t.
Jolly myasthenic reaction t.
Jones tendon t.
Kelikian metatarsal push-up t.
Kemp spinal t.
Kleiger ankle t.
Kleinman shear carpal ligament t.
knee-drop t.
knee flexion stress t.
knee instability t.
knee jerk reflex t.
knee laxity t.
kneeling bench t.
Knox Cube Imitation T.
Lachman knee ligamentous instability t.
Laguere sacroiliac t.
Lam inversion tarsal tunnel t.
Lasègue rebound herniated nucleus pulposus t.
Lasègue sitting t.
Lasègue straight leg raising t.
lateral and anteroposterior rib compression thoracic spine t.
lateral block t.
lateral elbow epicondyle t.
lateral pivot shift knee ligamentous instability t.
lateral scapular slide t. (LSST)
lateral squeeze t.

leaning hop t.
LEAP monofilament t.
1-leg hop for distance t.
1-leg stance t.
Lewin-Gaenslen sacroiliac lesion t.
Lewin punch referred back pain t.
Lewin reverse Lasègue t.
Lewin snuff disc rupture t.
Lewin standing hamstring t.
Lewin supine ankylosing spinal lesion t.
Lewis-Prusik capillary circulation t.
Lichtman midcarpal shift t.
lift-off subscapularis t.
ligamentous instability t.
light touch t.
Lippman biceps tendinopathy t.
Litroff t.
load and shift shoulder t.
locking-position t.
long bone compression t.
Losee knee instability t.
Lovett muscle strength t.
Lovett spring balance muscle t.
Ludington shoulder t.
lumbar extension t.
lumbar lateral flexion t.
lumbar protective mechanism t.
lumbar rotation t.
lunotriquetral ballottement t.
lunotriquetral shear t.
MacIntosh lateral pivot shift knee t.
Magnuson low back pain site t.
Maigne vertebrobasilar insufficiency t.
Maitland slump neural tissue tension t.
manual muscle t. (MMT)
matchstick t.
match to sample t.
mathematical processing t.
Maudsley tennis elbow t.
Maximum Voluntary Efforts T.
McCarthy t.
McMurray meniscal tear t.
medial elbow epicondyle t.
medial/lateral grind knee t.
Mennell 2–stage lower back t.
Michele t.
middle finger t.
military brace position shoulder t.
military posture t.
milk t.
Mills elbow t.
Minnesota Manual Dexterity T.
Minnesota Rate of Manipulation t. (MRMT)
Minnesota Spatial Relations T.
6-minute walk functional capacity t.

Moberg ninhydrin t.
Moberg Picking Up T.
monofilament pressure t.
Morton interdigital neuroma t.
movement coordination t.
MyoForce t.
Naffziger nerve root
  compression t.
navicular drop t.
Neer shoulder impingement t.
nerve compression t. (NCT)
nerve conduction velocity t.
nerve function t.
Neviaser t.
89-newton t.
ninhydrin print sweat t.
Nobel knee t.
nondynamometric trunk
  performance t.
Noyes flexion rotation drawer
  knee t.
Ober iliotibial band t.
oblique retinacular ligament
  tightness t.
O'Brien shoulder active
  compression t.
O'Connor finger dexterity t.
O'Connor tweezer dexterity t.
O'Donoghue cervical muscle
  strain t.
O'Driscoll posterolateral pivot t.
T. of Everyday Attention (TEA)
T. of Everyday Attention for
  Children (TEA-Ch)
T. of Infant Motor Performance
  (TIMP)
T. of Oral and Limb Apraxia
  (TOLA)
T. of Orientation for Rehabilitation
  Patients (TORP)
T. of Playfulness (ToP)
T. of Visual-Motor Skills (TVMS)
T. of Visual-Motor Skills: Upper
  Level Adolescents and Adults
  (TVMS:UL)
T. of Visual-Perception Skills
  (TVPS)
T. of Visual-Perceptual Skills: Upper
  Level Adolescents and Adults
  (TVPS:UL)
opposition t.
Ortolani pediatric hip dislocation t.
OsteoGram bone density t.
Osteomark bone-loss urine t.
Osteopatch bone density t.
overhead exercise t.
Paced Auditory Serial Addition t.
  (PASAT)
Paget tumor t.

pain, asymmetry, range, tone,
  special t. (PARTS)
pain provocation t.
palm-up t.
parachute t.
2-part Apley t.
passive accessory motion t.
passive patellar glide t.
passive patellar tilt t.
passive physiological t.
passive tennis elbow t.
patellar apprehension t.
patellar glide t.
patellar grind t.
patellar inhibition t. (PIT)
patellar retraction t.
patellar tap knee swelling t.
patella tap t.
patella tendon and patella ligament
  length t.
Patrick/fabere t.
Patrick hip joint disease t.
peak torque t.
pectoralis major shoulder
  contraction t.
pelvic rock t.
pencil t.
percussion elbow t.
peroneal tunnel compression t.
Perthes tourniquet t.
Phalen wrist flexion t.
Physical Ability T. (PAT)
pick-up t.
pinch grip t.
pinprick hyperalgesia t.
piriformis t.
pivot-shift t.
pivot-shift knee t.
plantar flexion-inversion t.
plica t.
2-point discrimination t.
posterior apprehension t.
posterior apprehension shoulder t.
posterior drawer knee t.
posterior sag knee t.
posterior shoulder impingement t.
posterior stress t.
posterior subluxation t.
posterolateral drawer t.
posterolateral pivot t.
posteromedial pivot-shift t.
probe t.
probe-to-bone t.
prone extension t.
prone external rotation t.
prone knee-bend t.
prone knee flexion t.
prone rectus t.
proximal compression t.

T

test (*continued*)

pseudostability t.
pulse status-pull t.
push-pull t.
push-up t.
quadrant hip scouring t.
quadriceps active t.
quadriceps contraction t.
quadriceps inhibition t.
Quantitative Sudomotor Axon Reflex T. (QSART)
Queckenstedt spinal stenosis t.
Queckenstedt-Stookey subarachnoid channel block t.
Quick Neurological Screening T. (QNST)
RA t.
recurvatum t.
rekindling t.
relocation t.
resisted straight leg raise t.
resistive tennis elbow t.
reverse Lachman t.
reverse Lasègue t.
reverse Phalen t.
reverse pivot-shift knee t.
Rivermead Behavioral Memory T. (RBMT)
Romberg dorsal column of spinal cord t.
Roos overhead exercise shoulder t.
rotary drawer t.
rotary instability t.
rotation drawer t.
rotation recurvatum t.
sacroiliac joint fixation t.
sacroiliac joint stress t.
sag t.
sagittal stress t.
saline acceptance t.
saline load t.
scaphoid lift t.
scaphoid shift t.
scapular approximation t.
scapular elevation t.
Schober lumbar spine range of motion t.
scratch t.
seated flexion t.
seated root t.
Seddon coin tactile t.
Semmes-Weinstein monofilament pressure t.
Sensory Integration and Praxis t. (SIPT)
Sensory Organization T. (SOT)
Sharp-Purser cervical cord compression t.
shear t.

Sherman block t.
shift t.
shoulder abduction t.
shoulder depression t.
shuck carpal ligament t.
shuttle walking t. (SWT)
side-glide t.
side-jump t.
side-lying iliac compression t.
Silfverskiöld tight calf t.
Simmonds Achilles tendon rupture t.
Simmonds-Thompson Achilles tendon rupture t.
simple knee t. (SKT)
single-heel rise t.
sit-and-reach t.
sitting duct stretch t.
sitting flexion t.
sitting root lumbar spine t.
sit-to-stand t.
sit-up t.
skin-gliding t.
skin resistance t.
skin wrinkling t.
Slocum ALRI t.
Slocum anterior rotary drawer knee t.
Slocum lateral pivot-shift knee t.
Slocum rotary instability of knee t.
SLR t.
SLR with Bragard t.
SLR with external rotation t.
SLR with Kernig t.
slump lumbar spine t.
Smith and Ross central slip tenodesis t.
Smith and Ross early boutonnière deformity t.
somatosensory t.
Soto-Hall spine pain t.
Speed shoulder t.
spinal extension t.
sponge t.
spring lumbar spine t.
Spurling cervical nerve root impingement t.
Spurling cervical spine t.
square-shaped wrist t.
squat t.
squatting t.
squeeze t.
Stagnara intraoperative wake-up t.
Staheli pediatric hip extension t.
Staheli pediatric lower extremity t.
stair running t.
standing apprehension t.
standing arm elevation t.
standing flexion t.

standing Gillet sacroiliac joint motion t.
starch t.
Star Excursion Balance T. (SEBT)
station t.
Steinmann meniscal injury t.
Steinman tenderness displacement t.
Sternberg memory t.
sternoclavicular joint stress t.
t. stimulus
Stinchfield resisted hip flexion t.
stork t.
stork standing lumbar spine t.
straight leg raising t.
stress t.
stretch t.
stroke t.
stroke knee t.
Stroop word color identification t.
subtalar inversion t.
sudomotor activity t.
sulcus t.
supine iliac gapping t.
supine long sitting t.
supine straight leg raising t.
suprapatellar plica snap t.
suprascapular nerve entrapment t.
supraspinatus isolation t.
supraspinatus rotator cuff tear t.
surprise shoulder t.
sweat t.
sweep knee t.
swing ankle/foot t.
Tack t.
Tack T.
taking off shoe t. (TOST)
talar tilt eversion t.
talar tilt inversion t.
tandem gait t.
tap elbow t.
tarsal twist t.
tennis elbow t.
tenodesis t.
Tensilon t.
tensing t.
thenar weakness t.
Thomasen ankle tendinitis t.
Thomas hip contracture t.
Thompson ruptured Achilles tendon t.
thumbnail t.
thumb-to-forearm t.
tibiotalar shuck t.
tight retinacular ligament t.
tilt-up t.
timed Allen hand revascularization t.
Tinel elbow t.
Tinel nerve lesion t.
tissue compression t.

Toglia Category Assessment T. (TCAT)
tourniquet t.
transverse humeral ligament t.
TRAP t.
treadmill t.
Trendelenburg dislocated hip t.
Trendelenburg gluteus medius weakness t.
Trendelenburg leg vein valve t.
triangular fibrocartilage complex stability t.
triceps jerk reflex t.
triceps skinfold t.
triple-jump t.
tripod hip tightness t.
Trömner corticospinal pathways disease t.
Trömner digital reflex t.
true leg-length discrepancy t.
trunk incurvation t.
ulnar collateral t.
ulnar grind t.
unilateral standing t.
upper limb neurodynamic t. (ULNT)
upper limb tension t. (ULTT)
valgus stress t.
valgus stress wrist t.
Valpar Whole Body Range of Motion Work Sample T.
Valsalva cervical spine and lumbar t.
varus stress t.
varus stress wrist t.
vertebral artery t. (VAT)
vertical compression t.
vertical suspension t.
vibration threshold t.
vibrometer t.
volitional muscle action t.
Voshell knee t.
Waddell functional overlay t.
wake-up t.
Waldron knee chondromalacia t.
walk t.
Wallenberg vertebral artery t.
Ward femoral neck t.
water acceptance t.
Watson scaphoid shift t.
Watson scapholunate instability t.
Weber foot t.
Weber hearing t.
Weber 2-point discrimination t.
Weinstein enhanced sensory t.
well-leg straight-leg raising lumbar spine t.
Wilson knee t.
Wingate anaerobic power t.

T

test (*continued*)
    wipe t.
    wipe knee t.
    Wolf motor function t.
    Wright-Adson thoracic outlet t.
    Wright thoracic outlet t.
    wrinkle t.
    wrist flexion t.
    Yeager t.
    Yeoman sacroiliac joint t.
    Yergason bicipital tenosynovitis t.

tester
    Artscan 200 arthroscopic cartilage stiffness t.
    Cybex t.
    grip t.
    GripTrack Commander strength t.
    Jamar grip t.
    MicroFET2 muscle t.
    Nicholas manual muscle t.
    OSI laxity t.
    West nerve t.

testing
    active motion t. (AMT)
    active movement t.
    angle isometric t.
    aquatic cardiac evaluation and t. (ACET)
    arthrometer t.
    axial closed-loop hydraulic mechanical t.
    biomechanical t.
    biothesiometer t.
    blunt pressure t.
    brush-evoked pain t.
    compression t.
    computerized adaptive t.
    confirmatory t.
    Cybex t.
    Disk-Criminator sensory t.
    dynametric t.
    enzyme-based lactic acid blood t.
    exercise t.
    face validity of rehabilitation t.
    isokinetic t.
    isometric motor t.
    isometric strength t.
    isotonic motor t.
    manual muscle t. (MMT)
    mobility t.
    motion t.
    motor neglect t.
    MRI t.
    muscle t.
    nerve involvement t.
    neurological t.
    Omnitron exercise t.
    palpation t.
    passive intervertebral motion t.

    passive mobility t.
    pincer t.
    PIVM t.
    premanipulative t.
    quantitative mechanical pain t.
    quantitative sensory t. (QST)
    range of motion t.
    ratio scale in rehabilitation t.
    reciprocal isokinetic t.
    rotation t.
    segmental mobility t.
    segmental motion t.
    sensory organization t. (SOT)
    shear t.
    strength t.
    stress t.
    susceptibility t.
    Tacticon quantitative sensory t.
    vertebral motion t.

testosterone
    synthetic t.

tetanic contraction

tetanolysin

tetanospasmin

tetanus
    t. immune globulin
    t. prophylaxis

tetany

tethered
    t. cord syndrome (TCS)
    t. patellar tendon syndrome
    t. spinal cord

tethering
    t. effect
    rib t.
    spinal cord t.

tetracaine and dextrose

tetracalcium phosphate

tetracycline

tetraphasic action potential

tetraplegia
    International Classification for Surgery of the Hand in T.
    traumatic t.

tetrapolar

Teufel cervical brace

Teuffer
    T. Achilles tendon repair technique
    T. tendo calcaneus repair

Teurlings wrist brace

TEV
    talipes equinovarus

Tevdek suture

Texas
    T. Scottish Rite Hospital (TSRH)
    T. Scottish Rite Hospital wrench
    T. T incision

Texon sole

textured allograft bone graft

TF
  tibiofemoral
TFA
  thigh-foot angle
  tibiofemoral angle
TFB-PS
  tibial fracture brace proximal support
TFC
  threaded fusion cage
  triangular fibrocartilage
  TFC tear
T-finger splint
T-Fix absorbable meniscal repair device
TFL
  tensor fasciae latae
TFM
  transverse friction massage
T-Foam
  T-F. bed pad
  T-F. cushion
  T-F. mattress
  T-F. pillow
T-Gel cushion
TGF
  transforming growth factor
TGN
  Trigeminal neuralgia
THA
  total hip arthroplasty
Thackray
  T. hip prosthesis
  T. low friction arthroplasty
thalamic
  t. fracture of calcaneum
  t. fragment of calcaneal fracture
thalassaemia (*var. of* thalassemia)
thalassanemia (*var. of* thalassemia)
thalassemia, thalassanemia, thalassaemia
thalidomide
thallium (TI)
  radioisotope t.
  t. scan
Than anaerobic threshold
T-handle
  T-h. curette
  T-h. elevator
  ratcheting T-h.
  T-h. Zimmer chuck
T-handled
  T-h. awl
  T-h. hook
  T-h. nut wrench
  T-h. reamer
  T-h. screw wrench
  T-h. trocar
tharies
  total hip arthroplasty with internal eccentric shells

total hip articular replacement by internal eccentric shells
  tharies femoral resurfacing component
  tharies hip component
  tharies hip replacement
  tharies hip replacement operation
  tharies hip replacement prosthesis
Thatcher
  T. nail
  T. screw
The
  T. Backstroke
  T. Experience of Leisure Scale (TELS)
  T. Healthy Back System
  T. Heeler inflatable heel protector
  T. Institute for Rehabilitation Research (TIRR)
  T. Jacknobber II
  T. Knee Society clinical-rating scale
  T. Painless One acupuncture needle
  T. Rope stretch-and-traction device
  T. Rope stretching device
  T. Unloader
  T. Wedge bioresorbable interference-fit implant
theater, theatre
  t. ache
  t. sign
theatre (*var. of* theater)
theca, *pl.* **thecae**
  digital t.
  t. tendinis
thecae (*pl. of* theca)
thecal
  t. abscess
  t. injection
  t. sac
  t. whitlow
themoplastic ankle-foot orthosis
thenar
  t. area
  t. atrophy
  t. branch
  t. creaking
  t. eminence
  t. fascia
  t. flap
  t. muscle
  t. palmar crease (TPC)
  t. palsy
  t. space
  t. weakness test
theory
  beam t.
  Burnet clonal selection t.
  closed-form bar t.
  3-column spine t.

773

theory (*continued*)
 craniosacral t.
 Denis Browne 3-column spine t.
 kinetic energy t.
 Maisel congenital hand transverse
  deficiency suppression t.
 QLV t.
 quasilinear viscoelastic t.
Thera
 T. Cane
 T. Cane massager
 T. Cane shoulder exerciser
Thera-Back back support
Thera-Band
 T.-B. Aqua Belt
 T.-B. Assist exerciser
 T.-B. exercise ball
 T.-B. Exercise System for Golfers
 T.-B. hand exerciser
 T.-B. handle
 T.-B. Max resistive exercise
 T.-B. progressive weight
 T.-B. resistive exerciser
 T.-B. resistive therapy system
 T.-B. strip
 T.-B. system of progressive
  resistance
 T.-B. tubing
Therabath paraffin heat therapy system
TheraBeads microwaveable moist heat
pack
Thera-Boot bandage
Thera-Ciser
 T.-C. light exercise system
 T.-C. therapeutic exercise system
Theracloud pillow
TheraCool cold therapy
Therafectin
Thera-Fit
Theraflex wrist exerciser
Therafoam padding
Theraform Selectives
Thera-Gesic cream
Theragloves
Theragym ball
Ther-A-Hoop exerciser
TheraKnit electrode glove
Thera-Loop exerciser
Thera-Med cold pack
Thera-Medic shoe
Theramini 1, 2 electrotherapy stimulator
therapeutic
 t. appliance
 t. conservatism
 t. exercise
 t. lifestyle change (TLC)
 t. light
 t. orthosis
 t. requirement

 t. shoe
 t. spinal support
 t. splint
 t. ultrasound
 t. ultrasound for tendon healing
therapeutics
 Journal of Manipulative and
  Physiological T.
 T. Sleeping Pillow
Thera-P exercise bar
therapist
Thera-Plast putty
Therap-Loop
 T.-L. door anchor
 T.-L. door handle
Thera-Pos elbow orthosis
Therapress pressure point release tool
TheraPulse bed
Thera-Putty CTS exerciser
therapy
 ablative laser t.
 active-assistive motion t.
 Acu-Magnet t.
 amplitude-summation interferential
  current t. (ASICT)
 animal-assisted t. (AAT)
 anticoagulant t.
 anticonvulsant t.
 antisense gene t.
 antithrombotic t.
 aquatic t.
 bee venom t.
 Biodex Unweighing System partial
  weight t.
 Bragg-peak photon-beam t.
 brisement t.
 carpal tunnel syndrome injection t.
 T. Carrot finger contracture orthosis
 T. Carrot Finger Orthosis
 cell t.
 chelation t.
 chiropractic manipulative t. (CMT)
 cold t.
 Coldflo cold t.
 compression t.
 conservative t.
 Cool-Aid continuous controlled
  cold t.
 corrective t.
 corticosteroid t.
 craniosacral t. (CST)
 deep muscle t.
 diet t.
 diversified chiropractic
  manipulative t.
 dry heat t.
 edema heat t.
 electrical stimulation t.
 electric differential t.

Electri-Cool continuous controlled cold t.
t. electroconvulsive therapy
electron-beam t.
ETPS t.
Exogen 2000+ noninvasive ultrasound t.
extended code t. (ECT)
extracorporeal shock wave t.
fad t.
flexion-distraction t.
fomentation t.
frequency-difference interferential current t. (FDICT)
geriatric physical t.
gold t.
HBO t.
heat t.
herbal t.
high-voltage t. (HVT)
hot fomentation t.
hyperbaric oxygen t.
hypnotic t.
IFC t.
immunosuppressive t. (IST)
inferential t.
inferential current t.
infrared t.
injection t.
interferential t.
intradiscal electrothermal t. (IDET)
intraosseous t.
intravenous t.
Kelsey unloading exercise t.
LaserPen laser t.
Livingstone t.
maggot debridement t.
magnetic t.
manipulative t.
manual t.
massage t. (MT)
McKenzie back pain and neck pain t.
meridian t.
microcurrent t.
mind-body t.
mirror box t.
mirror box pain management t.
moist heat t.
motion t.
moxa t.
negative pressure wound t. (NPWT)
neurological physical t.
neuromuscular electrical stimulation t.
NMES t.
occupational t. (OT)

orthomolecular medicine/ megavitamin t.
ortho physical t.
osteoinductive t.
osteomanipulative t. (OMT)
osteopathic manipulative t. (OMT)
outpatient physical t.
oxygen t.
pancreatic enzyme t.
parachute t.
paraffin heat t.
pediatric physical t.
perioperative antibiotic t.
physical t. (PT)
piperacillin/tazobactam t.
pneumatic compression t.
Polar Wrap cold t.
pool t.
positional release t.
postoperative t.
pressure t.
ProFlo vascular compression t.
proliferation t.
prophylactic antibiotic t.
Psoralen-UVA t.
pulsed short-wave t.
T. Putty
qi gong t.
radiation t.
range of motion t.
recreational t. (RT)
reflex t.
Rolfing t.
ROM t.
sedation t.
shockwave t. (SWT)
silastic ball t.
somatic t.
spinal injection t.
spinal manipulative t. (SMT)
spinal manual t.
splinting t.
steroid t.
Supartz joint fluid t.
SwimEx aquatic t.
Swiss ball t.
Synvisc injection t.
t. tank
Task Force on Standards of Physical T.
TENS t.
TheraCool cold t.
tonification t.
transfusion t.
transverse friction t.
trial of conservative t.
trigger point t. (TPT)
tumor t.

T

therapy (*continued*)
    ultrasound t.
    vacuum-assisted t.
    vasoconstrictive t.
    whirlpool t.
Ther-A-Shapes positioner
Therasleep Cervical Pillow
Therasound transducer
Theratouch 4.7 stimulator
Thera-Wedge system
TheriLok bone void filler
Thermadrene
thermal, thermic
    t. agent
    t. anesthesia
    t. capsulorrhaphy
    t. energy
    t. modality
    t. necrosis
    T. Pack
    t. sleeve
thermalator
    T. heating unit
    Whitehall t.
ThermalSoft hot & cold packs
Thermapad pad
Thermasonic gel warmer
Thermassage
    Aqua T.
ThermaStim
    T. muscle stimulator
    T. muscle warming device
thermic (*var. of* thermal)
Thermo
    T. Fusion
    T. hand comforter
    T. HK/Rohadur orthotic
    T. HK/Tepefom orthotic
    T. knee comforter
thermocoagulate
thermocoagulation
ThermoCork orthotic
thermocouple
    t. instrument
    low impedance t.
    t. skin temperature device
ThermoFlex
    Maramed T.
thermoforming
thermogram
thermographic
    t. examination
    t. finding
    t. scanner
thermography
    chiropractic t.
    infrared t.
    liquid crystal t. (LCT)
thermolabile plastic

Thermold heat moldable shoe lining
thermomassage
thermomechanical implant metal prosthesis
thermomoldable
    t. insert
    t. material
Thermophore
    T. hot pack
    T. moist heat pad
thermoplastic
    DynaPrene splinting t.
    t. elastomer (TPE)
    t. heating unit
    t. splint
    t. template
thermoregulate
thermoregulation
    localized t.
thermoregulatory sign
Thermoskin
    T. arthritic knee wrap
    T. brace
    T. heat retainer
    T. U wrist wrap
    T. 4-way elastic knee support
ThermoSKY orthotic material
Thermosport hot/cold wrap
thermotherapy
Thero-Skin gel padding
thickened synovial membrane
thickening
    cortical t.
    heel pad t.
    lamellar t.
    ligamentous t.
    tendon t.
thickness
    cortical t.
    t. of heel pad
    rim enhancement t.
thick patella sign
Thiemann disease
Thiersch
    T. medium split free graft
    T. thin split free graft
thigh
    t. atrophy
    t. corset
    t. cuff
    t. holder
    t. shell
    t. tourniquet
thigh-foot angle (TFA)
thigh-shank plane
thimerosal
thin
    t. disc
    t. glenoid retractor

t. osteotome
t. pin fixation
Thinline uncovered orthotic
THINSite dressing
thin-wire Ilizarov fixator
thiomalate
gold sodium t.
thiopental sodium
thioridazine
thiosulfate, thiosulphate
sodium t.
thiosulphate (*var. of* thiosulfate)
T28 hip prosthesis
third
distal t. (D/3, distal/3)
t. fibular muscle
t. metacarpal
middle t. (M/3)
proximal t. (P/3)
Steel rule of t.'s
third-generation
t.-g. cementing technique
t.-g. nail
THKAFO
trunk-hip-knee-ankle-foot orthosis
Thomas
T. buckle sling
T. cervical collar brace
T. classification
T. collar
T. collar cervical orthosis
T. extrapolated bar graft
T. fixator
T. frame
T. full-ring splint
T. heel
T. heel orthosis
T. hinged splint
T. hip contracture test
T. knee splint
T. Kodel sling
T. leg splint
T. needle
T. posterior splint
T. procedure
T. rigid collar
T. scaphoid-lunate gap sign
T. splint with Pearson attachment
T. suspension splint
T. traction
T. walking brace
T. walking caliper
T. wrench
Thomasen ankle tendinitis test
Thomas-Thompson procedure
Thomas-Thompson-Straub
T.-T.-S. external oblique transfer
T.-T.-S. rotational transfer of vastus
lateralis technique

Thompson
T. Achilles tendon test sign
T. anterolateral hip approach
T. anteromedial shoulder approach
T. arthroplasty
T. femoral neck prosthesis
T. frame
T. hemiarthroplasty hip prosthesis
T. hip endoprosthesis system
T. hip prosthesis forceps
T. leg check system
T. modification
T. modification of Denis Browne
splint
T. nail
T. posterior radial approach
T. quadricepsplasty
T. rasp
T. resection
T. ruptured Achilles tendon test
T. telescoping V osteotomy
Thompson-Epstein posterior hip fracture
dislocation classification (I-V)
Thompson-Parkridge-Richards (TPR)
T.-P.-R. implant
T.-P.-R. prosthesis
Thompson-Terwilliger terminal Syme
operation for ingrown toenail
procedure
Thomsen disease
thoraces (*pl. of* thorax)
thoracic (T)
t. approach
t. bone
t. curve
t. curve scoliosis
t. discography
t. duct
t. duct injury
t. epidural injection
t. extension component
t. facet fusion
t. gearshift
t. hemivertebrae
t. hyperkyphosis
t. hypokyphosis
t. inclination
t. inlet syndrome
t. insufficiency
t. insufficiency syndrome
t. kyphosis
t. lymphatic pump technique
t. manual traction
t. microtrauma
t. nerve
t. nerve injury
t. nerve palsy
t. orthosis
t. outlet syndrome (TOS)

T

thoracic (*continued*)
t. pedicle
t. pedicle marker
t. plane
t. spinal fusion
t. spine (T-spine)
t. spine biopsy
t. spine decompression
t. spine fracture
t. spine kyphotic deformity
t. spine lordosis
t. spine orthosis
t. spine pedicle diameter
t. spine scoliotic deformity
t. spine vertebral osteosynthesis
t. vertebrae 1-12 (T1-T12)
thoracis (*gen. of thorax*)
thoracoabdominal
t. approach
t. artery injury
t. incision
thoracoacromial artery
thoracodorsal
t. artery transfer
t. nerve
t. nerve injury
thoracoepigastric flap
thoracogenic scoliosis
thoracolumbar
t. burst fracture
t. corset
t. curve
t. curve pattern
t. erector spinae
t. fusion
t. hypertonus
t. idiopathic scoliosis
t. injury severity score (TLISS)
t. junction
t. junction alignment
t. junction surgical exposure
t. junction transitional zone
t. kyphoscoliosis
t. kyphosis
t. orthosis
t. pedicle screw
t. retroperitoneal approach
t. spinal injury
t. spine
t. spine anterior exposure
t. spine decompression
t. spine flexion-distraction injury
t. spine fracture-dislocation
t. spine scoliosis
t. spine stabilization
t. spine vertebral osteosynthesis
t. spondylosis
t. spondylosis surgical technique

t. standing orthosis brace
t. trauma
thoracolumbosacral (TLS)
t. orthosis (TLSO)
t. plate
t. spine
t. strain
thoracoplasty
thoracoscapular arthrodesis
thoracoscopic
t. approach
t. instrumentation
thoracotomy
t. approach
left-sided t.
right-sided t.
standard t.
thorax, *pl.* **thoraces,** *gen.* **thoracis**
barrel-shaped t.
Thorlo socks
Thornhill offset proximal femoral elevator
Thornton
T. bar
T. nail
T. nail plate
T. screw
thorny radiation
THORP
titanium hollow-screw osseointegrating reconstruction plate
THORP system
THR
total hip replacement
thread
cancellous screw t.
threaded
t. cancellous screw
t. cortical dowel
t. fusion cage (TFC)
t. guidepin
t. rod
t. spinal fusion cage
t. Steinmann pin
t. suture anchor
t. titanium acetabular prosthesis (TTAP)
t. titanium alloy prosthesis (TTAP)
t. titanium alloy prosthesis smooth threaded (TTAP-ST)
t. wire
threaded-hole-first technique
three-quarters prone position
threshold
anaerobic t. (AT)
bone conduction t.
cutaneous pressure t. (CPT)
experimental t.

lactate t.
lactic acidosis t.
mechanical pain t.
pressure t.
reflex t.
t. stimulus
Than anaerobic t.
vibration perception t.
(VPT)
thrombectomy
thrombin powder
thrombin-soaked Gelfoam
thrombocytopenia, thrombopenia
thrombocytopenia-absent
t.-a. radius (TAR)
t.-a. radius
thromboembolic
t. disease (TED)
t. stockings
thromboembolism
thromboembolus
thrombogenesis
thrombopenia (*var. of* thrombocytopenia)
thrombophilia
thrombophlebitis
femoroiliac t.
thrombosed
thromboses (*pl. of* thrombosis)
thrombosis, *pl.* **thromboses**
deep venous t. (DVT)
effort t.
effort-induced t.
iliofemoral t.
t. radial artery
silent t.
venous t.
Thrombostat topical hemostatic
through-and-through
t.-a.-t. fracture
t.-a.-t. tear
t.-a.-t. V-shaped horizontal
osteotomy
through-range feel
through stance
through-the-knee amputation
thrower's
t. elbow
t. exostosis
t. fracture
throwing
t. function
t. injury
thrust
adjustive t.
double-thumb t.
lateral-to-medial t.
t. manipulation
pattern of t.
t. plate prosthesis (TPP)

thumb
abducted t.
adducted t.
adductor sweep of t.
Bennett fracture dislocation of t.
Bennett fracture of basal joint of t.
bifid t.
bowler's t.
breakdancer's t.
clasped t.
congenital clasped t.
cortical t.
t. deformity
duplicate t.
t. duplication
t. extensor tendon
t. flexor tendon
floating t.
t. forceps
gamekeeper's t.
hitchhiker's t.
hypoplastic t.
t. instability
t. interphalangeal extension assist
jeweler's t.
laparoscopic surgeon's t.
t. loop
low-set t.
mallet t.
t. metacarpal
t. metacarpophalangeal joint
approach
t. opposition
t. pinch power
t. polydactyly
t. post
pouce flottant t.
proximal anular pulley of t.
t. reconstruction
t. screw
short t.
skier's t.
t. sling
spatulate t.
t. spica
t. spica cast
t. spica splint
spring swivel t.
supernumerary t.
surgeon's t.
tennis t.
trigger t.
triphalangeal t.
t. web
t. web splint
thumb-in-palm deformity
thumbkeeper
Freedom t.
T. splint

T

thumbnail test
thumb-pinch grasp
thumb-to-forearm test
thumb-wrist immobilizer
Thumper device
ThumSaver
    T. CMC Long splint
    T. CMC Short splint
    T. MP splint
ThumSling
    Action T.
ThumWrap
    FoamWrap T.
ThumZ'Up thumb splint
Thurston-Holland
    T.-H. fragment
    T.-H. fragment fracture
    T.-H. sign
thyroid
    t. cartilage
    t. gland
thyrotropin-releasing hormone (TRH)
TI
    thallium
Ti
    titanium
Ti-Bac
    T.-B. acetabular component
    T.-B. II hip prosthesis
tibia, *pl.* **tibiae**
    absent t.
    t. bone
    t. coordinate system
    corticotomy of proximal t.
    distal t.
    dysplastic t.
    facies articularis malleolus medialis
      tibiae
    groove distal t.
    lip of t.
    medial malleolus of t.
    osteochondrosis deformans tibiae
    Phemister medial approach to t.
    proximal t.
    saber t.
    transmetaphysial amputation
      of t.
    t. valga
    t. vara
tibiae (*pl. of* tibia)
tibial
    t. acceleration
    t. adamantinoma
    t. aimer
    t. aligner
    t. artery
    t. axial load injury
    t. base plate
    t. bolt

t. bone defect regeneration
t. bone graft
t. bowing
t. channel
t. collateral ligament (TCL)
t. collateral ligament bursitis
t. collet
t. component
t. condyle
t. crest
t. cutting block
t. cutting guide
t. defect
t. deformity
t. diaphysial shortening
t. drill guide
t. driver
t. eminence
t. endoprosthesis
t. epiphysis
t. footprint
t. fracture brace proximal support
  (TFB-PS)
t. guidepin
t. hallux sesamoid
t. head screw
t. hemimelia
t. hindfoot osteomusculocutaneous
  rotationplasty
t. insert
t. insertion site
t. jig
t. lengthening
t. lift-off
t. longitudinal deficiency
t. malleolus
t. medullary canal
t. metaphysis
t. mortise
t. muscle
t. nerve
t. nerve injury
t. phenomenon
t. pin
t. plafond
t. plafond fracture
t. plateau
t. plateau fracture
t. plateau fracture-dislocation
t. plateau prosthesis
posterior t. (PT)
t. pseudarthrosis
t. punch
t. resector
t. retractor
t. retroflexion
t. retrotorsion
t. retroversion
t. rim

t. sag
t. sesamoid
t. sesamoid ligament
t. sesamoid position (TSP)
t. slope
t. spacer
t. stress fracture
t. stylus
t. talar tilt (TTT)
t. tendon
t. torsion
t. torsion system
t. track holder
t. track template
t. tray
t. tubercle
t. tubercle avulsion
t. tubercle prominence
t. tuberosity
t. tuberosity fractures in children
   classification
t. tuberosity osteotomy
t. tunnel
t. tunnel enlargement
t. tunnel widening
t. varus
t. vein
t. wedge

tibialis
t. anterior
t. anterior muscle
t. anterior tendon
apophysitis t.
t. posterior dislocation
t. posterior function
t. posterior muscle
t. posterior tendon
t. sign

tibia-pro-fibula screw
tibioadductor reflex
tibiocalcaneal
t. arthrodesis
t. fusion
t. joint complex
t. ligament
t. medullary nailing
t. space

tibiofemoral (TF)
t. alignment
t. angle (TFA)
t. articulation
t. interaction
t. joint

tibiofibular
t. articulation
t. clear space
t. cyst
t. diastasis
t. fracture

t. fusion
t. joint
t. joint dislocation
t. joint instability
t. joint reduction
t. ligament
t. line
t. overlap
t. overlap measurement
t. pain syndrome
t. rotation
t. sprain
t. subluxation
t. synchondrosis
t. syndesmosis
t. synostosis

tibionavicular ligament
tibiospring ligament
tibiotalar
t. angle
t. arthritis
t. clear space
deep anterior t. (DATT)
deep posterior t. (DPTT)
t. diastasis
t. fusion
t. impingement
t. instability
t. joint
t. joint primary arthrodesis
t. shuck test
t. stability
superficial t. (STT)
t. tilt (TTT)

tibiotalocalcaneal
t. ankle fusion
t. arthrodesis

Tibone posterior shoulder
capsulorrhaphy
Tib-Transformer orthosis
tic
articulatory t.

ticarcillin and clavulanate
potassium
ticarcillin/clavulanate
ticlike pain
Ti/CoCr alloy hip prosthesis
Ti-Con prosthesis
tidemark
tie
free t.
table t.

Tiemann nail elevator
tie-over bolster
tier
Harris wire t.

Tietze syndrome
Ti-Fit total hip system
Tiger shaver blade

tight
t. retinacular ligament test
t. spinal canal trefoil canal
tightener
Charnley wire t.
Kirschner t.
Sklar wire t.
wire t.
tightness
adductor hamstring t.
hamstring t.
Tikhoff-Linberg
T.-L. bone and soft tissue tumors
procedure
T.-L. radical arm procedure
T.-L. shoulder girdle resection
tile
T. acetabular fracture classification
T. pelvic injury classification
T. pelvic inlet and outlet view
t. plate facet replacement
T. polytrauma algorithm
Tillaux anterolateral tibial epiphysis fracture
Tillaux-Chaput
T.-C. anterolateral tibial epiphysis
fracture
T.-C. tibial tubercle
Tillman prosthesis
tilt
T. and Turn Paragon bed
angular t.
anterior pelvic t.
anteroposterior t.
cock-robin head t.
innominate t.
manual talar t.
mediolateral t.
palmar t.
pelvic lateral t.
posterior pelvic t.
sacral t.
subtalar t.
superoinferior t.
t. table
talar t.
tibial talar t. (TTT)
tibiotalar t. (TTT)
varus t.
t. wrist
tilting
coronal t.
t. frame wheelchair
t. reflex
Tilt-In-Space wheelchair conversion
tilt-up test
tiludronate disodium
TIME
Toddler and Infant Motor Evaluation

time
activated partial thromboplastin t.
(aPTT)
capillary filling t. (CFT)
capillary refill t. (CRT)
conduction t.
cycle t.
double support t.
echo t.
floating t.
intercritical t.
loading t.
operating t.
pain-free walking t. (PFWT)
partial thromboplastin t. (PTT)
procedure t.
prothrombin t. (PT)
reaction t.
repetition t. (TR)
rise t.
simple reaction t. (SRT)
step t.
stride t.
swing t.
tincture of t. (TOT)
t. to stabilization
total end-range t. (TERT)
total tourniquet t. (TTT)
tourniquet t.
warm ischemic t.
timed Allen hand revascularization test
Timentin
1-time sharp débridement tray
TiMesh implantable hardware fixation
timing
right/left t.
timolol
TIMP
Test of Infant Motor Performance
tincture
t. of belladonna
t. of benzoin
t. of time (TOT)
opium t.
tinea
t. cruris
t. gladiatorum
t. pedis
t. versicolor
Tineacide antifungal lotion
Tinel
T. elbow test
T. nerve lesion test
T. sign
Tinel-Hoffmann sign
Tinetti
T. Assessment tool
T. gait assessment
Tiobi transfer

tip
>acromionizer t.
>Cloward cervical drill t.
>Fragmatome t.
>Frazier suction t.
>t. of medial malleolus
>t. pinch
>sacral bone t.
>screw t.
>suction t.
>Woodruff t.

tip-pinch dynamometry
tiptoe gait
tip-to-tip pinch
TIRR
>The Institute for Rehabilitation Research
>TIRR foot-ankle orthosis

Tisseel fibrin glue
tissue
>adipose t. (AT)
>t. anchor guide (TAG)
>bursal t.
>capsular support t.
>capsuloligamentous t.
>cartilaginous t.
>t. closure
>t. compression test
>connective t.
>Coonrad-Bugg posterior tibial tendon trapping and interposition of soft t.
>t. debris
>devitalized t.
>t. elongation
>t. expander
>exuberant granulation t. (EGT)
>fatty t.
>fibroadipose t.
>fibrocartilaginous t.
>fibroconnective t.
>fibrofatty t.
>fibrous scar t.
>t. forceps
>granulation t.
>hypertrophic granulation t.
>t. inhibitor
>t. inhibitor of metalloproteinase-1
>intervening connective t.
>ligamentous support t.
>t. mandrel implant material
>muscular t.
>necrotic t.
>neural t.
>t. nutrition
>osseous t.
>periarticular t.
>perineural t.
>periosteal t.

>pharyngeal t.
>t. pressure
>t. pressure measurement
>pressure-sensitive t.
>pressure-tolerant t.
>t. protector
>t. repair
>replacement t.
>residual disc t.
>revascularized t.
>scar t.
>t. scissors
>skeletal t.
>t. slack
>soft t.
>t. sterilization
>subcutaneous t.
>t. texture abnormality (TTA)
>tissue-engineered meniscal t.
>t. transfer
>t. transplant
>vascular t.
>viable t.
>viscoelastic t.
>weak bony t.

tissue-engineered meniscal tissue
tissue-level response
TissueTak corkscrew implant
tissue-type plasminogen activator
Titan
>T. Apollo electric flexion table
>T. cemented hip prosthesis
>T. Meridian intersegmental traction table
>T. Nova manual flexion-extension multiflex table

titanium (Ti)
>t. alloy
>t. alloy cancellous bone screw
>t. alloy hip prosthesis
>t. alloy implant metal
>t. alloy implant metal prosthesis
>t. cable
>t. circumferential grommet
>t. elastic nail
>t. geometric device
>t. half pin
>t. hip prosthesis
>t. hollow-screw osseointegrating reconstruction plate (THORP)
>t. hollow-screw plate system
>t. implant
>t. implant material
>t. implant prosthesis
>t. mandibular plate
>t. microsurgical bipolar forceps
>t. nail
>plasma-sprayed t.

T

titanium (*continued*)
    t. rod and buttress prosthesis
    t. screw
    t. spacer
titer
    antistreptolysin O t. (ASOT)
Ti-Thread prosthesis
tizanidine
TJA
    total joint arthroplasty
TJR
    total joint replacement
TKA
    total knee arthroplasty
    trochanter-knee-ankle
TKR
    total knee replacement
TLC
    therapeutic lifestyle change
TLISS
    thoracolumbar injury severity
      score
TLS
    thoracolumbosacral
      TLS strain
TLSO
    thoracolumbosacral orthosis
      TLSO brace
      CASH TLSO
TMA
    tarsometatarsal amputation
      TMA prosthesis
TMJ
    temporomandibular joint
      TMJ syndrome
TMT
    tarsometatarsal
TN
    talonavicular
      TN joint
T-nail
TNS
    tension night splint
Toad finger splint
tobramycin
tobramycin-impregnated PMMA implant
Tobruk splint
Todd gait
Toddler and Infant Motor Evaluation (TIME)
toddler's fracture
Todd-Wells stereotactic arc guide
toe
    t. alignment
    t. alignment splint
    t. amputation
    Astroturf t.
    t. block anesthesia

t. box
Butler procedure to correct overlapping t.'s
t. cap
Clanton turf t.
claw t.
t. clawing
clubbed t.
cock-up deformity of t.
t. comb
t. crest
crossover second t.
curly t.
t. disarticulation
distal tuberosity of t.
downgoing t.'s
t. drop
DuVries technique for overlapping fifth t.
t. extensor
t. extensor muscle
t. extensor tendon
extra t.
flail t.
t. flexion
t. flexor
t. flexor muscle
floating t.
floppy t.
t. gait
great t.
t. gripping exercise
t. implant
t. index
jogger's t.
lesser t.
t. loop
mallet t.
marathoner's t.
medial crossover t.
medial deviation of second t.
Morton t.
overlapping fifth t.
overriding fifth t.
over-straight t.
painful t.
t. phalanx transplant
t. phenomenon
t. plate
t. plate extension
t. pressure
t. prosthesis
push-off by great t.
t. raise exercise
t. range of motion
t. reflex
runner's t.
sand t.

sausage t.
t. separator
set angle of t.
t. spacer
spacer between t.'s
t. spica cast
splaying of t.
sportsman's t.
t. spread sign
stiff t.
striatal t.
supernumerary t.
tennis t.
turf t. (I-III)
underlapping t.
unilaterally upgoing t.
upgoing t.'s
varus t.
V-Y plasty correction of varus t.
t. walk
t. walking
webbed t.
t. wedge
Toe-Aid dressing
toe-drop brace
toe-ground purchase
toe-heel gait
toeing
t. in
t. out
toeing-in gait
toeing-out gait
toenail
dystrophic t.
gryphotic t.
ingrowing t.
ingrown t.
onychomycotic t.
Toennis tumor forceps
toe-off
t.-o. phase
t.-o. phase of gait
ToeOFF orthosis
toe-out angle
toe-straight device
toe-toe gait
toe-to-groin
t.-t.-g. cast
t.-t.-g. modified Jones dressing
toe-to-hand transfer
toe-to-midthigh cast
toe-touch weightbearing
toe-walker
idiopathic t.-w. (ITW)
toe-walking gait
Tofranil
toggle
screw t.
t. sign

toggle-recoil adjustment
Toglia Category Assessment Test (TCAT)
Tohen tendon technique
Tokuhashi
T. metastatic spine tumor
preoperative scoring system
T. metastatic spine tumor prognostic
evaluation system
TOLA
Test of Oral and Limb Apraxia
tolazoline
tolcapone
Tolectin DS
tolerance
fatigue t.
pressure t.
tolerated
weightbearing as t. (WBAT)
tolerogenic immunosuppression
tolmetin
tolnaftate
Tommy trapeze bar
tomogram, planogram, planigram
tomography, planigraphy, planography
computed t. (CT)
computerized axial t. (CAT)
conventional t.
emission t.
helical computed t. (HCT)
hypocycloidal ankle t.
positron emission t. (PET)
preoperative t.
quantitative computed t. (QCT)
single photon emission computed t.
(SPECT)
transpiral t.
trispiral t.
Tom Smith arthritis
tone
muscle t.
sphincter t.
tone-inhibiting leg cast
tone-reducing ankle-foot orthosis
(TRAFO)
tongs
Barton t.
Böhler t.
cervical fracture t.
Cone-Barton skull traction t.
cranial t.
Crutchfield-Raney cervical traction t.
Gardner-Wells t.
Raney-Crutchfield cervical traction t.
skull t.
traction t.
Trippi-Wells extraction fixation
traction t.
Vinke skull traction t.
tongue fracture of calcaneus

T

tongue-in-groove
  t.-i.-g. advancement
  t.-i.-g. recession
tonic
  t. muscle
  t. neck reflex
tonicity
  symmetric t.
tonification therapy
tonus
  myogenic t.
tool
  Acuforce 7.0 therapy t.
  AcuPressor myotherapy t.
  Adolescent and Pediatric Pain T.
    (APPT)
  ArthroWand t.
  Backnobber II massage t.
  Gore smoother crucial t.
  1-handed kitchen t.
  Index Knobber II massage t.
  Magnassager massage t.
  Original Backnobber massage t.
  Original Index Knobber II
    massage t.
  OsteoStat disposable power t.
  tang distractor t.
  Therapress pressure point
    release t.
  Tinetti Assessment t.
too many toes sign
tooth, *pl.* **teeth**
  Hutchinson teeth
  t. sign
toothed
  t. cutter
  t. tissue forceps
  t. washer
ToP
  Test of Playfulness
top
  circular laminar hook with
    offset t.
topaz
  T. manual flexion table
  T. MicroDebrider
top-entry hook
tophaceous
  t. deposit
  t. disease
  t. gout
tophectomy
tophi (*pl. of* tophus)
tophus, *pl.* **tophi**
  t. formation
  gouty t.
topical
  Achromycin T.
  Akne-Mycin T.
  A/T/S T.
  Baciguent T.
  BactoShield T.
  Caldesene T.
  Del-Mycin T.
  Dyna-Hex T.
  Elase T.
  Elase-Chloromycetin T.
  Emgel T.
  EryDerm T.
  Erygel T.
  Erymax T.
  E-Solve-2 T.
  ETS-2% T.
  Exelderm T.
  Flutex T.
  Garamycin T.
  G-myticin T.
  Hibiclens T.
  Hibistat T.
  Hydrocort T.
  MetroGel T.
  Micatin T.
  Monistat-Derm T.
  Mycifradin Sulfate T.
  Mycitracin T.
  NeoDecadron T.
  Neomixin T.
  Oxistat T.
  Pedi-Pro T.
  Polysporin T.
  Staticin T.
  terbinafine, t.
  Topicycline T.
  Triple Antibiotic T.
  T-Stat T.
Topicycline Topical
top-loading screw and rod system
topography
  internal t.
Toposar Injection
TOPS
  total posterior element system
  TOPS implant
Toradol
  T. injection
  T. Oral
Torg
  T. fifth metatarsal fracture
    classification (I-III)
  T. Jones fracture repair technique
  T. knee reconstruction
  T. tarsal navicular stress fracture
    repair technique
tori (*pl. of* torus)
torn
  t. ligament
  t. meniscus
tornado injury

Toronto
- T. brace
- T. Medical CPM exerciser
- T. parapodium orthosis
- T. pelvic fracture classification
- T. splint

TORP
Test of Orientation for Rehabilitation Patients

torque
- t. curve
- t. force
- frictional t.
- t. heel shoe
- t. load
- peak t.
- peak dorsiflexion t.
- plantarflexion t.
- t. production
- rotatory t.
- screw t.
- t. screwdriver
- supination t.
- t. wrench

torque-meter
Compudriver digital t.-m.

torsion
- angle of t.
- t. bar
- t. bar splint
- t. dystonia
- external tibial t.
- femoral t.
- femorotibial t.
- t. fracture
- internal tibial t. (ITT)
- internal tibiofibular t.
- medial t.
- t. neurosis
- tibial t.
- t. unit
- t. wedge fracture nonunion

torsional
- t. abnormality
- t. alignment
- t. deformity
- t. fracture
- t. gripping strength
- t. load
- t. overload
- t. rigidity
- t. stiffness
- t. stress

torsionometer
torticollis
- acquired t.
- congenital t.
- dermatogenic t.
- fixed t.

- intermittent t.
- mental t.
- muscular t.
- myogenic t.
- neurogenic t.
- nonspasmodic t.
- spasmodic t.
- spurious t.
- symptomatic t.

tortipelvis
torus, *pl.* **tori**
- T. external fixation system
- t. fracture
- regeneration t.

TOS
thoracic outlet syndrome

TOST
taking off shoe test

TOT
tincture of time

total
- t. active motion (TAM)
- t. anatomical hinge knee brace
- t. ankle arthroplasty (TAA)
- t. ankle replacement (TAR)
- t. arthrodesis of wrist
- t. articular replacement arthroplasty (TARA)
- t. articular replacement arthroplasty prosthesis
- t. articular resurfacing arthroplasty (TARA)
- t. body movement
- t. body water (TBW)
- t. bone matrix (TBM)
- t. cervical disc replacement (TCDR)
- t. cervical range of motion (TCROM)
- T. Concept ankle/foot prosthesis
- t. condylar III fully constrained prosthesis
- t. condylar knee
- t. condylar knee prosthesis
- T. Condylar Knee system
- t. condylar prosthesis (III)
- t. condylar semiconstrained tricompartmental prosthesis
- t. contact bivalve ankle-foot orthosis
- t. contact cast (TCC)
- t. contact casting (TCC)
- t. contact orthosis (TCO)
- t. contact shell ankle-foot orthotic
- t. contact socket
- t. elastic suspension (TES)
- t. elbow arthroplasty (TEA)
- t. end-range time (TERT)
- T. Environment Control (TEC)
- t. eversion range of motion

T

total (*continued*)
    t. extraperitoneal repair
    T. Gym
    T. Gym rehabilitation system
    t. hip arthroplasty (THA)
    t. hip arthroplasty with internal
      eccentric shells (tharies)
    t. hip articular replacement by
      internal eccentric shells
      (tharies)
    t. hip replacement (THR)
    t. hip replacement prosthesis
    t. hip revision
    t. hip stabilization orthosis
    t. joint arthroplasty (TJA)
    t. joint replacement (TJR)
    t. joint replacement prosthesis
    t. knee arthroplasty (TKA)
    T. Knee for Children prosthetic
    t. knee implant
    t. knee instrumentation
    T. Knee 2100 prosthetic knee
    t. knee replacement (TKR)
    t. knee replacement prosthesis
    t. matricectomy
    t. maxillary osteotomy
    t. meniscectomy
    t. mesenteric apron method
    t. necrosis
    t. parenteral nutrition (TPN)
    t. passive motion (TPM)
    t. patellectomy
    t. patellofemoral joint arthroplasty
    t. posterior element system (TOPS)
    t. range of motion (TROM)
    t. replacement joint
    t. rotating knee (TRK)
    t. sacrectomy
    T. Shock shock-absorbing prosthetic
      unit
    t. shoulder arthroplasty (TSA)
    t. talus fracture
    t. tourniquet time (TTT)
    t. transfer
    t. wrist arthroplasty (TWA)
TotalGym Exercise Program
totalis
    rachischisis t.
totally implantable lengthening device
Toti trephine drill
toto
    in t.
tottering gait
touchdown weightbearing (TDWB)
touch sensation
Touch-Test sensory evaluator
toughness
    fracture t.
Tourni-cot exsanguinating tourniquet

tourniquet
    Accuflate t.
    arthroscopic t.
    Bodenstab t.
    t. control
    Digikit finger t.
    digital t.
    double t.
    Esmarch t.
    finger t.
    forearm t.
    t. gauge
    t. ischemia
    t. palsy
    t. paralysis
    pneumatic t.
    pneumatic ankle t.
    t. pressure
    Profex arthroscopic t.
    t. test
    thigh t.
    t. time
    Tourni-cot exsanguinating t.
    upper arm t.
towel
    Charnley t.
    t. clamp
    t. clip
    t. exercise
    t. roll
    sterile t.
Townley
    T. anatomic knee system
    T. bone graft screw
    T. femur caliper
    T. horizontal platform
      prosthesis
    T. TARA prosthesis
    T. tibial plateau plate
    T. total articular resurfacing
      arthroplasty prosthesis
    T. total knee prosthesis
Townsend
    T. Air brace
    T. Premier brace
    T. Rebel convertible brace
    T. Reliever brace
Townsend-Gilfillan
    T.-G. plate
    T.-G. screw
toxaemia (*var. of* toxemia)
toxemia, toxicemia, toxaemia
toxicemia (*var. of* toxemia)
toxicity
    aluminum t.
    methotrexate t.
toxicodendron
    Rhus t.
Toygar angle

TPC
thenar palmar crease
TPE
thermoplastic elastomer
TPE ankle-foot orthosis
TPE biomechanical foot
orthosis
T-pin handle
T-plasty modification of Bankart shoulder operation
T-plate
ASIF T-p.
Association for the Study of Internal Fixation T-p. (ASIF T-plate)
dorsal T-p.
palmar T-p.
TPM
total passive motion
TPN
total parenteral nutrition
TPP
thrust plate prosthesis
TPP hip endoprosthesis
TPR
Thompson-Parkridge-Richards
TPR ankle prosthesis
TPT
trigger point therapy
TR
repetition time
TR-28
TR-28 hip prosthesis
TR-28 total hip replacement
trabecula, *gen.* and *pl.* **trabeculae**
naked t.
osseous t.
partially necrotic osseous t.
trabeculae (*gen.* and *pl. of* trabecula)
trabecular
t. bone
t. index of Singh
t. traction
trabeculation
Trac
T. II knee implant
T. II knee prosthesis
trace
tracer catheter
tracheal injury
trachelomastoid muscle
tracheostomy
tracheotomy tube
tracing
nerve t.
track
Frenkel t.
pin t.
track-bound joint

tracker
T. knee brace
Palumbo patella t.
patella t.
tracking
patellar t.
Trackmaster treadmill
Tracrium
tract
anterior spinocerebellar t.
anterior spinothalamic t.
corticospinal t.
gastrointestinal t.
iliotibial t. (ITT)
lateral corticospinal t.
sinus t.
spinal cord t.
spinocerebellar t.
spinothalamic t.
urinary t.
vestibulospinal t.
traction
ambulatory t.
American Orthopaedic Association halo cervical t.
t. anchor
Anderson t.
AOA halo cervical t.
Apley t.
t. apophysitis
t. application
t. atrophy
autologous t.
axial t.
axis t.
Baker trabecular t.
balanced skeletal t.
balanced suspension t.
banjo t.
t. bar
bidirectional t.
bipolar vertebral t.
Böhler tong t.
Borchgrevink t.
t. bow
t. bow nut
Bremer halo cervical t.
Bryant t.
Buck t.
calcaneal pin t.
Carpal Trac t.
t. cast
cervical AOA halo t.
cervical halter t.
cervical manual t.
C-Flex supine cervical t.
Chattanooga t.
continuous mechanical t.
Cotrel t.

traction (*continued*)
  Crile head t.
  Crutchfield skeletal tong t.
  t. device
  device for transverse t. (DTT)
  Dunlop t.
  Econo-Cerv supine cervical t.
  Econo 90 lumbar home t.
  ElastaTrac lumbar t.
  elastic t.
  t. epiphysis
  Exo-Static t.
  t. exostosis
  external t.
  finger trap t.
  floating t.
  t. footpiece
  t. fracture
  Freiberg t.
  Frejka t.
  Gallo t.
  Gardner-Wells tong t.
  gentle t.
  Georgiade visor cervical t.
  Graham t.
  Granberry t.
  halo cervical t.
  halo-dependent t.
  halo-femoral t.
  halo-pelvic t.
  halo-wheelchair t.
  halter t.
  Hamilton t.
  Hamilton-Russell t.
  t. handle
  Handy-Buck t.
  Hare t.
  head-halter t.
  high-dose t.
  Hoke-Martin t.
  Holter t.
  HomeStretch lumbar t.
  t. hook
  Houston halo cervical t.
  Hoyer t.
  Ingebrightsen t.
  inhibitive t.
  intermittent cervical t.
  internal t.
  isometric t.
  isotonic t.
  Jones suspension t.
  Kessler t.
  King cervical t.
  Kirschner skeletal t.
  Kuhlman t.
  leg t.
  Logan t.
  longitudinal t.

low-dose t.
low-profile halo t.
lumbar t.
lumbosacral t.
Lyman-Smith t.
LymphaPress t.
manual t.
McBride tripod pin t.
metatarsal t.
Miami Acute collar cervical t.
Miami J collar cervical t.
Necktrac t.
Neufeld roller t.
t. neurapraxia
Ortho-Vent t.
overhead olecranon t.
Pease-Thomson t.
pelvic hyperextension t.
Perkins t.
Peterson t.
Philadelphia collar cervical t.
t. pin
3-point skeletal t.
pound of t.
Pronex home t.
Pronex pneumatic cervical t.
Pugh t.
pulp t.
Quantum 400 t.
Quigley t.
Raney-Crutchfield tong t.
t. response
Roger Anderson t.
rubber band t.
Russell skeletal t.
Saunders t.
Sayre suspension t.
sequential pneumatic pump t.
simple shoulder test thermal
 alteration Thomas t.
skeletal t.
skin t.
skull t.
snug t.
t. splint
split Russell skeletal t.
t. spur
static t.
Steinmann t.
t. stirrup
sugar-tong t.
supine C-Trax t.
suspension t.
Syms t.
tape t.
Thomas t.
thoracic manual t.
t. tongs
t. tongs screw

trabecular t.
transverse t.
vertical t.
Vinke tong t.
Watson-Jones t.
weight t.
well-leg t.
Whitman t.
Zimfoam splint t.
tractograph
Tracto-Halter training
tractor
    Hamilton pelvic traction
      screw t.
    Syms t.
    Zim-Trac traction splint t.
tractotomy
TRAFO
    tone-reducing ankle-foot orthosis
Trager method
Tragerwork
trailer
    leaders and t.'s
train
    near-constant frequency t.
trainer
    athletic t.
    Biodex Gait T.
    Biodex target balance t.
    dynamic stabilization t.
    Gator gait t.
    impulse inertial exercise t.
    Kinesthetic Ability T. (KAT)
    Monark Rehab T.
    Posture Pump Spine T.
    Shuttle Balance t.
    Sprint cross t.
training
    activity t. (AT)
    ankle disc t.
    balance board t.
    bowel t.
    daily adjusted progressive resistance
      exercise strength t.
    DAPRE strength t.
    t. diet
    eccentric muscle t.
    endurance t.
    fartlek t.
    flexibility t.
    functional t.
    functional integrated t. (FIT)
    gait t.
    graded exposures t. (GET)
    hypertrophic strength t.
    interval t.
    isometric t.
    isotonic t.
    light intensity t.

neural strength t.
neurodevelopmental t.
periodization of t.
physical t. (PT)
progression of t.
progressive resistance t.
proprioceptive t.
propriosensory t.
prosthetic t.
prosthetic gait t.
relaxation t.
resistance t.
t. room
sensory-motor t.
speed play t.
stabilization t.
strength t.
Tracto-Halter t.
variable resistance t.
weight t.
TRAM
    transverse rectus abdominis
    myocutaneous
    TRAM flap
tramadol
    t. HCl
    t. hydrochloride
trampoline injury
tranexamic acid
trans
    t. fat elaidic acid
    T. Fix ACL fixation device
    t. unsaturated fatty acid
transacromial
    t. approach
    t. coracoacromial ligament
    repair
transaminase
    glutamic-oxaloacetic t.
    glutamic-pyruvic t. (GPT)
transarticular
    t. pin
    t. screw
    t. screw fixation
    t. wire fixation
transaxillary approach
transbone plasty
transbrachioradialis approach
transcalcaneal approach
transcapitate
    t. fracture
    t. fracture-dislocation
transcapitellar
    t. pin
    t. wire fixation
transcarpal amputation
transcervical femoral fracture
transchondral fracture
transclavicular approach

T

transcondylar
- t. amputation
- t. axis (TCA)
- t. fracture

transcortical contrast extravasation
transcranial motor-evoked potential (TcMEP)
transcutaneous
- t. crush injury
- t. electrical nerve stimulation (TENS)
- t. electrical nerve stimulation unit
- t. oxygen
- t. oxygen level
- t. oxygen monitor (TCOM)
- t. oxygen tension determination

transdermal
- Alora T.
- Climara T.
- Duragesic T.
- Esclim T.
- Vivelle T.

transducer
- differential variable reluctance t. (DVRT)
- ergonomically designed t.
- force t.
- FT03C t.
- Hall-effect strain t.
- in-shoe t.
- linear variable differential t.
- magnetic motion t.
- multifrequency t.
- pressure t.
- rotatory-variable-differential t.
- Therasound t.

transection, transsection
- step-cut t.

transepicondylar axis
transepiphysial
- t. fracture
- t. separation

transfemoral
- t. alignment
- t. amputation
- t. amputee
- t. modular prosthesis
- t. suspension

transfer
- t. aid
- anterior t.
- anteromedial tubercle t.
- autogenous osteocartilage t.
- Baker lateral semitendinosus t.
- Barr tibialis posterior t.
- bed-to-chair t.
- biceps brachialis muscle t.
- t. board
- bone t.

Boyes finger tendon t.
brachioradialis t.
Brown fibular t.
Buncke toe to hand t.
Camitz palmaris longus tendon t.
Campbell t.
Chandler tendon t.
Chaves pectoralis major t.
Chaves pectoralis minor muscle t.
Clark pectoralis major t.
Columbus McKinnon assist for lifting or t.
composite free tissue t.
coracoacromial ligament t.
crossed intrinsic t.
Dickson vascularized bone t.
distal t.
double tendon t.
Drennan hip adductor posterior t.
dynamic muscle t.
Eggers biceps femoris tendon t.
epicondylar resection and anconeus muscle t.
extensor digitorum t.
extensor hallucis longus t.
extensor tendon t.
fibular t.
Flatt tendon t.
flexor digitorum longus tendon t.
flexor-to-extensor tendon t.
Fowler tendon t.
free flap t.
free gracilis muscle t.
free tissue t.
free toe t.
Gage distal rectus femoris t.
Ganley extensor hallucis brevis t.
gastrocnemius tendon t.
Girdlestone flexor to extensor tendon t.
Green tendon t.
Haas trapezius muscle t.
T. Handle support handle
Harmon tendon t.
Hiroshima free muscle t.
Hoffer split tendon t.
Huber abductor digiti minimi t.
Ikuta free muscle t.
iliopsoas t.
iliotibial band t.
independent t.
ipsilateral vascularized fibula t. (IVFT)
Kessler tendon t.
Lamb muscle t.
lateral t.
t. lesion
Littler-Cooley abductor digiti minimi t.

Littler-Cooley tendon t.
load t.
magnetization t.
Manktelow pectoralis major
  muscle t.
McLaughlin subscapularis tendon t.
Menelaus triceps t.
t. metatarsalgia
microvascular osseous t.
Moberg deltoid-to-triceps elbow
  reconstruction t.
Moberg free muscle t.
muscle t.
Mustard iliopsoas muscle t.
neuromuscular t.
Ober anterior tendon t.
opponens t.
patellar tendon t. (PTT)
pedicled fibular t.
peroneus brevis t.
posterior deltoid-to-triceps t.
posterior tibial tendon t.
semitendinosus tendon t.
Sever-L'Episcopo tendon t.
Sharrard psoas tendon t.
single-stage tissue t.
SPLATT t.
split anterior tibialis tendon t.
  (SPLATT)
static tendon t.
stress t.
subscapularis tendon t.
Sutherland lateral t.
tendon t.
Thomas-Thompson-Straub external
  oblique t.
thoracodorsal artery t.
Tiobi t.
tissue t.
toe-to-hand t.
total t.
vascularized osseous t.
Vastamäki muscle t.
Whitman muscle t.
wraparound neurovascular composite
  free tissue t.
wraparound toe t.
transfer/augmentation
  FHL tendon t./a.
transfibular
  t. approach
  t. arthrodesis
  t. fusion
transfix
  T. ACL system
  T. ACL system fixation
  T. femoral fixation system
transfixation amputation
transfixing pin

transfixion
  t. bolt
  t. screw
transformation
  fibrous t.
transforming
  t. growth factor (TGF)
  t. growth factor beta (TGF beta)
transfusion
  autologous blood t.
  blood t.
  t. therapy
transglenoid suture repair
transhamate
  t. fracture
  t. fracture-dislocation
transhumeral amputation
transient
  t. bone marrow edema
  t. bone marrow edema syndrome
  bone remodeling t.
  t. clonus
  t. compressive creep
  t. epiphysitis
  t. lesion
  t. neurapraxia
  t. osteopenia
  t. osteoporosis
  t. quadriplegia
  t. synovitis
transiliac
  t. amputation
  t. bar technique
  t. fracture
  t. lengthening
  t. rod fixation
transition
  cervicothoracic t.
transitional vertebra
translaminar
  t. facet screw
  t. facet screw construct
translating and congruent mobile-bearing
knee
translation
  anterior t.
  anterior lumbar t.
  anterior talar t. (ATT)
  anteroposterior t.
  caudal t.
  cephalad t.
  coronal plane deformity sagittal t.
  dorsal t.
  t. injury
  t. mobility
  t. motion
  obligate t.
  posterior t.
  sagittal t.

T

translation (*continued*)
    ulnar t.
    vertebral body t.
    vertical t.
translational
    t. correction
    t. displacement
    t. osteotomy
    t. parameter
    t. position
translatory
    t. force
    t. motion
translocation
    ulnar t.
translumbar amputation
transmalleolar
    t. ankle
    t. ankle arthrodesis
    t. drilling
    t. portal
transmetacarpal amputation
transmetaphysial
    t. amputation
    t. amputation of tibia
transmetatarsal capsulotomy
transmission
    t. electron microscopy
    impulse-based nerve t.
    nerve t.
    nociceptive t.
    nonimpulsed base nerve t.
transmitter
    chest-band t.
transmitter-receiver
    Itrel programmed t.-r.
transolecranon
    anconeus flap t. (AFT)
    t. approach
transoral
    t. atlantoaxial reduction plate
    (TARP)
    t. odontoid resection
transosseous suture
transparent
    t. adhesive dressing
    t. template
transpatellar tendon portal
transpedal
    t. multiplanar wedge fusion
    t. multiplanar wedge osteotomy
transpedicular
    t. approach
    t. fixation
    t. fixation effective pedicle diameter
    t. fixation system design
    t. screw
    t. wedge resection osteotomy
    procedure

transpedicularly implanted anterior spinal support device
transpelvic amputation
transperitoneal
    t. approach
    t. exposure
transphalangeal amputation
transpiral tomography
Transpire wrist orthosis
transplant, transplantation
    allograft t.
    t. antigen
    autogenous cartilage t.
    autologous osteochondral t.
    Bosworth femoroischial t.
    d'Aubigné patellar t.
    Elmslie-Trillat total tendon t.
    femoroischial t.
    fibular t.
    free vascularized bone t.
    meniscal autograft t.
    muscle-tendon t.
    one-half patellar tendon t.
    osteoarticular allograft t.
    patellar t.
    pedicled t.
    pes anserinus t.
    Pierrot and Murphy tendo Achillis insertion t.
    Silfverskiöld heads of origin of gastrocnemius t.
    Slocum pes anserinus t.
    tendon t.
    tissue t.
    toe phalanx t.
    vascularized bone t.
    whole bone t.
    whole fibular t.
transplantation (*var. of* transplant)
transport
    anterograde axoplasmic t.
    axoplasmic t. (AXT)
    bulk flow axoplasmic t.
    fast axoplasmic t.
    slow axoplasmic t.
transposing index ray
transposition
    Dellon ulnar nerve t.
    dorsal subcutaneous nerve t.
    t. flap
    intermuscular neuroma t.
    intramuscular nerve t.
    intraosseous nerve t.
    MacKinnon modification of Dellon ulnar nerve t.
    nerve t.
    plantar t.
    subcutaneous anterior t.
    subfascial t.

tendon t.
ulnar nerve t.
transpositional
transradial prosthesis
transsacral
t. block
t. fracture
transscaphoid
t. dislocation fracture
t. perilunate dislocation
transsection (*var. of* transection)
transsphenoidal dissector
transsternal approach
transsyndesmotic screw fixation
transtendocalcaneus portal
transtentorial brainstem
transthoracic
t. approach
t. lateral view
transtibial
t. amputation
t. immediate postoperative prosthesis
transtriquetral
t. fracture
t. fracture-dislocation
transtrochanteric
t. approach
t. rotational osteotomy
t. valgus osteotomy (TVO)
transversalis fascia
transversarium
foramen t.
transverse
t. abdominis
t. acetabular ligament
t. amputation
t. approach
t. arch stress
t. atlantal ligament
t. axis
t. axis knee flexion
t. capsulotomy
t. carpal ligament (TCL)
t. chevron osteotomy
t. connector
t. deficiency
t. diaphysial osteotomy
t. disc
t. divergent dislocation of elbow
t. fixation
t. fixator application
t. friction massage (TFM)
t. friction therapy
t. humeral ligament test
t. incision
t. intertarsal ligament
t. ligament of knee
t. ligament rupture

t. line of Park
t. loading device
t. metatarsal ligament
t. metatarsal osteotomy
t. myelopathy
t. pedicle angle
t. pedicle diameter
t. plane
t. plane alignment
t. plane motion insufficiency
t. process
t. process fracture
t. process of sacrum
t. process of vertebra
t. rectus abdominis muscle flap
t. rectus abdominis myocutaneous (TRAM)
t. retinacular ligament
t. scapular ligament
t. screw
t. spinal ligament
t. supracondylar osteotomy
t. tarsal articulation
t. tarsal joint
t. tear
t. tenotomy
t. tibiofibular ligament
t. traction
transversectomy
transversely
transversoplanus
talipes t.
transversospinalis syndrome
transversum
Caput t.
transversus abdominis muscle
Tranxene
TRAP
tartrate resistant acid phosphatase
trap
finger t.
T. test
trapdoor
trapeze bar
trapezial
t. area
t. arthrosis
t. prosthesis
t. ridge
trapezia, trapeziums
trapeziectomy
trapeziodeltoid interval
trapeziometacarpal
t. capsule
t. fusion
t. joint
t. joint replacement prosthesis
trapeziotrapezoidal joint

trapezium, *pl.* **trapezia, trapeziums**
    t. bone
    Burton-Pellegrini excision
      of t.
    t. fracture
    t. implant prosthesis
    t. ossification
trapeziums
trapezius
    t. fiber analysis
    t. muscle
    t. myofascial pain syndrome
trapezoid
    t. bone
    t. bone of Henle
    t. bone of Lyser
    t. ligament
    t. line
    t. ossification
trapezoidal
    t. imaging
    t. resection osteotomy
Trapezoidal-28
    Trapezoidal-28 hip prosthesis
    Trapezoidal-28 internal
      prosthesis
trapped meniscus
trapper
    FoamWrap finger t.
trapping
    Coonrad-Bugg posterior tibial
      tendon t.
    optical t.
    tendon t.
trauma, *pl.* **traumata, traumas**
    arterial t.
    awakening t.
    birth t.
    cervical spine t.
    craniospinal t.
    geriatric t.
    high-energy t.
    hyperextension t.
    hyperflexion t.
    lumbar spine t.
    multiple t.'s
    musculoskeletal t.
    nonosseous tissue t.
    nonunion fracture t.
    repetitive t.
    t. score
    skin t.
    thoracolumbar t.
    t. view
    whiplash t.
trauma-induced membrane
TraumaJet wound debridement
 system
traumas (*pl. of* trauma)

traumata (*pl. of* trauma)
traumatic
    t. abscess
    t. amputation
    t. anterior instability
    t. anterior shoulder instability
    t. arthritis
    t. bone cyst
    t. brain injury (TBI)
    t. brain injury-related ataxia
    t. brain injury-related neglect
    t. burn injury
    t. cervical disc herniation
    t. cervical discopathy
    t. compartment syndrome
    t. dislocation
    t. displacement
    t. heel wound
    t. hemarthrosis
    t. hemiplegia
    t. neuroma
    t. osteoarthritis
    t. paraplegia
    t. prepatellar neuralgia
    t. sinus
    t. spondylolisthesis
    t. synovitis
    t. tetraplegia
    t. unidirectional Bankart lesion
      surgery
    t. unidirectional instability and
      Bankart lesion
traumatized ligament
traumatologist
Traumeel
Travase ointment
traverse amputation
TraXis
    T. Ti alloy spacer
    T. Vue alloy spacer
tray
    Alcon Instrument Delivery
      System t.
    Bucky x-ray t.
    Denis Browne t.
    glenoid metal t.
    PFC offset tibial t.
    surgical hand t.
    tibial t.
    1-time sharp débridement t.
    x-ray t.
trazodone
treadmill
    Aquaciser underwater t.
    AquaGaiter t.
    Cateye T220 t.
    Lifestride t.
    Orbiter t.
    t. running

t. test
Trackmaster t.
Woodway t.
treatment
acid t.
active t.
adjustive t.
bipartite patella operative t.
bone cyst t.
Boyd-Ingram-Bourkhard t.
Carrel t.
Chapman point t.
closed t.
cold laser t.
compression rod t.
CyberKnife t.
distraction-compression scoliosis t.
dual compression scoliosis t.
intradiscal electrothermal t. (IDET)
IonGuard orthopaedic surface t.
Kenny t.
low-friction ion t. (LFIT)
manual t.
McKenzie back and neck pain t.
microendoscopic surgical t.
neurodevelopmental t. (NDT)
neuromuscular reflex t.
neuromuscular scoliosis orthotic t.
nonoperative t.
osteopathic manipulative t.
Parabath paraffin heat t.
paraffin t.
poliomyelitis t.
rehabilitation t.
ReJuveness scar t.
Rolfing t.
Sakellarides calcaneal fracture t.
shock t.
spasticity t.
surgical t.
ulcer t.
viscosupplementation t.
Tredex
Universal T.
tree
BTE Assembly T.
Finger Blocking T.
pinch t.
pipe t.
trellis formation
tremor
action t.
contraction t.
essential t.
intention t.
pill rolling t.
postural t.
resting t.
tremulor

tremulousness
trench foot
Trendelenburg
T. dislocated hip test
T. gait
T. gluteus medius weakness test
T. leg vein valve test
T. limp
T. lurch
T. pelvis sign
T. position
Trental
trepan (*var. of* trephine)
trephine, trepan
t. autologous bone harvesting system
bone t.
Castroviejo t.
t. drill
hollow bone t.
Michele vertebral t.
t. needle biopsy
Phemister biopsy t.
trepidans
abasia t.
Trevor disease
Trevor-Fairbank disease
TRH
thyrotropin-releasing hormone
Triacet
triacetin
triad
Charcot t.
female athlete t. (FAT)
t. knee repair
t. of O'Donoghue
T. prosthesis
Virchow t.
Waddell t.
triage
sidelines t.
trial
t. acetabular cup
t. base plate
clinical t.
component t.
t. driver
t. femoral component
t. fit
Fracture Intervention T. (FIT)
t. implant
lower hook t.
t. of conservative therapy
t. prosthesis
radial t.
t. range of motion
t. reduction
t. seating
t. spacer

trial (*continued*)
 t. stem
 ulnar t.
 upper hook t.
trialkylphosphine gold complex
Triam-A
triamcinolone
 t. acetate
 t. acetonide
Triam Forte
triamterene/hydrochlorothiazide
triangle
 Achilles t.
 Alsberg t.
 anal t.
 anterior t.
 aponeurotic t.
 t. blade system
 Bryant iliofemoral t.
 Burow t.
 cervical t.
 clavipectoral t.
 Codman tumor-normal bone t.
 iliofemoral t.
 IMP knee positioning t.
 infraclavicular t.
 Innovative Medical Products knee
  positioning t.
 intern's t.
 Kager Achilles tendon t.
 Kanavel palm t.
 knee positioning t.
 Langenbeck hip joint t.
 metal measuring t.
 Middeldorpf splint t.
 neutral t.
 Petit inferior lumbar t.
 posterior t.
 sacral t.
 urogenital t.
 Volkmann posterolateral corner of
  tibia t.
 von Weber t.
Tri-Angle shoulder abduction brace
triangular
 t. advancement flap
 t. ankle fusion frame
 t. arm sling
 t. bandage
 t. base transverse bar configuration
 t. bone reamer
 t. compression device
 t. defect
 t. disc of wrist
 t. external ankle fixation
 t. fibrocartilage (TFC)
 t. fibrocartilage complex
 t. fibrocartilage complex stability
  test

 t. fibrocartilage tear
 t. fibrocartilage tear syndrome
 t. ligament
 t. medullary nail
 t. muscle
 t. pillow splint
 t. rasp
 t. working zone
 t. wrist bone
triangulated pedicle screw
triangulate triple frame
triangulating
triangulation
 indirect t.
 t. technique
 t. technique for arthroscope
Triathlon knee system
triaxial
 t. motion
 T. prosthesis
 t. semiconstrained elbow prosthesis
 t. total elbow arthroplasty
Triax monotube external fixation system
triazolam
tribology
tricalcium phosphate
tricepses, *pl.* **triceps, tricepses**
 t. brachii muscle
 t. brachii tendon
 t. jerk
 t. jerk reflex test
 t. skinfold test
 t. surae jerk
 t. surae muscle
 t. surae reflex
 t. surae release
 t. tendinitis
triceps (*pl. of* triceps)
tricepsplasty
triceps-splitting approach
trichloromonofluoromethane
 dichlorodifluoromethane and t.
Trichophyton
 T. mentagrophytes
 T. rubrum
trichterbrust
tricipital muscle
trick
 t. knee
 t. movement
Tricodur
 T. compression support bandage
 T. Epi compression bandage
 T. Epi compression dressing
 T. Omos compression bandage
 T. Omos compression dressing
 T. Omos elastic bandage
 T. Talus compression bandage
 T. Talus compression dressing

tricompartmental
    t. implant
    t. knee prosthesis
    t. replacement
Tricon component
Tricon-M
    T.-M component
    T.-M cruciate-sparing prosthesis
    T.-M patellar prosthesis
Tricore cervical support pillow
tricorrectional bunionectomy
tricortical
    t. iliac crest bone graft
    t. ilial strip graft
tricyclic antidepressant (TCA, TCAD)
trident hand
triethanolamine salicylate
triethiodide
    gallamine t.
triflanged
    t. Lottes nail
    t. medullary nail
Tri-Flex auxiliary suspension belt
Tri-Float pressure reduction mattress
trifluoperazine
trifurcation
trigeminal neuralgia (TGN)
Trigen
    T. femoral antegrade nailing
    T. Intertan femoral fracture nail
    T. Meta-Nail tibial nail system
    T. Peri-Loc periarticular locked plating device
    T. TAN antegrade femoral nail
    T. third generation knee nail
trigger
    t. digit
    t. finger
    t. finger release
    t. finger syndrome
    t. point (TrP)
    t. point injection
    t. point therapy (TPT)
    t. thumb
    t. thumb release
TriggerWheel
    T. muscle therapy device
    T. Wand
trigonum
Trilafon
trilaminate cushion
trilateral knee-ankle-foot orthosis
trileaflet prosthesis
Trilisate
Trillat
    T. osteotomy
    T. shoulder bone block procedure
    T. total knee arthroplasty

Tri-Lock
    T.-L. bone preservation stem hip prosthesis
    T.-L. press-fit prosthesis
    T.-L. total hip prosthesis with Porocoat
trilogy
    T. AB acetabular prosthesis
    T. acetabular cup system
    T. prosthesis
Trilon multilayered material
trimalleolar
    t. ankle fracture
    t. fracture
Trimed system for fracture of distal radius
Trimedyne Omnipulse holmium laser
trimethoprim sulfamethoxazole
trimipramine
Trim-It
    T.-I. drill pin
    T.-I. screw system
    T.-I. Spin Pin
Trimline knee immobilizer
trimmer
    motorized t.
Tri-Motion Knee System
Trinion meniscus screw
Trinity multipotential cellular bone matrix
Trinkle
    T. bone drill
    T. brace
    T. brace and adapter
    T. chuck adapter
    T. power drill
    T. screwdriver
    T. Super-Cut twist drill
trio
    T. arthroscope
    T. medialized rod system
triode
Trio-Stim neuromuscular stimulator
tri-panel knee immobilizer
tripartite
    t. bone
    t. muscle origin
triphalangeal
    t. thumb
    t. thumb deformity
triphase technetium scintigraphy
triphasic action potential
Tripier foot amputation
triplanar
    t. protractor
    t. protractor apparatus
triplane
    t. construct

T

triplane (*continued*)
    t. motion
    t. osteotomy
    t. stretch
    t. tibial fracture
triple
    T. Antibiotic Topical
    t. arthrodesis
    t. bundle technique
    t. discharge
    t. envelope system
    t. frame
    t. hemisection
    t. innominate osteotomy
    t. ligamentous repair
    t. reamer
    t. tarsal fusion
    t. tenodesis
triple-frequency probe
triplegia
triple-injection cinearthrography
triple-jump test
triple-phase isotope bone scan
triple-wire
    t.-w. fusion
    t.-w. procedure
    t.-w. technique
triploscope
tripod
    t. cane
    t. foot
    t. hip tightness test
    McBride t.
    t. sign
tripoding gait
Trippi-Wells extraction fixation traction tongs
tripsis
triquetral fracture
triquetrolunate
    t. dislocation
    t. instability
triquetrum
    t. bone
    t. ossification
triquetrum-lunate arthrodesis
triradial, triradiate
    t. acetabular extensile approach
    t. cartilage
    t. incision
    t. resector blade
    t. transtrochanteric approach
triradiate (*var. of* triradial)
trisalicylate
    choline magnesium t.
triscaphe
    t. arthrodesis
    t. fusion
    t. joint

trismus
trispiked
trispiral tomography
TriStander
Tristoject
Tritin
triton tumor
trivector retaining approach
Tri-Wedge total hip system
Tri W-G table
TRK
    total rotating knee
trocar
    blunt t.
    sharp t.
    T-handled t.
trochanter
    greater t.
    t. holder
    lesser t.
trochanter-holding clamp
trochanterian (*var. of* trochanteric)
trochanteric, trochanterian
    t. advancement
    t. band
    t. bolt
    t. bursa
    t. bursitis
    t. migration
    t. osteotomy
    t. pin
    t. reamer
    t. shift
    t. slide
    t. spine
    t. syndrome
    t. wire
trochanter-knee-ankle (TKA)
trochanterplasty
trochlea peronealis
trochlear
    t. defect
    t. groove
    t. notch
trochoid
    t. articulation
    t. joint
troika
    aponeurotic t.
trolley
    Bolero lift bath t.
    t. track sign
    Tupper t.
TROM
    total range of motion
    TROM knee brace
tromethamine
    ketorolac t.

Trömner
- T. corticospinal pathways disease test
- T. digital reflex test
- T. percussion hammer

Tronzo
- T. elevator
- T. intertrochanteric fracture classification (1-3)
- T. total hip prosthesis

trophic
- t. change
- t. fracture
- t. joint disorder
- t. ulcer
- t. ulceration

trophoneurosis
- muscular t.

tropism
- facet t.
- negative t.
- positive t.

tropocollagen
tropometer
trough
- bone t.
- t. line
- t. line sign

trousers
- military antishock t. (MAST)

Trousseau spinous process point
Trowbridge
- T. Terra-Round accessory foot
- T. Terra-Round sports limb
- T. T5 Terra-Round

TrP
- trigger point

true
- t. acetabular region
- t. acetabulum
- t. ankylosis
- T. Blue exercise band
- t. lateral view
- t. leg-length discrepancy test
- t. metatarsus adductus
- t. rib
- t. spacer
- t. vertebra

True/Fit femoral intramedullary rod system
True/LOK
- T. external fixation system
- T. external fixator

TruePoint PET-CT technology
Tru-Fit
- T.-F. brace
- T.-F. custom-molded shoe

Trumble
- T. hip arthrodesis
- T. talectomy

Trümmerfeld
- T. scurvy line
- T. zone

Tru-Mold shoe
truncal dysmetria
truncated
- t. tarsometatarsal wedge arthrodesis
- t. wedge tarsometatarsal arthrodesis

trunk
- anatomic nerve t.
- t. control
- t. curl
- t. incurvation test
- t. loading
- t. righting
- t. shift
- t. stabilization rehabilitation program
- sympathetic t.

Trunkey pelvic fracture classification (I-III)
trunk-hip-knee-ankle-foot orthosis (THKAFO)
trunnion-bearing hip prosthesis
TruStep foot prosthesis
Tru-Support
- T.-S. EW bandage
- T.-S. SA bandage

Truswell-Hansen disease
TruWedge
- T. BGS osteotomy wedge
- T. bone graft substitute osteotomy wedge

Trypanosoma gambiense
trypsin, balsam peru, and castor oil
TSA
- total shoulder arthroplasty

Tsai-Stillwell distal radioulnar joint repair procedure
Tscherne
- T. closed femur fracture (0-III)
- T. soft tissue injury in closed fracture classification

T-score of bone mineral density
T-shaped
- T-s. AO plate
- T-s. capsulotomy
- T-s. fracture
- T-s. incision
- T-s. inserter

TSP
- tibial sesamoid position

T-spine
- thoracic spine

TSRH
- Texas Scottish Rite Hospital
- TSRH buttressed laminar hook

T

TSRH (*continued*)
    TSRH circular laminar hook
    TSRH corkscrew device
    TSRH crosslink
    TSRH crosslink stabilization
    TSRH crosslink system
    TSRH double-rod construct
    TSRH eyebolt spreader
    TSRH fixation system
    TSRH hook holder
    TSRH hook inserter
    TSRH hook-rod
    TSRH implant
    TSRH instrumentation
    TSRH L-bolt
    TSRH mini-corkscrew device
    TSRH pedicle hook
    TSRH pedicle screw
    TSRH pedicle screw-laminar claw
      construct
    TSRH plate
    TSRH rod fixation
    TSRH spinal implant system
    TSRH trial hook
    TSRH universal spinal
      instrumentation system
    TSRH wrench
T-Stat Topical
T-Stick adhesive
T-strap
    medial T-s.
Tsuge
    T. macrodactyly debulking
    T. tendon repair
Tsuji laminaplasty
T1-T12
    thoracic vertebrae 1-12
TTA
    tissue texture abnormality
TTAP
    threaded titanium acetabular
      prosthesis
    threaded titanium alloy prosthesis
TTAP-ST
    threaded titanium alloy prosthesis
      smooth threaded
      TTAP-STacetabular cup
T4-T8 kyphosis
TT Pylon prosthesis
TTR
    tarsal tunnel release
TTS
    tarsal tunnel syndrome
TTT
    tibial talar tilt
    tibiotalar tilt
    total tourniquet time
tube, tubing
    Adson suction t.

    Baron suction t.
    chest t. (CT)
    Chinese fingertrap t.
    Dawson-Yuhl suction t.
    digit t.
    Dynamic digit extensor t.
    endoneural t.
    Esmarch t.
    Exerband Pak bilateral t.
    Exerband Pak unilateral t.
    Ferguson-Frazier suction t.
    finger trap t.
    t. flap graft
    t. foam
    Gillquist suction t.
    t. guide
    Hemovac suction t.
    irrigation t.
    Jergesen t.
    stockinette t.
    suction t.
    tracheotomy t.
    vent t.
TubeGauz bandage
tuber angle
tubercle
    adductor t.
    anterior tibial t.
    articular bone t.
    t. avulsion
    Chaput tibial t.
    Chassaignac 6th cervical vertebra t.
    conoid t.
    Gerdy tibial t.
    lateral tibial t.
    Lisfranc scalene t.
    Lister dorsal radius t.
    medial calcaneal t.
    t. osteotomy
    talus lateral t.
    tibial t.
    Tillaux-Chaput tibial t.
    Wagstaff malleolar t.
tubercula (*pl. of* tuberculum)
tubercular granuloma
tuberculoma
    bone t.
tuberculosis (TB)
    diaphysial t.
    extraarticular t.
    metaphysial t.
    Mycobacterium t.
    t. of hip
    osteoarticular t.
    skeletal t.
    spinal t.
tuberculous
    t. arthritis
    t. dactylitis

t. lesion
t. peroneal tenosynovitis
t. rheumatism
t. sequestrum
t. spinal osteomyelitis
t. spondylitis
t. synovitis
t. trochanteric bursitis
t. vertebral osteomyelitis
tuberculum, *pl.* **tubercula**
t. arthriticum
t. conoideum
tuber-joint angle
tuberosity
adductor t.
t. avulsion fracture
bicipital t.
calcaneal t.
coracoid t.
cuboidal t.
distal t.
femoral t.
t. fragment
greater t.
iliac t.
infraglenoid t.
ischial t. (IT)
t. joint angle
lateral t.
lesser t.
navicular t.
t. of calcaneus
t. of carpal bone
t. of clavicle
t. of cuboid bone
parietal t.
patellar t.
posterior t.
radial t.
sacral t.
supraglenoid t.
tibial t.
ulnar t.
ungual t.
ununited tibial t.
tuberous
t. sclerosis
t. xanthoma
Tubex gauze dressing
Tubigrip
T. bandage
T. dressing
T. glove
tubing (*var. of* tube)
Dakin t.
elastic t.
Exerband t.
Fit-Lastic therapy t.
foam t.

gel t.
medullary vent t.
PVC t.
Silipos mesh t.
Thera-Band t.
Tubsider Kneeling Seat
tubular
t. bone plate
t. elastic bandage
t. punch
t. retractor
t. stockinette
tubularization of graft
tubulization of nerve
tucker
tendon t.
tuck sign
Tudor-Edwards bone-cutting forceps
Tuf Nex neck exerciser
Tuf-Skin tape adherent
TufStuf II cast tape
tuft
distal t.
finger t.
t. fracture
tuftal resorption
tufted phalanx
Tuinal
Tuke saw
Tuli
T. Pro heel cup
T. rubber heel cup
TuliGel heel cup
tulip pedicle screw
Tullos technique
tumble
T. Forms feeder
T. Forms roll
T. Forms Vestibulator
tumbler graft
tumbling bullet sign
tumefaction
tumefactive synovial osteochondromatosis
tumor, tumour
Abrikossoff t.
aggressive t.
ball-valve t.
benign t.
blood vessel t.
bone-forming t.
bone marrow t.
brown-fat t.
calcaneal t.
calcaneal t.
cartilaginous t.
cerebellopontine angle t.
Codman bone t.
cortical desmoid t.
cystic t.

T

tumor (*continued*)
 desmoid t.
 dumbbell t.
 Enneking staging (IA, IB, IIA, IIB, III) of malignant bone and soft tissue t.'s
 epidermal cell t.
 epiphysial chondromatous giant cell t.
 Ewing family of t.'s
 extraabdominal desmoid t.
 fatty tissue t.
 fibroblastic t.
 fibroid t.
 fibrous t.
 giant cell t. (GCT)
 glomus t.
 Gubler wrist t.
 histiocytic t.
 hyperparathyroidism t.
 intraosseous t.
 lipid t.
 lumbar t.
 malignant soft tissue t.
 mesenchymal t.
 metastatic spinal t.
 nerve sheath t.
 neural t.
 neuroectodermal t.
 occult primary malignant t.
 paraspinous t.
 plexiform fibrohistiocytic t.
 pluripotential mesenchymal t.
 posterolateral decompression for spine t.
 Pott puffy t.
 primary t.
 t. resection
 Schwann t.
 soft tissue t.
 spinal t.
 superior sulcus t.
 synovial t.
 tenosynovial giant cell t.
 t. therapy
 triton t.
 vascular t.
 vertebral body t.
 t. vessel
 xanthomatous giant cell t.
tumoral calcinosis
tumor-bearing bone
tumor-grasping forceps
tumorous
 t. condition
 t. involvement
 t. mass

tumor-replacement endoprosthesis
tumour (*var. of* tumor)
Tums
 T. E-X Extra Strength Tablet
 T. Extra Strength Liquid
tunnel
 bone t.
 bottleneck femoral t.
 carpal t. (CT)
 cubital t.
 t. drill guide
 femoral t.
 femoral drill t.
 fibroosseous t.
 t. locator guide
 t. of Guyon syndrome
 osseous t.
 peroneal t.
 radial t.
 release of fibroosseous t.
 subsartorial t.
 talar neck t.
 tarsal t.
 tibial t.
 ulnar t.
 t. view
tunnel-and-sling fixation
tunneler
 tendon t.
TunneLoc bone mulch screw
Tunturi hand exerciser
Tuohy lumbar puncture needle
Tupman femur fracture plate
Tupper
 T. hand-holder and retractor
 T. palmar plate interposition arthroplasty
 T. trolley
turbinated bone
Turco
 T. clubfoot posteromedial release
 T. clubfoot release
 T. clubfoot release technique
 T. oblique posteromedial incision
 T. repair of talipes equinovarus
turf
 t. toe (I-III)
 t. toe injury
turgor
Turkel bone marrow biopsy
TurnAide therapeutic system
turnbuckle
 t. ankle brace
 t. cast
 t. distractor
 t. elbow splint
 t. jack
 t. knee brace
 t. wrist orthosis

turn-down tendon flap
Turn-Easy transfer aid
turned-up pulp deformity
turner
    T. pin
    T. prosthesis
    rotating t.
    T. syndrome
Turning Board Exercise System
turn out
turnover
    bone t.
turnstile casting stand (TCS)
turret exostosis
turtle neck nail
Turvy internal screw fixation
Turyn back pain sign
Tutofix cortical pin
Tutoplast process
Tuxedo collar
TVMS
    Test of Visual-Motor Skills
TVMS:UL
    Test of Visual-Motor Skills: Upper
    Level Adolescents and Adults
TVO
    transtrochanteric valgus osteotomy
TVPS
    Test of Visual-Perception Skills
TVPS:UL
    Test of Visual-Perceptual Skills: Upper
    Level Adolescents and Adults
TWA
    total wrist arthroplasty
tweezers
    Kaprelian easy-access t.
    (KEAT)
T2-weighted dual-echo sequence
twelfth rib syndrome
Twilite Oral
twin-blade oscillating saw
Twin Cities Lo-Profile halo

twins
    craniopagus t.
twist
    t. drill
    t. drill point
    t. hook
    t. maneuver
twisted plate
twister
    Axel wire t.
    Batzdorf cervical wire t.
    t. cable
    cerclage wire t.
    Cooley-Baumgarten wire t.
    DMP wire t.
    Miltex wire t.
    orthotic coiled spring t.
    Shifrin wire t.
    wire t.
Twist-Off Screw
twitch muscle
Tworek screw guide
TX-1–TX-15 traction table
Tycron suture
tying forceps
Tylenol
    T. Extended Relief
    T. With Codeine
Tylok high-tension cable system
tyloma
Tylox
tympanic bone
type
    contraction t.
    epidermolysis bullosa dermal t.
    epidermolysis bullosa epidermal t.
    epidermolysis bullosa junctional t.
    foot t.
    frequency, intensity, time, t. (FITT)
    rectus foot t.
    sleeve t.
typhoid osteomyelitis

T

U
   upper
      U Luque vertebral rod
      U osteotomy
      U wrench
UBC
   University of British Columbia
      UBC brace
      UBC orthosis
UBE
   uniaxial balance evaluation
   upper body ergometer
UBIS
   ultrasound bone imaging system
      UBIS 5000 quantitative ultrasound
      bone sonometer
      UBIS 5000 ultrasound bone
      sonometer
UBP
   universal bone plate
      UBP system
UCB
   University of California Berkeley
      UCB foot orthosis
      UCB shoe insert
UCBL
   University of California Berkeley
   Laboratory
      UCBL foot plate
      UCBL orthosis
UCI
   University of California Irvine
      UCI ankle prosthesis
      UCI unconstrained prosthesis
UCL
   ulnar collateral ligament
UCLA
   University of California Los
   Angeles
      UCLA anatomic shoulder
      arthroplasty
      UCLA functional long leg brace
      UCLA Shoulder Rating scale
UCLC
   ulnar collateral ligament complex
UCOheal orthotic
UCOlite orthosis
UCR
   University of California Riverside
      UCR thoracolumbar fusion posterior
      fixation pedicle screw
UDV
   under direct vision
UE
   upper extremity

Ueba release
UEFI
   upper extremity functional index
Uematsu shoulder arthrodesis
U/F
   Fulvicin U/F
UFO
   Universal plantar fasciitis orthosis
   Universal Plantar Fasciitis Orthotic
      Orthomerica UFO
UFOS
   universal frame outer socket
UHMWPE
   ultrahigh molecular weight polyethylene
      UHMWPE prosthesis
UHR
   universal head replacement
      UHR locking ring mechanism
Uhthoff
      U. multiple sclerosis sign
      U. syndrome
UID
   unilateral interfacetal dislocation
UKA
   unicompartmental knee
   arthroplasty
ulcer
      decubitus u.
      diabetic neurotrophic u.
      diabetic plantar hallux u.
      u. dressing
      high-grade u.
      ischemic u.
      low-grade u.
      mal perforans u.
      moderate-grade u.
      neuropathic u.
      neurotrophic food u.
      peptic u.
      plantar u.
      pressure u. (grade I-IV)
      recalcitrant neuropathic u.
      stasis u.
      supramalleolar venous u.
      target u.
      u. treatment
      trophic u.
ulceration
      neuropathic forefoot u.
      neurotrophic u.
      pinpoint u.
      sublesional u.
      trophic u.
ulcerative mutilating acropathy
Ullmann spondylolisthesis line

U

Ullrich
U. drill
U. drill guard
ulna, *gen.* and *pl.* **ulnae**
absent u.
u. bone
distal u.
femur, fibula, u. (FFU)
Milch cuff resection of u.
Monteggia fracture-dislocation
of u.
proximal u.
proximal third of radius and u.
synostosis between radius
and u.
ulnae (*gen.* and *pl. of* ulna)
ulnar
u. anlage
u. antebrachial region
u. artery
u. artery injury
u. bearing
u. brace
u. bursa
u. carpal collateral ligament
u. clubhand
u. collateral ligament (UCL)
u. collateral ligament complex
(UCLC)
u. collateral ligament injury
u. collateral ligament rupture
u. collateral nerve of Krause
u. collateral test
u. column
u. convexity
u. creaking
u. cubital tunnel syndrome
u. deviation
u. deviation deformity
u. dimelia
u. drift
u. drift deformity
u. extensor
u. grind test
u. gutter splint
u. head
u. head excision
u. head implant prosthesis
u. hemiresection interposition
arthroplasty
u. impaction syndrome
u. lengthening
u. malleolus
midcarpal u. (MCU)
u. minus variance
u. motor neurectomy
u. nerve (UN)
u. nerve block
u. nerve entrapment

u. nerve injury
u. nerve motor/sensory
electromyogram
u. nerve palsy
u. nerve paralysis
u. nerve release
u. nerve transposition
u. nerve transposition surgery
u. neuropathy
u. notch
u. rasp
u. recession
u. reflex
u. ruler
u. sesamoid bone
u. side grip
u. styloid bone
u. styloid fracture
u. styloid impaction syndrome
u. synovial recess
u. translation
u. translocation
u. trial
u. tuberosity
u. tunnel
u. tunnel syndrome
u. wrist extensor tendinitis
ulnaris
extensor carpi u. (ECU)
flexor carpi u. (FCU)
malleolus u.
ulnarward
ulnocarpal
u. abutment
u. abutment syndrome
u. arthrodesis
u. impaction syndrome
u. impingement
u. joint
u. ligament
ulnohumeral
u. angle
u. joint
ulnolunate
u. abutment syndrome
u. articulation
u. ligament
ulnomeniscotriquetral joint
ulnotriquetral ligament
ulnotriquetrum articulation
ULNT
upper limb neurodynamic test
ULO
upper limb orthosis
ULP
upper limb prosthesis
Ulrich
U. bone-holding clamp
U. bone-holding forceps

Ulrich-St. Gallen forceps
Ulson fixator system
Ultec thin dressing
Ultima
    U. calcar stems
    U. C femoral component
    U. Fx stems
    U. hip replacement system
    U. total hip system
ultimate
    U. Cold N' Hot Pack
    U. Hand Helper strengthening
      program
    U. knee prosthesis
    u. strength
**Ultimax distal femoral intramedullary
rod system**
Ultiva
ultra
    Grisactin U.
    U. Mide 25 lotion
    U. Stim silver electrode
Ultrabrace
    U. brace
    U. knee orthosis
Ultra-Cut instrument
Ultra-Drive
    U.-D. bone cement removal
      system
    U.-D. plug puller
    U.-D. ultrasonic revision system
ultraendurance
UltraFix
    U. MicroMite anchor suture
    U. MicroMite suture anchor
    U. RC implant
    U. RC suture anchor
    U. RC suture anchor system
    U. rotator cuff repair implant
Ultraflex
    U. dynamic joint
    U. orthopaedic bed
Ultra-Guard
    U.-G. FS hip bracing system
    U.-G. hip orthosis system
**ultrahigh molecular weight polyethylene
(UHMWPE)**
Ultra-Light athletic tape
Ultram
UltraPower drill system
Ultraprin
UltraSling
ultrasonic
    u. aspirator
    u. mobility aid
    u. probe
ultrasonography
    compression u.
    duplex Doppler u.

ultrasonometer
    QUS-2 calcaneal u.
UltraSorb suture anchor
ultrasound
    Amrex therapeutic u.
    u. bone imaging system
      (UBIS)
    compression u.
    Doppler u.
    duplex u.
    u. electrotherapy
    Exogen 2000+ noninvasive u.
    Mysono 201 portable u.
    u. phonophoresis
    pulsed u.
    quantitative u. (QUS)
    therapeutic u.
    u. therapy
ultrasound-guided
    u.-g. echo biopsy
    u.-g. stereotactic biopsy
ultrasound/stimulator
    SynchroSonic U/HVG50 u.
UltraStep orthotic
ultraviolet (UV)
    u. light
Ultra-X external fixation system
ULTT
    upper limb tension test
Umbau zone
umbilical tape
UMS
    upper fossa active, medial knee pain,
    and short leg on side ipsilateral to
    weak fossa
UN
    ulnar nerve
unassisted locking-suture technique
Unasyn
unbalanced
    u. depolymerization
    u. hemivertebra
    u. wrist syndrome
uncemented femoral component
unciform
    u. bone
    u. fracture
    u. process
uncinate
    u. bone
    u. hypertrophy
    u. process fracture
uncommitted metaphysial lesion
uncompensated rotary scoliosis
unconditional stimulus
unconstrained
    u. shoulder arthroplasty
    u. tricompartmental knee prosthesis
uncoordinated gait

U

uncovertebral
    u. arthrosis
    u. joint
    u. spur
undecylenic acid
underarm
    u. body jacket
    u. brace
    u. cast
    u. orthosis
under direct vision (UDV)
undergrowth
underlapping toe
undermined skin
underscoring
undersurface of patella
underwater Bovie
underwear
    HipSaver protective u.
undetermined
    etiology u.
undifferentiated oligoarthritis
undisplaced fracture
undyed suture
ungual
    u. process
    u. tuberosity
unguarded osteotome
unguis
    u. aduncus
    u. incarnatus
unhappy triad of O'Donoghue
uniarticular
uniaxial
    u. balance evaluation (UBE)
    u. joint
    u. strain gauge
    u. structure
unicameral bone cyst
Uni-Clip staple
unicompartmental
    u. knee arthroplasty (UKA)
    u. knee implant
    u. knee prosthesis
    u. knee replacement
    u. knee system
unicondylar
    u. fracture
    U. Geomedic hemi-knee system
    u. prosthesis
unicortical screw
Uniflex
    U. calibrated step drill
    U. dressing
    U. drill bushing
    U. humeral nail
    U. intramedullary nail
    U. nailing system
Unigraft bone graft material

Unilab
    U. Surgibone
    U. Surgibone bone replacement
    material
    U. Surgibone surgical implant
unilateral
    u. acute radicular syndrome
    u. calcaneal brace
    u. chronic radicular syndrome
    u. facet subluxation
    u. interfacetal dislocation (UID)
    u. interfacetal subluxation
    u. pedicle cannulation
    u. posterior-anterior movement
    u. sacroiliac approach
    u. spastic leg
    u. standing test
    u. variable screw placement
    system
unilaterally upgoing toe
Unilink system for hand surgery
unilocular joint
uninhibited
    u. ankle motion
    u. flexion
union
    bony u.
    u. broach retention drill
    u. broach retention pin
    callous bone u.
    delayed fracture u.
    European Chiropractic U.
    faulty u.
    fibrous u.
    osteonal bone u.
    Osteotron stimulator for
    bone u.
    primary bone u.
    secondary bone u.
    slow u.
    vicious u.
Uni-Patch electrode gel
Unipen
    U. Injection
    U. Oral
unipennate muscle
Uniplane rocker
unipolar
    u. bearing
    u. cauterization
    u. cautery
    u. needle electrode
    u. release
uniportal
    u. arthroscopic microdiskectomy
    U. fascial release system
    u. plantar fasciotomy
unisegmental mobility
UniSyn modular hip system

unit

> AME microcurrent TENS u.
> Austin Medical Equipment microcurrent TENS u.
> Autoflex II, III CPM u.
> Back Bubble gravity traction u.
> Back Revolution traction/exercise u.
> basic multicellular remodeling u.
> BioMed TENS u.
> bone metabolic u.
> bone remodeling u.
> Bovie coagulating u.
> C-arm fluoroscopy u.
> Cybex Torso Rotation Testing and Rehabilitation U.
> Cybex Trunk Extension Flexion u.
> Dynasplint knee extension u.
> Eclipse TENS u.
> Econo 90 traction u.
> E-2 hydrocollator heating u.
> ElastaTrac home lumbar traction u.
> electromyography retrainer biofeedback u.
> EMG retrainer biofeedback u.
> Exo-Bed traction u.
> Exo-Overhead traction u.
> functional spinal u. (FSU)
> G5 Fleximatic massage/percussion u.
> G5 Vibramatic massage/percussion u.
> Gymmy exercise u.
> home cervical traction u. (HCTU)
> Hydra-Cadence gait-control u.
> hydraulic knee u.
> hydrocollator heating u.
> intervertebral motor u.
> Jace hand continuous passive motion u.
> Magnatherm SSP electromagnetic therapy u.
> MENS u.
> microcurrent electrical neuromuscular stimulator u.
> motor u.
> musculotendinous u.
> myofascial u.
> myotatic u.
> Orthodyne Enhancer u.
> Orthotic Research and Locomotor Assessment U. (ORLAU)
> over-the-door traction u.
> Pebax counter u.
> postanesthesia care u. (PACU)
> rotator u.
> single-axis knee u.
> sit-to-stand training parallel bar u.
> Solitens transcutaneous electrical nerve stimulation u.
> u. spinal rod
> TENS u.
> Thermalator heating u.
> thermoplastic heating u.
> torsion u.
> Total Shock shock-absorbing prosthetic u.
> transcutaneous electrical nerve stimulation u.
> vertebral motion u. (VMU)
> wrist flexion u.

unitary plastic

united

> U. States (U.S.)
> U. States Manufacturing Company (USMC)

Unitek steel crown

unitunnel technique

unity

> U. 51 lumbosacral fixation plate
> U. lumbosacral fixation system

univalve cast

univalved

universal

> u. acromioclavicular splint
> U. AerobiCycle
> u. bone grafting/impacting forceps
> u. bone plate (UBP)
> u. bone plate system
> u. canvas body restraint
> u. coronal movement
> u. distal radius fracture classification
> u. drill point
> u. femoral head prosthesis
> U. Fitstep
> u. fixation screw
> u. frame outer socket (UFOS)
> u. full-circle manual goniometer
> u. gutter splint
> u. head replacement (UHR)
> u. hex screwdriver
> u. hip prosthesis
> u. (I, II) prosthesis
> u. incision
> u. knee positioner
> u. lateral positioner
> U. Minimally Invasive Assistant Free hip surgery instruments
> U. modular femoral hip component extractor
> u. nail
> U. plantar fasciitis orthosis (UFO)
> U. Plantar Fasciitis Orthotic (UFO)
> u. precautions
> U. Proximal Femur (UPF)
> u. radial component
> u. sacral spine instrumentation
> u. sling
> u. sling and swathe shoulder immobilizer
> u. 2-speed hand drill

U

universal (*continued*)
  u. spine classification (type A-C)
  U. Spine System
  u. support splint
  U. Tredex
  u. tri-panel knee immobilizer
  u. wire clamp
Uni-Versatil sling
university
  Louisiana State U. (LSU)
  New York U. (NYU)
  U. of British Columbia (UBC)
  U. of British Columbia brace
  U. of British Columbia Orthosis
  U. of California Berkeley (UCB)
  U. of California Berkeley
    Laboratory (UCBL)
  U. of California Berkeley
    Laboratory orthosis
  U. of California Berkeley Orthosis
  U. of California Biomechanics
    Laboratory heel cup
  U. of California cuff suspension
    PTB socket
  U. of California Irvine (UCI)
  U. of California Los Angeles
    (UCLA)
  U. of California Riverside (UCR)
  U. of Florida LINAC
  Western Ontario and McMaster U.
    (WOMAC)
  Xtra Depth U. (XDU)
unknown
  etiology u.
unleveling
  pelvic u.
unloader
  U. ADJ OA knee brace
  U. Bi-ComPF knee brace
  U. brace
  U. Express OA knee brace
  U. Select OA knee brace
  U. Spirit knee brace
  The U.
unlocking spiral technique
unmineralized osteoid
unmyelinated
Unna
  U. boot
  U. boot cast
  U. boot wrap
  U. paste
  U. paste boot
  U. paste shell
Unna-Flex Plus venous ulcer kit
unopposed
unplanned valgus osteotomy
unrectified socket
unreduced dislocation

unremodeled defect
unremovable plaster cast
unrestricted closed and open chain knee extension exercise
unsegmented vertebral bar
unsound ankylosis
unstable
  u. cervical spine injury
  u. fracture
  u. fracture-dislocation
  u. joint
  u. pelvic ring
unsteadiness of gait and station
unsteady gait
unstriated muscle, unstriped muscle
unstriped muscle
unsustained clonus
unsynchronous growth
unthreaded wire
ununited
  u. bone
  u. fracture
  u. tibial tuberosity
unwinding
  myofascial u.
up
  U. and About system
  press u.
up-angle hook
upbiting
  u. basket forceps
  u. rongeur
upcurved punch forceps
upcut rongeur
UPF
  Universal Proximal Femur
upgoing toes
6U portal
upper (U)
  u. arm tourniquet
  u. body cycle
  u. body ergometer (UBE)
  u. cervical spine anterior construct
  u. cervical spine anterior exposure
  u. cervical spine fusion
  u. cervical spine posterior construct
  u. cervical spine procedure
  u. extremity (UE)
  u. extremity functional index
    (UEFI)
  u. extremity myoelectric prosthesis
  u. fossa active, medial knee pain,
    and short leg on side ipsilateral
    to weak fossa (UMS)
  u. hand retractor
  U. 7 head halter
  u. hook trial
  u. limb neurodynamic test (ULNT)
  u. limb orthosis (ULO)

u. limb prosthesis (ULP)
u. limb tension test (ULTT)
u. limits of normal
u. motor neuron disease
u. motor neuron lesion
u. thoracic kyphosis
u. thoracic spine
uppermost instrumented vertebra
Uppsala screw
upright
adjustable posterior u. (APU)
orthosis overlapped u.'s
u. skeletal radiography
u. view
upright-Y incision
uptake
maximal oxygen u. (VO$_2$max)
maximum oxygen u. (VO$_2$max)
upward-cutting triangular knife
urarthritis
Urbaniak
U. neurovascular free flap
U. scapular flap
Urban Walkers shoe
urea
Ureacin-20
Ureacin-20 cream
Ureacin-20 creme
Ureacin-20
Ureacin-10 lotion
urethane
Poron cellular u.
Urias
U. air splint
U. pressure splint
uric acid crystal
uricosuric agent
urinary
u. incontinence
u. nitrogen
u. output
u. tract

urine culture
urogenital
u. diaphragm
u. triangle
urologic
u. complication
u. disturbance
U.S.
United States
U.S. Army bone chisel
U.S. Army gouge
U.S. Army osteotome
U-shaped
U-s. incision
U-s. retractor
Uslenghi
U. drill guide
U. plate
USMC
United States Manufacturing Company
USMC luxury liner
USMC multiaxis ankle
USMC stance locking safety knee
USP
USP 2-0 (3) size suture
USP 3-0 (2) size suture
USP 4-0 (1.5) size suture
USP 5-0 (1) size suture
USP #1, #2, #3 suture
U-splint splint
ustilaginea
necrosis u.
U-stirrup splint
Utah
U. artificial arm
U. artificial limb
utensil
Good Grips u.
swivel u.
Utrata forceps
UV
ultraviolet

U

V

vanadium
vertebra
   V blade plate
   V capsulotomy
   Grifulvin V
   V nail plate
   V osteotomy
   V sign

v

vein

V40

   V40 femoral head implant
     component
   V40 forged femoral head

VA

vertebral artery

V-A alignment rod

VABS

Vineland Adaptive Behavior Scales,
Revised

V.A.C.

   V.A.C. Freedom wound-healing
     system
   V.A.C. GranuFoam heel dressing

VAC

vacuum-assisted closure
   Wound VAC

Vac

Sani V.

vacant glenoid sign

Vac-Lok immobilization cushion

Vac-Pac

   V.-P. pad
   V.-P. positioner

Vacumix vacuum pump

vacuolar myelopathy

vacuum

   v. cement mix technique
   v. disc
   facet joint v.
   M-Pact cast v.
   v. phenomenon
   v. phenomenon sign
   v. pump

vacuum-assisted

   v.-a. closure (VAC)
   v.-a. therapy

vagal reaction

vaginal

   v. hand ligament
   v. ligament of hand
   v. pack
   v. synovitis

vagoglossopharyngeal neuralgia

Vainio metacarpal joint arthroplasty

Valenti

   V. arthroereisis device
   V. first metatarsophalangeal joint
     arthroplasty
   V. hallux limitus/rigidus procedure
   V. metatarsophalangeal arthroplasty

Valentine splint

Valeo back support

valga

   coxa v.
   manus v.
   tibia v.

valgization osteotomy

valgoid

valgum

   genu v.
   idiopathic genu v. (IGV)

valgus

   v. angle
   v. angulation
   v. bar
   calcaneal v.
   congenital convex pes plano v.
   v. contracture
   convex pes v.
   v. corrective ankle strap
   cubitus v.
   digitus v.
   v. extension osteotomy
   v. extension overload syndrome
   flexible pes v.
   v. foot
   forefoot v.
   hallux v. (HV)
   heel v.
   v. heel deformity
   v. high tibial osteotomy
   hindfoot v.
   idiopathic hallux v.
   v. instability
   v. intertrochanteric-wedge
     osteotomy
   juvenile hallux v.
   v. knee
   v. knee control pad
   v. knee motion
   v. laxity
   Mayday distal first metatarsal
     osteotomy for hallux v.
   metatarsus quintus v.
   pes planus et v.
   physiologic v.
   rearfoot v.
   senile hallux v.

V

valgus (*continued*)
    v. stress
    v. stress test
    v. stress wrist test
    v. subtrochanteric osteotomy
    talipes v.
    v. tilt of talus
    v. wedge osteotomy
    v. Y-shaped osteotomy
validation
    symptom v.
validity
    face v.
Valium Oral
Valleix
    V. entrapment neuropathy sign
    V. phenomenon
Valls hip prosthesis
Valls-Ottolenghi-Schajowicz bone
  neoplasm needle biopsy
Valorin
    V. Extra
    V. Super
Valpar
    V. Component Work Samples
    V. Component Work Sample series
    V. Whole Body Range of Motion
      Work Sample Test
valproate
valproic acid
Valsalva
    V. cervical spine and lumbar test
    V. maneuver
value
    mean v.
    Tanner-Whitehouse bone-age
      reference v.
    V. Walker brace
valvae (*pl. of* valve)
valve, *pl.* **valvae**
    bulb and thumb screw v.
    Heyer-Schulte bur hole v.
    Quadtro cushion with Isoflap v.
vamp of shoe
van
    V. Arsdale triangular splint
    V. Beek nerve approximator
    v. Buchem disease
    v. Buren sequestrum forceps
    v. der Hoeve brittle bones
      syndrome
    v. der Hoeve-de Klyn brittle bones
      syndrome
    v. der Hoeve disease
    V. Neck disease
    v. Ness lower limb amputation with
      foot reversal procedure
    v. Ness rotational arthroplasty
    v. Ness rotationplasty

vanadium (V)
Vancocin
Vancoled
vancomycin
Vanderbilt Pain Management Inventory
Vanghetti limb prosthesis
Vanguard
    V. complete knee system
    V. Uni unicompartmental knee
      replacement
Vanore modification of
  Youngswick-Austin osteotomy
Vantage Performance monitor
Vanzetti sciatica sign
VAPC
    Veterans Administration Prosthetic
    Center
    VAPC dorsiflexion assist orthosis
vapocoolant spray and stretch
Vapr
    V. coagulation and cautery device
    V. system
vara
    adolescent tibia v.
    coxa v.
    developmental coxa v.
    false coxa v.
    infantile tibia v. (ITV)
    manus v.
    tibia v.
variabilis
    Dermacentor v.
variable
    v. axis knee system
    v. circumference suprapatellar socket
      (VCSPS)
    v. flexion overhinge
    metabolic v.
    v. resistance training
    v. screw placement (VSP)
    v. screw placement plate
    v. screw placement system
    v. screw placement system
      instrumentation
    v. screw placement
      system-instrumented lumbar spine
    v. screw plate (VSP)
    v. spinal plating (VSP)
variance
    negative ulnar v. (NUV)
    positive ulnar v. (PUV)
    ulnar minus v.
Vari-Angle
    V.-A. clip applier
    V.-A. screw
variant
    Becker v.
    Neuhauser v.
    4-part v.

variation
>hindfoot anatomic v.
>postural v.

vari-balance board set

varices (*pl. of* varix)

varicosity
>superficial v.

Vari-Duct hip and knee orthosis

Vari-Firm Medicine Ball

VariFix spinal implant device

Vari-Flex prosthetic foot

VariGrip spinal implant device

Varikopf hip prosthesis

VariLock socket lock

varix, *pl.* **varices**

Varney
>V. acromioclavicular brace
>V. pin

Varni-Thompson Pediatric Pain Questionnaire

varum
>genu v.

varus
>calcaneal v.
>v. contracture
>v. corrective ankle strap
>cubitus v.
>v. derotational osteotomy (VDO)
>v. derotational osteotomy with adolescent pediatric hip screw
>digitus v.
>dynamic hallux v.
>forefoot v.
>v. habitus
>hallux v.
>heel v.
>v. hindfoot
>v. hindfoot deformity
>v. knee
>v. knee control pad
>v. laxity
>v. malalignment
>v. malunion
>metatarsus v. (MTV)
>metatarsus primus v. (MPV)
>v. MTP angle
>pes v.
>v. plafond
>rearfoot v.
>v. rotational osteotomy (VRO)
>v. rotation shortening osteotomy
>v. stress test
>v. stress wrist test
>subtalar v.
>v. supramalleolar osteotomy
>talipes v.
>tibial v.
>v. tilt
>v. toe

varus-valgus
>v.-v. adjustment screw
>v.-v. angulation
>v.-v. instability
>knee v.-v.
>v.-v. lift-off
>v.-v. plane
>v.-v. stress
>v.-v. stress of elbow

VAS
>visual analog scale

vascular
>v. accident
>v. assessment
>v. bundle implantation
>v. bundle implantation into bone
>v. endothelium
>v. forceps
>v. gangrene
>v. inflow
>v. injury
>v. invasion
>v. metaphysial bone
>v. nonunion
>v. surgery
>v. tissue
>v. tumor

vasculare
>heloma v.

vascularity
>femoral head v.
>tenuous v.

vascularized
>v. bone graft (VBG)
>v. bone transplant
>v. fibular graft
>v. free flap
>v. osseous transfer
>v. osteoseptocutaneous fibular autogenous graft
>v. rib strut graft

vasculature

vasculitis
>mesenteric v.
>rheumatoid v.

vasculopathy

vasoconstrictive therapy

vasocoolant spray

vasodilatation (*var. of* vasodilation)

vasodilation, vasodilatation
>flow-mediated v. (FMV)

vasodilator

vasodilatory effect

vasogenic shock

vasomotor
>v. disorder
>v. technique

vasopneumatic intermittent compression

vasopressor

V

vasospasm
vasospastic ischemia
Vastamäki
    V. muscle transfer
    V. pectoralis major tendon transfer technique
    V. wrist arthroscopy technique
vastus
    v. intermedius (VI)
    v. intermedius muscle
    v. lateralis (VL)
    v. lateralis muscle
    v. lateralis ridge
    v. medialis (VM)
    v. medialis advancement (VMA)
    v. medialis muscle
    v. medialis obliquus (VMO)
    v. medialis obliquus exercise
    v. medialis obliquus retraining
    v. medialis obliquus to vastus lateralis
VAT
    vertebral artery test
VATER
    vertebral anomaly, anal atresia, tracheoesophageal fistula, renal anomalies, radial dysplasia
    VATER syndrome
vault
    plantar v.
VAX-D
    vertebral axial decompression
    VAX-D therapy table
VBG
    vascularized bone graft
VBI
    vertebrobasilar insufficiency
VBR
    vertebral body replacement
    Cambria thoracolumbar fusion interbody VBR
    Hollywood thoracolumbar fusion interbody VBR
    Pacifica thoracolumbar fusion interbody VBR
    Redondo thoracolumbar fusion interbody VBR
    STALIF TT VBR
    Ventura thoracolumbar fusion interbody VBR
    Zuma thoracolumbar fusion interbody VBR
VCF
    vertebral [body] compression fracture
VCL
    volar carpal ligament
VCSPS
    variable circumference suprapatellar socket

VD
    video densitometry
VDA
    video-dimensional analysis
VDDR
    vitamin D-dependent rickets
VDO
    varus derotational osteotomy
VDRR
    vitamin D-resistant rickets
VDS
    ventral derotation spondylodesis
    VDS compression rod
    VDS hex nut
    VDS screw
    VDS wrench
VE
    vocational evaluation
vector
    V. intertrochanteric nail
    V. low back analysis system
    major injury v. (MIV)
    v. point
    v. quantity
vectored adjustment
Vectra Genisys laser system device
vehicle
    all-terrain v.
Veillonella
vein (v), vena
    anterior jugular v.
    axillary v.
    Boyd communicating perforation v.
    brachiocephalic v.
    carotid v.
    cephalic v.
    Cockett communicating perforating v.'s
    common iliac v.
    grafting v.
    iliac v.
    iliolumbar v.
    innominate v.
    intercostal v.
    intermetatarsal v.
    internal iliac v.
    internal jugular v.
    lingual v.
    lumbar v.
    middle sacral v.
    middle thyroid v.
    v. of Batson
    peroneal v.
    popliteal v.
    saphenous v.
    subclavian v.
    superficial temporal v.
    superior thyroid v.

tibial v.
vertebral v.
vela (*pl. of* velum)
velar
fronting of v.
Velcro
V. closure
V. extenders splint
V. fitting
V. Hand Exerboard
V. immobilization
V. immobilizer
V. strap
Velcro-Lock mat platform
Veleanu-Rosianu-Ionescu obturator neurectomy technique
velocity
conduction v.
curve progression v.
free-walking v.
maximum conduction v.
maximum eversion v.
maximum inversion v.
mean flow v.
motion v.
motor conduction v.
motor nerve conduction v. (MNCV)
muscle fiber conduction v.
nerve conduction v. (NCV)
orthodromic v.
peak height v. (PHV)
propagation v.
push-off v.
sensory nerve conduction v. (SNCV)
stretching v.
Velocor footbed
Velpeau
V. axillary lateral shoulder view
V. axillary radiograph
V. bandage
V. cast
V. deformity
V. dressing
V. plaster
V. shoulder immobilizer
V. shoulder sling
V. sling-dressing
V. stockinette
V. wrap
velum, *pl.* **vela**
vena (*var. of* vein)
v. cava
Venable
V. plate
V. screw
Venable-Stuck nail
venlafaxine
Venn-Watson polydactyly classification
Venodyne boot

venography
epidural v.
intraosseous v.
magnetic resonance v. (MRV)
Venosan
V. support hose
V. support sock
venous
v. cleft
v. compression
v. foot pump
v. stasis dermatitis
v. thromboembolic disease (VTED)
v. thrombosis
ventral
v. derotating spinal wrench
v. derotation spondylodesis (VDS)
ventriculography
ventroflexion
vent tube
Ventura thoracolumbar fusion interbody VBR
VEP
visual evoked potential
VePesid
V. Injection
V. Oral
VEPTR
vertical expandable prosthetic titanium rib
verapamil
Verbrugge
V. bone clamp
V. bone-holding forceps
V. needle
Verbrugge-Hohmann bone retractor
Verdan
V. intrasynovial flexor tendon technique
V. osteoplastic thumb reconstruction
Verebelyi-Ogston decancellation procedure
Veress needle
Verhoeff stain
Verlow brace
Vermont
V. Interdependent Services Team Approach (VISTA)
V. pedicle fixation system
V. spinal fixator (VSF)
V. spinal fixator articulation
V. spinal fixator clamp
vernier
v. caliber gauge
v. caliper
verruca, *pl.* **verrucae**
v. cryotherapy
mosaic plantar v.
single plantar v.
verrucae (*pl. of* verruca)

V

Verruca-Freeze freezing system
verruciformis
    epidermodysplasia v.
verrucous lesion
Versaback
    V. back system
    V. gym ball
VersaBond medium-viscosity bone
  cement
VersaClimber RX exercise machine
VersaFlex tubing kit
Versa-Fx
    V.-F. femoral fixation
    V.-F. femoral hip fixation system
Versa-Helper floor stand
Versalok low back fixation system
VersaPulse holmium laser
Versa-Stim self-adhering electrode
versatility
    attachment v.
Versa-Trainer exerciser
VersaWrist wrist splint
versicolor
    tinea v.
version
    external v.
    femoral neck v.
    internal v.
    Rivermead Behavioral Memory
      Test-Extended V. (RBMT-E)
Versi-Splint carry bag
Verstreken computed-aided closed
  medullary nailing
VerSys
    V. fiber metal taper
    V. hip system
    V. prosthesis
VertAlign spinal support system
vertebra (V), *gen.* and *pl.* **vertebrae**
    apex v.
    apical v.
    basilar v.
    biconcave v.
    block v.
    body of v.
    butterfly v.
    caudal v.
    cervical spine vertebrae 1-7 (C1-C7)
    cleft v.
    coccygeal v.
    codfish v.
    displaced v.
    dorsal v.
    end v.
    false v.
    first cervical v.
    fish v.
    fractured v.
    fused v.

    hourglass v.
    ivory v.
    last normal v. (LNV)
    lumbar v.
    lumbar (spine) vertebrae 1-5
      (L1-L5)
    lumbosacral v.
    malposed v.
    midbody of v.
    neural tube defect-related anomaly
      of v.
    olisthetic v.
    pear-shaped v.
    v. plana
    v. prominens reflex
    sacral v.
    scalloping of v.
    second cervical v.
    stable v.
    subluxed v.
    thoracic vertebrae 1-12 (T1-T12)
    transitional v.
    transverse process of v.
    true v.
    uppermost instrumented v.
    wasp-waist v.
    wedge-shaped v.
    wedging of olisthetic v.
vertebrae (*gen.* and *pl. of* vertebra)
vertebral
    v. adjustment
    v. angiography
    v. ankylosis
    v. anomaly, anal atresia,
      tracheoesophageal fistula, renal
      anomalies, radial dysplasia
      (VATER)
    v. arch
    v. arteriography
    v. artery (VA)
    v. artery test (VAT)
    v. arthritis
    v. axial decompression (VAX-D)
    v. bar
    v. body
    v. body anterior cortex
    v. body collapse
    v. [body] compression fracture
      (VCF)
    v. body corpectomy
    v. body decompression
    v. body endplate
    v. body fracture
    v. body height loss
    v. body impactor
    v. body replacement (VBR)
    v. body stapling wedge resection
    v. body translation
    v. body tumor

v. body wedge fracture
v. bone
v. border
v. canal
v. canal stenosis
v. column
v. column cleft
v. column resection
v. compression
v. compression fracture
v. compression fracture
  vertebroplasty
v. derangement
v. end plate
v. exposure
v. fascia
v. formula
v. fusion
v. hydatidosis
v. instability
v. lesion
v. level
v. medicine
v. motion segment
v. motion testing
v. motion unit (VMU)
v. nerve
v. neural reflection
v. notch
v. osteomyelitis
v. osteosynthesis
v. osteosynthesis fusion rate
v. pedicle
v. plana fracture
v. polyarthritis
v. rib
v. ring apophysis
v. rotation
v. scalloping
v. segmentation anomaly
v. space tang
v. stable burst fracture
v. steal phenomenon
v. steal syndrome
v. stripe
v. subluxation
v. subluxation complex (VSC)
v. subluxation syndrome
v. vein
v. wedge angle
v. wedge compression fracture
v. wedging
v. wrist block
vertebrectomy
Bohlman anterior cervical v.
cervical v.
cervical spondylotic myelopathy v.
microsurgical thoracoscopic v.
partial cervical v.

vertebrobasilar
v. injury
v. insufficiency (VBI)
vertebrocostal rib
vertebrogenic interference
vertebropelvic ligament
vertebroplastic cement
vertebroplasty
percutaneous v.
vertebral compression fracture v.
vertebrosternal rib
VerteFill implant
Verteflex
V. arthrotonic stabilizer
V. Intersegmental Traction Table
Vertetrac ambulatory traction system
vertical
anatomical v.
v. axis
v. capsulotomy
v. compression
v. compression test
v. expandable prosthetic titanium rib
  (VEPTR)
v. foot board
v. ground reaction force
  (VGRF)
v. loading
v. longitudinal tear
v. loop suture technique
v. loop suture technique for
  meniscus repair
v. mattress suture
v. pedicle diameter
v. plane
v. sacral compaction
v. sagittal split osteotomy (VSO)
v. septum
v. shear
v. shear fracture
v. shock pylon
v. subsidence
v. suspension reflex
v. suspension response
v. suspension test
v. symphysial mobility
v. talus
v. talus foot deformity
v. traction
v. translation
verticality control
**VertiGraft textured allograft bone
 graft**
VertiLok spinal orthosis
vesalianum
v. bone
os v.
Vesalius bone
Vesely splint

V

vessel
    v. clamp
    v. dilator
    endosteal v.
    great v.
    haversian v.
    v. hook
    humeral circumflex v.
    lymph v.
    milking of v.
    periosteal v.
    popliteal v.
    v. shifting
    tumor v.

vest
    Bremer AirFlo halo v.
    halo v.
    Minerva v.
    Ortho-Trac pneumatic v.
    Standard E-Z-On V.
    Vitrathene v.
    weighted v.

vestibular
    v. balance control
    v. ball
    v. postural control

Vestibulator
    Tumble Forms V.

vestibulocerebellar ataxia

vestibulospinal
    v. reflex
    v. tract

vestigial muscle

Veterans Administration Prosthetic Center (VAPC)

VGRF
    vertical ground reaction force

V-groove hollow-ground connection design

V1 halo ring

VI
    vastus intermedius

viability

viable tissue

Vibram
    V. rockerbottom shoe
    V. sole

Vibramat

Vibramycin

vibration
    v. glove
    v. perception threshold (VPT)
    v. sensation
    v. sense
    v. sensitivity
    v. synovitis
    v. threshold test
    v. white finger syndrome
    whole-body v.

vibrative, vibratory

vibrator
    v. hand syndrome
    Magic Wand v.

vibratory (*var. of* vibrative)
    v. massage

vibrogram
    digital v.

vibromasseur

vibrometer test

vibrotactile
    v. device
    v. feedback
    v. sensory prosthesis

vibrotherapeutics

vicious union

Vicodin
    V. ES
    V. HP

Vicon 3-dimensional gait analysis system

Vicoprofen

Vicryl suture

Victorian brace

Vidal-Adrey
    V.-A. femoral fracture technique
    V.-A. modified Hoffman external fixation device apparatus
    V.-A. modified Hoffmann external fixation device
    V.-A. modified Hoffmann fixation

video
    v. densitometry (VD)
    videofluoroscopic v.

video-assisted
    v.-a. lumbar surgery
    v.-a. thoracic spine surgery

video-dimensional analysis (VDA)

videofluoroscopic video

videofluoroscopy

video-gate analysis

videoradiography

Videx

vidian neuralgia

Vi-Drape
    V.-D. dressing
    Ioban V.-D.

view
    abdominal v.
    abduction and external rotation v.
    ABER v.
    Adams shoulder v.
    Alexander acromioclavicular joint v.
    anterior v.
    anterior drawer stress x-ray v.
    anteroposterior v.
    anteroposterior supine v.
    apical lordotic v.
    AP supine v.

Arcelin petrous temporal v.
axial calcaneus v.
axial sesamoid v.
axillary lateral v.
ball-catcher's v.
baseline v.
bicipital tuberosity v.
Böhler calcaneal v.
Böhler lumbosacral v.
Breuerton MCP joint v.
Broden subtalar joint (I-II) v.
Bucky abdominal v.
calcaneal axial v.
Canale-Kelly talar neck v.
Canale talus v.
carpal tunnel v.
Carter Rowe shoulder v.
cine v.
clenched fist v.
coalition v.
coned-down v.
cross-table lateral v.
 (CTLV)
dens x-ray v.
Didiee shoulder v.
dorsiflexion v.
dorsoplantar radiographic v.
dynamic stress x-ray v.
erect v.
false profile v.
FCS v.
Ferguson sacroiliac v.
Ficat v.
frog-leg lateral v.
full cervical spine v.
Garth shoulder v.
Gaynor-Hart carpal tunnel v.
Grashey shoulder v.
Harris axial heel v.
Harris-Beath axial calcaneus v.
Hermodsson internal rotation
 shoulder v.
Hermodsson tangential shoulder v.
Hill-Sachs AP shoulder v.
hip-to-ankle v.
Hobb sternoclavicular joint v.
Hughston patella v.
iliac oblique v.
infrapatellar v.
inlet v.
intraoperative v.
inversion ankle stress v.
Jones elbow in flexion v.
Judet oblique acetabulum v.
lateral bending v.
lateral monopodal stance v.
lateral oblique v.
lateral tilt stress ankle v.
Laurin patella v.

Laurin tangential patella v.
Lawrence lateral proximal
 humerus v.
Lawrence transthoracic lateral
 humerus v.
Löwenstein frog-leg lateral hips v.
magnification v.
Merchant patella v.
mortise v.
Neer lateral shoulder v.
Neer transscapular v.
nonstanding lateral oblique v.
nonweightbearing v.
Norgaard both hands v.
notch v.
oblique v.
obturator oblique v.
odontoid x-ray v.
outlet v.
patellar skyline v.
plantar axial v.
plantarflexion stress v.
prayer v.
push-pull ankle stress v.
push-pull hip v.
radial head-capitellum v.
Robert true AP thumb v.
Rosenberg knee v.
Rowe shoulder v.
scapulolateral v.
semisupinated oblique v.
serendipity v.
skijump v.
skyline v.
spot v.
standing dorsoplantar v.
standing lateral v.
standing weightbearing v.
Stenver petrous temporal v.
Stenver temporal bone v.
stress v.
Stryker notch humeral head v.
sunrise knee x-ray v.
sunset knee x-ray v.
swimmer's v.
tangential x-ray v.
Tile pelvic inlet and outlet v.
transthoracic lateral v.
trauma v.
true lateral v.
tunnel v.
upright v.
Velpeau axillary lateral shoulder v.
von Rosen hip v.
weightbearing dorsoplantar v.
West Point axillary lateral
 shoulder v.
White leg length v.
x-ray v.

V

view (*continued*)
    Y scapular v.
    Zanca acromioclavicular joint v.
Vigilon dressing
vigorimeter
Viking postoperative shoe
Viladot
    V. arthroereisis device
    V. implant
    V. prosthesis
    V. subtalar arthrocrisis technique
Vilex
    V. cannulated screw system
    V. F-Series dual-thread screw
    V. Ouchless Hook
    V. screw system
villonodular
    v. pigmented tenosynovitis
    v. synovitis (VNS)
    v. tenosynovitis
villosa
    polyarthritis chronica v.
villose (*var. of* villous)
villous, villose
    v. lipomatous proliferation of
      synovial membrane
    v. synovitis
    v. tenosynovitis
villusectomy
Vincasar PFS Injection
vincula (*pl. of* vinculum)
vinculum, *pl.* **vincula**
    v. breve
    intertendinous v.
    vincula longa
**Vineland Adaptive Behavior Scales,
Revised (VABS)**
Vinertia implant metal prosthesis
Vinke
    V. skull traction tongs
    V. tong traction
Vioform
violet monofilament suture
viral
    v. monarthritis
    v. myositis
viral-associated arthritis
Virchow triad
Virgin hip screw
Virtual hip joint
Virtullene brace material
visceral tendon sheath
visceroptosia (*var. of* visceroptosis)
visceroptosis, visceroptosia
viscerosomatic reflex
viscerospinal syndrome
viscoelastic
    v. creep
    v. heel insert

    v. insole
    v. material
    v. polymer
    quasilinear v. (QLV)
    v. tissue
viscoelasticity
Viscoheel
    V. K heel cushion
    V. K, N orthosis
    V. N cushion
    V. SofSpot viscoelastic heel cushion
Viscolas
    V. Blue Dot heel cup
    V. heel orthosis
    V. heel spur cushion
    V. orthosis
    V. standard heel cup
ViscoPed
    V. S insole
    V. S support
viscosity
    blood v.
    cement v.
ViscoSpot
    V. heel cushion
    V. support
viscosupplementation treatment
viscous
vise
    allograft bone v.
    AlloGrip bone v.
    pin v.
    Starrett pin v.
viselike pain
VISI
    volar flexed intercalated segment
    instability
vision
    V. Epic wheelchair
    under direct v. (UDV)
visor
    v. halo fixation device
    v. osteotomy
visor/sandwich osteotomy
VISTA
    Vermont Interdependent Services Team
    Approach
Vistacon
Vistaril
Vistazine
Vistec x-ray-detectable sponge
visual
    v. analog scale (VAS)
    v. analog scale of handicap
    v. closure
    v. evoked potential (VEP)
    v. evoked response
    v. neglect
    v. orientation

v. perception
v. postural control
visual-motor integration (VMI)
visual-spatial ability impairment
Vita ADE cream
vitalism
vitallium
v. cup arthroplasty
v. humeral replacement prosthesis
v. implant
v. implant material
v. implant metal
v. Küntscher nail
v. Luhr plate
v. screw
v. staple
vitallium-W implant metal prosthesis
Vitalock
V. cluster acetabular component
V. solid-back acetabular component
vitamin
Catalyn v.
v. C, D, K deficiency
v. D-dependent rickets (VDDR)
v. D receptor gene serum assay
v. D-resistant rickets (VDRR)
v. E emollient
Vitoss
V. Scaffold synthetic cancellous
bone void filler
V. synthetic bone
Vitox
HIP V.
Vitrathene
V. jacket
V. vest
Vivatek treatment system
Vivelle Transdermal
VL
vastus lateralis
Vladimiroff-Mikulcz foot
amputation
VM
vastus medialis
VMA
vastus medialis advancement
VMC
void metal composite
V-medullary nail
VMI
visual-motor integration
VMO
vastus medialis obliquus
VMO exercise
VMO retraining
VMU
vertebral motion unit
VNS
villonodular synovitis

VO
voluntary opening
VO$_2$
aerobic capacity
vocal cord
vocational
v. assessment
v. evaluation (VE)
v. feasibility
v. rehabilitation
Vogue arm sling
void
v. metal composite
(VMC)
signal v.
Vojta reaction
volar
v. angulation deformity
v. antebrachial region
v. approach
v. aspect
v. beak ligament
v. capsule
v. carpal ligament (VCL)
v. compartment syndrome
v. condyle
v. digital artery
v. epineurolysis
v. flexed intercalated segment
instability (VISI)
v. flexion
v. glide
v. intercalary wrist instability
v. midline oblique incision
v. osteotomy
v. plaster splint
v. plate arthroplasty
v. plate repair
v. semilunar wrist dislocation
v. shear fracture
v. surface
v. synovectomy
v. T plate
v. ulnar sling
v. wrist
v. zigzag finger incision
volarly
volarward approach
volitional
v. activation
v. activity
v. contraction
v. exercise
v. fatigue
v. muscle action test
v. resisted flexion
v. resisted flexion and
extension
volitionally

V

Volkmann
V. bone curette
V. bone hook
V. canal
V. clawhand
V. clawhand deformity
V. contracture
V. ischemia
V. ischemic contracture
V. ischemic paralysis
V. posterior tibia fracture
V. posterolateral corner of tibia triangle
V. rake retractor
V. splint
V. subluxation

Volkov-Oganesian
V.-O. elbow distraction device
V.-O. external fixation
V.-O. external fixation apparatus
V.-O. external fixation device

volley of pain
Volpicelli functional ambulation scale
Voltaren
V. Ophthalmic
V. Oral

Voltaren-XR Oral
Voltz wrist implant
volume
cartilage v.
v. conduction
stroke v.

volumeter
Ableware V.
foot v.
hand v.
v. set

volumetric wear rate
voluntary
v. activity
v. closing
v. closing terminal device
v. control
v. control 4-bar knee
v. muscle
v. opening (VO)
v. opening terminal device

Volz
V. total wrist arthroplasty
V. wrist implant
V. wrist prosthesis

VO₂max
aerobic capacity
maximal oxygen uptake
maximum oxygen uptake

vomer bone
von
v. Bekhterev reflex
v. Gies joint
v. Hippel-Lindau syndrome
v. Lackum transection shift jacket
v. Lackum transection shift jacket brace
v. Langenbeck periosteal elevator
v. Mises stress
v. Recklinghausen neurofibromatosis disease
v. Rosen abduction splint
v. Rosen cruciform splint
v. Rosen hip view
v. Rosen splint hip orthosis
v. Saal medullary pin
v. Schwann law
v. Weber triangle

Von-Loc personal ice pack
Voorhoeve disease
Voshell
V. knee test
V. medial collateral ligament bursa

Vostal radial head fracture
V-osteotomy
Japas V-o.

VPT
vibration perception threshold

VRO
varus rotational osteotomy

Vrolik
V. brittle bones recessive syndrome
V. disease

VSC
vertebral subluxation complex

VSF
Vermont spinal fixator
VSF fixation system
VSF rod
VSF screw

V-shaped
V-s. fracture
V-s. incision
V-s. osteotomy
V-s. rotator cuff tear

VSO
vertical sagittal split osteotomy

VSP
variable screw placement
variable screw plate
variable spinal plating
VSP fixation
VSP plate
VSP plate instrumentation
VSP system

VTED
venous thromboembolic disease

Vulpian atrophy
Vulpian-Bernhardt spinal muscular atrophy

Vulpius
    V. Achilles tendon reconstruction
    V. equinus deformity operation
    V. gastrocnemius muscle lengthening
    V. lengthening of gastrocnemius
      muscle procedure
**Vulpius-Stoffel gastrocnemius
intramuscular aponeurotic recession
procedure**

VuRyser monitor lift
V-Y
    V-Y advancement flap
    V-Y Kutler fingertip flap
    V-Y lengthening of Achilles tendon
    V-Y plasty
    V-Y plasty correction
    V-Y plasty correction of varus toe
    V-Y quadricepsplasty

V

W
  west
  width
WACH
  wedge adjustable cushioned heel
  WACH orthopaedic shoe
wad
  flexor w.
  mobile w.
Waddell
  W. functional overlay test
  W. nonorganic back pain sign
  W. triad
wadding
  cotton sheet w.
  shot w.
waddle
  duck w.
waddling gait
Wadsworth
  W. elbow approach
  W. posterolateral approach
  W. triceps tendon release technique
  W. unconstrained elbow prosthesis
wafer
  w. distal ulna resection
  w. procedure
Wagdy double-V osteotomy
Wagner
  W. acetabular reamer
  W. closed pinning
  W. device external fixator
  W. diabetic foot disease
   classification
  W. diabetic foot ulcer grade
  W. distraction device
  W. distractor
  W. external fixation apparatus
  W. external fixation device
  W. femoral lengthening
  W. femoral metaphysial shortening
  W. fixation
  W. fixator
  W. frame
  W. leg-lengthening apparatus
  W. limb lengthening method
  W. modification of Syme amputation
  W. multiple K-wire osteosynthesis
  W. open reduction technique
  W. profundus advancement
  W. prosthesis
  W. retractor
  W. revision hip system
  W. skin incision
  W. 2-stage Syme amputation

  W. tibial lengthening
  W. transfemoral total hip approach
  W. trochanteric advancement
Wagner-Schanz
  W.-S. screw
  W.-S. screw apparatus
  W.-S. screw device
wagon
  dumbbell w.
  w. wheel fracture
Wagoner
  W. cervical spine technique
  W. posterior cervical spinal
   approach
Wagstaffe fracture
Wagstaffe-Le Fort fracture
Wagstaff malleolar tubercle
Wainwright plate
WAIS
  Wechsler Adult Intelligence Scale
waist
  w. fracture
  w. of anatomical structure
  w. of phalanx
  w. of scaphoid
  w. suspension belt
wakeboarding
wake-up test
Waldenström
  W. classification
  W. pediatric femoral head fracture
   sign
  W. staging
  W. syndrome
Waldron knee chondromalacia test
WALK
  weight-activated locking knee
walk
  heel w.
  heel-and-toe w.
  lift-off of heel in w.
  nonweightbearing crutch w.
  w. test
  toe w.
Walkabout
  W. orthosis
  W. walker
WalkAide system
Walkamatic walker
walkaway
WalkCare slippers
walker
  air w.
  Aircast pneumatic w.
  Ato w.

W

walker (*continued*)
  w. basket
  Body Armor short leg w.
  Cam W. II
  Cam Walker ankle w.
  cast w.
  Castaway ankle w.
  Castaway leg w.
  Charcot restraint orthotic w.
    (CROW)
  Comfy w.
  controlled ankle w.
  Darco Body Armor short
    leg w.
  Delta w.
  DH pressure relief w.
  EasyStep pressure relief w.
  Equalizer air w.
  Guardian Red Dot w.
  Hi-Top foot/ankle w.
  Hi-Top II adjustable w.
  Lumex w.
  Maddacrawler prone support w.
  Merry W.
  Moon W.
  obese w.
  ORLAU swivel w.
  4-point w.
  Roll-A-Bout 4-wheel w.
  Rollator Nova w.
  rubber sole cast w.
  rubber wedge w.
  W. ruptured disc curette
  short leg w.
  w. skis
  w. sleds
  swivel w.
  Walkabout w.
  Walkamatic w.
  3-wheel w.
  Zimmer w.
**Walker-Murdoch Marfan syndrome
  sign**
walking
  w. adjunct
  aerobic w.
  w. aid
  w. biomechanics
  bipedal w.
  w. boot cast
  w. brace
  crutch w.
  w. cycle
  w. footprints classification
  w. heel
  heel-and-toe w.
  idiopathic toe w. (ITW)
  w. mechanics
  nonweightbearing crutch w.

  w. pole
  w. program
  stance phase w.
  w. stirrup
  w. task
  toe w.
  w. without support
  w. with support
Walk-'n-Tone exerciser
Walk-Rite device
wall
  medial w.
**Walldius vitallium mechanical knee
  prosthesis**
Wallenberg
  W. syndrome
  W. vertebral artery test
wallerian degeneration
wallet neuritis
Wallis
  W. interspinous implant
  W. interspinous process stabilization
    device
wall-slide exercise
Wal-Pil-O neck pillow
Walsh
  protocol of W.
Walther hip fracture
Walton
  W. acromioclavicular joint pain
    maneuver
  W. cartilage clamp
  W. meniscal clamp
  W. scissors
  W. wire-pulling forceps
Walton-Liston forceps
Wanchik
  W. neutral position splint
  W. writer
wand
  ArthroCare w.
  ArthroWand disposable surgical w.
  extensor w.
  nucleoplasty w.
  TriggerWheel W.
Wangensteen needle holder
waning discharge
ward
  W. femoral neck test
  W. periosteal elevator
warfarin sodium
warm
  w. and form
  w. and form cast
  w. and form insert
  w. ischemia
  w. ischemic time
  W. 'n' Form lumbosacral corset
  W. Springs brace

warmer
> gel w.
> Thermasonic gel w.

warmth
> joint w.

WarmTouch patient warming system

Warm-Up active wound therapy system

Warner-Farber ankle fixation technique

Warren-White open sliding Achilles tendon lengthening

wart
> mosaic w.
> plantar w.
> W. stick plantar wart remover

Wartenberg
> W. little finger abduction sign
> W. pinwheel
> W. ulnar paralysis sign

washboard syndrome

washer
> C w.
> contoured w.
> w. crimper
> female w.
> w. holder
> male w.
> oval w.
> plate spacer w.
> spiked ligament w.
> Synthes ligament w.
> toothed w.

WasherLoc device

wash mitt

wasp-waist vertebra

Wassel
> W. classification of thumb polydactyly (I-VI)
> W. thumb duplication classification (I-VI)
> W. thumb duplication (I-VI)

Wasserstein
> W. external fixation device
> W. limb lengthening

wasting
> w. palsy
> w. paralysis
> quadriceps w.

Watanabe
> W. costal pin
> W. discoid meniscus classification
> W. pin holder
> W. retractor

watch crystal nail

Watco
> W. ankle brace
> W. knee immobilizer

water
> w. acceptance test
> Essential Energy W.
> total body w. (TBW)

water-cooled power bur

Waterman hallux limitus osteotomy

WaterPik irrigation

Waterpillow
> Mediflow W.

water-soluble contrast agent

Watkins
> W. intertransverse process lumbar spine fusion technique
> W. spinal fusion

Watson
> W. scaphoid shift test
> W. scapholunate instability test
> W. scaphotrapeziotrapezoidal fusion
> W. wrist maneuver
> W. wrist salvage technique

Watson-Cheyne wedge excision of toenail technique

Watson-Jones
> W.-J. ankle tenodesis
> W.-J. anterolateral total hip approach
> W.-J. bone gouge
> W.-J. fracture repair
> W.-J. frame
> W.-J. guidepin
> W.-J. hip arthrodesis
> W.-J. incision
> W.-J. nail
> W.-J. navicular fracture
> W.-J. navicular fracture classification
> W.-J. procedure
> W.-J. reconstruction
> W.-J. spinal fracture classification
> W.-J. tibial fracture classification
> W.-J. traction

Watson-Williams intervertebral disc rongeur

Waugh
> W. knee prosthesis
> W. total ankle replacement prosthesis

wave
> A w.
> double flexion w.
> H w.
> w. keyboard
> M w.
> OssaTron shock w.
> positive sharp w.
> W. Web

waveform
> biphasic w.
> bipolar IF w.
> electrical stimulator w.

W

waveform (*continued*)
>   micro w.
>   monophasic w.
>   Russian w.

wax
>   bone w.
>   Horsley bone w.

way
>   giving w.
>   W.'s of Coping checklist

Wayfarer modifiable foot prosthesis

Wayne
>   W. County General Hospital reduction
>   W. County intertrochanteric fracture reduction

WBAT
>   weightbearing as tolerated

WBC
>   white blood cell count

WC
>   writer's cramp

WCS-90
>   Clorpactin WCS-90

WDWN
>   well-developed, well-nourished

weak
>   w. bony tissue
>   w. foot

weakness
>   breakaway w.
>   give-way w.
>   motor w.
>   overstretch w.
>   progressive w.
>   ratchety w.

wear
>   abnormal shoe w.
>   accelerated chondral w.
>   asymmetric w.
>   backside w.
>   3-body w.
>   w. debris
>   eccentric w.
>   shoe w.
>   SoftFlex Wrist W.

wear-and-tear degeneration
wear-resistant surface
weather ache
weave
>   bob and w.

Weaver-Dunn
>   W.-D. acromioclavicular joint stabilization procedure
>   W.-D. acromioclavicular operation
>   W.-D. acromioclavicular technique
>   W.-D. distal clavicle resection

Weaver rockerbottom shoe
weaver's bottom

web
>   w. area
>   w. area of hand
>   w. border
>   w. border of hand
>   w. contracture
>   w. corn
>   finger w.
>   w. space
>   thumb w.
>   Wave W.

Webb
>   W. bolt nail
>   W. fixation
>   W. pin
>   W. procedure
>   W. stove bolt

webbed
>   w. finger
>   w. toe

Weber
>   W. (A, B, C) fracture
>   W. (A, B, C) fracture classification
>   W. anterior talofibular ligament reconstruction procedure
>   W. antiglide plate
>   W. foot test
>   W. hearing test
>   W. hip implant
>   W. humeral osteotomy
>   W. 2-point discrimination test
>   W. static 2-point discrimination
>   W. subcapital rotation osteotomy
>   W. syndrome

Weber-Danis ankle injury (A, B, C) classification

Weber-Vasey
>   W.-V. olecranon tension band wiring technique
>   W.-V. traction-absorption wiring of olecranon fracture technique

Webril
>   W. bandage
>   W. cotton padding
>   W. dressing
>   W. immobilization

webspace, web space
>   w. creep
>   w. flap
>   w. incision
>   w. infection
>   interdigital w.

Webster
>   W. meniscectomy scissors
>   W. needle holder

Wechsler
>   W. Adult Intelligence Scale (WAIS)
>   W. Memory Scale

Weck
- W. clip
- W. knife
- W. microsuture cutting scissors
- W. osteotome

Wedeen wire passer

wedge
- abduction w.
- w. adjustable cushioned heel (WACH)
- w. adjustable cushioned heel shoe
- bed w.
- bone w.
- bumper w.
- cast w.
- closing base w.
- compensatory w.
- w. compression fracture
- Duo-Cline dual support contoured bed w.
- w. fixation
- w. flexion-compression fracture
- Good 'N Bed w.
- w. graft
- Hapad heel w.
- heel w.
- heel-to-toe medial shoe w.
- inner heel w.
- lateral w.
- w. matrix resection (WMR)
- medial heel w.
- medial heel-and-sole w.
- medial sole w.
- metaphysial w.
- w. nonunion
- open w.
- w. osteotomy
- Positex knee w.
- w. posting
- w. resection
- roof w.
- Saunders mobilization w.
- seating w.
- self-adhering varus/valgus w.
- shoe w.
- super w.
- w. TAG suture anchor system
- tibial w.
- toe w.
- TruWedge BGS osteotomy w.
- TruWedge bone graft substitute osteotomy w.

wedge-and-groove joint

wedged shoe

wedge-shaped
- w.-s. uncomminuted fragment
- w.-s. uncomminuted tibial plateau fracture
- w.-s. vertebra

wedging
- w. cast
- navicular w.
- w. of olisthetic vertebra
- w. of vertebral interspace
- vertebral w.

WeeFIM
- WeeFIM II 0-3 module

weekend athlete

Wegener granulomatosis

Wegner
- W. disease
- W. line

weight
- w. acceptance
- w. and pulley
- ankle w.
- body w.
- w. boot
- cutting w.
- distal segment w.
- handheld w. (HHW)
- lean body w. (LBW)
- progressive w.
- Thera-Band progressive w.
- w. traction
- w. training

weight-activated locking knee (WALK)

weightbearing
- w. acetabular dome
- w. as tolerated (WBAT)
- w. axis
- w. brace
- w. crutch
- w. dorsoplantar radiograph
- w. dorsoplantar view
- full w. (FWB)
- w. ground reaction force
- w. joint
- pain with w.
- partial w. (PWB)
- progression to full w.
- progressive w.
- protective w.
- w. rotation injury
- w. surface
- w. symmetry
- w. tangential radiograph
- toe-touch w.
- touchdown w. (TDWB)
- w. x-ray

weight/composition
- body w./c.

weighted
- w. glove
- w. pen
- w. vest
- w. walking stick

W

weightlifter's
    w. clavicle
    w. shoulder
weightlifting
weight-relieving
    w.-r. caliper
    w.-r. Forte harness
    w.-r. orthosis
weight-training program
Weil
    W. implant
    W. modified Swanson implant
    W. MTP joint osteotomy
    W. osteotomy
    W. pelvic sling
    W. splint
    W. type Swanson-design hammertoe
    implant
Weiland
    W. chronic osteomyelitis
    classification
    W. harvesting
    W. iliac crest bone graft
Weil-Blakesley intervertebral disc rongeur
Weinraub joint and calcaneal spreader
Weinstein enhanced sensory test
Weinstock desyndactylization
WEIS
    Work Environment Impact Scale
Weiss
    W. amputation saw
    W. jack screw
    W. spring
Weissman intraoperative therapeutic intensity score classification
Weitbrecht
    W. foramen
    W. ligament
    W. retinaculum
Weitlaner
    W. retractor
    W. self-retaining retractor
Welander distal myopathy
weld
    callus w.
    cold w.
    hot w.
    spot w.
well-developed, well-nourished (WDWN)
well-differentiated myxoid liposarcoma
Weller
    W. cartilage forceps
    W. cartilage scissors
    W. total hip joint prosthesis
well-leg
    w.-l. cast
    w.-l. holder

    w.-l. raising
    w.-l. splint
    w.-l. straight-leg raising lumbar
    spine test
    w.-l. support
    w.-l. traction
Wellmerling femoral neck fracture technique
well-nourished
    well-developed, w.-n. (WDWN)
well-padded splint
well-seated prosthesis
Wenger plate
Werdnig-Hoffmann
    W.-H. disease
    W.-H. spinal muscular atrophy
    W.-H. syndrome
Werenskiold physial separation sign
Wertheim-Bohlman
    W.-B. occipitocervical fusion
    technique
    W.-B. posterior cervical technique
Wertheim splint
west (W)
    W. and Soto-Hall patella operation
    W. and Soto-Hall patellectomy
    W. bone chisel
    W. bone gouge
    W. hand dissector
    W. nerve tester
    W. osteotome
    W. Point Ankle Grading System
    W. Point axillary lateral radiograph
    W. Point axillary lateral shoulder
    view
    W. Shur cartilage clamp
Westergren sedimentation rate (WSR)
western
    W. Ontario and McMaster
    University (WOMAC)
    W. Ontario and McMaster
    University osteoarthritis index
    W. Ontario Instability Index
    (WOSI)
    W. Ontario Rotator Cuff (WORC)
    W. Ontario Rotator Cuff index
Westfield-style
    W.-s. acromioclavicular immobilizer
    W.-s. envelope sling
Westhaven Yale Multidimensional Pain Inventory (WHYMPI)
Westin tendo Achillis tenodesis
Weston shelf procedure
Westphal phenomenon
wet
    w. gangrene
    w. globe temperature
    w. leather sign
wet-to-dry dressing

WFE
Williams flexion exercise
WFL
within functional limits
Wheaton
W. brace
W. bunion splint
W. Pavlik harness
WHECS
wrist hand extension compression
support
WHECS glove
wheel
carborundum grinding w.
w. chair seating component
pin w.
shoulder w.
wheelchair
Action Jr. w.
Amigo mechanical w.
antitipper w.
Applause Super-Hemi w.
AquaTrek W.
w. chain
w. confinement
w. cushion
electric w.
Epic w.
folding frame w.
Gendron bariatric w.
Invacare manual w.
Jay J2 w.
Kuschkin Ace w.
Landeez all-terrain w.
Lumex lightweight w.
manual w.
Navigator power w.
Nitro w.
power w.
Quickie Carbon w.
Quickie EX w.
Quickie GPS w.
Quickie GP Swing-Away w.
Quickie GPV w.
Quickie Kidz w.
Quickie Recliner w.
Quickie Shark pediatric w.
Quickie Ti w.
reclining frame w.
rigid frame w.
self-propelling w.
Skil-Care reclining w.
Slam'r w.
sling seat w.
tilting frame w.
W. User's Shoulder Pain Index
(WUSPI)
Vision Epic w.
4XP Tilt System w.

Zippie 2 w.
Zippie P500 w.
3-wheel walker
whiplash
acute w.
chronic w.
w. injury
reflex rebound component of w.
w. syndrome
w. trauma
whiplash-associated disorder
whiplash-shaken infant syndrome
whirlpool
w. bath
w. therapy
whiskering
whistling face syndrome
white
W. and Panjabi cervical spine
criteria
w. band on degenerated
implant
w. blood cell count (WBC)
w. blood cell scan
W. chisel
W. epiphysiodesis
W. leg length view
w. matter
w. muscle
W. posterior ankle fusion
W. posterior occipitocervical
arthrodesis
W. screwdriver
W. slide lengthening of tendo
Achillis
W. slide lengthening of tendo
Achillis procedure
W. tendo calcaneus lengthening
Whitecloud-LaRocca
W.-L. cervical arthrodesis
W.-L. fibular strut graft
Whitehall
W. Glacier Pack
W. thermalator
Whiteside
W. intraarticular infusion
technique
W. Ortholoc modular knee system
Whitesides
W. intracompartmental tissue
pressure technique
W. line
W. tissue pressure determination
**Whitesides-Kelly lateral retropharyngeal
cervical spine technique**
Whitfield's Ointment
whitlow
herpetic w.
thecal w.

W

Whitman
- W. arch support
- W. femoral neck reconstruction
- W. frame
- W. maneuver
- W. muscle transfer
- W. osteotomy
- W. paralysis
- W. plate
- W. talectomy procedure
- W. traction

Whitney single-use plastic curette

WHO
- World Health Organization
- wrist-hand orthosis

WHO/ILAR
- World Health Organization/International League Against Rheumatism

whole
- w. bone fresh-frozen allograft
- w. bone transplant
- w. fibular transplant
- w. fresh-frozen calcaneal allograft

whole-body vibration

whorled pattern

WHYMPI
- Westhaven Yale Multidimensional Pain Inventory

Wiberg
- angle of W.
- W. center-edge angle
- center-edge angle of W.
- W. fracture angle
- W. fracture staple
- W. patella classification (I-III)
- W. patellar contour (I-III)
- W. periosteal elevator

Wichman retractor

wick
- w. catheter technique
- w. technique

wicking catheter

wide
- w. excision
- w. periosteal elevator
- w. toe box
- w. toe box shoe

wide-based gait

wide-mesh petroleum gauze dressing

widening
- ankle mortise w.
- interpedicular distance widening joint w.
- tibial tunnel w.

width (W)
- step w.

Wiet
- W. cup forceps
- W. graft-measuring instrument

Wilde
- W. ethmoid forceps
- W. intervertebral disc rongeur
- W. rongeur forceps

Wiley-Galey Monteggia fracture-dislocation (1–3) classification

Wilkco ankle exercise machine

Wilke
- W. boot
- W. boot brace

Wilkinson knee synovectomy

William Harris hip prosthesis

Williams
- W. brace
- W. discectomy
- W. discectomy procedure
- W. discography
- W. flexion back exercise technique
- W. flexion exercise (WFE)
- W. interlocking Y-nail
- W. microlumbar disc excision
- W. nail
- W. orthosis
- W. rod
- W. screwdriver
- W. self-retaining retractor

Williams-Haddad femoral nerve block for hip fracture technique

Williger
- W. bone curette
- W. bone mallet
- W. periosteal elevator

willow fracture

Wilmington
- W. arthroscopic portal
- W. plastic jacket
- portal of W.
- W. scoliosis brace

Wilson
- W. angulation osteotomy for hallux valgus procedure
- W. ankle fusion
- W. approach
- W. bolt
- W. bone graft
- W. bunionectomy
- W. cone arthrodesis
- W. convex frame
- W. Cook prosthesis repositioner
- W. disease
- W. double oblique osteotomy
- W. fracture
- W. gonad retractor
- W. knee test
- W. muscle
- W. oblique displacement osteotomy
- W. osteochondritis dissecans sign
- W. plate

W. procedure for extraarticular
fusion of elbow
W. splint
W. technique
Wilson-Jacobs
W.-J. tibial fixation
W.-J. tibial fracture fixation
technique
Wiltberger anterior cervical approach
Wiltse
W. and Winter surgical treatment of
spondylolisthesis
W. angle
W. ankle osteotomy
W. bilateral lateral fusion
W. discectomy
W. fixator
W. osteotomy of ankle
W. paraspinal approach
W. pedicle screw
W. pedicle screw fixation system
W. screw rod
W. spinal fusion muscle-splitting
approach
W. system aluminum master rod
W. system cross bracing
W. system double-rod construct
W. system H construct
W. system single-rod construct
W. system spinal rod
W. varus supramalleolar
osteotomy
Wimberger bilateral metaphysial sign
Winberger line
Winco
W. adjusting bench
W. folding treatment table
wind
w. cold
w. heat
windblown
w. deformity
w. hand and whistling face
syndrome
w. hip
w. knee
windlass
w. mechanism
reverse w.
window
W. anterior cervical plate system
cast w.
cortical w.
femoral cortical w.
W. titanium and titanium alloy
anterior cervical plate
windowed cast
windowing
cortical w.

windshield
w. wiper effect
w. wiper sign
Windsor-Insall-Vince tissue grafting
technique
windswept
w. deformity
w. hip
windup
w. injury
w. phenomenon
wing
angel w.
Badgley resection of iliac w.
dorsal w.
w. excision of Littler
iliac w.
keel and w.
w. of ilium
w. of sphenoid
w. plate
Wingate anaerobic power test
winged
w. scapula
w. scapula syndrome
winging
w. motion
w. of scapula
w. scapula arthrosis
scapular w.
wink
anal w.
W. retractor
w. sign
Winkelmann femoral bone sarcoma
rotationplasty
winking
Gunn jaw w.
w. owl sign
Winograd
W. ingrown nail technique
W. nail plate removal
W. partial matricectomy
W. technique for ingrown nail
Winquist-Hansen
W.-H. classification (0–IV) of
femoral fracture
W.-H. femoral fracture (0-IV)
classification
winter
W. hemivertebrae convex
fusion
W. splint
W. spondylolisthesis reduction
technique
Winter-King-Moe scoliosis
wipe
w. knee test
w. test

W

wire

    w. and drill guide
    Babcock stainless steel w.
    band w.
    bayonet-point w.
    beaded transfixion w.
    bead-loaded w.
    w. bending pliers
    bind w.
    blocking w.
    bone suturing wire chisel-tip w.
    Brooker w.
    Bunnell pullout w.
    calibrated guide w.
    cerclage w.
    chisel-tip w.
    circular w.
    circumferential w.
    Compere fixation w.
    compression w.
    conical-point w.
    w. contour preparation
    w. crimper
    crossed Kirschner w.
    w. cutter
    Dall-Miles cerclage w.
    definitive cerclage w.
    diamond-point wire double-strand w.
    diamond tip w.
    double-looped cerclage w.
    double-stranded wire
      double-twisted w.
    w. drill
    w. driver
    Drummond w.
    encircling w.
    figure-of-8 w.
    w. fixation bolt
    w. frame collar
    w. grip finger splint
    w. grip toe splint
    guide w.
    Ilizarov w.
    interfragmentary w.
    intraosseous w.
    90-90 intraosseous wire Nitinol
      flexible w.
    Isola w.
    K w.
    Kirschner w. (K wire)
    w. knot
    Lengemann w.
    w. loop
    loop circumferential w.
    w. loop fixation
    Luque cerclage w.
    Magnuson w.
    Martin loop circumferential w.
    monofilament w.

    Nitinol flexible w.
    nonthreaded w.
    oblique w.
    olive w.
    Oppenheimer spring w.
    Outrigger w.
    over-tying w.
    w. passage
    w. passer
    w. penetration depth
    percutaneous K w.
    w. prosthesis-crimping forceps
    w. removal technique
    Schauwecker patellar tension band
      w.
    sharp-pointed w.
    small-diameter w.
    smooth transfixion w.
    spinous process w.
    w. stabilization
    stainless steel w.
    stay w.
    sublaminar w.
    w. suture
    temporary cerclage w.
    tension band w.
    threaded w.
    w. tightener
    w. traction bow
    trochanteric w.
    w. twister
    unthreaded w.
    Wisconsin button w.
    Wisconsin interspinous w.
    Wisconsin spinous w.

wire-cutting
    w.-c. forceps
    w.-c. scissors

wire-extracting forceps
wire-fixation buckle
Wire-Foam orthotic
wire-holding forceps
wire-pulling forceps
wire-tightening
    w.-t. clamp
    w.-t. forceps

4-wire trochanter reattachment
wire-twisting forceps
wiring
    cervical oblique facet w.
    circumferential w.
    compression w.
    facet fracture stabilization w.
    facet subluxation stabilization w.
    figure-of-8 w.
    Gallie atlantoaxial w.
    interfacet w.
    interspinous w.
    intraosseous w.

Luque w.
oblique facet w.
posterior interspinous w.
Schauwecker patellar w.
Scott lumbar spondylolysis direct
repair w.
spinous process w.
sublaminar w.
tension-band w.
Wisconsin w.

Wisconsin
W. button
W. button wire
W. interspinous segmental spinal
instrumentation
W. interspinous wire
W. segmental wire fixation through
spinous processes
W. spinal fracture system
W. spinous wire
W. wire fixation
W. wire technique
W. wiring
W. wiring scoliosis repair

Wissinger rod
within functional limits (WFL)
Wixson hip positioner
WMR
wedge matrix resection
WMSD
work-related musculoskeletal disorder
wobble
w. board
Wooden W.
Wohlfart-Kugelberg-Welander disease
wolf
W. arthroscope
W. blade plate ankle arthrodesis
W. full-thickness free graft
W. light source
W. motor function test
Wolfe hand surgery graft
Wolferman drill
Wolff
W. law
W. law of bone structure
wolffii
Acinetobacter w.
Wolin meniscoid lesion of ankle
Wolvek sternal approximator
WOMAC
Western Ontario and McMaster
University
WOMAC osteoarthritis index
women
Selsun Gold for W.
Wonder-Cup heel cup
Wonderflex silicone
Wonder-Spur heel cup

WonderZorb silicone shoe insert
wood
w. probe reflexology device
w. screw
wooden
w. postoperative clog
w. shoe
W. Wobble
Woodend intervertebral disc classification
wooden-soled shoe
Woodpecker total hip broaching system
Woodruff
W. screw
W. screwdriver
W. tip
Woodson
W. elevator
W. probe
Woodward
W. operation
W. release of high-riding scapula
procedure
W. scapula arthroplasty
W. scapula correction procedure
W. scapula correction technique
Woodway treadmill
Woofry-Chandler
W.-C. classification
W.-C. classification of
Osgood-Schlatter lesion
wool
lamb's w.
WORC
Western Ontario Rotator Cuff
WORC index
Woringer-Kolopp disease
work
concentric w.
w. conditioning
eccentric w.
W. Environment Impact Scale
(WEIS)
w. evaluation systems technology
w. hardening
w. hardening exercise
w. hardening program
manual w.
negative w.
physical w.
rhythmic handgrip w.
W. Seat driving simulator
sedentary w.
WorkAbout Carpal Mate wrist support
Worker Role Interview (WRI)
workgroup
National Arthritis Data W.
working
w. orthopaedic surgery film
w. zone

W

WorkMod back support
work-of-fracture
work-related musculoskeletal disorder
  (WMSD)
world
  W. Health Organization (WHO)
  W. Health Organization/International
    League Against Rheumatism
    (WHO/ILAR)
wormian bone
Worth disease
WOSI
  Western Ontario Instability Index
wound
  chronic heel w.
  w. cleanser
  closed w.
  w. closure
  w. closure system
  w. culture
  w. dehiscence
  w. dressing
  foot puncture w.
  w. gel
  gunshot w. (GSW)
  Gustilo classification of puncture w.
  incised w.
  w. irrigation
  joint w.
  w. measuring guide
  open w.
  w. packing
  puncture w.
  stab w.
  traumatic heel w.
  W. VAC
Wound-Evac drain
woven
  w. bone
  w. gastrocnemius aponeurosis
W-plasty
wrap
  Ace w.
  Action elbow w.
  Action wrist w.
  ankleRAP postsurgical wound
    w.
  BodyIce cold pack w.
  boot w.
  Coban elastic w.
  Co-Flex self-adherent w.
  Coopercare Lastrap support w.
  digit w.
  Dura-Kold reusable compression
    ice w.
  Dura-Soft soft-compression reusable
    ice or heat w.
  Elasto-Gel hot/cold therapy w.

Elasto-Gel shoulder therapy w.
Elasto-Link joint w.
Electro-Link joint w.
FoamWrap Final Flexion w.
gauze w.
gel w.
Gelocast Unna boot compression
  w.
Goode w.
Ice Wedge hot/cold therapy w.
joint w.
Kerlix w.
Kold W.
loop-over w.
neck w.
Nylatex w.
orthoRAP backRAP postsurgical
  wound w.
orthoRAP hipRAP postsurgical
  wound w.
orthoRAP kneeRAP w.
orthoRAP postsurgical wound w.
orthoRAP shoulderRAP postsurgical
  wound w.
orthoRAP wristRAP postsurgical
  wound w.
PneuGel ankle w.
PneuGel shoulder w.
Scott wrist w.
snug w.
Sorbothane w.
Stimprene w.
super w.
Thermoskin arthritic knee w.
Thermoskin U wrist w.
Thermosport hot/cold w.
Unna boot w.
Velpeau w.
wraparound
  w. flap bone graft
  w. neurovascular composite free
    tissue transfer
  w. neurovascular free flap
  w. splint
  w. toe transfer
wrapping
  compressive centripetal w.
  nerve w.
  stump w.
wrench
  Allen w.
  beaded-pin w.
  box-end w.
  cannulated w.
  conical nut w.
  Fox w.
  Harrington flat w.
  hex w.

key-lock w.
locknut w.
Mueller w.
open-end w.
w. pin
socket w.
Texas Scottish Rite Hospital w.
T-handled nut w.
T-handled screw w.
Thomas w.
torque w.
TSRH w.
U w.
VDS w.
ventral derotating spinal w.

wrenched knee
wrestler's elbow
WRI
Worker Role Interview
Wright
W. knee prosthesis
W. maneuver
W. Medical bone anchor
W. monoblock titanium implant
W. plate
W. syndrome
W. thoracic outlet test
W. titanium prosthesis
W. Universal brace
Wright-Adson thoracic outlet test
Wrightington Frusto-Conical hip cup and stem system
Wrightlock posterior spinal fixation device
wringer
w. arm
w. injury
wrinkle test
Wrisberg
W. cartilage
W. lesion
W. ligament
ligament of W.
wrist
w. and finger flexor stretch
w. arthroscopy
w. block
w. bone
w. brace
w. capsule
w. contracture
w. creaking
w. curl
w. deformity
w. disarticulation
dorsal arch of w.
w. drop
w. extension

w. extensor
w. extensor strengthening
w. extensor stretch
w. extensor tendinitis
w. extensor tendon
w. first
w. flexion reflex
w. flexion test
w. flexion unit
w. flexor strengthening
w. flexor tendinitis
w. fracture
w. gauntlet
golfer's w.
gymnast's w.
w. hand extension compression support (WHECS)
w. immobilizer
w. instability
w. joint
w. joint implant prosthesis
w. motion
w. motion splint
oarsman's w.
w. pain syndrome
palmar w.
w. rest splint
w. sign
slack w.
w. spasticity
w. speed profile
w. stretch exercise
w. subluxation
sulcus of w.
tilt w.
total arthrodesis of w.
triangular disc of w.
volar w.
wrist-driven
w.-d. flexor hinge orthosis
w.-d. lateral prehension orthosis
w.-d. wrist-hand orthosis
wrist-hand orthosis (WHO)
Wristiciser exerciser
WrisTimer
W. carpal tunnel syndrome support
W. CTS support
W. PM CTS support
WristJack wrist splint
wristlet
elastic w.
Freedom USA w.
writer
Wanchik w.
writer's
w. cramp (WC)
w. paralysis

W

writing
> Children's Handwriting Evaluation Scale for Manuscript W. (CHES-M)
> w. hand

wry neck, wryneck

wryneck (*var. of* wry neck)

WSR
> Westergren sedimentation rate

Wu bunionectomy

Wurzburg
> W. plate
> W. screw

WUSPI
> Wheelchair User's Shoulder Pain Index

Wygesic

Wylie lumbar bulldog clamp

X

X clamp
X plate
X Stop interspinous process
decompression device
X, Y, Z axis
Xact ACL graft-fixation system
X-Act podiatric marker
Xanax
xanthogranuloma
juvenile x.
xanthoma
Achilles tendon x.
fibrous x.
malignant fibrous x.
tuberous x.
xanthomatous giant cell tumor
X-10 Crosslink plate
XDU
Xtra Depth University
Xenophor femoral prosthesis
Xerac
Xercise
X. Band
X. Band exercise device
Xeroform gauze dressing
xerography
xeroradiography, xerography
xerotic
Xertube
XFCS
x-ray fluorescence correlation
spectroscopy
Xia hook system
XIP
x-ray in plaster
xiphisternal joint
xiphodynia syndrome
xiphoid
x. bone
x. cartilage
x. process
x. process of sternum
xiphoiditis
XiScan
X. fluoroscope
X. fluoroscopy
X. mini-C-arm
X. portable fluoroscopic C-arm
XL
Lodine XL
Procardia XL
X-long cement forceps

XLS
Polysorb meniscal stapler XLS
Xomed drill
XOP
x-ray out of plaster
XPand R radiolucent corpectomy
spacer
Xpanse
X. bone insert
X. R bone insert
X. S bone insert
XPE foot orthosis
4XP Tilt System wheelchair
x-ray
artifact on x-r.
dorsal planar x-r.
dorsiflexion stress ankle x-r.
dynamic motion x-r.
FCS x-r.
x-r. fluorescence correlation
spectroscopy (XFCS)
full cervical spine x-r.
Harris-Beath axial hindfoot x-r.
hip-to-ankle x-r.
x-r. in plaster (XIP)
intraoperative x-r.
lateral tilt stress ankle x-r.
nonweightbearing x-r.
x-r. out of plaster (XOP)
x-r. overlay
penciling of ribs on x-r.
x-r. photogrammetry
plantar stress ankle x-r.
x-r. position
postreduction x-r.
sagittal stress x-r.
x-r. series
x-r. sign silver dollar
stress x-r.
x-r. tray
x-r. view
weightbearing x-r.
Xsensibles shoe
X-shaped plate
X-Static silver fiber diabetic
shoe
Xtra
X. Depth University (XDU)
X. Depth University pedorthic
educational facility
XY
frontal plane XY
Xylocaine with epinephrine

X

Y
Y bone plate
Y fracture
Y incision
Y line
Y osteotomy
Y scapular view
Yale brace
Yamada myelotomy knife
Yancey osteotomy
Yankauer suction
Yasargil
Y. elevator
Y. Leyla retractor
Y. Leyla retractor arm
Y. ligature carrier
Y. ligature guide
Y. micro rasp
Y. needle holder
Y. spring hook
Y-axis translatory displacement
Yeager test
year
disability adjusted life y. (DALY)
Yee posterior shoulder approach
yellow
y. cartilage
y. ligament
y. marrow
y. nail syndrome
Yeoman sacroiliac joint test
Yergason
Y. biceps tendon injury sign
Y. bicipital tenosynovitis test
yield strength

Y-knot tying system
Y-nail
Williams interlocking Y-n.
Yochum chiropractic software
yoga
yoked muscle
yoke transposition procedure
Y-osteotomy
young
Y. hinged knee prosthesis
Y. medial approach
Y. modulus
Y. pelvic fracture classification
Youngswick
Y. metatarsal head procedure
Y. osteotomy
Youngswick-Austin metatarsal head procedure
Yount
Y. fasciotomy
Y. gluteal-iliotibial fasciotomy procedure
Y. knee flexion contracture release procedure
Y-shaped
Y-s. incision
Y-s. plate
Y-strap knee immobilizer
Y-T fracture
Yuan screw
yucca wood splint
Yu osteotomy
Y-V
Y-V plasty
Y-V plasty incision

Z
- Z band
- Z bunionectomy
- Z disc
- Z fixation nail
- Z foot
- Z foot deformity
- Z line
- Z pin
- Z retractor

Zachary sensory grade

Zadik
- Z. foot operation
- Z. foot procedure
- Z. total matricectomy
- Z. total nail bed ablation

Zahn
- line of Z.

Zaias nail biopsy

Zanca acromioclavicular joint view

Zancolli
- Z. biceps tendon rerouting
- Z. biceps tendon rerouting technique
- Z. biceps tendon transfer procedure
- Z. capsuloplasty
- Z. clawhand deformity procedure
- Z. flexion capsulodesis
- Z. lasso procedure
- Z. procedure for clawhand deformity
- Z. upper limb reconstruction

Zang
- Z. metatarsal cap
- Z. metatarsal cap implant

Zarins-Rowe
- Z.-R. ACL reconstruction technique
- Z.-R. semitendinosus and iliotibial band knee repair procedure

Zarontin

Zeasorb-AF powder

zebra body myopathy

Zefazone

Zeichner implant

Zeier transfer technique

Zelicof orthopaedic awl

Zel-X

zenith
- Z. chiropractic table
- Z. Electrotherapy ultrasound system
- Z. Hylo table
- Z. stationary table
- Z. Thompson table
- Z. VertiLift table

Zenith-Cox flexion/distraction table

Zenker
- Z. degeneration
- Z. necrosis

Zephir anterior cervical plate system

Zickel
- Z. fracture
- Z. fracture classification
- Z. fracture classification system
- Z. medullary apparatus
- Z. nail fixation
- Z. nailing
- Z. rod
- Z. subcondylar nail
- Z. subtrochanteric fracture fixation
- Z. subtrochanteric fracture operation
- Z. subtrochanteric nail
- Z. supracondylar device
- Z. supracondylar fixation apparatus
- Z. supracondylar medullary nail

zidovudine-induced myopathy

Ziehen-Oppenheim
- Z.-O. disease
- Z.-O. syndrome

Zielke
- Z. bifid hook
- Z. derotator bar
- Z. distraction device
- Z. gouge
- Z. instrumentation for scoliosis spinal fusion
- Z. pedicular instrumentation
- Z. rod
- Z. technique

zigzag
- z. approach
- z. compensatory deformity
- z. finger incision

Zimaloy
- Z. femoral head prosthesis
- Z. implant metal
- Z. implant metal prosthesis
- Z. staple

Zimeldine

Zimfoam
- Z. head halter
- Z. pad
- Z. pin
- Z. splint
- Z. splint traction

Zimmer
- Z. airplane splint
- Z. anatomic hip system
- Z. antiembolism stockings
- Z. bone cement
- Z. bone stem

Zimmer (*continued*)
- Z. cartilage clamp
- Z. chuck
- Z. clavicular cross splint
- Z. collarless polished taper hip system
- Z. compression hip screw
- Z. continuous anatomical passive exerciser
- Z. CPT 12/14 hip system
- Z. crossover instrumentation system
- Z. dermatome
- Z. extractor
- Z. femoral canal broach
- Z. femoral condyle blade-plate
- Z. fracture frame
- Z. goniometer
- Z. gouge
- Z. hand drill
- Z. head halter
- Z. hip implant system
- Z. hip prosthesis
- Z. impaction screw-plate
- Z. knee immobilizer
- Z. laminectomy frame
- Z. low-viscosity adhesive
- Z. low-viscosity cement
- Z. microsaw
- Z. minimally invasive solutions hip procedure
- Z. MIS 2-incision posterior hip
- Z. NexGen LPS knee femoral component
- Z. orthopaedic device
- Z. oscillating saw
- Z. pin
- Z. PMMA precoat process
- Z. postoperative shoe
- Z. protractor
- Z. Pulsavac wound débridement system
- Z. reamer brace
- Z. rotary bur
- Z. screwdriver
- Z. shoulder prosthesis
- Z. side plate
- Z. skin graft mesher
- Z. snare
- Z. Statak anchor
- Z. telescoping nail
- Z. tharies surface arthroplasty system
- Z. tibial bolt
- Z. tibial nail cap
- Z. tibial prosthesis
- Z. unicompartmental high-flex knee system
- Z. universal drill

- Z. walker
- Z. Y plate

Zimmer-Gigli saw blade
Zimmer-Hall drive system
Zimmer-Hoen forceps
Zimmer-Hudson shank
Zimmer-Kirschner hand drill
Zimmerlin atrophy
Zimmerman pericyte
Zimmer-Schlesinger forceps
Zim-Trac
- Z.-T. traction splint
- Z.-T. traction splint tractor

Zinacef injection
zinc (Zn)
- Dermagran wound cleanser with z.
- z. supplementation

Zinco
- Z. Air Cam brace
- Z. ankle orthosis
- Z. Cam Walker II brace
- Z. Castaway II brace
- Z. Hi-Top brace

zipper cast
Zippie
- Z. P500 wheelchair
- Z. 2 wheelchair

zirconia
- z. femoral head prosthesis
- z. orthopaedic prosthesis
- z. orthopaedic prosthetic head

zirconium (Zr)
- z. oxide arthroplasty material
- z. oxide ceramic prosthesis
- oxidized z.

Z-lengthening
- Achilles tendon Z-l.
- Z-l. of biceps tendon

ZMC
- zygomatic-malar complex
- ZMC fracture

ZMR hip system
ZMS intramedullary fixation system
Zn
- zinc

Zohar shoe
Zolicef
Zollinger
- Z. legholder
- Z. splint

Zollner rasp
Zoloft
zolpidem
zona
- z. dermatica
- z. epithelioserosa

zonal
- z. fifth metatarsal classification
- z. sclerosis

Zonas porous tape
zone
    autonomous z.
    bilaminar z.
    cornuradicular z.
    cut-back z.
    dorsal root entry z. (DREZ)
    elastic z.
    endplate z.
    z. (1–3) fifth metatarsal fracture
      classification
    fracture z.
    growth z.
    Gruen z.
    hyperintense z.
    hypertrophic z.
    isolated z.
    Kambin triangular working z.
    Lissauer z.
    Looser z.
    maturation z.
    neutral z.
    z. of Ranvier
    orbicular z.
    paraphysiologic z.
    peripolar z.
    polar z.
    proliferating z.
    red-red meniscal z.
    red-white meniscal z.
    resting z.
    Z. Specific II meniscal repair
      system
    thoracolumbar junction
      transitional z.
    triangular working z.
    Trümmerfeld z.
    Umbau z.
    working z.
zone-specific cannula
zonography
Zoradol
Zorbacel shock-absorbing material
Zoroc plaster
ZORprin
Z-osteotomy
    inverted scarf Z-o.
Zostrix
Zostrix-HP
Z-plasty
    Z-p. approach
    Broadbent-Woolf 4-limb Z-p.
    Cozen-Brockway Z-p.
    double-opposing Z-p.
    4-flap Z-p.
    frontal plane Z-p.
    Gudas scarf Z-p.

    Z-p. incision
    4-limb Z-p.
    Z-p. local flap graft
    Peet Z-p.
    Z-p. release
    scarf Z-p.
    sliding Z-p.
    Z-p. tenotomy
Zr
    zirconium
Z-score of bone mineral density
Z-shaped plate
Z-slide
    Z-s. lengthening
    Z-s. lengthening in hallux
      limitus
Z-stent prosthesis
Z-step cut
Z-Stim
ZTT
    ZTT acetabular cup
    ZTT (I, II) acetabular cup
      prosthesis
    ZTT (I, II) cup
Zuckerkandl dehiscence
Zucker splint
Zuelzer
    Z. awl
    Z. hook
    Z. hook plate
    Z. screw
Zuma thoracolumbar fusion interbody
VBR
Zuni
    Z. exercise system
    Z. gym
    Z. harness
Zweymüller
    Z. cementless hip prosthesis
    Z. hip system
Zwipp
    Z. fracture classification
    Z. subtalar joint instability
      measurement
Zydone
zygapophyseal (*var. of* zygapophysial)
zygapophysial, zygapophyseal
    z. arthrology
    z. articulation
    z. joint
    z. joint injection
zygodactyly
zygomatic bone
zygomatic-malar complex (ZMC)
Zyloprim
Zymderm collagen implant
Zyranox femoral head

Z

Contents: The Appendices

Appendix 1

Anatomical Illustrations

Anatomic Planes

Frontal (coronal) plane: A vertical plane at right angles to a sagittal plane, dividing the body into anterior and posterior portions, or any plane parallel to the central coronal plane.

Longitudinal plane: Running lengthwise; in the direction of the long axis of the body or any of its parts.

Median (midsagittal) plane: A plane vertical in the anatomic position, through the midline of the body that divides the body into right and left halves.

Sagittal plane: Plane parallel to the median plane; sagittal planes are vertical planes in the anatomic position.

Subcostal plane: A transverse plane passing through the inferior limits of the costal margin, i.e., the 10th costal cartilages; it marks the boundary between the hypochondriac and epigastric regions superiorly and the lateral and umbilical regions inferiorly.

Transpyloric plane: A transverse plane midway between the superior margins of the manubrium sterni and the symphysis pubis; the pylorus may be located on this plane in the supine or prone positions, but in the erect (anatomic) position it descends to a lower level.

Transverse plane: A plane across the body at right angles to the coronal and sagittal planes; transverse planes are perpendicular to the long axis of the body or limbs, regardless of the position of the body or limb; in the anatomic position, transverse planes are horizontal planes; otherwise the two terms are not synonymous.

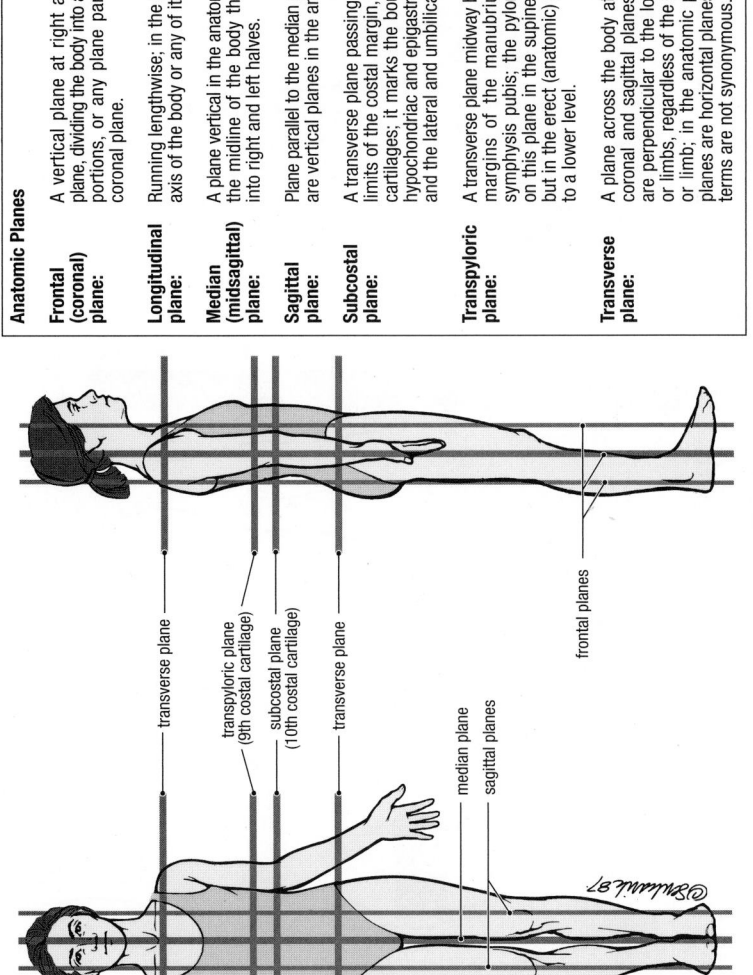

transverse plane

transpyloric plane (9th costal cartilage)

subcostal plane (10th costal cartilage)

transverse plane

frontal planes

median plane

sagittal planes

terms of relationship: anatomic planes

A1

Anterior: The front surface of the body; often used to indicate the position of one structure relative to another, i.e., situated nearer the front part of the body.

Posterior: The back surface of the body; often used to indicate the position of one structure relative to another, i.e., nearer the back of the body.

Proximal: Nearest the trunk or the point of origin; said of part of a limb, of an artery or a nerve, etc., so situated.

Distal: Situated away from the center of the body, or from the point of origin; specifically applied to the extremity or distant part of a limb or organ.

Medial: Relating to the middle or center; nearer to the median or midsagittal plane.

Lateral: Farther from the median or midsagittal plane.

Superior: Situated nearer the vertex of the head in relation to a specific reference point.

Inferior: Situated nearer the soles of the feet in relation to a specific reference point.

terms of relationship: body part terminology

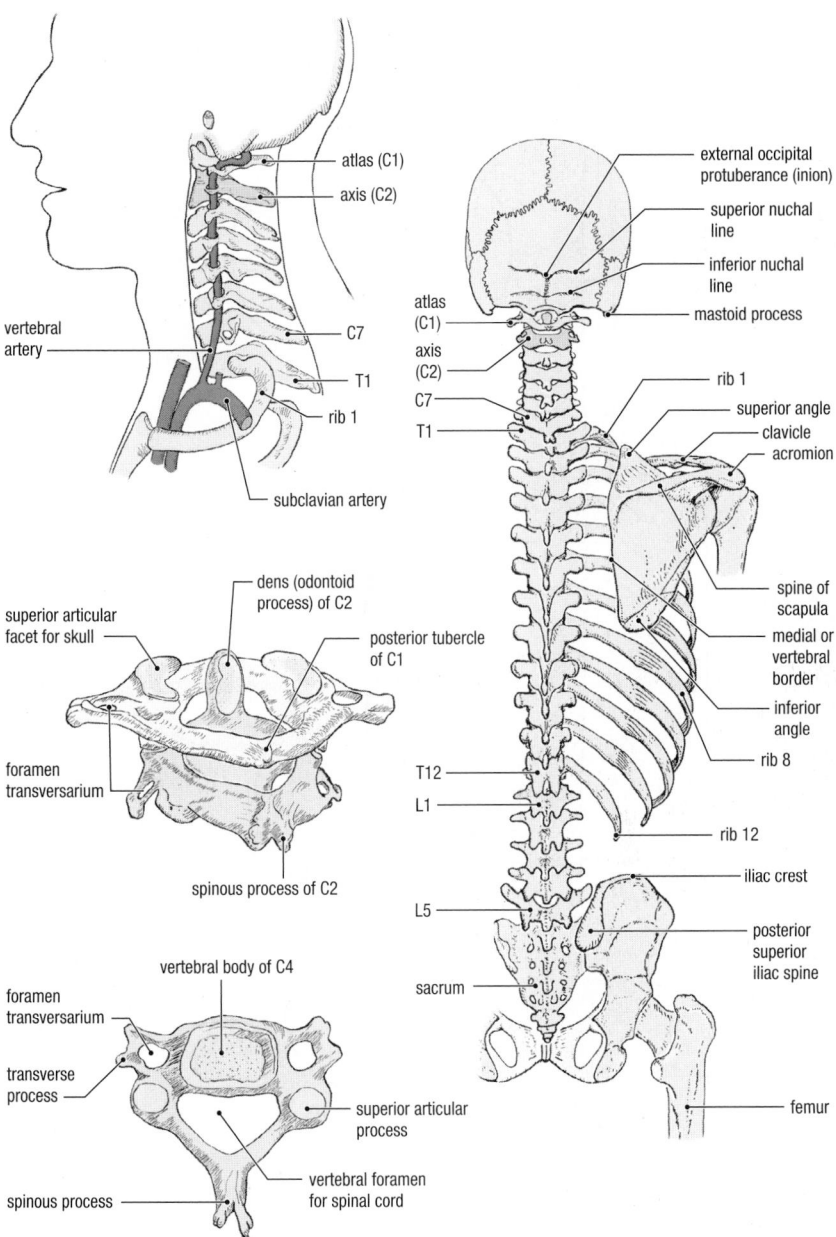

bony landmarks of the back and vertebral column

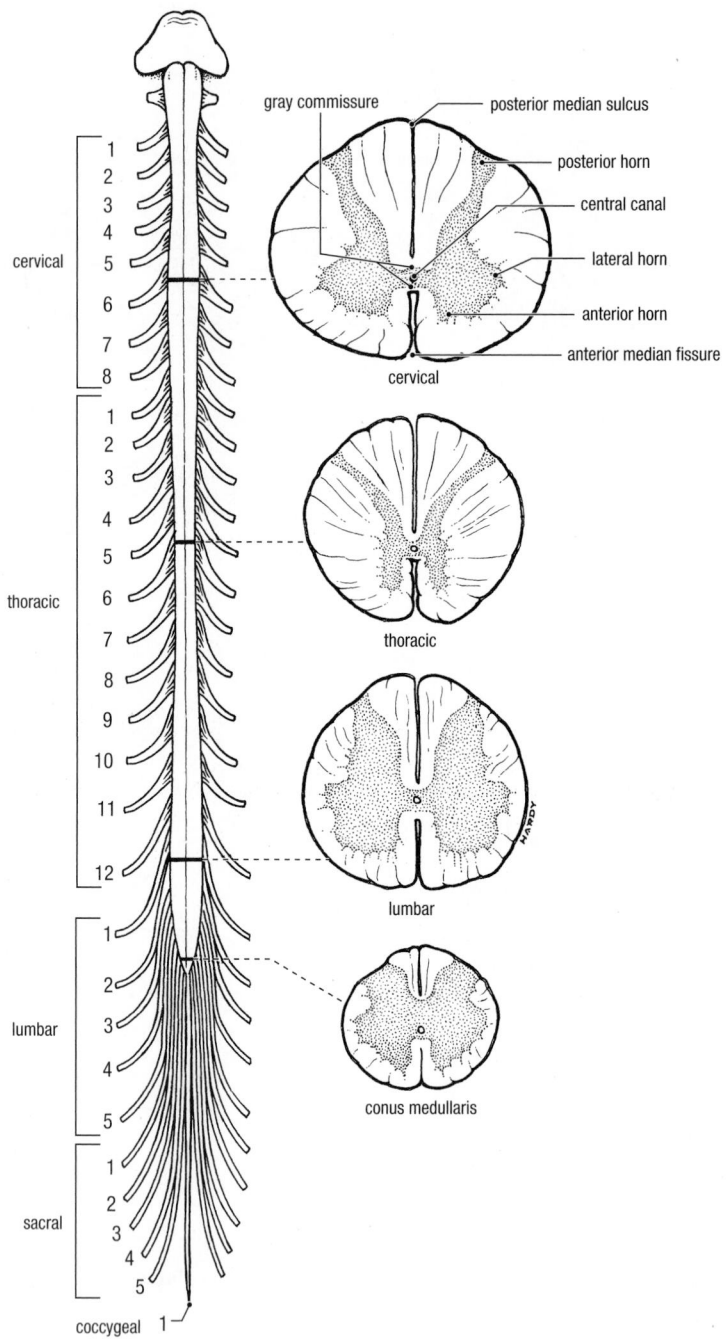

spinal cord showing cross-sections at various levels

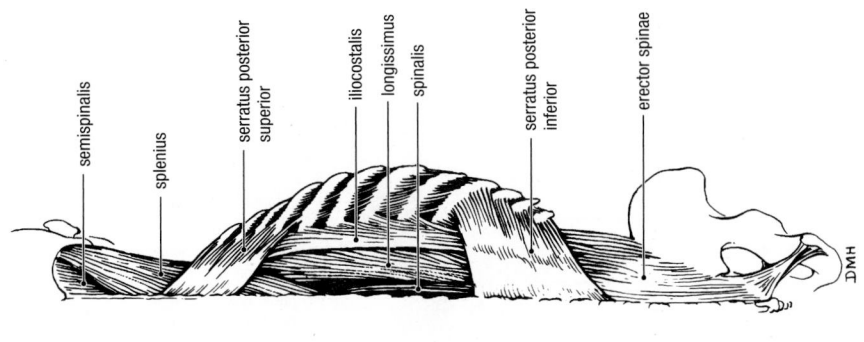

semispinalis
splenius
serratus posterior superior
iliocostalis
longissimus
spinalis
serratus posterior inferior
erector spinae

DMH

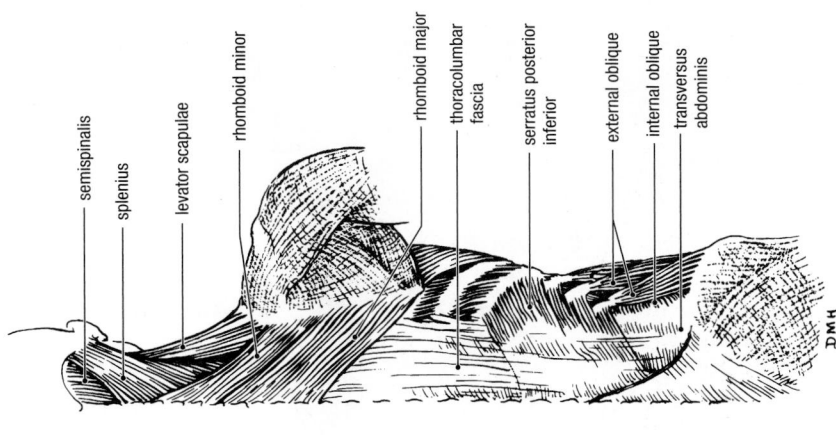

semispinalis
splenius
levator scapulae
rhomboid minor
rhomboid major
thoracolumbar fascia
serratus posterior inferior
external oblique
internal oblique
transversus abdominis

DMH

extrinsic and intrinsic muscles of the back

sternocleidomastoid
splenius
levator scapulae
trapezius
rhomboid major
latissimus dorsi
external oblique

D.M. Hutchinson

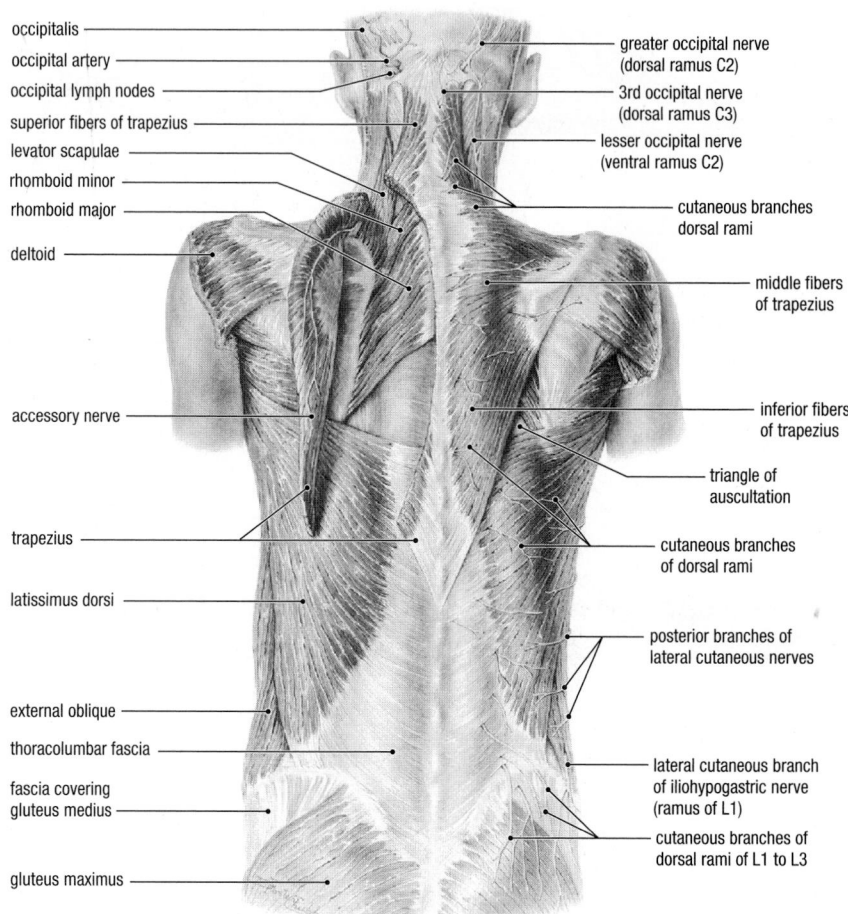

occipitalis

occipital artery

occipital lymph nodes

superior fibers of trapezius

levator scapulae

rhomboid minor

rhomboid major

deltoid

accessory nerve

trapezius

latissimus dorsi

external oblique

thoracolumbar fascia

fascia covering
gluteus medius

gluteus maximus

greater occipital nerve
(dorsal ramus C2)

3rd occipital nerve
(dorsal ramus C3)

lesser occipital nerve
(ventral ramus C2)

cutaneous branches
dorsal rami

middle fibers
of trapezius

inferior fibers
of trapezius

triangle of
auscultation

cutaneous branches
of dorsal rami

posterior branches of
lateral cutaneous nerves

lateral cutaneous branch
of iliohypogastric nerve
(ramus of L1)

cutaneous branches of
dorsal rami of L1 to L3

superficial muscles of the back, posterior view

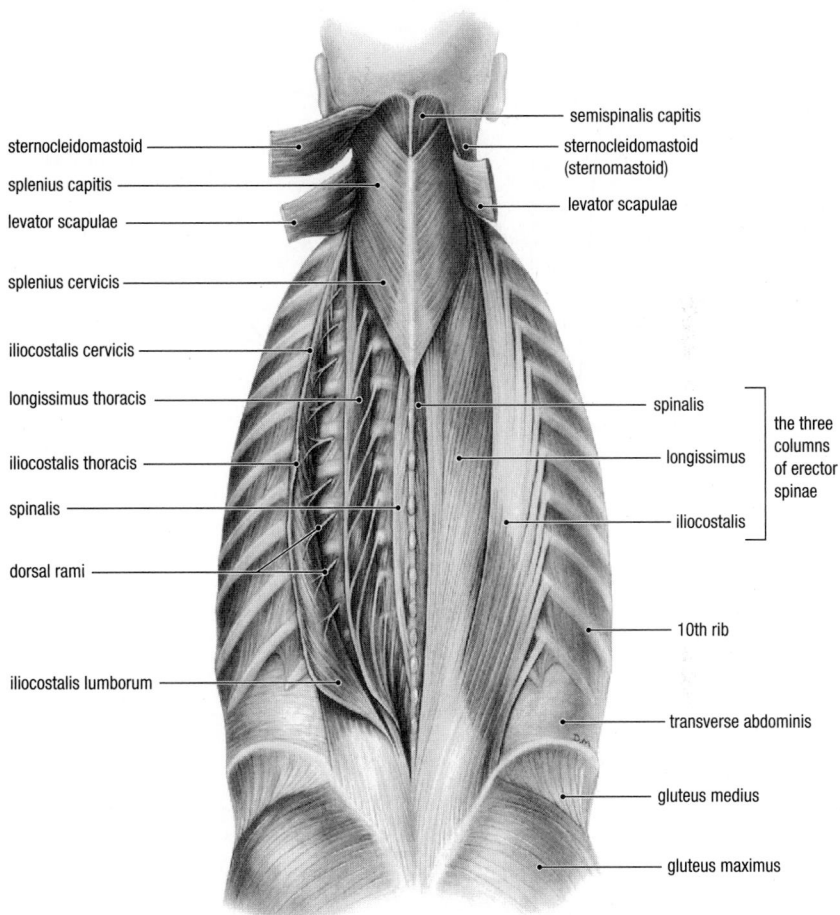

sternocleidomastoid

splenius capitis

levator scapulae

splenius cervicis

iliocostalis cervicis

longissimus thoracis

iliocostalis thoracis

spinalis

dorsal rami

iliocostalis lumborum

semispinalis capitis

sternocleidomastoid
(sternomastoid)

levator scapulae

spinalis

longissimus

iliocostalis

the three
columns
of erector
spinae

10th rib

transverse abdominis

gluteus medius

gluteus maximus

deep muscles of the back, posterior view

Appendix 1

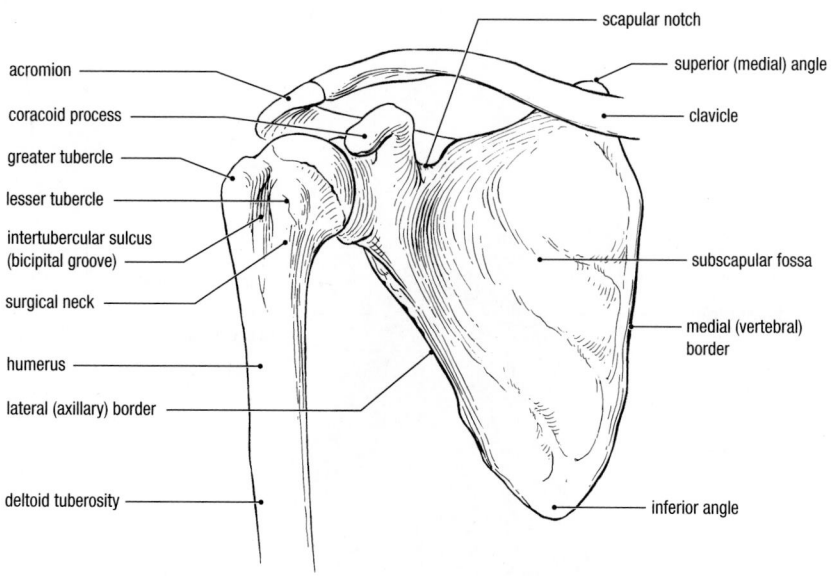

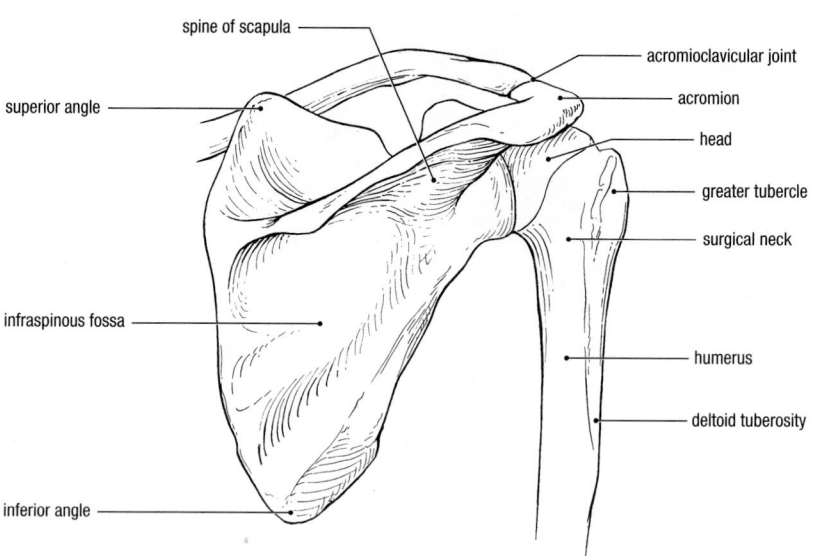

pectoral girdle and humerus: (top) anterior view; (bottom) posterior view

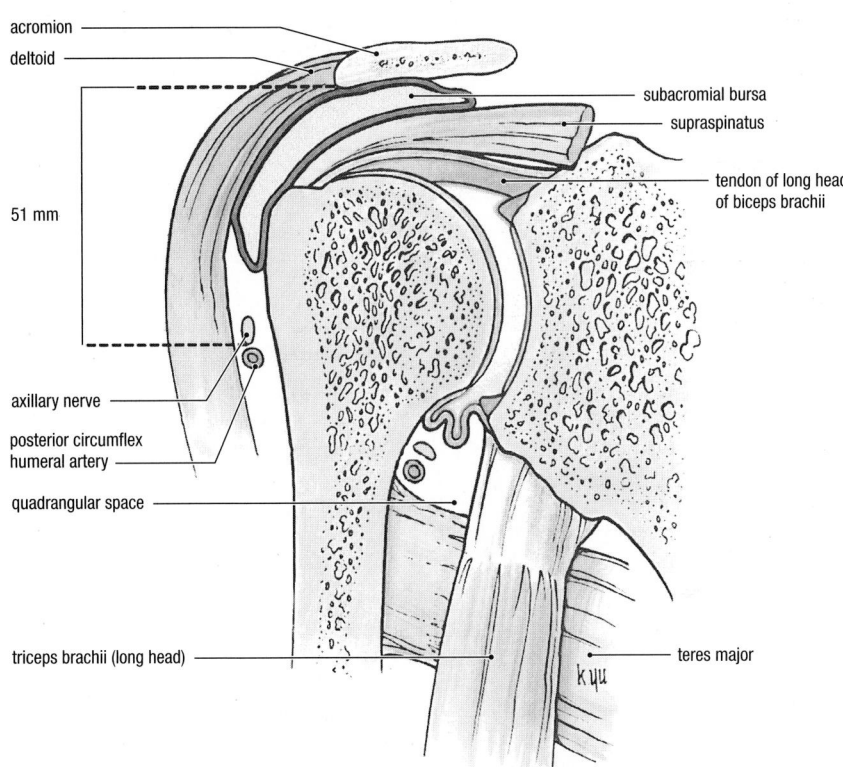

acromion

deltoid

subacromial bursa

supraspinatus

tendon of long head
of biceps brachii

51 mm

axillary nerve

posterior circumflex
humeral artery

quadrangular space

triceps brachii (long head)

teres major

coronal section of the shoulder joint, posterior view

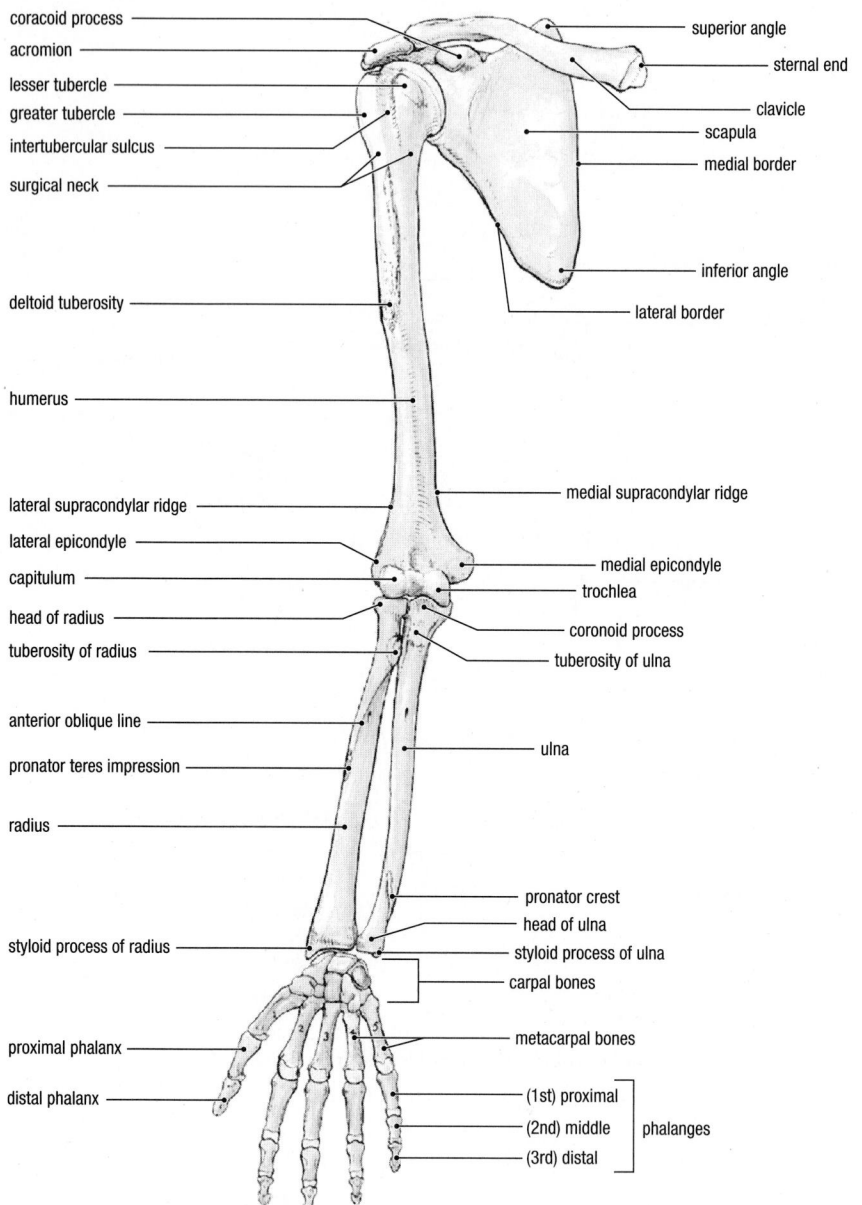

coracoid process — superior angle
acromion — sternal end
lesser tubercle — clavicle
greater tubercle — scapula
intertubercular sulcus — medial border
surgical neck —

deltoid tuberosity — inferior angle
lateral border

humerus —

lateral supracondylar ridge — medial supracondylar ridge
lateral epicondyle — medial epicondyle
capitulum — trochlea
head of radius — coronoid process
tuberosity of radius — tuberosity of ulna

anterior oblique line — ulna
pronator teres impression —

radius —

pronator crest
head of ulna
styloid process of radius — styloid process of ulna
carpal bones

proximal phalanx — metacarpal bones

distal phalanx — (1st) proximal
(2nd) middle   phalanges
(3rd) distal

bones of the upper limb, anterior view

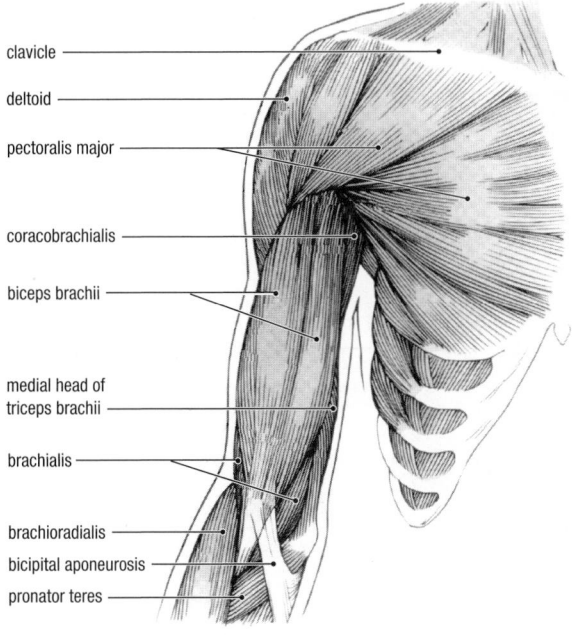

clavicle
deltoid
pectoralis major
coracobrachialis
biceps brachii
medial head of triceps brachii
brachialis
brachioradialis
bicipital aponeurosis
pronator teres

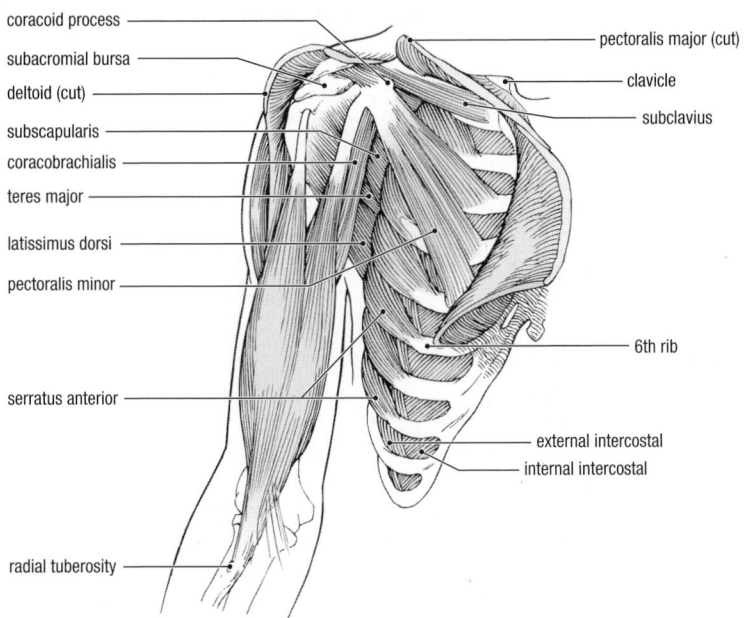

coracoid process
subacromial bursa
deltoid (cut)
subscapularis
coracobrachialis
teres major
latissimus dorsi
pectoralis minor
serratus anterior
radial tuberosity

pectoralis major (cut)
clavicle
subclavius
6th rib
external intercostal
internal intercostal

superficial (top) and deep (bottom) muscles of the shoulder and chest

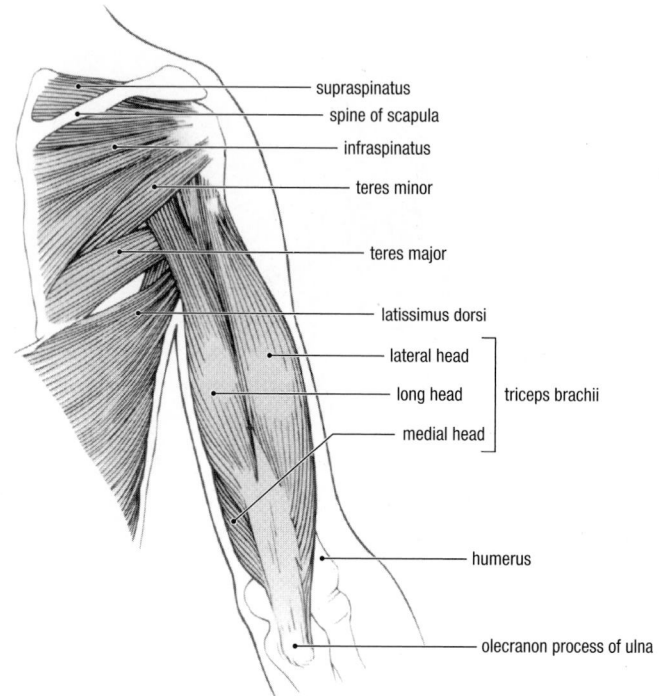

muscles of the arm, posterior view

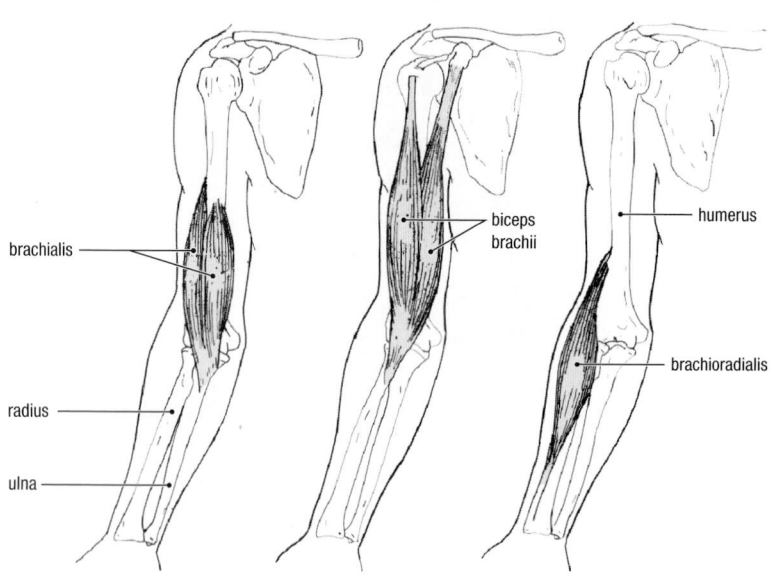

muscles of the arm, anterior view

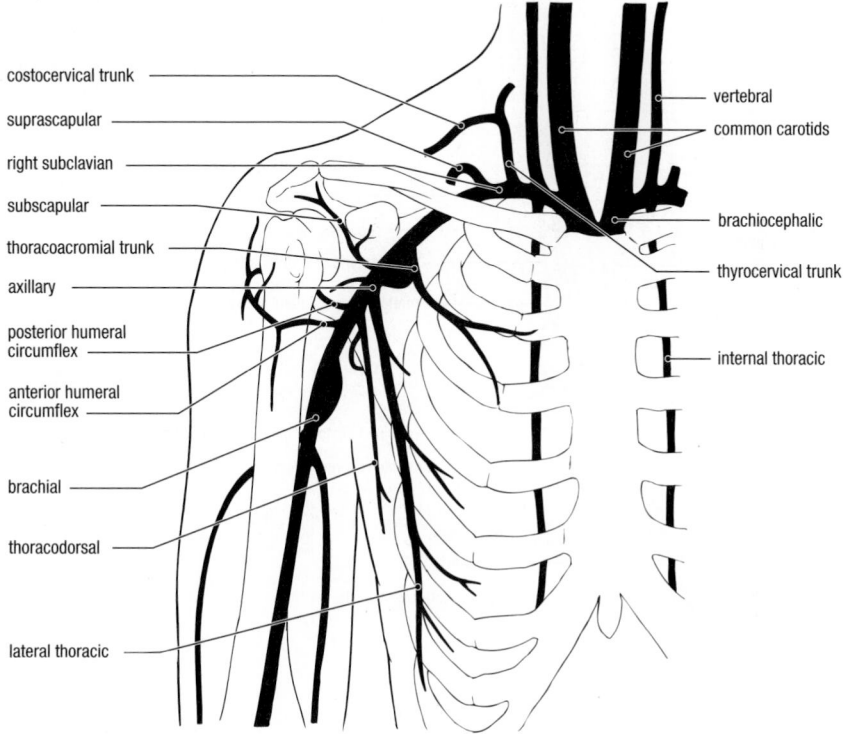

costocervical trunk

suprascapular

right subclavian

subscapular

thoracoacromial trunk

axillary

posterior humeral
circumflex

anterior humeral
circumflex

brachial

thoracodorsal

lateral thoracic

vertebral

common carotids

brachiocephalic

thyrocervical trunk

internal thoracic

blood supply to the shoulder

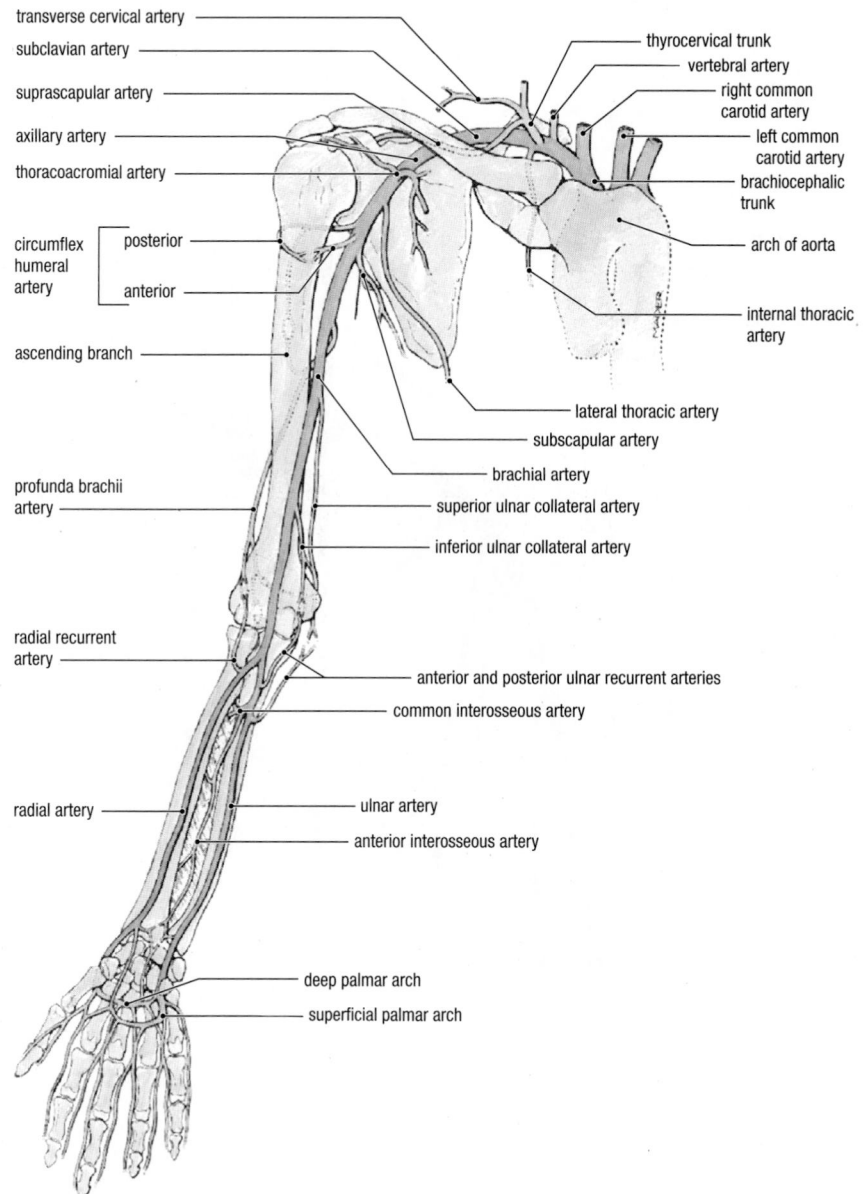

transverse cervical artery

subclavian artery

suprascapular artery

axillary artery

thoracoacromial artery

circumflex humeral artery
— posterior
— anterior

ascending branch

profunda brachii artery

radial recurrent artery

radial artery

thyrocervical trunk

vertebral artery

right common carotid artery

left common carotid artery

brachiocephalic trunk

arch of aorta

internal thoracic artery

lateral thoracic artery

subscapular artery

brachial artery

superior ulnar collateral artery

inferior ulnar collateral artery

anterior and posterior ulnar recurrent arteries

common interosseous artery

ulnar artery

anterior interosseous artery

deep palmar arch

superficial palmar arch

arteries of the upper limb, anterior view

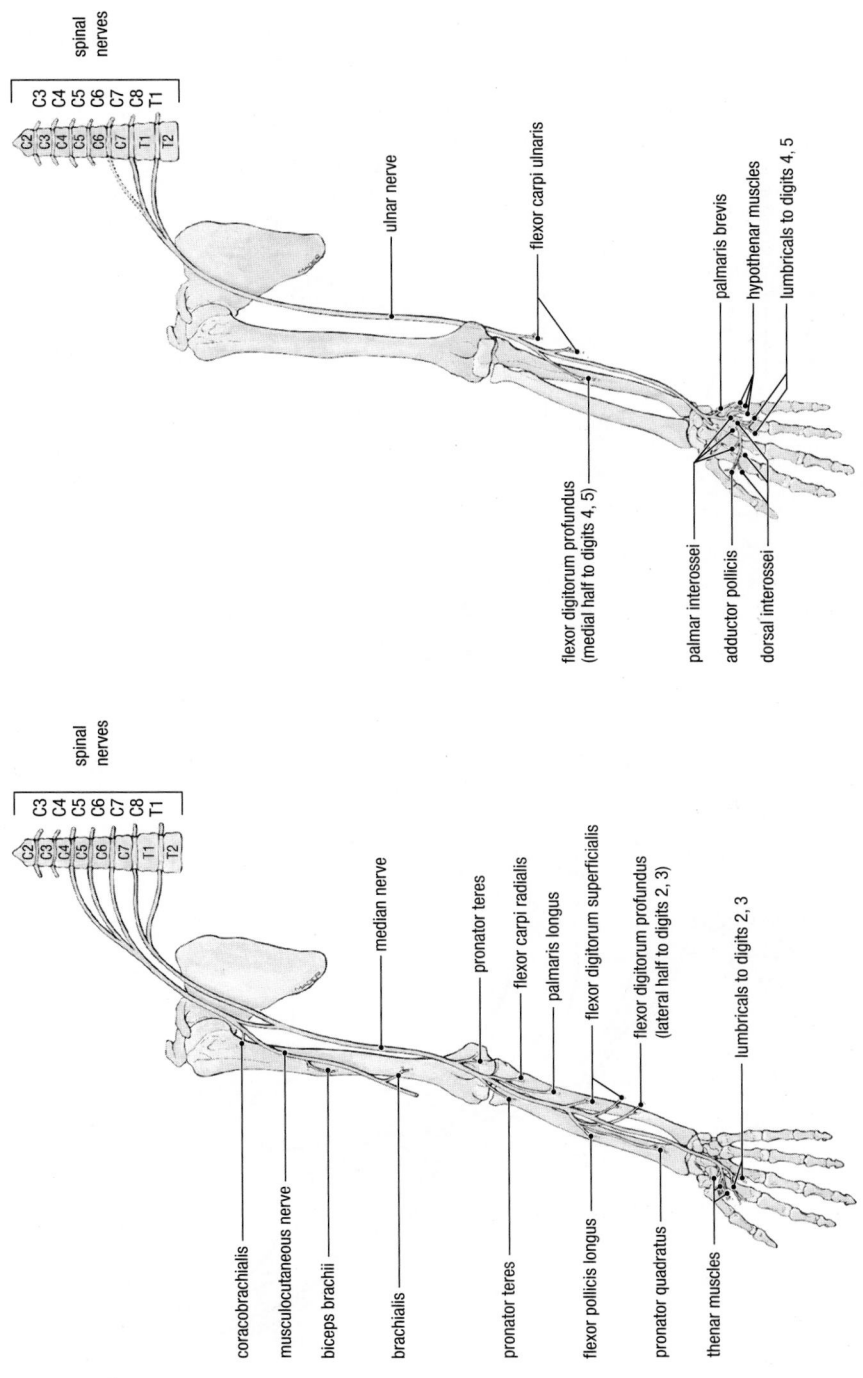

nerves that innervate the muscles of the upper limb: (left) median and musculocutaneous; (right) ulnar nerve

spinal nerves

C3 C4 C5 C6 C7 C8 T1

C2 C3 C4 C5 C6 C7 T1 T2

ulnar nerve

flexor carpi ulnaris

flexor digitorum profundus (medial half to digits 4, 5)

palmaris brevis

hypothenar muscles

lumbricals to digits 4, 5

palmar interossei

adductor pollicis

dorsal interossei

spinal nerves

C3 C4 C5 C6 C7 C8 T1

C2 C3 C4 C5 C6 C7 T1 T2

median nerve

pronator teres

flexor carpi radialis

palmaris longus

flexor digitorum superficialis

flexor digitorum profundus (lateral half to digits 2, 3)

lumbricals to digits 2, 3

coracobrachialis

musculocutaneous nerve

biceps brachii

brachialis

pronator teres

flexor pollicis longus

pronator quadratus

thenar muscles

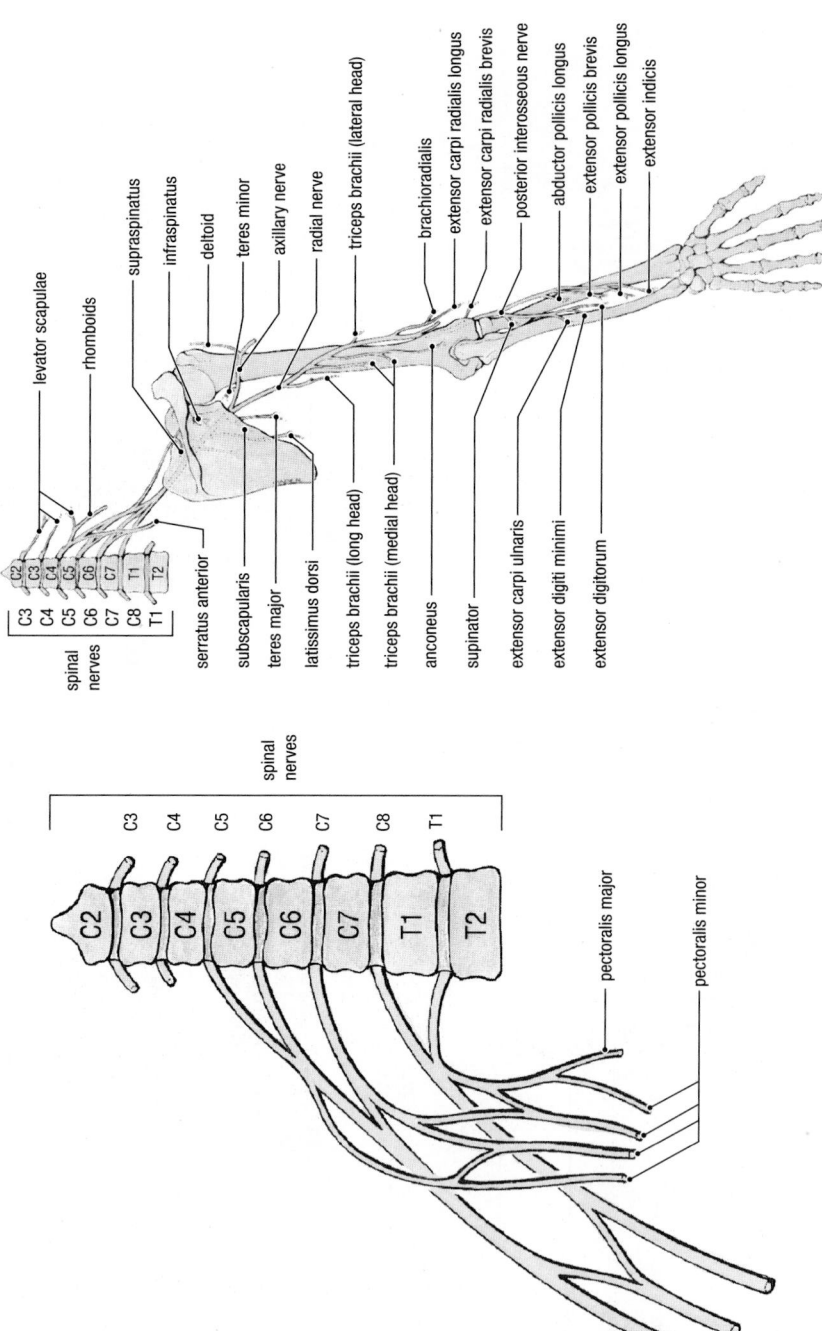

nerves that innervate the muscles of the upper limb: (left) medial and lateral pectoral nerves; (right) radial nerve

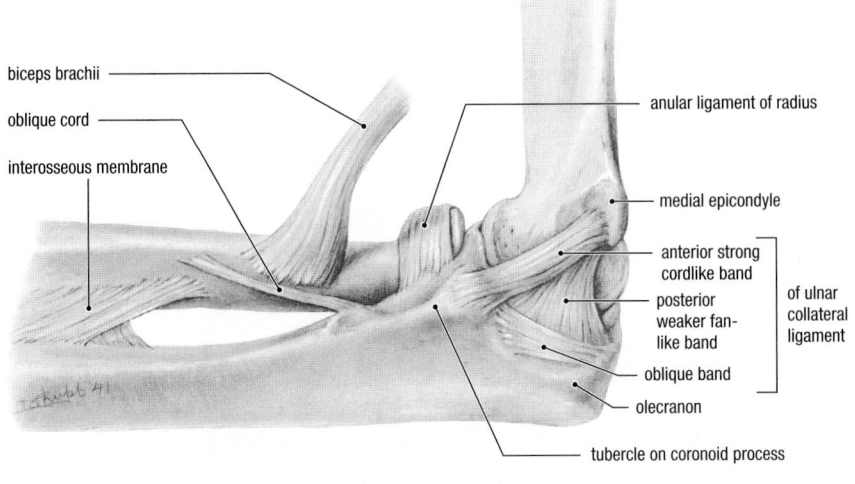

biceps brachii

oblique cord

interosseous membrane

anular ligament of radius

medial epicondyle

anterior strong cordlike band

posterior weaker fan-like band

of ulnar collateral ligament

oblique band

olecranon

tubercle on coronoid process

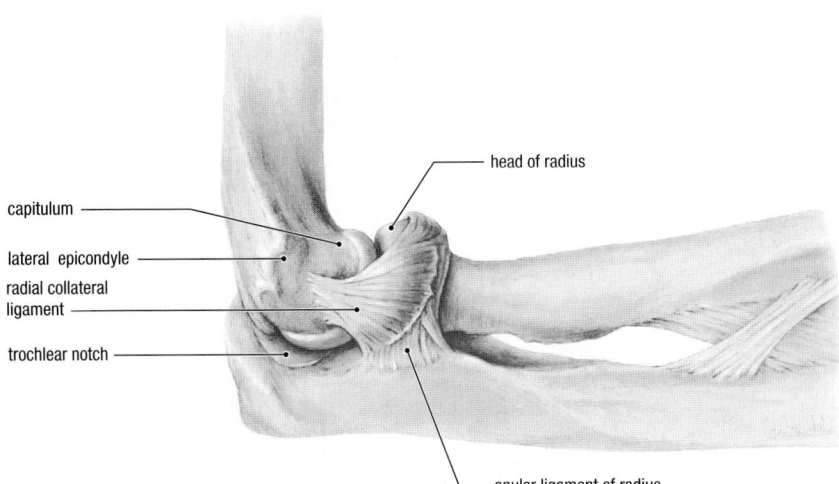

head of radius

capitulum

lateral epicondyle

radial collateral ligament

trochlear notch

anular ligament of radius

collateral ligaments of the elbow: (top) medial view; (bottom) lateral view

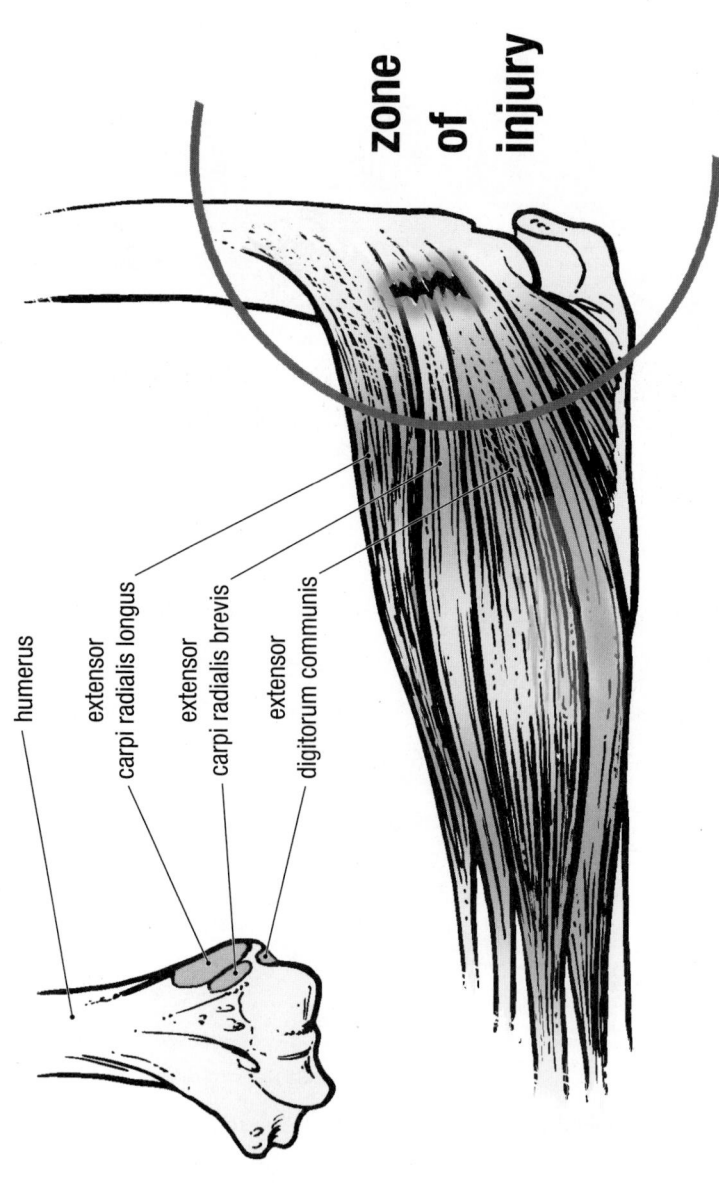

tennis elbow release: the forearm extensor muscles originate as a conjoined tendon from the lateral epicondyle of the elbow; note critical zone of injury

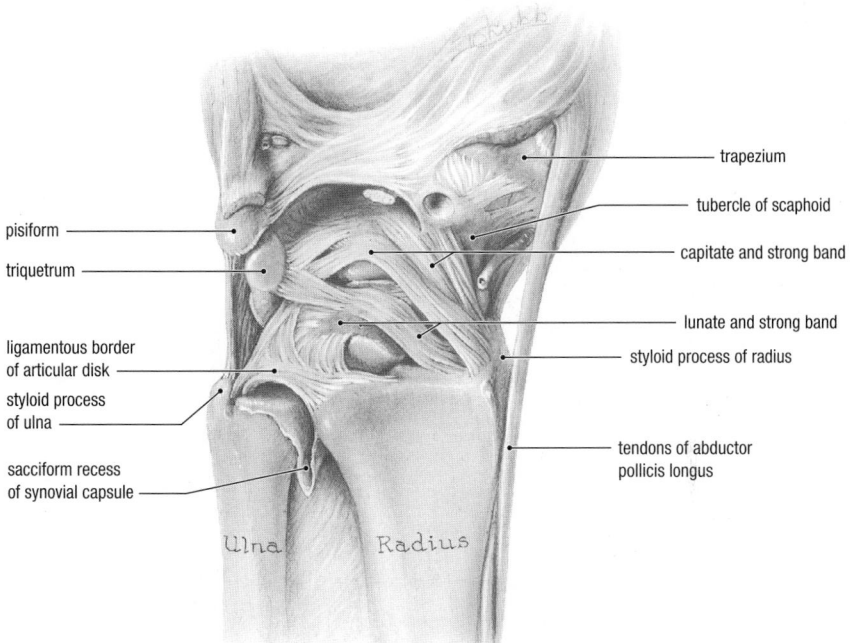

pisiform

triquetrum

ligamentous border
of articular disk

styloid process
of ulna

sacciform recess
of synovial capsule

trapezium

tubercle of scaphoid

capitate and strong band

lunate and strong band

styloid process of radius

tendons of abductor
pollicis longus

Ulna

Radius

ligaments of the distal radioulnar, radiocarpal, and intercarpal joints

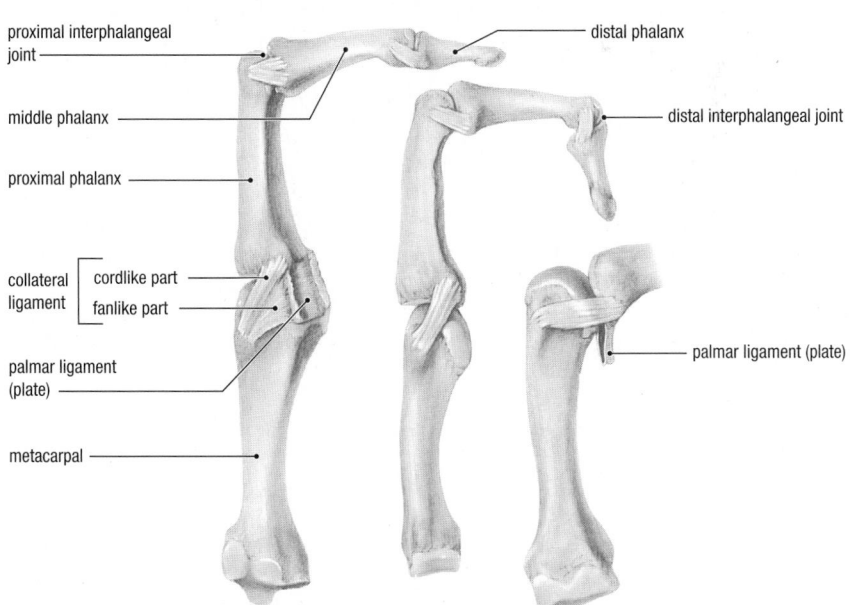

proximal interphalangeal
joint

middle phalanx

proximal phalanx

collateral | cordlike part
ligament | fanlike part

palmar ligament
(plate)

metacarpal

distal phalanx

distal interphalangeal joint

palmar ligament (plate)

ligaments of metacarpophalangeal and interphalangeal joints

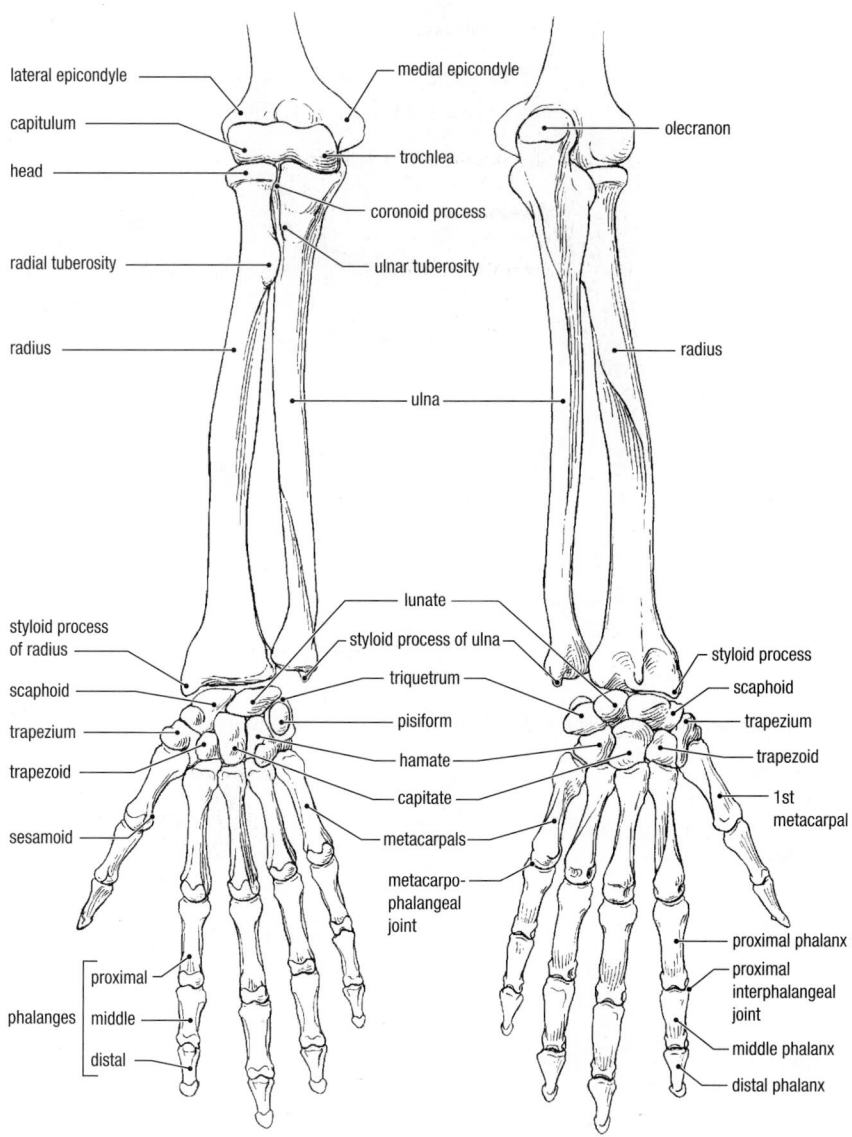

bones of the forearm and hand: (left) anterior view; (right) posterior view

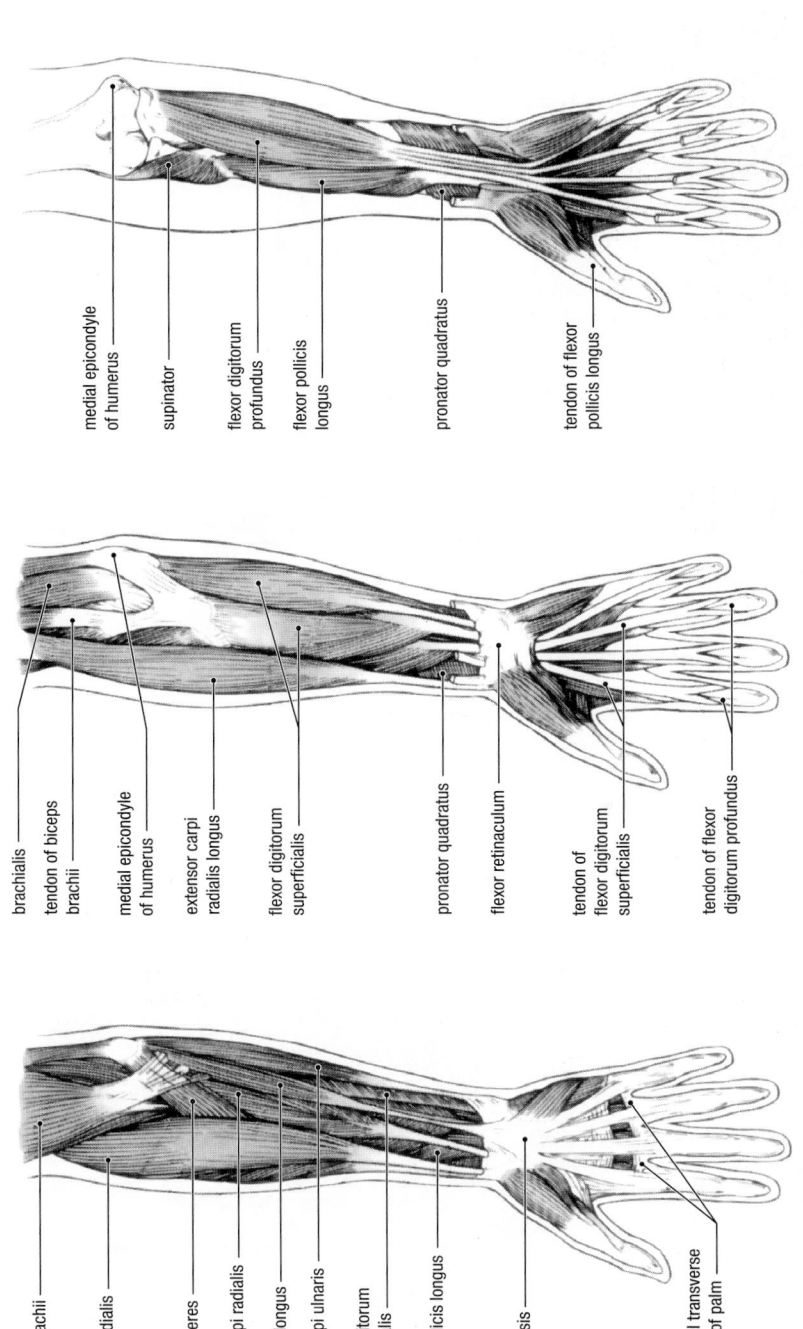

muscles of the wrist and hand, anterior view: (left) superficial; (middle) mid-level; (right) deep

medial epicondyle of humerus

supinator

flexor digitorum profundus

flexor pollicis longus

pronator quadratus

tendon of flexor pollicis longus

brachialis

tendon of biceps brachii

medial epicondyle of humerus

extensor carpi radialis longus

flexor digitorum superficialis

pronator quadratus

flexor retinaculum

tendon of flexor digitorum superficialis

tendon of flexor digitorum profundus

biceps brachii

brachioradialis

pronator teres

flexor carpi radialis

palmaris longus

flexor carpi ulnaris

flexor digitorum superficialis

flexor pollicis longus

palmar aponeurosis

superficial transverse ligament of palm

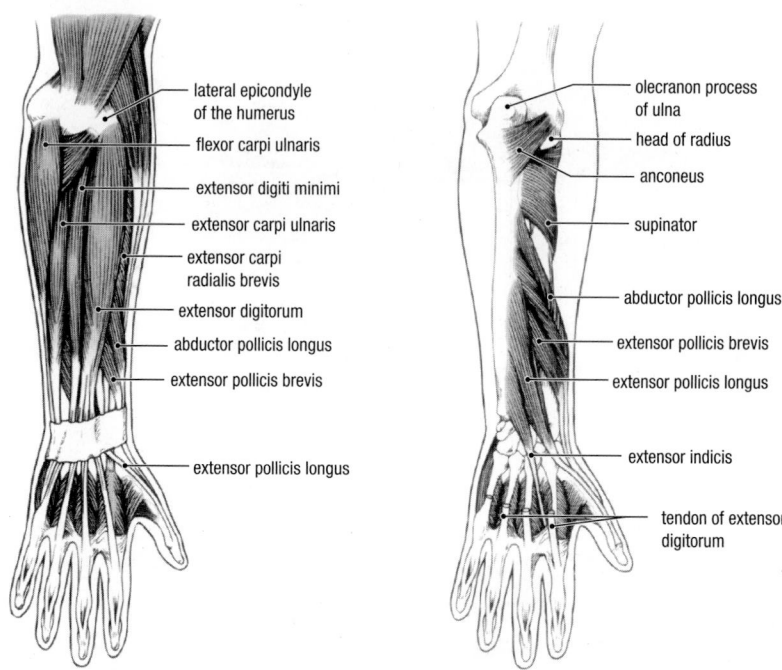

- lateral epicondyle of the humerus
- flexor carpi ulnaris
- extensor digiti minimi
- extensor carpi ulnaris
- extensor carpi radialis brevis
- extensor digitorum
- abductor pollicis longus
- extensor pollicis brevis
- extensor pollicis longus

- olecranon process of ulna
- head of radius
- anconeus
- supinator
- abductor pollicis longus
- extensor pollicis brevis
- extensor pollicis longus
- extensor indicis
- tendon of extensor digitorum

muscles of the wrist and hand, posterior view: (left) superficial; (right) deep

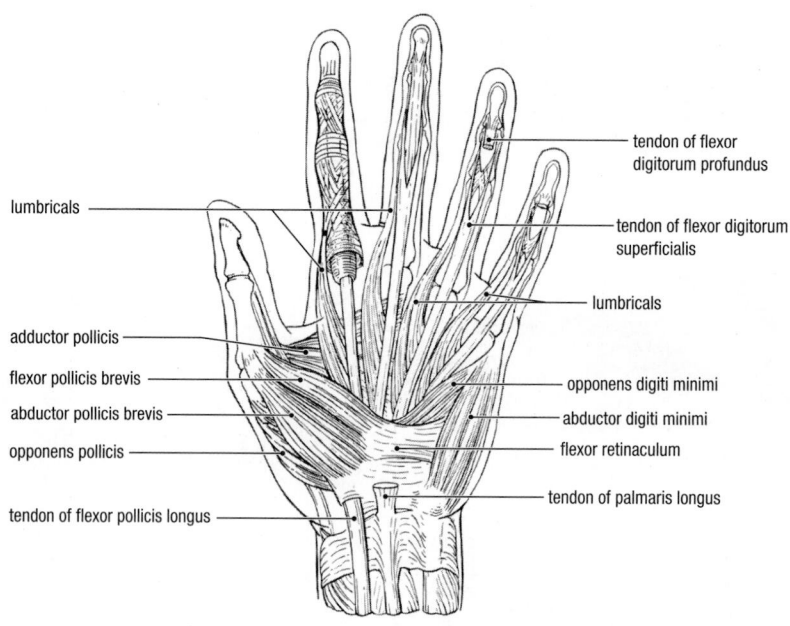

- lumbricals
- adductor pollicis
- flexor pollicis brevis
- abductor pollicis brevis
- opponens pollicis
- tendon of flexor pollicis longus

- tendon of flexor digitorum profundus
- tendon of flexor digitorum superficialis
- lumbricals
- opponens digiti minimi
- abductor digiti minimi
- flexor retinaculum
- tendon of palmaris longus

muscles of the hand, anterior (palmar) view

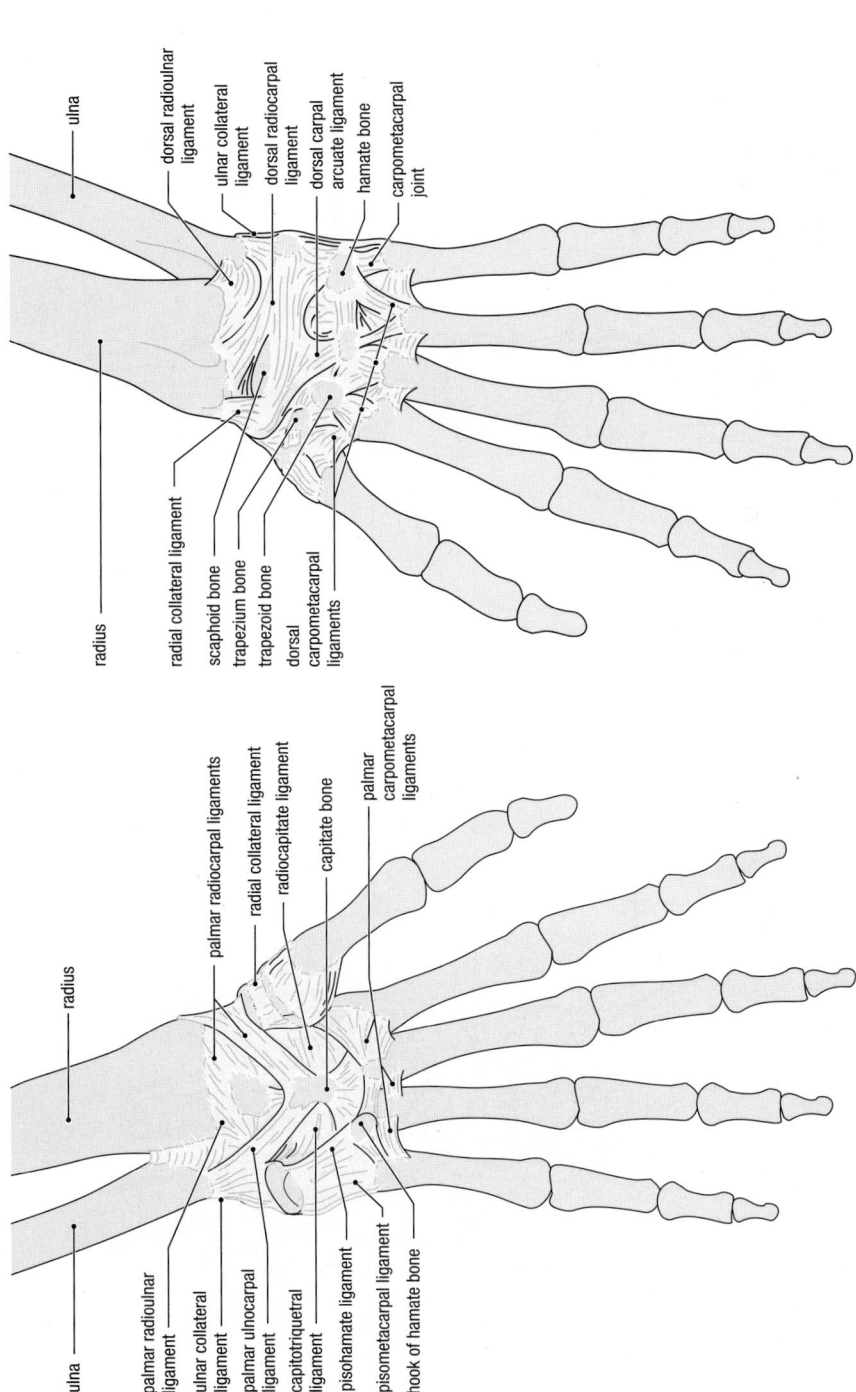

wrist showing relative positions of skeletal structures and ligaments: (left) anterior (palmar) view of left hand; (right) posterior (dorsal) view of left hand

blood supply to the hand: (left) anterior view; (right) lateral view

posterior interosseous artery

anterior interosseous artery

dorsal carpal arterial arch

perforating branches

dorsal metacarpal arteries

dorsal digital arteries

anterior interosseous artery

palmar carpal artery

deep palmar arch

palmar metacarpal arteries

superficial palmar arch

common palmar digital arteries

palmar digital arteries

MADER

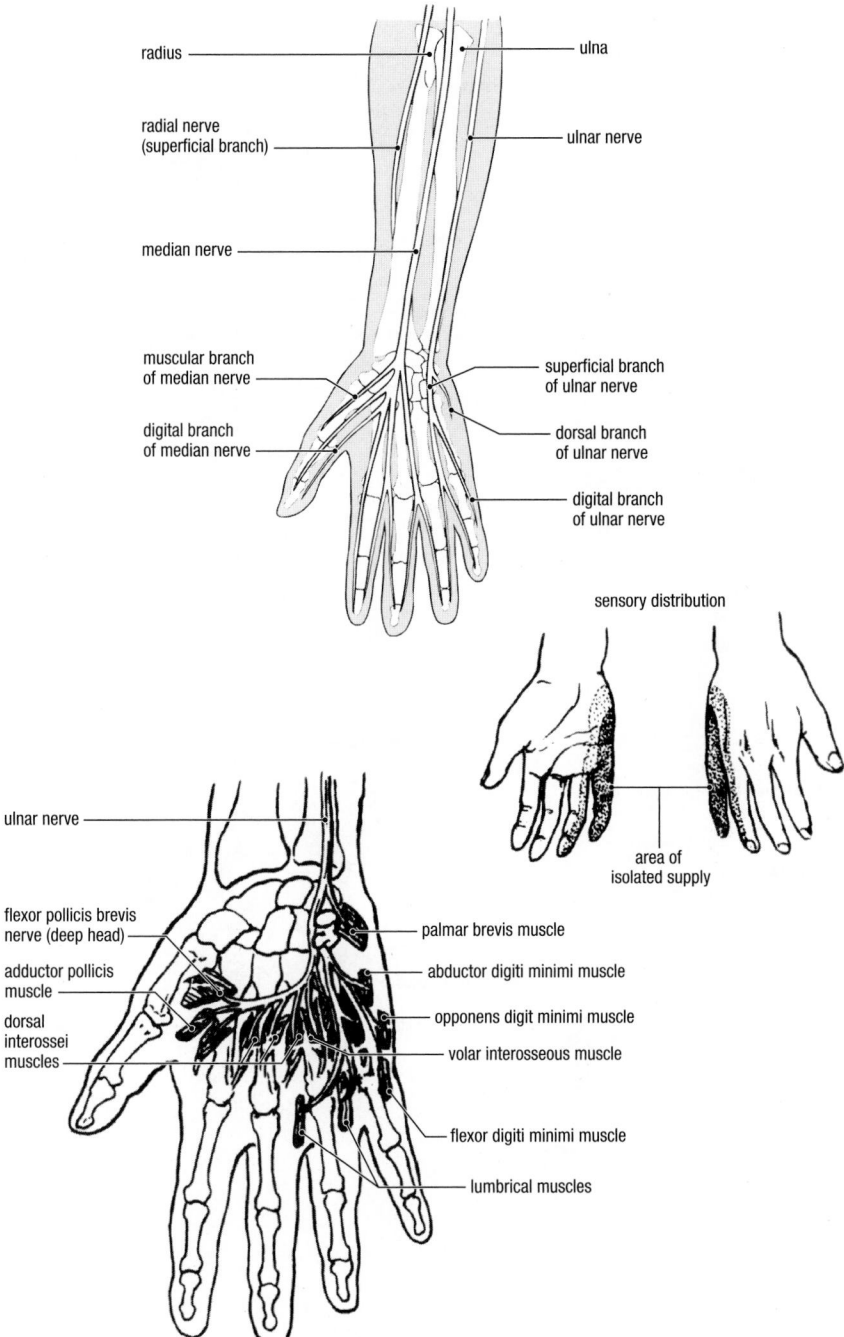

radius

ulna

radial nerve
(superficial branch)

ulnar nerve

median nerve

muscular branch
of median nerve

superficial branch
of ulnar nerve

digital branch
of median nerve

dorsal branch
of ulnar nerve

digital branch
of ulnar nerve

sensory distribution

ulnar nerve

area of
isolated supply

flexor pollicis brevis
nerve (deep head)

palmar brevis muscle

adductor pollicis
muscle

abductor digiti minimi muscle

dorsal
interossei
muscles

opponens digit minimi muscle

volar interosseous muscle

flexor digiti minimi muscle

lumbrical muscles

nerves of the hand, sensory distribution

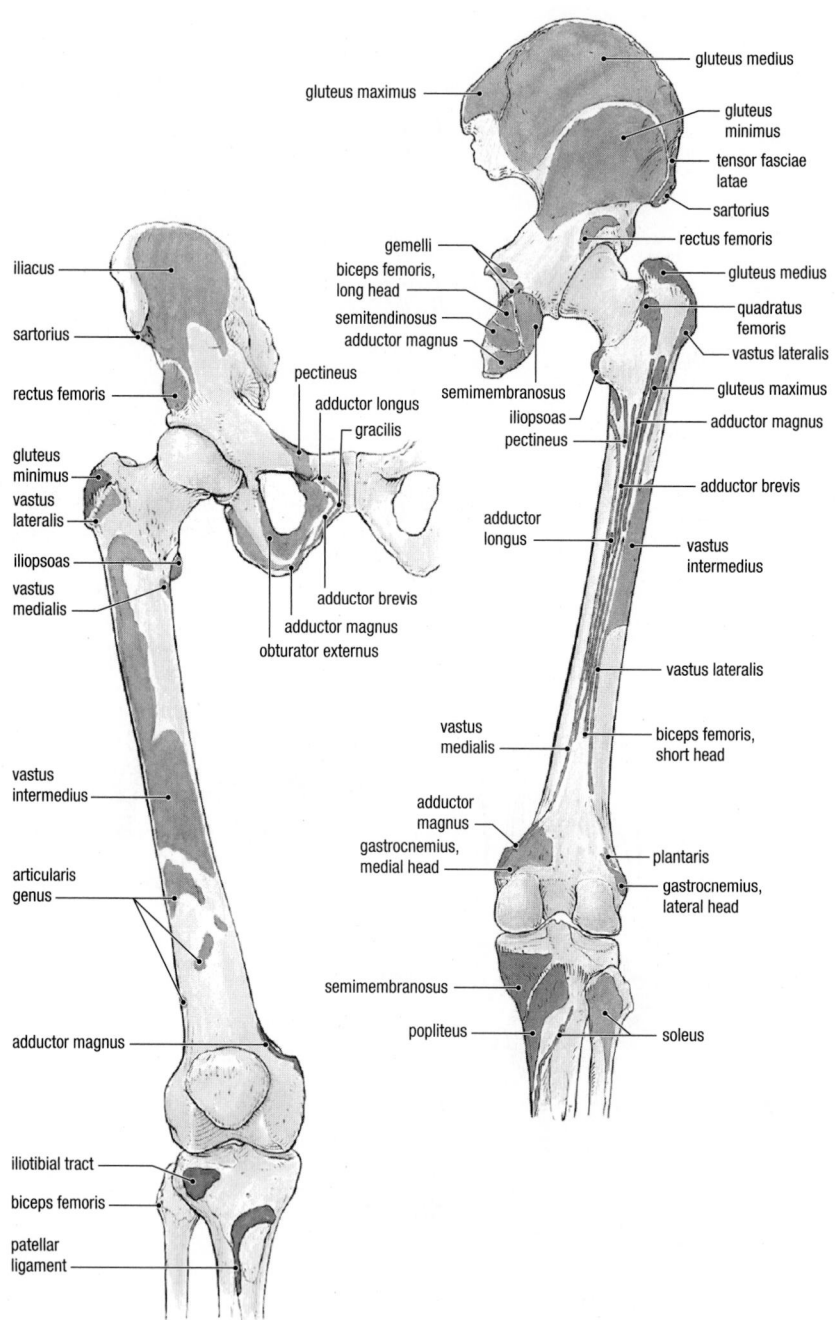

bones of the lower limbs showing muscle attachments: (left) anterior view; (right) posterior view

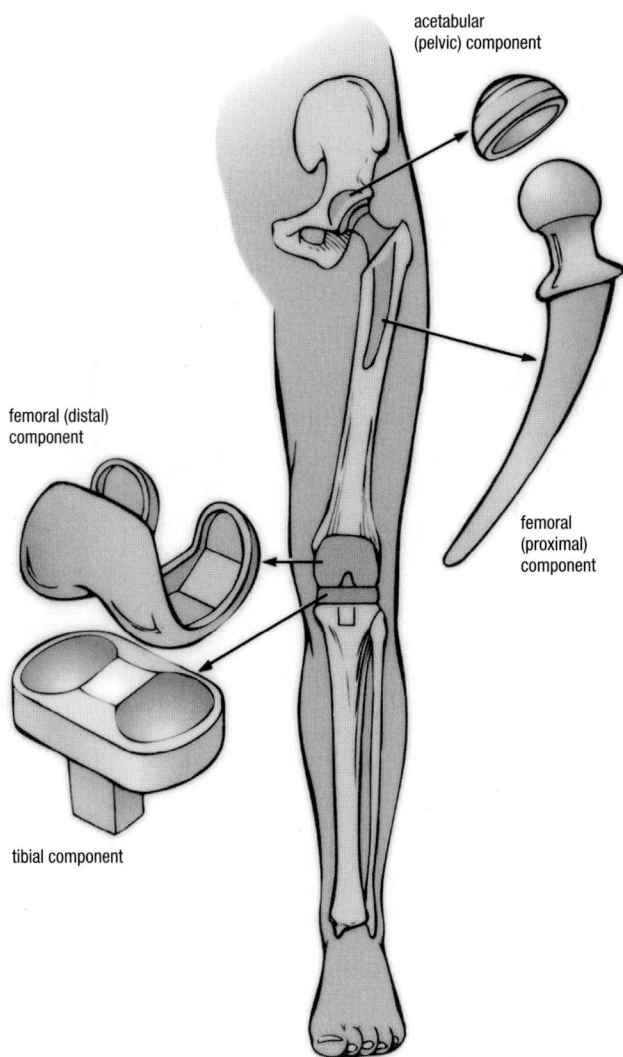

acetabular
(pelvic) component

femoral (distal)
component

femoral
(proximal)
component

tibial component

hip and knee replacement

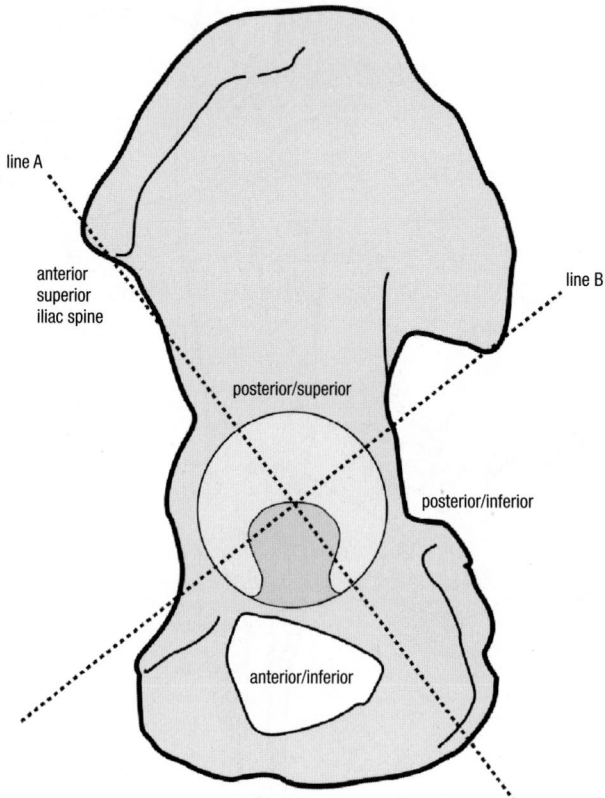

hybrid total hip arthroplasty: quadrant system for safe placement of acetabular screws

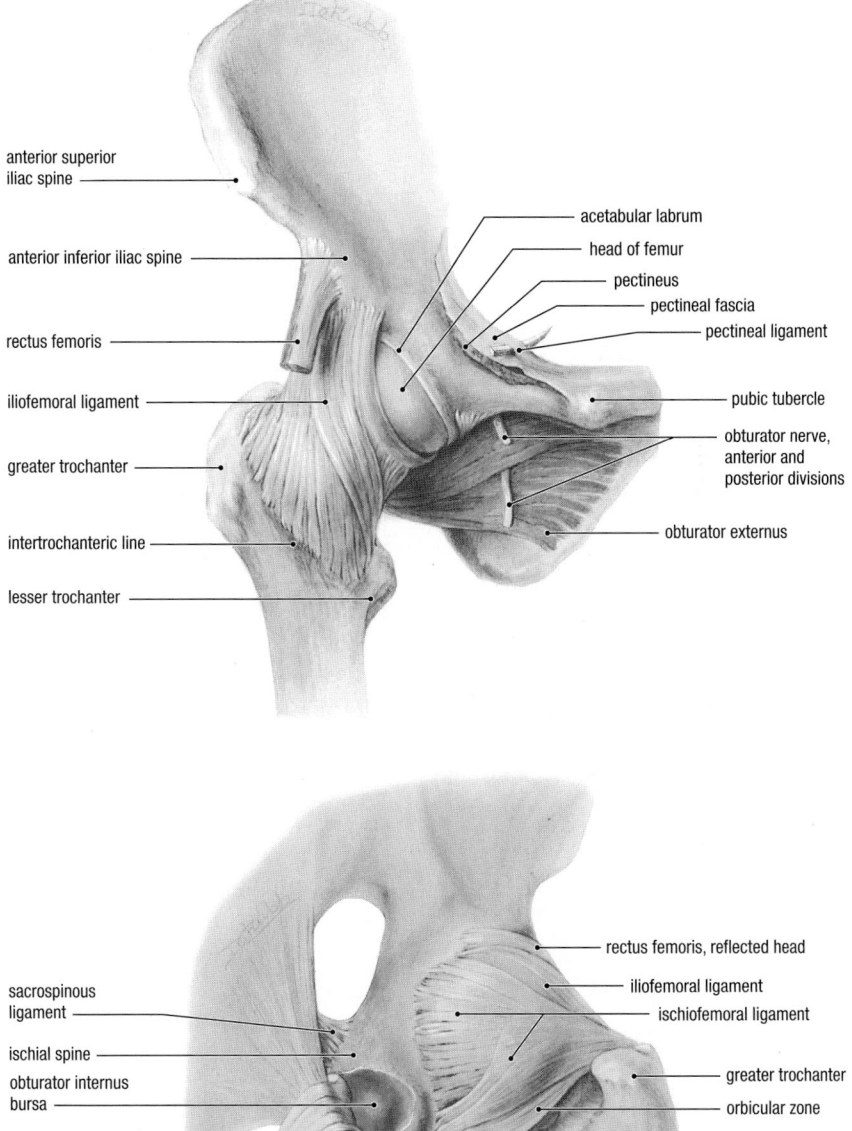

anterior superior iliac spine

anterior inferior iliac spine

rectus femoris

iliofemoral ligament

greater trochanter

intertrochanteric line

lesser trochanter

acetabular labrum

head of femur

pectineus

pectineal fascia

pectineal ligament

pubic tubercle

obturator nerve, anterior and posterior divisions

obturator externus

sacrospinous ligament

ischial spine

obturator internus bursa

obturator internus

rectus femoris, reflected head

iliofemoral ligament

ischiofemoral ligament

greater trochanter

orbicular zone

neck of femur

synovial protrusion

lesser trochanter

psoas major

hip joint: (top) anterior view; (bottom) posterior view

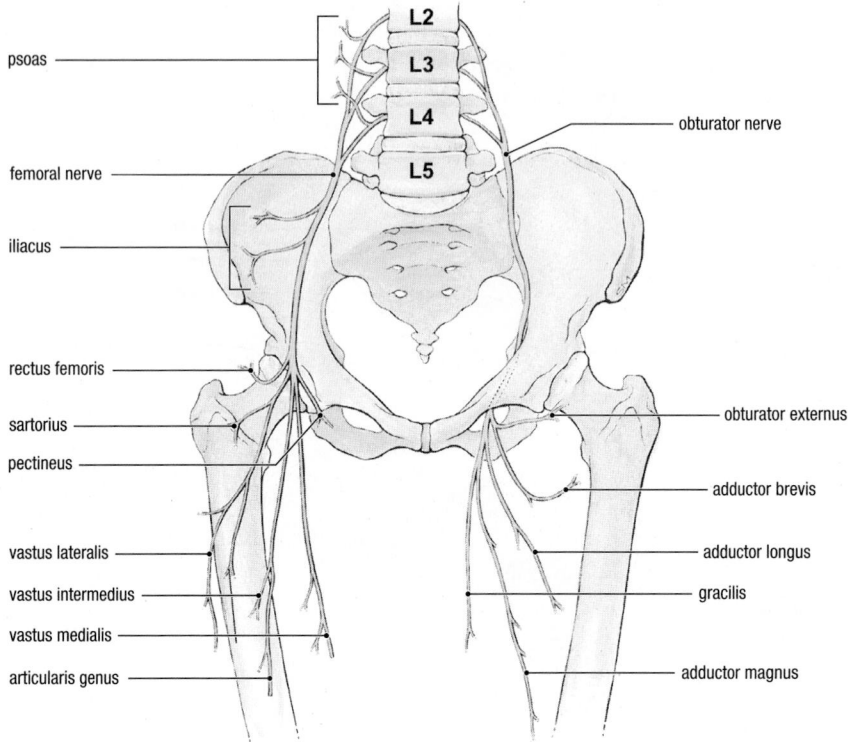

psoas

femoral nerve

iliacus

rectus femoris

sartorius

pectineus

vastus lateralis

vastus intermedius

vastus medialis

articularis genus

L2

L3

L4

L5

obturator nerve

obturator externus

adductor brevis

adductor longus

gracilis

adductor magnus

femoral and obturator nerves

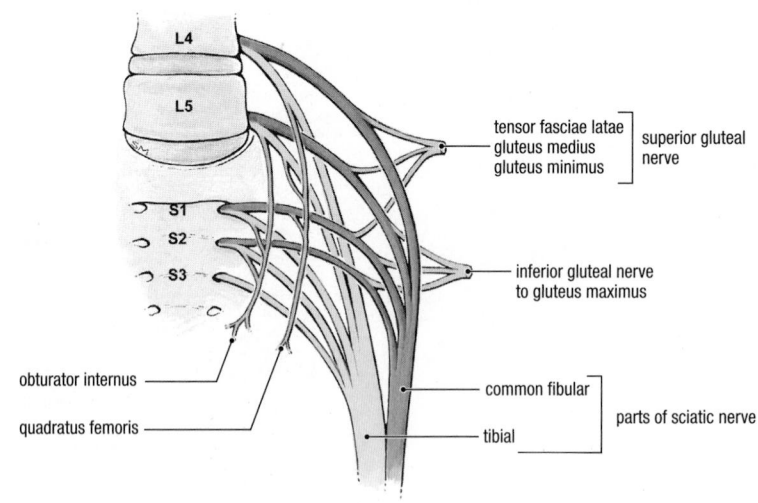

L4

L5

S1

S2

S3

tensor fasciae latae
gluteus medius
gluteus minimus

superior gluteal
nerve

inferior gluteal nerve
to gluteus maximus

obturator internus

quadratus femoris

common fibular

tibial

parts of sciatic nerve

formation of the sciatic nerve in the pelvis

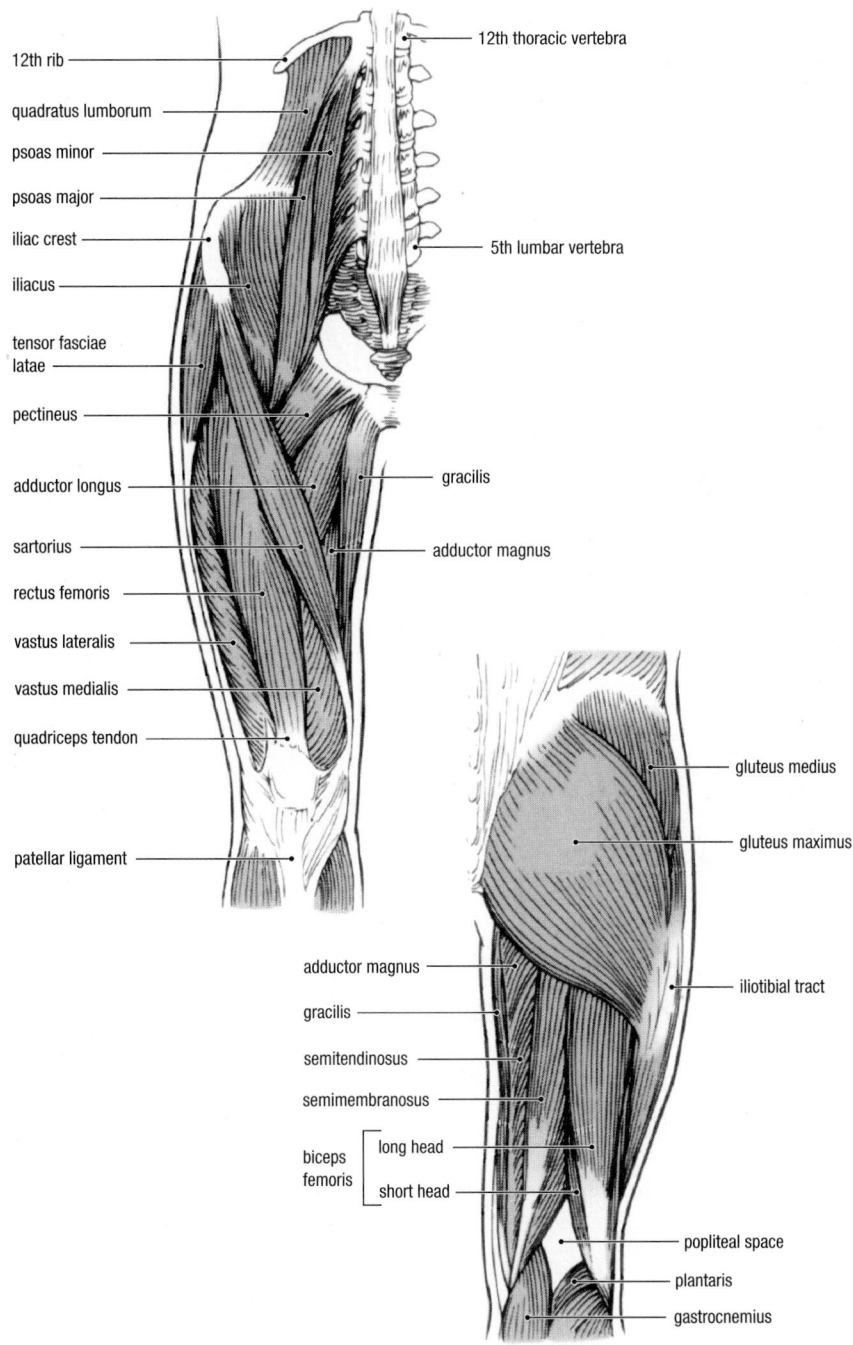

12th rib

quadratus lumborum

psoas minor

psoas major

iliac crest

iliacus

tensor fasciae latae

pectineus

adductor longus

sartorius

rectus femoris

vastus lateralis

vastus medialis

quadriceps tendon

patellar ligament

12th thoracic vertebra

5th lumbar vertebra

gracilis

adductor magnus

gluteus medius

gluteus maximus

adductor magnus

gracilis

semitendinosus

semimembranosus

biceps femoris

long head

short head

iliotibial tract

popliteal space

plantaris

gastrocnemius

superficial muscles of the hip and thigh: (left) anterior view; (right) posterior view

Pain	Numbness	Weakness	Atrophy	Reflexes
L4 lower back, hip, posterolateral thigh, anterior leg	anteromedial thigh and knee	quadriceps	quadriceps	knee jerk diminished
L5 over sacroiliac joint, hip, lateral thigh, and leg	lateral leg, web of great toe	dorsiflexion of great toe and foot; difficulty walking on heels; foot drop may occur	minor	changes uncommon (absent or diminished posterior tibial reflex)
S1 over sacroiliac joint, hip, posterolateral thigh, and leg to heel	back of calf; lateral heel, foot, and toe	plantar flexion of foot and great toe may be affected; difficulty walking on toes	gastrocnemius and soleus	ankle jerk diminished or absent

intervertebral disc herniation (nerves compressed: L4, L5, and S1)

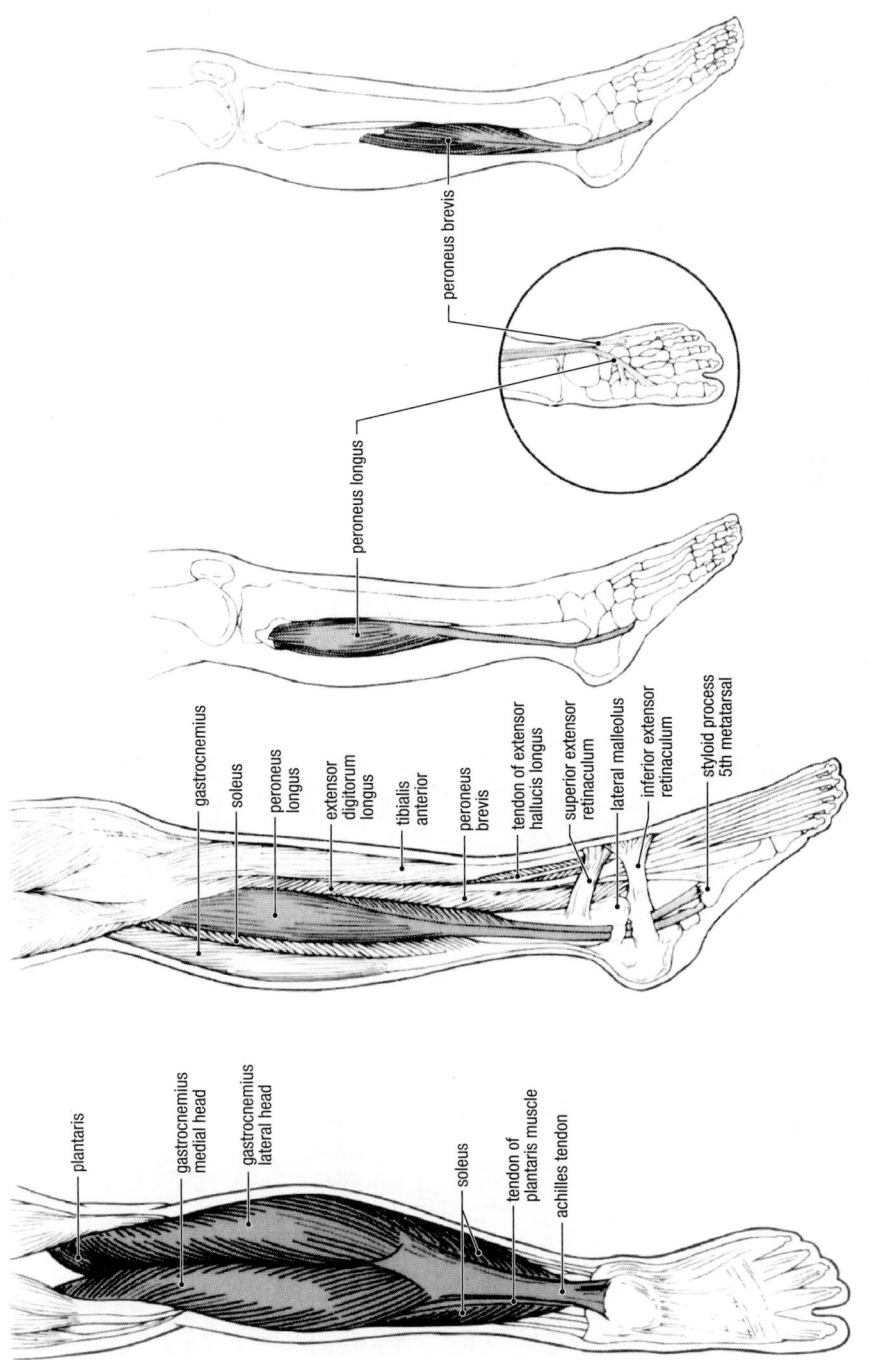

peroneus brevis

peroneus longus

gastrocnemius

soleus

peroneus longus

extensor digitorum longus

tibialis anterior

peroneus brevis

tendon of extensor hallucis longus

superior extensor retinaculum

lateral malleolus

inferior extensor retinaculum

styloid process 5th metatarsal

plantaris

gastrocnemius medial head

gastrocnemius lateral head

soleus

tendon of plantaris muscle

achilles tendon

muscles of the lower leg: (left) superficial compartment, posterior view; (middle and right) lateral compartment

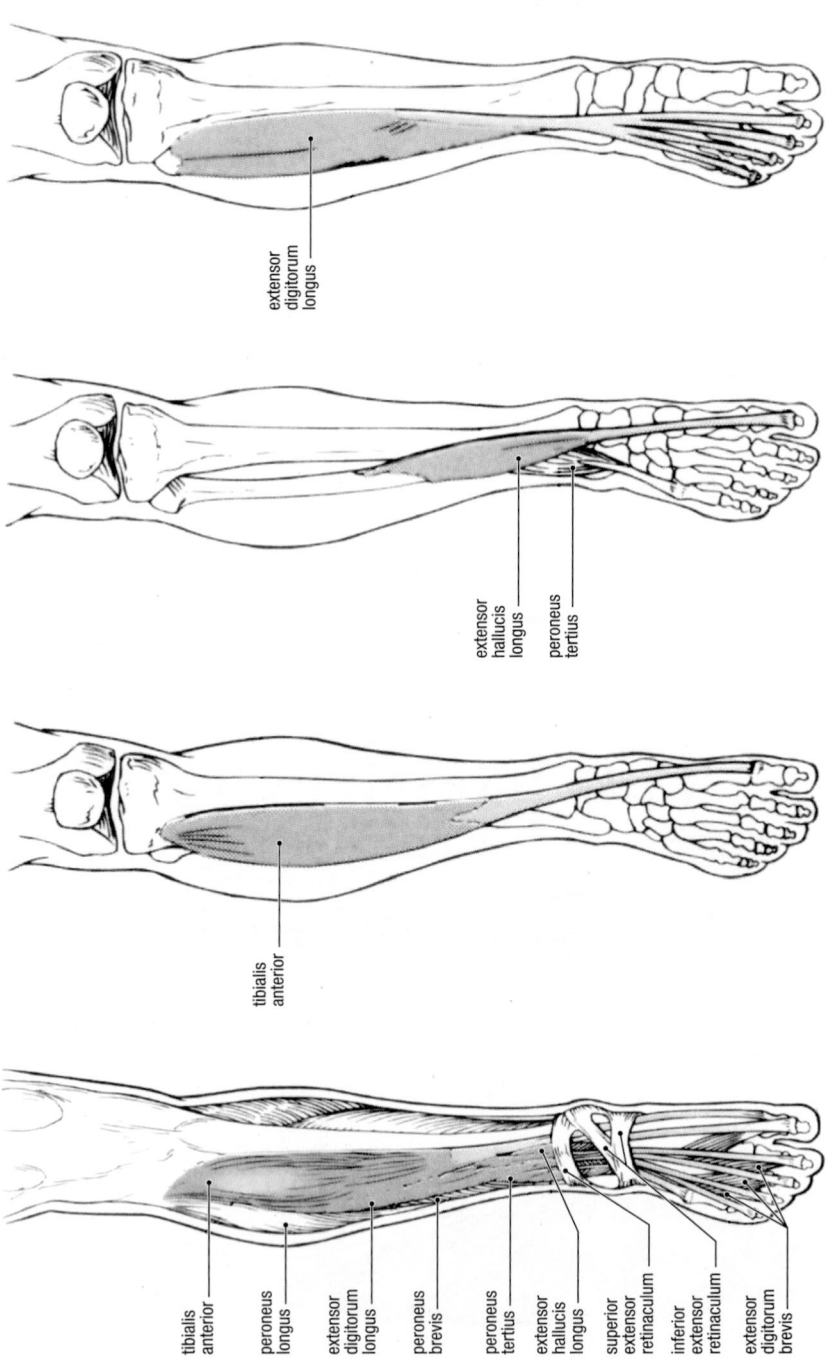

extensor
digitorum
longus

extensor
hallucis
longus

peroneus
tertius

tibialis
anterior

tibialis
anterior

peroneus
longus

extensor
digitorum
longus

peroneus
brevis

peroneus
tertius

extensor
hallucis
longus

superior
extensor
retinaculum

inferior
extensor
retinaculum

extensor
digitorum
brevis

muscles of the lower leg, anterior compartment

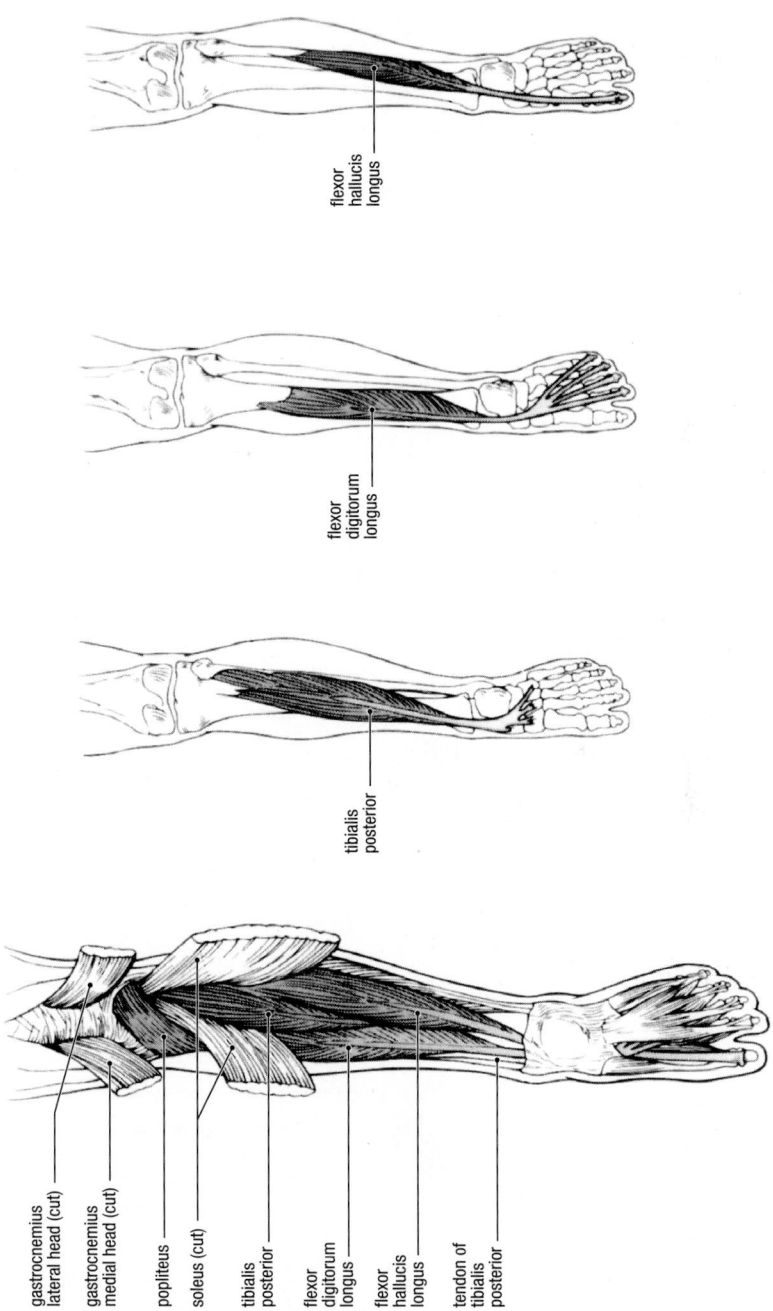

flexor
hallucis
longus

flexor
digitorum
longus

tibialis
posterior

gastrocnemius
lateral head (cut)

gastrocnemius
medial head (cut)

popliteus

soleus (cut)

tibialis
posterior

flexor
digitorum
longus

flexor
hallucis
longus

tendon of
tibialis
posterior

muscles of the lower leg, deep compartment, posterior view

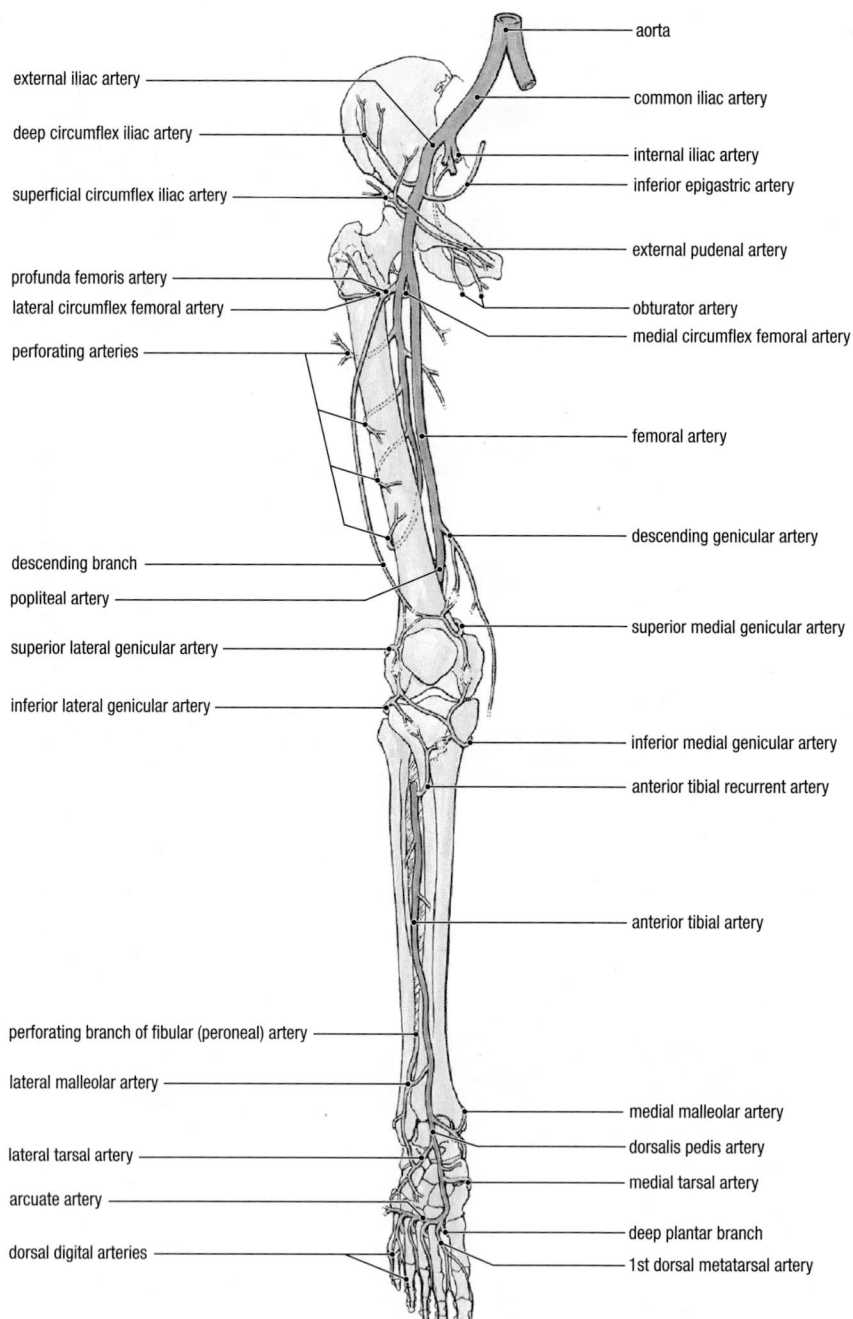

aorta

external iliac artery

common iliac artery

deep circumflex iliac artery

internal iliac artery

inferior epigastric artery

superficial circumflex iliac artery

external pudenal artery

profunda femoris artery

obturator artery

lateral circumflex femoral artery

medial circumflex femoral artery

perforating arteries

femoral artery

descending genicular artery

descending branch

popliteal artery

superior medial genicular artery

superior lateral genicular artery

inferior lateral genicular artery

inferior medial genicular artery

anterior tibial recurrent artery

anterior tibial artery

perforating branch of fibular (peroneal) artery

lateral malleolar artery

medial malleolar artery

dorsalis pedis artery

lateral tarsal artery

medial tarsal artery

arcuate artery

deep plantar branch

dorsal digital arteries

1st dorsal metatarsal artery

arteries of the lower limb, anterior view

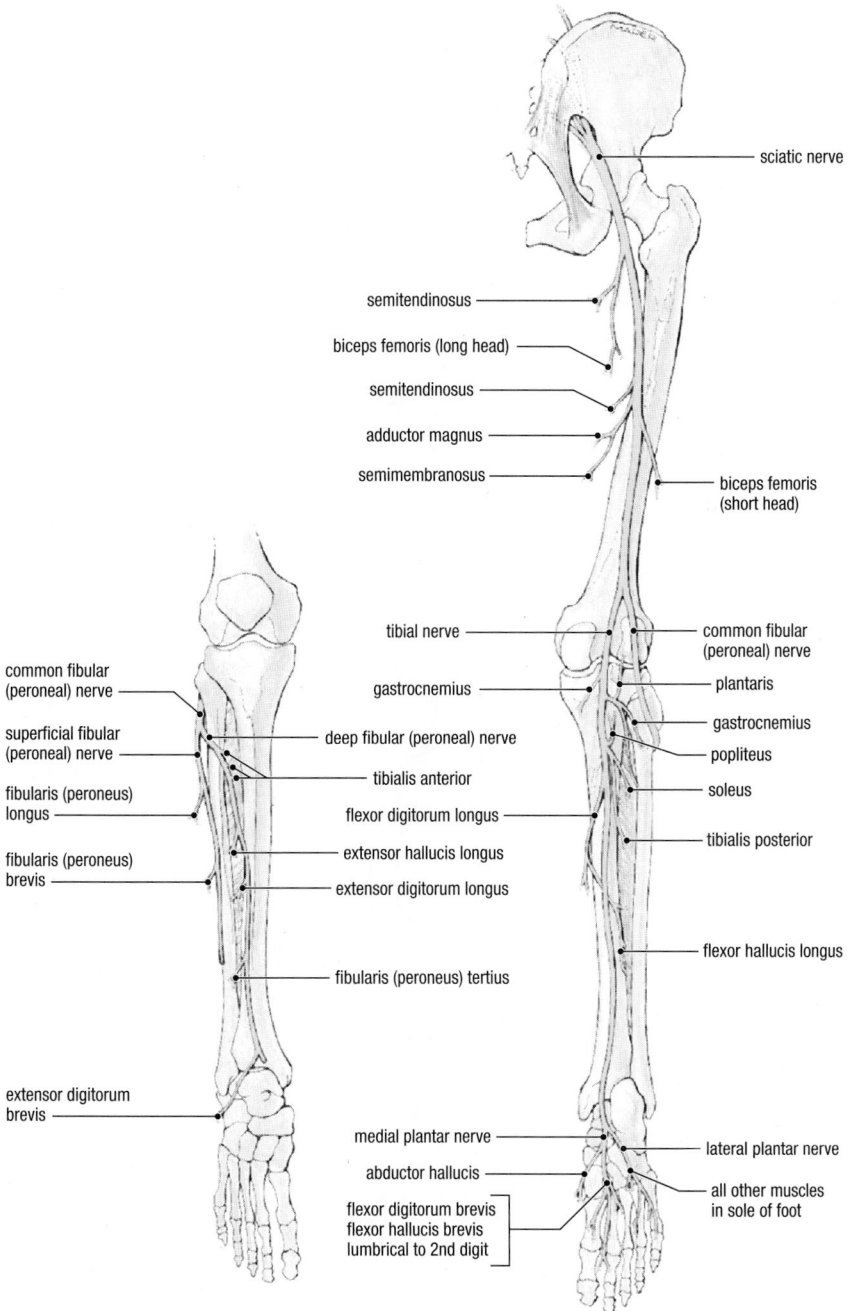

sciatic nerve

semitendinosus

biceps femoris (long head)

semitendinosus

adductor magnus

semimembranosus

biceps femoris (short head)

tibial nerve

common fibular (peroneal) nerve

common fibular (peroneal) nerve

plantaris

gastrocnemius

gastrocnemius

superficial fibular (peroneal) nerve

deep fibular (peroneal) nerve

popliteus

fibularis (peroneus) longus

tibialis anterior

soleus

flexor digitorum longus

tibialis posterior

fibularis (peroneus) brevis

extensor hallucis longus

extensor digitorum longus

flexor hallucis longus

fibularis (peroneus) tertius

extensor digitorum brevis

medial plantar nerve

lateral plantar nerve

abductor hallucis

all other muscles in sole of foot

flexor digitorum brevis
flexor hallucis brevis
lumbrical to 2nd digit

motor distribution of the nerves of the lower limb: (left) common fibular (peroneal) nerve; (right) sciatic nerve

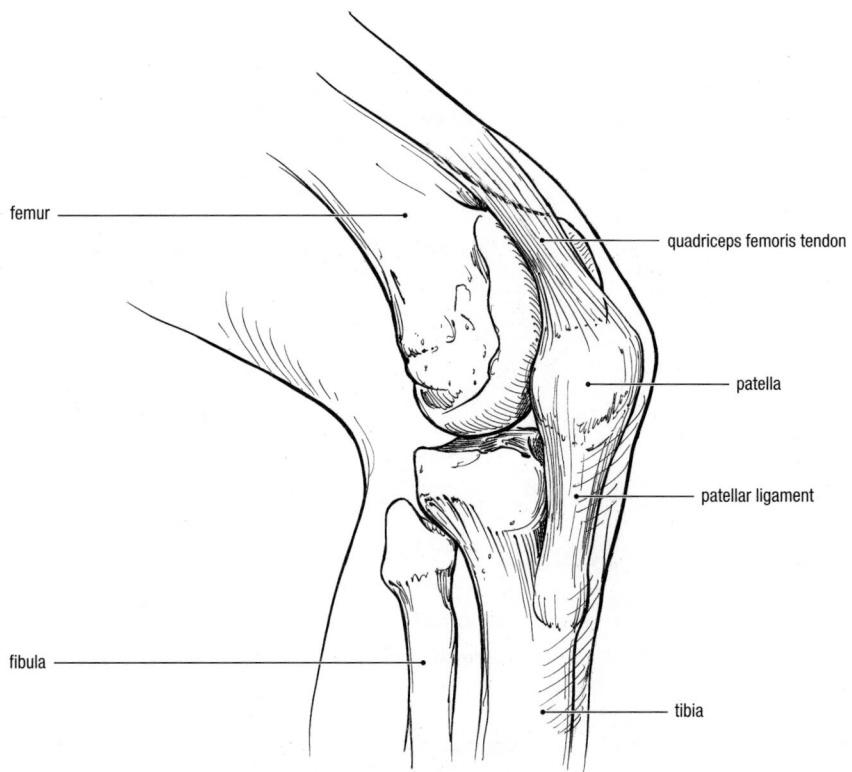

femur

quadriceps femoris tendon

patella

patellar ligament

fibula

tibia

the bones of the knee joint

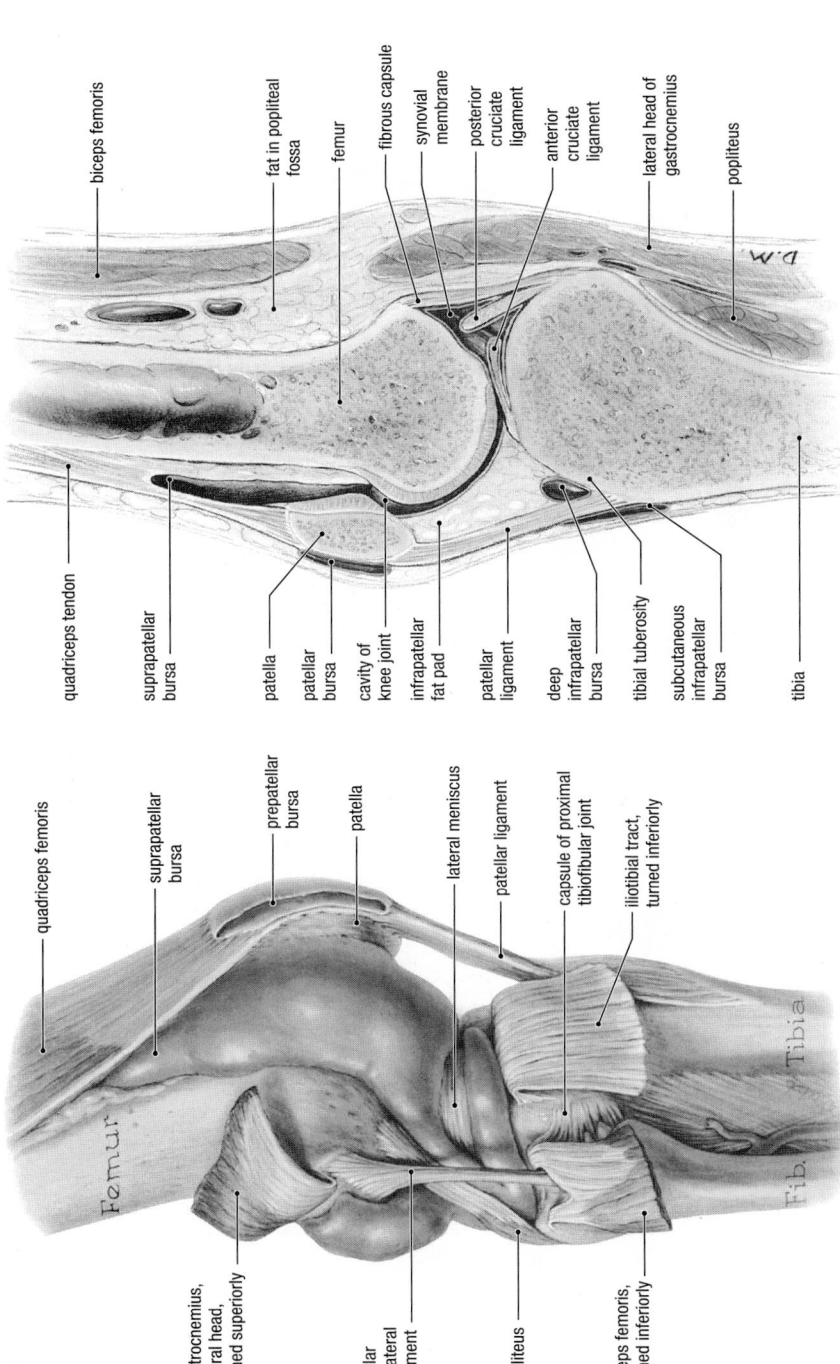

biceps femoris

fat in popliteal fossa

femur

fibrous capsule

synovial membrane

posterior cruciate ligament

anterior cruciate ligament

lateral head of gastrocnemius

popliteus

quadriceps tendon

suprapatellar bursa

patella

patellar bursa

cavity of knee joint

infrapatellar fat pad

patellar ligament

deep infrapatellar bursa

tibial tuberosity

subcutaneous infrapatellar bursa

tibia

sagittal section through lateral aspect of intercondylar notch of femur

quadriceps femoris

suprapatellar bursa

prepatellar bursa

patella

lateral meniscus

patellar ligament

capsule of proximal tibiofibular joint

iliotibial tract, turned inferiorly

gastrocnemius, lateral head, turned superiorly

fibular collateral ligament

popliteus

biceps femoris, turned inferiorly

distended knee joint, lateral view

A39

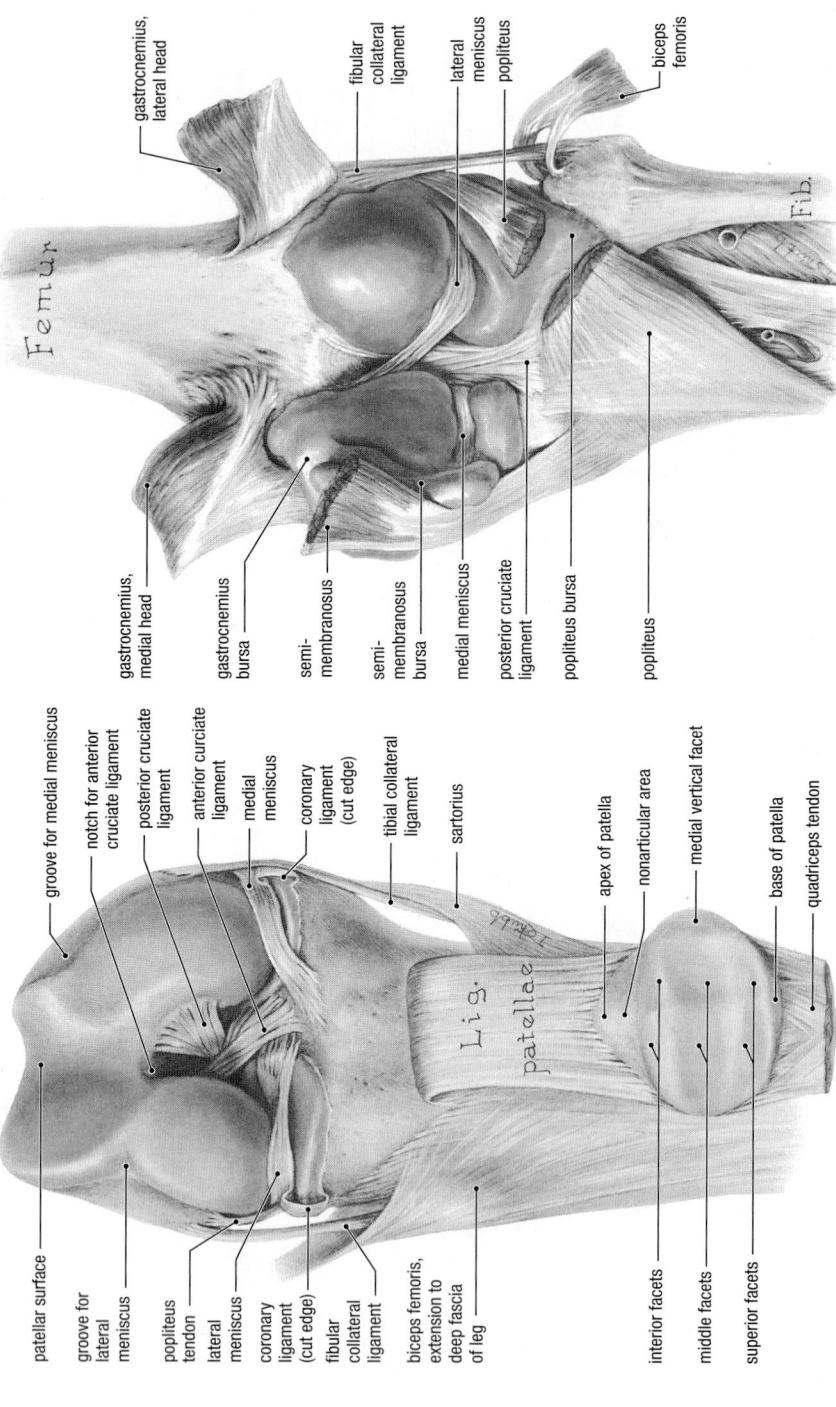

articular surfaces and ligaments of the knee joint: (left) anterior view; (right) posterior view

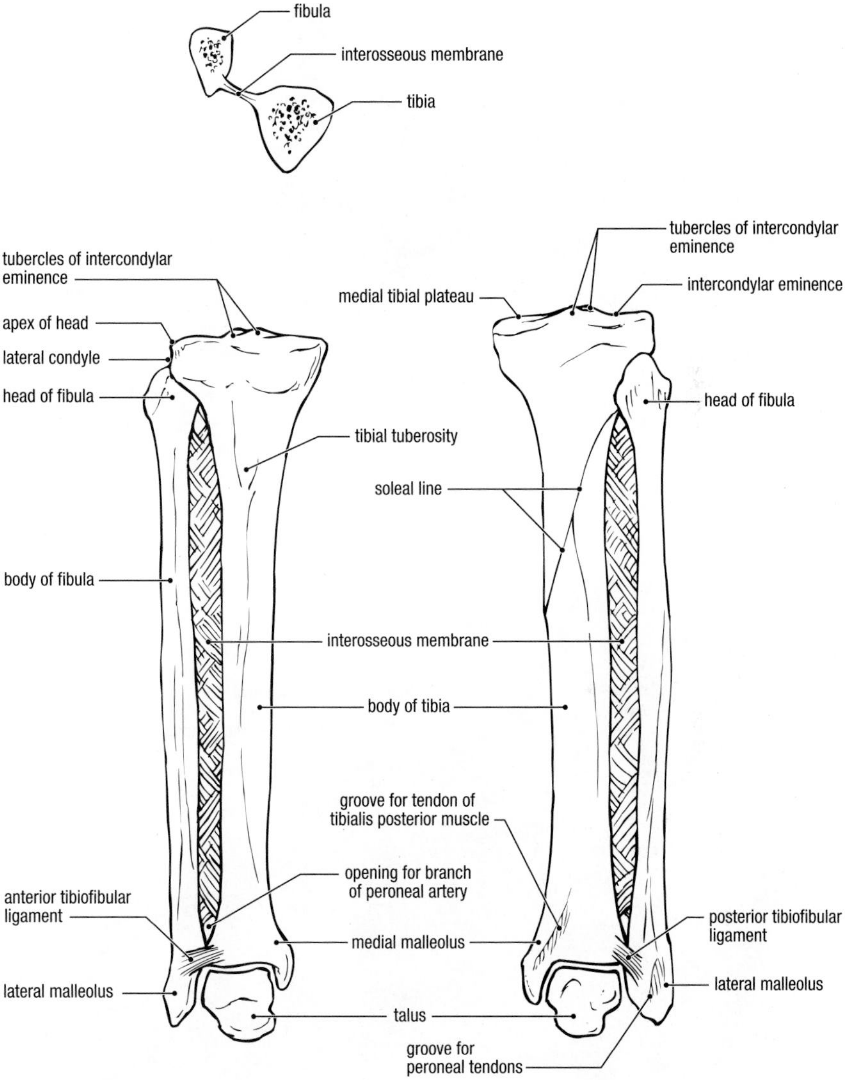

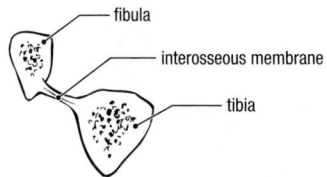

fibula

interosseous membrane

tibia

tubercles of intercondylar eminence

tubercles of intercondylar eminence

intercondylar eminence

medial tibial plateau

apex of head

lateral condyle

head of fibula

head of fibula

tibial tuberosity

soleal line

body of fibula

interosseous membrane

body of tibia

groove for tendon of tibialis posterior muscle

opening for branch of peroneal artery

anterior tibiofibular ligament

posterior tibiofibular ligament

medial malleolus

lateral malleolus

lateral malleolus

talus

groove for peroneal tendons

bones of lower leg: (left) anterior view; (right) posterior view; (top) cross-section

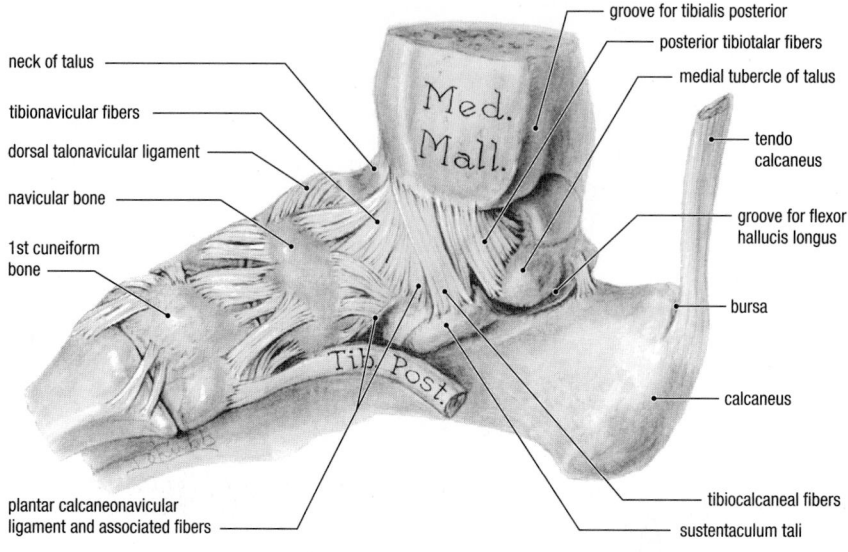

neck of talus

tibionavicular fibers

dorsal talonavicular ligament

navicular bone

1st cuneiform bone

plantar calcaneonavicular ligament and associated fibers

groove for tibialis posterior

posterior tibiotalar fibers

medial tubercle of talus

Med. Mall.

Tib. Post.

tendo calcaneus

groove for flexor hallucis longus

bursa

calcaneus

tibiocalcaneal fibers

sustentaculum tali

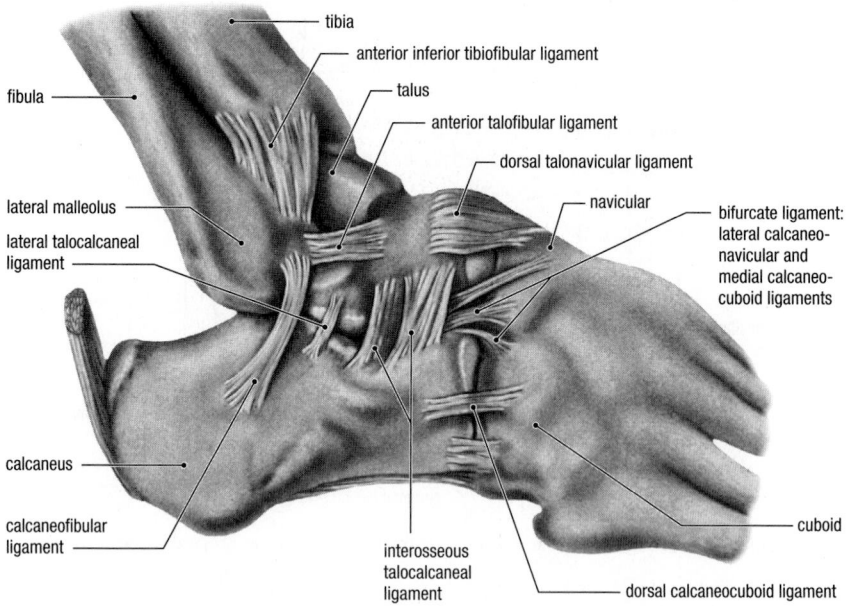

tibia

anterior inferior tibiofibular ligament

fibula

talus

anterior talofibular ligament

dorsal talonavicular ligament

navicular

lateral malleolus

lateral talocalcaneal ligament

bifurcate ligament: lateral calcaneo-navicular and medial calcaneo-cuboid ligaments

calcaneus

calcaneofibular ligament

interosseous talocalcaneal ligament

dorsal calcaneocuboid ligament

cuboid

ligaments of the ankle: (top) medial view; (bottom) lateral view

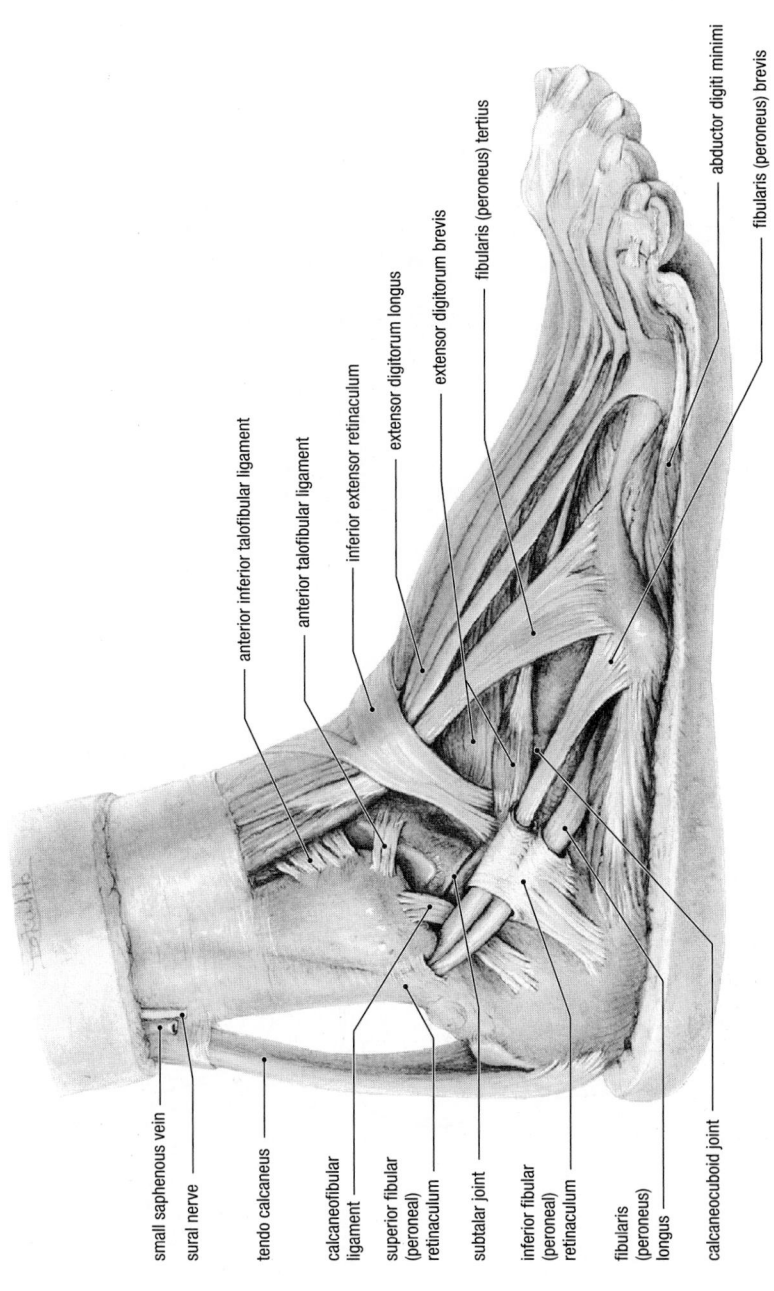

small saphenous vein

sural nerve

tendo calcaneus

calcaneofibular ligament

superior fibular (peroneal) retinaculum

subtalar joint

inferior fibular (peroneal) retinaculum

fibularis (peroneus) longus

calcaneocuboid joint

anterior inferior talofibular ligament

anterior talofibular ligament

inferior extensor retinaculum

extensor digitorum longus

extensor digitorum brevis

fibularis (peroneus) tertius

abductor digiti minimi

fibularis (peroneus) brevis

tendons of the ankle, lateral view

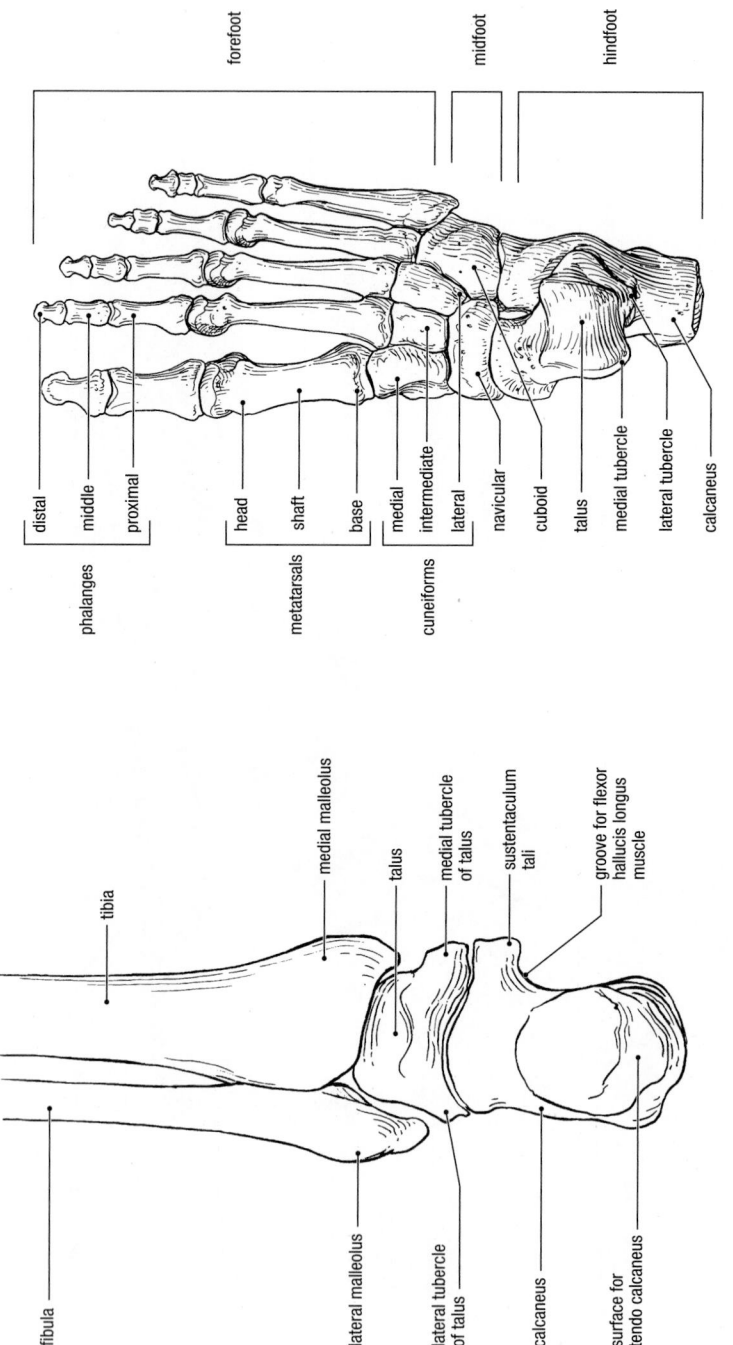

bones of the ankle and foot: (left) posterior view; (right) dorsal view

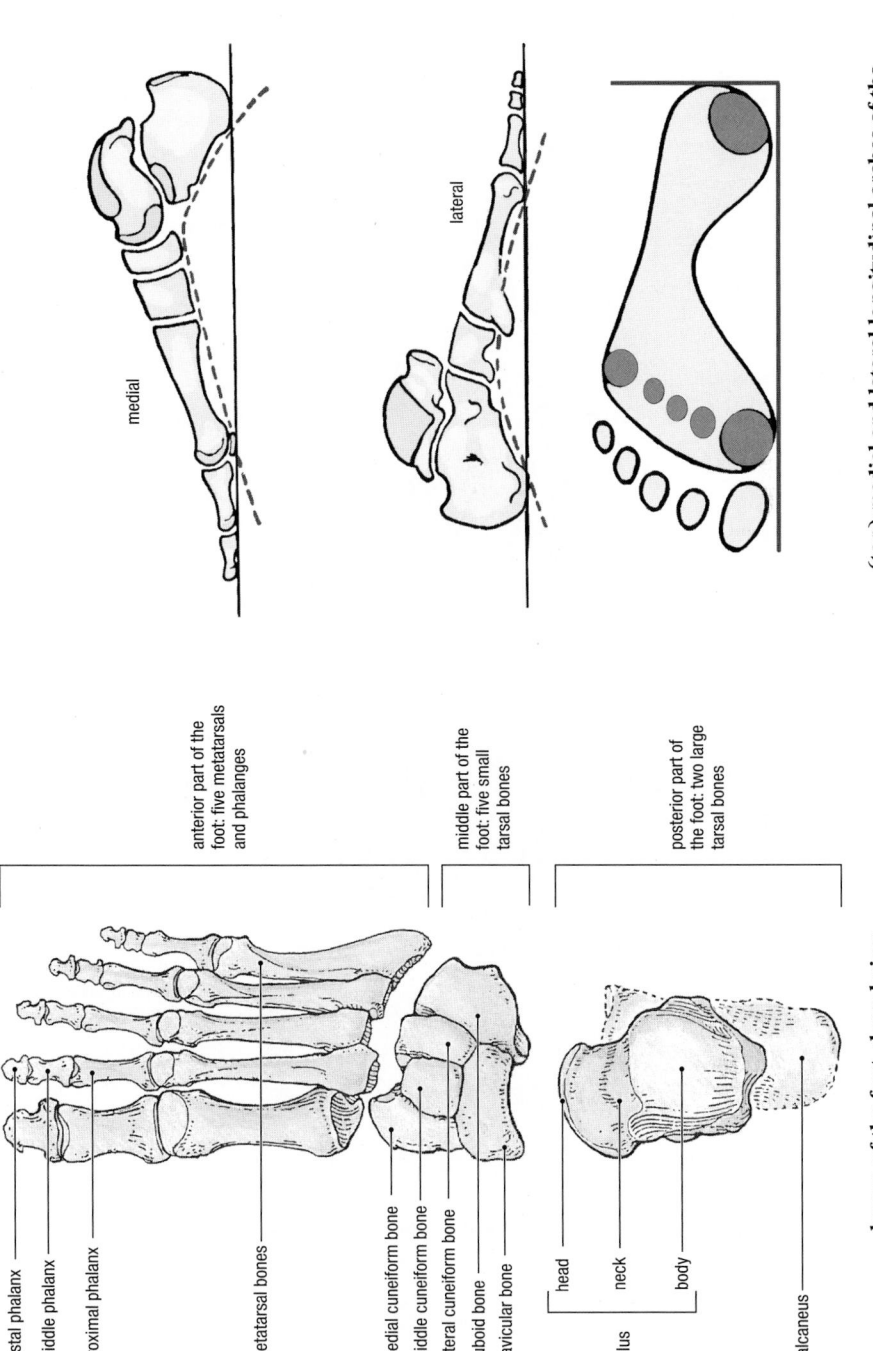

medial

lateral

(top) medial and lateral longitudinal arches of the foot; (bottom) bearing points of the foot

anterior part of the foot: five metatarsals and phalanges

middle part of the foot: five small tarsal bones

posterior part of the foot: two large tarsal bones

bones of the foot, dorsal view

distal phalanx
middle phalanx
proximal phalanx

metatarsal bones

medial cuneiform bone
middle cuneiform bone
lateral cuneiform bone
cuboid bone
navicular bone

head
neck
body

talus

calcaneus

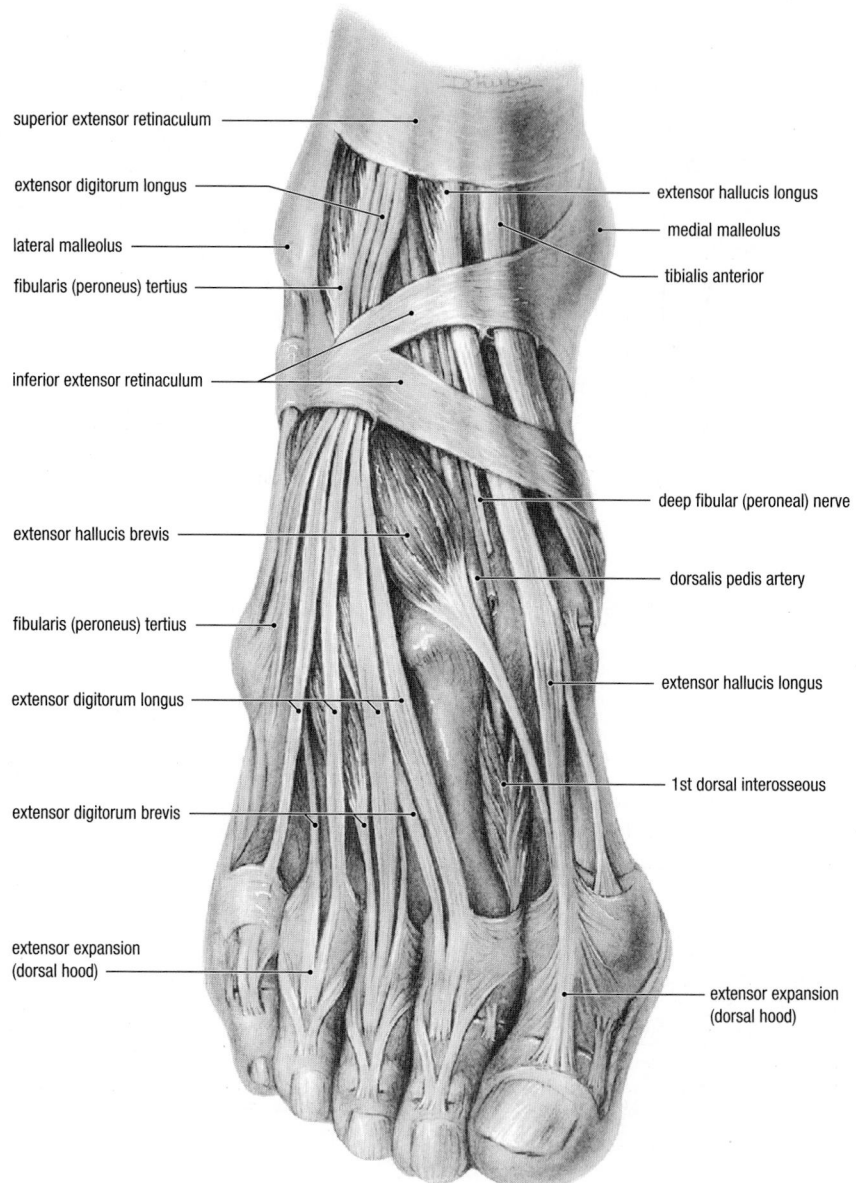

superior extensor retinaculum

extensor digitorum longus

lateral malleolus

fibularis (peroneus) tertius

inferior extensor retinaculum

extensor hallucis brevis

fibularis (peroneus) tertius

extensor digitorum longus

extensor digitorum brevis

extensor expansion
(dorsal hood)

extensor hallucis longus

medial malleolus

tibialis anterior

deep fibular (peroneal) nerve

dorsalis pedis artery

extensor hallucis longus

1st dorsal interosseous

extensor expansion
(dorsal hood)

muscles of the dorsum of the foot

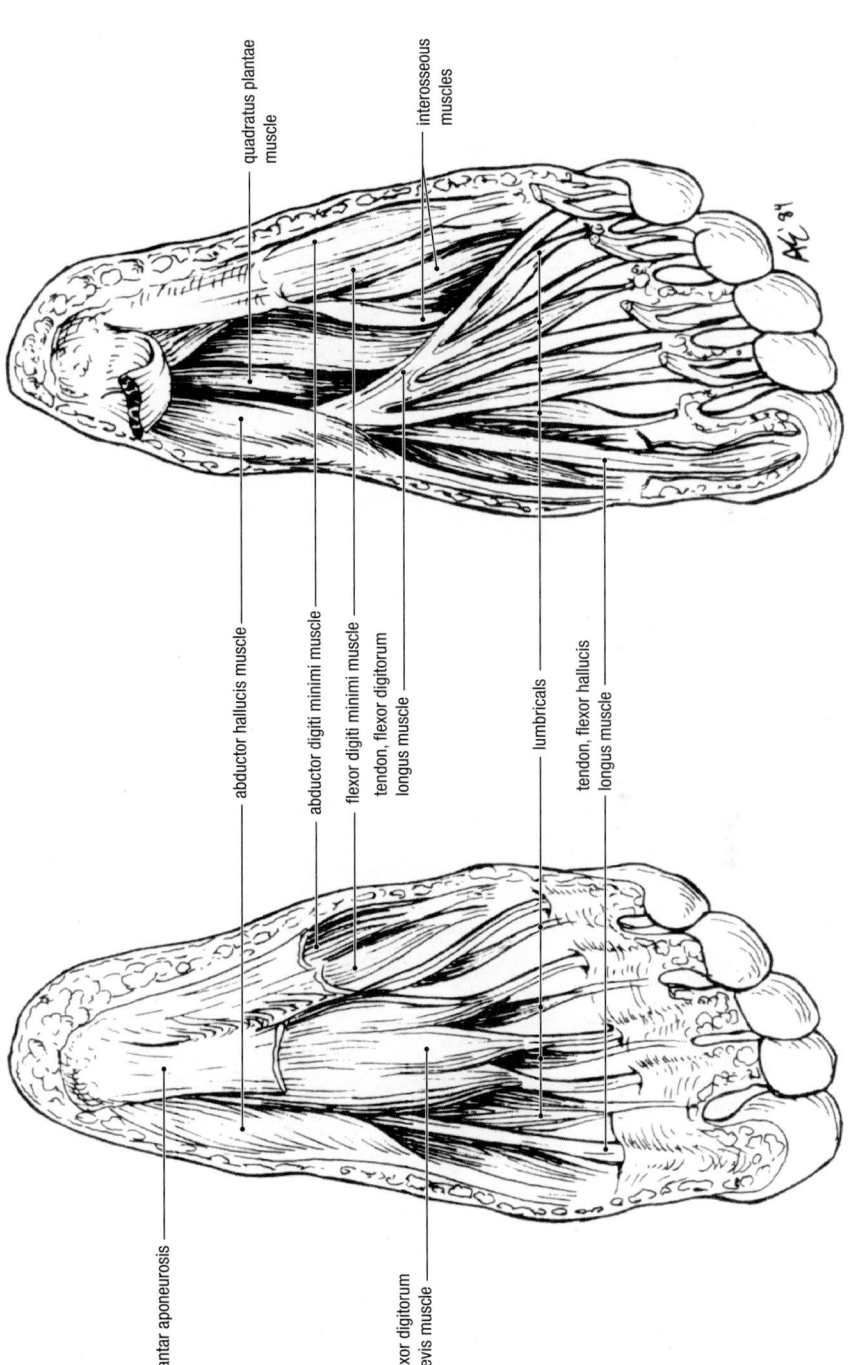

quadratus plantae muscle

interosseous muscles

abductor hallucis muscle

abductor digiti minimi muscle

flexor digiti minimi muscle

tendon, flexor digitorum longus muscle

lumbricals

tendon, flexor hallucis longus muscle

plantar aponeurosis

flexor digitorum brevis muscle

superficial muscles of the plantar foot: (left) first layer; (right) second layer

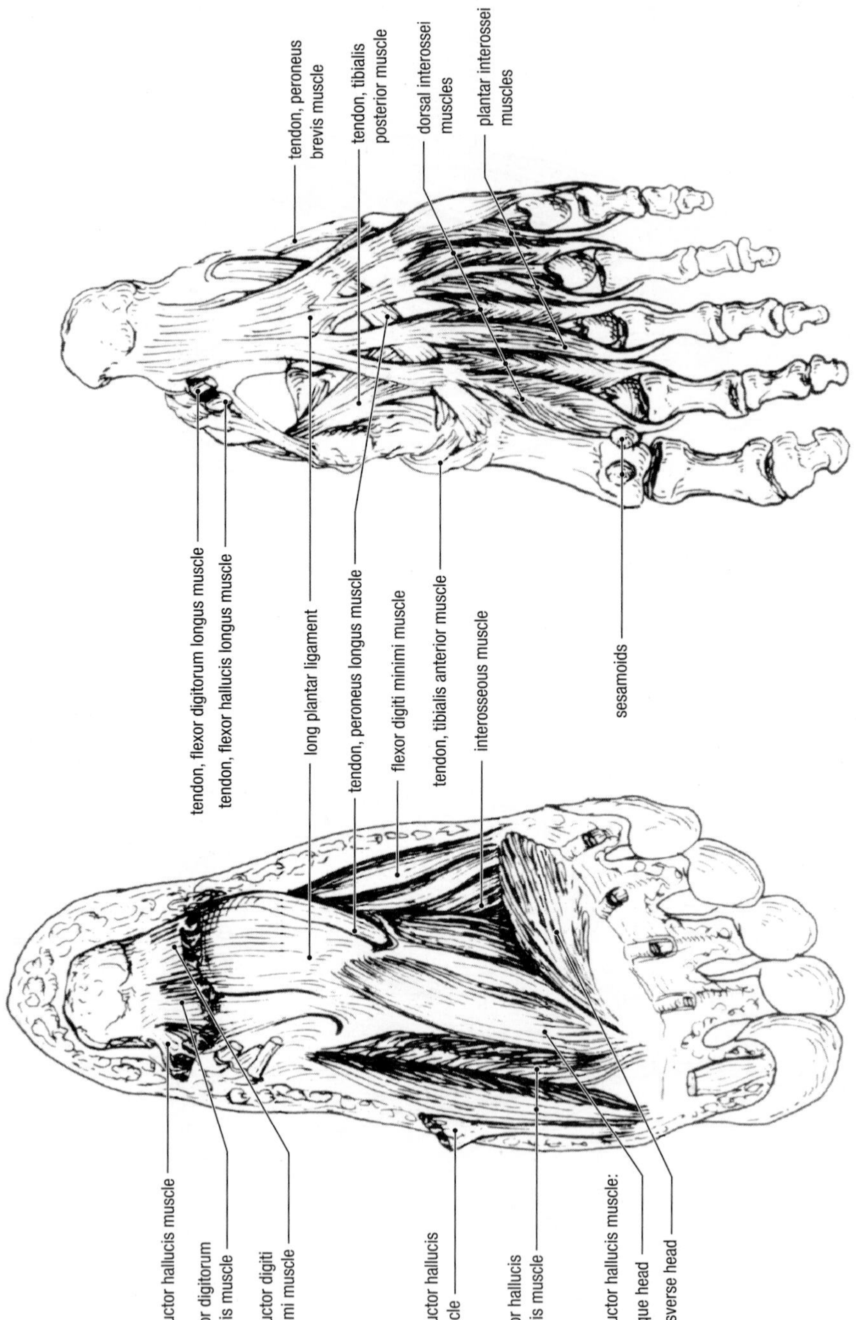

abductor hallucis muscle
flexor digitorum brevis muscle
abductor digiti minimi muscle
abductor hallucis muscle
flexor hallucis brevis muscle
adductor hallucis muscle:
oblique head
transverse head
tendon, flexor digitorum longus muscle
tendon, flexor hallucis longus muscle
long plantar ligament
tendon, peroneus longus muscle
flexor digiti minimi muscle
tendon, tibialis anterior muscle
interosseous muscle
sesamoids
tendon, peroneus brevis muscle
tendon, tibialis posterior muscle
dorsal interossei muscles
plantar interossei muscles

deep muscles of the plantar foot: (left) third layer; (right) fourth layer with deep ligaments

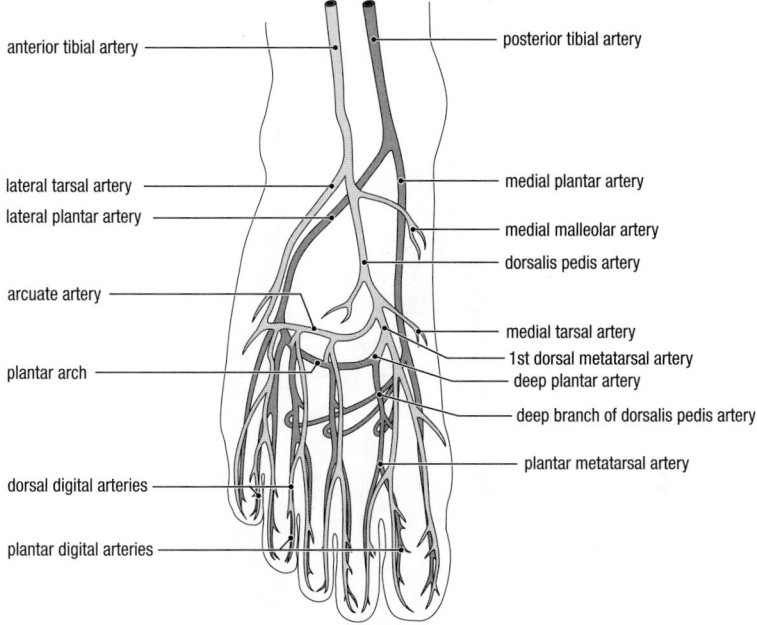

anterior tibial artery

posterior tibial artery

lateral tarsal artery

lateral plantar artery

arcuate artery

plantar arch

dorsal digital arteries

plantar digital arteries

medial plantar artery

medial malleolar artery

dorsalis pedis artery

medial tarsal artery

1st dorsal metatarsal artery

deep plantar artery

deep branch of dorsalis pedis artery

plantar metatarsal artery

dorsum of the foot showing the arterial circulation

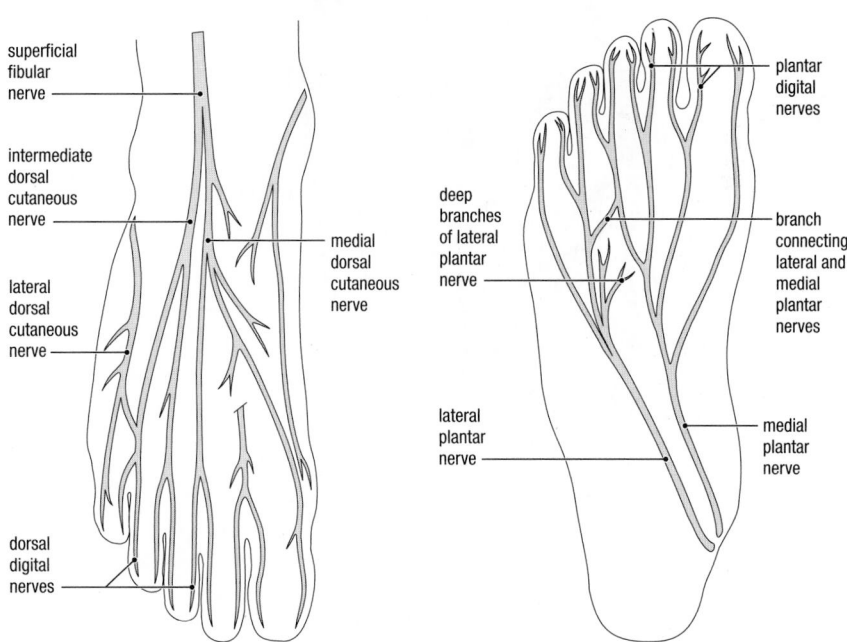

superficial fibular nerve

intermediate dorsal cutaneous nerve

lateral dorsal cutaneous nerve

dorsal digital nerves

medial dorsal cutaneous nerve

deep branches of lateral plantar nerve

lateral plantar nerve

plantar digital nerves

branch connecting lateral and medial plantar nerves

medial plantar nerve

innervation of the foot: (left) dorsal view; (right) plantar view

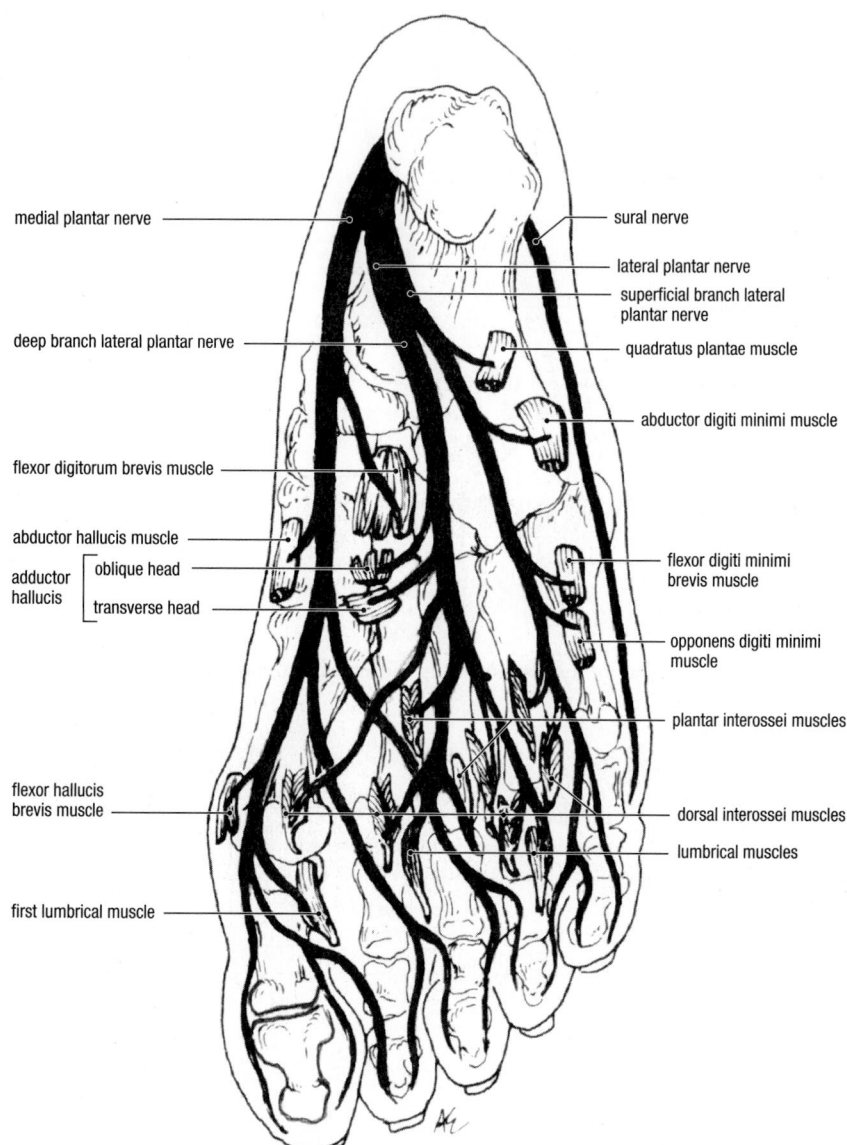

distribution of the tibial nerve in the foot

medial plantar nerve

sural nerve

lateral plantar nerve

superficial branch lateral plantar nerve

deep branch lateral plantar nerve

quadratus plantae muscle

abductor digiti minimi muscle

flexor digitorum brevis muscle

abductor hallucis muscle

adductor hallucis — oblique head

transverse head

flexor digiti minimi brevis muscle

opponens digiti minimi muscle

plantar interossei muscles

flexor hallucis brevis muscle

dorsal interossei muscles

lumbrical muscles

first lumbrical muscle

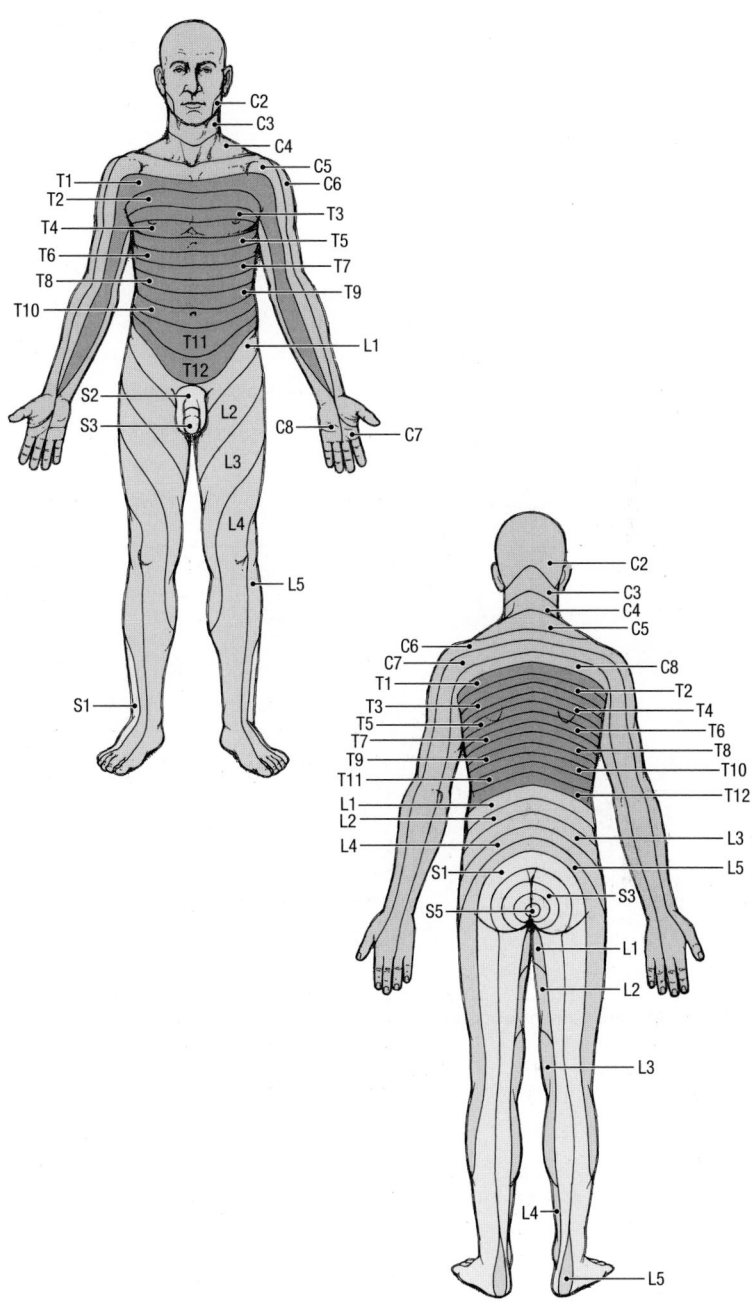

dermatomes

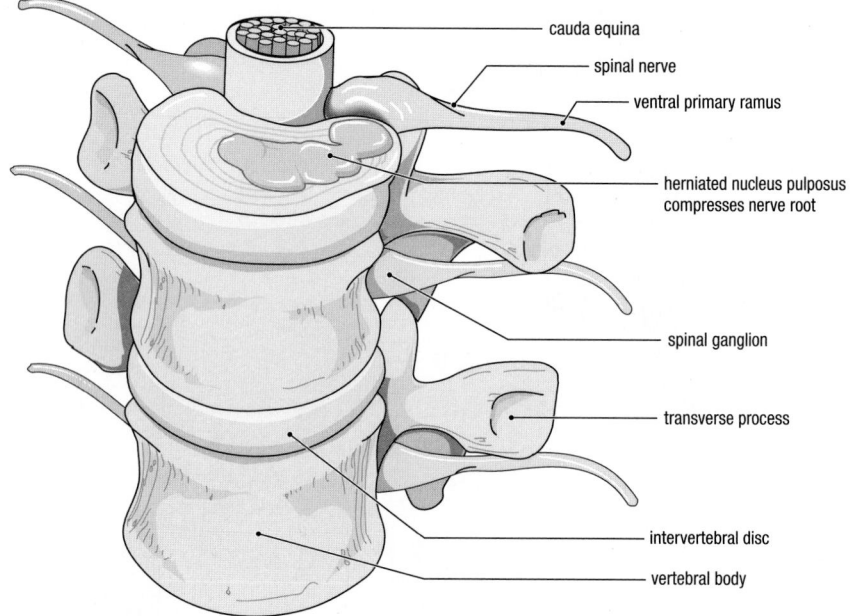

- cauda equina
- spinal nerve
- ventral primary ramus
- herniated nucleus pulposus compresses nerve root
- spinal ganglion
- transverse process
- intervertebral disc
- vertebral body

anterosuperior view of portion of spinal column showing a herniation of the intervertebral disc

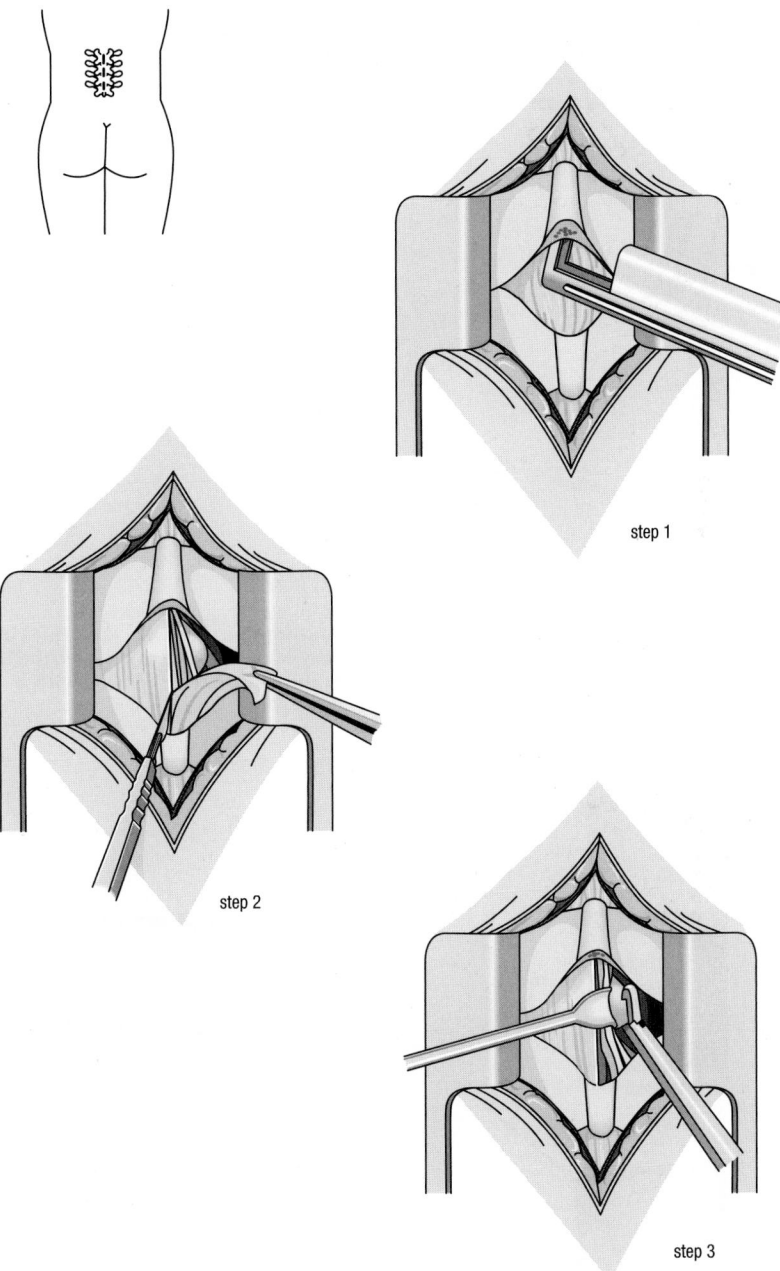

step 1

step 2

step 3

surgical procedure, shown in 3 steps, of the excision of an intervertebral disc during discectomy

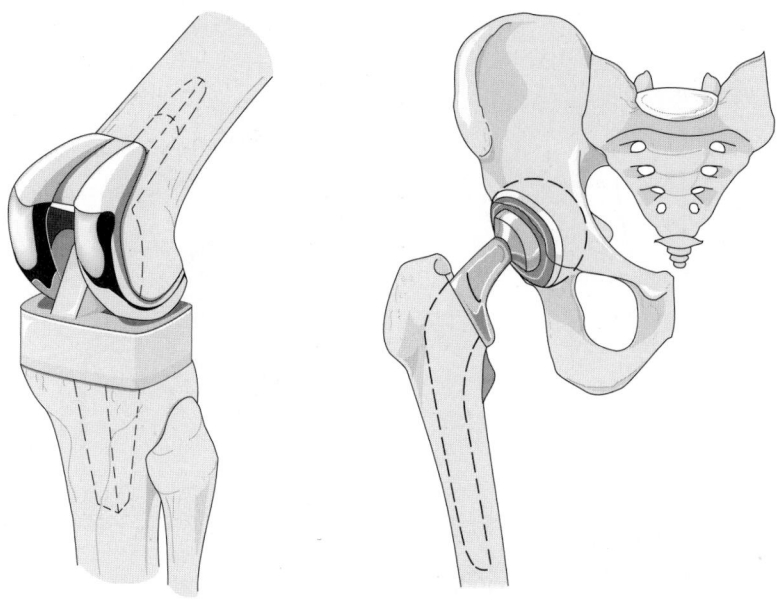

(left) anterolateral view of knee where bones that comprise the hinge joint have been replaced with a prosthetic knee; (right) anterior view of pelvic skeleton where the bones that comprise the ball and socket joint of the hip have been replaced with a prosthetic hip

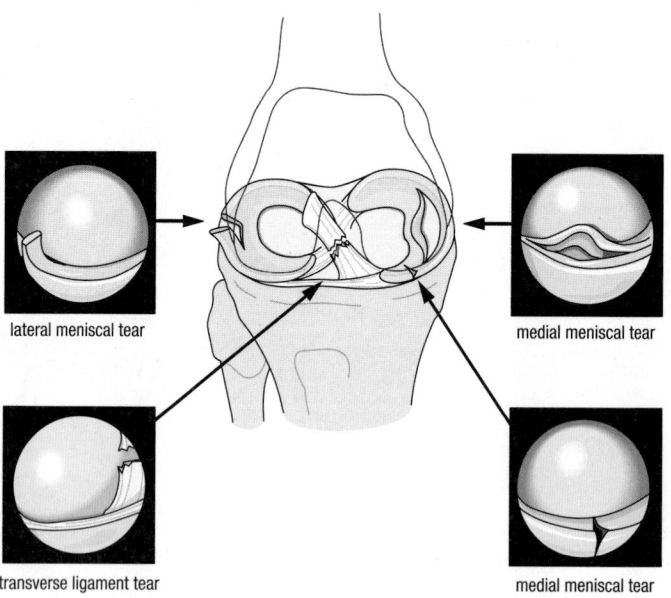

lateral meniscal tear

medial meniscal tear

transverse ligament tear

medial meniscal tear

anterior view of knee joint surrounded by arthroscopic views of tears

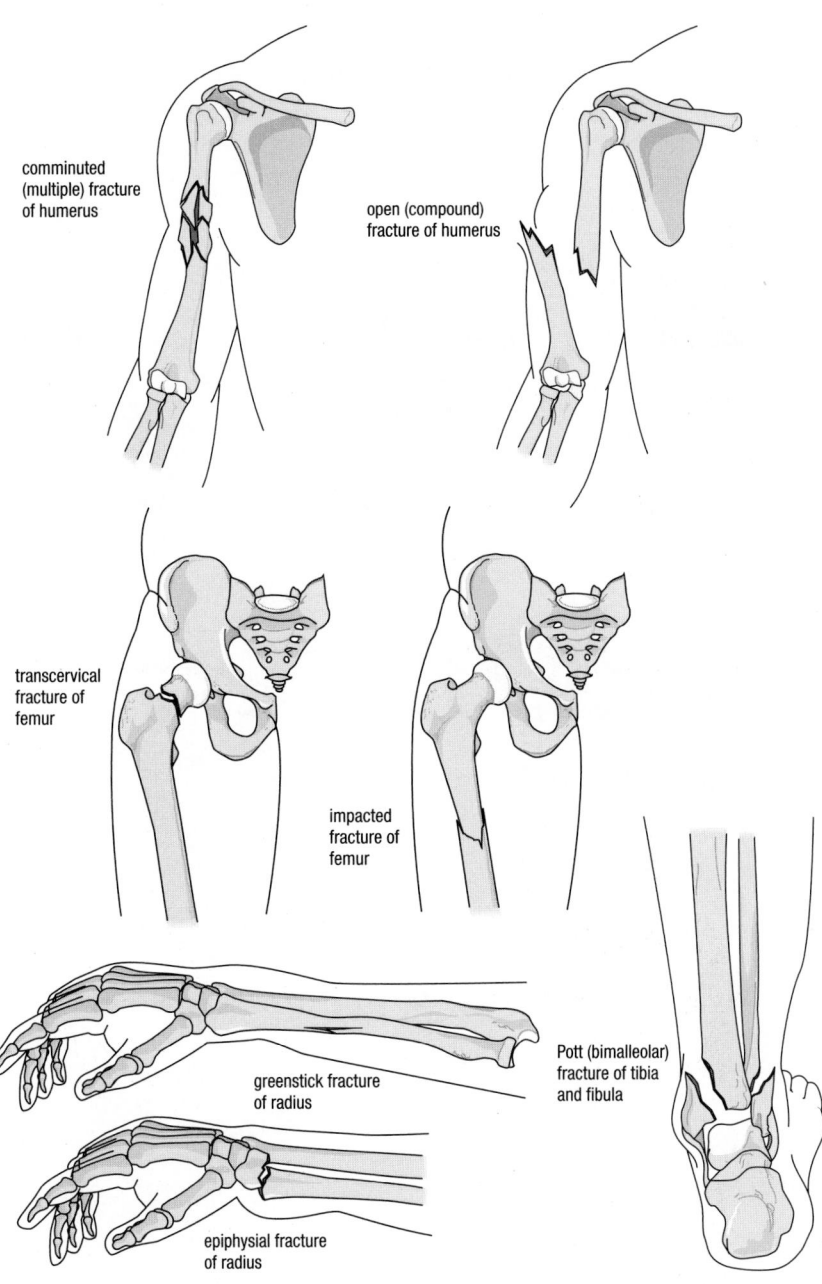

comminuted (multiple) fracture of humerus

open (compound) fracture of humerus

transcervical fracture of femur

impacted fracture of femur

greenstick fracture of radius

epiphysial fracture of radius

Pott (bimalleolar) fracture of tibia and fibula

types of fractures

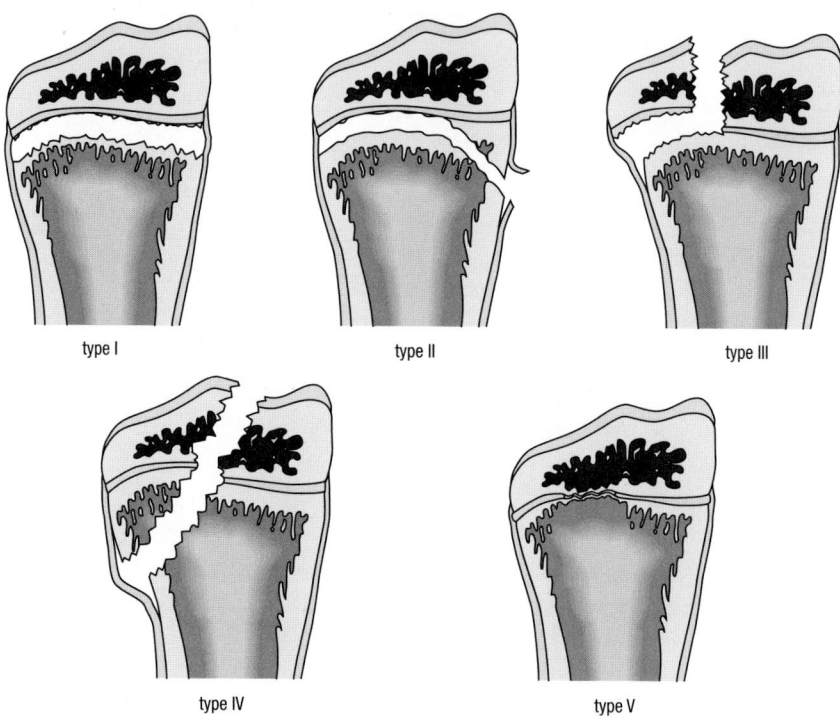

five groups of the Salter-Harris classification of epiphysial plate injuries

Direction of Fracture Lines

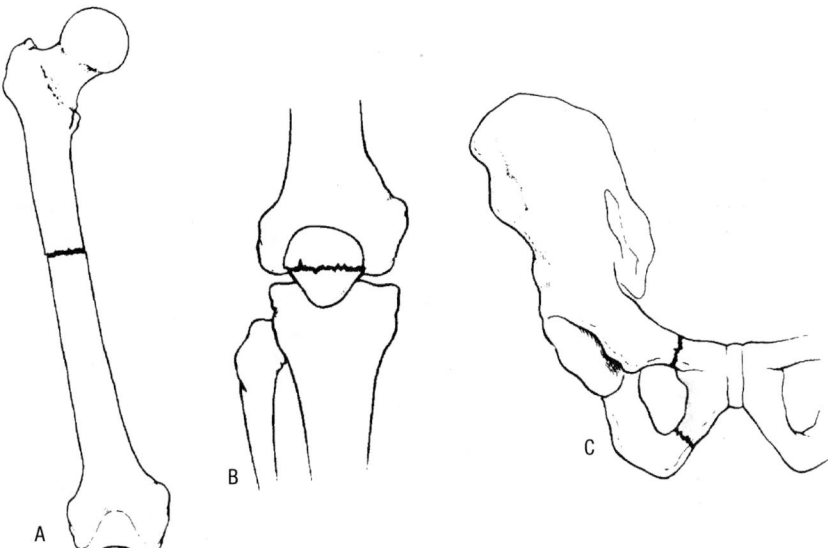

transverse fractures: (A) transverse fracture of the middle third of femur; (B) transverse fracture of midpatella; (C) transverse fracture of superior and inferior pubic rami

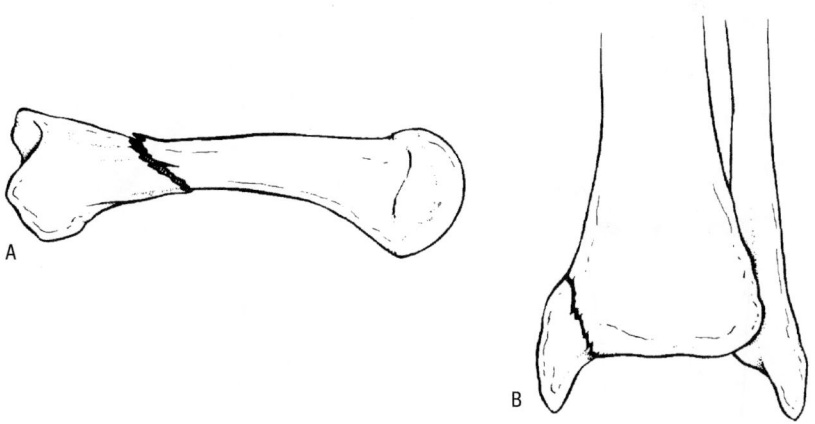

oblique fractures: (A) oblique fracture of proximal third of metacarpal; (B) oblique fracture of medial malleolus

Spinal Fractures

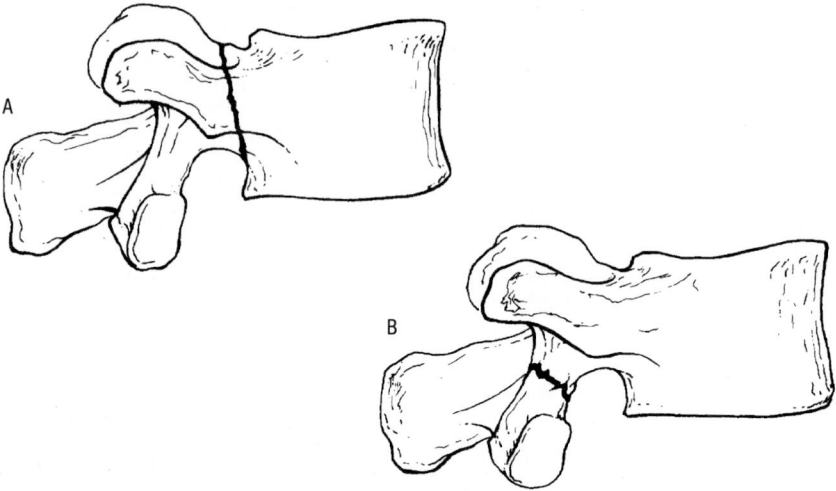

(A) fracture through the pedicle; (B) fracture through the pars interarticularis

Shoulder Fractures

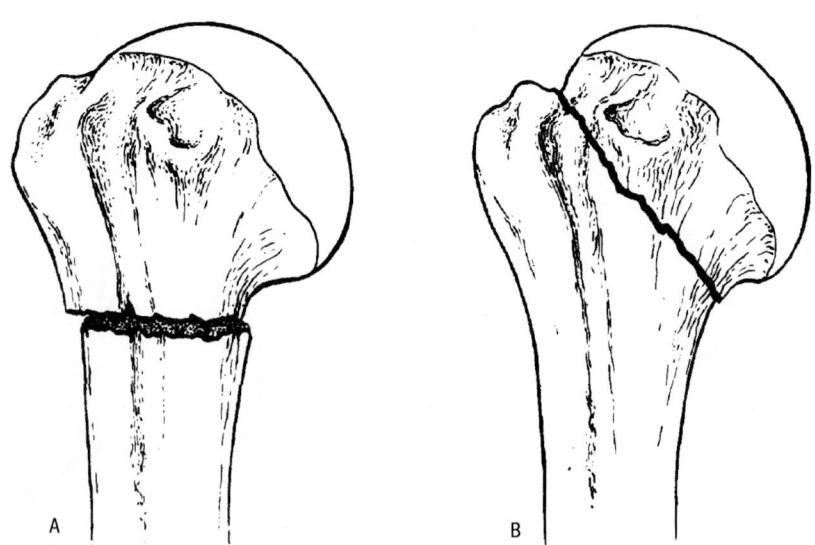

(A) transverse fracture of the surgical neck of the humerus; (B) fracture of the anatomic neck of the humerus

Elbow Fractures

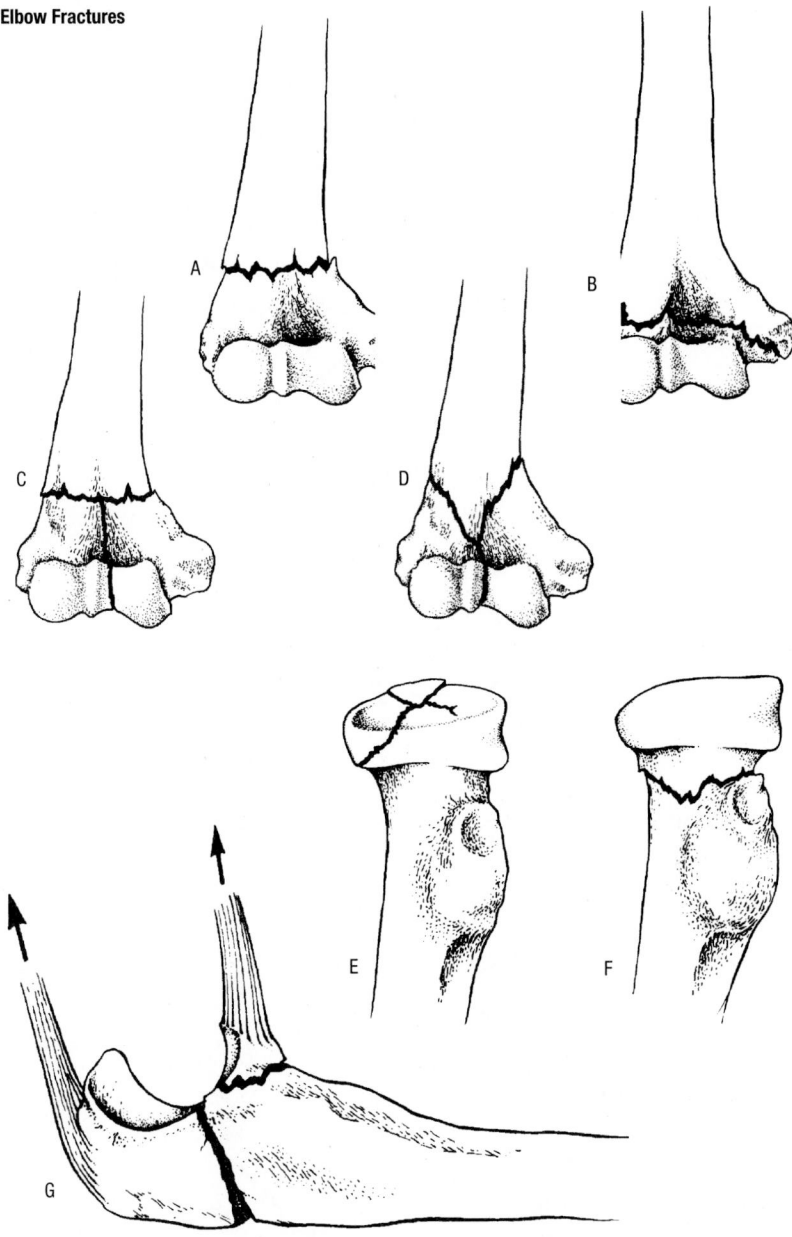

(A) supracondylar fractures are fractures that occur above the level of the condyles; (B) transcondylar fracture; note that the fracture extends through both condyles; (C) T-shaped fracture; (D) Y-shaped fracture; (E) comminuted fracture of the head of the radius; (F) transverse nondisplaced fracture of the neck of the radius; (G) fracture of the olecranon and coronoid process; muscle contraction can cause distraction of fracture fragments

Pelvic Fractures

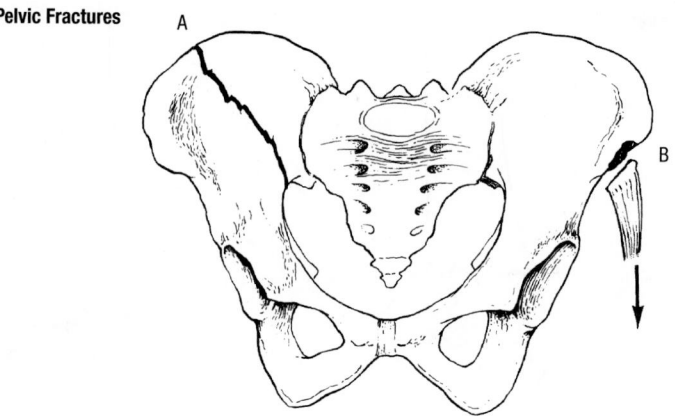

fractures of the ilium: (A) oblique fracture through the wing of the ilium; (B) avulsion fracture of the anteroinferior iliac spine

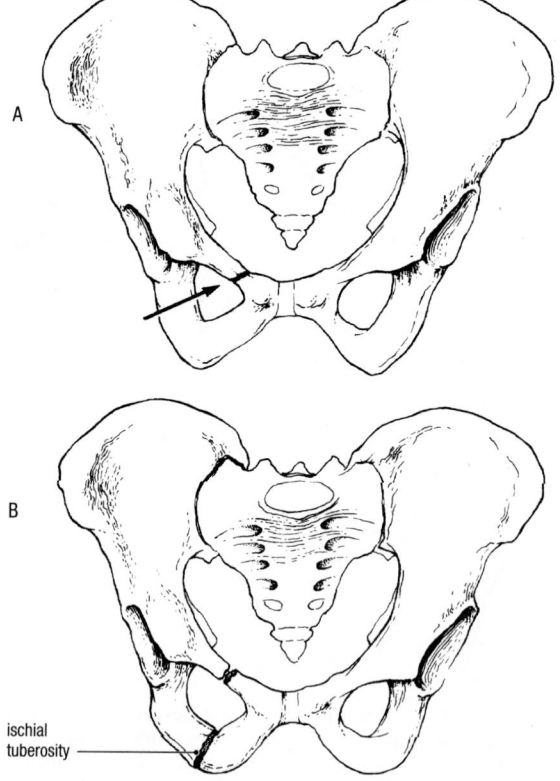

ischial tuberosity

(A) oblique fracture of the superior pubic ramus; (B) transverse fractures of the inferior ischial ramus and superior pubic ramus

Hip Fractures

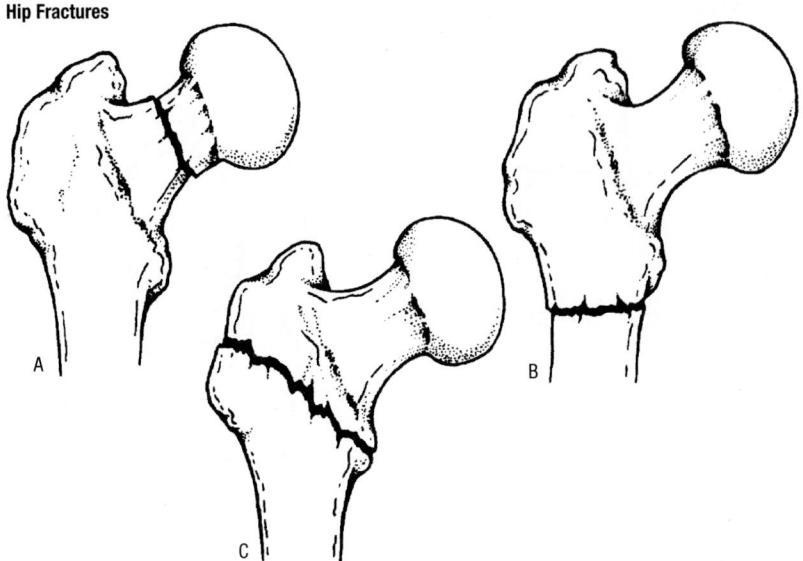

fractures of the hip are described by the location in which they occur: (A) transverse intracapsular fracture; (B) oblique intertrochanteric fracture; (C) transverse subtrochanteric fracture

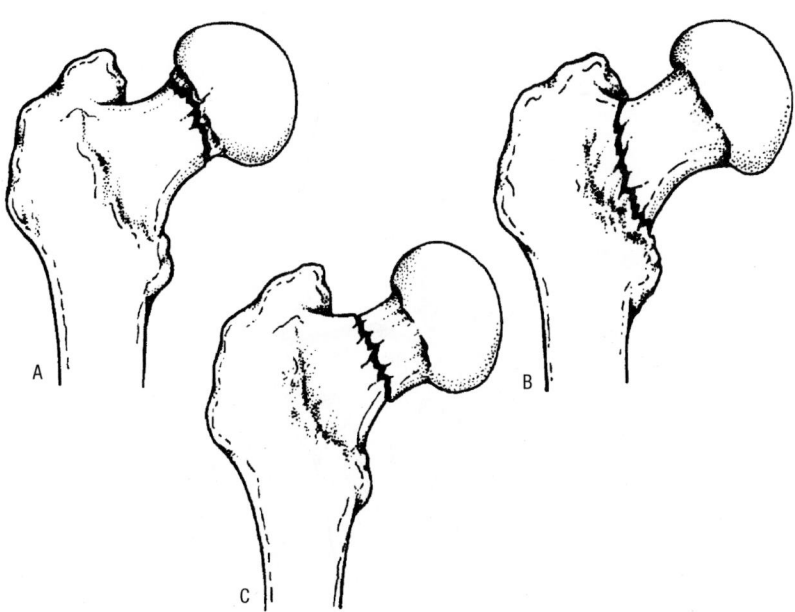

subclassification of intracapsular fractures: (A) subcapital fracture; (B) transcervical fracture; (C) base of neck fracture

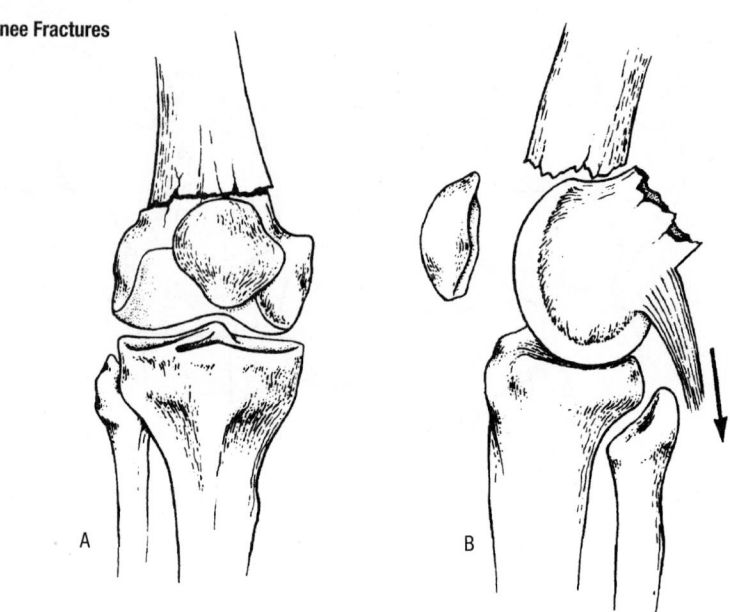

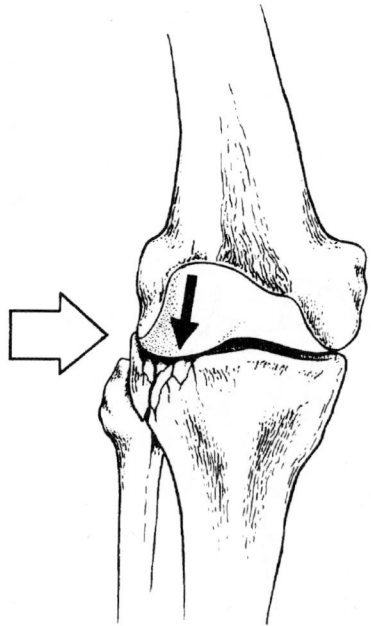

Knee Fractures

supracondylar fracture: transverse supracondylar fracture of the femur (note the pull of the gastrocnemius muscle, causing the distal fragment to be rotated posteriorly)

a valgus force applied to the knee causes the hard femoral condyle to be driven into the softer tibial plateau, resulting in depression of the tibial plateau

Ankle Fractures

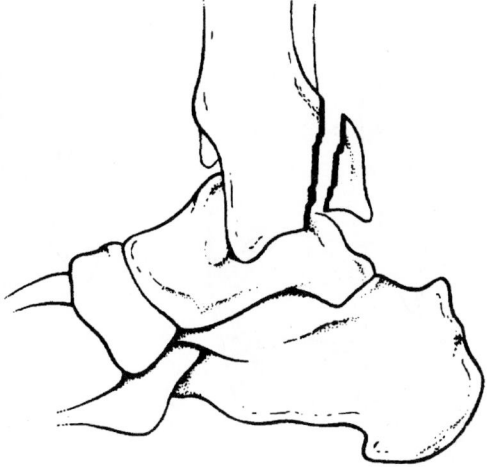

fracture of the posterior malleolus

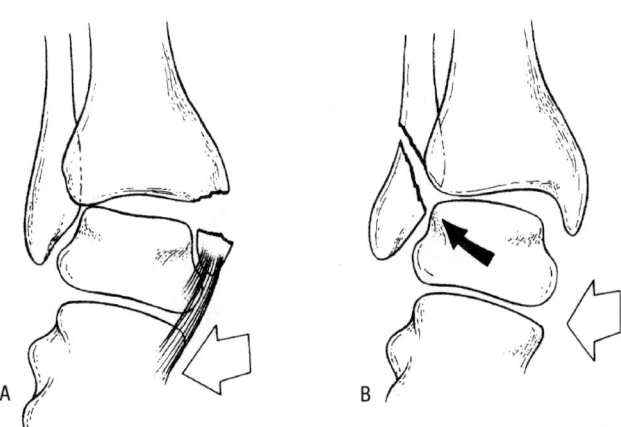

(A) avulsion fracture of the medial malleolus; (B) oblique fracture of the lateral malleolus

Ankle Fractures

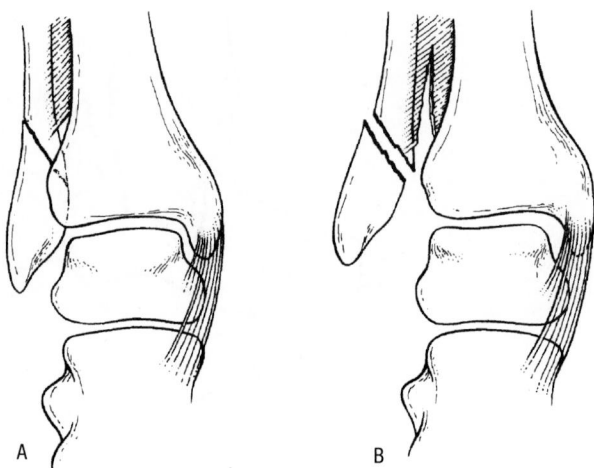

(A) fractures of the lateral malleolus occurring above its articular surface; thus, the ankle mortise is not involved; (B) similar fracture as in (A), above the articular surface with disturbance of the mortise due to separation of the syndesmosis

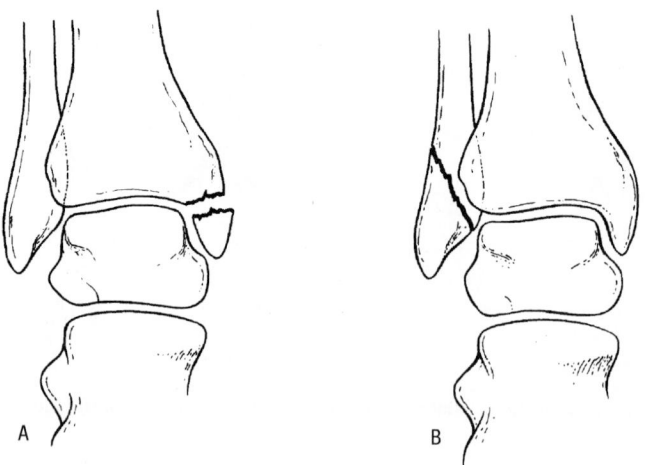

fractures of the malleoli: (A) transverse fracture of the medial malleolus; (B) oblique fracture of the lateral malleolus

Ankle Fractures

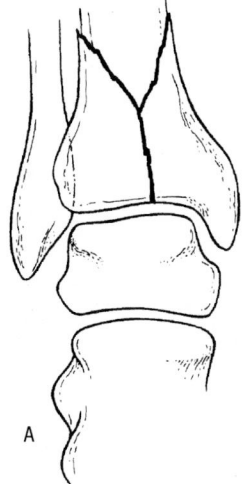 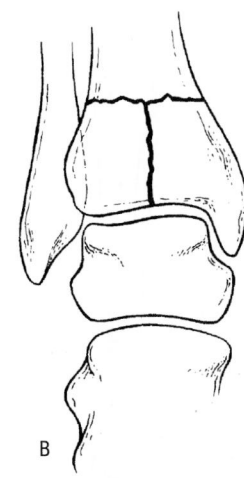

(A) Y-shaped comminuted intraarticular fracture of the distal tibia; (B) T-shaped comminuted intraarticular fracture of the distal tibia

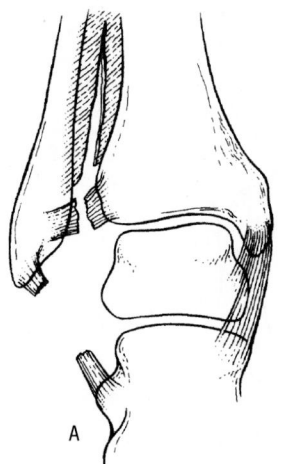 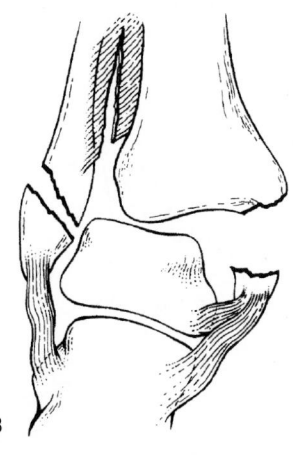

separation of the distal tibiofibular syndesmosis: (A) separation of the tibiofibular syndesmosis without an accompanying fracture; (B) separation of the syndesmosis associated with fracture of the medial and lateral malleoli

Leg Fractures

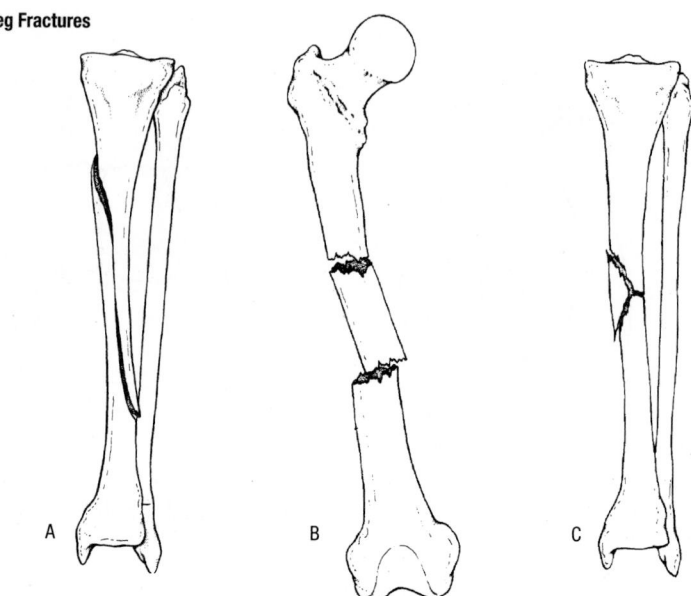

(A) spiral fractures of the middle third of the tibia; (B) segmental fracture of the femur; (C) butterfly fragment

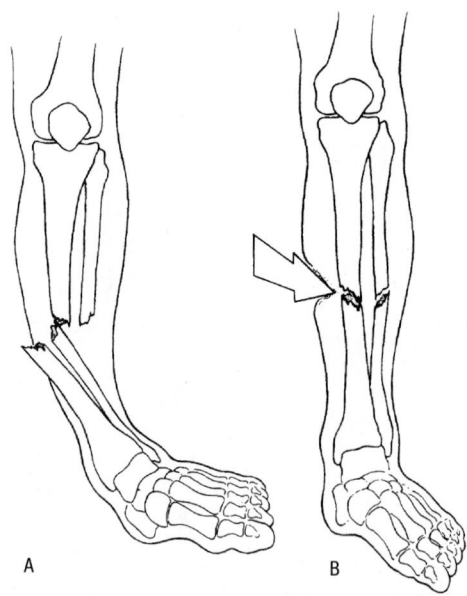

(A) compound fracture caused by an inside-out injury where the skin defect is caused, following the fracture, by the bone perforating the skin from within; (B) outside-in compound fracture where the skin defect is produced by the fracturing agent entering from without

Foot Fractures

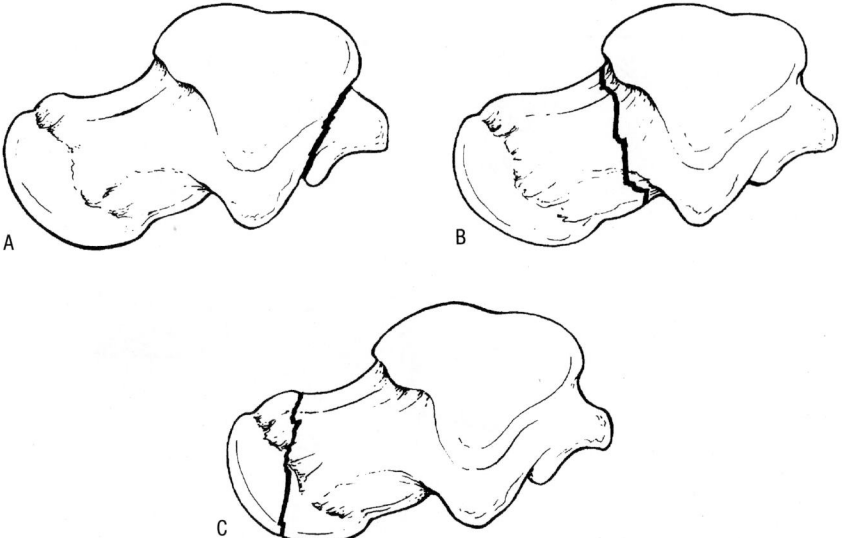

(A) fractures of the talus can be described by the anatomic area involved: (A) fracture of the posterior process; (B) fracture of the body; (C) fracture of the head

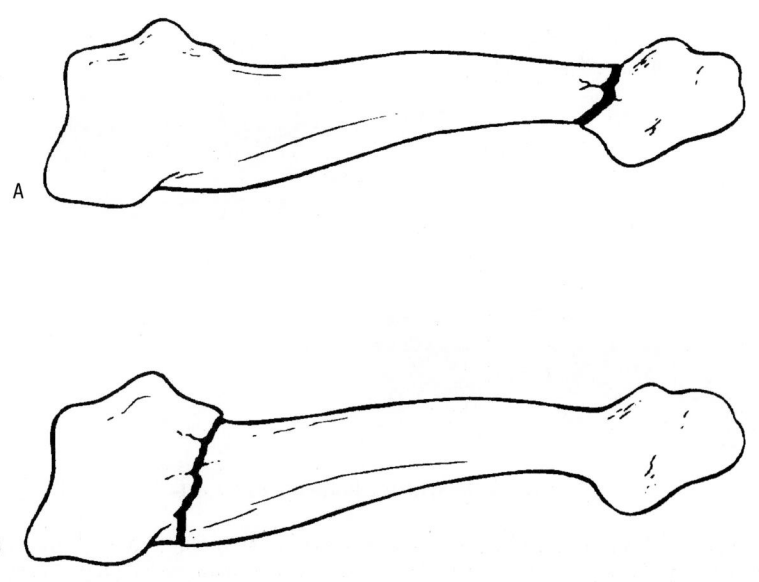

(A) fracture of the head of a metatarsal; (B) fracture of the base of a metatarsal

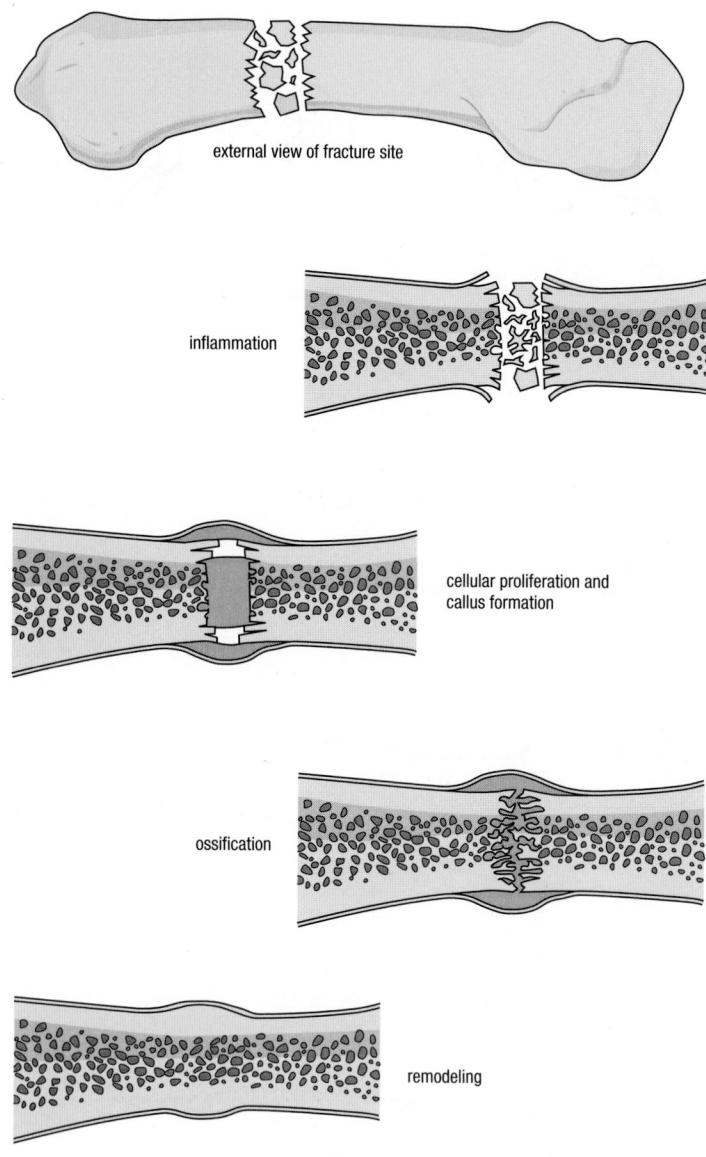

external view of fracture site

inflammation

cellular proliferation and
callus formation

ossification

remodeling

the process by which a bone fracture heals

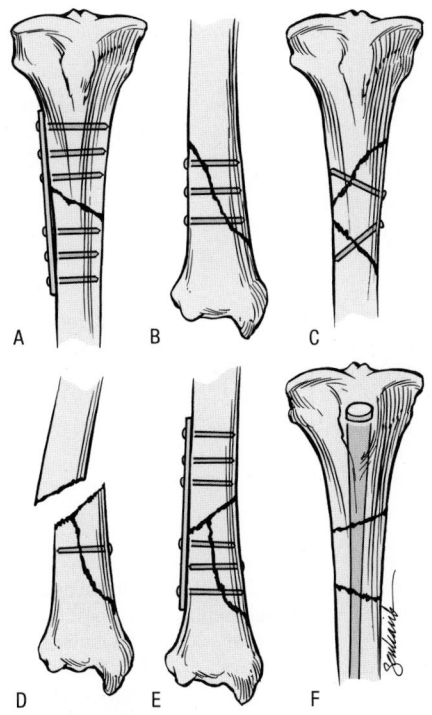

internal fixation: (A) plate and 6 screws for a transverse or short oblique fracture; (B) screws for a long oblique or spiral fracture; (C) screws for a long butterfly fragment; (D, E) plate and 6 screws for a short butterfly fragment; (F) medullary nail for a segmental fracture

Table of Muscles and Cranial Nerves

1. Muscles of the Shoulder

Muscle	Origin	Insertion	Nerve	Action
Deltoid	Lateral 3rd of clavicle, acromion, and spine of scapula	Deltoid tuberosity of humerus	Axillary, C5, C6	Abducts, adducts, flexes, extends, and rotates arm medially
Infraspinatus	Infraspinous fossa of scapula	Middle facet of greater tubercle of humerus	Suprascapular, C5, C6	Rotates arm laterally; helps to hold humeral head in glenoid cavity of scapula
Latissimus dorsi	Spines of T7-T12 thoracolumbar fascia; iliac crest; ribs 9-12	Floor of bicipital groove of humerus	Thoracodorsal, C6, C7, C8	Extends, adducts, and medially rotates humerus; raises body toward arms during climbing
Pectoralis major	Clavicular head; anterior surface of medial half of clavicle	Lateral lip of intertubercular groove of humerus	Lateral and medial pectoral nerves; clavicular head, C5, C6; sternocostal head, C7, C8, T1	Abducts, medially rotates humerus; draws scapula anteriorly and inferiorly
Pectoralis minor	3rd to 5th ribs near the costal cartilages	Medial border and superior surface of coracoid process of scapula	Medial pectoral nerve, C8, T1	Stabilizes scapula against thoracic wall
Subscapularis	Subscapular fossa	Lesser tubercle of humerus	Upper and lower subscapular, C5, C6, C7	Medially rotates arm and adducts it; helps to hold humeral head in glenoid cavity

1. Muscles of the Shoulder

Muscle	Origin	Insertion	Nerve	Action
Supraspinatus	Supraspinous fossa of scapula	Superior facet of greater tubercle of humerus	Suprascapular, C4, C5, C6	Initiates and assists deltoid in abduction of arm and acts with rotator cuff muscles
Teres major	Dorsal surface of inferior angle of scapula	Medial lip of intertubercular groove of humerus	Lower subscapular, C6, C7	Adducts and rotates arm medially
Teres minor	Superior portion of lateral border of scapula	Inferior facet of greater tubercle of humerus	Axillary, C5, C6	Laterally rotates arm; helps to hold humeral head in glenoid cavity of scapula

2. Muscles of the Arm

Muscle	Origin	Insertion	Nerve	Action
Anconeus	Lateral epicondyle of humerus	Lateral surface of olecranon and superior part of posterior surface of ulna	Radial, C7, C8, T1	Assists triceps in extending forearm; abducts ulna during pronation
Biceps brachii	Long head, supraglenoid tubercle; short head, coracoid process	Radial tuberosity of radius	Musculocutaneous, C5, C6	Flexes arm and forearm; supinates forearm
Brachialis	Distal anterior surface of humerus	Coronoid process of ulna and ulnar tuberosity	Musculocutaneous, C5, C6	Flexes forearm in all positions
Coracobrachialis	Tip of coracoid process of scapula	Middle 3rd of medial surface of humerus	Musculocutaneous, C5, C6, C7	Flexes and adducts arm

Muscles and Cranial Nerves

A71

2. Muscles of the Arm

Muscle	Origin	Insertion	Nerve	Action
Triceps	Long head, infraglenoid tubercle; lateral head, superior to radial groove of humerus; medial head to radial groove	Posterior surface of olecranon process of ulna	Radial, C6, C7, C8	Chief extensor of forearm at elbow

3. Muscles of the Anterior Forearm

Muscle	Origin	Insertion	Nerve	Action
Flexor carpi radialis	Medial epicondyle of humerus	Bases of 2nd and 3rd metacarpals	Median, C6, C7	Flexes forearm; flexes and abducts hand
Flexor carpi ulnaris	Humeral head, medial epicondyle of humerus; ulnar head; olecranon and posterior border of ulna	Pisiform bone, hook of hamate, and base of 5th metacarpal	Ulnar, C7, C8	Flexes and adducts hand; flexes forearm
Flexor digitorum profundus	Anteromedial surface of ulna; interosseous membrane	Base of distal phalanges of medial 4 fingers	Ulnar and median, C8, T1	Flexes distal interphalangeal joints and hand
Flexor digitorum superficialis	Medial epicondyle, coronoid process of ulna, superior anterior border of radius	Middle phalanges of finger	Median, C7, C8, T1	Flexes proximal interphalangeal joints; flexes hand at wrist
Flexor pollicis longus	Anterior surface of radius; interosseous membrane; coracoid process	Base of distal phalanx of thumb	Median, C8, T1	Flexes thumb

3. Muscles of the Anterior Forearm

Muscle	Origin	Insertion	Nerve	Action
Palmaris longus	Medial epicondyle of humerus	Distal half of flexor retinaculum, palmar aponeurosis	Median, C7, C8	Flexes hand at wrist and forearm
Pronator quadratus	Anterior surface of distal ulna	Anterior surface of distal radius	Anterior interosseous nerve from median, C8, T1	Pronates forearm; helps hold radius and ulna together
Pronator teres	Medial epicondyle of humerus and coracoid process of ulna	Middle of lateral surface of radius	Median, C6, C7	Pronates and flexes arm at elbow

4. Muscles of the Posterior Forearm

Muscle	Origin	Insertion	Nerve	Action
Abductor pollicis longus	Interosseous membrane, middle 3rd of posterior surface of radius and ulna	Lateral surface of base of 1st metacarpal	Radial, deep branch, posterior interosseous nerve, C7, C8	Abducts thumb and hand
Articularis cubiti	Distal portion of posterior aspect of shaft of humerus	Posterior fibrous capsule of elbow joint	Radial, C7, C8	Retracts posterior joint capsule during extension of elbow
Brachioradialis	Lateral supracondylar ridge of humerus	Base of radial styloid process	Radial, C5, C6, C7	Flexes forearm
Extensor carpi radialis brevis	Lateral epicondyle of humerus	Posterior base of 3rd metacarpal	Radial, deep branch, C7, C8	Extends fingers and abducts hands at wrist

Muscles and Cranial Nerves

4. Muscles of the Posterior Forearm

Muscle	Origin	Insertion	Nerve	Action
Extensor carpi radialis longus	Lateral supracondylar ridge of humerus	Dorsum of base of 2nd metacarpal	Radial, C6, C7	Extends and abducts hand at wrist and joint
Extensor carpi ulnaris	Lateral epicondyle and posterior surface of ulna	Base of 5th metacarpal	Radial, deep branch, posterior interosseous nerve, C7, C8	Extends and abducts hand at wrist joint
Extensor digiti minimi	Common extensor tendon and interosseous membrane	Extensor expansion, base of middle and distal phalanges	Radial, deep branch, posterior interosseous nerve, C7, C8	Extends little finger
Extensor digitorum	Lateral epicondyle of humerus	Extensor expansion, base of middle and digital phalanges	Radial, deep branch, posterior interosseous nerve, C7, C8	Extends fingers and hand at wrist
Extensor indicis	Posterior surface of ulna and interosseous membrane	Extensor expansion of index finger	Radial, deep branch, posterior interosseous nerve, C7	Extends index finger; helps extend hand
Extensor pollicis brevis	Interosseous membrane and posterior surface of middle 3rd of radius	Base of proximal phalanx of thumb	Radial, deep branch, posterior interosseous nerve, C7, C8	Extends proximal phalanx of thumb and abducts hand
Extensor pollicis longus	Interosseous membrane, middle 3rd of posterior surface of ulna	Base of distal phalanx of thumb	Radial, deep branch, posterior interosseous nerve, C7, C8	Extends distal phalanx of thumb and abducts hand
Supinator	Lateral epicondyle of humerus; radial collateral and annular ligaments; crest of ulna	Lateral side of upper part of radius	Radial, deep branch, C5, C6	Supinates forearm

5. Muscles of the Hand

Muscle	Origin	Insertion	Nerve	Action
Abductor digiti minimi	Pisiform; pisohamate ligament; flexor retinaculum	Medial side of base of proximal phalanx of little finger	Ulnar, deep branch, C8, T1	Abducts little finger
Abductor pollicis brevis	Flexor retinaculum; scaphoid; trapezium	Lateral side of base of proximal phalanx of thumb	Median, recurrent branch, C8, T1	Abducts thumb
Adductor pollicis	Capitate and bases of 2nd and 3rd metacarpals, (oblique head); palmar surface of 3rd metacarpal (transverse head)	Medial side of base of proximal phalanx of the thumb	Ulnar, deep branch, C8, T1	Adducts thumb toward middle digit
Dorsal interossei (4)	Adjacent sides of metacarpal bones	Extensor expansions and bases of phalanges of digits 2-4	Ulnar, deep branch, C8, T1	Abducts fingers; flexes metacarpopha-langeal joints; extends inter-phalangeal joints
Flexor digiti minimi brevis	Flexor retinaculum and hook of hamate	Medial side of base of proximal phalanx of little finger	Ulnar, deep branch, C8, T1	Flexes proximal phalanx of little finger
Flexor pollicis brevis	Flexor retinaculum and trapezium	Base of proximal phalanx of thumb	Median, recurrent branch, C8, T1	Flexes thumb

Muscles and Cranial Nerves

5. Muscles of the Hand

Muscle	Origin	Insertion	Nerve	Action
Lumbricals (4)	1-2 lateral, 3-4 medial side of tendons of flexor digitorum profundus	Lateral side of extensor expansion	Median (2 lateral), ulnar (2 medial)	Flexes metacarpophalangeal joints, extends interphalangeal joints
Opponens digiti minimi	Flexor retinaculum and hook of hamate	Medial side of 5th metacarpal	Ulnar, deep branch, C8, T1	Opposes little finger with thumb
Opponens pollicis	Flexor retinaculum and tubercles of scaphoid and trapezium	Lateral side of 1st metacarpal	Median, recurrent branch, C8, T1	Opposes thumb to other digits
Palmar interossei (3)	Palmar surfaces of 2nd, 4th, and 5th metacarpals (unipennate muscles)	Bases of proximal phalanges in same sides as their origins; extensor expansion	Ulnar, deep branch, C8, T1	Adducts fingers; flexes metacarpophalangeal joints; extends interphalangeal joints
Palmaris brevis	Ulnar side of flexor retinaculum, palmar aponeurosis	Skin of ulnar side of hand	Ulnar, superficial, T1	Wrinkles skin on palmar side of hand

6. Anterior Muscles of the Thigh

Muscle	Origin	Insertion	Nerve	Action
Abductor brevis/minimus	Inferior pubic ramus	Pectineal line; uppermost linea aspera of femur	Obturator, L2, L3, L4	Adducts, flexes, rotates thigh
Adductor longus	Body of pubis inferior to pubic crest	Middle 3rd of linea aspera of femur	Obturator, branch of anterior division, L2, L3, L4	Adducts, flexes, rotates thigh laterally

6. Anterior Muscles of the Thigh

Muscle	Origin	Insertion	Nerve	Action
Adductor magnus	Ischiopubic ramus; ischial tuberosity	Linea aspera; medial supracondylar line; adductor tubercle	Obturator, L2, L3, L4; sciatic L4	Adducts, flexes, and extends thigh
Gracilis	Body of inferior ramus of pubis	Superior part of medial surface of tibia	Obturator, L2, L3	Adducts and flexes thigh; flexes and rotates leg medially
Iliacus	Iliac crest, iliac fossa; ala of sacrum	Lesser trochanter, psoas major tendon	Femoral, L2, L4	Flexes and rotates thigh medially with psoas major
Obturator externus	Margin of obturator foramen and obturator membrane	Trochanteric fossa of femur	Obturator, L3, L4	Rotates thigh laterally
Pectineus	Pectineal line of pubis	Pectineal line of femur	Femoral, L3, L4; obturator	Adducts and flexes thigh; helps with rotation
Rectus femoris	Anterior-inferior iliac spine; ilium rim of acetabulum	Base of patella; tibial tuberosity	Femoral, L2, L3, L4	Extends leg at knee joint; stabilizes hip; helps iliopsoas flex thigh
Sartorius	Anterior-superior iliac spine, superior part of notch inferior to it	Upper medial side of tibia	Femoral, L2, L3	Flexes, abducts, rotates thigh at hip laterally; flexes, rotates leg at knee joint

Muscles and Cranial Nerves

6. Anterior Muscles of the Thigh

Muscle	Origin	Insertion	Nerve	Action
Vastus intermedius	Upper shaft of femur; lower lateral intermuscular septum	Base of patella; by patellar ligament to tibial tuberosity	Femoral	Extends leg at knee joint
Vastus lateralis	Intertrochanteric line; greater trochanter; linea aspera; gluteal tuberosity; lateral intermuscular septum	Lateral side of patella; tibial tuberosity	Femoral, L2, L3, L4	Extends leg at knee joint
Vastus medialis	Intertrochanteric line; linea aspera; medial intermuscular septum	Medial side of patella; tibial tuberosity	Femoral, L2, L3, L4	Extends leg at knee joint

7. Medial Muscles of the Thigh

Muscle	Origin	Insertion	Nerve	Action
Abductor brevis	Body and inferior ramus of pubis	Pectineal line and proximal part of linea aspera of femur	Obturator, L2, L3, L4	Adducts thigh; aids in flexion
Adductor longus	Body of pubis inferior to pubic crest	Middle 3rd of linea aspera of femur	Obturator L2, L3, L4	Adducts thigh
Adductor magnus	Ischiopubic ramus; ischial tuberosity	Linea aspera; medial supracondylar line; adductor tubercle	Obturator and sciatic	Adducts, flexes, and extends thigh
Gracilis	Body of inferior pubic of ramus	Superior part of medial surface of tibia	Obturator, L2, L3	Adducts thigh; flexes leg; helps rotate thigh medially

7. Medial Muscles of the Thigh

Muscle	Origin	Insertion	Nerve	Action
Obturator externus	Margin of obturator foramen and obturator membrane	Trochanteric fossa of femur	Obturator, L3, L4	Laterally rotates thigh; steadies head of femur in acetabulum
Pectineus	Pectineal line of pubis	Pectineal line of femur	Femoral L2 and L3; branch of obturator	Adducts and flexes thigh; aids in medial rotation of thigh

8. Muscles of the Gluteal Region

Muscle	Origin	Insertion	Nerve	Action
Coccygeus (ischiococcygeus)	Ischial spine	Inferior end of spine	Branches of S4 and S5 nerves	Forms small part of pelvic diaphragm that supports pelvic viscera and flexes coccyx
Gluteus maximus	Ilium; sacrum; coccyx; sacrotuberous ligament	Gluteal tuberosity; iliotibial tract	Inferior gluteal, L5, S1, S2	Extends and rotates thigh laterally
Gluteus medius	Ilium between iliac crest and anterior and posterior gluteal lines	Greater trochanter	Superior gluteal, L5, S1	Abducts and rotates thigh medially; helps keep pelvis level
Gluteus minimus	Ilium between anterior and posterior gluteal lines	Greater trochanter	Superior gluteal, L5, S1	Abducts and rotates thigh medially; helps keep pelvis level
Inferior gemellus	Ischial tuberosity	Obturator internus tendon	Nerve to quadratus femoris	Rotates thigh laterally

Muscles and Cranial Nerves

8. Muscles of the Gluteal Region

Muscle	Origin	Insertion	Nerve	Action
Obturator internus	Ischiopubic rami; obturator membrane	Greater trochanter	Nerve to obturator internus, L5, S1	Abducts and rotates thigh laterally
Piriformis	Pelvic surface of sacrum; sacrotuberous ligament	Superior border of greater trochanter	Sacral, S1, S2	Rotates thigh medially
Quadratus femoris	Ischial tuberosity	Intertrochanteric crest	Nerve to quadratus femoral, L5, S1	Rotates thigh laterally

9. Posterior Muscles of the Thigh*

Muscle	Origin	Insertion	Nerve	Action
Biceps femoris	Long head from ischial tuberosity; short head from linea aspera and upper supracondylar line	Lateral side of head of fibula; tendon split here by fibular collateral ligament of knee	Tibial (long head), common peroneal; division of sciatic nerve, L5, S1, S2	Flexes leg medially; extends thigh
Semimem-branosus	Ischial tuberosity	Medial condyle of tibia	Tibial portion of sciatic, L5, S1, S2	Extends thigh; rotates leg medially; helps raise trunk of body against gravity
Semitendinosus	Ischial tuberosity	Medial surface of superior part of tibia	Tibial division of sciatic nerve, L5, S1, S2	Extends thigh; flexes leg; rotates knee medially when flexed

*These 3 muscles collectively are called hamstrings.

10. Muscles of the Anterior and Lateral Leg

Muscle	Origin	Insertion	Nerve	Action
Anterior				
Articularis genus	Distal portion of anterior aspect of shaft of femur	Synovial membrane of suprapatellar bursa of knee joint	Femoral, L2-L4	Retracts synovial membrane during extension of the knee
Extensor digitorum longus	Lateral tibial condyle; upper two thirds of fibula	Bases of middle and distal phalanges	Deep peroneal, L5, S1	Extends great toe; dorsiflexes ankle
Extensor hallucis longus	Middle half of anterior surface of fibula; interosseous membrane	Base of distal phalanx of great toe	Deep peroneal, L5, S1	Extends great toe; dorsiflexes and inverts foot
Peroneus tertius	Distal 3rd of fibula; interosseous membrane	Base of 5th metatarsal	Deep peroneal	Dorsiflexes and inverts foot
Tibialis anterior	Lateral tibial condyle; interosseous membrane	1st cuneiform; 1st metatarsal	Deep peroneal, L4, L5	Dorsiflexes and inverts foot
Lateral				
Peroneus brevis	Lower lateral side of fibula; interosseous membrane	Base of 5th metatarsal	Superficial peroneal	Everts and plantar flexes foot
Peroneus longus	Lateral tibial condyle; head and upper lateral side of fibula	Base of 1st metatarsal; medial cuneiform	Superficial peroneal	Everts and plantar flexes foot

Muscles and Cranial Nerves

11. Posterior Muscles of the Leg

Muscle	Origin	Insertion	Nerve	Action
Superficial group				
Gastrocnemius	Lateral (head) and medial (head) femoral condyle	Posterior aspect of calcaneus via tendo calcaneus	Tibial, S2, S2	Flexes knee; plantar flexes ankle when knee extended
Plantaris	Lower lateral supracondylar line and oblique popliteal ligament	Posterior surface of calcaneus	Tibial, S1, S2	Assist gastrocnemius in plantar flexing ankle and flexing knee
Soleus	Upper fibular head; soleal line on tibia	Posterior aspect of calcaneus via tendo calcaneus	Tibial, S1, S2	Plantar flexes foot and ankle
Deep group				
Flexor hallucis longus	Inferior two thirds of posterior surface of fibula and interior part of interosseous membrane	Base of distal phalanx of great toe	Tibial, S2, S3	Flexes great toe at all joints; weakly plantar flexes ankle; supports medial longitudinal arches of foot
Flexor digitorum longus	Medial portion of posterior surface of tibia inferior to soleal line	Base of distal phalanges of lateral 4 digits	Tibial, S2, S3	Flexes lateral 4 digits; plantar flexes ankle; supports arches of foot
Popliteus	Lateral surface of lateral condyle of femur and lateral meniscus	Posterior surface of tibia, superior to soleal line	Tibial, L4, L5, S1	Weakly flexes knee and unlocks knee

11. Posterior Muscles of the Leg

Muscle	Origin	Insertion	Nerve	Action
Tibialis posterior	Interosseous membrane; posterior surface of tibia inferior to soleal line; posterior surface of fibula	Tuberosity of navicular cuneiform and cuboid; base of 2-4 metatarsals	Tibial, L4, L5	Plantar flexes ankle; inverts foot

12. Muscles of the Foot

Muscle	Origin	Insertion	Nerve	Action
Dorsum of foot				
Extensor digitorum brevis	Dorsal surface of calcaneus	Lateral side of long extensor tendons with slips to proximal phalanges 2-4 toes	Deep peroneal, L5, S1	Assist in extending middle 3 toes
Extensor hallucis brevis	Dorsal surface of calcaneus	Base of proximal phalanx of great toe	Deep peroneal, L5, S1	Extends great toe
Sole of foot				
Abductor digiti minimi	Medial and lateral tubercles of calcaneus, plantar aponeurosis and intermuscular septa	Lateral side of base of proximal phalanx of 5th digit	Lateral plantar, S2, S3	Abducts and flexes 5th digit
Abductor hallucis	Medial tubercle of calcaneus; flexor retinaculum and plantar aponeurosis	Medial side of base of proximal phalanx of 1st digit	Medial plantar, S2, S3	Abducts and flexes great toe

12. Muscles of the Foot

Muscle	Origin	Insertion	Nerve	Action
Adductor hallucis; oblique head	Base of metatarsals 2-4	Proximal phalanx of great toe	Deep branch of lateral plantar, S2, S3	Adducts great toe; assists in maintaining transverse arch
Adductor hallucis; transverse head	Capsule of lateral 4 metatarsophalangeal joints	Tendon of head attached to lateral sides of base of proximal phalanx of 1st digit	Deep branch of plantar, S2, S3	Adducts great toe; assists in maintaining transverse arch
Dorsal interossei (4)	Adjacent shafts of metatarsals	Proximal phalanges of 2nd toe medial and lateral sides; 3rd and 4th toes lateral sides	Lateral plantar, S2, S3	Abducts toes; flexes and extends proximal and distal phalanges
Flexor digitorum brevis	Medial tubercle of calcaneus, plantar aponeurosis and intermuscular septa	Middle phalanges of lateral 4 toes	Medial plantar, S2, S3	Flexes middle phalanges of lateral 4 toes
Flexor digiti minimi brevis	Base of 5th metatarsal	Proximal phalanx of 5th toe	Lateral plantar, S2, S3	Flexes 5th toe
Flexor hallucis brevis	Cuboid; 3rd cuneiform	Proximal phalanx of great toe	Medial plantar, S2, S3	Flexes great toe
Lumbricals (4)	Tendons of flexor digitorum longus	Proximal phalanges; extensor expansion	1st by medial plantar nerve; lateral 3 by lateral plantar nerve, S2, S3	Flexes metatarsophalangeal joints and extends interphalangeal joints

12. Muscles of the Foot

Muscle	Origin	Insertion	Nerve	Action
Plantar interossei (3)	Medial sides of metatarsals 3-5	Medial side of base of proximal phalanges 3-5	Lateral plantar, S2, S3	Adducts toes; flexes proximal and extends distal phalanges
Quadratus plantae	Medial and lateral side of calcaneus	Tendons of flexor digitorum longus	Lateral plantar, S2, S3	Assists in flexing toes

13. Muscles of the Thoracic Wall

Muscle	Origin	Insertion	Nerve	Action
External intercostals	Lower border of ribs	Upper border of rib below	Intercostal	Elevates rib in inspiration
Internal intercostals	Lower border of ribs	Upper border of rib below	Intercostal	Depresses ribs; interchondral part elevates ribs
Levator costarum	Tips of transverse processes of C7 and T7-T11 vertebrae	Subjacent ribs between tubercle and angle	Dorsal primary rami of C8-T11	Elevates ribs; assists with lateral bending
Subcostals	Inner surface of lower ribs near their angles	Upper borders of ribs 2 or 3 below	Intercostal	Elevates ribs
Transverse thoracic	Posterior surface of lower sternum and xiphoid	Inner surface of costal cartilages 2-6	Intercostal	Depresses ribs

Muscles and Cranial Nerves

14. Muscles of the Anterior Abdominal Wall

Muscle	Origin	Insertion	Nerve	Action
External oblique	External surface of lower 8 ribs, 5-12	Anterior half of iliac crest; anterior-superior iliac spine; pubic tubercle; linea alba	Intercostal, T7-T11; subcostal, T12	Compresses abdomen; flexes trunk; assists in forced expiration
Internal oblique	Lateral two thirds of inguinal ligament; iliac crest; thoracolumbar fascia	Lower 4 costal cartilages; lineal alba; pubic crest; pectineal line	Intercostal, T7-T11; subcostal T12; iliohypogastric and ilioinguinal, L1	Compresses abdomen; flexes trunk; assists in forced expiration
Pyramidalis	Pubic body	Linea alba	Subcostal, T12	Tenses linea alba
Rectus abdominis	Pubic crest and pubic symphysis	Xiphoid process and costal cartilages 5-7	Intercostal, T7-T12	Depresses ribs; flexes trunk
Transverse abdominis	Lateral 3rd of inguinal ligament; iliac crest; thoracolumbar fascia; lower 6 costal cartilages	Linea alba; pubic crest; pectineal line	Intercostal, T7-T12; subcostal, T12; iliohypogastric and ilioinguinal, L1	Compresses abdomen; depresses ribs

15. Muscles of the Posterior Abdominal Wall

Muscle	Origin	Insertion	Nerve	Action
Psoas major	Sides of T12-L5 vertebra and disc; transverse processes	Lesser trochanter of femur	Anterior rami of L1, L2, and L3	Flexes and rotates thigh laterally at hip; flexes lumbar vertebral column anteriorly and laterally

15. Muscles of the Posterior Abdominal Wall

Muscle	Origin	Insertion	Nerve	Action
Psoas minor	Sides of T12-L1 vertebra and intervertebral disc	Pectineal line, iliopectineal eminence via iliopectineal arch	Anterior rami of L1, L2	Works conjointly with psoas major to flex thigh at hip; stabilizes joint
Quadratus lumborum	Medial half of inferior border of 12th rib and tips of lumbar transverse processes	Iliolumbar ligament and internal tip of iliac crest	Ventral branches of T12, L1-L4	Extends, laterally flexes vertebral column; flexes 12th rib during inspiration

16. Superficial Muscles of the Back

Muscle	Origin	Insertion	Nerve	Action
Erector spinae	Arises by a broad tendon from posterior part of iliac crest, posterior surface of sacrum, sacral and inferior lumbar spinous processes and supraspinous ligament	Iliocostalis lumborum, thoracis and cervicis; longissimus thoracis, cervicis and capitis; spinalis thoracis, cervicis and capitis	Posterior rami of spinal nerves	Extend vertebral column and head
Interspinales	Superior surface of spinous processes of cervical and lumbar vertebrae	Inferior surface of spinous process of vertebrae superior to vertebrae of origin	Posterior rami of spinal nerves	Assist in extension and rotation of vertebral column

16. Superficial Muscles of the Back

Muscle	Origin	Insertion	Nerve	Action
Intertransversarii	Transverse process of cervical and lumbar vertebrae	Transverse process of adjacent vertebrae	Posterior and anterior rami of spinal nerves	Assists in lateral bending of vertebral column; stabilizes vertebral column
Latissimus dorsi	Spines of T5-T12	Floor of bicipital groove	Thoracodorsal	Adducts, extends, and rotates arm medially
Levator scapulae	Transverse process of C1-C4	Superior part of medial border of scapula	Dorsal scapular, C5; cervical, C3-C4	Elevates scapula
Rhomboid major	Spines of T2-T5	Medial border of scapula	Dorsal scapular, C4, C5	Adducts scapula
Rhomboid minor	Spines of C7-T1	Root of spine of scapula	Dorsal scapular, C4, C5	Adducts scapula
Serratus anterior	External surface of lateral parts of 1-8 ribs	Anterior surface of medial border of scapula	Long thoracic nerve, C5, C6, C7	Protracts and rotates scapula
Serratus posterior inferior	Spinal processes of T11 to L2 vertebrae	Inferior border of 8-12 ribs near their angles	Intercostal, 9-12	Depresses ribs
Serratus posterior superior	Ligamentum nuchae, supraspinal ligament and spines of C7-T3	Superior borders of 2-4 ribs	Intercostal, 1-4	Elevates ribs

16. Superficial Muscles of the Back

Muscle	Origin	Insertion	Nerve	Action
Transversospinal	Transverse process of C4-T12 vertebrae; multifidus arises from sacrum, ilium, transverse process of T1-T3 and articular process of C4-C7	Thoracis, cervicis, and capitis	Spinal, posterior rami	Extends and rotates vertebral column; stabilizes vertebrae during movement
Trapezius	External occipital protuberance, superior nuchal line, ligamentum nuchae, spines of C7-T12	Lateral 3rd of clavicle, acromion, and spine of scapula	Spinal accessory, C3-C4	Adducts, rotates, elevates, and depresses scapula

17. Suboccipital Muscles

Muscle	Origin	Insertion	Nerve	Action
Obliquus capitis inferior	Spine of axis C2	Transverse process of atlas, C1	Suboccipital	Extends and laterally rotates head
Obliquus capitis superior	Transverse process of atlas, C1	Occipital bone above inferior nuchal line	Suboccipital	Extends, rotates, and laterally flexes head
Rectus capitis posterior major	Spine of axis, C2	Lateral portion of inferior nuchal line	Suboccipital	Extends, rotates, and laterally flexes head
Rectus capitis posterior minor	Posterior tubercle of atlas, C1	Occipital bone below inferior nuchal line	Suboccipital	Extends, rotates, and laterally flexes head

Muscles and Cranial Nerves

18. Muscles of the Neck

Muscle	Origin	Insertion	Nerve	Action
Cervical muscles				
Platysma	Superficial fascia over upper part of deltoid and pectoralis major	Mandible; skin and muscles over the mandible and angle of mouth	Facial, CN 7	Depresses lower jaw and lip and angle of mouth; wrinkles skin of neck
Sternoclei-domastoid	Lateral surface of mastoid process of temporal bone and lateral half of superior nuchal line	Mastoid process and lateral one half of superior nuchal line	Spinal accessory, C2-C3	Tilts head; laterally flexes and rotates face to opposite side; raises thorax
Suprahyoid muscles				
Digastric	Anterior belly from digastric fossa of mandible posterior belly from mastoid notch	Intermediate tendon attached to body of hyoid	Anterior belly: mylohyoid nerve, branch of alveolar nerve; posterior belly: facial nerve, CN 7	Depresses mandible and elevates hyoid and tongue
Geniohyoid	Genial tubercle of mandible	Body of hyoid	C1 via the hypoglossal nerve	Pulls hyoid bone anterosu-periorly, shortens floor of mouth; widens pharynx
Mylohyoid	Mylohyoid line of mandible	Median raphe and body of hyoid bone	Mylohyoid and trigeminal, CN 3	Elevates hyoid and tongue; depresses mandible
Styloid	Styloid process	Body of hyoid	Facial, CN 7	Elevates and retracts hyoid

18. Muscles of the Neck

Muscle	Origin	Insertion	Nerve	Action
Infrahyoid muscles				
Omohyoid	Inferior belly from medial lip of suprascapular notch and suprascapular ligament; superior belly from intermediate tendon	Inferior belly to intermediate tendon; superior belly to body of hyoid	Ansa cervicalis, C1-C3	Depresses and retracts hyoid and larynx
Sternohyoid	Manubrium sterni and medial end of clavicle	Body of hyoid	Ansa cervicalis, C1-C3	Depresses hyoid and larynx
Sternothyroid	Manubrium sterni; 1st costal cartilage	Oblique line of thyroid cartilage	Ansa cervicalis, C1-C3	Depresses thyroid cartilage and larynx
Thyrohyoid	Oblique line of thyroid cartilage	Body and greater horn of hyoid	C1 via hypoglossal nerve	Depresses and retracts hyoid and larynx

19. Prevertebral Muscles

Muscle	Origin	Insertion	Nerve	Action
Lateral vertebral				
Anterior scalene	Transverse process of C3-C6 vertebrae	1st rib	Cervical, C4, C5, C6	Elevates 1st rib; laterally flexes and rotates neck
Middle scalene	Posterior tubercles of transverse processes of C2-C6 vertebrae	Superior surface of 1st rib, posterior groove for subclavian artery	Cervical spine, anterior rami	Elevates 1st rib during forced inspiration; flexes neck laterally

19. Prevertebral Muscles

Muscle	Origin	Insertion	Nerve	Action
Posterior scalene	Posterior tubercles of transverse processes of C4-C6 vertebrae	External border of 2nd rib	Anterior rami of cervical spine, C7, C8	Elevates 2nd rib during forced inspiration; flexes neck laterally
Anterior vertebral				
Longus capitis	Anterior tubercles of transverse processes of C3-C6 vertebrae	Basilar process of occipital bone	Spinal, anterior rami, C1-C3	Flexes
Longus colli	Anterior tubercle of C2 vertebra; bodies of C1-C3 and transverse processes of C3-C6 vertebrae	Bodies of C5-T3 vertebrae, transverse processes of C3-C5 vertebrae	Spinal, anterior rami, C2-C6	Flexes and rotates head to opposite side
Rectus capitis anterior	Anterior surface of lateral mass of atlas, C1	Base of skull, anterior to occipital condyle	C1 and C2	Flexes head
Rectus capitis lateralis	Transverse processes of C1	Jugular process of occipital bone	C1 and C2	Flexes head; helps stabilize head
Rectus capitis posterior	Spinous processes of C2 vertebra	Middle of inferior nuchal line of occipital bone	Suboccipital	Extends head

19. Prevertebral Muscles

Muscle	Origin	Insertion	Nerve	Action
Splenius capitis et cervicis	Inferior half of ligamentum nuchae; spinous processes of C7-T3 of T4 vertebrae	Splenius capitis: superolaterally to mastoid process of temporal bone, lateral 3rd of superior nuchal line of occipital bone; Splenius cervicis: posterior tubercles of transverse C1-C3 or C4 vertebrae		

20. Muscles of Facial Expression

Muscle	Origin	Insertion	Nerve	Action
Auricularis anterior, posterior, and superior	Epicranial aponeurosis and mastoid part of temporal bone	Auricle (external ear)	Facial	Protraction, retraction, and elevation of external ear
Buccinator	Mandible; pterygo-mandibular raphe; alveolar processes	Angle of mouth	Facial, CN 7	Presses cheek against molar teeth to aid in chewing
Corrugator supercilii	Medial supraorbital margin	Skin of medial eyebrow	Facial, CN 7	Draws eyebrow medially and inferiorly producing vertical wrinkles above nose

20. Muscles of Facial Expression

Muscle	Origin	Insertion	Nerve	Action
Depressor anguli oris	Oblique line of mandible	Angle of mouth	Facial, CN 7	Depresses angle of mouth
Depressor labii inferioris	Mandible below mental foramen	Orbicularis oris and skin of lower lip	Facial, CN 7	Depresses lower lip
Depressor septi	Incisor fossa of maxilla	Mobile part of nasal septum	Facial	Helps dilate nostril during inspiration; depresses nasal septum
Levator anguli oris	Canine fossa of maxilla	Angle of mouth	Facial, CN 7	Elevates angle of mouth medially
Levator labii superioris	Maxilla above infraorbital foramen	Skin of upper lip and alar cartilage of nose	Facial, CN 7	Elevates upper lip; dilates nose
Levator labii superioris alaeque nasi	Frontal process of maxilla	Skin of upper lip	Facial	Elevates ala of nose and upper lip
Mentalis	Incisor fossa of mandible	Skin of chin	Facial, CN 7	Elevates and protrudes lower lip
Nasalis	Maxilla lateral to incisor fossa	Nasal cartilages	Facial, CN 7	Draws ala (side) of nose toward nasal septum
Occipitofrontalis	Superior nuchal line; upper orbital margin	Epicranial aponeurosis	Facial, CN 7	Elevates eyebrows; wrinkles forehead
Orbicularis oculi	Medial orbital margin; medial palpebral ligament; lacrimal bone	Skin and rim of orbit; tarsal plate; lateral palpebral raphe	Facial, CN 7	Closes and/or squints eyelids

20. Muscles of Facial Expression

Muscle	Origin	Insertion	Nerve	Action
Procerus	Nasal bone and cartilage	Skin between eyebrows	Facial, CN 7	Depresses medial end of eyebrow; produces wrinkles over nose
Zygomaticus major	Zygomatic arch	Angle of mouth	Facial, CN 7	Draws angle of mouth backward and upward
Zygomaticus minor	Zygomatic arch	Angle of mouth	Facial, CN 7	Elevates upper lip

21. Muscles of Mastication

Muscle	Origin	Insertion	Nerve	Action
Lateral pterygoid	Superior head from infratemporal surface of sphenoid; inferior head from lateral surface of lateral pterygoid plate	Neck of mandible; articular disk and capsule of temporo-mandibular joint	Trigeminal, CN V3	Protracts and depresses mandible; produces side-to-side movements of mandible
Masseter	Lower border and medial surface of zygomatic arch	Lateral surface of coronoid process, ramus and angle of mandible	Trigeminal, CN V3	Elevates mandible
Medial pterygoid	Tuber of maxillary; medial surface of lateral pterygoid plate; pyramidal process of palatine bone	Medial surface of angle and ramus of mandible	Trigeminal, CN V3	Protracts, protrudes and elevates mandible; closes jaw; produces grinding motion

Muscles and Cranial Nerves

22. Muscles of Eye Movement

Muscle	Origin	Insertion	Nerve	Action
Ciliary	Scleral spur	Meridional, radial, and circular fibers are intrinsic to ciliary body	Parasympathetic fibers of oculomotor nerve and ciliary ganglion	Relieve tension on lens of eye, allowing it to become more convex for near vision
Inferior oblique	Floor of orbit lateral to lacrimal groove	Sclera beneath lateral rectus	Oculomotor, CN 3	Rotates eyeball upward and laterally; elevates adducted eye
Inferior rectus	Common tendinous ring	Sclera just behind cornea	Oculomotor, CN 3	Depresses, adducts, and rotates eyeball medially
Lateral rectus	Common tendinous ring	Sclera just behind cornea	Abducens, CN 6	Abducts eyeball
Levator palpebrae superioris	Lesser wing of sphenoid above and anterior to optic canal	Tarsal plate and skin of upper eyelid	Oculomotor, CN 3	Elevates upper eyelid
Medial rectus	Common tendinous ring	Sclera just behind cornea	Oculomotor, CN 3	Adducts eyeball
Superior oblique	Body of sphenoid bone above optic canal	Sclera beneath superior rectus	Trochlear, CN 4	Abducts, depresses and medially rotates eyeball
Superior rectus	Common tendinous ring	Sclera just behind cornea	Oculomotor, CN 3	Elevates, adducts, and rotates eye medially

23. Muscles of the Palate

Muscle	Origin	Insertion	Nerve	Action
Levator veli palatini	Petrous part of temporal bone; cartilage of auditory tube	Aponeurosis of soft palate	Vagus via pharyngeal plexus, CN 10, 11	Elevates soft palate
Musculus uvulae	Posterior nasal spine of palatine bone; palatine aponeurosis	Mucous membrane of uvula	Vagus nerve via pharyngeal plexus, CN 10, 11	Elevates uvula
Palato-pharyngeus	Hard palate and palatine aponeurosis	Lateral wall of pharynx	Cranial part of accessory nerve CN 11 through pharyngeal branch of vagus nerve CN 10 via pharyngeal plexus	Tenses soft palate; moves walls of pharynx superiorly, anteriorly, and medially during swallowing
Tensor veli palatini	Scaphoid fossa; spine of sphenoid; cartilage of auditory tube	Palatine aponeurosis	Mandibular branch nerve, CN V3, via otic ganglion	Tenses soft palate and opens auditory tube during swallowing and yawning

24. Muscles of the Tongue

Muscle	Origin	Insertion	Nerve	Action
Genioglossus	Superior part of mental spine of mandible	Dorsum of tongue and body of hyoid bone	Hypoglossal, CN 12	Depresses tongue; pulls tongue anteriorly for protrusion
Hyoglossus	Body of greater horn of hyoid bone	Side and inferior aspect of tongue	Hypoglossal, CN 12	Depresses and retracts tongue

Muscles and Cranial Nerves

24. Muscles of the Tongue

Muscle	Origin	Insertion	Nerve	Action
Inferior long muscle of tongue	Root of tongue and body of hyoid bone	Apex of tongue	Hypoglossal, CN 12	Curls tip of tongue inferiorly and shortens tongue
Palatoglossus	Palatine aponeurosis	Side of tongue	Cranial part of accessory nerve CN 12 through pharyngeal branch of vagus nerve CN 10 via pharyngeal plexus	Elevates posterior tongue and draws soft palate onto tongue
Superior long muscle of tongue	Submucous fibrous layer and median fibrous septum	Margins of tongue and mucous membrane	Hypoglossal, CN 12	Curls tip and sides of tongue superiorly and shortens tongue
Transverse muscle of tongue	Median fibrous septum	Fibrous tissue at margins of tongue	Hypoglossal, CN 12	Narrows and elongates tongue; aids in protrusion of tongue
Vertical muscle of tongue	Superior surface of borders of tongue	Inferior surface of borders of tongue	Hypoglossal, CN 12	Flattens tongue; aids in protrusion of tongue

25. Muscles of the Pharynx

Muscle	Origin	Insertion	Nerve	Action
Circular muscles				
Cricopharyngeus	Posterolateral cricoid cartilage on 1 side	Posterolateral cricoid cartilage of other side	Vagus, CN 10	Serves as upper esophageal sphincter

25. Muscles of the Pharynx

Muscle	Origin	Insertion	Nerve	Action
Geniohyoid	Inferior mental spine of mandible	Body of hyoid bone	C1 via hypoglossal	Pulls hyoid bone superiorly; shortens floor of mouth; widens pharynx
Inferior constrictor	Arch of cricoid and oblique line of thyroid cartilage	Median raphe of pharynx	Vagus via pharyngeal plexus; recurrent and external laryngeal, CN 10, 11	Constricts lower pharynx
Middle constrictor	Greater and lesser horns of hyoid; stylohyoid ligament	Median raphe	Vagus via pharyngeal plexus, CN 10, 11	Constricts lower pharynx
Superior constrictor	Medial pterygoid plate; pterygoid hamulus; pterygomandibular raphe; mylohyoid line of mandible; side of tongue	Median raphe and pharyngeal tubercle of skull	Vagus via pharyngeal plexus	Constricts upper pharynx
Longitudinal muscles				
Palatopharyngeus	Hard palate; aponeurosis of soft palate	Thyroid cartilage and muscles of the pharynx	Vagus via pharyngeal plexus, CN 10, 11	Elevates pharynx and closes nasopharynx
Salpingopharyngeus	Cartilage of auditory tube	Muscles of the pharynx	Vagus via pharyngeal plexus	Elevates nasopharynx; opens auditory tube
Stylopharyngeus	Styloid process	Thyroid cartilage and muscles of the pharynx	Glossopharyngeal, CN 9	Elevates pharynx and larynx

Muscles and Cranial Nerves

26. Muscles of the Larynx

Muscle	Origin	Insertion	Nerve	Action
Aryepiglottic	Apex of arytenoid cartilage	Side of epiglottic cartilage	Recurrent laryngeal	Adducts
Cricothyroid	Arch of cricoid cartilage	Inferior horn and lower lamina of thyroid cartilage	External laryngeal	Tenses and stretches vocal fold
Lateral cricoarytenoid	Arch of cricoid cartilage	Muscular process of arytenoid cartilage	Recurrent laryngeal, CN 10	Adducts
Oblique arytenoid	Muscular process of arytenoid cartilage	Apex of opposite arytenoid	Recurrent laryngeal, CN 10	Closes inter-cartilaginous portion of rima glottidis
Posterior cricoarytenoid	Posterior surface of lamina of cricoid cartilage	Muscular process of arytenoid cartilage	Recurrent laryngeal, CN 10	Abducts
Thyroarytenoid	Inner surface of thyroid lamina	Anterolateral surface of arytenoid cartilage	Recurrent laryngeal, CN 10	Adducts; relaxes vocal fold
Thyroepiglottic	Anteromedial surface of lamina of thyroid cartilage	Lateral margin of epiglottic cartilage	Recurrent laryngeal, CN 10	Adducts
Transverse arytenoid	Posterior surface of arytenoid cartilage	Opposite arytenoid cartilage	Recurrent laryngeal, CN 10	Adducts

26. Muscles of the Larynx

Muscle	Origin	Insertion	Nerve	Action
Vocalis	Anteromedial surface of lamina of thyroid cartilage	Vocal process	Recurrent laryngeal, CN 10	Relaxes posterior vocal ligaments; maintains tension of anterior part of ligament

27. Summary of Autonomic Ganglia of the Head and Neck

Ganglion	Location	Parasympathetic Fibers	Sympathetic Fibers	Chief Distribution
Ciliary	Behind eyeball between optic nerve and lateral rectus muscle	Inferior division oculomotor nerve via short ciliary nerves	Internal carotid artery; long ciliary nerve	Ciliary muscle and sphincter pupillae (parasympathetic); dilator pupillae and tarsal muscle (sympathetic)
Otic	Below foramen ovale	Glossopharyngeal nerve, its tympanic branch, lesser petrosal nerve	Plexus on middle meningeal	Parotid gland
Pterygopalatine	In pterygopalatine fossa below maxillary nerve, lateral to the sphenopalatine foramen and anterior pterygoid canal	Facial nerve, greater petrosal nerve, and pterygoid nerve	Internal carotid plexus	Nasal, palatine, and lacrimal glands via maxillary, zygomatic, and lacrimal nerves
Submandibular	Lateral surface of hypoglossus muscle, deep to the mylohyoid muscle, suspended from the lingual nerve	Facial nerve, chorda tympani and lingual nerve	Plexus on facial artery	Submandibular and sublingual glands

28. Muscles of the Ears

Muscle	Origin	Insertion	Nerve	Action
Stapedius	Internal walls of pyramidal eminence of posterior wall of tympanic cavity	Neck of the stapes	Facial, CN V2	Dampens vibrations of stapes reflexively in response to loud nose
Tensor tympani	Canal for tensor tympani of petrous part of temporal bone and cartilage of pharyngotym-panic (auditory) tube	Handle of malleus	Branch of mandibular nerve, CN V3 via otic ganglion	Tenses tympanic membrane to dampen excessive vibration

29. Cranial Nerves (CN)

Nerve	Cranial Exit	Cell Bodies	Components	Chief Function
I: Olfactory	Cribriform plate	Nasal mucosa	SVA	Smell
II: Optic	Optic canal	Ganglion cells of retina	SSA	Vision
III: Oculomotor	Superior orbital fissure	Nucleus CN III (midbrain)	GSE	Eye movements (superior, inferior, and medial recti, inferior oblique, and levator palpebrae superioris muscles)
		Edinger-Westphal nucleus (midbrain)	GVE	Constriction of pupil (sphincter pupillae muscle) and accommoda-tion (ciliary muscle)

29. Cranial Nerves (CN)

Nerve	Cranial Exit	Cell Bodies	Components	Chief Function
IV: Trochlear	Superior orbital fissure	Nucleus CN IV (midbrain)	GSE	Eye movements (superior oblique muscle)
V: Trigeminal	Superior orbital fissure; foramen rotundum and foramen ovale	Motor nucleus CN V (pons)	SVE	Muscles of mastication, (mylohyoid, anterior belly of digastric, tensor veli palatini, and tensor tympani muscles)
		Trigeminal ganglion	GSA	Sensation in head (skin and mucous membranes of face and head)
VI: Abducens	Superior orbital fissure	Nucleus CN VI (pons)	GSE	Eye movement (lateral rectus muscle)
VII: Facial	Stylomastoid foramen	Motor nucleus CN VII (pons)	SVE	Muscle of facial expression (posterior belly of digastric stylohyoid and stapedius muscles)
		Salivatory nucleus (pons)	GVE	Lacrimal and salivary secretion
		Geniculate ganglion	SVA	Taste from anterior two thirds of tongue and palate

29. Cranial Nerves (CN)

Nerve	Cranial Exit	Cell Bodies	Components	Chief Function
		Geniculate ganglion	GVA	Sensation from palate
		Geniculate ganglion	GSA	Sensation from external acoustic means
VIII: Vestibulo-cochlear	Does not leave skull	Vestibular ganglion	SSA	Equilibrium, hearing
IX: Glosso-pharyngeal	Jugular foramen	Nucleus ambiguus (medulla)	SVE	Elevation of pharynx (sty-lopharyngeus muscle)
		Dorsal nucleus (medulla)	GVE	Secretion of saliva (parotid gland)
		Inferior ganglion	GVA	Sensation in carotid sinus and body, tongue, and pharynx
		Inferior ganglion	SVA	Taste from posterior 3rd of tongue
		Inferior ganglion	GSA	Sensation in external and middle ear
X: Vagus	Jugular foramen	Nucleus ambiguus	SVE	Muscles of movements of pharynx, larynx, and palate
		Dorsal nucleus (medulla)	GVE	Involuntary muscle and gland control in thoracic and abdominal viscera

29. Cranial Nerves (CN)

Nerve	Cranial Exit	Cell Bodies	Components	Chief Function
		Inferior ganglion	GVA	Sensation in pharynx, larynx, and other viscera
		Inferior ganglion	SVA	Taste from root of tongue and epiglottis
		Superior ganglion	GSA	Sensation in external ear and external acoustic meatus
XI: Accessory	Jugular foramen	Spinal cord (foramen)	SVE	Movement of head and shoulder (sternocleido-mastoid and trapezius muscles)
XII: Hypoglossal	Hypoglossal canal	Nucleus CN XII (medulla)	GSE	Muscles of movements of tongue

Muscles and Cranial Nerves

CN	cranial nerve
CNI–CNXII	cranial nerves I–XII
C1–C7	cervical vertebrae
C1–C8	cervical nerve
T1–T12	thoracic nerve, vertebrae
L1–5	lumbar nerve, vertebrae
GSA	general somatic afferent
GSE	general somatic efferent
SVA	special visceral afferent
SVE	special visceral efferent
V1, V2, V3	divisions of CN V, trigeminal nerve

Ligaments and Tendons

Latin name	English name	Articulation
Shoulder/Upper Arm		
Lm. acromio-claviculare	acromioclavicular l.	Connects acromion to clavicle; strengthens articular capsule
Lm. anulare radii	anular l. of radius	Connects head of radius in radial notch
Lm. collaterale ulnare	collateral ulnar l.	Connects medial epicondyle to humerus and coronoid process of ulna and olecranon
Lm. conoideum	conoid l.	Connects coracoid process of scapula to clavicle
Lm. coracoacromiale	coracoacromial l.	Connects coracoid process to acromion
Lm. coraco-claviculare	coracoclavicular l.	Connects coracoid process of scapula to clavicle
Lm. coracohumerale	coracohumeral l.	Connects coracoid process of scapula to humerus
Lm. costoclaviculare	costoclavicular l.	Connects 1st costal cartilage to clavicle
La. glenohumeralia	glenohumeral ligs.	Connects articular capsule of humerus to glenoid cavity and anatomical neck of humerus
Lm. interclaviculare	interclavicular l.	Connects clavicle to opposite clavicle
Lm. Orbiculare radii	anular l. of radius	L. that encircles and holds head of radius in radial notch of ulna
La. sternoclaviculare anterius	anterior sternoclavicular l.	Fibrous band that reinforces sternoclavicular joints anteriorly
La. sternoclavicular posterius	posterior sternoclavicular l.	Fibrous band that reinforces sternoclavicular joints posteriorly
Lm. suspensorium axillae	suspensory l.	Connects between clavipectoral fascia downward to axillary fascia

Latin name	English name	Articulation
Lm. transversum humeri	transverse humeral l.	Connects obliquely from greater to lesser tuberosity of humerus
Lm. transversum scapulae inferius	inferior transverse l.	Connects scapula to glenoid cavity; creates foramen of scapula for vessels/nerves
Lm. transversum scapulae superius	superior transverse l.	Connects coracoid process to scapular notch of scapula
Lm. trapezoideum	trapezoid l.	Connects coracoid process to clavicle
Hand/Forearm		
Lm. anulare radii	anular l. of radius	Connects radius to ulna
Lm. carpi radiatum	radiate l. of wrist	Multiple fibrous bands on palmar surface of metacarpal joints
Lm. carpi transversum	transverse carpal l.	Continuous with antebrachial fascia
Lm. carpi volare	transverse carpal l.	Reinforcing fibers in antebrachial fascia, palmar surface of wrist
La. carpo-metacarpalia dorsalia	dorsal carpometacarpal ligs.	Joins carpal bones to bases of metacarpals
La. carpo-metacarpalia palmaria	palmar carpometacarpal ligs.	Joins carpal bones to metacarpals ligs.
Lm. collateralia articulationum interphalangealium manus	collateral ligs. of of interphalangeal articulations	Fibrous bands on each side of interphalangeal joints of fingers
Lm. collateralia articulationum metacarpopha-langealium	collateral ligs. of metacarpopha-langeal articulations	Fibrous bands on sides of each metacarpophalangeal joints
Lm. collaterale carpi radiale	radial carpal collateral l.	Connects styloid process of radius to scaphoid

Latin name	English name	Articulation
Lm. collaterale carpi ulnare	ulnar carpal collateral l.	Connects styloid process of ulna to triquetral and pisiform bones
Lm. collaterale radiale	collateral radial l.	Connects lateral epicondyle of humerus to anular l. of radius
Lm. intercarpalia dorsalia	dorsal intercarpal ligs.	Connects carpal bones together
Lm. intercarpalia interossea	interosseous intercarpal ligs.	Connects various carpal bones
Lm. intercarpalia palmaria	palmar intercarpal ligs.	Connects various carpal bones
La. metacarpalia dorsalia	dorsal metacarpal ligs.	Interconnects bases of metacarpal bones
La. metacarpalia interossea	interosseous metacarpal ligs.	Interconnects bases of metacarpal bones
La. metacarpalia palmaria	palmar metacarpal ligs.	Interconnects bases of metacarpals
Lm. metacarpeum transversum profundum	deep transverse metacarpal l.	Interconnects heads of metacarpals
Lm. metacarpale transversum superficiale	superficial transverse metacarpal l.	Between longitudinal bands of palmar aplurosis.
Lm. natatorium	superficial transverse metacarpal l	Thickening of deep fascia in most distal part of base of triangular palmar aponeurosis
La. palmaria	palmar l.	Connects anterior aspect of each metacarpophalangeal and interphalangeal joints of hand
La. palmaria articulationis interphalangeae manus	palmar ligs. of interphalangeal joints of hand	Interphalangeal articulations of hand between collateral articulations

Latin name	English name	Articulation
La. palmaria articulationis metacarpophalangeae	palmar ligs. of metacarpal joints	Connects metacarpophalangeal joints to collateral ligs.
Lm. pisohamatum	pisohamate l.	Connects pisiform bone to hook of hamate bone
Lm. pisometacarpeum	pisometacarpal l.	Connects pisiform bone to bases of metacarpals
Lm. quadratum	quadrate l.	Connects radial notch of ulna to neck of radius
Lm. radiocarpale dorsale	dorsal radiocarpal l.	Connects radius to carpal bones
Lm. radiocarpale palmare	palmar radiocarpal l.	Connects radius to lunate, triquetral, capitate, and hamate bones
Lm. ulnocarpale palmare	palmar ulnocarpal l.	Connects styloid process of ulna to carpal bones
Head/Neck		
Lm. anulare stapedis	anular l. of stapes	Connects stapes to fenestra vestibuli
La. anularia	anular l. of trachea	Connects adjacent tracheal cartilages
Lm. articulare anterius	anterior l. of auricle	Connects zygomatic process to helix
Lm. articulare posterius	anterior l. of auricle	Connects mastoid process to conchal eminence
Lm. articulare superius	superior l. of auricle	Connects osseous external acoustic meatus to helix
Lm. cerato-cricoideum	ceratocricoid l.	1 of 3 ligs. reinforcing cricothyroid articulation capsule
Lm. corni-culopharyngeal	cricopharyngeal l.	Connects corniculate cartilage and cricoid cartilage
Lm. crico-arytenoideum posterius	cricoarytenoid l.	Connects arytenoid cartilage to lamina of cricoid cartilage

Latin name	English name	Articulation
Lm. crico-pharyngeum	cricopharyngeal l.	Connects tip of corniculate cartilage and lamina of cricoid cartilage
Lm. cricotracheale	cricotracheal l.	Connects cricoid cartilage with 1st ring of trachea
Lm. hyaloideo-capsulare	hyalocapsular l.	Connects vitreous body to posterior surface of lens of eye
Lm. hyoepiglotticum	hyoepiglottic l.	Connects epiglottis to upper border of hyoid bone
Lm. hyothyroideum laterale	lateral thyroid l.	Connects superior horn of thyroid cartilage to tip of greater horn of hyoid cartilage
Lm. hyothyroideum medium	median thyroid l.	Central portion of thyroid membrane.
Lm. incudis posterius	posterior l. of incus	Ligamentous band extending from short crus of incus
Lm. incudis superius	superior l. of incus	Connects body of incus with root at tympanic recess
La. intracapsularia	intrascapular l.	Ligs. located within and separate from articular capsule of synovial joints
Lm. jugale	cricopharyngeal l.	Connects tip at corniculate cartilage and lamina at cricoid cartilage and pharyngeal mucosa
Lm. laterale articulationis temporomandibularis	lateral l. of temporomandibular joints	Capsular l. that passes down and backward across lateral surface of temporomandibular joints
Lm. mallei anterius	anterior l. of malleus	Connects base of anterior process to spine of sphenoid
Lm. mallei laterale	lateral l. of malleus	Connects posterior half of tympanic notch to neck of malleus
Lm. mallei superius	superior l. of malleus	Connects from head of malleus to epitympanic recess

Latin name	English name	Articulation
Lm. mediale articulationis temporomandibularis	medial l. of temporomandibular joints	Strengthens medial part of articular capsule
La. ossiculorum auditus tympanic cavity	l. of auditory ossicles	Connects ear bones with each other and with walls of
Lm. palpebrale externum	lateral palpebral l.	Connects tarsal plates to orbital eminence of zygomatic bone
Lm. palpebrale laterale	lateral palpebral l.	Connects tarsal plates to orbital eminence of zygomatic bone
Lm. palpebral mediale	medial palpebral l.	Connects medial ends of tarsal plates to maxilla at medial orbital margin
Lm. sphenomandibulare	sphenomandibular l.	Connects from spine to sphenoid bone to lingula of mandible
Lm. spirale cochleae	spiral l. of cochlear duct	Forms outer wall of cochlear duct to which basal lamina attaches
Lm. spirale ductus cochlearis	spiral l. of cochlear duct	Forms outer wall of cochlear duct to which basal lamina attaches
Lm. stylohyoideum	stylohyoid l.	Connects from tip of styloid process to lesser cornu of hyoid bone
Lm. stylomandibulare	stylomandibular l.	Connects from tip of styloid process to temporal bone
Lm. suspensorium bulb	suspensory l.	Connects between lateral and medial orbital margins
Lm. suspensorium glandulae thyroideae	suspensory l.	Connects from sheath of thyroid gland to thyroid and cricoid cartilages
Lm. tarsale externum	lateral palpebral l.	Connects tarsal plates to orbital eminence of zygomatic bone
Lm. tarsale internum	medial palpebral l.	Connects between medial ends of tarsal plates to maxilla at medial orbital margin

Latin name	English name	Articulation
Lm. temporo-mandibular	lateral temporomandi-bular l.	Capsular l. that passes obliquely down and backward across lateral surface of temporomandibular joints
Lm. thyroepiglotticum	thyroepiglottic l.	Connects petiole of epiglottis to interior of thyroid cartilage
Lm. thyrohyoideum laterale	lateral thyroid l.	Connects superior horn of thyroid cartilage to tip of greater horn of hyoid cartilage
Lm. thyrohyoideum medium	median thyrohyoid l.	Central thickened portion of thyroid membrane
La. trachealia	anular l.	Connects adjacent tracheal cartilages
Lm. ventriculare	vestibular l.	Inferior border of quadrangular membrane that underlies ventricular fold of larynx
Lm. vestibulare	vestibular l.	Inferior border of quadrangular membrane that underlies ventricular fold of larynx
Lm. vocale	vocal l.	Connects on either side from thyroid cartilages to vocal process of arytenoid cartilages

Thorax/upper abdomen

Latin name	English name	Articulation
Lm. colli costae	costotransverse l.	Connects neck of rib to corresponding transverse process
Lm. costo-transversarium anterius	superior costotransverse l.	Connects transverse rib to next highest vertebra
Lm. costo-transversarium laterale	lateral costotransverse l.	Connects tip of transverse process to neck of rib
Lm. costo-transversarium posterius	lateral costotransverse l.	Connects tip of process to neck of ribs

Latin name	English name	Articulation
Lm. costotransversarium superius	superior costotransverse l.	Connects neck of ribs to transverse process of next higher vertebrae
Lm. costoxiphoideum	costoxiphoid l.	Connects xiphoid process to 7th and often 6th cartilages
Lm. pulmonale	pulmonary l.	2-layered fold formed as pleura of mediastinum is reflected onto lung inferior to root of lung
Lm. sternocostale intraarticulare	intraarticular sternocostal l.	Connects between a costal cartilage and sternum within articular capsule
La. sternocostalia radiata	radiate sternocostal l.	Fibers of articular capsule that radiate from costal cartilages to anterior surface of sternum
La. sternopericardiaca	sternopericardial l.	Connects from pericardium to sternum
La. suspensoria mammaria	suspensory l. of breast	Connects from fibrous stroma of mammary gland to overlying skin
Lm. tuberculi costae	lateral costotransverse l.	Connects tip of transverse process to posterior surface of neck and rib
Lm. vena cava sinistrae	left vena caval l.	Connects from left brachiocephalic vein to oblique vein of left atrium

Spine

Latin name	English name	Articulation
Lm. alaria	alar l.	Connects axis to occiput; limits rotation of head
Lm. apicis dentis axis	apical dental l.	Connects axis to occiput
Lm. atlantooccipitale laterale	lateral atlantooccipital l.	Connects occiput to atlas
Lm. capitis costae intraarticulare	interarticular l. of head of rib	Connects crest of rib to intervertebral disc
Lm. capitis costae radiatum	radiate l. of head of rib	Connects head of rib to adjacent vertebrae/discs

Latin name	English name	Articulation
Lm. caudale integumenti communis	caudal retinaculum	Forms coccygeal foveola
Lm. costo-transversarium	costotransverse l.	Connects neck of rib to transverse process of corresponding vertebra
Lm. costo-transversarium laterale	lateral costotransverse l.	Connects transverse process of vertebra to corresponding rib
Lm. costotransversarium superius	superior costotransverse l.	Connects neck of rib to transverse process of vertebra above
Lm. cruciforme atlantis	cruciform l. of atlas	Connects transverse l. of atlas to longitudinal fascicles
La. flava	yellow ligs.	Joins laminae of 2 adjacent vertebrae
Lm. iliofemorale	iliofemoral l.	Connects anterior/inferior iliac spine and intertrochanteric femur
Lm. iliolumbale	iliolumbar l.	Connects L4-L5 to iliac crest
Lm. interspinalia	interspinal ligs.	Interconnects spinous processes
Lm. intertransversaria	intertransverse ligs.	Interconnects vertebral transverse processes
Lm. longitudinale anterius	ant. longitudinal l.	Extends from occiput/atlas to sacrum
Lm. longitudinale posterius	post. longitudinal l.	Extends from occiput to coccyx
Lm. lumbocostale	lumbocostal l.	Connects 12th rib to transverse processes of L1-L2
Lm. nuchae	radiate l.	Connects head of each rib to bodies of 2 vertebrae with which it articulates
Lm. sacrococcygeum anterius	anterior sacrococcygeal l.	Connects sacrum to coccyx

Latin name	English name	Articulation
Lm. sacrococcygeum laterale	lateral sacrococcygeal l.	Connects 1st coccygeal vertebra to sacrum; completes foramen of S5
Lm. sacrococcygeum posterius profundum	deep posterior sacrococcygeal l.	Terminal portion of posterior longitudinal l.; unites S5 and profundum coccyx
Lm. sacrococcygeum posterius	superficial posterior superficiale sacrococcygeal l.	Connects sacral hiatus to coccyx
La. sacroiliaca anteriora	anterior sacroiliac ligs.	Connects sacrum to ilium
La. sacroiliaca interossea	interosseous sacroiliac ligs.	Numerous bundles connecting tuberosities of sacrum to those of ilium
La. sacroiliaca posteriora	posterior sacroiliac ligs.	Connects ilium and iliac spines to sacrum
Lm. sacrospinalum	sacrospinal l.	Connects ischium to lateral margins of sacrum
Lm. sacrotuberale	sacrotuberal l.	Connects ischial tuberosity to sacrum and coccyx and iliac spine
Lm. supraspinale	supraspinal l.	Interconnects tips of spinous processes of vertebrae
Lm. transversum atlantis	transverse l. of atlas	Horizontal portion of cruciform l. of atlas
Abdominal/Pelvic		
Lm. arcuatum laterale	lateral arcuate l.	Connects 1st lumbar vertebrae and 12th rib to diaphragm
Lm. arcuatum mediale	medial arcuate l.	Connects body of 1st lumbar vertebra to transverse process
Lm. arcuatum medianum	median arcuate l.	Connects crura of diaphragm that arches over aorta
Lm. arcuatum pubis	inferior pubic l.	Arches across pubic symphysis

Latin name	English name	Articulation
Lm. cardinale	cardinale l.	Connects uterine, cervix and vault of lateral fornix of vagina
Lm. coronarium hepatis	coronary l. of liver	Connects perit1al reflections to diaphragm at margins of bare area of liver
Lm. duodenorenale	duodenorenal l.	Connects termination of hepatoduodenal to front of right kidney
Lm. falciforme	falciform process of sacrotuberous l.	Passes from ischial tuberosity to ilium, sacrum, and coccyx
Lm. falciforme hepatis	falciform l. of liver	Connects liver to diaphragm and anterior abdominal wall
Lm. fundiforme clitoris	fundiform l. of clitoris	Connects linea alba with fascia of clitoris
Lm. fundiforme penis	fundiform l. of penis	Connects linea alba with fascia of penis
Lm. gastrophrenicum	gastrocolic l.	Connects stomach with transverse colon
Lm. gastrophrenicum	gastrophrenic l.	Connects greater curvature of stomach with inferior surface of diaphragm
Lm. gastrosplenicum	gastrosplenic l.	Connects greater curvature of stomach with ilium of spleen
Lm. genitoinguinale	genitoinguinal l.	In a fetus, a fold of mesorchium containing gubernaculum testis
Lm. hepatocolicum	hepatocolic l.	Connects hepatoduodenal l. to transverse colon
Lm. hepatoesophageum	hepatoesophageal l.	Connects between liver and part of esophagus
Lm. hepatogastricum	hepatogastric l.	Connects liver to lesser curvature of stomach

Latin name	English name	Articulation
Lm. hepatorenale	hepatorenal l.	A prolongation of coronary ligs. downward over right kidney
Lm. ischiocapsulare	ischiofemoral l.	Connects from ischium upward and laterally over femoral neck
Lm. lacunare	lacunar l.	Connects from medial end of inguinal l. to pectineal line
Lm. laterale vesicae	lateral bladder l.	Passes from 1 side of bladder to blend with pelvic fascia
Lm. pectineale	pectineal l.	Strong fibrous band that passes laterally from lacunar l. along pectineal line of pubis
Lm. phrenicocolicum	phrenicocolic l.	Connects from left flexure of colon to diaphragm
Lm. phrenicolienal	phrenosplenic l.	Connects between diaphragm and spleen
Lm. phrenicosplenicum	phrenicosplenic l.	Connects between diaphragm and spleen
Lm. pubicum inferius	inferior pubic l.	Arches across inferior aspect of pubic symphysis
Lm. pubicum superius	superior pubic l.	Passes transversely above pubic symphysis
Lm. pubofemorale	pubofemoral l.	Connects from superior ramus of pubis to intertrochanteric femur
Lm. puboprostaticum	puboprostatic l.	Anchors prostate and neck of bladder to pubis on each side
Lm. puboprostaticum mediale	puboprostatic l.	Anchors prostate and neck of bladder to pubis on each side
Lm. pubovesicale	pubovesical l. (female)	Fascial thickening comparable with puboprostatic l.
Lm. pubovesicale	pubovesical l. (male)	Connects between lower part of pubic symphysis and prostate and bladder

Latin name	English name	Articulation
Lm. sacrodurale	sacrodural l.	Connects between midline of inferior part of dorsal sac to posterior longitudinal l. of sacrum.
Lm. sacroiliacum posterius	posterior sacroiliac l.	Connects from ilium to sacrum posterior to sacroiliac joints
Lm. sacrospinale	sacrospinal l.	Connects between ischial spine and sacrum and coccyx
Lm. serosum	serous l.	Connects certain viscera to abdominal wall or to each other
Lm. splenorenale	suspensory l.	Connects from pubic symphysis to deep fascia of clitoris
Lm. suspensorium ovarii	suspensory l.	Extends upward from upper pole of ovary
Lm. suspensorius penis	suspensory l.	Connects from pubic symphysis to deep fascia of penis
Lm. teres hepatis	round l.	Connects from umbilicus to liver where it continues to origins of left portal vein
Lm. teres uteri	round l.	Attached to uterus on either side of front and below opening of uterine tube and connects to labium majus
Lm. transversale cervicis	cardinal l.	Connects uterine cervix and vault of lateral fornix of vagina
Lm. transversum pelvis	transverse perineal l.	Thickened anterior border of perineal membrane
Lm. triangulare dextrum hepatis	right triangular l.	Connects from right lobe of liver to diaphragm
Lm. triangulare sinistrum hepatis	left triangular l.	Connects from left lobe of liver to diaphragm

Hip/Thigh

Lm. capitis femoris	l. of head of femur	Connects femur, acetabular notch, and transverse l. of acetabulum

Latin name	English name	Articulation
Lm. inguinale	inguinal l.	Connects ilium to pubis
Lm. ischiofemorale	ischiofemoral l.	Connects ischium to femur
Lm. transversum acetabuli	transverse l. of acetabulum	Connects acetabular lip of hip joints to acetabular notch

Knee/Calf

Latin name	English name	Articulation
Lm. capitis fibulae anterius	anterior l. of head of fibula	Connects head of fibula to lateral condyle of tibia
Lm. capitis fibulae posterius	posterior l. of head of fibula	Connects head of fibula to lateral condyle of tibia
Lm. collaterale fibulare	collateral fibular l.	Connects lateral epicondyle of femur to head of fibula
Lm. collateral tibiale	collateral tibial l.	Connects medial epicondyle of femur to medial meniscus and tibia
Lm. cruciatum anterius genus	anterior cruciate l. of knee.	Connects lateral condyle of femur to condylar eminence of tibia
La. cruciata genus	cruciate ligs. of knee	Bundles in knee joints between condyles of femur
Lm. cruciatum posterius genus	posterior cruciate l. of knee	Connects medial condyle of femur to intercondylar area of tibia
Lm. menisci lateralis	posterior meniscofemoral l.	Connects between medial condyle of femur to posterior crus of lateral meniscus
Lm. meniscofemorale anterius	anterior meniscofemoral l.	Connects lateral meniscus to posterior cruciate l.
Lm. meniscofemorale posterius	posterior meniscofemoral l.	Connects lateral meniscus to medial condyle of femur
Lm. patellae	patellar l.	Connects patella to tibial tuberosity
Lm. popliteum arcuatum	arcuate popliteal l.	Connects fibula to articular capsule

Latin name	English name	Articulation
Lm. popliteum obliquum	oblique popliteal l.	Connects medial condyle of tibia to lateral epicondyle of femur
Lm. teres femoris	head of femur l.	Connects from fovea in head of femur to borders of acetabular notch
Lm. tibiofibulare anterius	anterior tibiofibular l.	Connects tibia to fibula
Lm. tibiofibulare medium	interosseous membrane	
Lm. tibiofibulare posterius	posterior tibiofibular l.	Connects tibia to distal fibula
Lm. tibionaviculare	medial l.	Connects from medial malleolus of tibial downward to tarsal bones
Lm. transversum genus	transverse l. of knee	Connects lateral meniscus to medial meniscus
Foot and Ankle		
Lm. bifurcatum	bifurcate l.	Dorsum of foot; comprises calcaneonavicular and calcaneocuboid ligs.
Lm. calcaneo-cuboideum	calcaneocuboid l.	Connects calcaneus to cuboid
Lm. calcaneo-cuboideum plantare	plantar calcaneocuboid l. short plantar l.	Connects calcaneus to cuboid
Lm. calcaneo-fibulare	calcaneofibular l.	Connects fibula to calcaneus
Lm. calcaneona-viculare	calcaneonavicular l.	Connects calcaneus to navicular bone
Lm. calcaneona-viculare dorsale	dorsal calcaneonavicular l.	Connects calcaneus to navicular bone
Lm. calcaneona-viculare plantare	plantar calcaneonavicular l.	Connects sustentaculum tali to navicular; supports talus

Latin name	English name	Articulation
Lm. calcaneotibiale	calcaneotibial l.	Connects medial malleolus to sustentaculum tali of calcaneus
Lm. collateralia articulationum	collateral ligs. of metatarsopha-langeal articulations	Fibrous bands on sides of each metatarsophalangeal joints
Lm. cruciatum cruris	inferior extensor of foot	Joins malleolus to dorsum of foot
La. cuboideonaviculare dorsale	dorsal cuboideonavicular l.	Connects cuboid and navicular bones
La. cuboideonaviculare plantare	plantar cuboideonavicular l.	Connects cuboid and navicular bones
Lm. cuneocuboideum dorsale	dorsal cuneocuboid l.	Connects cuboid and lateral cuneiform bones
Lm. cuneocuboideum interosseum	interosseus cuneocuboid l.	Connects cuboid and lateral cuneiform bones
Lm. cuneocuboideum plantare	plantar cuneocuboid l.	Connects cuboid and lateral cuneiform bones
La. cuneometatarsalia interossea	interosseous cuneometatarsal ligs.	Connects cuneiform and metatarsal bones
La. cuneonavicularia dorsalia	dorsal cuneonavicular ligs.	Connects navicular and cuneiform bones
La. cuneonavicularia plantaria	plantar cuneonavicular ligs.	Connects navicular to cuneiform bones
La. intercuneiformia dorsalia	dorsal intercuneiform ligs.	Connects dorsal surfaces of cuneiform bones
La. intercuneiformia interossea	interosseous intercuneiform ligs.	Connects adjacent cuneiform bones
La. intercuneiformia plantaria	plantar intercuneiform ligs.	Joins plantar surfaces of cuneiform bones

Latin name	English name	Articulation
Lm. laterale articulationis talocruralis	lateral l. of ankle joints	Lateral side of ankle joints
Lm. mediale articulationis talocruralis	medial l. of ankle	Connects medial malleolus of tibia to tarsal bones
La. meniscofemoralia	meniscofemoral ligs.	Connects from posterior part of lateral meniscus to lateral surface of medial meniscus
Lm. metatarsale transversum profundum	deep transverse metatarsal l.	Joins heads of metatarsals
Lm. metatarsale transversum superficiale	superficial transverse metatarsal l.	Lies on sole of foot beneath heads of metatarsals
La. metatarsalia dorsalia	dorsal metatarsal ligs.	Interconnects bases of metatarsal bones
La. metatarsalia interossea	interosseous metatarsal ligs.	Interconnects bases of metatarsal bones
La. metatarsalia plantaria	plantar metatarsal ligs.	Plantar surface of metatarsal bones
La. plantaria articulationum interphalangealium pedis	plantar ligs. of interphalangeal articulations	Interphalangeal articulations of foot between collateral ligs.
La. plantaria articulationum metatarsophalangeal	plantar ligs. of metatarsopha-langeal articulations	Plantar surface of metatarsophalangeal articulations between collateral ligs.
Lm. plantare longum	long plantar l.	Connects calcaneus to bases of metatarsal bones
Lm. talocalcaneare laterale	lateral talocalcaneal l.	Connects talus to calcaneus
Lm. talocalcaneare mediale	medial talocalcaneal l.	Connects tubercle of talus to sustentaculum tali of calcaneus

Latin name	English name	Articulation
Lm. talocalcaneum	talocalcaneal l.	Connects talus and calcaneus
Lm. talocalcaneum interosseum	interosseous talocalcaneal l.	Connects calcaneus to talus
Lm. talofibulare anterius	anterior talofibular l.	Connects lateral malleolus of fibula to posterior process of talus.
Lm. talonaviculare	talonavicular l.	Connects neck of talus to navicular bone
Lm. talotibiale	medial tibiotalar l.	Connects downward from medial malleolus of tibia of tarsal bones.
La. tarsi	ligs. of tarsus	Connects bones of tarsus
La. tarsi dorsalia	dorsal ligs. of tarsus	Collectively, bifurcate, dorsal cuboideonavicular, cuneocuboid, cuneonavicular, intercuneiform, and talonavicular ligs.
La. tarsi interossea	interosseous ligs. of tarsus	Collectively, interosseous, cuneocuboid, intercuneiform, and talocalcaneal ligs.
La. tarsi plantaria	plantar ligs. of tarsus	Inferior ligs. of foot (long plantar, plantar calcaneocuboid, calcaneonavicular, cuneonavicular, cuboideonavicular, intercuneiform, cuneocuboid)
La. tarsometatarsalia dorsalia	dorsal tarsometatarsal ligs.	Connects bases of metatarsals to dorsal cuboid and cuneiform bones
La. tarsometatarsalia plantaria	plantar tarsometatarsal ligs.	Connects metatarsal bones to cuboid and cuneiform bones
Lm. transversum cruris	superior extensor retinaculum of foot	Connects tibia to fibula; holds extensor tendons in place
Tendo calcaneus	Achilles tendon calcaneal tendon	Connects triceps surae muscle to tuberosity of calcaneus

Abbreviations used: l., ligament; Lm., ligamenta; ligs., ligaments; Lm., ligamentum.

Appendix 4
Professional Organizations, Associations, and Titles

Professional Organizations and Associations

Academy of Forensic and Industrial Chiropractic Consultants (AFICC)
American Academy of Neurological and Orthopaedic Surgeons (AANOS)
American Association of Orthopaedic Medicine (AAOM)
American Academy of Orthopaedic Surgeons (AAOS)
American Academy of Orthotists and Prosthetists (AAOP)
American Academy of Physical Medicine and Rehabilitation (AAPM&R)
American Academy of Podiatric Sports Medicine (AAPSM)
American Arthritis Foundation (AAF)
American Arthritis Society (AAS)
American Association for Hand Surgery (AAHS)
American Association of Hip and Knee Surgeons (AAHKS)
American Association of Orthopaedic Foot and Ankle Surgeons (AAOFAS)
American Association of Tissue Banks (AATB)
American Back Society (ABS)
American Board for Certification (ABC)
American Board for Certification in Orthotics, Prosthetics, and Pedorthics (ABCOP)
American Board of Orthopaedic Surgery (ABOS)
American Board of Physical Therapy Specialties (ABPTS)
American Chiropractic Association (ACA)
American College of Chiropractic Consultants (ACCC)
American College of Chiropractic Orthopedists (ACCO)
American College of Foot & Ankle Orthopedics & Medicine (ACFAOM)
American College of Foot and Ankle Surgeons (ACFAS)
American College of Occupational and Environmental Medicine (ACOEM)
American College of Rheumatology (ACR)
American College of Sports Medicine (ACSM)
American Congress of Rehabilitation Medicine (ACRM)
American Health Care Association (AHCA)
American Institute of Orthopaedic and Sports Medicine (AIOSM)
American Knee Society (AKS)
American Medical Society for Sports Medicine (AMSSM)
American Occupational Therapy Association (AOTA)
American Orthopaedic Foot and Ankle Society (AOFAS)
American Orthopaedic Society (AOS)
American Orthopaedic Society for Sports Medicine (AOSSM)
American Orthotic and Prosthetic Association (AOPA)
American Osteopathic Academy for Sports Medicine (AOASM)
American Osteopathic Academy of Orthopedics (AOAO)
American Osteopathic Association (AOA)

American Osteopathic Board of Orthopedic Surgery (AOBOS)
American Osteopathic College of Occupational & Preventive Medicine (AOCOPM)
American Physical Therapy Association (APTA)
American Podiatric Medical Association (APMA)
American Rheumatism Association (ARA)
American Shoulder and Elbow Surgeons (ASES)
American Society for Bone and Mineral Research (ASBMR)
American Society for Testing and Materials (ASTM)
American Society of Orthopaedic Physician's Assistants (ASOPA)
American Spinal Injury Association (ASIA)
Arthroscopy Association of North America (AANA)
Association of Academic Physiatrists (AAP)
Association for the Study of Internal Fixation (ASIF)
Association of Bone and Joint Surgeons (ABJS)
Association of Chiropractic Colleges (ACC)
Association of Rehabilitation Nurses (ARN)
British Orthopaedic Association (BOA)
Canadian Academy of Sport Medicine (Académie Canadienne de Médecine du
    Sport) (CASM-ACMS)
Canadian Association of Physical Medicine and Rehabilitation (CAPMR)
Canadian Athletic Therapists Association (CATA)
Canadian Orthopaedic Nurses Association (CONA)
Canadian Physiotherapy Association (CPA)
Chiropractic Rehabilitation Association (CRA)
Commission on Accreditation of Rehabilitation Facilities (CARF)
Council on Chiropractic Education (CCE)
Council on Chiropractic Education International (CCEI)
European Society of Foot and Ankle Surgeons (ESFAS), now European Foot and
    Ankle Society (EFAS)
Federation of Chiropractic Licensing Boards (FCLB)
Fitness Safety Standards Committee (FSSC)
Foundation for Chiropractic Education and Research (FCER)
International Cartilage Repair Society (ICRS)
International Chiropractors Association (ICA)
International Headache Society (IHS)
International Knee Documentation Committee (IKDC)
International Society for Prosthetics and Orthotics (ISPO)
International Society of Arthroscopy, Knee Surgery, and Orthopaedic Sports
    (ISAKOS)
Mid-America Orthopaedic Association (MAOA)
Musculoskeletal Transplant Foundation (MTF)
National Academy of Sports Medicine (NASM)
National Association of Medical Equipment Suppliers (NAMES)
National Association of Orthopaedic Nurses (NAON)

Professional Organizations

National Association of Orthopaedic Technologists (NAOT)
National Athletic Trainers' Association (NATA)
National Board of Chiropractic Examiners (NBCE)
National Center for Assisted Living (NCAL)
National Institute of Arthritis and Musculoskeletal and Skin Diseases (NIAMS)
National Rehabilitation Association (NRA)
North American Spine Society (NASS)
Occupational Injury Prevention Rehabilitation Society (OIPRS)
Occupational Safety and Health Administration (OSHA)
Orthopaedic Trauma Association (OTA)
Visiting Nurse Association (VNA)

Professional Titles

Athletic Trainer Certified (ATC)
Certified Chiropractic Sports Physician (CCSP)
Certified Occupational Therapy Assistant (COTA)
Certified Orthopaedic Physician's Assistant (OPA-C)
Certified Orthotist (CO)
Certified Pedorthist (CPed)
Certified Prosthetist (CP)
Certified Prosthetist/Orthotist (CPO)
Doctor of Chiropractic (DC)
Doctor of Occupational Therapy (OTD)
Doctor of Osteopathy (DO)
Doctor of Physical Therapy (DPT)
Doctor of Podiatric Medicine (DPM)
Doctor of Podiatry (DP)
Fellow of the American College of Foot Orthopedics (FACFO)
Fellow of the American College of Sports Medicine (FACSM)
Fellow of the American Occupational Therapy Association (FAOTA)
Fellow of the American Physical Therapy Association (FAPTA)
Industrial Physical Therapist (IPT)
Master of Physical Therapy (MPT)
Occupational Therapist (OT)
Occupational Therapist (Canadian) (OT-C)
Occupational Therapist, Licensed (OTL)
Occupational Therapist, Licensed (Canadian) (OT-L)
Occupational Therapist, Registered (OTR)
Occupational Therapist, Registered (Canadian) (OT-R)
Orthopaedic Certified Specialist (OCS)
Orthopaedic Physician's Assistant (OPA)
Orthopaedic Nurse Certified (ONC)
Physical Therapist (PT)
Physical Therapy Assistant (PTA)
Sports Certified Specialist (SCS)

Sample Reports

ANKLE FRACTURE OFFICE CONSULTATION

SUBJECTIVE: This is a middle-aged female who injured her right ankle yesterday. She was seen in the emergency room where she was evaluated, treated, splinted. She is seen in my office today in followup. She is noted to have a Weber B distal fibula fracture with medial joint space widening and tenderness over her deltoid ligament. It is subsequently determined that she has an unstable right ankle fracture. Her past medical history is positive for carpal tunnel syndrome. She had a carpal tunnel release 1 year ago. She currently takes no medications and says she has no medication allergies. She does have a long history of smoking.

OBJECTIVE: She has a minimal amount of swelling over her right ankle. She has tenderness medially and laterally. Overall alignment is good. The skin is intact. She is neurovascularly intact to motor and sensory grossly in all distributions. I reviewed the x-rays, 3 views of the right ankle. They reveal a Weber B distal fibula fracture with slight angulation. There is widening of the medial joint space.

ASSESSMENT: This is an SER IV equivalent fracture in a middle-aged female smoker.

PLAN: The plan is to get preoperative laboratory studies this afternoon, including CBC, chemistries, coagulation studies, EKG, chest x-ray, and urinalysis. She will be scheduled for outpatient surgery tomorrow. The patient should be n.p.o. after midnight. She should be strict nonweightbearing with elevation overnight.

The patient was informed regarding the risks and benefits of surgery. These include, but are not limited to, bleeding, infection, nerve damage, painful hardware, need for reoperation including hardware removal, delayed union, malunion, and nonunion especially given the fact that the patient is a smoker. She could have chronic pain that changes with weather, and other chronic issues including paresthesias. The patient could have anesthetic complications and could even suffer a sudden death should there be complications associated with the anesthesia. The patient understands the risks and benefits as described to her. All questions have been answered in detail. The patient would like to proceed with the above-mentioned procedure. The informed consent was signed by the patient and myself. I think she will do quite well with this injury, but with her smoking history she is at risk for increased complications.

CALCIFIC TENOSYNOVITIS HISTORY AND PHYSICAL

CHIEF COMPLAINT: The patient is a female with a complaint of pain and enlargement in the posterior aspect of her right heel.

HISTORY OF PRESENT ILLNESS: The patient has had this pain for almost 2 years. The enlarged area protrudes out and rubs in her shoes. She has difficulty walking up and down stairs. She does not recall any trauma to this area. She has found that Icy Hot and some athletic rubs have been helpful but do not reduce her symptoms completely. She has tried immobilization and physical therapy without relief of symptoms.

PAST SURGICAL HISTORY: She has had an anterior cervical disc surgery.

CURRENT MEDICATIONS

1. Albuterol inhaler.
2. Indapamide.
3. Accolate.
4. Vytorin.
5. FemHRT hormone replacement therapy.
6. Lunesta.

ALLERGIES: Adhesive tape causes a skin rash.

SOCIAL HISTORY: She does not use tobacco. Denies alcohol use. Never been treated for drug or alcohol addiction. She is a retired school teacher.

FAMILY HISTORY: Diabetes in maternal grandmother.

REVIEW OF SYSTEMS: Positive for asthma, hypertension, type 2 diabetes which is diet controlled, high cholesterol. She denies any cardiovascular issues. Denies any previous anesthesia problems. Denies any stomach, intestinal, gallbladder disease.

PHYSICAL EXAMINATION

Vital signs: Blood pressure is 135/75, temperature 98.8 orally, pulse 72 beats per minute, and respirations 15 per minute. Height is 5 feet 7 inches, weight 220 pounds.
Skin: Redness and swelling around the posterior aspect of the right heel. Otherwise normal skin and nails.
Heent: Normal.
Neck: Normal.
Lungs: Normal chest sounds are present.
Heart: Rate and rhythm are normal.
Extremities: Both feet have normal vascularization. Dorsalis pedis and posterior tibial pulses are palpable and normal. Capillary refill is less than 3 seconds. The patient has a painful enlargement of the posterior aspect of the right heel near the insertion of Achilles tendon. There is pain with palpation. Dorsiflexion is slightly reduced and painful in the ankle joint. Subtalar joint range of motion is normal. Digital range of motion is normal.

Neurologic: Sensation to light touch is intact. Deep tendon reflexes are 2+ and symmetric in bilateral lower extremities.

DIAGNOSTIC IMAGING: Radiographic examination in the lateral weightbearing view demonstrates a large bony spurring at the insertion of the Achilles tendon that measures 1 cm in length; on the calcaneal view this measures 1.2 cm in width. Otherwise, normal bone and joint formation of the right foot, and ankle joint space is normal.

IMPRESSION: Right heel calcific tenosynovitis.

PLAN: Surgical excision of the calcific tenosynovitis.

CERVICAL MYELOPATHY REHABILITATION HISTORY AND PHYSICAL

CHIEF COMPLAINT: Cervical myelopathy status post laminectomy.

HISTORY OF PRESENT ILLNESS: The patient is an elderly female with a history of hypothyroidism, hypertension, diabetes, and rheumatoid arthritis. The patient has had previous lumbar back surgery with complication of residual right foot drop. The patient says she has been able to ambulate short distances but over the past several months has had a significant decline in her function. The patient was planning to move to senior housing with elevator accessibility. The patient most recently had been transferring out of bed into her power wheelchair. Of late she has complained of more weakness of the hands and some numbness. The patient also has complaints of radicular pain down the left leg. The patient was referred to a local neurosurgeon.

The patient has undergone radiographic studies which reveal her to have significant degenerative changes at multiple levels. The patient has spinal stenosis from C4 through C7. A diagnosis of cervical myelopathy was made. The patient elected to undergo a decompressive laminectomy. Status post surgery the patient has had decreased pain in the left leg. The patient has less numbness of the fingers. She has started to mobilize with the physical therapist. The patient is felt to have potential for improvement, and ultimately she may not have to rely so heavily on her power wheelchair.

The patient is now being admitted for inpatient rehabilitation. The goal is to improve her overall function so she can be more independent in caring for herself.

CURRENT MEDICATIONS
1. Diltiazem 240 mg daily.
2. Lipitor 40 mg at bedtime.
3. Prednisone 10 mg daily.
4. Levothroid 0.05 mg daily.

5. Folic acid 1 mg daily.
6. Multivitamin with mineral one p.o. daily.
7. NovoLog 15 units t.i.d.
8. Lantus 40 units subcutaneously in the morning and 30 units subcutaneously at bedtime.
9. Diovan 160 mg b.i.d.
10. Clonidine 0.15 mg t.i.d.
11. Allopurinol 100 mg daily.
12. Leflunomide 20 mg daily.
13. Lasix 80 mg daily.
14. Flexeril 10 mg p.r.n. spasm.
15. Reglan 10 mg before meals and at bedtime.
16. Hydrocodone p.r.n. pain.

ALLERGIES: Lisinopril.

SOCIAL HISTORY: The patient is widowed. She resides in an apartment building that has an elevator. She has her own walker and power wheelchair. She denies tobacco and rarely drinks alcohol.

REVIEW OF SYSTEMS: The patient feels less numbness in her fingers. She has less pain down the left leg. The patient still has a right foot drop. She denies any shortness of breath. There is no chest pain. The patient is continent of bowel and bladder.

PHYSICAL EXAMINATION
General: Well-developed, well-nourished female in no acute distress.
Heent: Normocephalic, atraumatic. Sclerae anicteric. Pupils equal, round, and reactive to light and accommodation. Extraocular movements intact. Negative for nystagmus. Moist oral mucosa.
Neck: Supple. Full, active range of motion.
Lungs: Clear to auscultation and percussion.
Heart: Regular S1 and S2 without murmurs, rubs, or gallops.
Abdomen: Normoactive bowel sounds. Soft and nontender.
Genitourinary: Normal female genitalia.
Musculoskeletal: The patient has a right foot drop. The hands reveal some moderate joint deformities secondary to rheumatoid arthritis. Good movement across the shoulders. Trace pedal edema.
Rectal: Deferred.
Neurologic: The patient is pleasant and is speaking well. Alert and oriented. She has intact cranial nerves II through XII. Manual muscle testing shows 4/5 strength in the upper extremities and 3/5 strength at the hip flexors. She has an obvious right foot drop. There is good movement of the left ankle. Sensation to light touch

is intact in the fingers. Muscle stretch reflexes are trace throughout. Toes are not responsive.

Functional: The patient is at minimum assistance for transfers. She is able to ambulate up to 40 feet with a front-wheeled walker.

IMPRESSION

1. Status post decompressive cervical laminectomy.
2. History of spinal stenosis, C4 through C7.
3. Right foot drop.
4. Rheumatoid arthritis.
5. Diabetes.
6. Hypertension.

PLAN: The patient is status post decompressive laminectomy for cervical myelopathy with spinal stenosis. She is doing fairly well at this point and has good potential for improvement. We will try to get her more functional with aggressive PT and OT. The patient will continue to be monitored for pain. We will monitor for any neurological symptoms, especially in the lower extremities. The patient apparently wears some type of brace on her right foot. We will evaluate this and make adjustments as needed. She should do fairly well. We anticipate she will be here for less than a week.

CHRONIC PAIN REHABILITATION CONSULTATION

REASON FOR CONSULTATION: Chronic pain with deconditioning after renal failure.

HISTORY OF PRESENT ILLNESS: The patient is a right-handed white male who is under treatment for chronic pain. His past medical history is significant for morbid obesity, diabetes, hypertension, and lumbar radiculopathy with bilateral footdrop. He has been using bilateral AFOs. The patient was doing fairly well but then developed flulike symptoms which were followed by confusion. He was brought to the hospital, and his CBG at the time of admission was 25. The patient had a significantly elevated BUN and creatinine, 88 and 10 respectively. He was admitted to the intermediate care unit and underwent dialysis. He is now making some improvement, and consultation is requested for determination of need for rehabilitation.

CURRENT MEDICATIONS

1. Tylenol p.r.n. pain.
2. Lantus 10 units subcutaneous at bedtime.
3. Nicotine 14 mg patch daily.
4. Lopressor 2.5 mg q.8 h.

5. Procrit 10,000 units after hemodialysis.
6. Norvasc 10 mg daily.
7. Hydralazine 50 mg q.6 h.
8. Protonix 40 mg daily.
9. Zosyn 2.25 g IV q.8 h.

ALLERGIES: No known drug allergies.

SOCIAL HISTORY: The patient lives at home with his wife. His home entrance has 3 steps. He has bilateral ankle-foot orthoses and uses a cane for ambulation.

REVIEW OF SYSTEMS: The patient has chronic pain. He has poor sensation in the feet. Denies any chest pain. No shortness of breath.

PHYSICAL EXAMINATION

General: Well-developed, well-nourished white male in no acute distress, sitting up in his bed.

Musculoskeletal: The patient has trace pedal edema. He has spontaneous movement in all 4 extremities. The patient is lacking dorsiflexion bilaterally. He has no gross deformities.

Neurologic: The patient is alert and oriented x3. Speech is clear. Cognition is grossly normal. Cranial nerves II through XII are grossly intact. Manual muscle testing is about 4+ in the upper extremities, about 4/5 in the lower extremities, and trace with dorsiflexion bilaterally. Sensation is diminished in a stocking distribution in the lower extremities. Muscle stretch reflexes are trace throughout. Toes are not responsive.

Functional: The patient is at minimum assist for transfers. He is ambulatory with the therapist up to about 180 feet using a front-wheeled walker.

ASSESSMENT AND PLAN: This patient developed flulike symptoms then went into encephalopathy due to electrolyte imbalance with very low blood sugar. He subsequently developed renal insufficiency, was admitted to the hospital and received dialysis. The patient's electrolytes have normalized. He has undergone diabetic teaching, and his glucose levels have been followed. The patient has chronic pain. He states that he has been on Lortab in the past. At this point he is felt to have components of peripheral neuropathy in his lower extremities. He will be started on Lyrica 75 mg b.i.d., to be increased as needed. The patient was reminded that he should not accept any narcotic medication from the hospitalist on discharge since he is followed in the community for chronic pain. The patient should do fairly well, and I do not see the need for the patient undergo inpatient rehabilitation.

Thank you very much for this interesting consult.

CLOSED REDUCTION AND PERCUTANEOUS PINNING OF SALTER I FRACTURE

PREOPERATIVE DIAGNOSIS: Displaced Salter I fracture, right proximal humerus.

POSTOPERATIVE DIAGNOSIS: Displaced Salter I fracture, right proximal humerus.

PROCEDURE

1. Closed reduction with manipulation.
2. Percutaneous pinning with 2 Schanz pins, 2.5 mm in size.

ANESTHESIA: General.

ESTIMATED BLOOD LOSS: Less than 10 mL.

FLUIDS: Total of 300 mL of Plasma-Lyte A.

DESCRIPTION OF PROCEDURE: The patient was brought to the operating room. General anesthetic was administered. The patient's right shoulder was examined under fluoroscopy. The shoulder reduced nicely with abduction and rotation. We visualized this on both the AP and lateral views. It was relatively stable in this position with abduction and about 45 degrees of internal rotation. We then prepped and draped the arm. A pin was placed in the AP view, and we marked it with a marking pen, then in the axillary view with a marking pen, and then at the intersection of these 2 lines we made a small stab incision with dissection carried bluntly down to the bone. We then used a drill guide and a terminally threaded Schanz pin and drilled 1 pin across the physis in both AP and lateral projections and axillary view. This pin was somewhat anterior. A 2nd pin was placed more posterior and central. With the 2 pins in place, we had excellent stability. This was examined in multiple views, and the pins were contained within the head. We then injected the soft tissues with a total of about 8 mL of 0.5% Marcaine with epinephrine. After cutting the pins, we closed them beneath the skin with 4-0 nylon suture. Sterile dressing was applied, followed by an axillary pad and an arm sling. The patient was then taken to the recovery room.

CLOSED REDUCTION BOTH-BONE FOREARM FRACTURE

PREOPERATIVE DIAGNOSIS: Left distal both-bone forearm fracture.

POSTOPERATIVE DIAGNOSIS: Left distal both-bone forearm fracture.

PROCEDURE: Closed reduction and long arm casting of the left distal both-bone forearm fracture.

ANESTHESIA: General anesthesia.

FLUIDS: Per anesthesia service record.

ESTIMATED BLOOD LOSS: None.

DRAINS: None.

SPECIMENS: None.

FINDINGS: As mentioned below.

COMPLICATIONS: There were no complications.

DESCRIPTION OF PROCEDURE: After informed consent was signed by the patient's father, he was taken to the operating room. General anesthesia was given. Once the patient was fully sedated and relaxed, gentle manipulation was carried out. It was quite difficult to achieve reduction of the distal radius in bayonet apposition. Subsequently the finger traps were used and the forearm was hung with weights from an IV pole. After approximately 5 minutes, gentle manipulation was continued. The fracture was accentuated and the fragments brought out to length. It was difficult to get full translation of the diaphysial components to abut. Nevertheless, on AP view using the mini C-arm, the radius was not out to length, as was the distal ulna. On the lateral view, the alignment was excellent. There was still 50% translation in a dorsal direction; however, the overall alignment and angulation was anatomic.

The forearm was then left to hang for another 5 minutes, with 5 pounds of weight from the elbow. Cast padding was applied up to the elbow. Fiberglass rolls were used to apply a circumferential fiberglass short arm cast. This was allowed to dry. As it dried, it was well molded over the fracture itself. An interosseous mold and a mold-holding 3-point fixation were then carried out.

Additional fluoroscopic views were taken. The overall alignment in AP and lateral planes was perfect. The 50% translation dorsally persisted. It appeared that the ends of the fracture fragment on the distal radius locked in this position, and to unlock them and translate them in a volar direction was not only extremely difficult but was also unnecessary. A well-padded long arm fiberglass cast was then over-wrapped, taking great care to pad the elbow area. This was placed with the elbow in 90 degrees of flexion and the forearm in neutral rotation. Final fluoroscopic views were taken, printed and placed in the chart.

The patient was aroused from anesthesia, transferred to a stretcher, and taken to the recovery room. The patient was noted to be in stable condition, having tolerated the procedure very well. There were no complications. The findings were as noted above.

The postoperative plan will be admission to the inpatient unit overnight for neurovascular checks and pain control. I would like them to monitor for compartment syndrome. If the patient does well with p.o. pain medications, he will be discharged to home in the morning. The patient is to use a sling only for ambulation; otherwise, the arm should be elevated above the heart at all times for the next 72 to 96 hours. The patient will follow up in the office in 7 to 10 days for x-ray evaluation and further instructions.

Given the patient's age and robust healing potential, combined with the fact that this was achieved through closed means, I think he will show significant callus formation within 3 weeks' time. If robust callus formation does exist at that time, I would recommend a long arm cast for about 4 to 6 weeks, followed by a short arm cast and then a removable cock-up wrist splint.

EXPLORATION AND REPAIR OF CAPSULAR LIGAMENT

PREOPERATIVE DIAGNOSIS: Laceration of left index finger extensor mechanism and metacarpophalangeal joint.

POSTOPERATIVE DIAGNOSIS: Laceration of left index finger extensor mechanism and metacarpophalangeal joint.

PROCEDURE: Exploration and repair of capsular ligament and irrigation of joint.

ANESTHESIA: Local with sedation.

TOTAL TOURNIQUET TIME: 11 minutes.

FLUIDS: 800 mL.

ESTIMATED BLOOD LOSS: Less than 10 mL.

DESCRIPTION OF PROCEDURE: The patient was brought to the operating room, and sedation and local anesthesia were administered. The left arm was prepped and draped in the usual fashion. The limb was elevated, exsanguinated, and the tourniquet inflated to 250 mmHg. The patient had a proximal-based flap tear over the radial aspect of the metacarpophalangeal joint. It went through the capsule on the radial side of the extensor tendon and down to the capsule of the MCP joint with just a very small pinpoint opening. I opened this just a little bit and irrigated the joint. There was no purulent fluid encountered. The wound was quite clean. After irrigation, the soft tissue was injected with a small amount of 0.5% Marcaine. The capsular ligament was then closed with interrupted 4-0 PDS suture. This approximated the extensor hood quite nicely. The finger was put through a range of motion, and there was no significant tension on the capsule. The tourniquet was released, and hemostasis was obtained with pressure. One subcuticular Vicryl suture was placed and then 3 nylon sutures around the flap, and Dermabond was used to hold the flap down. A gauze wrap was applied, buddy tapping the index finger to the long finger. The patient was taken to the recovery room, having tolerated the procedure well.

EXPLORATION, IRRIGATION, AND DÉBRIDEMENT OF HAND WOUND

PREOPERATIVE DIAGNOSIS: Open wound of left thumb and index finger from gunshot.

POSTOPERATIVE DIAGNOSES

1. Open wound with volar fracture of interphalangeal joint of left thumb.
2. Soft tissue injury of tip of index finger.

PROCEDURE: Exploration, irrigation, and débridement of skin and subcutaneous tissue, and removal of small bone fragments.

ANESTHESIA: General.

TOTAL TOURNIQUET TIME: 20 minutes.

ESTIMATED BLOOD LOSS: Less than 25 mL.

FLUIDS: 900 mL.

DESCRIPTION OF PROCEDURE: The patient was brought to the operating room. General anesthetic was administered. The left arm was examined, then cleaned, prepped, and draped in the usual fashion with a tourniquet on the arm. The limb was elevated, exsanguinated, and the tourniquet inflated to 275 mmHg. We first irrigated the index finger and the thumb. The index finger showed an 8 mm to 10 mm area at the pulp that appeared to be either a powder burn or impact point. It did not involve the bone and was only into the subcutaneous tissue. This was irrigated, and we lightly débrided some skin at the edges.

The thumb showed a fairly large flap of tissue distally involving a somewhat stellate injury at the volar side of the interphalangeal joint. This appeared to have disrupted the neurovascular bundle on the radial side. There was, however, good capillary fill distally.

We inspected and débrided some of the skin and subcutaneous tissue, particularly the tissue that had powder burns. Some bone fragments were also removed. We inspected down to the IP joint volarly; there was a communication with the joint, and 1 small volar radial aspect of the bone from the distal phalanx at the articular surface that was partially intact was sutured with a 4-0 Vicryl suture. We irrigated the joint and irrigated the soft tissue. The flexor pollicis longus tendon was intact. We then loosely approximated some of the subcutaneous tissue over the bone. We released the tourniquet, and hemostasis was obtained with pressure. We had good capillary fill, and the distal tuft appeared to have good circulation. I closed a portion of the skin; approximately half of what was open. There was a section that will have to granulate in due to loss of skin from the injury. Xeroform gauze was applied to both the thumb and the index finger, and tube gauze dressings were applied. The patient was then taken to the recovery room.

FINGER AMPUTATION

PREOPERATIVE DIAGNOSIS: Gangrene of right index finger.

POSTOPERATIVE DIAGNOSIS: Gangrene of right index finger.

PROCEDURE: Amputation of right index finger through the proximal phalanx.

ANESTHESIA: General.

ESTIMATED BLOOD LOSS: Less than 10 mL.

FLUIDS: 500 mL.

DESCRIPTION OF PROCEDURE: The patient was brought to the operating room. A general anesthetic was administered. The right hand was prepped and draped in the usual fashion. We used a Penrose drain along the base of the finger as a tourniquet. The incision line was drawn out, and an elliptical incision was made. Dissection was carried sharply through the skin and down through the tendon. The vessels of the finger were calcified. The nerves were transected sharply. We disarticulated the finger at the proximal interphalangeal joint, removing the gangrenous tip of the finger. We then smoothed the edges of the proximal phalanx, removing the articular surface to shorten the bone sufficiently to be able to get soft tissue closure without tension. We irrigated and then released the Penrose tourniquet. There was no arterial bleeding. There was good capillary bleeding. We accomplished hemostasis with pressure. The soft tissue was closed over the bone with 4-0 Vicryl suture to approximate the subcutaneous tissue, and the skin was closed with interrupted 4-0 and 5-0 nylon suture, followed by placement of a sterile dressing. The patient was taken to the recovery room.

FOREARM FASCIOTOMY

PREOPERATIVE DIAGNOSIS: Left forearm compartment syndrome.

POSTOPERATIVE DIAGNOSIS: Left forearm compartment syndrome.

PROCEDURE: Left forearm volar compartment fasciotomy.

ANESTHESIA: General.

ESTIMATED BLOOD LOSS: Minimal.

DRAINS: Penrose drains, 2 in number.

DESCRIPTION OF PROCEDURE: The patient was brought to the operating room. General anesthetic was administered. The left arm was prepped and draped in the usual fashion. The limb was elevated, exsanguinated, and tourniquet inflated to 275 mmHg. A longitudinal incision was made in the volar forearm, incorporating the patient's longitudinal stab wound which was about 1.5 cm long and in the mid volar forearm. Dissection was carried down sharply through the skin and bluntly through the subcutaneous tissue, protecting the superficial nerves and veins. Both the superficial and deep compartments were released. Culture was taken at the level of the wound. There was no sign of purulence. We irrigated briefly with peroxide and then with saline, released the tourniquet, and did not identify any significant arterial bleeders. Hemostasis was obtained. Partial closure was obtained with a combination of 3-0 and 4-0 Vicryl suture. Penrose drains were placed in the deep tissue. A sterile dressing was applied, followed by a sugar-tong splint for the forearm, and the patient was taken to the recovery room.

HIP REPLACEMENT FOR AVASCULAR NECROSIS DISCHARGE SUMMARY

ADMISSION DIAGNOSIS: Left hip replacement for arthritis and avascular necrosis.

DISCHARGE DIAGNOSIS: Arthritis left hip secondary to avascular necrosis.

PROCEDURE: Left hip replacement.

HISTORY OF PRESENT ILLNESS: The patient is an elderly female with fairly sudden onset of pain in her left hip that became progressive and quite disabling. She was admitted for a left hip replacement secondary to avascular necrosis and arthritis. The cause of her avascular necrosis is felt to be idiopathic.

HOSPITAL COURSE: On the day of admission, the patient was taken to the operating room. Under a general anesthetic plus a fascia iliaca block, a left hip replacement was performed, along with platelet-rich plasma autograft. A Stryker Accolade system was used with a 46 cup, a 36 head with a polyethylene liner and a #1 Accolade stem, 127-degree angle.

Postoperatively, she was treated with prophylactic antibiotics for 24 hours, DVT prophylaxis with Coumadin, foot pumps, and TED hose. She made good progress with physical therapy. She did not require a transfusion. Her dressing was changed at the time of discharge, and the incision was clean and dry. She was discharged to home. She will continue on Coumadin and will have this followed in the Coumadin Clinic.

DISCHARGE MEDICATIONS

1. Resume previous medications.
2. OxyContin 10 mg one q.12 h. for pain.
3. Hydrocodone for breakthrough pain.
4. Coumadin 4 mg daily.
5. Surfak as a stool softener.

PLAN/DISPOSITION: She will follow up with me in the office 10 to 12 days post discharge.

ISCHEMIC GANGRENE OF LEG CONSULTATION

REASON FOR CONSULTATION: Evaluation and treatment of right leg ischemic gangrene.

HISTORY OF PRESENT ILLNESS: This patient has multiple medical problems, including coronary artery disease status post CVA and severe peripheral vascular disease. She was admitted for an angioplasty of the lower extremities to hopefully provide better blood flow to the right lower extremity to treat nonhealing ischemic ulcers. She has had ischemic ulcers for the past 2 to 3 weeks. They have been getting larger, more painful, and have been preventing her from walking and from sleeping. The patient was initially admitted 2 weeks ago for an angioplasty procedure; however, they were unable to open the vessels at that time because they were completely calcified. The patient then had a consultation with the vascular surgeon and was offered arterial bypass to revascularize the lower extremity, but she declined the procedure because it was too high risk.

Two weeks ago the patient developed a large blister on the right heel. That turned into an ulcer that did not heal, and it developed a black spot in that area. The black spot grew larger very rapidly over a 2-week period. Since development of that spot, she has not been able to walk on it. She went to the emergency room a number of times and received IV antibiotics. Eventually she was referred to the interventional radiologist who planned to perform an angioplasty of the lower extremity arteries. As stated before, this procedure was attempted, but the angioplasty was not able to be accomplished because it was too clotted and calcified.

Today the patient requested an amputation of the lower extremity because it was painful, and she refused to be discharged from the hospital with later return as an outpatient.

PAST MEDICAL HISTORY

1. Hypertension.
2. History of a stroke.
3. Diverticulosis.
4. Iron-deficiency anemia.
5. Osteoporosis.
6. Hyperlipidemia.

PAST SURGICAL HISTORY

1. Three-vessel bypass.
2. Hip replacement surgery.

CURRENT MEDICATIONS

1. Potassium.
2. Lasix.
3. Vitamins.
4. Aggrenox.
5. Metoprolol.
6. Benazepril.
7. Crestor.
8. Chromagen.
9. Clarinex.
10. Os-Cal.

ALLERGIES

1. Sulfa.
2. Lasix.

HABITS: The patient does drink but does not smoke.

SOCIAL HISTORY: The patient lives alone, but she has a daughter and grand-daughter living close by, and they have been helping her out.

REVIEW OF SYSTEMS
Cardiovascular: No chest pain or shortness of breath.
Gastrointestinal: No vomiting or diarrhea.
Musculoskeletal: No upper extremity pain. Right leg pain is the only pain. It starts by the ankle and heel area and then radiates proximally.

PHYSICAL EXAMINATION
General: No acute distress. Alert and oriented.
Vital Signs: Temperature 97.7, heart rate 89, blood pressure 175/91, respirations 18, saturation 98% on 3 L.
Lungs: Clear to auscultation but very faint breath sounds.
Heart: Regular rate and rhythm. Heart sounds are very faint also.
Abdomen: Soft, nontender.
Extremities: The right lower extremity is very thin and looks emaciated. There is redness about halfway up the leg and throughout the whole ankle and foot area, consistent with ischemia. All the blood vessels are very prominent in the right lower extremity. There is hardly any bulk to the muscles, and there are no pulses palpable in the foot at all. Perfusion has decreased significantly in the heel. There is a large blister, and there is a black gangrenous area measuring approximately 5 × 4 cm. There is redness ascending proximally up the leg to about midcalf. The ankle can be moved without pain. The knee joint is painless, and the lower extremity is cool. There is no redness or swelling in the right thigh area.

LABORATORY DATA: Sodium 136, potassium 4.6, BUN 42, creatinine 1.8. CBC is pending. PT, INR, and PTT are pending. Type and crossmatch are pending.

DIAGNOSTIC IMAGING: X-rays of the foot taken earlier show severe osteopenia with vascular calcification all the way down to the distal aspect of the forefoot, meaning there is fairly severe arteriosclerotic peripheral vascular disease. An ABI showed significant severe peripheral vascular disease.

ASSESSMENT
1. Right leg ischemic gangrene with ischemic nonhealing ulcers.
2. Right leg ischemic pain.
3. Right leg severe peripheral vascular disease with failed angioplasty. The patient refuses a revascularization procedure.
4. Coronary artery disease status post 3-vessel coronary artery bypass grafting procedure.

RECOMMENDATION
1. I discussed the issues involved with the interventional radiologist, and he updated me regarding the patient's condition and the decision-making involved. The patient

has refused any type of vascularization procedure and wants amputation of the leg because it is just too painful.

2. The patient requested an orthopedic consultant to consider amputation of the leg.
3. I am familiar with the patient because I have taken care of her for a multitude of other problems. She preferred to have the amputation provided by someone she is familiar with instead of another surgeon.
4. I spoke with the patient and the patient's daughter, counseling them regarding the issues. At this point in time they do not want a revascularization procedure, and they do not want to just leave the leg alone. Even with the risk of having a procedure that may cause a heart attack, stroke, or death, because it is so painful and she cannot sleep, cannot get up, cannot walk, cannot sit up, and has the constant need for pain medicines, the patient still requests the procedure.
5. The plan is to proceed with scheduling an amputation procedure, if possible, and this will most likely be an above-knee amputation.

OPEN REDUCTION AND INTERNAL FIXATION OF RIGHT INTERTROCHANTERIC HIP FRACTURE

PREOPERATIVE DIAGNOSIS: Right intertrochanteric hip fracture.

POSTOPERATIVE DIAGNOSIS: Right intertrochanteric hip fracture.

PROCEDURE: Open reduction and internal fixation of right intertrochanteric hip fracture.

ANESTHESIA: General.

FLUIDS

1. Two units packed red blood cells.
2. Two units FFP.
3. One liter crystalloid.

ESTIMATED BLOOD LOSS: 500 mL.

DRAIN: 1 Hemovac drain.

SPECIMENS: None.

COMPLICATIONS: None.

INDICATIONS: The patient is an elderly male who had a fall that resulted in right hip pain. Emergency room evaluation showed a displaced hip fracture. The pros and cons of operative management were discussed with the patient and family, and operative management was selected.

DESCRIPTION OF PROCEDURE: The consent was reviewed, and the right lower extremity was verified as the correct extremity. After induction of general anesthesia, the patient was placed on the fracture table without difficulty. Manipulation under fluoroscopy was performed, and the fracture was unable to be anatomically reduced with closed manipulation. Therefore, the decision was made to place a Synthes sliding hip screw after open reduction.

The right lower extremity was prepped and draped in a standard sterile fashion for orthopedic surgery. A standard lateral approach was made. The IT band was incised, and the vastus lateralis was lifted off with control of bleeding vessels. The lateral wall of the femur was identified. Attempts were made to reduce the fragment, but this was difficult secondary to the pull of the psoas muscle on the proximal fragment. Using a Verbrugge-type clamp, the fracture was reduced, and a cable was placed to maintain the reduction. A 135 guide was then placed on the femur, and a guide pin was placed into the femoral head after verification of correct position in AP and lateral views. The measured length was 95 mm.

The DHS triple reamer was used to open the lateral wall as well as the femoral neck and head. Fluoroscopy was used to verify there was no migration of the pin. The 95 mm screw was placed into the head and verified in good position on AP and lateral views. A 4-hole side plate was selected, and large fragment screws were used to secure the plate to the side. The cable was tensioned, tightened and cut and left for additional fixation. Using fluoroscopy, reduction was again verified on AP and lateral views. The wound was irrigated. Bleeding vessels were cauterized. The vastus lateralis was closed using 0 Vicryl. A medium Hemovac drain was placed. The skin was closed with 2-0 Vicryl suture and staples. The patient was awakened from anesthesia without difficulty. The sponge and needle counts were correct at the end of the case.

POSTOPERATIVE PLAN: The patient will be returned to the surgical floor for continued medical monitoring. It is anticipated he will be able to weight bear as tolerated with physical therapy tomorrow. An INR and CBC will be ordered to verify his blood levels as well as his Coumadin level for DVT prophylaxis. He will restart the Coumadin tonight and may start on heparin if his Coumadin level is low on the INR evaluation.

PROXIMAL HUMERUS FRACTURE EMERGENCY ROOM CONSULTATION

REASON FOR CONSULTATION: Right shoulder proximal humerus fracture. Requested by ER physician for evaluation and treatment.

HISTORY OF PRESENT ILLNESS: The patient has recently moved to this region. She is right-hand dominant. She fell in a local park when she was pulled down by her dog and dragged for some distance. She subsequently sustained a fracture of the right shoulder and also fractures of the left ribs. No other associated injuries, according to the patient.

PAST MEDICAL HISTORY

1. Hypertension.
2. Depression.
3. Left foot surgery.
4. Appendectomy.
5. Total abdominal hysterectomy and bilateral salpingo-oophorectomy.
6. Scoliosis.
7. Low back pain.
8. Hypertension.

MEDICATIONS

1. Zoloft.
2. Trazodone.
3. Atenolol.

ALLERGIES: Sulfa.

HABITS: Nonsmoker. She does drink alcohol occasionally.

REVIEW OF SYSTEMS: The patient does have chest pain related to the location of the rib fractures and has shortness of breath when she takes a deep breath. She has pain in the right shoulder but none in the left. No pain in the lower extremities. No back or neck pain.

PHYSICAL EXAMINATION
General: She has acute distress when her shoulder is moved or she takes a deep breath. She is alert and oriented x3.
Vital signs: Normal.
Neck: Nontender, supple.
Back: Nontender to palpation.
Lungs: Clear to auscultation.
Heart: Regular rate and rhythm.
Abdomen: Soft, nontender. Positive bowel sounds.
Chest: Tenderness in the ribs just below the left breast and anteriorly.
Pelvic: Nontender pelvic rock.

EXTREMITIES: Palpation of the lower extremities reveals no deformities or areas of tenderness or pain. The right elbow area is mildly tender, appears to be over the radial head area. She also is mildly tender around the proximal humerus. There is no breakdown of the skin. The patient has intact radial and ulnar nerves. The median nerve was not tested. Perfusion appears to be normal. The patient is comfortable when she is not being moved.

DIAGNOSTIC IMAGING: Right shoulder x-rays show a surgical neck fracture of the proximal humerus that is nondisplaced and also a greater tuberosity fracture with less than 5 mm of displacement. X-ray of the humerus shows the shoulder joint is not displaced.

ASSESSMENT

1. Right proximal humerus surgical neck fracture that is mildly impacted with the greater tuberosity slightly displaced.
2. Left anterior rib fractures.
3. Right elbow occult radial head fracture.

PLAN

1. X-rays were reviewed with the patient, and we discussed the implications of the treatment.
2. Conservative measures will be employed at this time. She is aware if displacement occurs or there are other issues, such as discovery of a rotator cuff tear or the fragment displaces further, surgery will be necessary.
3. I provided the patient with a pillow sling to help protect the shoulder better and give some more aeration around the axilla.
4. I obtained elbow x-rays. They were read by me and showed no obvious fractures, although the patient could have a radial head fracture that is nondisplaced.
5. Pain medications will be prescribed by the ER physician. I recommend a narcotic plus Vistaril and also a stool softener.
6. I recommend the patient sit up in a chair for at least the next couple of weeks because that is usually the most comfortable position for patients with proximal humeral fractures.
7. Follow up with an orthopaedist in 10 to 14 days.
8. I recommend using ice on the area to help reduce the pain and the swelling.

RADIUS FRACTURE, LIGAMENT TEAR, CARPAL TUNNEL REPAIR

PREOPERATIVE DIAGNOSES

1. Left wrist perilunate dislocation of the carpus.
2. Left distal radius intraarticular fracture.
3. Median nerve compression.

POSTOPERATIVE DIAGNOSES

1. Left wrist perilunate dislocation of the carpus.
2. Left distal radius intraarticular fracture.
3. Median nerve compression.

PROCEDURES

1. Open reduction and percutaneous pinning of left distal radius fracture.
2. Closed reduction and percutaneous pinning of left wrist perilunate dislocation.
3. Lunotriquetral ligament repair.
4. Carpal tunnel release.

ANESTHESIA: General anesthesia with local infiltration of 0.5% Marcaine plain.

FLUIDS: Per anesthesia record.

ESTIMATED BLOOD LOSS: Less than 20 mL.

DRAINS: None.

SPECIMENS: None.

FINDINGS

1. Perilunate dislocation of the carpus in the dorsal direction.
2. Lunotriquetral ligament disruption.
3. Radial styloid was fractured in a crushing fashion, with comminution.
4. There was an articular surface fracture line of less than 1 mm with no major depression.
5. There was an intact scapholunate ligament.
6. There was a thickened transverse carpal ligament.

INDICATIONS: This male was in a motor vehicle accident. All history was obtained from the family, due to patient sedation. Consent was signed by the patient's wife, and he underwent closed reduction and internal fixation with a long intramedullary nail to stabilize his left hip and femur. This was successful. At the same time he underwent placement of a short arm cast on his left wrist in order to stabilize it.

Today the patient began complaining of significant left wrist pain. A CT scan revealed the patient had a perilunate dislocation of the left wrist. It appeared that the force occurred with extreme dorsiflexion to the left wrist. This caused a radial styloid and articular surface fracture in a compressive fashion. The force was transmitted in a perilunate direction, causing a dorsal dislocation of the carpus with complete disruption of the lunotriquetral ligament.

After the CT scan, the patient was consented for performance of closed reduction of the left carpus with the possibility of open reduction and internal fixation with pins, if needed. We also planned to repair any obvious ligament disruption and achieve bony stability at this time. The primary goal was the reduction and maintenance of the reduction with percutaneous pinning, if necessary. Referral to a hand specialist will be made for recommendation of future treatment options. All this was explained to the patient, and all questions were answered. Risks and benefits were discussed including the need for further surgeries. The informed consent was signed and placed in the chart.

DESCRIPTION OF PROCEDURE: The patient was taken to the operating room and underwent induction of general anesthesia. Once the patient was fully anesthetized and relaxed, the left upper extremity was placed in finger traps, and weights were hung from the elbow. A closed reduction was attempted, but this was unsatisfactory as noted on mini-C-arm fluoroscopy, after which the case was converted to an open procedure.

A tourniquet was placed on the left upper extremity, after which the left upper extremity was prepped and draped in the usual sterile fashion. A hand table was used. An Esmarch bandage was used to exsanguinate the limb, and the tourniquet was inflated to 250 mmHg. Total tourniquet time was 65 minutes. The plan was to perform a dorsal approach to the left wrist with open relocation and reduction of the carpus and maintenance of this reduction with cross-pinning. This was to be followed by a median nerve decompression through a volar approach with carpal tunnel release. These procedures were performed.

After inflation of the tourniquet, a longitudinal incision was made centered over the left wrist. Dissection was carried out through the soft tissues. Hemostasis was achieved. Neurovascular structures were avoided. The 4th extensor compartment was entered. The tendons were retracted in an ulnar direction. The capsule was subsequently incised over the carpus in a longitudinal fashion. The carpal bones were exposed at this time, as was the distal radius. The distal radius, dorsal aspect, was comminuted. The radiocarpal joint was explored. There was an intraarticular split depression fracture noted. The stepoff, however, was less than 1 mm. The radial styloid was visualized and noted to be extensively comminuted. The distal radius was then stabilized in this position with 2 K-wires through the tip of the radial styloid into the distal radial metaphysis.

We next turned our attention to the carpus. The scapholunate ligament was largely intact. There was some subluxation of the lunocapitate joint, and this was reduced into place. The lunotriquetral ligament was completely disrupted. Subsequently the wound was thoroughly irrigated, and all bony fragments were removed. The lunotriquetral ligament was repaired using 4-0 Ethibond figure-of-8 stitches ×4. This created a nice repair of these 2 bones; however, I still felt the carpus was unstable. Consequently, a single K-wire was placed through the scaphoid and into the body of the capitate. Subsequently the scaphoid, the capitate, the lunate and the triquetrum were all fixed together either through ligamentous repair or through K-wire fixation.

Mini-C-arm fluoroscopy was used to assess the reduction and stability of the repair. In AP and lateral planes, the radius lined up with the lunate, the capitate, and the 3rd metacarpal. The overall alignment of the distal radius was within anatomic limits, and the configuration of the carpus was anatomic.

Next our attention focused on the volar side. The patient had complained of numbness and tingling in the thumb, index finger, and long finger on the palmar aspect. It appeared the carpal dislocation put significant pressure on the carpal tunnel of the left wrist. It was felt that in order to alleviate this pressure, reduction of the carpus was necessary, and an open carpal tunnel release would be performed to prevent any more significant swelling within the confined space of the carpal tunnel.

A small 1-inch incision was made in the palmar crease in a longitudinal direction. Dissection was carried out through the soft tissues. The neurovascular structures were avoided. The palmar fascia was cut and spread. The transverse carpal ligament was identified. Using a 15 blade, the transverse carpal ligament was transected, and great care was taken to avoid all neurovascular structures including the motor branch of the thenar musculature. The transverse carpal ligament was completely transected in half, and the carpal tunnel was explored. The median nerve did appear somewhat injected, as if it had been traumatized. The floor of the carpal tunnel was palpated and noted to be smooth.

At this point final pictures were taken, printed, and placed in the chart. The wounds were thoroughly irrigated with normal saline, and the tourniquet was released. The skin on the volar side was reapproximated using 3-0 nylon vertical mattress sutures. On the dorsal side the capsule over the carpus was reapproximated using 0 Vicryl suture. The extensor tendons of the 4th compartment were allowed to lay back into their native bed, and the extensor retinaculum was repaired over the top of them with 0 Vicryl suture. The wrist was put through a range of motion. Excursion was noted to be smooth and easy. Subsequently the subcutaneous tissue was closed using 2-0 Vicryl buried simple suture, and 3-0 nylon suture was used for an everted skin closure.

Three K-wires were bent and left percutaneously. Xeroform was applied around all wounds, followed by sterile gauze and Webril. A well-padded posterior splint with sugar tong was applied to stabilize and keep the arm with the elbow in 90 degrees of flexion and the forearm in neutral rotation.

The patient was awakened from anesthesia and transferred to a stretcher. He was then taken to the recovery room and noted to be in stable condition, having tolerated the procedure very well. There were no complications.

POSTOPERATIVE PLAN: Readmission back to the intermediate care unit, and we will observe him overnight. If he continues to do well, we will transfer him to the orthopaedic floor and start physical therapy. If he has no mental status changes, and the subarachnoid bleed is not worsening, we will start him on DVT prophylaxis. In the meantime TED hose and SCDs will be utilized. The patient will be given Ancef in the postoperative period. He will have neurovascular checks of his upper and lower extremities. We will resume a diet very slowly. I will consult with a hand specialist who will consult on him early next week. The patient will likely be in the hospital for approximately 5 days post procedure, with a goal of mobilization with a platform walker prior to discharge. He may need further surgery on his wrist, to be determined by a hand specialist. He will be 50% weightbearing on his left lower extremity until callus is noted on followup x-rays.

REHABILITATION DISCHARGE, DECONDITIONING

DISCHARGE DIAGNOSES

1. Anoxic encephalopathy.
2. Deconditioned.
3. Diabetic foot ulcer.
4. Diabetes.
5. Peripheral vascular disease.
6. Myocardial infarction.

HISTORY OF PRESENT ILLNESS: The patient is a 68-year-old female with a history of congestive heart failure, diabetes, renal insufficiency, and peripheral vascular disease. The patient, unfortunately, had developed a diabetic foot ulcer of the right foot. She has failed outpatient management. She was started on IV antibiotic but then had a severe reaction to the antibiotic and became obtunded. She was seen by a neurologist and found to have encephalopathy due to the medication. The patient has had medication switched by the Infectious Disease Service and has had improvement. She had become significantly deconditioned and weak due to the encephalopathy. She has some cognitive deficit as well with stabilization but ongoing difficulty. The patient will be admitted for inpatient rehabilitation.

HOSPITAL COURSE: The patient remained afebrile, and vital signs remained stable. She continued her antibiotic treatment plan. She was eating and sleeping well on the rehabilitation unit. She continued with Wound VAC to the right foot. She denied significant pain. She was continent of bowel and bladder. The patient made significant improvement with her cognition. She did develop worsening of her anemia, and she was given 2 units of packed red blood cells.

The patient did fairly well. She was aware of the needed precautions on the right leg. She continued with Wound VAC care. At the time of discharge, she was independent for transfers. Once up, she was able to ambulate for about 50 feet, which is the goal for her while having the Wound VAC. She was pushing a wheelchair quite adequately. She was doing her ADLs fairly independently for feeding, grooming, and total body dressing. The patient had made significant improvement in her cognition. She had fairly intact cognition at the time of discharge, although she did have occasional word-finding difficulties. With completion of goals, the patient was discharged home. She will have outpatient antibiotic treatment.

LABORATORY DATA: Electrolytes were followed serially to adjust for any abnormalities. Complete blood count was followed to monitor her white count and hemoglobin. Her CBG was followed serially to adjust for insulin needs.

DISCHARGE MEDICATIONS

1. Hydralazine 50 mg t.i.d.

2. Aspirin 325 mg every day.
3. Paroxetine 10 mg every day.
4. Nitro-Dur 0.2 mg/h patch.
5. Toprol-XL 50 mg b.i.d.
6. Clonidine 0.1 mg q.6 h.
7. Cozaar 50 mg b.i.d.
8. Lantus insulin 10 units subcutaneous at bedtime.
9. Novolin insulin 4 units subcutaneous before meals.
10. Labetalol 200 mg q.8 h.
11. Calcium carbonate 500 mg t.i.d.
12. Carafate 1 g before meals and at bedtime.
13. Prevacid 30 mg every day.
14. Lasix 20 mg every day.
15. Metolazone 2.5 mg every day.
16. Ceftazidime 1 g IV q.24 h.

DISCHARGE DIET: An 1800-calorie ADA diet.

PLAN AND DISPOSITION: The patient has done well with inpatient rehabilitation. She is mobile and independent with her ambulation. She will continue with wound care. The patient will have outpatient IV antibiotic treatment. She will continue seeing the Infectious Disease Service, and she will have home health services.

SUBDURAL HEMATOMA REHABILITATION CONSULTATION

REASON FOR CONSULTATION: Subdural hematoma with bleed.

HISTORY OF PRESENT ILLNESS: The patient is a 58-year-old male with a history of seizures since childhood, hypertension, and previous head trauma ×3 after a motor vehicle accident. He actually wears a helmet on a regular basis. The patient recently developed diabetes. He apparently suffered a seizure at home. There is no history of falls.

After the seizure, the patient was brought to the hospital, where a CT scan showed him to have an acute right-sided subdural hematoma. He had left-sided weakness with complaint of headache. He was admitted and underwent craniotomy for hematoma evacuation. He had significantly elevated blood pressure requiring ICU care prior to transfer to the intermediate care unit. He has begun acute therapy, and he is hoping to improve, such that he can return home with his wife. Consultation is being obtained at this point to evaluate the patient's rehabilitation needs and potentials.

CURRENT MEDICATIONS

1. Depakote 500 mg q.i.d.
2. Lamictal 100 mg t.i.d.

3. Valium 2 mg t.i.d.
4. Hydrocodone p.r.n. pain.
5. Norvasc 5 mg every day.
6. Lisinopril 20 mg b.i.d.
7. Colace 100 mg b.i.d.

SOCIAL HISTORY: The patient lives at home with his wife. He has 3 steps to negotiate to get into the house.

REVIEW OF SYSTEMS: He denies any previous history of bowel or bladder problems. He denies any chest pain. There is no shortness of breath.

PHYSICAL EXAMINATION
General: Well-developed, well-nourished male in no distress.
Heent: The patient's craniotomy incision is intact. Staples are in place. There are no signs of drainage.
Extremities: The patient is without pedal edema. He has spontaneous movement of all 4 extremities. Passive range of motion is fairly intact. He is without any gross deformities.
Neurologic: The patient is alert and is speaking quite well. Manual muscle testing reveals the patient to have at least 4/5 muscle power throughout. Sensation is intact to light touch and pinprick. Muscle stretch reflexes are 1+ and symmetrical. Toes are upgoing on the left but downgoing on the right. On functional testing, the patient is transferring with mild assistance.

ASSESSMENT AND PLAN: The patient is status post seizure activity with fall, resulting in subdural hematoma. He is status post right-sided craniotomy and is still weak at this point. He requires mild assistance for his transfers. He will be a good inpatient rehabilitation candidate. He should do fairly well with inpatient treatment. We will need to do family training as well.

Common Terms by Procedure

ANKLE FRACTURE OFFICE CONSULTATION

alignment
angulation
ankle
deltoid ligament
distribution
hardware
malunion
medial joint space
motor
nonunion
paresthesia
sensory
SER IV fracture
supination-external rotation (SER)
Weber B distal fibula fracture
x-ray

CALCIFIC TENOSYNOVITIS HISTORY AND PHYSICAL

Achilles tendon
ankle joint space
bone formation
bony spurring
calcaneal view
calcific tenosynovitis
capillary refill
disc surgery
digital range of motion
dorsalis pedis pulse
dorsiflexion
heel
insertion
joint formation
joint space
immobilization
lateral weightbearing
posterior tibial pulse
radiographic examination

range of motion
subtalar joint
tenosynovitis
vascularization
surgical excision
weightbearing

CERVICAL MYELOPATHY REHABILITATION HISTORY AND PHYSICAL

ambulate
back surgery
cervical myelopathy
continent of bowel and bladder
cranial nerves II through XII
decompressive laminectomy
degenerative change
footdrop
front-wheeled walker
hip flexor
inpatient rehabilitation
laminectomy
manual muscle testing
minimum assistance (min-assist)
mobilize
multiple levels
muscle stretch reflex
myelopathy
numbness
occupational therapy (OT)
physical therapist
physical therapy (PT)
power wheelchair
radicular pain
radiographic study
rheumatoid arthritis
sensation to light touch
spinal stenosis
transfer
weakness

CHRONIC PAIN REHABILITATION CONSULTATION

ambulation
ambulatory
ankle-foot orthosis (AFO)
capillary blood glucose (CBG)
chronic pain
cognition
cranial nerves II through XII
deconditioning
diabetes
dorsiflexion
footdrop
gross deformity
hypertension
inpatient rehabilitation
intermediate care unit
Lortab
lower extremity
Lyrica
manual muscle testing
minimum assist
morbid obesity
muscle stretch reflex
narcotic medication
pedal edema
peripheral neuropathy
radiculopathy
rehabilitation
sensation
spontaneous movement
stocking distribution
therapist
upper extremity

CLOSED REDUCTION AND PERCUTANEOUS PINNING OF SALTER I FRACTURE

abduction
anteroposterior (AP)
AP view
arm sling
axillary pad
axillary view
closed reduction
displaced
dissection
drill guide
fluoroscopy
general anesthetic
internal rotation
lateral view
manipulation
0.5% Marcaine with epinephrine
marking pen
4-0 nylon suture
percutaneous pinning
physis
pin
Plasma-Lyte A
projection
proximal humerus
rotation
Salter I fracture
Schanz pin
shoulder
stab incision
sterile dressing

CLOSED REDUCTION BOTH-BONE FOREARM FRACTURE

abut
alignment
anatomic
angulation
anteroposterior (AP)
AP plane
AP view
bayonet apposition
both-bone forearm fracture
callus formation
cast padding
closed reduction
compartment syndrome
diaphysial component

distal radius
distal ulna
dorsal direction
elbow
fiberglass roll
finger trap
fluoroscopic view
forearm fracture
fracture fragment
fragment
general anesthesia
interosseous mold
lateral plane
lateral view
long arm cast
long arm fiberglass cast
manipulation
mini C-arm
mold-holding 3-point fixation
neurovascular check
neutral rotation
pain control
radius
reduction
removable cock-up wrist splint
short arm cast
sling
translation
volar direction
weights

EXPLORATION AND REPAIR OF CAPSULAR LIGAMENT

capsular ligament
capsule
Dermabond
exploration and repair
exsanguinate
extensor hood
extensor mechanism
extensor tendon
finger
gauze wrap

hemostasis
index finger
interrupted 4-0 PDS suture
irrigation
laceration
limb
local anesthesia
0.5% Marcaine
MCP joint
metacarpophalangeal (MCP)
nylon suture
pinpoint opening
proximal-based flap tear
purulent fluid
range of motion
sedation
soft tissue
subcuticular Vicryl suture
tourniquet
wound

EXPLORATION, IRRIGATION, AND DÉBRIDEMENT OF HAND WOUND

articular surface
bone fragment
capillary fill
capillary refill
circulation
débridement
distal phalanx
distal tuft
exploration
exsanguinate
flap
flexor pollicis longus tendon
general anesthetic
granulate
hemostasis
index finger
interphalangeal (IP)
interphalangeal joint
IP joint

irrigation
neurovascular bundle
open wound
pulp
skin
soft tissue injury
stellate injury
subcutaneous tissue
thumb
tourniquet
tube gauze dressing
4-0 Vicryl suture
volar fracture
volar side
Xeroform gauze

FINGER AMPUTATION

amputation
arterial bleeding
articular surface
calcified
capillary bleeding
disarticulate
dissection
elliptical incision
gangrene
general anesthetic
hemostasis
incision line
index finger
interrupted 4-0 and 5-0 nylon suture
nerve
Penrose drain
Penrose tourniquet
PIP joint
proximal interphalangeal (PIP)
proximal phalanx
sterile dressing
subcutaneous tissue
tendon
tourniquet
transect
vessel
4-0 Vicryl suture

FOREARM FASCIOTOMY

arterial bleeder
compartment syndrome
culture
deep compartment
dissection
exsanguinate
fasciotomy
general anesthetic
hemostasis
irrigate
longitudinal stab wound
Penrose drain
peroxide
purulence
saline
sterile dressing
subcutaneous tissue
sugar-tong splint
superficial compartment
superficial nerve
superficial vein
tourniquet
3-0 and 4-0 Vicryl suture
volar compartment fasciotomy
volar forearm

HIP REPLACEMENT FOR AVASCULAR NECROSIS DISCHARGE SUMMARY

Accolade stem
arthritis
avascular necrosis
Coumadin
DVT prophylaxis
fascia iliaca block
foot pump
general anesthetic
hip replacement
hydrocodone
idiopathic
OxyContin
physical therapy
platelet-rich plasma autograft

polyethylene liner
prophylactic antibiotic
Stryker Accolade system
Surfak
TED hose
transfusion

ISCHEMIC GANGRENE OF LEG CONSULTATION

above-knee amputation
amputation
failed angioplasty
ankle
ankle-brachial index (ABI)
arterial bypass
arteriosclerotic peripheral vascular disease
black spot
blister
bulk
blood vessel
calcified
clotted
coronary artery disease
emaciated
extremity pain
foot
forefoot
gangrenous
heel
interventional radiologist
ischemia
ischemic gangrene
ischemic ulcer
IV antibiotic
knee joint
lower extremity
midcalf
muscle
nonhealing ischemic ulcer
osteopenia
palpable
perfusion
peripheral vascular disease (PVD)

prominent
proximally
pulse
pulses palpable
revascularization
thigh area
ulcer
vascular calcification
vascularization
x-ray

OPEN REDUCTION AND INTERNAL FIXATION OF RIGHT INTERTROCHANTERIC HIP FRACTURE

anatomically reduced
anteroposterior (AP)
AP view
as tolerated
bleeding vessel
cable
cauterized
closed manipulation
complete blood count (CBC)
crystalloid
Coumadin
deep vein thrombosis (DVT)
DHS triple reamer
displaced hip fracture
DVT prophylaxis
femoral head
femoral neck
femur
fixation
fluoroscopy
fracture table
fragment
fragment screw
fresh frozen plasma (FFP)
general anesthesia
135 guide
guide pin

Hemovac drain
heparin
4-hole side plate
iliotibial (IT)
international normalized ratio (INR)
intertrochanteric hip fracture
irrigate
IT band
lateral view
lateral wall of the femur
lower extremity
manipulation under fluoroscopy
medical monitoring
migration
open reduction
open reduction and internal fixation
 (ORIF)
operative management
orthopedic surgery
packed red blood cells
physical therapy
psoas muscle
screw
standard lateral approach
staple
Synthes sliding hip screw
vastus lateralis
Verbrugge-type clamp
0 Vicryl
2-0 Vicryl suture
weight bear

PROXIMAL HUMERUS FRACTURE EMERGENCY ROOM CONSULTATION

acute distress
aeration
axilla
chest pain
conservative measures
displacement
elbow
elbow occult radial head fracture
fragment

greater tuberosity
humerus
impacted
median nerve
narcotic
nondisplaced
occult
pain medication
palpation
perfusion
pillow sling
proximal humerus
radial head
radial nerve
rotator cuff tear
shoulder
shoulder joint
stool softener
surgery
surgical neck fracture
swelling
tenderness
ulnar nerve
Vistaril
x-ray

RADIUS FRACTURE, LIGAMENT TEAR, CARPAL TUNNEL REPAIR

alignment
anatomic
Ancef
anteroposterior (AP)
AP plane
articular surface
15 blade
bony fragment
bony stability
callus
capitate
capsule
carpal bone
carpal tunnel
carpal tunnel release

carpus
closed reduction and internal fixation
closed reduction and percutaneous
    pinning
comminuted
comminution
4th compartment
compression
compressive fashion
configuration
cross-pinning
crushing fashion
CT scan
decompression
depression
disruption
dissection
distal radial metaphysis
distal radius
distal radius intraarticular fracture
dorsal approach
dorsal aspect
dorsal direction
dorsal dislocation
dorsiflexion
DVT prophylaxis
elbow
Esmarch bandage
4-0 Ethibond figure-of-8 stitch
everted skin closure
excursion
exsanguinate
4th extensor compartment
extensor retinaculum
extensor tendon
femur
finger trap
flexion
fracture line
general anesthesia
hand table
hand specialist
hemostasis
hip

index finger
intraarticular
K-wire
K-wire fixation
lateral plane
ligament disruption
ligamentous repair
local infiltration
long finger
long intramedullary nail
longitudinal direction
longitudinal fashion
longitudinal incision
lower extremity
lunate
lunocapitate joint
lunotriquetral ligament
lunotriquetral ligament disruption
lunotriquetral ligament repair
maintenance of reduction
0.5% Marcaine plain
median nerve
median nerve compression
median nerve decompression
metacarpal
metaphysis
mini-C-arm fluoroscopy
mobilization
motor branch
native bed
neurovascular check
neurovascular structure
neutral rotation
normal saline
3-0 nylon suture
3-0 nylon vertical mattress suture
open carpal tunnel release
open procedure
open reduction and percutaneous
    pinning
open relocation and reduction
palmar aspect
palmar crease
palmar fascia

palpate
percutaneous pinning
perilunate
perilunate dislocation
pictures
pin
platform walker
radial styloid
radiocarpal joint
radius
range of motion
readmission
reapproximated
reduction
scaphoid
scapholunate ligament
sequential compression device
   (SCD)
short arm cast
splint with sugar tong
stepoff
sterile gauze
subarachnoid bleed
subcutaneous tissue
subluxation
sugar tong
TED hose
tendon
thenar musculature
thumb
tourniquet
tourniquet time
transect
transverse carpal ligament
traumatized
triquetrum
tunnel
ulnar direction
ulnar fashion
upper extremity
vertical mattress suture
0 Vicryl suture
2-0 Vicryl buried simple suture
volar approach

volar side
Webril
weightbearing
weights
wound
wrist
wrist perilunate dislocation of the
   carpus
Xeroform

REHABILITATION DISCHARGE, DECONDITIONING

activities of daily living (ADLs)
ADA diet
afebrile
ambulate
ambulation
American Dietetic Association
   (ADA)
anoxic encephalopathy
antibiotic treatment plan
capillary blood glucose (CBG)
cognition
cognitive deficit
deconditioned
diabetes
diabetic foot ulcer
electrolytes
encephalopathy
home health services
independent
independent for transfer
inpatient rehabilitation
IV antibiotic
mobile
myocardial infarction
obtunded
outpatient management
peripheral vascular disease
stabilization
word-finding difficulty
wound care
Wound VAC

SUBDURAL HEMATOMA REHABILITATION CONSULTATION

acute right-sided subdural hematoma
acute therapy
bleed
craniotomy
CT scan
drainage
elevated blood pressure
evacuation
family training
functional testing
gross deformity
head trauma
headache
hematoma evacuation
inpatient treatment
intensive care unit (ICU)
intermediate care unit
left-sided weakness
manual muscle testing
mild assistance (mild assist)
muscle stretch reflex
passive range of motion
pedal edema
pinprick
potentials
rehabilitation
right-sided cranitomy
sensation to light touch
spontaneous movement
staple
subdural hematoma
transfers

Common Chiropractic Terms

abduction stress test
activator
activator adjusting instrument
acupressure
acupuncture
Adam sign
adduction stress test
adjustment
Adson maneuver
Allen test
Amoss sign
anterior foot draw sign
anterior innominate test
Apley test
atlas orthogonal technique (AOT)
Babinski reflex
Bakody sign
Barge analysis
Bechterew test
biceps reflex
Bikele sign
Bio Energetic synchronization
    technique (BEST)
biokinetic
biokinetics
Blair upper cervical technique
Bonnet sign
bowstring sign
brachial plexus tension test
Bragard sign
Buerger test
Burns bench test
Carver technique
cavitation
cervical distraction test
chest expansion test
Childress duck waddle test
chiropractic biophysics (CBP)
Codman sign
concept therapy
contact reflex analysis (CRA)

contour analysis
Cox flexion-distraction technique
Cox sign
Cozen test
Dawbarn sign
degeneration
Dejerine sign
Demianoff sign
Derefield leg check
Deyerle sciatic tension test
diathermy
directional non-force technique (DNFT)
distraction
diversified
diversified chiropractic technique
double leg raise test
Dreyer sign
Duchenne sign
Dugas test
dynamic thrust
electrical galvanic stimulation (EGS)
electromyogram (EMG)
electrotherapy
Ely heel-to-buttock test
Ely sign
Erichsen sign
faber test
fabere test
fadir test
fadire test
Fajersztajn sign
finger-thumb reflex
finger-to-finger test
finger-to-nose test
flexion-distraction technique
Forestier bowstring sign
full-spine technique
Gaenslen test
George test
Gillis test
Goldthwait sign

Gonstead technique
Gordon reflex
Grostic procedure
Hamilton ruler test
heel-knee test
heel-toe test
heel-walk test
Hennequin sign
Hibb test
hip abduction stress test
Hoffa sign
hole-in-one (HIO)
HIO method
Homan sign
Hoover sign
Huntington sign
iliac compression test
impingement sign
infraspinatus reflex
interferential electrotherapy
intersegmental traction
inverted radial reflex
iontophoresis
Jackson compression test
Kale method
Kemp test
kinesiology
Kleist hooking sign
Klippel-Weil sign
Laguerre sign
Lasègue differential sign
Lasègue sitting test
Leander method
leg-length test
Lewin punch test
Lewin snuff test
Lewin standing test
Lewin supine test
Lewin-Gaenslen test
Lhermitte sign
Lindner sign
locked spinal joint
Logan basic technique
long-lever manipulation

low-force technique
lumbopelvic technique
lumbosacral stress test
Magnuson test
Maisonneuve sign
manipulation
manipulation under anesthesia (MUA)
manual percussion test
massage
Mennell test
Mercy Guidelines
metatarsal test
Mill maneuver
mobilization
moiré contour analysis
Morquio sign
Moszkowicz test
motion palpation
Murphy punch test
Nachlas test
Naffziger test
National Upper Cervical Chiropractic
   Association (NUCCA)
Néri bowling sign
nerve conduction velocity (NCV)
Nervo-Scope
neural organization technique (NOT)
Neuro Emotional Technique (NET)
neurocalometer
Nimmo technique
non-force method
NUCCA/Grostic technique
O'Connell test
Oppenheim sign
orthogonal method
PAL technique
Palmer method
Patrick test
pectoral reflex
percussion test
Pettibon technique
Phalen sign
phonophoresis
Pierce-Stillwagon method

platysma sign
positive anatomical length (PAL)
radial reflex
Romberg sign
sacral-occipital technique (SOT)
sacroiliac resisted abduction test
sacroiliac stretch test
shoulder compression test
shoulder depression test
Sicard sign
sitting root test
Smith-Peterson test
snout reflex
sonography
Soto-Hall test
spinal adjustment
spinal analysis
spinal compression test
spinal manipulation
spinal manipulative therapy
 (SMT)
spinal percussion
Spurling maneuver
straight leg raise
stressology
Strümpell tibialis anterior sign
Strunsky sign
subluxation
supraspinatus press test
surface electromyography (SEMG)

sweat method
thermography
thermotherapy
Thomas test
Thompson table technique
Thompson terminal point technique
Thompson test
Tinel sign
toe-walk test
Toftness technique
toggle recoil technique
total body modification (TBM)
Trendelenburg test
trepidation sign
trigger point
trigger point therapy
tripod sign
Turyn sign
ulnar reflex
ultrasound
Valsalva maneuver
vertebral axial decompression (Vax-D)
vertebral subluxation complex
Wartenberg test
Webster technique
well-leg-raising test of Fajersztajn
Wright test
yeoman test
Yergason test
zygomatic reflex

Appendix 8
Pain Management Terms

ablative surgery
acupressure
acupuncture
addiction
adjuvant analgesic drug
anxiolysis
anxiolytic
behavioral technique
biofeedback training
breakthrough pain
conscious sedation
counterirritant
cryoanalgesia
cryotherapy
deafferentation pain
distraction
dysesthesia
epidural
equianalgesic
eutectic mixture of local anesthetics (EMLA)
hyperpathia
iatrogenic
incident pain
intrapleural
intrathecal
lancinating
local nerve block
meditation
mixed opioid agonist-antagonist
movement-related pain
mucositis
myofascial pain
neurolytic block
neuropathic pain
nociception
nonsteroidal anti-inflammatory drug (NSAID)
opiate receptor
opioid agonist
opioid partial agonist

pain threshold level
palliative therapy
paradoxical reaction
patient controlled analgesia (PCA)
peridural
perineural
physical dependence
progressive muscle relaxation
pseudoaddiction
pseudotolerance
psychosocial intervention
spinal cord stimulator
tactile strategies
TENS unit
transcutaneous electrical nerve stimulation (TENS)
tolerance

COMPLEMENTARY AND ALTERNATIVE MEDICINE PAIN MANAGEMENT TERMS

Aikido
aromatherapy
breath work
Chi Kung (Qi Gong)
cognitive reappraisal
crystal therapy
electromagnetism
energy field work
Feng Shui
flower remedies
guided imagery
homeopathy
hypnotherapy
Jin Shin Jutsu
light and color therapy
magnetic therapy
Reiki
sound therapy
yoga

Common Physical Therapy and Sports Medicine Terms

abduction
adduction
analgesic
anterior
anterior compartment syndrome
antiinflammatory
apophysis
aquatic therapy
arthroscopy
atrophy
avascular
avulsion
body mechanics
bursa
bursitis
cold pack
collagen
concentric
constant passive motion (CPM)
corticosteroid injection
crepitation
crepitus
cryokinetics
cryotherapy
deep tendon reflex
dislocation
distal
dorsiflexion
eccentric
ecchymosis
edema
electrical galvanic stimulation (EGS)
electrical stimulation
electromyogram (EMG)
epidural steroid injection (ESI)
epiphysis
ethyl chloride cold spray therapy
eversion
exostosis
extension

fibrocartilage
flexibility
flexibility exercise
flexion
fracture
ganglion
genu valgum
genu varum
hemarthrosis
hematoma
hot pack
hydrarthrosis
hydrotherapy
hyperextension
hypermobility
hypertrophy
ice massage
infrared cold laser
intermittent compression pump
inversion
iontophoresis
isokinetic exercise
isometric
isotonic
joint capsule
joint mobilization
kinesthesis
kyphosis
land-based therapy
lordosis
luxation
manual muscle testing
manual therapy
manual traction
massotherapy
mechanical traction
modality
myofascial stretching
myositis ossificans
neoprene sleeve

osteoarthritis
osteochondral
overtraining
passive modality
pes cavus
pes planus
posture
pressure release
progressive resistance exercise (PRE)
proprioceptive neuromuscular
   facilitation (PNF)
proximal
range of motion
range-of-motion exercise

scoliosis
splint
steroid injection
strengthening program
stretch
subluxation
suprapatellar reflex
thermotherapy
ultrasound
ultraviolet light
valgus
varus
volar
whirlpool bath

Drugs by Indication

ACROMEGALY
Ergot Alkaloid and Derivative
  Apo-Bromocriptine® [Can]
  bromocriptine
  Parlodel® [US/Can]
  pergolide (Canada only)
  Permax® [Can]
  PMS-Bromocriptine [Can]
Growth Hormone Receptor Antagonist
  pegvisomant
  Somavert® [US]
Somatostatin Analog
  lanreotide
  octreotide
  Octreotide Acetate Injection [Can]
  Octreotide Acetate Omega [Can]
  Sandostatin® [US/Can]
  Sandostatin LAR® [US/Can]
  Somatuline® Autogel® [Can]
  Somatuline® Depot [US]

ANESTHESIA (GENERAL)
Barbiturate
  Brevital® [Can]
  Brevital® Sodium [US]
  methohexital
General Anesthetic
  Amidate® [US/Can]
  Compound™ [US]
  desflurane
  Diprivan® [US/Can]
  enflurane
  Ethrane® [US]
  etomidate
  Forane® [US/Can]
  halothane
  isoflurane
  Ketalar® [US/Can]
  ketamine
  Ketamine Hydrochloride Injection,
    USP [Can]

propofol
sevoflurane
Sevorane™ [Can]
Suprane® [US/Can]
Terrell™ [US]
Ultane® [US]

ANESTHESIA (LOCAL)
Local Anesthetic
  Alcaine® [US/Can]
  Americaine® [US-OTC]
  Ametop™ [Can]
  Anestacon® [US]
  Anusol® Ointment [US-OTC]
  articaine and epinephrine
  Astracaine® with epinephrine [Can]
  Astracaine® with epinephrine forte
    [Can]
  Band-Aid® Hurt-Free™ Antiseptic
    Wash [US-OTC]
  benzocaine
  benzocaine, butamben, and tetracaine
  Benzodent® [US-OTC]
  Betacaine® [Can]
  bupivacaine
  bupivacaine and epinephrine
  Carbocaine® [US/Can]
  Carbocaine® 2% with
    Neo-Cobefrin® [US]
  Cetacaine® [US]
  cetylpyridinium
  chloroprocaine
  Citanest® Plain [US/Can]
  cocaine
  Curasore [US-OTC]
  Cylex® [US-OTC]
  Detane® [US-OTC]
  dibucaine
  Diocaine® [Can]
  Duocaine™ [US]
  dyclonine

ethyl chloride
ethyl chloride and
  dichlorotetrafluoroethane
Exactacain™ [US]
Flucaine® [US]
Fluoracaine® [US]
Fluro-Ethyl® [US]
Foille® [US-OTC]
Gebauer's Ethyl Chloride® [US]
hexylresorcinol
Hurricaine® [US-OTC]
L-M-X™ [US-OTC]
L-M-X™ [US-OTC]
Lanacane® [US-OTC]
LidaMantle® [US]
lidocaine
lidocaine and bupivacaine
lidocaine and epinephrine
Lidodan™ [Can]
Lidoderm® [US/Can]
LidoSite™ [US]
LTA® [US]
Marcaine® [US/Can]
Marcaine® Spinal [US]
Marcaine® with Epinephrine [US]
mepivacaine
mepivacaine and levonordefrin
Mycinettes® [US-OTC]
Naropin® [US/Can]
Nesacaine® [US]
Nesacaine®-CE [Can]
Nesacaine®-MPF [US]
Novocain® [US]
Nupercainal® [US-OTC]
Polocaine® [US/Can]
Polocaine® 2% and Levonordefrin
  1:20,000 [Can]
Polocaine® MPF [US]
Pontocaine® [US/Can]
Pontocaine® Niphanoid® [US]
pramoxine
Prax® [US-OTC]
Premjact® [US-OTC]
prilocaine

procaine
proparacaine
proparacaine and fluorescein
ropivacaine
Sarna® Sensitive [US-OTC]
Sensorcaine® [US/Can]
Sensorcaine®-MPF [US]
Sensorcaine®-MPF Spinal [US]
Sensorcaine®-MPF with Epinephrine
  [US]
Sensorcaine® with Epinephrine
  [US/Can]
Septanest® N [Can]
Septanest® SP [Can]
S.T. 37® [US-OTC]
Tanac® [US-OTC]
tetracaine
Topicaine® [US-OTC]
Trocaine® [US-OTC]
Tronolane® [US-OTC]
Ultracaine® D-S [Can]
Ultracaine® D-S Forte [Can]
Xylocaine® [US/Can]
Xylocaine® MPF [US]
Xylocaine® MPF With Epinephrine
  [US]
Xylocaine® Viscous [US]
Xylocaine® With Epinephrine
  [US/Can]
Xylocard® [Can]
Zilactin® [Can]
Zilactin-L® [US-OTC]
Zilactin®-B [US-OTC/Can]
Zilactin Baby® [Can]
Zorcaine™ [US/Can]

ARTHRITIS
Analgesic, Topical
  Capsagel® [US-OTC]
  capsaicin
  Capzasin-HP® [US-OTC]
  Capzasin-P® [US-OTC]
  Zostrix® [US-OTC/Can]
  Zostrix®-HP [US-OTC/Can]

Antiinflammatory Agent
  Apo-Leflunomide® [Can]
  Arava® [US/Can]
  leflunomide
  Novo-Leflunomide [Can]
Gold Compound
  auranofin
  gold sodium thiomalate
  Myochrysine® [US/Can]
  Ridaura® [US/Can]
Immunosuppressant Agent
  Alti-Azathioprine [Can]
  Apo-Azathioprine® [Can]
  Azasan® [US]
  azathioprine
  cyclosporine
  Gen-Azathioprine [Can]
  Gengraf® [US]
  Imuran® [US/Can]
  Neoral® [US/Can]
  Novo-Azathioprine [Can]
  Restasis® [US]
  Rhoxal-cyclosporine [Can]
  Sandimmune® [US]
  Sandimmune® I.V. [Can]
  Sandoz-Cyclosporine [Can]
Monoclonal Antibody
  adalimumab
  Humira® [US/Can]
Nonsteroidal Antiinflammatory Drug
  (NSAID)
  Advil® [US-OTC/Can]
  Advil® Children's [US-OTC]
  Advil® Infants™ [US-OTC]
  Advil® Junior [US-OTC]
  Advil® Migraine [US-OTC]
  Albert® Tiafen [Can]
  Aleve® [US-OTC]
  Alti-Flurbiprofen [Can]
  Amigesic® [US/Can]
  Anaprox® [US/Can]
  Anaprox® DS [US/Can]
  Ansaid® [Can]
  Apo-Diclo® [Can]

Apo-Diclo Rapide® [Can]
Apo-Diclo SR® [Can]
Apo-Diflunisal® [Can]
Apo-Flurbiprofen® [Can]
Apo-Ibuprofen® [Can]
Apo-Indomethacin® [Can]
Apo-Keto® [Can]
Apo-Keto-E® [Can]
Apo-Keto SR® [Can]
Apo-Nabumetone® [Can]
Apo-Napro-Na® [Can]
Apo-Napro-Na DS® [Can]
Apo-Naproxen® [Can]
Apo-Naproxen EC® [Can]
Apo-Naproxen SR® [Can]
Apo-Oxaprozin® [Can]
Apo-Piroxicam® [Can]
Apo-Sulin® [Can]
Apo-Tiaprofenic® [Can]
Asaphen [Can]
Asaphen EC [Can]
Ascriptin® [US-OTC]
Ascriptin® Maximum Strength
  [US-OTC]
Aspercin [US-OTC]
aspirin
Aspirtab [US-OTC]
Bayer® Aspirin Extra Strength
  [US-OTC]
Bayer® Aspirin Regimen Adult Low
  Dose [US-OTC]
Bayer® Aspirin Regimen Children's
  [US-OTC]
Bayer® Aspirin Regimen Regular
  Strength [US-OTC]
Bayer® Genuine Aspirin [US-OTC]
Bayer® Plus Extra Strength
  [US-OTC]
Bayer® Women's Aspirin Plus
  Calcium [US-OTC]
Buffasal [US-OTC]
Bufferin® [US-OTC]
Bufferin® Extra Strength [US-OTC]
Buffinol [US-OTC]

Cataflam® [US/Can]
choline magnesium trisalicylate
Clinoril® [US]
Daypro® [US/Can]
diclofenac
diflunisal
Doan's® Extra Strength [US-OTC]
Dom-Tiaprofenic® [Can]
Easprin® [US]
EC-Naprosyn® [US]
Ecotrin® [US-OTC]
Ecotrin® Low Strength [US-OTC]
Ecotrin® Maximum Strength
    [US-OTC]
ElixSure™ IB [US-OTC]
Entrophen® [Can]
Feldene® [US]
fenoprofen
flurbiprofen
Froben® [Can]
Froben-SR® [Can]
Genacote™ [US-OTC]
Gen-Nabumetone [Can]
Gen-Naproxen EC [Can]
Gen-Piroxicam [Can]
Genpril® [US-OTC]
Halfprin® [US-OTC]
Ibu-200 [US-OTC]
ibuprofen
Indocid® PDA [Can]
Indocin® [US/Can]
Indo-Lemmon [Can]
indomethacin
Indotec [Can]
I-Prin [US-OTC]
ketoprofen
Keygesic [US-OTC]
lansoprazole and naproxen
magnesium salicylate
meclofenamate
Meclomen® [Can]
Momentum® [US-OTC]
Motrin® [US]
Motrin® Children's [US-OTC/Can]

Motrin® IB [US-OTC/Can]
Motrin® Infants™ [US-OTC]
Motrin® Junior Strength [US-OTC]
nabumetone
Nalfon® [US/Can]
Naprelan® [US]
Naprosyn® [US/Can]
naproxen
Naxen® [Can]
Naxen® EC [Can]
NeoProfen® [US]
Novasal™ [US]
Novasen [Can]
Novo-Difenac [Can]
Novo-Difenac K [Can]
Novo-Difenac-SR [Can]
Novo-Diflunisal [Can]
Novo-Flurprofen [Can]
Novo-Keto [Can]
Novo-Keto-EC [Can]
Novo-Methacin [Can]
Novo-Nabumetone [Can]
Novo-Naproc EC [Can]
Novo-Naprox [Can]
Novo-Naprox Sodium [Can]
Novo-Naprox Sodium DS [Can]
Novo-Naprox SR [Can]
Novo-Pirocam [Can]
Novo-Profen [Can]
Novo-Sundac [Can]
Novo-Tiaprofenic [Can]
Nu-Diclo [Can]
Nu-Diclo-SR [Can]
Nu-Diflunisal [Can]
Nu-Flurprofen [Can]
Nu-Ibuprofen [Can]
Nu-Indo [Can]
Nu-Ketoprofen [Can]
Nu-Ketoprofen-E [Can]
Nu-Naprox [Can]
Nu-Pirox [Can]
Nu-Sundac [Can]
Nu-Tiaprofenic [Can]
Oruvail® [Can]

oxaprozin
Pennsaid® [Can]
Pexicam® [Can]
piroxicam
Proprinal [US-OTC]
Relafen® [Can]
Rhodacine® [Can]
Rhodis™ [Can]
Rhodis-EC™ [Can]
Rhodis SR™ [Can]
Rhoxal-nabumetone [Can]
Riva-Diclofenac [Can]
Riva-Diclofenac-K [Can]
Riva-Naproxen [Can]
Salflex® [Can]
salsalate
Sandoz-Nabumetone [Can]
Solaraze® [US]
St. Joseph® Adult Aspirin [US-OTC]
sulindac
Surgam® [Can]
Tiaprofenic- [Can]
tiaprofenic acid(Canada only)
Tolectin® [US]
tolmetin
Ultraprin [US-OTC]
Voltaren® [US/Can]
Voltaren Rapide® [Can]
Voltaren®-XR [US]
ZORprin® [US]
Nonsteroidal Antiinflammatory Drug
    (NSAID), COX-2 Selective
Celebrex® [US/Can]
celecoxib
GD-Celecoxib [Can]

ARTHRITIS (RHEUMATOID)
Antirheumatic, Disease Modifying
    abatacept
    Orencia® [US]

BACK PAIN (LOW)
Analgesic, Narcotic
    codeine
    Codeine Contin® [Can]

Analgesic, Nonnarcotic
    Asaphen [Can]
    Asaphen EC [Can]
    Ascriptin® [US-OTC]
    Ascriptin® Maximum Strength
        [US-OTC]
    Aspercin [US-OTC]
    Aspergum® [US-OTC]
    aspirin
    Aspirtab [US-OTC]
    Bayer® Aspirin Extra Strength
        [US-OTC]
    Bayer® Aspirin Regimen Adult Low
        Dose [US-OTC]
    Bayer® Aspirin Regimen Children's
        [US-OTC]
    Bayer® Aspirin Regimen Regular
        Strength [US-OTC]
    Bayer® Genuine Aspirin
        [US-OTC]
    Bayer® Plus Extra Strength
        [US-OTC]
    Bayer® Women's Aspirin Plus
        Calcium [US-OTC]
    Buffasal [US-OTC]
    Bufferin® [US-OTC]
    Bufferin® Extra Strength
        [US-OTC]
    Buffinol [US-OTC]
    Easprin® [US]
    Ecotrin® [US-OTC]
    Ecotrin® Low Strength [US-OTC]
    Ecotrin® Maximum Strength
        [US-OTC]
    Entrophen® [Can]
    Genacote™ [US-OTC]
    Halfprin® [US-OTC]
    Novasen [Can]
    St. Joseph® Adult Aspirin
        [US-OTC]
    ZORprin® [US]
Skeletal Muscle Relaxant
    methocarbamol
    Robaxin® [US/Can]

BEHÇET SYNDROME

Immunosuppressant Agent
Alti-Azathioprine [Can]
Apo-Azathioprine® [Can]
Azasan® [US]
azathioprine
cyclosporine
Gen-Azathioprine [Can]
Gengraf® [US]
Imuran® [US/Can]
Neoral® [US/Can]
Novo-Azathioprine [Can]
Restasis® [US]
Rhoxal-cyclosporine [Can]
Sandimmune® [US]
Sandimmune® I.V. [Can]
Sandoz-Cyclosporine [Can]

BURSITIS

Nonsteroidal Antiinflammatory Drug
(NSAID)
Advil® [US-OTC/Can]
Advil® Children's [US-OTC]
Advil® Infants™ [US-OTC]
Advil® Junior [US-OTC]
Advil® Migraine [US-OTC]
Aleve® [US-OTC]
Anaprox® [US/Can]
Anaprox® DS [US/Can]
Apo-Ibuprofen® [Can]
Apo-Indomethacin® [Can]
Apo-Napro-Na® [Can]
Apo-Napro-Na DS® [Can]
Apo-Naproxen® [Can]
Apo-Naproxen EC® [Can]
Apo-Naproxen SR® [Can]
Asaphen [Can]
Asaphen EC [Can]
Ascriptin® [US-OTC]
Ascriptin® Maximum Strength
[US-OTC]
Aspercin [US-OTC]
Aspergum® [US-OTC]
aspirin

Aspirtab [US-OTC]
Bayer® Aspirin Extra Strength
[US-OTC]
Bayer® Aspirin Regimen Adult Low
Dose [US-OTC]
Bayer® Aspirin Regimen Children's
[US-OTC]
Bayer® Aspirin Regimen Regular
Strength [US-OTC]
Bayer® Genuine Aspirin [US-OTC]
Bayer® Plus Extra Strength
[US-OTC]
Bayer® Women's Aspirin Plus
Calcium [US-OTC]
Buffasal [US-OTC]
Bufferin® [US-OTC]
Bufferin® Extra Strength [US-OTC]
Buffinol [US-OTC]
choline magnesium trisalicylate
Easprin® [US]
EC-Naprosyn® [US]
Ecotrin® [US-OTC]
Ecotrin® Low Strength [US-OTC]
Ecotrin® Maximum Strength
[US-OTC]
ElixSure™ IB [US-OTC]
Entrophen® [Can]
Genacote™ [US-OTC]
Gen-Naproxen EC [Can]
Genpril® [US-OTC]
Halfprin® [US-OTC]
Ibu-Tab ® [US-OTC]
ibuprofen
Indocid® PDA [Can]
Indocin® [US/Can]
Indocin® I.V. [US]
Indo-Lemmon [Can]
indomethacin
Indotec [Can]
I-Prin [US-OTC]
lansoprazole and naproxen
Motrin® [US]
Motrin® Children's [US-OTC/Can]
Motrin® IB [US-OTC/Can]

Motrin® Infants™ [US-OTC]
Motrin® Junior Strength [US-OTC]
Naprelan® [US]
Naprosyn® [US/Can]
naproxen
Naxen® [Can]
Naxen® EC [Can]
NeoProfen® [US]
Novasen [Can]
Novo-Methacin [Can]
Novo-Naproc EC [Can]
Novo-Naprox [Can]
Novo-Naprox Sodium [Can]
Novo-Naprox Sodium DS [Can]
Novo-Naprox SR [Can]
Novo-Profen [Can]
Nu-Ibuprofen [Can]
Nu-Indo [Can]
Nu-Naprox [Can]
Proprinal [US-OTC]
Rhodacine® [Can]
Riva-Naproxen [Can]
St. Joseph® Adult Aspirin [US-OTC]
Ultraprin [US-OTC]
ZORprin® [US]

CACHEXIA
Progestin
    Apo-Megestrol® [Can]
    Megace® [US/Can]
    Megace® ES [US]
    Megace® OS [Can]
    megestrol
    Nu-Megestrol [Can]

CLAUDICATION
Blood Viscosity Reducer Agent
    Albert® Pentoxifylline [Can]
    Apo-Pentoxifylline SR® [Can]
    Nu-Pentoxifylline SR [Can]
    pentoxifylline
    Pentoxil® [US]
    ratio-Pentoxifylline [Can]
    Trental® [US/Can]

DÉBRIDEMENT OF CALLOUS TISSUE
Keratolytic Agent
    Tri-Chlor® [US]
    Trichlor Fresh Pac™ [US]
    trichloroacetic acid

DÉBRIDEMENT OF ESCHAR
Protectant, Topical
    Granulex® [US]
    Optase™ [US]
    trypsin, balsam peru, and castor oil
    Xenaderm™ [US]

DECUBITUS ULCER
Enzyme
    collagenase
    Santyl® [US]
Enzyme, Topical Débridement
    Accuzyme® [US]
    Allanzyme [US]
    Allanzyme [US]
    Ethezyme™ [US]
    Ethezyme™ [US]
    Gladase® [US]
    Kovia® [US]
    papain and urea
Protectant, Topical
    Granulex® [US]
    Optase™ [US]
    trypsin, balsam peru, and castor oil
    Xenaderm™ [US]

DEEP VEIN THROMBOSIS (DVT)
Anticoagulant (Other)
    Apo-Warfarin® [Can]
    Coumadin® [US/Can]
    dalteparin
    danaparoid(Canada only)
    enoxaparin
    Enoxaparin Injection [Can]
    Fragmin® [US/Can]

Gen-Warfarin [Can]
Hepalean® [Can]
Hepalean® Leo [Can]
Hepalean®-LOK [Can]
heparin
HepFlush®- [US]
Hep-Lock® [US]
Hep-Lock U/P [US]
Innohep® [US/Can]
Jantoven™ [US]
Lovenox® [US/Can]
Lovenox® HP [Can]
Novo-Warfarin [Can]
Orgaran® [Can]
Taro-Warfarin [Can]
tinzaparin
warfarin
Factor Xa Inhibitor
Arixtra® [US/Can]
fondaparinux
Low Molecular Weight Heparin
Fraxiparine™ [Can]
Fraxiparine™ Forte [Can]
nadroparin (Canada only)

DWARFISM

Growth Hormone
Genotropin® [US]
Genotropin Miniquick® [US]
Humatrope® [US/Can]
Norditropin® [US]
Norditropin® NordiFlex® [US]
Nutropin® [US]
Nutropin AQ® [US/Can]
Nutropine® [Can]
Omnitrope™ [US]
Saizen® [US/Can]
Serostim® [US/Can]
somatropin
Tev-Tropin® [US]
Zorbtive® [US]

EPICONDYLITIS

Nonsteroidal Antiinflammatory Drug
(NSAID)

Advil® [US-OTC/Can]
Advil® Children's [US-OTC]
Advil® Infants™ [US-OTC]
Advil® Junior [US-OTC]
Advil® Migraine [US-OTC]
Aleve® [US-OTC]
Anaprox® [US/Can]
Anaprox® DS [US/Can]
Apo-Ibuprofen® [Can]
Apo-Indomethacin® [Can]
Apo-Napro-Na® [Can]
Apo-Napro-Na DS® [Can]
Apo-Naproxen® [Can]
Apo-Naproxen EC® [Can]
Apo-Naproxen SR® [Can]
EC-Naprosyn® [US]
ElixSure™ IB [US-OTC]
Gen-Naproxen EC [Can]
Genpril® [US-OTC]
Ibu-200 [US-OTC]
ibuprofen
Indocid® PDA [Can]
Indocin® [US/Can]
Indocin® I.V. [US]
Indo-Lemmon [Can]
indomethacin
Indotec [Can]
I-Prin [US-OTC]
lansoprazole and naproxen
Midol® Cramp and Body Aches
  [US-OTC]
Midol® Extended Relief [US]
Motrin® [US]
Motrin® Children's [US-OTC/Can]
Motrin® IB [US-OTC/Can]
Motrin® Infants™ [US-OTC]
Motrin® Junior Strength [US-OTC]
Naprelan® [US]
Naprosyn® [US/Can]
naproxen
Naxen® [Can]
Naxen® EC [Can]
NeoProfen® [US]
Novo-Methacin [Can]

Novo-Naproc EC [Can]
Novo-Naprox [Can]
Novo-Naprox Sodium [Can]
Novo-Naprox Sodium DS [Can]
Novo-Naprox SR [Can]
Novo-Profen [Can]
Nu-Ibuprofen [Can]
Nu-Indo [Can]
Nu-Naprox [Can]
Proprinal [US-OTC]
Rhodacine® [Can]
Riva-Naproxen [Can]
Ultraprin [US-OTC]

FIBROMYOSITIS

Antidepressant, Tricyclic (Tertiary
   Amine)
  amitriptyline
  Apo-Amitriptyline® [Can]
  Levate® [Can]
  Novo-Triptyn [Can]
  PMS-Amitriptyline [Can]

FUNGUS (DIAGNOSTIC)

Diagnostic Agent
  Candida albicans (Monilia)
  Candin® [US]
  Trichophyton skin test

GOUT

Antigout Agent
  colchicine
  colchicine and probenecid
Nonsteroidal Antiinflammatory Drug
  (NSAID)
  Advil® [US-OTC/Can]
  Advil® Children's [US-OTC]
  Advil® Infants™ [US-OTC]
  Advil® Junior [US-OTC]
  Advil® Migraine [US-OTC]
  Aleve® [US-OTC]
  Anaprox® [US/Can]
  Anaprox® DS [US/Can]
  Apo-Diclo® [Can]
  Apo-Diclo Rapide® [Can]

Apo-Diclo SR® [Can]
Apo-Ibuprofen® [Can]
Apo-Indomethacin® [Can]
Apo-Napro-Na® [Can]
Apo-Napro-Na DS® [Can]
Apo-Naproxen® [Can]
Apo-Naproxen EC® [Can]
Apo-Naproxen SR® [Can]
Apo-Sulin® [Can]
Cataflam® [US/Can]
Clinoril® [US]
diclofenac
EC-Naprosyn® [US]
ElixSure™ IB [US-OTC]
Gen-Naproxen EC [Can]
Genpril® [US-OTC]
Ibu-200 [US-OTC]
ibuprofen
Indocid® PDA [Can]
Indocin® [US/Can]
Indo-Lemmon [Can]
indomethacin
Indotec [Can]
I-Prin [US-OTC]
Motrin® [US]
Motrin® Children's [US-OTC/Can]
Motrin® IB [US-OTC/Can]
Motrin® Infants™ [US-OTC]
Motrin® Junior Strength [US-OTC]
Naprelan® [US]
Naprosyn® [US/Can]
naproxen
Naxen® [Can]
Naxen® EC [Can]
NeoProfen® [US]
Novo-Difenac [Can]
Novo-Difenac K [Can]
Novo-Difenac-SR [Can]
Novo-Methacin [Can]
Novo-Naproc EC [Can]
Novo-Naprox [Can]
Novo-Naprox Sodium [Can]
Novo-Naprox Sodium DS [Can]
Novo-Naprox SR [Can]

Novo-Profen [Can]
Novo-Sundac [Can]
Nu-Diclo [Can]
Nu-Diclo-SR [Can]
Nu-Ibuprofen [Can]
Nu-Indo [Can]
Nu-Naprox [Can]
Nu-Sundac [Can]
Pennsaid® [Can]
PMS-Diclofenac [Can]
PMS-Diclofenac SR [Can]
Proprinal [US-OTC]
Rhodacine® [Can]
Riva-Diclofenac [Can]
Riva-Diclofenac-K [Can]
Riva-Naproxen [Can]
Solaraze® [US]
sulindac
Ultraprin [US-OTC]
Voltaren® [US/Can]
Voltaren Rapide® [Can]
Voltaren®-XR [US]
Uricosuric Agent
Apo-Sulfinpyrazone® [Can]
Benuryl™ [Can]
Nu-Sulfinpyrazone [Can]
probenecid
sulfinpyrazone
Xanthine Oxidase Inhibitor
Alloprin® [Can]
allopurinol
Aloprim™ [US]
Apo-Allopurinol® [Can]
Novo-Purol [Can]
Zyloprim® [US/Can]

GRAM-NEGATIVE INFECTION

Aminoglycoside (Antibiotic)
AKTob® [US]
Alcomicin® [Can]
amikacin
Amikacin Sulfate Injection, USP [Can]
Amikin® [US/Can]
Diogent® [Can]
Garamycin® [Can]
Gentak® [US]
gentamicin
Gentamicin Injection, USP [Can]
kanamycin
Kantrex® [US/Can]
PMS-Tobramycin [Can]
SAB-Gentamicin [Can]
Sandoz-Tobramycin [Can]
TOBI® [US/Can]
tobramycin
Tobramycin Injection, USP [Can]
Tobrex® [US/Can]
Antibiotic, Carbapenem
ertapenem
Invanz® [US/Can]
Antibiotic, Irrigation
polymyxin B
Poly-Rx [US]
Antibiotic, Lincosamide
Lincocin® [US/Can]
lincomycin
Antibiotic, Miscellaneous
Apo-Nitrofurantoin® [Can]
Azactam® [US/Can]
aztreonam
colistimethate
Coly-Mycin® M [US/Can]
Furadantin® [US]
Macrobid® [US/Can]
Macrodantin® [US/Can]
nitrofurantoin
Novo-Furantoin [Can]
polymyxin B
Poly-Rx [US]
Antibiotic, Quinolone
gatifloxacin
Iquix® [US]
Levaquin® [US/Can]
levofloxacin
Novo-Levofloxacin [Can]
Quixin™ [US]

Tequin® [Can]
Zymar™ [US/Can]
Carbapenem (Antibiotic)
  imipenem and cilastatin
  meropenem
  Merrem® [Can]
  Merrem® I.V. [US]
  Primaxin® [US/Can]
  Primaxin® I.V. [Can]
Cephalosporin (1st Generation)
  Apo-Cefadroxil® [Can]
  Apo-Cephalex® [Can]
  cefadroxil
  cefazolin
  cephalexin
  Duricef® [US/Can]
  Keflex® [US]
  Keftab® [Can]
  Novo-Cefadroxil [Can]
  Novo-Lexin [Can]
  Nu-Cephalex [Can]
Cephalosporin (2nd Generation)
  Apo-Cefaclor® [Can]
  Apo-Cefoxitin® [Can]
  Apo-Cefprozil® [Can]
  Apo-Cefuroxime® [Can]
  Ceclor® [Can]
  cefaclor
  cefoxitin
  cefpodoxime
  cefprozil
  Ceftin® [US/Can]
  cefuroxime
  Cefzil® [US/Can]
  Mefoxin® [US]
  Novo-Cefaclor [Can]
  Nu-Cefaclor [Can]
  PMS-Cefaclor [Can]
  Raniclor™ [US]
  ratio-Cefuroxime [Can]
  Vantin® [US/Can]
  Zinacef® [US/Can]
Cephalosporin (3rd Generation)
  Cedax® [US]

Cefizox® [US/Can]
cefotaxime
ceftazidime
ceftibuten
ceftizoxime
ceftriaxone
Claforan® [US/Can]
Fortaz® [US/Can]
Rocephin® [US/Can]
Tazicef® [US]
Cephalosporin (4th Generation)
  cefepime
  Maxipime® [US/Can]
Genitourinary Irrigant
  neomycin and polymyxin B
  Neosporin® GU Irrigant [US]
  Neosporin® Irrigating Solution [Can]
Macrolide (Antibiotic)
  Akne-Mycin® [US]
  Apo-Azithromycin® [Can]
  Apo-Erythro Base® [Can]
  Apo-Erythro E-C® [Can]
  Apo-Erythro-ES® [Can]
  Apo-Erythro-S® [Can]
  Azasite™ [US]
  azithromycin
  Biaxin® [US/Can]
  Biaxin® XL [US/Can]
  clarithromycin
  CO Azithromycin [Can]
  Diomycin® [Can]
  Dom-Azithromycin [Can]
  EES® [US/Can]
  Erybid™ [Can]
  Eryc® [Can]
  Eryderm® [US]
  Erygel® [US]
  EryPed® [US]
  Ery-Tab® [US]
  Erythrocin® [US]
  erythromycin
  erythromycin and sulfisoxazole
  GMD-Azithromycin [Can]
  Novo-Azithromycin [Can]

Novo-Rythro Estolate [Can]
Novo-Rythro Ethylsuccinate [Can]
Nu-Erythromycin-S [Can]
PCE® [US/Can]
Pediazole® [Can]
PHL-Azithromycin [Can]
PMS-Azithromycin [Can]
PMS-Erythromycin [Can]
ratio-Azithromycin [Can]
ratio-Clarithromycin [Can]
Romycin® [US]
Sandoz-Azithromycin [Can]
Sans Acne® [Can]
Zithromax® [US/Can]
Zmax™ [US]

Penicillin

Alti-Amoxi-Clav [Can]
Amoclan [US]
amoxicillin
amoxicillin and clavulanate
  potassium
Amoxil® [US]
ampicillin
ampicillin and sulbactam
Apo-Amoxi® [Can]
Apo-Amoxi-Clav® [Can]
Apo-Ampi® [Can]
Apo-Pen VK® [Can]
Augmentin® [US/Can]
Augmentin ES-600® [US]
Augmentin XR® [US]
Bicillin® L-A [US/Can]
Bicillin® C-R [US]
Bicillin® C-R 900/300 [US]
carbenicillin
Clavulin® [Can]
Gen-Amoxicillin [Can]
Geocillin® [US]
Lin-Amox [Can]
Novamoxin® [Can]
Novo-Ampicillin [Can]
Novo-Clavamoxin [Can]
Novo-Pen-VK [Can]
Nu-Amoxi [Can]

Nu-Ampi [Can]
Nu-Pen-VK [Can]
penicillin V potassium
penicillin G benzathine
penicillin G benzathine and penicillin
  G procaine
penicillin G procaine
Pfizerpen-AS® [Can]
PHL-Amoxicillin [Can]
piperacillin
piperacillin and tazobactam sodium
Piperacillin for Injection, USP [Can]
pivampicillin(Canada only)
PMS-Amoxicillin [Can]
Pondocillin® [Can]
ratio-Aclavulanate [Can]
Tazocin® [Can]
Ticar® [US]
ticarcillin
ticarcillin and clavulanate potassium
Timentin® [US/Can]
Unasyn® [US/Can]
Wycillin® [Can]
Zosyn® [US]

Quinolone

Apo-Ciproflox® [Can]
Apo-Norflox® [Can]
Apo-Oflox® [Can]
Apo-Ofloxacin® [Can]
Ciloxan® [US/Can]
Cipro® [US/Can]
Cipro® XL [Can]
ciprofloxacin
Cipro® XR [US]
CO Ciprofloxacin [Can]
CO Norfloxacin [Can]
Floxin® [US/Can]
Gen-Ciprofloxacin [Can]
norfloxacin
Norfloxacine® [Can]
Noroxin® [US/Can]
Novo-Ciprofloxacin [Can]
Novo-Norfloxacin [Can]
Novo-Ofloxacin [Can]

Ocuflox® [US/Can]
ofloxacin
PMS-Ciprofloxacin [Can]
PMS-Norfloxacin [Can]
PMS-Ofloxacin [Can]
Proquin® XR [US]
RAN™ Ciprofloxacin [Can]
ratio-Ciprofloxacin [Can]
Rhoxal-ciprofloxacin [Can]
Riva-Norfloxacin [Can]
Sandoz-Ciprofloxacin [Can]
Taro-Ciprofloxacin [Can]
Sulfonamide
Apo-Sulfatrim® [Can]
Apo-Sulfatrim® DS [Can]
Apo-Sulfatrim® Pediatric [Can]
Bactrim™ [US]
Bactrim™ DS [US]
erythromycin and sulfisoxazole
Gantrisin® [US]
Novo-Soxazole [Can]
Novo-Trimel [Can]
Novo-Trimel DS [Can]
Nu-Cotrimox [Can]
Pediazole® [Can]
Septra® [US]
Septra® DS [US]
Septra® Injection [Can]
sulfadiazine
sulfamethoxazole and trimethoprim
sulfisoxazole
Sulfizole® [Can]
Tetracycline Derivative
Adoxa® [US]
Alti-Minocycline [Can]
Apo-Doxy® [Can]
Apo-Doxy Tabs® [Can]
Apo-Minocycline® [Can]
Apo-Tetra® [Can]
Doryx® [US]
Doxy-100® [US]
Doxycin [Can]
doxycycline
Doxytec [Can]

Dynacin® [US]
Gen-Minocycline [Can]
Minocin® [Can]
Minocin® PAC [US]
minocycline
Monodox® [US]
Myrac™ [US]
Novo-Doxylin [Can]
Novo-Minocycline [Can]
Nu-Doxycycline [Can]
Nu-Tetra [Can]
Oracea™ [US]
oxytetracycline
Periostat® [US/Can]
PMS-Minocycline [Can]
Rhoxal-minocycline [Can]
Sandoz-Minocycline [Can]
Solodyn™ [US]
Terramycin® [Can]
tetracycline
Vibramycin® [US]
Vibra-Tabs® [US/Can]

GUILLAIN-BARRÉ SYNDROME
Immune Globulin
Carimune™ NF [US]
Flebogamma® [US]
Gamimune® N [Can]
Gammagard® Liquid [US/Can]
Gammagard® S/D [US/Can]
Gammar®-P I.V. [US]
Gamunex® [US/Can]
immune globulin (intravenous)
Iveegam EN [US]
Iveegam Immuno® [Can]
Octagam® [US]
Panglobulin® NF [US]
Polygam® S/D [US]

INFLAMMATION (NONRHEUMATIC)
Adrenal Corticosteroid
Apo-Dexamethasone® [Can]

Apo-Prednisone® [Can]
Aristospan® [US/Can]
Betaject™ [Can]
betamethasone (systemic)
Bubbli-Pred™ [US]
Celestone® [US]
Celestone® Soluspan® [US/Can]
Cortef® [US/Can]
corticotropin
cortisone acetate
Decadron® [US]
Depo-Medrol® [US/Can]
Dexamethasone Intensol® [US]
dexamethasone (systemic)
Dexasone® [Can]
DexPak® TaperPak® [US]
Diodex® [Can]
Diopred® [Can]
HP Acthar® Gel [US]
Hydeltra TBA® [Can]
hydrocortisone (systemic)
Kenalog-10® [US]
Kenalog-40® [US]
Medrol® [US/Can]
methylprednisolone
Methylprednisolone Acetate
  [Can]
Novo-Prednisolone [Can]
Novo-Prednisone [Can]
Oracort [Can]
Orapred® [US]
Pediapred® [US/Can]
PMS-Dexamethasone [Can]
prednisolone (systemic)
prednisone
Prednisone Intensol™ [US]
Prelone® [US]
Sab-Prenase [Can]
Solu-Cortef® [US/Can]
Solu-Medrol® [US/Can]
Sterapred® [US]
Sterapred® DS [US]
triamcinolone (systemic)
Winpred™ [Can]

INTERMITTENT CLAUDICATION
Platelet Aggregation Inhibitor
  cilostazol
  Pletal®[US/Can]

EG CRAMP
Blood Viscosity Reducer Agent
  Albert® Pentoxifylline [Can]
  Apo-Pentoxifylline SR® [Can]
  Nu-Pentoxifylline SR [Can]
  pentoxifylline
  Pentoxil® [US]
  ratio-Pentoxifylline [Can]
  Trental® [US/Can]

MARFAN SYNDROME
Rauwolfia Alkaloid reserpine

MUSCLE SPASM
Skeletal Muscle Relaxant
  Apo-Cyclobenzaprine® [Can]
  carisoprodol
  carisoprodol and aspirin
  carisoprodol, aspirin, and codeine
  chlorzoxazone
  cyclobenzaprine
  Fexmid™ [US]
  Flexeril® [US/Can]
  Flexitec [Can]
  Gen-Cyclobenzaprine [Can]
  metaxalone
  methocarbamol
  Mivacron® [Can]
  mivacurium
  Norflex™ [US/Can]
  Norgesic™ [Can]
  Norgesic™ Forte [Can]
  Novo-Cycloprine [Can]
  Nu-Cyclobenzaprine [Can]
  Orphenace® [Can]
  orphenadrine
  orphenadrine, aspirin, and caffeine
  Parafon Forte® [Can]

Rhoxal-orphendrine [Can]
Robaxin® [US/Can]
Skelaxin® [US/Can]
Soma® [US/Can]
Soma® Compound [US]
Soma® Compound w/Codeine
  [US]
Strifon Forte® [Can]

MYCOSIS (FUNGOIDES)

Psoralen
  methoxsalen
  8-MOP® [US/Can]
  Oxsoralen® [US/Can]
  Oxsoralen-Ultra® [US/Can]
  Ultramop™ [Can]
  Uvadex® [US/Can]

NERVE BLOCK

Local Anesthetic
  Ametop™ [Can]
  Anestacon® [US]
  Band-Aid® Hurt-Free™ Antiseptic
    Wash [US-OTC]
  Betacaine® [Can]
  bupivacaine
  Carbocaine® [US/Can]
  chloroprocaine
  Citanest® Plain [US/Can]
  L-M-X™ 4 [US-OTC]
  L-M-X™ 5 [US-OTC]
  LidaMantle® [US]
  lidocaine
  lidocaine and epinephrine
  Lidodan™ [Can]
  Lidoderm® [US/Can]
  LidoSite™ [US]
  LTA® 360 [US]
  Marcaine® [US/Can]
  Marcaine® Spinal [US]
  mepivacaine
  Nesacaine® [US]
  Nesacaine®-CE [Can]
  Nesacaine®-MPF [US]
  Novocain® [US]

Polocaine® [US/Can]
Polocaine® Dental [US]
Polocaine® MPF [US]
Pontocaine® [US/Can]
Pontocaine® Niphanoid® [US]
Premjact® [US-OTC]
prilocaine
procaine
Sensorcaine® [US/Can]
Sensorcaine®-MPF [US]
Sensorcaine®-MPF Spinal [US]
tetracaine
Topicaine® [US-OTC]
Xylocaine® [US/Can]
Xylocaine® MPF [US]
Xylocaine® MPF With Epinephrine
  [US]
Xylocaine® Viscous [US]
Xylocaine® With Epinephrine
  [US/Can]
Xylocard® [Can]
Zilactin® [Can]
Zilactin-L® [US-OTC]

NEURALGIA

Analgesic, Nonnarcotic
  Asaphen [Can]
  Asaphen EC [Can]
  Ascriptin® [US-OTC]
  Ascriptin® Maximum Strength
    [US-OTC]
  Aspercin [US-OTC]
  Aspergum® [US-OTC]
  aspirin
  Aspirtab [US-OTC]
  Bayer® Aspirin Extra Strength
    [US-OTC]
  Bayer® Aspirin Regimen Adult Low
    Dose [US-OTC]
  Bayer® Aspirin Regimen Children's
    [US-OTC]
  Bayer® Aspirin Regimen Regular
    Strength [US-OTC]
  Bayer® Genuine Aspirin [US-OTC]

Bayer® Plus Extra Strength [US-OTC]
Bayer® Women's Aspirin Plus Calcium [US-OTC]
Buffasal [US-OTC]
Bufferin® [US-OTC]
Bufferin® Extra Strength [US-OTC]
Buffinol [US-OTC]
Easprin® [US]
Ecotrin® [US-OTC]
Ecotrin® Low Strength [US-OTC]
Ecotrin® Maximum Strength [US-OTC]
Entrophen® [Can]
Genacote™ [US-OTC]
Halfprin® [US-OTC]
Novasen [Can]
St. Joseph® Adult Aspirin [US-OTC]
ZORprin® [US]
Analgesic, Opioid
acetaminophen, codeine, and doxylamine (Canada only)
Mersyndol® With Codeine [Can]
Analgesic, Topical
Antiphlogistine Rub A-535 No Odour [Can]
Aspercreme® [US-OTC]
Capsagel® [US-OTC]
capsaicin
Capzasin-HP® [US-OTC]
Capzasin-P® [US-OTC]
Flex-Power [US-OTC]
Mobisyl® [US-OTC]
Myoflex® [US-OTC/Can]
Sportscreme® [US-OTC]
trolamine
Zostrix® [US-OTC/Can]
Zostrix®-HP [US-OTC/Can]

ONYCHOMYCOSIS

Antifungal Agent
Grifulvin® V [US]
griseofulvin
Gris-PEG® [US]

Lamisil® Oral [US/Can]
terbinafine (oral)

OSTEOARTHRITIS

Nonsteroidal Antiinflammatory Drug (NSAID)
Advil® [US-OTC/Can]
Advil® Children's [US-OTC]
Advil® Infants™ [US-OTC]
Advil® Junior [US-OTC]
Advil® Migraine [US-OTC]
Albert® Tiafen [Can]
Aleve® [US-OTC]
Amigesic® [US/Can]
Anaprox® [US/Can]
Anaprox® DS [US/Can]
Apo-Diclo® [Can]
Apo-Diclo Rapide® [Can]
Apo-Diclo SR® [Can]
Apo-Diflunisal® [Can]
Apo-Etodolac® [Can]
Apo-Ibuprofen® [Can]
Apo-Indomethacin® [Can]
Apo-Keto® [Can]
Apo-Keto-E® [Can]
Apo-Keto SR® [Can]
Apo-Meloxicam® [Can]
Apo-Nabumetone® [Can]
Apo-Napro-Na® [Can]
Apo-Napro-Na DS® [Can]
Apo-Naproxen® [Can]
Apo-Naproxen EC® [Can]
Apo-Naproxen SR® [Can]
Apo-Oxaprozin® [Can]
Apo-Piroxicam® [Can]
Apo-Sulin® [Can]
Apo-Tiaprofenic® [Can]
Asaphen [Can]
Asaphen EC [Can]
Ascriptin® [US-OTC]
Ascriptin® Maximum Strength [US-OTC]
Aspercin [US-OTC]
aspirin

Aspirtab [US-OTC]
Bayer® Aspirin Extra Strength [US-OTC]
Bayer® Aspirin Regimen Adult Low Dose [US-OTC]
Bayer® Aspirin Regimen Children's [US-OTC]
Bayer® Aspirin Regimen Regular Strength [US-OTC]
Bayer® Genuine Aspirin [US-OTC]
Bayer® Plus Extra Strength [US-OTC]
Bayer® Women's Aspirin Plus Calcium [US-OTC]
Buffasal [US-OTC]
Bufferin® [US-OTC]
Bufferin® Extra Strength [US-OTC]
Buffinol [US-OTC]
Cataflam® [US/Can]
choline magnesium trisalicylate
Clinoril® [US]
CO Meloxicam [Can]
Daypro® [US/Can]
diclofenac
diflunisal
Doan's® Extra Strength [US-OTC]
Dom-Tiaprofenic® [Can]
Easprin® [US]
EC-Naprosyn® [US]
Ecotrin® [US-OTC]
Ecotrin® Low Strength [US-OTC]
Ecotrin® Maximum Strength [US-OTC]
ElixSure™ IB [US-OTC]
Entrophen® [Can]
etodolac
Feldene® [US]
fenoprofen
Genacote™ [US-OTC]
Gen-Meloxicam [Can]
Gen-Nabumetone [Can]
Gen-Naproxen EC [Can]
Gen-Piroxicam [Can]
Genpril® [US-OTC]

Halfprin® [US-OTC]
Ibu-200 [US-OTC]
ibuprofen
Indocid® PDA [Can]
Indocin® [US/Can]
Indo-Lemmon [Can]
indomethacin
Indotec [Can]
I-Prin [US-OTC]
ketoprofen
Keygesic [US-OTC]
lansoprazole and naproxen
Lodine® [Can]
magnesium salicylate
meclofenamate
Meclomen® [Can]
meloxicam
Mobic® [US/Can]
Mobicox® [Can]
Momentum® [US-OTC]
Motrin® [US]
Motrin® Children's [US-OTC/Can]
Motrin® IB [US-OTC/Can]
Motrin® Infants™ [US-OTC]
Motrin® Junior Strength [US-OTC]
nabumetone
Nalfon® [US/Can]
Naprelan® [US]
Naprosyn® [US/Can]
naproxen
Naxen® [Can]
Naxen® EC [Can]
NeoProfen® [US]
Novasal™ [US]
Novasen [Can]
Novo-Difenac [Can]
Novo-Difenac K [Can]
Novo-Difenac-SR [Can]
Novo-Diflunisal [Can]
Novo-Keto [Can]
Novo-Keto-EC [Can]
Novo-Meloxicam [Can]
Novo-Methacin [Can]
Novo-Nabumetone [Can]

Novo-Naproc EC [Can]
Novo-Naprox [Can]
Novo-Naprox Sodium [Can]
Novo-Naprox Sodium DS [Can]
Novo-Naprox SR [Can]
Novo-Pirocam [Can]
Novo-Profen [Can]
Novo-Sundac [Can]
Novo-Tiaprofenic [Can]
Nu-Diclo [Can]
Nu-Diclo-SR [Can]
Nu-Diflunisal [Can]
Nu-Ibuprofen [Can]
Nu-Indo [Can]
Nu-Ketoprofen [Can]
Nu-Ketoprofen-E [Can]
Nu-Naprox [Can]
Nu-Pirox [Can]
Nu-Sundac [Can]
Nu-Tiaprofenic [Can]
Oruvail® [Can]
oxaprozin
Pennsaid® [Can]
Pexicam® [Can]
piroxicam
PMS-Diclofenac [Can]
PMS-Diclofenac SR [Can]
PMS-Meloxicam [Can]
PMS-Tiaprofenic [Can]
Proprinal [US-OTC]
Relafen® [Can]
Rhodacine® [Can]
Rhodis™ [Can]
Rhodis-EC™ [Can]
Rhodis SR™ [Can]
Rhoxal-nabumetone [Can]
Riva-Diclofenac [Can]
Riva-Diclofenac-K [Can]
Riva-Naproxen [Can]
Salflex® [Can]
salsalate
Sandoz-Nabumetone [Can]
Solaraze® [US]
St. Joseph® Adult Aspirin [US-OTC]

sulindac
Surgam® [Can]
Tiaprofenic- [Can]
Tiaprofenic- [Can]
tiaprofenic acid(Canada only)
Tolectin® [US]
tolmetin
Ultraprin [US-OTC]
Utradol™ [Can]
Voltaren® [US/Can]
Voltaren Rapide® [Can]
Voltaren®-XR [US]
ZORprin® [US]
Nonsteroidal Antiinflammatory Drug
   (NSAID), COX-2 Selective
   Celebrex® [US/Can]
   celecoxib
   GD-Celecoxib [Can]
   lumiracoxib(Canada only)
   Prexige® [Can]

OSTEODYSTROPHY
Vitamin D Analog
   Calciferol™ [US]
   Calcijex® [US/Can]
   calcitriol
   Drisdol® [US/Can]
   ergocalciferol
   Ostoforte® [Can]
   Rocaltrol® [US/Can]

OSTEOMALACIA
Vitamin D Analog
   Calciferol™ [US]
   Drisdol® [US/Can]
   ergocalciferol
   Ostoforte® [Can]

OSTEOMYELITIS
Antibiotic, Miscellaneous
   Alti-Clindamycin [Can]
   Apo-Clindamycin® [Can]
   Cleocin® [US]
   Cleocin HCl® [US]
   Cleocin Pediatric® [US]

Cleocin Phosphate® [US]
Cleocin T® [US]
Clindagel® [US]
ClindaMax™ [US]
clindamycin
Clindamycin Injection, USP [Can]
Clindesse™ [US]
Clindoxyl® [Can]
Dalacin® C [Can]
Dalacin® T [Can]
Dalacin® Vaginal [Can]
Evoclin™ [US]
Novo-Clindamycin [Can]
Riva-Clindamycin [Can]
Taro-Clindamycin [Can]
Vancocin® [US/Can]
vancomycin
Antifungal Agent, Systemic
Fucidin® [Can]
Fucithalmic® [Can]
fusidic acid(Canada only)
Carbapenem (Antibiotic)
imipenem and cilastatin
meropenem
Merrem® [Can]
Merrem® I.V. [US]
Primaxin® [US/Can]
Primaxin® I.V. [Can]
Cephalosporin (1st Generation)
cefazolin
Cephalosporin (2nd Generation)
Apo-Cefoxitin® [Can]
Apo-Cefuroxime® [Can]
cefoxitin
Ceftin® [US/Can]
cefuroxime
Mefoxin® [US]
ratio-Cefuroxime [Can]
Zinacef® [US/Can]
Cephalosporin (3rd Generation)
Cefizox® [US/Can]
cefotaxime
ceftazidime
ceftizoxime

ceftriaxone
Claforan® [US/Can]
Fortaz® [US/Can]
Rocephin® [US/Can]
Tazicef® [US]
Penicillin
ampicillin and sulbactam
dicloxacillin
Dycill® [Can]
nafcillin
Nallpen® [Can]
oxacillin
Pathocil® [Can]
ticarcillin and clavulanate potassium
Timentin® [US/Can]
Unasyn® [US/Can]
Unipen® [Can]
Quinolone
Apo-Ciproflox® [Can]
Ciloxan® [US/Can]
Cipro® [US/Can]
Cipro® XL [Can]
ciprofloxacin
Cipro® XR [US]
CO Ciprofloxacin [Can]
Gen-Ciprofloxacin [Can]
Novo-Ciprofloxacin [Can]
PMS-Ciprofloxacin [Can]
Proquin® XR [US]
RAN™ Ciprofloxacin [Can]
ratio-Ciprofloxacin [Can]
Rhoxal-ciprofloxacin [Can]
Sandoz-Ciprofloxacin [Can]
Taro-Ciprofloxacin [Can]

OSTEOPOROSIS

Bisphosphonate Derivative
Actonel® and Calcium [US]
alendronate
alendronate and cholecalciferol
Apo-Alendronate® [Can]
Aredia® [US/Can]
Bondronat® [Can]
Boniva® [US]

CO Alendronate [Can]
Didrocal™ [Can]
Didronel® [US/Can]
etidronate and calcium
etidronate disodium
Fosamax® [US/Can]
Fosamax Plus D™ [US]
Fosavance [Can]
Gen-Alendronate [Can]
Gen-Etidronate [Can]
ibandronate
Novo-Alendronate [Can]
pamidronate
Pamidronate Disodium® [Can]
PMS-Alendronate [Can]
ratio-Alendronate [Can]
Rhoxal-pamidronate [Can]
risedronate and calcium
Riva-Alendronate [Can]
Sandoz Alendronate [Can]
Calcium Salt
Actonel® and Calcium [US]
calcium and vitamin D
Cal-CYUM [US-OTC]
Caltrate® +D [US-OTC]
Caltrate® + Soy™ [US-OTC]
Caltrate® ColonHealth™ [US-OTC]
Chew-Cal [US-OTC]
Didrocal™ [Can]
etidronate and calcium
Liqua-Cal [US-OTC]
Os-Cal® +D [US-OTC]
Oysco D [US-OTC]
Oysco +D [US-OTC]
Oyst-Cal-D [US-OTC]
Oyst-Cal-D 500 [US-OTC]
risedronate and calcium
Electrolyte Supplement, Oral
Calcionate [US-OTC]
calcium and vitamin D
calcium glubionate
calcium lactate
calcium phosphate (tribasic)
Cal-CYUM [US-OTC]

Caltrate® +D [US-OTC]
Caltrate® + Soy™ [US-OTC]
Caltrate® ColonHealth™ [US-OTC]
Chew-Cal [US-OTC]
Liqua-Cal [US-OTC]
Os-Cal® 500+D [US-OTC]
Oysco D [US-OTC]
Oysco 500+D [US-OTC]
Oyst-Cal-D [US-OTC]
Oyst-Cal-D [US-OTC]
Posture® [US-OTC]
Estrogen and Androgen Combination
Estratest® [US/Can]
Estratest® HS [US]
estrogens (esterified) and
methyltestosterone
Syntest DS [US]
Syntest HS [US]
Estrogen and Progestin Combination
estrogens (conjugated/equine) and
medroxyprogesterone
Premphase® [US/Can]
Premplus® [Can]
Prempro™ [US/Can]
Estrogen Derivative
Alora® [US]
Cenestin® [US/Can]
CES® [Can]
Climara® [US/Can]
Delestrogen® [US]
Depo®-Estradiol [US/Can]
Divigel® [US]
Elestrin™ [US]
Esclim® [US]
Estrace® [US/Can]
Estraderm® [US/Can]
estradiol
Estradot® [Can]
Estrasorb™ [US]
Estratab® [Can]
Estring® [US/Can]
EstroGel® [US/Can]
estrogens (conjugated A/synthetic)
estrogens (conjugated/equine)

estrogens (esterified)
Evamist® [US]
Femring® [US]
Femtrace® [US]
Gynodiol® [US]
Menest® [US/Can]
Menostar™ [US/Can]
Oesclim® [Can]
Premarin® [US/Can]
Sandoz-Estradiol Derm 50 [Can]
Sandoz-Estradiol Derm 75 [Can]
Sandoz-Estradiol Derm 100 [Can]
Vagifem® [US/Can]
Vivelle® [US]
Vivelle-Dot® [US]
Polypeptide Hormone
Apo-Calcitonin® [Can]
Calcimar® [Can]
calcitonin
Caltine® [Can]
Fortical® [US]
Miacalcin® [US]
Miacalcin® NS [Can]
Selective Estrogen Receptor Modulator
(SERM)
Evista® [US/Can]
raloxifene
Vitamin D Analog
alendronate and cholecalciferol
Fosamax Plus D™ [US]
Fosavance [Can]
Vitamin, Fat Soluble
calcium and vitamin D
Cal-CYUM [US-OTC]
Caltrate® 600+D [US-OTC]
Caltrate® 600+ Soy™ [US-OTC]
Caltrate® ColonHealth™ [US-OTC]
Chew-Cal [US-OTC]
Liqua-Cal [US-OTC]
Os-Cal® 500+D [US-OTC]
Oysco D [US-OTC]
Oysco 500+D [US-OTC]
Oyst-Cal-D [US-OTC]
Oyst-Cal-D 500 [US-OTC]

OSTEOSARCOMA
Antineoplastic Agent
Adriamycin® [US/Can]
Apo-Methotrexate® [Can]
cisplatin
doxorubicin
methotrexate
ratio-Methotrexate [Can]
Rheumatrex® Dose Pack® [US]
Trexall™ [US]

PAGET DISEASE OF BONE
Bisphosphonate Derivative
alendronate
Apo-Alendronate® [Can]
Aredia® [US/Can]
CO Alendronate [Can]
Didronel® [US/Can]
etidronate disodium
Fosamax® [US/Can]
Gen-Alendronate [Can]
Gen-Etidronate [Can]
Novo-Alendronate [Can]
pamidronate
Pamidronate Disodium® [Can]
PMS-Alendronate [Can]
ratio-Alendronate [Can]
Rhoxal-pamidronate [Can]
Riva-Alendronate [Can]
Sandoz Alendronate [Can]
Skelid® [US]
tiludronate
Polypeptide Hormone
Apo-Calcitonin® [Can]
Calcimar® [Can]
calcitonin
Caltine® [Can]
Fortical® [US]
Miacalcin® [US]
Miacalcin® NS [Can]

PAIN
Analgesic Combination (Narcotic)
propoxyphene, aspirin, and caffeine

Analgesic Combination (Opioid)
  acetaminophen, caffeine, and
    dihydrocodeine
  Panlor® DC [US]
  Panlor® SS [US]
  pentazocine and acetaminophen
  Talacen® [US]
  ZerLor™ [US]
Analgesic, Miscellaneous
  acetaminophen and tramadol
  Tramacet [Can]
  Ultracet™ [US]
Analgesic, Narcotic
  acetaminophen and codeine
  Actiq® [US/Can]
  Alfenta® [US/Can]
  alfentanil
  Alfentanil Injection, USP [Can]
  Anexsia® [US]
  Apo-Butorphanol® [Can]
  Ascomp® with Codeine [US]
  Astramorph/PF™ [US]
  Avinza® [US]
  Balacet 325™ [US]
  belladonna and opium
  B&O Supprettes® [US]
  Buprenex® [US/Can]
  buprenorphine
  butalbital, aspirin, caffeine, and
    codeine
  butorphanol
  Capital® and Codeine [US]
  codeine
  Codeine Contin® [Can]
  Co-Gesic® [US]
  Damason-P® [US]
  Darvocet A500™ [US]
  Darvocet-N® 50 [US/Can]
  Darvocet-N® 100 [US/Can]
  Darvon® [US]
  Darvon-N® [US/Can]
  Demerol® [US/Can]
  DepoDur™ [US]
  dihydrocodeine, aspirin, and caffeine

Dilaudid® [US/Can]
Dilaudid-HP® [US/Can]
Dilaudid-HP-Plus® [Can]
Dilaudid® Sterile Powder [Can]
Dilaudid-XP® [Can]
Dolophine® [US]
Duragesic® [US/Can]
Duramorph® [US]
Endocet® [US/Can]
Endodan® [US/Can]
ETH-Oxydose™ [Can]
fentanyl
Fentanyl Citrate Injection, USP [Can]
Fentora™ [US]
Fiorinal®-C 1/2 [Can]
Fiorinal®-C 1/4 [Can]
Fiorinal® With Codeine [US]
Hycet™ [US]
hydrocodone and acetaminophen
hydrocodone and aspirin
hydrocodone and ibuprofen
Hydromorph Contin® [Can]
Hydromorph-IR® [Can]
hydromorphone
Hydromorphone HP [Can]
Hydromorphone HP® 10 [Can]
Hydromorphone HP® 20 [Can]
Hydromorphone HP® 50 [Can]
Hydromorphone HP® Forte [Can]
Hydromorphone Hydrochloride
  Injection, USP [Can]
Infumorph® [US]
Ionsys™ [US]
Kadian® [US/Can]
Levo-Dromoran® [US]
levorphanol
Lorcet® 10/650 [US]
Lorcet® Plus [US]
Lortab® [US]
Magnacet™ [US]
Margesic® H [US]
Maxidone™ [US]
meperidine
meperidine and promethazine

Meperitab® [US]
M-Eslon® [Can]
Metadol™ [Can]
methadone
Methadone Diskets® [US]
Methadone Intensol™ [US]
Methadose® [US]
Morphine HP® [Can]
Morphine LP® Epidural [Can]
morphine sulfate
M.O.S.® 10 [Can]
M.O.S.® 20 [Can]
M.O.S.® 30 [Can]
M.O.S.-SR® [Can]
M.O.S.-Sulfate® [Can]
MS Contin® [US/Can]
MS-IR® [Can]
nalbuphine
Norco® [US]
Nubain® [US]
Opana® [US]
Opana® ER [US]
opium tincture
Oramorph SR® [US]
Oxycocet® [Can]
Oxycodan® [Can]
oxycodone
oxycodone and acetaminophen
oxycodone and aspirin
OxyContin® [US/Can]
OxyFast® [US]
Oxy.IR® [Can]
oxymorphone
paregoric
pentazocine
Percocet® [US/Can]
Percocet®-Demi [Can]
Percodan® [US/Can]
PMS-Butorphanol [Can]
PMS-Hydromorphone [Can]
PMS-Morphine Sulfate SR [Can]
PMS-Oxycodone-Acetaminophen
   [Can]
Pronap-100® [US]

propoxyphene
propoxyphene and acetaminophen
ratio-Emtec [Can]
ratio-Lenoltec [Can]
ratio-Morphine SR [Can]
remifentanil
Reprexain™ [US]
Roxanol™ [US]
Roxicet™ [US]
Roxicet™ 5/500 [US]
Roxicodone® [US]
Stadol® [US]
Stagesic® [US]
Statex® [Can]
Sublimaze® [US]
Subutex® [US/Can]
Sufenta® [US/Can]
sufentanil
Sufentanil Citrate Injection, USP
   [Can]
Supeudol® [Can]
Synalgos®-DC [US]
® Tablet [Can]
Talwin® [US/Can]
Talwin® NX [US]
Tecnal C 1/2 [Can]
Tecnal C 1/4 [Can]
Triatec-8 [Can]
Triatec-8 Strong [Can]
Triatec-30 [Can]
Tylenol® Elixir with Codeine [Can]
Tylenol® No. 1 [Can]
Tylenol® No. 1 Forte [Can]
Tylenol® No. 2 with Codeine [Can]
Tylenol® No. 3 with Codeine [Can]
Tylenol® No. 4 with Codeine [Can]
Tylenol® With Codeine [US]
Tylox® [US]
Ultiva® [US/Can]
Vicodin® [US]
Vicodin® ES [US]
Vicodin® HP [US]
Vicoprofen® [US/Can]
Xodol® 5/300 [US]

Xodol® 7.5/300 [US]
Xodol® 10/300 [US]
Zomorph® [Can]
Zydone® [US]
Analgesic, Nonnarcotic
Abenol® [Can]
Acephen™ [US-OTC]
Aceta-Gesic [US-OTC]
acetaminophen
acetaminophen and diphenhydramine
acetaminophen and phenyltoloxamine
acetaminophen and tramadol
acetaminophen, aspirin, and caffeine
Acular® [US/Can]
Acular LS™ [US/Can]
Acular® PF [US]
Advil® [US-OTC/Can]
Advil® Children's [US-OTC]
Advil® Infants™ [US-OTC]
Advil® Junior [US-OTC]
Advil® Migraine [US-OTC]
Aleve® [US-OTC]
Alpain [US]
Alti-Flurbiprofen [Can]
Amigesic® [US/Can]
Anaprox® [US/Can]
Anaprox® DS [US/Can]
Ansaid® [Can]
Apo-Acetaminophen® [Can]
Apo-Diclo® [Can]
Apo-Diclo Rapide® [Can]
Apo-Diclo SR® [Can]
Apo-Diflunisal® [Can]
Apo-Etodolac® [Can]
Apo-Flurbiprofen® [Can]
Apo-Ibuprofen® [Can]
Apo-Indomethacin® [Can]
Apo-Keto® [Can]
Apo-Keto-E® [Can]
Apo-Ketorolac® [Can]
Apo-Ketorolac Injectable® [Can]
Apo-Keto SR® [Can]
Apo-Mefenamic® [Can]
Apo-Nabumetone® [Can]

Apo-Napro-Na® [Can]
Apo-Napro-Na DS® [Can]
Apo-Naproxen® [Can]
Apo-Naproxen EC® [Can]
Apo-Naproxen SR® [Can]
Apo-Oxaprozin® [Can]
Apo-Piroxicam® [Can]
Apo-Sulin® [Can]
Apra Children's [US-OTC]
Asaphen [Can]
Asaphen EC [Can]
Ascriptin® [US-OTC]
Ascriptin® Maximum Strength
    [US-OTC]
Aspercin [US-OTC]
aspirin
Aspirin Free Anacin® Maximum
    Strength [US-OTC]
Aspirtab [US-OTC]
Atasol® [Can]
Bayer® Aspirin Extra Strength
    [US-OTC]
Bayer® Aspirin Regimen Adult Low
    Dose [US-OTC]
Bayer® Aspirin Regimen Children's
    [US-OTC]
Bayer® Aspirin Regimen Regular
    Strength [US-OTC]
Bayer® Genuine Aspirin [US-OTC]
Bayer® Plus Extra Strength
    [US-OTC]
Bayer® Women's Aspirin Plus
    Calcium [US-OTC]
Buffasal [US-OTC]
Bufferin® [US-OTC]
Bufferin® Extra Strength [US-OTC]
Buffinol [US-OTC]
Cataflam® [US/Can]
Cetafen® [US-OTC]
Cetafen Extra® [US-OTC]
choline magnesium trisalicylate
Clinoril® [US]
Comtrex® Sore Throat Maximum
    Strength [US-OTC]

Daypro® [US/Can]
diclofenac
diflunisal
Dologesic® [US]
Dom-Mefenamic Acid [Can]
Easprin® [US]
EC-Naprosyn® [US]
Ecotrin® [US-OTC]
Ecotrin® Low Strength [US-OTC]
Ecotrin® Maximum Strength
    [US-OTC]
ElixSure™ IB [US-OTC]
Entrophen® [Can]
etodolac
Excedrin® Extra Strength [US-OTC]
Excedrin® Migraine [US-OTC]
Excedrin® PM [US-OTC]
Feldene® [US]
Fem-Prin® [US-OTC]
fenoprofen
FeverAll® [US-OTC]
Flextra 650 [US]
Flextra-DS [US]
flurbiprofen
Froben® [Can]
Froben-SR® [Can]
Genaced™ [US-OTC]
Genacote™ [US-OTC]
Genapap™ [US-OTC]
Genapap™ Children [US-OTC]
Genapap™ Extra Strength [US-OTC]
Genapap™ Infant [US-OTC]
Genebs [US-OTC]
Genebs Extra Strength [US-OTC]
Genesec™ [US-OTC]
Gen-Nabumetone [Can]
Gen-Naproxen EC [Can]
Gen-Piroxicam [Can]
Genpril® [US-OTC]
Goody's® Extra Strength Headache
    Powder [US-OTC]
Goody's® Extra Strength Pain Relief
    [US-OTC]
Goody's PM® [US-OTC]

Halfprin® [US-OTC]
Hyflex-DS® [US]
Ibu-200 [US-OTC]
ibuprofen
Indocid® PDA [Can]
Indocin® [US/Can]
Indocin® I.V. [US]
Indo-Lemmon [Can]
indomethacin
Indotec [Can]
Infantaire [US-OTC]
I-Prin [US-OTC]
ketoprofen
ketorolac
Ketorolac Tromethamine Injection,
    USP [Can]
Lagesic™ [US]
Legatrin PM® [US-OTC]
Lodine® [Can]
Mapap [US-OTC]
Mapap Children's [US-OTC]
Mapap Extra Strength [US-OTC]
Mapap Infants [US-OTC]
meclofenamate
Meclomen® [Can]
Mefenamic-250 [Can]
mefenamic acid
Midol® Cramp and Body Aches
    [US-OTC]
Midol® Extended Relief [US]
Motrin® [US]
Motrin® Children's [US-OTC/Can]
Motrin® IB [US-OTC/Can]
Motrin® Infants™ [US-OTC]
Motrin® Junior Strength [US-OTC]
nabumetone
Nalfon® [US/Can]
Naprelan® [US]
Naprosyn® [US/Can]
naproxen
Naxen® [Can]
Naxen® EC [Can]
NeoProfen® [US]
Norgesic™ [Can]

Norgesic™ Forte [Can]
Nortemp Children's [US-OTC]
Novasen [Can]
Novo-Difenac [Can]
Novo-Difenac K [Can]
Novo-Difenac-SR [Can]
Novo-Diflunisal [Can]
Novo-Flurprofen [Can]
Novo-Gesic [Can]
Novo-Keto [Can]
Novo-Keto-EC [Can]
Novo-Ketorolac [Can]
Novo-Methacin [Can]
Novo-Nabumetone [Can]
Novo-Naproc EC [Can]
Novo-Naprox [Can]
Novo-Naprox Sodium [Can]
Novo-Naprox Sodium DS [Can]
Novo-Naprox SR [Can]
Novo-Pirocam [Can]
Novo-Profen [Can]
Novo-Sundac [Can]
Nu-Diclo [Can]
Nu-Diclo-SR [Can]
Nu-Diflunisal [Can]
Nu-Flurprofen [Can]
Nu-Ibuprofen [Can]
Nu-Indo [Can]
Nu-Ketoprofen [Can]
Nu-Ketoprofen-E [Can]
Nu-Mefenamic [Can]
Nu-Naprox [Can]
Nu-Pirox [Can]
Nu-Sundac [Can]
Ocufen® [US/Can]
orphenadrine, aspirin, and caffeine
Oruvail® [Can]
oxaprozin
Pain Eze [US-OTC]
Pain-Off [US-OTC]
Pamprin® Maximum Strength All
  Day Relief [US-OTC]
Pediatrix [Can]
Pennsaid® [Can]
Percogesic® [US-OTC]
Percogesic® Extra Strength
  [US-OTC]
Pexicam® [Can]
Phenagesic [US-OTC]
Phenylgesic [US-OTC]
piroxicam
PMS-Diclofenac [Can]
PMS-Diclofenac SR [Can]
PMS-Mefenamic Acid [Can]
Ponstan® [Can]
Ponstel® [US]
Prialt® [US]
Proprinal [US-OTC]
ratio-Ketorolac [Can]
Relafen® [Can]
RhinoFlex™ [US]
RhinoFlex 650 [US]
Rhodacine® [Can]
Rhodis™ [Can]
Rhodis-EC™ [Can]
Rhodis SR™ [Can]
Rhoxal-nabumetone [Can]
Riva-Diclofenac [Can]
Riva-Diclofenac-K [Can]
Riva-Naproxen [Can]
Salflex® [Can]
salsalate
Sandoz-Nabumetone [Can]
Silapap® Children's [US-OTC]
Silapap® Infants [US-OTC]
Solaraze® [US]
Staflex [US]
St. Joseph® Adult Aspirin
  [US-OTC]
sulindac
Tempra® [Can]
Tolectin® [US]
tolmetin
Toradol® [US/Can]
Toradol® IM [Can]
Tramacet [Can]
tramadol
Tycolene [US-OTC]

Tycolene Maximum Strength
[US-OTC]
Tylenol® [US-OTC/Can]
Tylenol® 8 Hour [US-OTC]
Tylenol® Arthritis Pain [US-OTC]
Tylenol® Children's [US-OTC]
Tylenol® Children's with Flavor
Creator [US-OTC]
Tylenol® Extra Strength [US-OTC]
Tylenol® Infants [US-OTC]
Tylenol® Junior [US-OTC]
Tylenol® PM [US-OTC]
Tylenol® Severe Allergy [US-OTC]
Ultracet™ [US]
Ultram® [US/Can]
Ultram® ER [US]
Ultraprin [US-OTC]
Utradol™ [Can]
Valorin [US-OTC]
Valorin Extra [US-OTC]
Vanquish® Extra Strength Pain
Reliever [US-OTC]
Voltaren® [US/Can]
Voltaren Ophtha® [Can]
Voltaren Ophthalmic® [US]
Voltaren Rapide® [Can]
Voltaren®-XR [US]
ziconotide
ZORprin® [US]
Zytram® XL [Can]
Analgesic, Opioid
acetaminophen, codeine, and
doxylamine (Canada only)
Combunox™ [US]
Mersyndol® With Codeine [Can]
oxycodone and ibuprofen

PAIN (BONE)
Radiopharmaceutical
Metastron® [US/Can]
strontium-89

PAIN (LUMBAR PUNCTURE)
Analgesic, Topical
EMLA® [US/Can]

lidocaine and prilocaine
Oraquix® [US]

PAIN (MUSCLE)
Analgesic, Topical
dichlorodifluoromethane and
trichloromonofluoromethane
Fluori-Methane® [US]

POLYMYOSITIS
Antineoplastic Agent
Apo-Methotrexate® [Can]
chlorambucil
cyclophosphamide
Cytoxan® [US/Can]
Leukeran® [US/Can]
methotrexate
Procytox® [Can]
ratio-Methotrexate [Can]
Rheumatrex® Dose Pack®
[US]
Trexall™ [US]
Immunosuppressant Agent
Alti-Azathioprine [Can]
Apo-Azathioprine® [Can]
Azasan® [US]
azathioprine
Gen-Azathioprine [Can]
Imuran® [US/Can]
Novo-Azathioprine [Can]

PSEUDOGOUT
Antigout Agent
colchicine
Nonsteroidal Antiinflammatory Drug
(NSAID)
Apo-Indomethacin® [Can]
Indocid® PDA [Can]
Indocin® [US/Can]
Indo-Lemmon [Can]
indomethacin
Indotec [Can]
Novo-Methacin [Can]
Nu-Indo [Can]
Rhodacine® [Can]

RHEUMATIC DISORDER
Adrenal Corticosteroid
Apo-Dexamethasone® [Can]
Apo-Prednisone® [Can]
Aristospan® [US/Can]
Betaject™ [Can]
betamethasone (systemic)
Bubbli-Pred™ [US]
Celestone® [US]
Celestone® Soluspan® [US/Can]
Cortef® [US/Can]
corticotropin
cortisone acetate
Decadron® [US]
Depo-Medrol® [US/Can]
Dexamethasone Intensol® [US]
dexamethasone (systemic)
Dexasone® [Can]
DexPak® TaperPak® [US]
Diodex® [Can]
Diopred® [Can]
HP Acthar® Gel [US]
Hydeltra TBA® [Can]
hydrocortisone (systemic)
Kenalog-10® [US]
Kenalog-40® [US]
Medrol® [US/Can]
methylprednisolone
Methylprednisolone Acetate [Can]
Novo-Prednisolone [Can]
Novo-Prednisone [Can]
Oracort [Can]
Orapred® [US]
Pediapred® [US/Can]
PMS-Dexamethasone [Can]
prednisolone (systemic)
prednisone
Prednisone Intensol™ [US]
Prelone® [US]
Sab-Prenase [Can]
Solu-Cortef® [US/Can]
Solu-Medrol® [US/Can]
Sterapred® [US]
Sterapred® DS [US]
triamcinolone (systemic)
Winpred™ [Can]

RHEUMATOID ARTHRITIS
Prostaglandin
Arthrotec® [US/Can]
diclofenac and misoprostol

RICKETS
Vitamin D Analog
Calciferol™ [US]
Drisdol® [US/Can]
ergocalciferol
Ostoforte® [Can]

SKELETAL MUSCLE RELAXANT (SURGICAL)
Skeletal Muscle Relaxant
Anectine® [US]
atracurium
Atracurium Besylate Injection [Can]
cisatracurium
doxacurium
Nimbex® [US/Can]
Norcuron® [Can]
Nuromax® [US]
pancuronium
Pancuronium Bromide® [Can]
Quelicin® [US/Can]
rocuronium
succinylcholine
vecuronium
Zemuron® [US/Can]

SKIN ULCER
Enzyme
collagenase
Santyl® [US]

SPINAL CORD INJURY
Skeletal Muscle Relaxant
Dantrium® [US/Can]
dantrolene

SPONDYLITIS (ANKYLOSING)

Nonsteroidal Antiinflammatory Drug (NSAID)
Apo-Diclo® [Can]
Apo-Diclo Rapide® [Can]
Apo-Diclo SR® [Can]
Apo-Piroxicam® [Can]
Cataflam® [US/Can]
diclofenac
Feldene® [US]
Gen-Piroxicam [Can]
Novo-Difenac [Can]
Novo-Difenac K [Can]
Novo-Difenac-SR [Can]
Novo-Pirocam [Can]
Nu-Diclo [Can]
Nu-Diclo-SR [Can]
Nu-Pirox [Can]
Pennsaid® [Can]
Pexicam® [Can]
piroxicam
PMS-Diclofenac [Can]
PMS-Diclofenac SR [Can]
Riva-Diclofenac [Can]
Riva-Diclofenac-K [Can]
Solaraze® [US]
Voltaren® [US/Can]
Voltaren Ophtha® [Can]
Voltaren Ophthalmic® [US]
Voltaren Rapide® [Can]
Voltaren®-XR [US]

SUDECK ATROPHY

Calcium Channel Blocker
Adalat® XL® [Can]
Adalat® CC [US]
Afeditab™ CR [US]
Apo-Nifed® [Can]
Apo-Nifed PA® [Can]
Nifediac™ CC [US]
Nifedical™ XL [US]
nifedipine
Novo-Nifedin [Can]

Nu-Nifed [Can]
Procardia® [US/Can]
Procardia XL® [US]

TINEA

Antidote
sodium thiosulfate
Versiclear™ [US]
Antifungal Agent
Aloe Vesta® 2-n-1 Antifungal [US-OTC]
Apo-Ketoconazole® [Can]
Baza® Antifungal [US-OTC]
Blis-To-Sol® [US-OTC]
butenafine
Canesten® Topical [Can]
Carrington Antifungal [US-OTC]
ciclopirox
Clotrimaderm [Can]
clotrimazole
Cruex® Cream [US-OTC]
DermaFungal [US-OTC]
Dermagran® AF [US-OTC]
Dermazole [Can]
DiabetAid™ Antifungal Foot Bath [US-OTC]
econazole
Ecostatin® [Can]
Exelderm® [US/Can]
Extina® [US]
Fungi-Guard [US-OTC]
Fungoid® Tincture [US-OTC]
Grifulvin® V [US]
griseofulvin
Gris-PEG® [US]
Gyne-Lotrimin® 3 [US-OTC]
ketoconazole
Ketoderm® [Can]
Kuric™ [US]
Lamisil® Topical [US/Can]
Loprox® [US/Can]
Lotrimin® AF Powder/Spray [US-OTC]

Lotrimin® Ultra™ [US-OTC]
Mentax® [US]
Micaderm® [US-OTC]
Micatin® [Can]
miconazole
Micozole [Can]
Micro-Guard® [US-OTC]
Mitrazol™ [US-OTC]
Mycelex® [US]
Mycelex®-7 [US-OTC]
Mycelex® Twin Pack [US-OTC]
Mycocide® NS [US-OTC]
naftifine
Naftin® [US]
Neosporin® AF [US-OTC]
Nizoral® [US]
Nizoral® A-D [US-OTC]
Novo-Ketoconazole [Can]
oxiconazole
Oxistat® [US/Can]
Penlac® [US/Can]
Pitrex [Can]
Podactin Cream [US-OTC]
Podactin Powder [US-OTC]
Q-Naftate [US-OTC]
Secura® Antifungal [US-OTC]
sodium thiosulfate
Spectazole® [US/Can]
Stieprox® [Can]

sulconazole
terbinafine (topical)
Tinactin® Antifungal [US-OTC]
Tinaderm [US-OTC]
Ting® Cream [US-OTC]
Ting® Spray Liquid [US-OTC]
tolnaftate
triacetin
undecylenic acid and derivatives
Versiclear™ [US]
Xolegel™ [US/Can]
Zeasorb®-AF [US-OTC]
Antifungal Agent, Topical
Ertaczo™ [US]
sertaconazole
Antifungal/Corticosteroid
betamethasone and clotrimazole
Lotriderm® [Can]
Lotrisone® [US]
Disinfectant
Dakin's Solution [US]
Di-Dak-Sol [US]
sodium hypochlorite solution

ULCER, DIABETIC FOOT OR LEG
Topical Skin Product
becaplermin
Regranex® [US/Can]